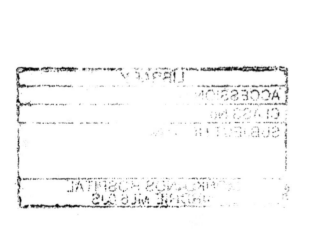

THE ESOPHAGUS

THE ESOPHAGUS

FOURTH EDITION

Editors

DONALD O. CASTELL, MD

Professor of Medicine and Director
Esophageal Disorders Program
Division of GI/Hepatology
Medical University of South Carolina
Charleston, South Carolina

JOEL E. RICHTER, MD

Chairman
Department of Gastroenterology and Hepatology
Cleveland Clinic Foundation and
Professor of Medicine
Cleveland Clinic Lerner College of Medicine of Case Western Reserve University
Cleveland, Ohio

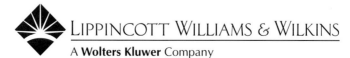

LIPPINCOTT WILLIAMS & WILKINS
A **Wolters Kluwer** Company
Philadelphia · Baltimore · New York · London
Buenos Aires · Hong Kong · Sydney · Tokyo

Acquisitions Editor: *Charles W. Mitchell*
Developmental Editor: *Michelle LaPlante*
Production Editor: *Patrick Carr*
Manufacturing Manager: *Colin Warnock*
Cover Designer: *David Levy*
Indexer: *Ann Blum*
Compositor: *Lippincott Williams & Wilkins Desktop Division*
Printer: *Maple Press*

Printed in the United States of America

9 8 7 6 5 4 3 2 1

Library of Congress Cataloging-in-Publication Data

The esophagus / editors, Donald O. Castell, Joel E. Richter.—4th ed.
  p. ; cm.
Includes bibliographical references and index.
ISBN 0-7817-4199-8
  1. Esophagus—Diseases I. Castell, Donald O. II. Richter, Joel E.
[DNLM: 1. Esophageal Diseases. WI 250 E792 2003]
RC815.7.E763 2003
616.3′2—dc22

2003056491

Care has been taken to confirm the accuracy of the information presented and to describe generally accepted practices. However, the authors, editors, and publisher are not responsible for errors or omissions or for any consequences from application of the information in this book and make no warranty, expressed or implied, with respect to the contents of the publication.

The authors, editors, and publisher have exerted every effort to ensure that drug selection and dosage set forth in this text are in accordance with current recommendations and practice at the time of publication. However, in view of ongoing research, changes in government regulations, and the constant flow of information relating to drug therapy and drug reactions, the reader is urged to check the package insert for each drug for any change in indications and dosage and for added warnings and precautions. This is particularly important when the recommended agent is a new or infrequently employed drug.

Some drugs and medical devices presented in this publication have Food and Drug Administration (FDA) clearance for limited use in restricted research settings. It is the responsibility of the health care provider to ascertain the FDA status of each drug or device planned for use in their clinical practice.

Dedication

To June Anne who continues to provide intellectual stimulation and personal support for my ventures in esophagology.

—*Donald O. Castell, MD*

To the loves of my life—Marci, Nicole, Steve, Mandy, and Jason. Thanks for your constant support as I pursue my clinical and research career in academic gastroenterology.

—*Joel E. Richter, MD*

CONTENTS

Color plate sections appear in Chapters 8 and 29.

CONTRIBUTING AUTHORS

Sami R. Achem, MD   Associate Professor, Department of Internal Medicine, Mayo School of Medicine, Mayo Clinic, Jacksonville, Florida

Edgar Achkar, MD   Vice Chairman, Department of Gastroenterology and Hepatology, The Cleveland Clinic Foundation, Cleveland, Ohio

Stanley B. Benjamin, MD   Division Chief, Professor of Medicine, Department of Gastroenterology, Georgetown University Medical Center, Washington, DC

Michael Camilleri, MD   Professor of Medicine and Physiology, Mayo Medical School, Consultant, Division of Gastroenterology, Mayo Clinic, Rochester, Minnesota

Charles Camisa, MD   Staff Dermatologist, Cleveland Clinic Florida, Naples, Florida, Affiliate Associate Professor, Department of Dermatology and Cutaneous Surgery, University of South Florida, Tampa, Florida

Donald O. Castell, MD   Professor of Medicine and Director, Esophageal Disorders Program, Division of Gastroenterology and Hepatology, Medical University of South Carolina, Charleston, South Carolina

Howard Y. Chang, MD   Associate Investigator, Department of Research and Development, Boston VA Healthcare System, West Roxbury, Massachusetts

Heather J. Chial, MD   Fellow in Gastroenterology, Mayo Clinic, Division of Gastroenterology, Rochester, Minnesota

Ian J. Cook, MD, FRACP   Professor, Faculty of Medicine, University of New South Wales, Kensington, New South Wales, Chief, Department of Gastroenterology, The St. George Hospital, Kogarah, Sydney , Australia

Kenneth R. DeVault, MD   Associate Professor, Associate Chair, Department of Medicine, Mayo Clinic, Jacksonville, Florida

Thomas R. Eubanks, DO   Portland Surgical Specialists, Portland, Oregon

Gary W. Falk, MD   Associate Professor and Director, Center for Swallowing and Esophageal Disorders, Department of Gastroenterology & Hepatology, The Cleveland Clinic Foundation, Cleveland, Ohio

Ronnie Fass, MD, FACP, FACG   Associate Professor of Medicine, University of Arizona, Director, Gastrointestinal Motility Laboratories, Southern Arizona VA Health Care System, Tucson, Arizona

Janice Freeman, RN   Digestive Disease Center, Medical University of South Carolina, Charleston, South Carolina

John R. Goldblum, MD   Chairman, Department of Anatomic Pathology, Cleveland Clinic Foundation, Cleveland, Ohio

Raj K. Goyal, MD   Mallinckrodt Professor of Medicine, Department of Medicine, Harvard Medical School, Boston, Massachusetts, Associate Chief of Staff, Department of Research and Development, VA Boston Healthcare System, West Roxbury, Massachusetts

Terry L. Gramlich, MD   The Cleveland Clinic Foundation, Cleveland, Ohio

Susan M. Harding, MD   Associate Professor of Medicine, Division of Pulmonary, Allergy, and Critical Care Medicine, Medical Director, University of Alabama at Birmingham Sleep–Wake Disorders Center, University of Alabama at Birmingham, Birmingham, Alabama

Robert C. Heading, BSc, MD, FRCP   Reader in Medicine, University of Edinburgh, Consultant Gastroenterologist, Royal Infirmary, Centre for Liver & Digestive Disorders, Royal Infirmary, Edinburgh, Scotland

Amine Hila, MD   Fellow , Department of Gastroenterology, Medical University of South Carolina, Charleston, South Carolina

Walter J. Hogan, MD   Professor of Medicine and Radiology, Medical College of Wisconsin, Department of Gastroenterology and Hepatology, Froedtert Memorial Lutheran Hospital, Milwaukee, Wisconsin

Anthony Infantolino, MD, FACP   Assistant Clinical Professor of Medicine, Division of Gastroenterology and Hepatology, Thomas Jefferson Medical College, Thomas Jefferson University Medical Center, Philadelphia, Pennsylvania

Jozef Janssens, M.D., Ph.D.   Professor of Medicine, Head, Department of Gastroenterology, Division of Internal Medicine, University Hospital Gasthuisberg, University of Leuven, Leuven, Belgium

Mark H. Johnston, MD   Associate Professor of Medicine, Uniformed Services University of the Health Sciences, Chief, Department of Gastroenterology, National Naval Medial Center, Bethesda, Maryland

Brian T. Johnston, MD   Consultant Gastroenterologist and Honorary Senior Lecturer, Royal Victoria Hospital, Grosvenor Road, Belfast, United Kingdom

Joseph L. Jorizzo, MD   Professor and Founding Chair, Department of Dermatology, Wake Forest University School of Medicine, Medical Center Blvd., Winston-Salem, North Carolina

Peter J. Kahrilas, MD   Chief, Division of Gastroenterology, Northwestern University, The Feinberg School of Medicine, Chicago, Illinois

Philip O. Katz, MD   Kimbel Professor and Chairman, Department of Medicine, Chief, Division of Gastroenterology, Graduate Hospital, Philadelphia, Pennsylvania

David A. Katzka, MD   Associate Professor, Division of Gastroenterology , Hospital of the University of Pennsylvania, Philadelphia, Pennsylvania

Seema Khan, MD   Assistant Professor of Pediatrics, Department of Pediatrics, University of Pittsburgh School of Medicine, Children's Hospital of Pittsburgh, Pittsburgh, Pennsylvania

James Walter Kikendall, MD   Associate Professor, Department of Medicine, Uniformed Services University of the Health Sciences, Bethesda, Maryland, Director of Clinical Gastrointestinal Services, Walter Reed Army Medical Center, Washington, DC

Marc S. Levine, MD   Professor of Radiology, Department of Radiology, Chief, Gastrointestinal Radiology Section, Hospital of the University of Pennsylvania, Philadelphia, Pennsylvania

Lars R. Lundell, MD, PhD   Professor of Surgery, Karolinska Institute, Huddinge University Hospital, Stockholm, Sweden

Ravinder K. Mittal, MD   Professor of Medicine, Department of Internal Medicine, University of California, San Diego, Staff Physician, Division of Gastroenterology, San Diego VA Medical Center, La Jolla, California

Joseph A. Murray, MD   Professor of Medicine, Division of Gastroenterology and Hepatology, Mayo Clinic, Rochester, Minnesota

E. Christian Noguera, MD   Fellow, Dept. of Gastroenterology, Georgetown University Medical Center, Gastroenterology Department, Washington, DC

Brant K. Oelschlager, MD   Assistant Professor, Department of Surgery, University of Washington, Attending Surgeon, Department of Surgery, University of Washington Medical Center, Seattle, Washington

Susan R. Orenstein, MD   Professor, Department of Pediatrics, University of Pittsburgh School of Medicine, Children's Hospital of Pittsburgh, Pittsburgh, Pennsylvania

Roy C. Orlando, MD   Professor of Medicine, Adjunct Professor of Physiology, Chief, Gastroenterology and Hepatology, Tulane University Health Sciences Center, New Orleans, Louisiana

John E. Pandolfino, MD   Assistant Professor of Medicine, Division of Gastroenterology and Hepatology, Department of Medicine, Northwestern University Medical School, Chicago, Illinois

Carlos A. Pellegrini, MD   Henry Harkins Professor and Chairman, Department of Surgery, University of Washington, Attending Surgeon, Department of Surgery, University of Washington Medical Center, Seattle, Washington

Madhu Prasad, MD   Assistant Professor, Department of Surgery, Harvard Medical School, Boston, Massachusetts, Department of Surgery, Boston VA Healthcare System, West Roxbury, Massachusetts

Thomas W. Rice, MD   Head of the Section of General Thoracic Surgery, Department of Cardiovascular Surgery, Cleveland Clinic Foundation, Cleveland, Ohio

Joel E. Richter, MD   Professor of Medicine, Division of Medicine, Lerner College of Medicine of Case Western Reserve University, Chairman, Department of Gastroenterology and Hepatology, Cleveland Clinic Foundation, Cleveland, Ohio

Stephen E. Rubesin, MD   Professor of Radiology, Department of Radiology, Hospital of the University of Pennsylvania, Philadelphia, Pennsylvania

Richard E. Sampliner, MD   Professor of Medicine, Universityof Arizona College of Medicine, Chief of Gastroenterology, Southern Arizona VA Health Care System, Tucson, Arizona

Robert Thayer Sataloff, MD, DMA   Chairman, Department of Otolaryngology—Head and Neck Surgery, Graduate Hospital, Philadelphia, Pennsylvania, Professor, Department of Otolaryngology—Head and Neck Surgery, Thomas Jefferson University, Philadelphia, Pennsylvania

Reza Shaker, MD   Professor of Medicine and Otolaryngology, Chief, Division of Gastroenterology and Hepatolog, Medical College of Wisconsin, Milwaukee, Wisconsin

Prateek Sharma, MD   Associate Professor of Medicine, University of Kansas School of Medicine, Veterans Affairs Medical Center, Kansas City, Missouri

Steven S. Shay, MD   Staff Gastroenterologist, Department of Gastroenterology, The Cleveland Clinic Foundation, Cleveland, Ohio

Harjot Sidhu, MD   Fellow, Division of Gastroenterology, Division of Gastroenterology and Hepatology, Medical College of Wisconsin, Milwaukee, Wisconsin

André J.P.M. Smout, MD, PhD   Professor, Department of Gastroenterology, University Medical Center, Utrecht, The Netherlands

Stuart Jon Spechler, MD   Chief, Division of Gastroenterology, Dallas VA Medical Center, Dallas, Texas

Joseph R. Spiegel, MD, FACS   Chairman, Department of Otolaryngology—Head and Neck Surgery, Graduate Hospital, Philadelphia, Pennsylvania

Jan Tack, MD, PhD   Associate Professor of Medicine, Department of Gastroenterology, Division of Internal Medicine, University Hospital Gasthuisberg, University of Leuven, Leuven, Belgium

Roland B. Ter, MD   Hawthorn East, Melbourne, Australia

George Triadafilopoulos, MD   Professor, Department of Medicine, Stanford University, Chief, Gastroenterology Section, Palo Alto VA Health Care System, Palo Alto, California

Radu Tutuian, MD   Fellow in Gastroenterology, Division of Gastroenterology and Hepatology, Medical University of South Carolina, Charleston, South Carolina

Michael F. Vaezi, MD, PhD   Staff Gastroenterologist, Department of Gastroenterology and Hepatology, Center for Swallowing and Esophageal Disorders, The Cleveland Clinic Foundation, Cleveland, Ohio

Marcelo F. Vela, MD   Fellow in Gastroenterology, The Cleveland Clinic Foundation, Cleveland, Ohi

Michael B. Wallace, MD, MPH   Assistant Professor of Medicine and Biometry, Medical University of South Carolina, Charleston, South Carolina

Bas L.A.M. Weusten, MD, PhD   Senior Consultant, Department of Gastroenterology, St. Antonius Ziekenhuis, Nieuwegein, The Netherlands

C. Mel Wilcox, MD   Professor, Department of Medicine, University of Alabama at Birmingham, Birmingham, Alabama

John M. Wo, MD   Associate Professor of Medicine and Director, Swallowing and Motility Center, Department of Medicine, University of Louisville School of Medicine, University of Louisville Hospital, Louisville, Kentucky

Roy K.H. Wong, MD   Professor of Medicine, Director, Division of Digestive Diseases, Uniformed Services University of the Health Sciences, Bethesda, Maryland, Chief of Gastroenterology, Walter Reed Army Medical Center, Washington, DC

Gregory Zuccaro, Jr., MD   Section Head, Gastrointestinal Endoscopy, Deptartment of Gastroenterology and Hepatology, Cleveland Clinic Foundation, Cleveland, Ohio

PREFACE

In this fourth edition of *The Esophagus* we have attempted to make appropriate changes in chapters and authors to achieve our goal of maintaining the high level of clinical utility and new information that was achieved in the three prior editions. In the process of planning the fourth edition, we have conscientiously revised old chapters to provide current and clinically relevant information and added new chapters where appropriate. Over half of the chapters have been revised by new authors and new chapters on endoscopic treatments of GERD, *H. pylori* and GERD, GERD in Children, and Multichannel Intraluminal Impedance appear for the first time in this edition. The new authors include many of international stature in the hope of continuing to provide a fresh and up-to-date discussion of each area of esophagology contained within this text. This is particularly true with esophageal surgery, where Drs. Rice and Lundell have joined the list of authors. We

are delighted to have the opportunity to continue to develop this textbook with a respected, reputable publishing company such as Lippincott Williams & Wilkins. This collaboration has allowed us to disseminate important information on esophageal function and disease more widely throughout the world. The preparation of the text material for *The Esophagus* remains a labor of love and an honest attempt to provide information that we believe is of clinical importance to those internists, gastroenterologists, and surgeons who frequently care for patients with esophageal disorders and often seek direction for diagnosis and treatment of perplexing clinical scenarios. It is our hope that you will find the material in this fourth edition as helpful and exciting as we do.

—DONALD O. CASTELL
JOEL E. RICHTER

THE ESOPHAGUS

1

FUNCTIONAL ANATOMY AND PHYSIOLOGY OF SWALLOWING AND ESOPHAGEAL MOTILITY

RAJ K. GOYAL
MADHU PRASAD
HOWARD Y. CHANG

The oral cavity, pharynx, and esophagus constitute the swallowing passage that transports food into the stomach. The oropharyngeal part of the swallowing passage is not a simple conduit in that it is a crossroad that is shared by a variety of vital functions, including respiration and swallowing. Oropharyngeal muscles make precise and split-second adjustments to allow its use by respiratory or swallowing functions because mixing of swallowing and respiration can be fatal. The swallowing passage also serves as a conduit for the backflow of digestive contents that may occur during vomiting and belching. During these activities, an abrupt conversion of the pharynx from a respiratory to a digestive conduit is required. The pharynx is also well armed to handle any mishaps that might occur if timely movement of food does not take place in the pharyngeal passage, by means of special local reflexes. The passage of food through the esophagus is less demanding than that through the pharynx. The upper esophageal sphincter (UES) also has an important task of stopping the backflow of gastric contents into the pharynx and larynx. The lower esophageal sphincter (LES) has to constantly guard against gastric acid moving up into the esophagus, opening only transiently to allow passage of the swallowed food into the stomach. Clearly, swallowing is one of the very demanding reflex activities. The details of this reflex are still not fully understood. Many general and more focused reviewers have summarized past research advances that are now taken for granted (1–13). There are also some excellent recent reviews that describe aspects of oropharyngeal and esophageal motility in detail (14–23). This chapter provides a general review of the physiology of swallowing and oropharyngeal and esophageal motility.

R. K. Goyal, M. Prasad, H. Y. Chang: Center for Swallowing and Motility Disorders, Brockton/West Roxbury VA Medical Center, West Roxbury, Massachusetts.

SWALLOWING REFLEX

The act of swallowing can be divided into voluntary and involuntary phases. The voluntary component of the oral stage of swallowing involves mastication and mixing of a food bolus with saliva and positioning of an appropriate-sized food bolus on the dorsum of the tongue. The involuntary component of the oral stage includes opening of the glossopalatal gate, which separates the oral cavity from the pharynx, and a wavelike contraction starting from the anterior part of the tongue and working backward to squeeze the bolus against the hard palate and propel it into the pharynx. Movement of the bolus through the pharynx and the UES constitutes the pharyngeal stage. After entering the esophagus, the food bolus is carried across the esophagus and LES into the stomach, which constitutes the esophageal stage. Oral, pharyngeal, and esophageal stages are the motor expression of the swallowing reflex. Normal human subjects swallow about 500 times during a 24-hour period (24). The onset of the swallowing reflex is marked by contraction of the mylohyoid muscle. The muscles involved in swallowing are shared by other complex reflexes, including mastication, gagging, retching, vomiting, belching, respiration, and speech (3).

Initiation

Stimulation of receptors at the base of the tongue, tonsils, anterior and posterior pillars of the fauces, soft palate, uvula, posterior pharyngeal wall, epiglottis, and larynx can elicit the swallowing reflex (3,25,26). Even though the nature of these receptors is unclear, they are apparently superficial in that when fluids of different chemical composition are applied to sensitive regions, the deglutition reflex is quickly activated (26). There are significant interspecies differences in the relative sensitivity of these areas in initiating deglutition. In humans, the anterior and posterior tonsillar pillars and posterior wall of the pharynx appear to be the most sensitive areas for initiating the reflex. The afferents initiating the deglutitive reflex are carried in the maxillary branch of the trigeminal nerve (cranial nerve V), the glossopharyngeal nerve (cranial nerve IX), and the superior laryngeal branch of the vagus nerve (cranial nerve X) (3,8).

Swallowing can also be initiated voluntarily from the cerebral cortex (19,27), but this requires some additional sensory input from the pharynx because voluntary deglutition is difficult when the pharynx is anesthetized or if there is no bolus present. In humans, stimulation of afferent cranial nerve fibers enhances cortically evoked swallowing pathways (28). Esophageal distention may also induce swallowing in humans, as does perfusion of the esophagus with a fluid of low pH and reflux of gastric acid (29,30).

Electrical stimulation of the superior laryngeal nerve (SLN) is a popular method of inducing swallowing in experimental animals (31–33). However, SLN stimulation elicits other reflexes as well, and a specific pattern and intensity of stimuli are necessary for eliciting swallowing. For example, higher intensities of electrical SLN stimulation elicit gagging, whereas lower intensities produce swallowing and even lower intensities produce only LES relaxation (34,35). In the opossum, contraction of the cricopharyngeus, which resembles gagging, is elicited after the onset of SLN stimulation. However, with continued stimulation, cricopharyngeal inhibition associated with the swallowing reflex is induced (34).

Central Organization

Peripheral afferent and cortical inputs activate swallowing center neurons to elicit the swallowing reflex (9–11,20,36). *Swallowing center* is an operational term that describes a complex of organizing and follower excitatory and inhibitory interneurons, which produce a patterned sequence of inhibitory and excitatory discharges for the motor neurons that innervate the muscles participating in the swallowing reflex. The complex of interneurons involved in the swallowing reflex is also called the swallowing pattern generator (SPG) because, once activated, it carries out the entire sequence of swallowing without additional sensory input.

Electrical recording of medullary neurons during swallowing has established that the swallowing center neurons are located in two main brainstem areas, namely, the nucleus tractus solitarius (NTS) and the adjacent reticular formation and the nucleus ambiguus (NA) and the adjacent reticular formation (37). These neurons exhibit a characteristic sequential firing pattern that closely correlates with the sequential motor pattern typical of deglutition. The areas in and around the NTS and NA are called *dorsal* and *ventral regions* of the swallowing center, respectively. Organization of swallowing has been reviewed by Jean (28).

The earliest neurons of the SPG are the organizing neurons that orchestrate the activities of other interneurons and the premotor neurons that provide sequential activation of motor neurons innervating the muscles involved in swallowing. The organizing neurons for the oropharyngeal phase of swallowing are located in the interstitial, intermediate, and ventral subnuclei of the NTS ($NTS_{int.}$, $NTS_{is.}$, and NTS_v), whereas those for the esophageal phase are located in the central subnucleus (NTS_c) (38). The organizing neurons for the oropharyngeal phase are closely connected with those for the esophageal phase, thereby linking oropharyngeal and esophageal phases of swallowing. Stimulation of oropharyngeal swallowing inhibits the esophageal phase and provides central contribution to the phenomenon of "deglutitive inhibition" (39).

Although it is not yet clear whether $NTS_{int.}$, $NTS_{is.}$, and NTS_v have distinct or overlapping roles in regulation of the oropharyngeal phase, the organizing neurons for oropharyngeal swallowing project onto a pool of excitatory and inhibitory interneurons located within the dorsal region and orchestrate sequential and patterned discharges from these interneurons. Output from these dorsal interneurons projects onto a second set of interneurons, which are located in the ventral region. These neurons have been called *switch neurons* because they relay patterned inhibitory and excitatory discharges to motor neurons involved in oropharyngeal swallowing. These premotor switch neurons for oropharyngeal swallowing project onto the motor nuclei of trigeminal (V), facial (VII), hypoglossal (XII), and the loose formation of the NA of glossopharyngeal (IX) and vagus (X) nerves (40–42).

The organizing neurons for the esophageal phase of swallowing project from the NTS_C in the dorsal complex to a group of inhibitory and excitatory interneurons in the ventral complex. The fiber tracts that connect the neurons in the NTS_C in the dorsal complex to the ventral complex neurons for the esophageal phase of swallowing pass through an area between the NTS and dorsal motor nucleus of vagus (DMNV). This is supported by the observation that while stimulation of the dorsal swallowing complex elicits both pharyngeal and esophageal phases of swallowing, lesion in the area between the NTS and DMNV abolishes the esophageal phase, leaving only pharyngeal swallow activity upon stimulation of the dorsal swallowing complex in the NTS. The premotor neurons from the ventral complex project onto the compact formation of the NA, which contains cell bodies of lower motor neurons carried in cranial nerves IX and X to the striated muscle portion of the esophagus (40). The DMNV contains cell bodies of vagal preganglionic motor neurons that provide innervation to excitatory cholinergic myenteric neurons in the smooth muscle portion of the esophagus. The DMNV also appears to contain preganglionic neurons for the myenteric inhibitory neurons innervating the esophageal smooth muscle (32,43). Recent studies using neural fiber tract tracing techniques lead to somewhat different conclusions regarding locations of the premotor neurons (44–46). Further studies will help reveal the complex neuronal network of the swallowing center.

The chemical mediators and neurotransmitters of the swallowing center are not well understood. Even though a variety of neurotransmitters (thyrotropin-releasing hormone, substance P, oxytocin, antidiuretic hormone, serotonin, norepinephrine) have been shown to generate rhythmic swallowing by activating the swallowing center, both deglutitive subcircuits appear to be activated primarily by glutamate release from primary afferent fibers of the vagus. Excitatory effects are mediated by the various classes of glutamate receptors (kainate, α-amino-3-hydroxy-5-methyl-4-isoxazolepropionic acid, NMDA, and metabotropic receptor subtypes). Excitatory cholinergic fibers in local circuit neurons of the SPG facilitate coordination between oropharyngeal and esophageal phases of swallowing via binding to muscarinic receptors (47,48). The physiologic significance of these findings is not yet clear. On the other hand, γ-aminobutyric acid (GABA), released by GABAergic interneurons, exerts a tonic inhibitory action on the swallowing center by binding to GABA$_A$ receptors so that inhibitors of GABAergic neurotransmitters stimulate the swallowing center (49). Some esophageal premotor neurons have nitric oxide synthase (NOS), suggesting their inhibitory influence on the lower motor neurons (50).

The activity of the swallowing center is intimately linked with that of other medullary centers, such as respiratory and cardiovascular centers, allowing for close integration of swallowing with other reflex activities (51,52). The swallowing centers in each half of the medulla are also well connected so that, in the event of destruction of the swallowing center on one side, the contralateral half of the center can execute the entire swallowing sequence (9).

The pattern of output by the swallowing center is programmed to be reproducible; however, it is not rigid and is modifiable. The pattern of swallowing reflex can be modified in several different ways. First, as mentioned earlier, oropharyngeal and esophageal stages can be dissociated so that either oropharyngeal or esophageal stages alone are expressed. Similarly, pharyngeal swallowing can occur without the oral phase (53). Moreover, evidence suggests that the esophageal vagal inhibitory pathway can be activated alone without the excitatory pathway, leading to deglutitive inhibition without esophageal peristaltic contraction. Second, the pattern of efferent swallowing discharge can be modified by the extensive sensory input from the pharynx and the esophagus (25,33). Finally, a variety of vagovagal reflexes that involve individual swallowing muscles can occur independently of the swallowing reflex. Some examples of these reflexes include transient LES relaxation, belching and vomiting reflexes, and UES and airway protective reflexes elicited by esophageal stimulation (22,54).

Cortical Influence

Although swallows can be elicited by cortical stimulation in experimental animals, recent studies show that transcranial magnetic stimulation of the motor cortex in humans does not initiate swallowing, probably because of the weakness of the applied stimulus (14). However, it evokes two distinct electromyographic (EMG) responses in the oropharyngeal and esophageal striated muscles (14,55). The nerve fibers mediating these cortical responses may pass through the SPG, but this is uncertain (56). Cortical topographic representation of muscles involved in the oropharyngeal and esophageal phases of swallowing can be obtained by three-dimensional magnetic resonance imaging (MRI) scans using transcranial magnetic stimulation (14,55,57,58). The swallowing muscles are bilaterally represented with somatotopic organization on the motor cortex. Positron emission tomography (PET) has demonstrated regional increases in blood flow to the multiple cortical regions activated by volitional swallowing (59). Responses of swallowing muscles to cortical stimulation are facilitated by stimulation of afferents that evoke swallowing. Cortical ischemic lesions that involve the dominant hemisphere for swallowing lead to dysphagia and reorganization of the contralateral hemisphere; this plasticity underlies the improvement in swallowing seen after cortical stroke (55,60).

OROPHARYNGEAL STAGE

General Description

The oral stage includes both voluntary and involuntary phases of swallowing. The voluntary stage includes components such as oral filling, chewing, mixing with saliva, loading of food bolus on the tongue, and voluntary shift of food toward the posterior part of the tongue. The involuntary phase involves glossopalatal expulsion and clearing of the food bolus. A food bolus loaded on the tongue is contained in a cavity that is closed on all sides by the peripheral edges of the tongue contracting against the hard palate, and the glossopalatal gate remains closed. As the glossopalatal gate opens, bulk volume of the food bolus is expelled into the pharyngeal cavity. This forceful expulsion of bulk volume is followed by clearing of residue by an anterior-posterior glossopalatal occluding contraction wave (61). Kahrilas and co-workers (61,62) have investigated the effect of bolus volume on the oral phase of swallowing. Larger volume boluses require greater loading times than smaller volume ones (61). The size of the bolus chamber on the dorsum of the tongue varies with the size of the ingested bolus. However, in general, the period of expulsion and oral clearance of a barium bolus is similar regardless of the volume, being around 0.5 second. Larger volumes are associated with a larger opening of the posterior glossopalatal gate as well as a faster change in volume of the bolus chamber on the dorsum of the tongue. Thus, the overall pattern of lingual motion is similar among bolus volumes; however, larger volume boluses are expelled into the pharynx more rapidly and more vigorously than smaller volume ones (61), but the clearance of residues of large- and small-volume boluses is similar. The oral phase of swallowing is generally investigated by videofluoroscopy, and disturbances in tongue contour have been investigated by sonography (63).

Just before the involuntary oral stage, in anticipation of the arrival of a food bolus, respiration is temporarily suppressed and the pharynx is converted from a respiratory to a swallowing pathway. Conversion of the pharynx to a swallowing pathway requires (a) closure of openings of the pharynx to nasal passages, oral cavity, and laryngeal vestibule (64); (b) opening of the UES; and (c) shortening and widening of the pharyngeal chamber.

A food bolus enters the pharynx close to the onset of swallowing, and as soon as the food enters the pharynx, pharyngeal emptying starts. Most of the pharyngeal emptying into the esophagus occurs before the start of the pharyngeal peristaltic contraction. Ergun and colleagues (65), using ultrafast computed tomography (CT), reported that, during filling, the pharyngeal chamber volume was estimated to be 4.6 cm² after 0.36 second and 1 cm² after 0.42 second following the onset of swallowing, around which time the pharyngeal contraction started. The pharyngeal propulsive peristaltic contraction begins by apposition of the soft palate and the contracting posterior pharyngeal wall (Passavant's ridge). It then proceeds toward the esophagus by sequential appositions of the posterior pharyngeal wall with the posterior surface of the tongue, epiglottis, laryngeal, arytenoid and interarytenoid muscles, and finally the posterior surface of the cricoid cartilage (2,66). The anatomy of the pharynx, the epiglottis, and cricoid cartilage effectively occlude the medial part of the swallowing chamber, splitting the bolus into two lateral halves before complete occlusion.

Pharyngeal clearance is also highly reproducible in timing and does not appear to vary much by the size of the bolus (Fig. 1.1). Larger volume boluses exit earlier and move with a greater velocity than smaller volume swallows. Kahrilas and colleagues (66) reported velocity of propagation to be 50 cm per second for a 10-mL swallow and only

15 cm per second for a 1-mL swallow. However, the craniocaudal velocity of propagation of the tail end of the bolus representing the velocity of propagation of pharyngeal contraction does not vary with the bolus volume. So that the early and rapid movement of large-volume boluses through the pharynx can be properly handled, the UES opens much earlier than the onset of pharyngeal contraction (66).

The pharyngeal stage of swallowing is usually investigated by videofluoroscopy. Pharyngeal pressures reveal marked radial and axial asymmetry because of the anatomy of the pharynx (67,68). Moreover, head position markedly affects the dynamics of the pharynx (69). Therefore, results of manometric studies of the pharynx are not reproducible and may not be helpful in clinical practice. Measurement of intrabolus pressure using swallowing videofluoroscopy and manometry is sometimes performed to evaluate resistance to the distal flow of a barium bolus.

Neuromuscular Control

Almost two dozen individual muscles innervated by branches of six cranial nerves (V, VII, IX, X, XI, and XII) with their motor neurons in the nucleus of cranial nerves V, VII, and XII and the NA (loose formation) participate to accomplish the wonder of oropharyngeal swallowing (18). EMG of individual key muscles during swallowing provides information regarding inhibition and excitation (70).

The hyoid bone is critically located at the posterior part of the base of the oral cavity and the upper part of the fibrocartilaginous anterior wall of the pharynx. Movement of the hyoid bone with its attached muscle therefore controls the critical junction where a swallowed food bolus takes a 90-degree downward turn as it flows from the oral to the pharyngeal cavity. Hyoid muscles are active throughout the oropharyngeal phase of swallowing. In the first half of oropharyngeal swallowing (about 0.5 second), which

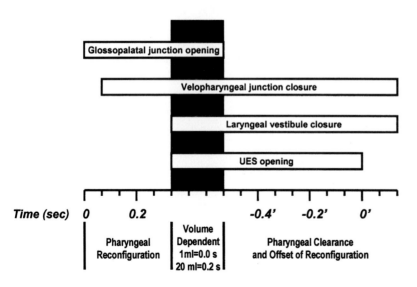

FIGURE 1.1. Time lines of 1- and 20-mL swallows showing volume-induced modifications in the timing of events within the pharyngeal swallow. Each horizontal bar depicts the period in which one of the oropharyngeal valves is in a swallow configuration as opposed to respiratory configuration. Events at the onset and offset of pharyngeal reconfiguration bear a fixed time relationship to each other regardless of swallow bolus volume. The stereotype of these phases is demonstrated by referencing onset of events from time 0 counting forward and offset events from time 0' counting forward or backward. This timing scheme defines the volume-dependent middle portion of the time line (*shaded*), which has a value of 0 for 1-mL swallows and 0.2 sec for 20-mL swallows. (From Kahrilas PJ, Lin S, Chen J, et al. Oropharyngeal accommodation to swallow volume. *Gastroenterology* 1996;111:297–306, with permission.)

includes the entire oral stage and filling and free flow of bolus through the pharynx, the hyoid bone moves up by 10 to 12 mm and forward by 10 to 12 mm (71). In the second half of the pharyngeal phase (also lasting about 0.5 second), the hyoid bone descends to its resting place (Fig. 1.2). The ascent of the hyoid bone is associated with raising of the floor of the mouth, which is important in accomplishing the oral phase. Elevation of the hyoid bone also brings the epiglottis from its vertical orientation to a horizontal one, which can provide a cover for the laryngeal opening during the passage of the food bolus, and shortens the length of the pharyngeal passage by more than 1 cm. Forward displacement of the hyoid bone is essential for opening up the angle where the food bolus makes a turn into the pharynx, widening the pharyngeal passage and the opening of the UES. The descent of the hyoid bone corresponds with the pharyngeal peristaltic contraction wave. Jacob and co-workers (71) have shown that movement of the hyoid during its ascent and descent does not follow the same path but describes an ellipse so that its path of descent is up to 5 mm anterior to its path of ascent. It rises rapidly to reach a maximum height in about 0.4 second. It then moves forward for only 0.2 second, descends for approximately 0.4 second, and finally moves back to its original position (Fig. 1.2).

The main muscles that cause elevation and forward movement of the hyoid include the mylohyoid, the anterior belly of the digastric (innervated by V), the stylopharyngeus (IX), and the geniohyoid (XII) muscles. Inhibition of activity in these muscles and contractions of infrahyoid muscles ensure orderly descent of the hyoid. The hyoid bone finally moves posteriorly to its natural resting position. The suprahyoid and infrahyoid muscles provide for a well-balanced movement of the hyoid bone during swallowing.

Just before the onset of the oral stage of swallowing, closure of the glossopalatal passage is ensured by elevation of the posterior surface of the tongue by styloglossus (innervated by XII) and palatoglossus (IX, X, and XI cranial nerve branches) muscles. The palatoglossus muscles play a particularly important role in the closure of this passage (Fig. 1.3). At the onset of the oral stage of swallowing, opening of the palatoglossal passage is facilitated by suppression of activities of the styloglossus and palatoglossus muscles and anterior pull on the hyoid bone and the posterior part of the tongue by geniohyoid muscle, supplied by cranial nerve XII. Elevation of the soft palate and uvula by levator veli palatini and uvular muscles, both innervated by cranial nerves X and XI, plays an important role in the opening of this passage.

A sequential anterior-posterior wave of apposition between the tongue and the palate move food residues from the oral cavity into the pharynx. This is brought about by activities of the hypoglossus and genioglossus muscles supplied by cranial nerve XII. As the contraction wave reaches the palatoglossal sphincter area, the palatoglossus, styloglossus, and posterior belly of digastric muscles contract to close the oral cavity from the pharynx once more.

The pharyngeal phase of swallowing consists of conversion of the pharynx from a respiratory to a swallowing passage, pharyngeal filling, passive transport, and active pharyngeal peristalsis. One of the important components of conversion of the pharynx from a respiratory passage to a food passage is closure of the nasopharynx, which is accomplished by mus-

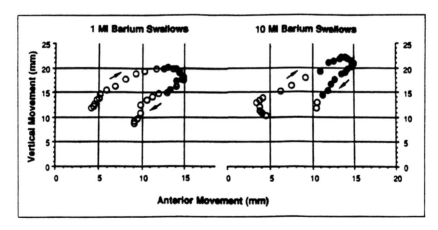

FIGURE 1.2. Movement patterns of the hyoid bone during 1- and 10-mL swallows. Each circle represents the hyoid position during a single video frame of the recorded fluoroscopic sequence (0.03-second interval). *Arrows* indicate the direction of movement. *Open circles* denote frames during which the sphincter was closed; *solid circles* indicate times at which the sphincter was open; *hatched circles* indicate times that it was variably open, depending on the subject. Sphincter opening and closing occurred at nearly identical hyoid coordinates among subjects and among volumes. Larger volume swallows were associated with persistence of the hyoid superior to and anterior to the opening coordinates. (From Jacob P, Kahrilas PJ, Logemann JA, et al. Upper esophageal sphincter opening and modulation during swallowing. *Gastroenterology* 1989;97: 1469–1478, with permission.)

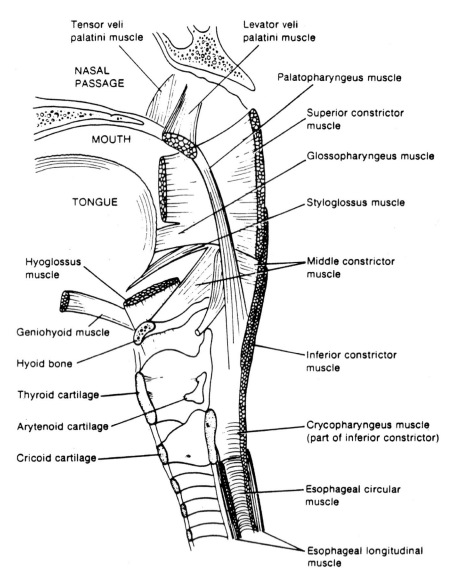

Tensor veli palatini muscle

Levator veli palatini muscle

NASAL PASSAGE

Palatopharyngeus muscle

MOUTH

Superior constrictor muscle

Glossopharyngeus muscle

TONGUE

Styloglossus muscle

Hyoglossus muscle

Middle constrictor muscle

Geniohyoid muscle

Hyoid bone

Inferior constrictor muscle

Thyroid cartilage

Arytenoid cartilage

Cricoid cartilage

Crycopharyngeus muscle (part of inferior constrictor)

Esophageal circular muscle

Esophageal longitudinal muscle

FIGURE 1.3. Schematic of pharyngeal musculature. The pharynx, bridging the nose and mouth on one end to the esophagus and trachea on the other, is responsible for separating food and air as they pass through this area. The exquisite motor control required for this task is reflected by the complexity of its structure. The pharynx consists of several distinct muscle groups and, in its lower portion, is supported anteriorly by arytenoid, cuneiform, corniculate, and cricoid cartilages. Traditionally, the pharynx has been divided into the nasopharynx, oropharynx, and hypopharynx. The nasopharynx, extending from the base of the skull behind the soft palate to the distal edge of the soft palate, is not part of the alimentary tract. Muscles in the nasopharynx, such as the tensor veli palatini, levator veli palatini, and others, contribute to elevating the soft palate and closing the nasopharyngeal passage during swallowing, preventing bolus entry into the nasal passage. The oropharynx extends from the soft palate above to the base of the tongue and the level of the hyoid bone below and contains the upper border of the epiglottis, called the *vallecula*. In this area, the respiratory and gastrointestinal tracts cross. Muscles in the oropharynx are responsible for bolus propulsion (e.g., middle constrictor) and for elevation (e.g., palatopharyngeus) and forward displacement (e.g., geniohyoid) of the pharynx. The hypopharynx extends from the vallecula at the base of the tongue to the lower border of the cricoid cartilage and contains the inferior constrictor muscle and the upper esophageal sphincter. (From Biancani P, Behar J. Esophageal motor function. In: Yamada T, ed. *Textbook of gastroenterology*. Philadelphia: JB Lippincott, 1995:158, with permission.)

cles attached to the soft palate (Fig. 1.4). These are levator veli palatini, tensor veli palatini, uvular, and palatopharyngeus muscles. These muscles, except tensor veli palatini, are innervated by motor fibers carried in the vagus and accessory nerves with cell bodies in the NA. Tensor veli palatini is innervated by motor fibers in the trigeminal (V) nerve.

Another important component of the pharyngeal phase is closure of the larynx. Elevation of the hyoid causes the epiglottis to assume a horizontal position, to direct the food bolus from entering the larynx. The laryngeal opening during swallowing is further protected by adduction of three tiers of thyroarytenoid muscle (72,73). The first level involves approximation of aryepiglottic folds to allow coverage of the superior inlet of the larynx by the epiglottic tubule anteriorly and the arytenoid cartilages posteriorly. This is brought about by contraction of the most superior division of the thyroarytenoid muscle. A second tier of protection occurs at the level of the false vocal folds that form the roof

of the laryngeal ventricle. Adduction of these folds is due to contraction of fibers of the thyroarytenoid muscles present in these folds. The third tier of protection occurs at the level of the true vocal cords. This is the most effective of the three barriers against aspiration. Adduction of the true vocal cords is brought about by contraction of the thyroarytenoid muscle. Thyroarytenoid receives its motor innervation from the recurrent laryngeal branch of the vagus. Other muscles of the larynx, namely, lateral and posterior cricoarytenoids, thyroarytenoid, and interarytenoid muscles (all innervated by the recurrent laryngeal nerve) and cricothyroid muscle (innervated by the external branch of the SLN), also help in adduction and closure of the vocal cords.

Apart from swallowing, a variety of protective reflexes against aspiration in response to afferent stimulation from the pharynx and esophagus have been identified (54, 74–76). These reflexes are important in avoiding respiratory complications of gastroesophageal reflux disease (23).

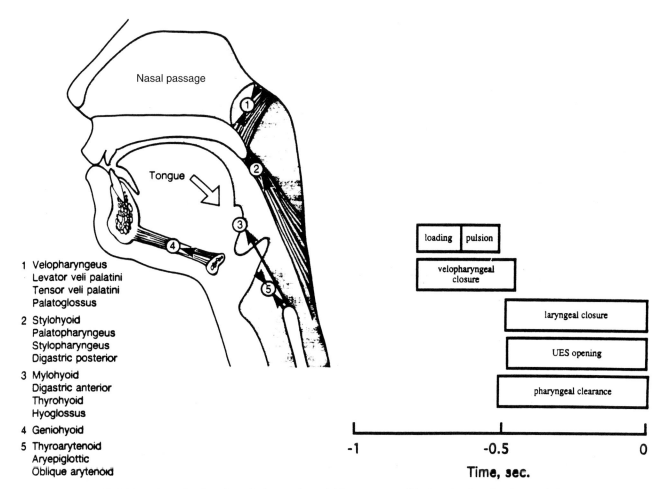

1 Velopharyngeus
  Levator veli palatini
  Tensor veli palatini
  Palatoglossus
2 Stylohyoid
  Palatopharyngeus
  Stylopharyngeus
  Digastric posterior
3 Mylohyoid
  Digastric anterior
  Thyrohyoid
  Hyoglossus
4 Geniohyoid
5 Thyroarytenoid
  Aryepiglottic
  Oblique arytenoid

FIGURE 1.4. Left: List of extrinsic muscles, which are responsible for altering the shape of the pharynx and closing the airways, and intrinsic muscles, which are responsible for collapsing the lumen of the pharynx and propelling the bolus. The extrinsic muscles, including the levator veli palatini, tensor veli palatini, and palatoglossus, are located in the nasopharynx; they raise and tense the soft palate and uvula and close the nasal passage, preventing pressure generated in the mouth from being dissipated through the nose. The stylohyoid, palatopharyngeus, stylopharyngeus, digastric posterior, and other muscles located posteriorly cause elevation; and the geniohyoid, mylohyoid, digastric anterior, thyrohyoid, and other muscles located anteriorly cause forward displacement of the larynx and pharynx and contribute to opening the upper esophageal sphincter (UES). The thyroarytenoid, aryepiglottic, and oblique arytenoid muscles and others close the larynx to prevent food from entering the trachea. **Right:** Time course of events during swallowing of a 1-mL liquid bolus: closure of the velopharyngeus to prevent reflux into the nose, closure of the larynx to prevent aspiration, pharyngeal peristalsis to clear the bolus out of the pharynx, laryngeal upward and forward displacement to move the larynx out of the path of the bolus and to force open the cricopharyngeal region, and opening of the UES. Time zero represents the end of the swallow, determined by the occurrence of UES closure. Velopharyngeal closure occurs as the bolus is gathered on the tongue (i.e., loading) and propelled forward (i.e., pulsion). Laryngeal closure and UES opening occur later, during the phase of pharyngeal clearance. (From Biancani P, Behar J. Esophageal motor function. In: Yamada T, ed. *Textbook of gastroenterology.* Philadelphia: JB Lippincott, 1995:158, with permission.)

Elevation of the hyoid bone by the suprahyoid muscle raises and shortens the anterior wall of the pharynx. The posterior and lateral muscular pharynx is shortened and elevated by the inner longitudinal muscles in the pharyngeal wall, that is, the stylopharyngeus and salpingopharyngeus muscles. Motor neurons innervating these muscles are located in the NA, and the motor fibers are carried along the vagus (for salpingopharyngeus) and glossopharyngeal (for stylopharyngeus) nerves. The duration of elevation of the hyoid bone during swallowing can be voluntarily augmented (as in the Mendelsohn maneuver) so as to increase the period of pharyngeal swallowing. This allows for behavioral modification by biofeedback therapy for oropharyngeal dysphagia (18).

The craniocaudal sequential contraction (peristaltic wave) begins at the level of the superior pharyngeal constrictor and the palatopharyngeus muscle and travels down the overlapping middle and inferior pharyngeal constrictor muscles (Fig. 1.3). The pharyngeal constrictors are also innervated by large motor neurons in the semicompact formation of the NA, and the lower motor neurons are carried in the pharyngeal branches of the vagus nerve (42).

Upper Esophageal Sphincter: Inferior Pharyngeal Sphincter

General Description

The UES refers to a zone of intraluminal high pressure that exists between the pharynx and the upper esophagus. Although it is generally called UES, it may be more justifiably called the *inferior pharyngeal sphincter*. Anatomically, the UES is comprised of the muscular cartilaginous hypopharynx along with the cricoid cartilage ventrally and the cricopharyngeus muscle both dorsally and laterally. The cricopharyngeus muscle has oblique and horizontal components. It is generally agreed that the horizontal portion of the cricopharyngeus is part of the UES. This muscle, however, is only 1 cm wide and therefore cannot itself account for the entire high-pressure zone, which measures between 2 and 4 cm (77). The inferior pharyngeal constrictor joins with the cricopharyngeus in forming the UES (77).

The cricopharyngeus muscle is structurally, biochemically, and mechanically different from the surrounding pharyngeal muscles (31). It is composed of striated muscle fibers of small average diameter (25 to 35 μm), which are not oriented in strict parallel fashion (78,79), and a large amount of connective tissue and no muscle spindles (78). The cricopharyngeus has both slow-twitch (type I) and fast-twitch (type II) muscle fibers; however, the predominant fiber is the slow-twitch type, which is more oxidative (80). The electromyographic properties of the human cricopharyngeus have been recently reviewed (81). Mechanically, the length at which the cricopharyngeus develops maximum tension is larger than usual (82). Innervation is also distinctive. Glycogen depletion studies have shown that it is innervated by both the pharyngeal nerve and the SLN (42). The cell bodies of lower motor neurons carried in these nerves are located in the NA and additional neurons are located outside this nucleus (42).

Basal Pressure

The closing pressure of the UES varies somewhat with the circumstances under which the measurements are made (69,83–85). The pressure profile of the UES shows axial asymmetry with a sharp ascent in its upper part and a more gradual decline in its lower part, as well as marked radial asymmetry (69,86). Welch and colleagues (86) constructed a three-dimensional pressure profile of the UES. The pressures are higher in the anterior-posterior than in the lateral orientation, but there is also a dissociation of peak pressures along the anterior and posterior aspects. Peak pressure occurs 1 cm below the upper border of the high-pressure zone anteriorly and 2 cm below the upper portion of the high-pressure zone posteriorly (Fig. 1.5). The radial and

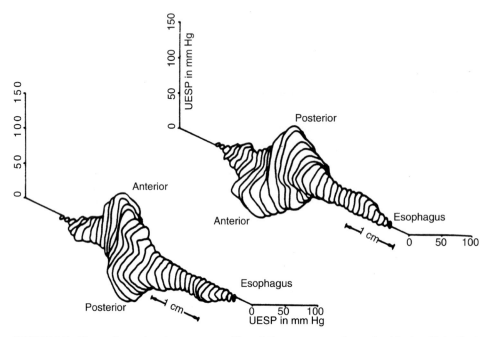

FIGURE 1.5. Three-dimensional pressure profiles of the upper esophageal sphincter. Note that pressures are higher in the anteroposterior orientation than on the sides. (From Welch RW, Gray JE. Influence of respiration on recordings of lower esophageal sphincter pressure in humans. *Gastroenterology* 1982;83:590–594, with permission.)

axial asymmetry is not observed after laryngectomy, indicating that the rigid cartilages of the larynx forming the anterior wall of the UES are responsible for the asymmetry (86). Reported resting UES pressures in normal subjects with low-compliance recording systems have ranged from 35 to 200 mm Hg (69,85,86). Pressure recorded with a laterally oriented manometric device is 33% of the magnitude of pressures recorded when the device is oriented in the anterior or posterior direction. Resting UES pressures may be lower in infancy, in the aged, and during sleep (87). The UES opens with each swallow to permit passage of the bolus into the esophagus. Pressure recordings demonstrate a decrease in UES pressure immediately after the onset of deglutition. Pressures at the nadir of relaxation may reach subatmospheric levels (2) but do not usually reach intraesophageal levels.

Several studies have demonstrated continuous electrical spike activity in the cricopharyngeus muscle (34,88–91) (Fig. 1.6). The significance of this activity, however, is a subject of debate. Doty (3) concluded that resting UES pressure is entirely due to passive forces caused by elasticity of the tissues and that tonic electrical spike activity is caused by reflex stimulation by the intraluminal manometry tube or other reflexes (31,82). Asoh and Goyal (34), in contrast, suggested that continuous electrical spike activity in both the cricopharyngeus and the caudal-most fibers of the inferior pharyngeal constrictor muscle combined with passive forces are responsible for the resting UES pressure. The activity of the UES muscles is depressed during deep sleep and during anesthesia and shows a phasic change in activity with inspiration (34,90).

Reflex increases in UES pressure occur with pharyngeal stimulation (54,92), esophageal distention (93), and intraesophageal acid infusion (94). The reflex increase in UES

pressure induced by acid infusion or balloon distention is less marked when the more distal, rather than the more proximal, esophageal segments are stimulated (31). The reflex increase in UES pressure caused by esophageal distention or acid infusion is largely mediated by vagal afferent pathways (95). Bilateral cervical vagosympathetic cooling does not change the resting UES pressure but partially antagonizes the increase in pressure caused by distention or acid infusion. UES pressure also increases with inspiration, glossopharyngeal breathing, and gagging and during the Valsalva maneuver when it is performed against a closed mouth and nose as opposed to a closed glottis (5).

Relaxation

Relaxation and opening of the UES occur during deglutition, rumination, vomiting, regurgitation, and belching (31,75). During swallow-induced relaxation of the UES, the continuous spike activity of the cricopharyngeus muscle ceases (34,90) (Fig. 1.6). This is due to inhibition of lower motor neurons in the brainstem that innervate the UES. The inhibition of tonic muscle activity is in itself not sufficient to open the UES because its closure due to passive factors persists even after cessation of all cricopharyngeal electrical activity. Elevation and anterior displacement of the larynx by the suprahyoid muscles, such as the geniohyoid muscle, are required to abolish this residual pressure and open the sphincter, although in experimental settings, contraction of the geniohyoid muscle may obliterate the UES high-pressure zone even when the cricopharyngeus continues to be active (34) (Figs. 1.7 and 1.8). Under normal circumstances, the cessation of activity in the cricopharyngeus and the contraction of the suprahyoid muscles are coordinated to ensure efficient opening of the UES (96,97). Paralysis of suprahyoid muscles, such

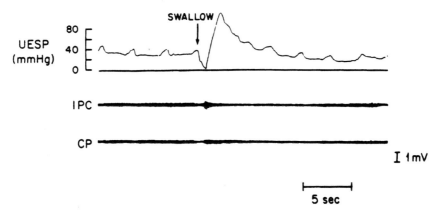

FIGURE 1.6. Simultaneous manometric and electromyographic recordings from opossum upper esophageal sphincter (UES). Sphincter pressure (UESP) decreases abruptly on swallowing; this is associated with cessation of tonic electrical spike activity in cricopharyngeus (CP) and inferior pharyngeal constrictor (IPC) muscles. UESP then recovers and increases to well above baseline (postrelaxation contraction). This corresponds to increased spike-burst activity in CP and IPC. (From Goyal RK, Cobb BW. Motility of the pharynx, esophagus, and esophageal sphincter. In: Johnson LR, ed. *Physiology of the gastrointestinal tract*. New York: Raven Press, 1981:359, with permission.)

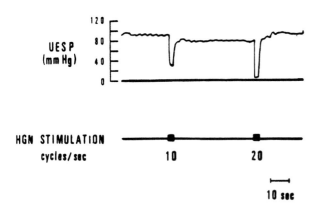

FIGURE 1.7. Effect of geniohyoid muscle contraction on upper esophageal sphincter pressure (UESP) in opossum. Electrical stimulation of a branch of the hypoglossal nerve (*HGN*) to the geniohyoid muscle causes contraction of the muscle and a precipitous decrease in UESP. This indicates that the suprahyoid muscles function to open UES independent of relaxation of the intrinsic UES muscles. (From Asoh R, Goyal RK. Manometry and electromyography of the upper esophageal sphincter in the opossum. *Gastroenterology* 1978;74:514–520, with permission.)

as the geniohyoid, significantly impairs UES opening even when the cricopharyngeus functions normally (34). On the other hand, contraction of the suprahyoid muscles may cause considerable opening of the UES despite impaired cricopharyngeal relaxation. Because UES opening is related to two factors, it is best to distinguish between cricopharyngeal relaxation and UES opening. The relaxation component is due to the cessation of tonic activity in the cricopharyngeal and inferior pharyngeal constrictor muscles, whereas the opening is due to contraction of the suprahyoid muscles. Impaired relaxation of the cricopharyngeus muscle or loss of its compliance

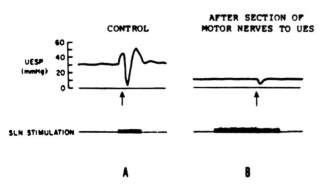

FIGURE 1.8. Effect of transecting motor nerves to the upper esophageal sphincter (UES) on resting pressures and deglutitive responses as evoked by superior laryngeal muscle (SLN) stimulation. During control period (*A*), resting UES pressure (UESP) is approximately 30 mm Hg. Stimulation of SLN causes initial transient UES contraction, followed by relaxation upon activation of deglutition reflex (*arrow*). After sectioning motor nerves to the UES (*B*), resting UESP decreases to about 10 mm Hg and deglutition, which is induced by SLN stimulation, causes a further decline in pressure as a result of opening of the UES by contraction of the suprahyoid muscles. (From Asoh R, Goyal RK. Manometry and electromyography of the upper esophageal sphincter in the opossum. *Gastroenterology* 1978;74:514–520, with permission.)

by fibrosis is responsible for the prominent cricopharyngeal bar or cricopharyngeal achalasia (25,96,98). In contrast, paralysis of the suprahyoid muscle and lack of opening of the UES are responsible for paralytic upper sphincter achalasia (77). Simultaneous EMG and manometric studies are useful for investigating dysfunction of the UES (89).

ESOPHAGEAL STAGE

General Description

In adults, the body of the esophagus, exclusive of the sphincters, is 18 to 22 cm long (12). The upper level of the esophageal body begins approximately 18 cm from the incisors and ends at 40 cm (range 26 to 50 cm) in men and at 37 cm (range 22 to 41 cm) in women. The esophageal wall, like other regions of the gut, consists of mucosa, submucosa, and muscularis propria; however, unlike the other regions, it has no serosal covering. The outer esophageal wall is bounded by a thin, poorly defined layer of connective tissue. The mucosa consists of stratified squamous epithelium in all regions except the LES, where esophageal squamous epithelium joins gastric columnar epithelium. Relatively few glands are present in the esophageal mucosa; hence, its secretory function is limited. The muscularis propria consists of inner circular and outer longitudinal muscle layers, in addition to a longitudinally oriented muscle layer called the *muscularis mucosa* located between the muscle layers and the mucosa.

During swallowing of liquid food, the food bolus enters the esophagus soon after it enters the pharynx. In the upright position, the head of a liquid barium bolus traverses the esophagus and enters the stomach within a few seconds from the onset of swallowing. The tail of the bolus is propelled by the esophageal peristaltic contraction. Thus, in the upright position, the head of the liquid bolus moves faster than its tail because of gravity. On the other hand, when the effect of gravity is removed, as in the recumbent position, the head and tail of the bolus move closely together. Normally, the esophagus is completely cleared of the ingested food bolus in 8 to 10 seconds (Fig. 1.9).

The esophageal peristaltic wave associated with swallowing is called *primary peristalsis* and is recognized by its association with pharyngeal peristaltic contraction, UES relaxation, and mylohyoid muscle activity. The peristaltic wave is produced by a lumen-occluding contraction of the esophageal muscle. The characteristics of this wave vary with the segment of esophagus in which it is measured (99). The duration of the pressure wave varies from 2 to 7 seconds and increases in an aboral direction. Recording peak pressures with an intraesophageal transducer system reveals values of 53.4 ± 9.0 mm Hg (mean ± SE) in the upper esophagus, 35.0 ± 6.4 mm Hg in the middle portion, and 69.5 ± 12.1 mm Hg in the lower esophagus. The lower pressures in the midesophagus correspond to the junction of striated and smooth muscle. The average peristaltic speed is approximately 4 cm

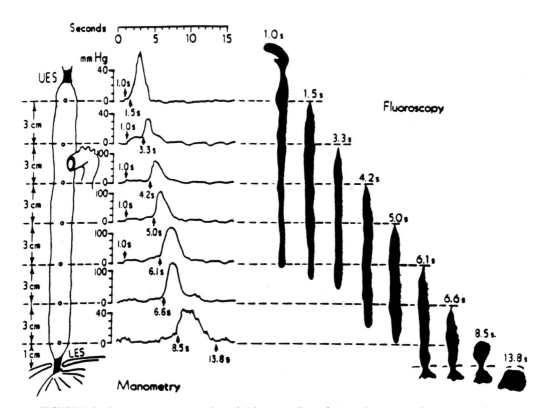

FIGURE 1.9. Concurrent manometric and video recording of a 5-mL barium swallow. Tracings from the video images of the fluoroscopic sequence on the right show the distribution of the barium column at the times indicated above the individual tracings and by arrows on the manometric record. In this example, a single peristaltic sequence completely cleared the barium bolus from the esophagus. Pharyngeal injection of barium into the esophagus occurs at the 1.0-second mark. The entry of barium causes distention and a slightly increased intraluminal pressure, indicated by the downward pointing arrows marked "1.0 s." Shortly thereafter, esophageal peristalsis is initiated. During esophageal peristalsis, luminal closure and, hence, the tail of the barium bolus passed each recording site concurrent with the onset of the manometric pressure wave. Thus, at 1.5 seconds, the peristaltic contraction had just reached the proximal recording site and barium had been stripped from the esophagus proximal to that point. Similarly, at 4.2 seconds, the peristaltic contraction was beginning at the third recording site and, correspondingly, the tail was located at the third recording site. Finally, after completion of the peristaltic contraction (time 13.8 seconds), all of the barium was cleared into the stomach. (From Kahrilas PJ, Dodds WJ, Dent J, et al. Upper esophageal sphincter function during deglutition. *Gastroenterology* 1988;95:52–62, with permission.)

per second; it is approximately 3 cm per second in the upper esophagus, accelerates to approximately 5 cm per second in the midregion, and then slows again to approximately 2.5 cm per second just above the LES (Fig. 1.10). The magnitude of maximal esophageal shortening is greatest at the most distal segment of the esophagus (100). Several factors may influence the amplitude, duration, and propagation velocity of the peristaltic wave. Within the same individual and with the same technique, peristaltic amplitude remains reasonably constant when examined serially and is unaffected by age (101). Amplitudes of esophageal contractions are less when recorded in the upright position, with velocity greater in the upper esophagus and decreasing in the mid to lower esophagus (102). Also, the duration and amplitude are increased and the velocity is decreased when a fluid bolus is swallowed as opposed to a dry bolus, that is, gulping air (103). Moreover, larger bolus volumes elicit stronger peristaltic contrac-

tions (104,105). Increases in intraabdominal pressure or outflow obstruction slow the speed of peristalsis. Warm boluses augment and cold boluses inhibit peristaltic contraction, but bolus osmolality is without significant effect (106,107). The esophageal peristaltic mechanism is not well developed in premature infants (108).

The amplitude (force) of peristalsis ensures that it completely sweeps the bolus without leaving any residue behind. However, weaker contractions can leave some residue behind. Moreover, if the bolus pressure is increased as a result of distal obstruction or reduced compliance of the lumen, the liquid bolus may appear to flow back through the ineffective peristaltic wave. Nonperistaltic contractions do not propel the food bolus but break it up into segments. On barium swallow examination, nonperistaltic contractions are responsible for a corkscrew or beaded appearance of the esophagus.

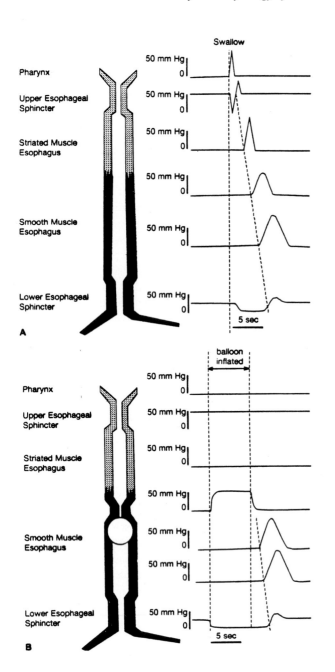

FIGURE 1.10. A: Manometric profile of a primary peristalsis. At rest, the normal esophagus is quiescent and the sphincters are tonically contracted. Swallow triggers relaxation of the upper and lower esophageal sphincters (LES) and gives rise to a peristaltic contraction traveling smoothly through the striated and then the smooth muscle portion of the esophagus. Each location along the esophageal axis contracts with a latency that increases gradually from the upper esophagus to the LES. The latencies are site dependent and reproducible. In the upper third of the esophagus, contraction occurs within 1 to 2 seconds after swallowing; in the middle third, within 3 to 5 seconds; in the lower third, between 5 and 8 seconds. The velocity of the peristaltic wave is slower in the striated muscle and faster in the smooth muscle segments of the esophagus. Contractions reach the smooth muscle segment within 2 seconds after the onset of the swallow, traveling at a speed of about 3 cm per second; in the smooth muscle segment, the velocity of propagation may be as fast as 5 cm per second. The contractions in the striated muscle segment are shorter (1 to 2 seconds), and in the smooth muscle segment, they are longer (4 to 7 seconds). Contractions in the distal one third of the esophagus are usually stronger (50 to 150 mm Hg) than those in the upper third (40 to 120 mm Hg), and both are stronger than those in the middle third (20 to 80 mm Hg), where they are relatively weak, probably occurring at the transition between the striated and smooth muscle esophagus. **B:** Manometric profile of a secondary peristalsis. Secondary peristalsis results when a bolus remains in the esophagus after an ineffective primary peristalsis or when gastric contents reflux into the esophagus. It is thought to be caused by distention and can be demonstrated by inflating a balloon in the esophagus. Upon inflation, the esophagus contracts proximal to and relaxes distal to the balloon, including the LES. When the balloon is deflated, peristalsis proceeds down the esophagus. (From Biancani P, Behar J. Esophageal motor function. In: Yamada T, ed. *Textbook of gastroenterology.* Philadelphia: JB Lippincott, 1995: 158, with permission.)

Food residue left behind in the esophagus by ineffective primary peristalsis is removed by the so-called secondary peristalsis. Secondary peristalsis is distinguished from primary peristalsis in that it is localized to the esophagus and not accompanied by pharyngeal peristalsis or UES relaxation. Experimentally, secondary peristalsis is elicited by transient esophageal distention and deflation of an intraluminal balloon (109) (Fig. 1.10). The peristaltic wave induced by balloon distention exhibits regional differences along different segments of the esophagus (46). Esophageal distention may induce primary peristalsis as well. Secondary peristalsis can also be triggered by air and water boluses. However, slow infusion of fluids into the esophagus elicits either peristaltic or simultaneous contractions. Patients with reflux esophagitis

have higher thresholds for eliciting a secondary peristalsis and reduced frequency of peristalsis (110,111); treatment of esophagitis with medications (112) or antireflux surgery (113) may not reverse these abnormalities. The amplitude and velocity of secondary peristaltic contractions resemble those of primary peristalsis (114), but there are some differences in the sensitivity to atropine (115).

Winship and Zboralske (116) reported that, if a balloon is inflated in the human esophageal body and prevented from moving distally, an aborally directed steady force of up to 200 g is exerted on the balloon, called the *esophageal propulsive force.* The esophageal propulsive force appears to increase with increasing bolus size and is greatest in the distal esophagus. During the period of fixed balloon distention, no contractions occur in the esophagus distal to the balloon; however, when restraints are removed from the balloon, the contraction producing the localized propulsive force is converted to a peristaltic sequence that progresses distally, pushing the balloon ahead of it (116). Williams and co-workers (117) have shown that this propulsive force is produced by phasic and tonic contractions of the circular and longitudinal muscles at and just above the balloon. These consist of simultaneous contractions that become multipeaked, repetitive, and associated with a sustained increase in the basal pressure with increasing distention volumes (117,118). Generation of the esophageal propulsive force appears to be reflexly mediated, involving both central and local, afferent and efferent pathways (119).

Normally, the esophagus responds on a one-to-one basis to each pharyngeal swallow. However, the time required for the pharyngeal stage of swallowing is much shorter than that for the esophageal stage (1 second versus 8 seconds). Moreover, during rapid drinking, successive oropharyngeal swallows are performed up to every 2 seconds. During the period of rapid successive swallowing, the esophageal activity is inhibited and only the last swallow of the swallowing train is associated with esophageal peristaltic contraction (120,121) (Fig. 1.11). This phenomenon of deglutitive inhibition has been quantified by investigating responses to paired swallows made at different time intervals (121–123). During normal food ingestion, when swallows are performed in rapid succession but irregularly, fewer peristaltic waves than swallows are observed. Moreover, the amplitudes are variable, presumably due to deglutitive inhibition (124). Mayrand and colleagues (125)

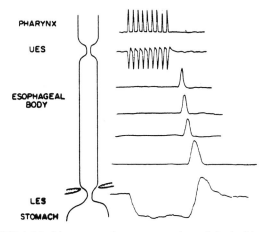

FIGURE 1.11. Diagrammatic representation of deglutitive inhibition. Swallows taken in rapid succession are marked by repeated phasic pressure changes recorded in the pharynx. The upper esophageal sphincter relaxes and recovers with each swallow on a one-to-one basis. However, peristalsis in the esophageal body does not ensue until after the last swallow. Also, the lower esophageal sphincter relaxes to first swallow and does not recover until after the peristaltic wave initiated by the last swallow has traversed the esophagus. (From Goyal RK, Paterson WG. Esophageal motility. In: Wood JD, Schultz SG, eds. *The gastrointestinal system*. Washington, DC: American Physiological Society, 1987:865, with permission.)

measured esophageal resting tone *in vivo* and Sifrim and co-workers (126,127) have demonstrated a wave of inhibition before peristaltic contraction motility. Deglutitive inhibition is critically important for the passage of swallowed food through the esophagus, and failing deglutitive inhibition is associated with esophageal motility disorders (127).

Striated Muscle (Cervical Esophagus)

The human cervical esophagus is composed of striated muscle in both the inner circular and outer longitudinal muscle layers. The longitudinal muscle fibers arise from the superior aspect of the median ridge on the dorsal surface of the cricoid cartilage and are joined by muscle bundles from the cricopharyngeus and posterolateral cricoid cartilage on each lateral aspect. Fibers course dorsally and caudally to join approximately 3 cm below the cricoid cartilage posteriorly. This arrangement leaves a triangular area devoid of longitudinal muscle that is called *Laimer's triangle*. Esophageal striated muscle develops from esophageal smooth muscle by a process of transdifferentiation (128). Approximately 4 cm (2 to 6 cm) of the proximal end of the esophageal body is constituted by striated muscle (12,129). Smooth and striated muscles are present in nearly equal amounts between 4 and 8 cm from the upper end. This mixture of striated and smooth muscle extends to a point 10 to 13 cm from the lower border of the cricopharyngeus. From that point distally, it is exclusively smooth muscle, so the distal one half to one third of the esophagus is entirely smooth muscle in both the inner circular and outer longitudinal coats. There have been rare reports of striated muscle extending the length of the entire esophagus in humans (7).

The somatic motor fibers to the striated muscles of the esophagus arise from lower motor neurons located in the nucleus retrofacialis and the compact formation of the NA (40) and contain choline acetyltransferase and calcitonin gene-related peptide (CGRP). Axons of the lower motor neurons projecting to the esophagus are carried in the vagus nerve. Nerve fibers to the striated muscle portion of the esophagus depart from the vagus in the upper part of the neck as the recurrent laryngeal nerve. Therefore, electrical stimulation of the vagus nerve in the midportion of the neck produces no response in the striated muscle segment of the esophagus. The lower motoneurons are myelinated and make direct contact with individual striated muscle fibers, which contain choline acetyltransferase and CGRP, via the motor endplate. Acetylcholine (ACh) is the excitatory neurotransmitter involved at the motor endplate, exerting its effects through stimulation of nicotinic cholinergic receptors (130). The role of CGRP is not known. The striated muscle portion of the esophagus also has a myenteric plexus with a large number of neurons that are NOS-positive (131–134). These neurons provide nitrergic innervation to the motor endplates that is unique to the esophageal striated muscle. Although exogenous application of the NOS antagonist L-NNA or the nitric oxide donor DEA-NO does not significantly alter striated muscle contraction induced by vagal stimulation (135), the physiologic role of these nitrergic neurons has yet to be determined. These nitrergic neurons may receive preganglionic input from the DMNV, but this remains to be documented as well.

Peristalsis in the striated muscle portion of the esophagus is mediated by the lower motoneurons, the fibers of which are carried in the vagus nerve, as evidenced by the fact that bilateral cervical vagotomy above the origin of the pharyngoesophageal branches abolishes peristalsis in the striated muscle esophagus (12,136). Andrew (137) suggested that sequential discharge of the motoneurons destined for progressively more distal levels was responsible for peristalsis. Roman and Gonella (10) performed experiments in which the central portion of a sectioned vagus (containing nerve fibers from lower motor neurons to the striated muscle portion of the esophagus) was sutured to the distal end of the motor nerve innervating the sternocleidomastoid and trapezius muscles, allowing vagal motor fibers to reinnervate these muscles. They then recorded EMG activity in muscle units in the neck in response to swallowing. It was found that activation of deglutition induced sequential contraction of the reinnervated muscles and that this coincided with esophageal peristaltic contractions. This observation further supported the view that sequential activation of vagal motoneurons elicited peristaltic activity. The esophageal sensory afferent input can quantitatively affect the peristaltic amplitude and velocity by modulating the central vagal efferent discharge.

Distention-induced peristalsis in the striated muscle segment of the dog and sheep esophagus is also entirely dependent on central vagal pathways. Thus, there is no difference between primary and secondary peristalsis in the striated muscle segments other than in the method of initiation and in the fact that the occurrence of the latter is independent of the oropharyngeal component. In humans, esophageal balloon distention has been reported to induce pharyngeal peristalsis that passes through the striated muscle segment and into the smooth muscle segment (122). The distention-induced secondary peristalsis and esophageal propulsion in the striated muscle portion are mediated by central reflexes. The deglutitive inhibition of the striated muscle esophagus is thought to be centrally mediated by inhibiting lower motoneurons in the compact formation of the NA (16). Whether the intramural NOS-positive neurons in the myenteric plexus within the striated muscle play a role in peristalsis and deglutitive inhibition is not known.

Smooth Muscle (Thoracic Esophagus)

The thoracic esophagus in humans is mostly composed of smooth muscle fibers that receive innervation from preganglionic neurons in the DMNV via the vagus (138). These fibers then branch to form the esophageal plexus and finally enter the esophagus at different levels. The preganglionic fibers travel within the esophageal wall for several centime-

ters before reaching the postganglionic neurons in the intramural plexuses. The smooth muscle portion of the esophagus also receives a sympathetic nerve supply that arises from the cell bodies in the intermediolateral cell columns of spinal segments T1 to T10. Preganglionic fibers enter the cervical sympathetic ganglia, ganglia in the thoracic sympathetic chain, and possibly the celiac ganglia. Most fibers to the lower esophagus travel in the greater splanchnic nerves to enter the celiac ganglia, where they synapse with postganglionic neurons (139). Postganglionic branches accompany the blood vessels, and a few fibers join the vagus to reach the esophagus. Most of the postganglionic axons terminate in the myenteric plexus (139,140) and submucosal plexus. Very few terminate directly on the muscle cells. The density of the adrenergic innervation is less in the lower sphincter than in the more proximal esophagus (139).

Intramural neural ganglia in the esophagus, like in other parts of the gut, are located in the myenteric and submucous plexuses. In the esophagus, the intramural neurons are fewer in number and more haphazard in arrangement than elsewhere in the gut (141,142). The esophageal neurons contain many different peptide and nonpeptide chemical markers (133,143–145). However, there are two predominant types of motor neuron: those staining for NOS and vasoactive intestinal polypeptide (VIP) and those that stain for substance P and choline acetyltransferase. Although indirect studies suggest that there are two populations of neurons that receive separate preganglionic projections, this has not yet been documented by morphologic studies.

The neurophysiology of primary peristalsis and other motor activities in the smooth muscle portion of the esophagus is more complicated. It is clear, however, that swallow-induced primary peristalsis in the smooth muscle portion of the esophagus is also dependent on activation of the swallowing center and the vagal pathways to the esophagus because bilateral cervical vagotomy or vagal cooling abolishes primary peristalsis in the esophagus (121,146–148). However, unlike the striated muscle, sequential firing of vagal efferent neurons destined for progressively more caudal smooth muscle esophageal segments is not essential to activate peristalsis. This is demonstrated experimentally by simultaneously stimulating all vagal efferent fibers with an electric current and observing that peristalsis is still induced (149–151).

It was initially proposed that esophageal peristalsis in the smooth muscle portion of the esophagus was also due to sequential cholinergic excitation. Tieffenbach and Roman (148), using recordings from baboon skeletal muscle that had been reinnervated by vagal preganglionic efferent fibers, detected a vagal efferent discharge that coincided with peristaltic activity in the smooth muscle esophagus. The pattern of this discharge was sequential, indicating that vagal preganglionic fibers destined for the smooth muscle esophagus are activated by a central sequencing mechanism in the same manner as is seen with the vagal lower motoneurons that supply the striated muscle esophagus.

Tieffenbach and Roman (148) suggested that these preganglionic efferent fibers synapse with postganglionic cholinergic fibers in the smooth muscle esophageal wall, which in turn produce the peristaltic contractions. This was consistent with the demonstration of atropine sensitivity of esophageal circular muscle contractions elicited by intramural nerve stimulation *in vitro*. According to this model, during swallowing, the esophageal circular muscle remains in its resting, quiescent state, responsible for the latency period, which is followed by contraction caused by sequential activation of excitatory cholinergic neurons (10).

This model of sequential activation of the cholinergic pathway leading to peristalsis was called into question when it was found that simultaneous electrical stimulation of vagal efferents elicits peristalsis rather than simultaneous contraction at all levels of the esophagus. These studies raised the possibility that vagal efferents to all levels of the smooth muscle portion of the esophagus may be activated simultaneously and pointed to a peripheral mechanism for peristalsis. Moreover, Rattan and co-workers (152) and others have reported that vagal efferent stimulation as well as swallowing cause a sequence of inhibition followed by contraction of the esophageal circular muscle. The sequence of mechanical inhibition (latency) and contraction correlated with the membrane potential changes of hyperpolarization followed by depolarization of esophageal circular smooth muscle (Fig. 1.12). Weisbrodt and Christensen (153) made the original observation that transmural stimulation of esophageal circular muscle strips produces a contraction after a period of latency and well after the end of the stimulus. They called it the "off" contraction. They also found that this contraction was not cholinergically mediated but was due to a nonadrenergic and noncholinergic inhibitory neurotransmitter. Electrophysiologic studies have shown that transmural stimula-

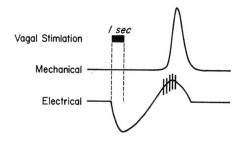

FIGURE 1.12. Schematic illustrating simultaneous mechanical and electrical potential changes recorded from opossum esophageal circular smooth muscle. Note that vagal stimulation elicited hyperpolarization (inhibitory junction potential [IJP], trough) followed by a rebound depolarization (excitatory junctional potential [EJP], crest) with superimposed spikes in the electrical activity trace. Mechanical trace shows a period of latency after vagal stimulation, followed by a contraction. The latency corresponds to the IJP and the contraction to EJP and spike activity. The neurotransmitter nitric oxide (NO) seems to be responsible for the hyperpolarization and associated latency of the smooth muscle, whereas the EJP and smooth muscle contraction seem to be due to a blend of NO-associated rebound and cholinergic excitation.

tion elicits membrane hyperpolarization followed by depolarization, which correlate with the latency period and "off" contractions, respectively, in mechanical studies (152). Both of these responses are noncholinergic and are thought to be mediated by the gaseous neurotransmitter nitric oxide (NO) (154). Furthermore, Weisbrodt and Christensen (153) reported that the latency of circular muscle contraction increased progressively in caudal segments of the esophageal circular smooth muscle and suggested that esophageal peristalsis was due to noncholinergic inhibitory nerves and that a gradient in their influence or a regional difference in smooth muscle was responsible for swallow-induced peristalsis (5). This model, however, could not account for the fact that the latency gradient elicited by vagal efferent stimulation did not match the slower velocity of swallow-induced peristalsis. Moreover, this model also could not account for the observed effect of atropine on primary peristalsis (155,156).

More recent studies suggest that both noncholinergic inhibitory and sequential cholinergic excitatory pathways are involved in esophageal peristalsis. The presence of two parallel pathways in the vagal efferents was suggested by studies of Gidda and Buyniski (157). They recorded swallow-evoked potentials from single cervical vagal efferent fibers of the opossum (Fig. 1.13) and found two types of preganglionic efferent fiber destined for the smooth muscle esophagus based on electrophysiologic characteristics and latency distributions (32). Short-latency fibers began firing within 1 second of the onset of swallowing, as recorded by mylohyoid activity. Long-latency fibers had latencies to onset of discharge that ranged between 1 and 5 seconds. The respective latency distributions indicate that short-latency discharges correlate with deglutitive inhibition and long-latency fibers correlate with peristaltic contractions. The swallow-evoked efferent discharge in each fiber lasts approximately 1 second with four to six spikes per discharge. These results were consistent with sequential activation of excitatory nerves during swallowing, as proposed by Roman and Gonella (10). However, Gidda and Buyniski (157) suggested the existence of a parallel inhibitory vagal pathway that is also activated during swallowing.

Evidence for both cholinergic and noncholinergic peripheral pathways was first furnished by Dodds and co-workers (158), who showed that, depending on the intensity of stimulus used, vagal efferent stimulation can elicit either a cholinergic or a noncholinergic contraction in the esophageal circular muscle, as evidenced by sensitivity to atropine. They also showed that with long trains of vagal stimulation, the cholinergic contraction occurred with the onset ("on" contraction) and the noncholinergic contraction occurred after the end ("off," or rebound, contraction) of the stimulus. Careful *in vitro* studies of circular smooth muscle strips also showed that, depending on the stimulus used, either cholinergic or noncholinergic contractions can be elicited. Moreover, long-train electrical stimuli also produced a cholinergic ("on") contraction near the onset and a noncholinergic ("off") contraction after the end of the stimulus (Fig. 1.14). Recent studies

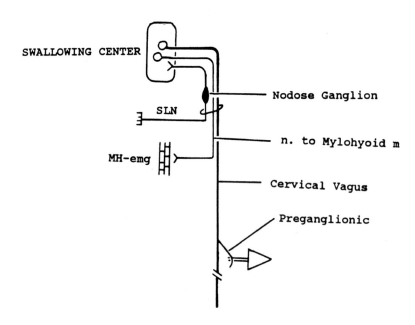

FIGURE 1.13. Schematic illustrating the setup used for recording swallow-evoked responses from single-unit efferent vagal fibers of opossums. The superior laryngeal nerve (SLN) was stimulated to evoke swallowing, and the mylohyoid muscle activity (EMG) was monitored as an index of swallowing.

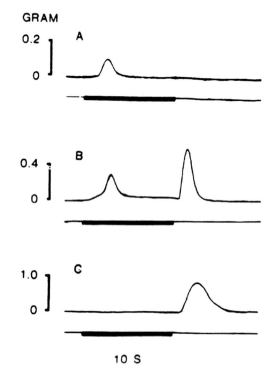

FIGURE 1.14. Main patterns of contraction seen with transmural electrical stimulation of opossum esophageal circular smooth muscle strips. Stimulus train duration and pulse width were constant at 10 seconds and 1 millisecond, respectively. **A:** Stimulus of 60 V and 40 Hz resulted in only an "on" contraction, occurring shortly after onset of stimulus. **B:** Stimulus 80 V and 20 Hz produced both "on" and "off"' contractions. "On" contractions were sensitive to cholinergic blockade with atropine, whereas "off" contractions were not sensitive to cholinergic or adrenergic blockade. **C:** Stimulus of 80 V and 10 Hz evoked only an "off" contraction, occurring after termination of stimulus. (From Hollerbach S, Kamath MV, Chen Y, et al. The magnitude of the central response to esophageal electrical stimulation is intensity dependent. *Gastroenterology* 1997;112:1137–1146, with permission.)

have shown that "off" contractions are blocked by chemical inhibitors of the enzyme NOS (159–161).

The aforementioned observations are consistent with the view that during short-train electrical vagal efferent or transmural stimulations, the contraction waves may be a blend of overlapping cholinergic and noncholinergic contractions. However, they do not explain the roles of cholinergic and noncholinergic nerves in esophageal peristalsis, that is, the latency gradient along the esophagus. It appears that peristalsis in the smooth muscle portion of the esophagus is due to the latency gradient that is determined both by noncholinergic inhibitory as well as cholinergic excitatory nerves.

Weisbrodt and Christensen (153) were the first to demonstrate a latency gradient along the esophagus resulting from noncholinergic inhibitory nerves. Studies of membrane potential recording also show that, on transmural stimulation of noncholinergic nerves, the duration of the inhibitory junction potential (IJP) is shorter in circular smooth muscle from proximal rather than distal sites (162,163). This may be due to increasing noncholinergic influence distally along the esophagus.

The cholinergic influence has been shown to decrease the latency of contraction (164). A craniocaudally decreasing cholinergic influence would have the effect of slowing the velocity of peristalsis, as seen during swallowing. Crist and colleagues (164) have reported that cholinergic motor influence was maximal in the proximal portion of the esophagus and decreased distally. This was evidenced by greater sensitivity to atropine of the contraction amplitude and latency elicited by transmural stimulation of the circular muscle strips from proximal than from distal esophageal segments. Studies of membrane potential recordings more clearly showed a greater expression of cholinergic influence in reducing the duration of the IJP at proximal rather than distal esophageal sites (163) (Fig. 1.15). These and other observations led Crist and colleagues (164) to suggest a model showing gradients of decreasing cholinergic and increasing noncholinergic influences distally along the esophagus. These gradients explain, at least in part, how vagal efferent or transmural nerve stimulation elicits the peristaltic sequence of esophageal contractions and how changing the intensity of electrical stimulation of the vagus nerve could change the velocity of esophageal peristalsis by altering the cholinergic and noncholinergic components in the peristaltic contractions (149). In addition to the peripheral mechanism of peristalsis explained by the regional gradients of noncholinergic and cholinergic nerves, central sequential activation of the cholinergic pathway during swallowing would further aid in the normal slow speed of primary peristalsis (Fig. 1.16). During swallowing, there is immediate, near simultaneous activation of the inhibitory pathway but a delayed and sequential activation of the cholinergic excitatory neural pathway in the vagus. The early and more prominent cholinergic activation in the proximal esophageal site would cause greater shortening of latencies of contraction at the more proximal sites, resulting in increased velocity of esophageal peristalsis.

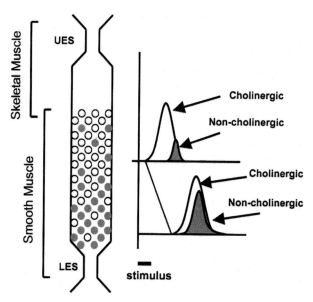

FIGURE 1.16. Schematic drawing illustrating gradients of cholinergic (*white*) and noncholinergic (*shaded*) nerve influence along the smooth muscle portion of the esophagus. Cholinergic influence is most prominent proximally and progressively decreases distally. In contrast, noncholinergic influence is most prominent distally and progressively decreases proximally. (From Crist J, Gidda JS, Goyal RK. Intramural mechanism of esophageal peristalsis: roles of cholinergic and noncholinergic nerves. *Proc Natl Acad Sci U S A* 1984;81:3595–3599, with permission.)

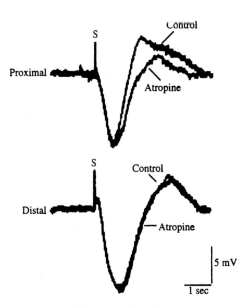

STUMULUS PULSE
1.0 m sec

FIGURE 1.15. Intracellular recording from opossum esophageal smooth muscle taken from proximal and distal esophageal sites. Note that transmural stimulation (at *S*) caused a hyperpolarization response in the smooth muscle cells from both sites. The control trace from the proximal site shows a shorter duration of hyperpolarization (inhibitory junctional potential [IJP]). However, following atropine treatment, the duration of IJP increased, suggesting cholinergic mediation in shortened duration of IJP. At the distal site, atropine had no marked effect, suggesting minimal cholinergic mediation. These observations illustrate that there is a gradient of cholinergic activity along the esophagus with the greatest influence at the proximal sites.

Successive vagal stimulation has been used to study whether the phenomenon of deglutitive inhibition in the esophageal circular muscle is also due to active peripheral inhibition by the noncholinergic inhibitory nerves (150). These studies show that, similar to successive swallows, vagal stimulation exerts an inhibitory effect on the esophagus and that a peripheral mechanism for inhibition exists in the smooth muscle esophagus. Studies also (a) show that the duration of deglutitive inhibition increases distally along the esophagus, (b) explain the phenomenon of rebound contraction, which is due to ongoing active inhibition throughout the period of vagal stimulation, and (c) reveal that esophageal peristaltic contractions are followed by a period of refractoriness (151).

The esophageal body circular muscle is a phasic muscle; it contracts transiently and does not develop sustained tone upon stimulation. This phasic property may be related to the composition of its contractile proteins. When compared with tonic sphincter muscle, esophageal phasic muscle contained less α-actin and a greater proportion of caldesmon, calmodulin, a unique seven amino acid–inserted myosin isoform, and an acidic essential light chain (LC17a) (165,166). A variety of ion channels, including potassium, chloride, calcium, and nonselective cations, have been identified in the esophagus. These channels modulate the membrane potential and influence calcium entry into the smooth muscle cells, thereby modifying contractility (167–169). Regional electrophysiologic differences resulting from ion channel diversity generate variations in the resting membrane potentials of smooth muscle cells along the esophageal body (170). These differences may contribute to differential muscular responses during peristalsis, but this has yet to be determined. In addition, the esophageal body circular muscle also exhibits different length-tension responses, with distal segments developing lower tension in response to stretch (171).

NO and ACh are the major inhibitory and excitatory neurotransmitters, respectively. The redox form of NO involved in inhibitory neurotransmission is the nitric oxide gas (NO$^\bullet$) (172), and its inhibitory effect is due to a wide variety of signaling pathways that lead to a decrease in intracellular Ca^{2+} and inhibition of contractile activity. One of the important actions of NO$^\bullet$ is to produce membrane hyperpolarization, thereby causing inhibition of voltage-dependent calcium entry in smooth muscle cells. Goyal and co-workers (172–174) have shown that this hyperpolarization is due to cyclic guanosine monophosphate (cGMP)-dependent inhibition of a resting chloride conductance. These chloride channels are regulated by myosin light-chain kinase (175). In contrast, others have suggested that nitrergic IJP is due to opening of potassium channels (176).

ACh affects many ionic currents in esophageal circular muscle (169,177). Carbachol activates a Ca^{2+}-sensitive chloride and nonselective cation currents (169). These currents appear to be activated by the release of Ca^{2+} from intracellular stores. Activation of the chloride currents would cause depolarization of the smooth muscle membrane, leading to Ca^{2+} entry into the cells by way of voltage-sensitive Ca^{2+} channels. The nonselective cation channels are also permeable to Ca^{2+} and other cations, but not to anions. The nonselective cation channels have a large conductance but are sparsely distributed on the smooth muscle membrane; therefore, single-channel currents can be observed. Their activation is not associated with significant depolarization. These channels may serve as a source for nonvoltage-dependent Ca^{2+} entry (178). ACh also inhibits a variety of potassium channels. These effects on potassium channels are most likely involved in the enhancement of the excitatory effect of ACh (177). The signaling cascade for ACh-induced contraction of the esophageal circular muscle is different from that in the LES (179–181). In the esophageal circular muscle, ACh acts on M_2 muscarinic receptors that are coupled to pertussis toxin sensitive G_i proteins or rho protein to activate phospholipase D (PLD), phosphatidyl-specific phospholipase C (PLC) via guanosine triphosphate (GTP)-binding protein (G_{i3}), and phospholipase A_2 (PLA$_2$) via an as yet unknown GTP-binding protein (182–184). Activation of these enzymes requires influx of extracellular Ca^{2+} (180). These phospholipases produce diacylglycerol (DAG) and arachidonic acid (AA). DAG and AA act synergistically to stimulate protein kinase C$_\Sigma$

(PKC$_\Sigma$) (180). Activated PKC$_\Sigma$ appears to act via mitogen-associated protein (MAP) kinase to inactivate actin-based inhibitory proteins such as caldesmon to cause muscle contraction. In experimental esophagitis, ACh-elicited contraction is not significantly affected (185). Inflammatory mediators may suppress esophageal contraction *in vivo* by inhibiting the release or action of ACh.

Muscarinic antagonists such as atropine suppress the amplitude of esophageal contractions and prolong the latency of contractions in the smooth muscle but have no effect on the striated muscle. This effect is more marked in proximal than in distal parts of the esophagus (156,164). Moreover, peristaltic contractions in certain species, such as cats, are more sensitive to atropine than those in opossums (157). Chemical blockers of NOS reduce the latency of contractions, particularly in the most distal parts of the esophagus, leading to simultaneous-onset contractions in response to swallowing (154,186). A combination of atropine and NOS blockers eliminates peristaltic contractions. Stroma-free hemoglobin solution binds and thereby scavenges released NO, resulting in effects on the esophageal peristalsis that are similar to those of NOS blockers used in animals (187,188). Esophageal peristalsis is also affected by agents that act centrally at neuronal synapses of esophageal neurons and directly at the smooth muscle.

The previous discussion has focused on the esophageal circular muscle. However, the esophageal longitudinal muscle, by causing esophageal shortening, also plays an important role in various reflex activities (189). Swallowing causes sequential activation of longitudinal muscle segments and is associated with inhibition and excitation, as seen in the esophageal circular muscle. The esophageal longitudinal muscle has prominent cholinergic and substance P innervation (190), and its pharmacology differs in some respects from that of the esophageal circular muscle. For example, NO donors and cGMP elicit a biphasic response of marked contraction preceded by transient relaxation. NO opens Ca^{2+}-activated Cl^- channels via a cGMP-dependent pathway, leading to extracellular Ca^{2+} entry through activation of L-type Ca^{2+} channels and contraction of the longitudinal smooth muscle (175). This contraction also is mediated by a tyrosine kinase-signaling pathway (191).

LOWER ESOPHAGEAL SPHINCTER

General Description

The LES can be readily identified by intraluminal manometry as a 2- to 4-cm zone of high pressure at the gastroesophageal junction. The manometrically defined LES is marked by a ring of thickened circular muscle (192,193). Ultrastructural studies of the sphincter muscle in the opossum suggest that muscle cells from the LES are of larger diameter and form fewer gap junctions than do those of the esophageal body. These sphincter muscle cells also have irregular surfaces and evaginations that are not seen in the esophageal body. The evaginations may be related to the tonically contracted state of the sphincter muscle (193). The LES can also be distinguished from the esophageal body by the presence of more numerous intermuscular spaces containing blood vessels and connective tissue (193). Mitochondria and the smooth endoplasmic reticulum mass are greater in the LES than in the esophageal body (194).

The LES is innervated by vagal preganglionic and sympathetic postganglionic efferents (195). Similar to the esophageal body, vagal preganglionic nerves to the LES regulate both inhibitory and excitatory responses. Preganglionic neurons forming the inhibitory pathway stem from caudal regions of the DMNV, whereas neurons conducting excitatory responses originate from rostral parts of the DMNV (43). These efferents largely innervate neurons in the myenteric plexus. The myenteric neurons contain many chemical markers (133,144,145). Two prominent populations of motor neurons are noteworthy: those that contain NOS and VIP are inhibitory motor neurons and those that contain choline acetyltransferase and substance P are excitatory motor neurons. The motor neurons supply innervation to the muscle layers, including the interstitial cells of Cajal (ICC), which may serve as intermediary to amplify actions of neurotransmitters on the smooth muscle cells (196–198).

Basal Pressure

The high-pressure zone caused by the LES shows axial as well as radial asymmetry (199). Axially, the LES pressure has a bell-shaped configuration with a total length of between 2 and 4 cm. Pressures tend to be higher in the more distal segment of the LES. The LES is radially symmetrical in its oral half, but in the aboral half, it shows higher pressures on the left side (200–202). The diaphragm makes an impression on the left side of the terminal esophagus. Thus, both diaphragmatic and gastric sling fibers that buttress the left side of the LES may help to create higher pressures in this region.

In humans, the pressures in the upper and lower halves of the LES are usually affected by respiration in opposite ways. In the lower part, inspiration causes an increase in LES pressure, whereas the opposite occurs in the upper part (202). This is thought to represent abdominal and thoracic influences at the distal and proximal locations, respectively. The point at which the respiratory pressure transition occurs is called the *point of respiratory reversal* or the pressure inversion point. This often occurs over a wide region that shows biphasic pressure changes with respiration. This zone is approximately 0.5 cm wide and is usually located in the middle of the high-pressure zone, but its precise location is

variable. The point of respiratory reversal may be related to the crura of the diaphragm, which separates thoracic from abdominal cavities and provides opposing pressure environments during respiration. It may also be related to the LES itself in that it separates intraesophageal from intragastric pressure or axial movement of the esophagus relative to the recording device. In addition, because of the position of the LES within the diaphragmatic hiatus, the sphincter pressure may be influenced by the respiratory contractions of the crural diaphragm (13,202–205). Slow phasic contractions in phase with the gastric component of the migrating myoelectrical complex (MMC) have been described in humans and animals (206–209).

The basal LES pressure is due to myogenic tone, which is normally modulated by excitatory and inhibitory neurohormonal influences. The hallmark of the sphincter muscle is its propensity to maintain tonic contraction (210). This ability distinguishes the LES from the esophageal body muscle. The cellular mechanisms involved in stress or tone maintenance in the LES are not fully understood. The tonic behavior of the LES muscle has been attributed to a depolarized state and the presence of spikes that cause influx of Ca^{2+} in the resting state of the muscle. Papasova and coworkers (211) found that the sphincter muscle exhibited tone in the absence of spike activity and that this spike-independent tone varied directly with the resting membrane potential. A relatively depolarized resting state of the sphincter muscle, which would result in increased tone, has been reported in studies with direct intracellular recordings. Zelcer and Weisbrodt (212) reported that resting membrane potential of the sphincter smooth muscle was approximately −40 mV, in contrast to the resting membrane potential of esophageal body circular muscle, which is −50 mV. Asoh and Goyal (213) showed that the opossum LES *in vivo* shows continuous spike activity. Moreover, increases in spike activity are associated with an increase in the maintained sphincter tone, and abolition of the spike activity is associated with a decrease (Fig. 1.17). Changes in spike activity may be regulated by K^+ and Ca^{2+}-activated Cl^- channels (214). Continuous spike activity has also been shown to be present in the cat LES (215). The depolarized state of the sphincter smooth muscle has been suggested to be due to resting chloride conductance (216).

Studies have also shown that sphincter muscles have higher resting intracellular Ca^{2+} levels than nonsphincteric muscles. Biancani and colleagues have proposed that there are two distinct contractile signal transduction pathways in LES smooth muscle cells and that the pathways are regulated by the concentration of intracellular Ca^{2+}. One pathway that contributes toward the maintenance of LES tone involves PKC-dependent mechanism of contraction. Spontaneously active PLC produces low levels of inositol 1,4,5-triphosphate (IP_3), which releases low levels of Ca^{2+} from intracellular stores. The mildly elevated intracellular Ca^{2+} levels are insufficient to activate calmodulin and myosin

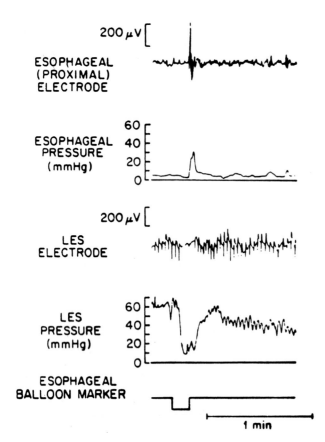

FIGURE 1.17. Influence of inflation of an intraluminal esophageal balloon on electrical activity and pressures of distal esophageal body and lower esophageal sphincter (LES). Balloon inflation causes cessation of tonic LES spike activity and simultaneous decrease in LES pressure. Balloon deflation causes spike activity that precedes contraction in the esophageal body; in LES, tonic spike activity reappears as LES pressure returns toward baseline. (From Asoh R, Goyal RK. Electrical activity of the opossum lower esophageal sphincter *in vivo.* Its role in the basal sphincter pressure. *Gastroenterology* 1978;74:835–840, with permission.)

light-chain kinase (MLCK). However, these $[Ca^{2+}]_i$ levels are sufficient to interact with DAG, generated by a phosphatidylcholine-specific PLC (PC-PLC) that is concurrently active, to generate tone through a PKC-dependent pathway (179,217–219). A second pathway involves maximal doses of ACh to stimulate phosphatidylinositol-specific PI-PLC, IP$_3$, and calmodulin. In this pathway, ACh activates M$_3$ muscarinic receptors linked to G$_{q/11}$-type G proteins to stimulate PI-PLC, which results in the formation of IP$_3$ and DAG. IP$_3$ subsequently releases a significant amount of Ca^{2+} from intracellular stores. The higher level of intracellular Ca^{2+} promotes the formation of calcium–calmodulin complex, leading to myosin light chain phosphorylation and muscle contraction (179). The level of intracellular Ca^{2+} available for contraction determines which of the two pathways will be activated, and a switch from one pathway to the other can occur (220).

Weisbrodt and Murphy (221) have studied the phosphorylation of myosin during force development and

maintenance in opossum LES. They found that the phosphorylation rate was approximately 4% of maximum during the relaxed state of the sphincter, increased to 33% during tone development, and then decreased to 16% during tone maintenance, supporting the role of the latch phenomenon in LES tone. Szymanski and co-workers (166) have reported that LES has a different contractile protein composition than the esophageal circular muscle. The LES muscle has proportionally more α-actin and basic essential light chains LC17b and less of a seven amino acid–inserted myosin isoform and caldesmon than esophageal body circular muscle. These differences in the contractile protein may determine the tonic phenotype of the LES muscle. The energy required to maintain sphincter tone is evidenced by its marked sensitivity to anoxia compared to that of esophageal body muscle (222,223). It has been reported that the LES has lower levels of cytochrome *c* oxidase activity than does the esophageal body (224). This may help to explain why the LES is more dependent on exogenous O$_2$.

The mechanical advantage afforded by the Laplace law to the tonic sphincter muscle *in vivo* explains the ability of the LES to stay closed at rest with a small tension requirement and to generate fairly stable pressures over a wide range of luminal diameters (192,225). Excitatory and inhibitory nerve activity on the myogenic tone of the sphincter can influence its resting pressure. However, it is clear that the major component of the resting basal pressure of the sphincter *in vivo* is not due to tonic excitatory nerve activity (226).

Relaxation

Deglutition causes relaxation of the LES, which may start with the onset of the deglutition. Usually, LES relaxation begins less than 2 seconds after the initiation of swallowing. At this time, the swallowed bolus is in the esophagus and the peristaltic contraction is oral to the bolus in the cervical esophagus. In the upright position, the swallowed bolus may reach the LES quickly because of gravity; when this happens, it may be transiently delayed at the sphincter before passage into the stomach. The LES normally relaxes to a pressure equal to or close to intragastric pressure. Relaxation of the LES may last for a total of 8 to 10 seconds and is followed in the oral part of the sphincter by an aftercontraction, which is in continuity with the peristaltic contraction in the esophageal body. The aftercontraction lasts 7 to 10 seconds. The lower part of the LES does not show aftercontractions, and the sphincter pressure simply returns to the resting level. Electrical recordings show that swallow-induced LES relaxation is associated with cessation of spike activity when present (213).

Relaxation of the LES is the most sensitive component of the swallowing reflex. Thus, it is possible to have LES relaxation without any other motor evidence of the swal-

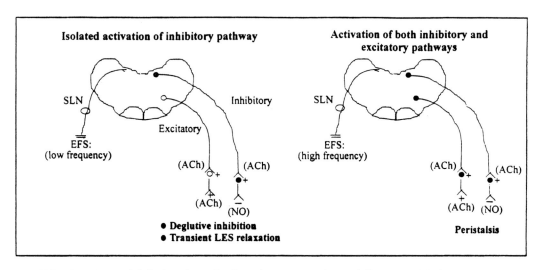

FIGURE 1.18. Model depicts the activation of neurons in the medulla responsible for peristalsis. Low-frequency stimulation of the superior laryngeal nerve activates only the inhibitory pathway, whereas high-frequency stimulation activates both the inhibitory and excitatory pathways.

lowing reflex (Fig. 1.18). Isolated LES relaxation can be induced experimentally by applying pharyngeal tactile stimulation, which is subthreshold for producing a full swallowing response. Similarly, electrical stimulation of the SLN with stimulus frequencies that fail to produce esophageal peristalsis causes isolated LES relaxation. Low-intensity stimulation of the swallowing center can also cause isolated LES relaxation (227). Modifying the stimulus from pharyngeal tactile stimulation to unilateral SLN stimulation decreases the relaxation reflex (228). When repeated swallows are made in succession, as during rapid drinking, the LES remains relaxed and returns to the baseline state of tone after the last swallow (1). The LES relaxation associated with primary peristalsis, as well as the isolated LES relaxation due to pharyngeal or SLN stimulation, is mediated by vagal efferent nerves and abolished by bilateral cervical vagal section or cooling (146,147).

Distention of either the striated or smooth muscle portion of the esophagus produces a reflex relaxation of the LES that is associated with secondary peristalsis in the esophageal body. During prolonged, localized esophageal distention, the LES may recover from relaxation despite ongoing distention (109,115). The sphincter relaxation due to distention in the striated muscle is centrally mediated and abolished by vagotomy, whereas the relaxation due to distention in the smooth muscle portion is mediated by intramural nerves and remains after bilateral vagotomy. However, recent studies have shown that the vagus nerves may exert a facilitative influence on LES relaxation evoked by balloon distention of the smooth muscle portion of the esophagus (109,146). As with primary peristalsis, LES relaxation is also the most sensitive component of secondary peristalsis. Thus, isolated LES

relaxation without esophageal contraction occurs with distentions that are subthreshold for activation of full secondary peristalsis.

Recently, it has been suggested that intramuscular types of ICC (ICC-IM) may play a role in transducing the effects of neurotransmitters released from nerve ending to smooth muscle cells (197,229). However, studies using nNOS-deficient mice and W/W^V mutant mice that lack ICC-IM show that the LES is achalasic in nNOS-deficient mice but hypotensive with normal relaxation in W/W^V mice (230) (Fig. 1.19). W/W^V mutant mice have a genetic abnormality that results in partial deficiency of *c-kit* and associated lack of ICC-IM. These findings suggest that ICC-IM may not serve as the mediator of inhibitory neurotransmission in the LES, but instead that deficiency in ICC-IM may impair the myogenic function of the LES. Further studies are needed to fully define the role of ICC-IM in inhibitory neurotransmission in the LES.

Transient Lower Esophageal Sphincter Relaxation

Apart from primary and secondary peristalsis, relaxation of the LES also occurs during belching, retching, vomiting, and rumination (1,12,231,232). During belching and vomiting, there is no esophageal contraction in association with LES relaxation (233). With rumination, LES relaxation is associated with reverse peristalsis. Dent and colleagues (29) performed long-term recording of LES pressure using a sleeve device and observed that normal volunteers showed esophageal reflux episodes that were related to transient relaxations of the LES, which were not associated with swallows. These relaxation episodes are also called *inappropriate relaxations*. These transient relax-

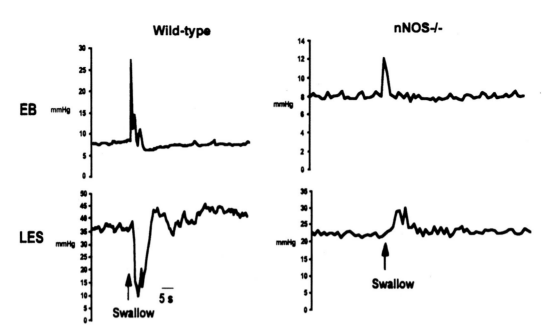

FIGURE 1.19. Esophageal motility in anesthetized wild-type and nNOS-deficient mice. Left panels show that, in the wild-type mouse, swallow induced by pharyngeal stimulation causes contraction in the esophageal body (EB) at 2 mm proximal to the lower esophageal sphincter (LES) and relaxation of the LES. Right panels show that in the nNOS-deficient mouse, swallow induced by pharyngeal stimulation causes contraction in the EB, but does not produce LES relaxation. Instead, a small contraction replaces the relaxation seen in the wild-type mouse.

ations cause a significant number of reflux episodes in normal subjects as well as in patients with reflux esophagitis. Transient LES (tLES) relaxations are frequently associated with reflux of gas and are a component of the belch reflex. However, not all tLES relaxations are accompanied by reflux episodes. The percentage of tLES relaxations accompanied by reflux varies, depending on experimental circumstances, from as few as 10% to 15% (234) to as many as 93% (29). The tLES relaxation is a vagally mediated reflex. The efferent arm of this reflex appears to involve vagal efferents that synapse on nitrergic postganglionic neurons, the same pathway that is involved in swallow-induced relaxation (Fig. 1.20). The tLES relaxations are facilitated by gastric distention with gas or after a meal. They are also facilitated by the presence of a nasogastric tube (22,235).

The neurotransmitters involved in the vagal inhibitory pathway to the LES have been investigated in some detail (236,237). This pathway consists of a chain of at least two neurons consisting of pre- and postgaglionic neurons. The preganglionic neurons are carried in the vagus and synapse on postganglionic inhibitory neurons present intramurally in the LES.

The preganglionic neurons release predominantly Ach, which activates the postgaglionic inhibitory neurons by stimulating both nicotinic and M_1 muscarinic receptors (236). There is also evidence that serotonin participates to a lesser degree in this synaptic transmission (238). However, the combination of M_1 and serotonergic antagonists does not modify LES relaxation due to electrical stimulation of intramural inhibitory nerves. These observations show that the effect of the antagonists is exerted at the synaptic site between pre- and postganglionic neurons (239). The intramural neural pathway involved in distention-induced LES relaxation is not known. Transient LES relaxation is also mediated via the vagal pathway because it is blocked by vagotomy or vagal cooling (22).

The inhibitory neurotransmitter released by the intramural inhibitory neurons remains unknown but is clearly not cholinergic or adrenergic in nature. Hence, this neurotransmitter is called *noncholinergic, nonadrenergic* (236, 240). However, strong evidence suggests that NO gas is the major inhibitory neurotransmitter for relaxation induced by swallowing, esophageal distention, or tLES relaxation (22,159,161,241,242). Chemical blockers of NO block transmurally stimulated relaxation of the LES *in vitro* (241) (Fig. 1.21) and swallow-induced relaxation in anesthetized animals (161) (Fig. 1.22). There is also evidence for the involvement of VIP in inhibitory neurotransmission (243, 244). In some systems, VIP serves as an intermediary agent

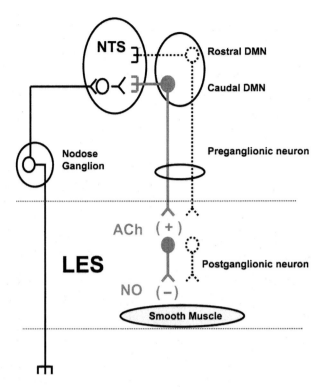

FIGURE 1.20. Neural circuitry for transient lower esophageal sphincter (tLES) relaxation. Afferent signals from the subdiaphragmatic vagus nerves are relayed sequentially to the nucleus of the solitary tract (NTS) and the dorsal motor nucleus of the vagus (DMN) in the medulla. The efferent arm involves vagal efferents that synapse on nitrergic postganglionic neurons and is the same pathway that is involved in swallow-induced relaxation. (From Rathmann W, Enck P, Frieling T, et al. Visceral afferent neuropathy in diabetic gastroparesis. *Diabetes Care* 1991;14:1086–1089, with permission.)

to release NO upon nerve stimulation (245–247). VIP may also act in parallel with NO to participate in inhibitory neurotransmission.

The cellular basis of reflex LES relaxation is not fully understood, although it is clear that it is an active process. It is associated with inhibition of continuous spike activity and hyperpolarization of the muscle cell membrane, which may be due to suppression of a resting chloride conductance by NO or activation of a potassium conductance. Smooth muscle hyperpolarization would cause muscle relaxation (electromechanical coupling) due to suppression of Ca^{2+} influx, leading to cessation of myosin phosphorylation. Both cyclic adenosine monophosphate and cGMP mediate LES relaxation (248–250) by activating protein kinases A and G, respectively. These signaling molecules can cause smooth muscle relaxation without causing membrane hyperpolarization (pharmacomechanical coupling). These kinases may lower the free intracellular Ca^{2+} for the enzyme MLCK.

Contraction

The upper part of the LES displays reflex contraction immediately after the peristalsis-related relaxation. This contraction occurs in continuity with the peristaltic wave of the esophageal body and may represent the response of esophageal body type: circular muscle mixed with the sphincter muscle. A similar behavior is seen in muscle strips

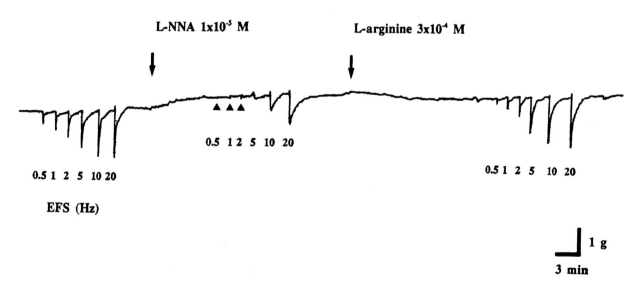

FIGURE 1.21. Nitric oxide (NO) mediates lower esophageal sphincter (LES) relaxation. Electrical field stimulation (EFS) causes frequency-dependent relaxation in the opossum LES circular smooth muscle. Pretreatment with the NO synthase inhibitor NW nitro-L-arginine (L-NNA) inhibits this response. Pretreatment with L-arginine, a competitive substrate to the enzyme and a precursor of NO, restores relaxatory responses to EFS.

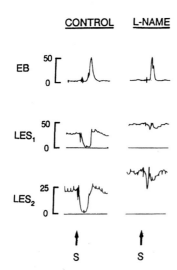

FIGURE 1.22. Effect of nitric oxide synthase blocker on swallow (S)-induced relaxation in the lower esophageal sphincter (LES). Note that nitro-L-arginine methyl ester (L-NAME) (20 mg/kg) markedly antagonized relaxation in both LES leads.

in vitro. This aftercontraction is somehow related to the level of baseline tone. Human LES circular muscle strips show prominent aftercontractions when basal tone is low, but as the tone increases, the aftercontraction is abolished.

Short-lived increases in LES pressure also occur as a result of increases in intraabdominal pressure. Considerable controversy exists as to whether this increase in LES pressure is due to reflex contraction or merely to a passive transmission of the increased intraabdominal pressure (251, 252). The studies that show this to be a true reflex also suggest that it is vagally mediated and dependent on cholinergic neurons. The LES also contracts transiently, in phase with stomach contractions. This is closely tied to the phasic antral contractions that occur during different stages of the MMC (206–208). During the first phase of the MMC, the LES pressure is stable, whereas during late phase II and throughout phase III, large-amplitude phasic contractions occur without there being a major change in the basal pressure. These MMC-related contractions are abolished by atropine and anesthesia (207,253). Studies suggest that they are initiated by the circulating hormone motilin (208). The effect of infused motilin is abolished by hexamethonium and markedly inhibited by atropine and the selective M_3 antagonist 4-DAMP. This indicates that motilin may stimulate preganglionic cholinergic fibers, which in turn activate nicotinic receptors on postganglionic cholinergic excitatory fibers. These latter neurons then release ACh.

The signaling pathway for ACh-induced contraction has been examined in detail by Biancani and colleagues (254). In the LES smooth muscle of cat, ACh stimulates M_3 muscarinic receptors that activate PLC via the GTP-binding protein (G_q) to produce IP_3. IP_3 causes release of Ca^{2+} from the sarcolemmal store. The released Ca^{2+} activates calmodulin, and Ca^{2+}= calmodulin activates MLCK, which phosphorylates myosin light chains (MLCs) to cause contraction. In experimental esophagitis, there is a change in the signaling cascade in that ACh causes contraction via the PKC-dependent pathway (185). Infusion of acid into the esophageal lumen also causes a neurally mediated reflex contraction of the LES. This reflex contraction involves substance P–containing nerves (215).

Pharmacology

Figure 1.23 represents three major factors that influence sphincter pressure. These are the myogenic tone (226) of the LES and the inhibitory (NO) (255–257) and excitatory (ACh) (253,258–260) influences. A multitude of endogenous compounds, hormones (261–264), and classic (239, 259,260,265,266) and putative neurotransmitters (187, 267–271) affect LES pressure in pharmacologic experiments by affecting one or more of these three mechanisms. However, the physiologic significance of their effect is not clear. Additionally, lifestyle and dietary habits affect LES activity (272,273). Table 1.1 summarizes the effect of some endogenous chemicals on LES function.

EXTERNAL LOWER ESOPHAGEAL SPHINCTER: DIAPHRAGMATIC CRURA

Mittal and colleagues (21,274) and others (203,275) have provided overwhelming evidence to suggest that the diaphragmatic crura of the esophageal hiatus acts on the external LES (Fig. 1.24). Manometric recordings of LES pressure are characterized by inspiratory spike-like increases in pressure that result from inspiratory contractions of the diaphragmatic crura that encircle the LES (21,203). The crural diaphragm acts independently of the costal diaphragm under certain gastrointestinal functions. For example, during vomiting and eructation, when the costal diaphragm shows marked electrical activity consistent with its contractile state, the esophageal crural diaphragm is inactive, consistent with its relaxation (276). Similarly, during esophageal distention, the crural diaphragm becomes inactive when the costal diaphragm is contracting. These observations indicate that the esophageal crural diaphragm relaxes during reflex relaxation of the smooth muscle LES (277). The crural diaphragm is also inhibited during other reflex activities that cause LES relaxation, such as swallowing and LES relaxation (234,278).

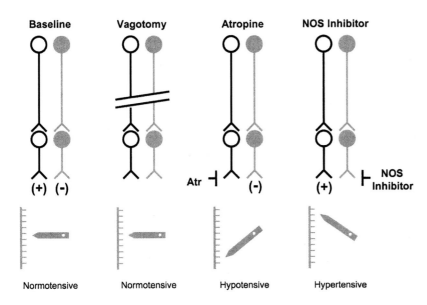

FIGURE 1.23. Effect of vagotomy and neural antagonists on the lower esophageal sphincter (LES) pressure. LES pressure is dependent on the balance among myogenic tone, vagal excitatory stimulus, and vagal inhibitory stimulus. When vagal excitatory and inhibitory neural influences are equal, bilateral vagotomy reveals underlying myogenic tone. Atropine selectively inhibits the vagal excitatory stimulus and reduces LES pressure. Conversely, nitric oxide synthase inhibitors selectively interrupt vagal inhibitory effects and increase LES pressure.

TABLE 1.1. EFFECTS OF SOME HORMONES AND PUTATIVE NEUROTRANSMITTERS ON THE LOWER ESOPHAGEAL SPHINCTER

Agent	Effect	Site of Action			Comments
		Circular Smooth Muscle	Inhibitory Neurons	Excitatory Neurons	
Bombesin	Contraction	√	—	√	Releases norepinephrine from adrenergic neurons
Calcitonin gene-related peptide	Relaxation	√	√	—	
Cholecystokinin	Biphasic	√	√	—	Inhibition overrides excitation, causes paradoxical excitation in achalasia patients
Dopamine	Relaxation (D$_2$)	√	—	—	
	Contraction (D$_1$)	√	—	—	
Galanin	Contraction	√	—	—	
Gastric inhibitory polypeptide	Relaxation	?	?	?	
Gastrin	Contraction	√	—	—	
Glucagon	Relaxation	√	—	—	Releases catecholamines from adrenal medulla
Histamine	Contraction	√ (H$_1$)	—	—	
Motilin	Contraction	√	—	√	
Neurotensin	Contraction	√	—	—	
Nitric oxide	Relaxation	√	—	—	
Pancreatic polypeptide	Contraction	√	—	√	
PGF$_{2\alpha}$	Contraction	√	—	—	
PGE$_{1,2}$	Relaxation	√	—	—	
Progesterone	Relaxation	—	—	—	
Secretin	Relaxation	√	—	—	
Serotonin	Contraction	√	—	—	
Somatostatin	Contraction	?	?	?	
Substance P	Contraction	√	—	√	
VIP	Relaxation	√	—	—	

PGE, prostaglandin E; PGF, prostaglandin F; VIP, vasoactive intestinal peptide.

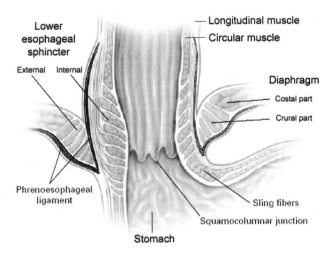

FIGURE 1.24. The anatomy at the region of the esophagogastric junction, showing the innermost fibers of the diaphragm around the esophageal hiatus. These fibers behave like a sphincter. (From Mittal RK, Balaban DH. The esophagogastric junction. *N Engl J Med* 1997;336:924–932, with permission.)

The crural diaphragm is composed of striated muscle, and it receives excitatory motor innervation by the phrenic nerve, similar to the costal diaphragm. Its inhibitory reflex activity could be mediated by unique, selective inhibition of lower motor neurons in the brainstem during such reflexes. Vagotomy abolishes the reflex inhibition of the crural diaphragm, indicating a role for the vagus in this reflex (279). This could represent a vagophrenic inhibitory reflex in which the afferent arc of the reflex is in the vagal afferents. It is also possible that vagal efferents provide inhibitory input to the crural striated muscle. Recent studies have shown that motor endplates of the crural striated muscle are innervated by nitrergic fibers. These nitrergic fibers may represent postganglionic fibers in the vagal inhibitory pathway. The nitrergic inhibitory vagal pathway may mediate reflex inhibition of the crural fibers. It has recently been shown that NO suppresses the excitatory potentials at the crural endplates (21). A part of the esophageal crural diaphragm develops from esophageal mesenchyma. It is possible that, like esophageal striated muscle, a part of the esophageal crural diaphragm develops from smooth muscle transdifferentiation. The presence of a peripheral mechanism of crural diaphragm inhibition has also been suggested recently (280). In cats with electrodes implanted on the crural diaphragm, electrical stimulation increases the pressure at the esophagogastric junction (EGJ). However, esophageal distention and bolus-induced secondary esophageal peristalsis cause relaxation of the EGJ despite neuromuscular stimulation through the electrodes. This relaxation occurs even after bilateral vagotomy, suggesting that the inhibition of the crural diaphragm transpires at the level of the neuromuscular junction.

The amplitude of inspiratory pressure increases with increased inspiratory effort, and the pressure augmentation observed during sustained inspiration corresponds with augmentation of the crural EMG activity both temporally and quantitatively. The inspiratory augmentations in pressure may play an important role in gastroesophageal reflux disease. The crural diaphragmatic contractions are involved only in inspiratory augmentation, and, therefore, end-expiratory pressure measurements reflect the intrinsic pressure of the LES (21,203).

ESOPHAGEAL SENSATIONS

Afferent fibers from the esophagus course along the vagal and splanchnic nerves. The vagal afferent fibers have their cell bodies in the nodose ganglion and project to the nucleus solitarius (281). Sympathetic afferents travel via dorsal root ganglia into the spinal cord at T1 to L2 (282).

Ultrastructural studies by Rodrigo and colleagues (283–287) reveal the presence of perivascular and free nerve endings in the esophageal submucosa of cats, as well as free intraepithelial nerve endings and peculiar tapelike nerve endings within the myenteric ganglia. The latter have been termed *intraganglionic* laminar endings (285) and are thought to be ideally located to serve as mechanoreceptors. The afferent nature of these endings has been confirmed by studies that show their degeneration after extirpation of the nodose ganglion (283,287). The intraepithelial nerve endings may serve as mechanoreceptors and as thermoreceptors, osmoreceptors, and chemoreceptors in the esophagus (106,288,289). The afferent receptors appear to be concentrated at the upper and the lower portions of the thoracic esophagus (285).

Esophageal mechanoceptors also transduce painful sensations (290). Esophageal distention with a compliant balloon in awake persons elicited three types of response depending on the degree of balloon distention. At small distention pressures, secondary esophageal peristalsis was produced without any sensory perception. At moderate distention pressures, the subjects experienced pressure sensation only; but at high distention pressures, they experienced chest discomfort and pain. According to the intensity theory of pain, all of these sensory responses were transduced by the same mechanoreceptor-afferent fiber so that the intensity of its stimulation determined whether discomfort or pain sensations were transduced. Sengupta and colleagues (291–293) showed that esophageal distention elicits spike activity in single vagal and splanchnic afferent fibers (units) (Fig. 1.25). They studied the quantitative stimulus intensity response relationship of single afferent units. Based on their findings, these units were classified as low-threshold mechanoreceptors (LTMs), wide dynamic range mechanonociceptors (WDR-MNs), and high-threshold mechanonociceptors (HTMNs) (291,292) (Fig. 1.26).

ESOPHAGEAL TENSION RECEPTORS

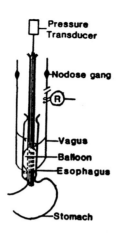

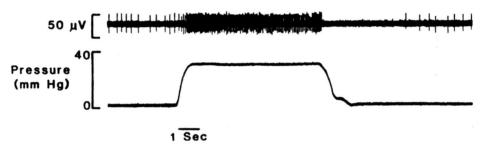

FIGURE 1.25. Esophageal tension-sensitive afferents increase their firing frequency to distention. The vagal fibers showed three broad phases in response to the esophageal distention (stimulus): a rapid increase in firing at the onset of distention; an adaptation to sustained distention by a decrease in frequency that was still far greater than the resting frequency; and, following withdrawal of distention, a decrease in frequency to a lower than resting level. The schematic diagram at the top represents the setup employed in this study.

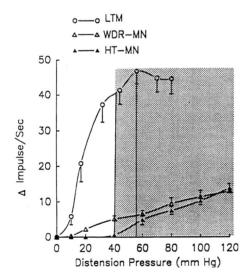

FIGURE 1.26. Stimulus-response relationships in the three types of esophageal, distention-sensitive unit. The esophageal distention-sensitive afferents were classified into three types based on the threshold pressure for activation and saturation pressure. Note that low-threshold mechanoceptors (LTMs) are saturated near the noxious threshold pressures. Wide dynamic range mechanonociceptors (WDR-MNs) had an intermediate activation threshold and showed no evidence of saturation. They were active in both innocuous and noxious stimulus ranges and had low discharge rates. On the other hand, high-threshold mechanoceptors (HTMNs) had a very high threshold pressure that was in the noxious range and showed no sign of saturation with very low discharge rates. Shaded area indicates noxious range of stimuli. (From Goyal RK, Sengupta JN, Saha JK. Properties of esophageal mechanosensitive receptors. In: Holle GE, ed. *Advances in the innervation of the gastrointestinal tract.* New York: Elsevier Science, 1992, with permission.)

These observations suggested that all afferent units were not homogenous and that distinct afferent units transduced different sensations and, therefore, supported the specificity theory of pain (290). Furthermore, it was shown that HTMNs were highly sensitive to the autacoid bradykinin (293). Properties of the three types of afferent unit are summarized in Table 1.2 (17).

These studies also showed that LTM units were present only in the vagus nerve, whereas WDR-MN and HTMN units were present in the splanchnic nerves. These observations are consistent with the view that the esophageal vagal afferents are involved in physiologic reflexes that occur without sensory perception, whereas the spinal splanchnic afferents transduce esophageal sensations and nociception. However, nociceptive pathways from the lower esophagus are not affected in patients with C6 or C7 spinal cord injury (294). These conclusions do not exclude a role for vagal afferents in the modulation of esophageal nociception in that they have been shown to suppress signal nociceptive mechanisms.

The vagal sensory units have their cell bodies in the nodose ganglia lying just below the jugular foramen. The nodose ganglia display rostrocaudal organization of the gut, with some neurons from the oropharynx and esophagus located superiorly (295). The central projections of the nodose ganglion cells terminate in the medial division of the NTS, where they also display rostrocaudal viscerotropic organization within the subnuclei (295). The NTS neurons project to different levels, including (a) neurons in the DMN and NA (containing swallowing neurons); (b) anteromediolateral cell column of the spinal cord (containing sympathetic pathway nerves); (c) neurons in the thalamus, hypothalamus, and limbic and insular cortical regions (which are concerned with autonomic, neuroendocrine, and behavioral functions); and (d) parabrachial nuclei, which are in turn connected to higher brain centers (14) (Fig. 1.27).

The splanchnic sensory units have the cell bodies in the dorsal root ganglia. They contain substance P and CGRP. The central projections of these neurons terminate in the spinal column and in the nucleus gracilis and cuneatus in the brainstem and then ascend to terminate in the thalamus. From the thalamus, projections ascend to primary somatosensory and insular cortical areas (14) (Fig. 1.27). Sensitization of nociceptors may play an important role in esophageal sensation (296).

Aziz and Thompson (14) have reviewed recent information on the projection of nerves conveying esophageal sensations to the brain in humans by studying cortical evoked potentials (CEPs), magnetoencephalography, PET, and functional magnetic resonance imaging (fMRI) following esophageal distention or electrical stimulation.

PET scan studies suggest that esophageal sensation, like somatic sensation, is processed in the primary somatosensory cortex (for sensoridiscriminative aspects) and the anterior cingulate cortex (for affective motivational aspects) and inhibits the medial prefrontal cortex (a region known for cognitive-evaluation aspects of sensation) (297). fMRI studies have found that parietooccipital and midparietal cortices were activated by distention of the distal and proximal esophagus, respectively. Moreover, esophageal distention and acid perfusion induces spatially and temporally distinct cortical activation. Painful stimuli induce activation in the same cortical area as nonpainful stimuli and cause activation of anterior cingulate gyri (14).

Mechanical and electrical stimuli of the esophagus also produce CEPs (298). Sensory perception is usually necessary to evoke CEPs, and there is a progressive increase in CEP magnitude with increasing perception scores. The magnitude of cortical response to esophageal electrical stimulation is intensity-dependent (299), and it has been suggested that CEPs might be mediated by stimulation of wide dynamic range mechanosensitive afferents that are carried in the splanchnic nerves (14). CEPs have been

TABLE 1.2. ESOPHAGEAL MECHANOSENSITIVE RECEPTORS

Characteristics	Low-Threshold Mechanoreceptors	Wide Dynamic Range Mechanononociceptors	High-Threshold Mechanononociceptors
Fiber type	Aδ, C	Aδ, C	Aδ, C
Mean threshold pressure for activation (mm Hg)	3	10	40
Mean saturation pressure (mm Hg)	50	>120	>120
Max. discharge rate	60	17	10
Resting activity	100%	73%	42%
Activity rate (impulses/sec)	~10	<1	<0.5
Response to physiologic peristalsis			
% responding	100%	100%	0%
Response rate as % maximum	100%	25%	0%
Activation by algogenic bradykinin	No	Yes	Yes (highly sensitive)
Anatomic course	Vagus	Splanchnic	Splanchnic
Physiologic role	Nonnoxious information	Nonnoxious to noxious information	Nociceptive information

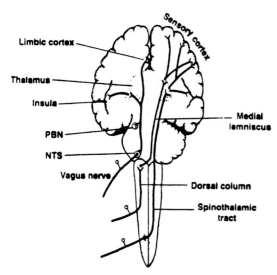

FIGURE 1.27. The bulbar and suprabulbar projections of vagal and spinal afferent pathways. Vagal afferents terminate in the nucleus tractus solitarius (NTS), from which projections ascend via the parabronchial nucleus (PBN) to the thalamus and the limbic and insular cortices. Spinal afferents ascend in the spinothalamic tract and the dorsal columns. The spinothalamic tracts ascend to the thalamus, and the dorsal columns ascend to the nuclei gracilis and cuneatus in the rostral medulla, from which they project to the thalamus via the medial lemniscus. From the thalamus, projections ascend to the primary somatosensory and insular cortices. (From Aziz Q, Thompson DG. Brain-gut axis in health and disease. *Gastroenterology* 1998;114: 559–578, with permission.)

used to determine the integrity of esophageal afferents (14,300).

REFERENCES

1. Code CF, Schlegel JF. Motor action of the esophagus and its sphincters. In: Code CF, ed. *Handbook of physiology*. Washington DC: American Physiology Society, 1968:1821–1840.
2. Cohen BR, Wolf BS. Cineradiographic and intraluminal correlations in the pharynx and esophagus. In: Code CF, ed. *Handbook of physiology*. Washington DC: American Physiology Society, 1968:841.
3. Doty RW, Bosma JF. Neural organization of deglutition. In: Code CF, ed. *Handbook of physiology*. Washington, DC: American Physiology Society, 1968:1861.
4. Goyal RK, Cobb BW. Motility of the pharynx, esophagus, and esophageal sphincter. In: Johnson LR, ed. *Physiology of the gastrointestinal tract*. New York: Raven Press, 1981:359.
5. Goyal RK, Paterson WG. Esophageal motility. In: Wood JD, Schultz SG, eds. *The gastrointestinal system*. Washington, DC: American Physiology Society, 1987: 865.
6. Goyal RK, Rattan S. Neurohumoral, hormonal, and drug receptors for the lower esophageal sphincter. *Gastroenterology* 1978;74:598–619.
7. Ingelfinger FJ. Esophageal motility. *Physiol Rev* 1958;38:533.
8. Jean A. Brainstem control of swallowing: localization and organization of the central pattern generator for swallowing. In: Taylor A, ed. *Neurophysiology of the jaws and teeth*. London: MacMillan Press, 1990.
9. Miller AJ. Deglutition. *Physiol Rev* 1982;62:129–184.
10. Roman C, Gonella J. Extrinsic control of digestive tract motility. In: Johnson LR, eds. *Physiology of the gastrointestinal tract*. New York: Raven Press, 1987:289.
11. Sessle BJ, Henry JL. Neural mechanisms of swallowing: neurophysiological and neurochemical studies on brain stem neurons in the solitary tract region *Dysphagia* 1989;4:61–75.
12. Vantrappen G, Hellemans J. *Diseases of the esophagus*. New York: Springer-Verlag, 1974.
13. Wolf BS. The inferior esophageal sphincter—anatomic, roentgenologic and manometric correlation, contradictions, and terminology. *Am J Roentgenol Radium Ther Nucl Med* 1970;110:260–277.
14. Aziz Q, Thompson DG. Brain-gut axis in health and disease. *Gastroenterology* 1998;114:559–578.
15. Biancani P, Behar J. Esophageal motor function. In: Yamada T, ed. *Textbook of gastroenterology*. Philadelphia: JB Lippincott, 1995:158.
16. Bieger D. Neuropharmacologic correlates of deglutition: lessons from fictive swallowing. *Dysphagia* 1991;6:147–164.
17. Goyal RK, Sengupta JN, Saha JK. Properties of esophageal mechanosensitive receptors. In: Holle GE, ed. *Advances in the innervation of the gastrointestinal tract*. New York: Elsevier Science, 1992.
18. Groher ME. *Dysphagia: diagnosis and management*. Boston; Butterworth-Heineman, 1997.
19. Martin RE, Sessle BJ. The role of the cerebral cortex in swallowing. *Dysphagia* 1993;8:195–202.
20. Miller AJ. The search for the central swallowing pathway: the quest for clarity. *Dysphagia* 1993;8:185–194.
21. Mittal RK, Balaban DH. The esophagogastric junction. *N Engl J Med* 1997;336:924–932.
22. Mittal RK, Holloway RH, Penagini R, et al. Transient lower esophageal sphincter relaxation. *Gastroenterology* 1995;109: 601–610.
23. Shaker R, Lang IM. Reflex mediated airway protective mechanisms against retrograde aspiration. *Am J Med* 1997;103: 64S–73S.
24. Lear CS, Flanagan JB, Moorrees CF. The frequency of deglutition in man. *Arch Oral Biol* 1965;10:83.
25. Ali GN, Laundl TM, Wallace KL, et al. Influence of mucosal receptors on deglutitive regulation of pharyngeal and upper esophageal sphincter function *Am J Physiol* 1994;267: G644–G649.
26. Shingai T, Shimada K. Reflex swallowing elicited by water and chemical substances applied in the oral cavity, pharynx, and larynx of the rabbit. *Jpn J Physiol* 1976;26:455–469.
27. Jean A, Car A. Inputs to the swallowing medullary neurons from the peripheral afferent fibers and the swallowing cortical area. *Brain Res* 1979;178:567–572.
28. Jean A. Brain stem control of swallowing: neuronal network and cellular mechanisms. *Physiol Rev* 2001;81:929–969.
29. Dent J, Dodds WJ, Friedman RH, Sekiguchi T, et al. Mechanism of gastroesophageal reflux in recumbent asymptomatic human subjects. *J Clin Invest* 1980;65:256–267.
30. Orr WC, Johnson LF, Robinson MG. Effect of sleep on swallowing, esophageal peristalsis, and acid clearance. *Gastroenterology* 1984;86:814–819.
31. Lang IM, Shaker R. Anatomy and physiology of the upper esophageal sphincter. *Am J Med* 1997;103:50S–55S.
32. Gidda JS, Goyal RK. Swallow-evoked action potentials in vagal preganglionic efferents *J Neurophysiol* 1984;52:1169–1180.
33. Beyak MJ, Collman PI, Valdez DT, et al. Superior laryngeal nerve stimulation in the cat: effect on oropharyngeal swallowing, oesophageal motility and lower oesophageal sphincter activity *Neurogastroenterol Motil* 1997;9:117–127.

34. Asoh R, Goyal RK. Manometry and electromyography of the upper esophageal sphincter in the opossum. *Gastroenterology* 1978;74:514–520.

35. Doty RW. Influence of stimulus pattern on reflex deglutition. *Am J Physiol* 1951;166:142.

36. Diamant NE. A glimpse at the central mechanism for swallowing? *Gastroenterology* 1995;109:1700–1702.

37. Jean A. Control of the central swallowing program by inputs from the peripheral receptors. A review. *J Auton Nerv Syst* 1984; 10:225–233.

38. Bieger D. Rhombencephalic pathways and neurotransmitters controlling deglutition. *Am J Med* 2001;111[Suppl 8A]: 85S–89S.

39. Bieger D. The brainstem esophagomotor network pattern generator: a rodent model. *Dysphagia* 1993;8:203–208.

40. Bieger D, Hopkins DA. Viscerotopic representation of the upper alimentary tract in the medulla oblongata in the rat: the nucleus ambiguus. *J Comp Neurol* 1987;262:546–562.

41. Kitamura S, Ogata K, Nishiguchi T, et al. Location of the motoneurons supplying the rabbit pharyngeal constrictor muscles and the peripheral course of their axons: a study using the retrograde HRP or fluorescent labeling technique. *Anat Rec* 1991;229:399–406.

42. Kobler JB, Datta S, Goyal RK, et al. Innervation of the larynx, pharynx, and upper esophageal sphincter of the rat. *J Comp Neurol* 1994;349:129–147.

43. Rossiter CD, Norman WP, Jain M, et al. Control of lower esophageal sphincter pressure by two sites in dorsal motor nucleus of the vagus. *Am J Physiol* 1990;259:G899–G906.

44. Bao X, Wiedner EB, Altschuler SM. Transsynaptic localization of pharyngeal premotor neurons in rat. *Brain Res* 1995;696: 246–249.

45. Barrett RT, Bao X, Miselis RR, et al. Brain stem localization of rodent esophageal premotor neurons revealed by transneuronal passage of pseudorabies virus. *Gastroenterology* 1994;107: 728–737.

46. Broussard DL, Lynn RB, Wiedner EB, et al. Solitarial premotor neuron projections to the rat esophagus and pharynx: implications for control of swallowing. *Gastroenterology* 1998;114: 1268–1275.

47. Jean A, Kessler JP, Tell F. *Nucleus tractus solitarii and deglutition: monoamines, excitatory amino acids and cellular properties.* Boca Raton, FL: CRC Press, 1994.

48. Lu WY, Bieger D. Vagovagal reflex motility patterns of the rat esophagus. *Am J Physiol* 1998;274:R1425–R1435.

49. Dong H, Loomis CW, Bieger D. Distal and deglutitive inhibition in the rat esophagus: role of inhibitory neurotransmission in the nucleus tractus solitarii. *Gastroenterology* 2000;118: 328–336.

50. Wiedner EB, Bao X, Altschuler SM. Localization of nitric oxide synthase in the brain stem neural circuit controlling esophageal peristalsis in rats. *Gastroenterology* 1995;108:367–375.

51. Shaker R, Li Q, Ren J, et al. Coordination of deglutition and phases of respiration: effect of aging, tachypnea, bolus volume, and chronic obstructive pulmonary disease. *Am J Physiol* 1992; 263:G750–G755.

52. Sumi T. The activity of brain stem respiratory neurons and spinal respiratory motoneuron during swallowing. *J Neurophysiol* 1963;26:466.

53. Shaker R, Ren J, Medda B, et al. Identification and characterization of the esophagoglottal closure reflex in a feline model. *Am J Physiol* 1994;266:G147–G153.

54. Shaker R, Ren J, Xie P, et al. Characterization of the pharyngo-UES contractile reflex in humans. *Am J Physiol* 1997;273: G854–G858.

55. Hamdy S, Aziz Q, Rothwell JC, et al. The cortical topography of human swallowing musculature in health and disease. *Nat Med* 1996;2:1217–1224.

56. Aziz Q, Rothwell JC, Hamdy S, et al. The topographic representation of esophageal motor function on the human cerebral cortex. *Gastroenterology* 1996;111:855–862.

57. Singh KD, Hamdy S, Aziz Q, et al. Topographic mapping of trans-cranial magnetic stimulation data on surface rendered MR images of the brain. *Electroencephalogr Clin Neurophysiol* 1997; 105:345–351.

58. Hartnick CJ, Rudolph C, Willging JP, et al. Functional magnetic resonance imaging of the pediatric swallow: imaging the cortex and the brainstem. *Laryngoscope* 2001;111: 1183–1191.

59. Hamdy S, Rothwell JC, Brooks DJ, et al. Identification of the cerebral loci processing human swallowing with H2(15)O PET activation *J Neurophysiol* 1999;81:1917–1926.

60. Hamdy S, Aziz Q, Thompson DG, et al. Physiology and pathophysiology of the swallowing area of human motor cortex. *Neural Plast* 2001;8:91–97.

61. Kahrilas PJ, Lin S, Logemann JA, et al. Deglutitive tongue action: volume accommodation and bolus propulsion. *Gastroenterology* 1993;104:152–162.

62. Kahrilas PJ, Lin S, Chen J, et al. Oropharyngeal accommodation to swallow volume. *Gastroenterology* 1996;111:297–306.

63. Wein B, Bockler R, Klajman S. Temporal reconstruction of sonographic imaging of disturbed tongue movements. *Dysphagia* 1991;6:135–139.

64. Dua KS, Ren J, Bardan E, et al. Coordination of deglutitive glottal function and pharyngeal bolus transit during normal eating. *Gastroenterology* 1997;112:73–83.

65. Ergun GA, Kahrilas PJ, Lin S, et al. Shape, volume, and content of the deglutitive pharyngeal chamber imaged by ultrafast computerized tomography. *Gastroenterology* 1993;105:1396–1403.

66. Kahrilas PJ, Logemann JA, Lin S, et al. Pharyngeal clearance during swallowing: a combined manometric and videofluoroscopic study. *Gastroenterology* 1992;103:128–136.

67. Castell JA, Dalton CB, Castell DO. Effects of body position and bolus consistency on the manometric parameters and coordination of the upper esophageal sphincter and pharynx. *Dysphagia* 1990;5:179–186.

68. Sears VW Jr, Castell JA, Castell DO. Radial and longitudinal asymmetry of human pharyngeal pressures during swallowing. *Gastroenterology* 1991;101:1559–1563.

69. Castell JA, Castell DO, Schultz AR, et al. Effect of head position on the dynamics of the upper esophageal sphincter and pharynx. *Dysphagia* 1993;8:1–6.

70. Doty RW, Bosma JF. An electromyographic analysis of reflex deglutition. *J Neurophysiol* 1956;19:44.

71. Jacob P, Kahrilas PJ, Logemann JA, et al. Upper esophageal sphincter opening and modulation during swallowing. *Gastroenterology* 1989;97:1469–1478.

72. Logemann JA, Kahrilas PJ, Cheng J, et al. Closure mechanisms of laryngeal vestibule during swallow. *Am J Physiol* 1992;262: G338–G344.

73. Sasaki CT, Weaver EM. Physiology of the larynx. *Am J Med* 1997;103:9S–18S.

74. Shaker R, Dodds WJ, Ren J, et al. Esophagoglottal closure reflex: a mechanism of airway protection. *Gastroenterology* 1992;102:857–861.

75. Shaker R, Ren J, Kern M, et al. Mechanisms of airway protection and upper esophageal sphincter opening during belching. *Am J Physiol* 1992;262:G621–G628.

76. Shaker R, Ren J, Zamir Z, et al. Effect of aging, position, and temperature on the threshold volume triggering pharyngeal swallows. *Gastroenterology* 1994;107:396–402.

77. Goyal RK, Martin SB, Shapiro J, et al. The role of cricopha-

ryngeus muscle in pharyngoesophageal disorders. *Dysphagia* 1993;8:252–258.

78. Bonington A, Mahon M, Whitmore I. A histological and histochemical study of the cricopharyngeus muscle in man *J Anat* 1988;156:27–37.

79. Brownlow H, Whitmore I, Willan PL. A quantitative study of the histochemical and morphometric characteristics of the human cricopharyngeus muscle. *J Anat* 1989;166:67–75.

80. Dick TE, van Lunteren E. Fiber subtype distribution of pharyngeal dilator muscles and diaphragm in the cat . *J Appl Physiol* 1990;68:2237–2240.

81. Ertekin C, Aydogdu I. Electromyography of human cricopharyngeal muscle of the upper esophageal sphincter. *Muscle Nerve* 2002;26:729–739.

82. Medda BK, Lang IM, Dodds WJ, et al. Correlation of electrical and contractile activities of the cricopharyngeus muscle in the cat. *Am J Physiol* 1997;273:G470–G479.

83. Castell JA, Dalton CB, Castell DO. Pharyngeal and upper esophageal sphincter manometry in humans. *Am J Physiol* 1990; 258:G173–G178.

84. Cook IJ, Dent J, Shannon S, et al. Measurement of upper esophageal sphincter pressure. Effect of acute emotional stress. *Gastroenterology* 1987;93:526–532.

85. Wilson JA, Pryde A, Cecilia A, et al. Normal pharyngoesophageal motility. A study of 50 healthy subjects. *Dig Dis Sci* 1989;34:1590–1599.

86. Welch RW, Luckmann K, Ricks PM, et al. Manometry of the normal upper esophageal sphincter and its alterations in laryngectomy. *J Clin Invest* 1979;63:1036–1041.

87. Kahrilas PJ, Dodds WJ, Dent J, et al. Effect of sleep, spontaneous gastroesophageal reflux, and a meal on upper esophageal sphincter pressure in normal human volunteers *Gastroenterology* 1987;92:466–471.

88. Elidan J, Shochina M, Gonen B, et al. Manometry and electromyography of the pharyngeal muscles in patients with dysphagia. *Arch Otolaryngol Head Neck Surg* 1990;116:910–913.

89. Elidan J, Shochina M, Gonen B, et al. Electromyography of the inferior constrictor and cricopharyngeal muscles during swallowing. *Ann Otol Rhinol Laryngol* 1990;99:466–469.

90. Shipp T, Deatsch WW, Robertson K. Pharyngoesophageal muscle activity during swallowing in man. *Laryngoscope* 1970;80: 1–16.

91. van Overbeek JJ, Wit HP, Paping RH, et al. Simultaneous manometry and electromyography in the pharyngoesophageal segment. *Laryngoscope* 1985;95:582–584.

92. Medda BK, Lang IM, Layman R, et al. Characterization and quantification of a pharyngo-UES contractile reflex in cats. *Am J Physiol* 1994;267:G972–G983.

93. Enzmann DR, Harell GS, Zboralske FF. Upper esophageal responses to intraluminal distention in man. *Gastroenterology* 1977;72:1292–1298.

94. Gerhardt DC, Shuck TJ, Bordeaux RA, et al. Human upper esophageal sphincter. Response to volume, osmotic, and acid stimuli. *Gastroenterology* 1978;75:268–274.

95. Freiman JM, El Sharkawy TY, Diamant NE. Effect of bilateral vagosympathetic nerve blockade on response of the dog upper esophageal sphincter (UES) to intraesophageal distention and acid. *Gastroenterology* 1981;81:78–84.

96. Cook IJ, Dodds WJ, Dantas RO, et al. Opening mechanisms of the human upper esophageal sphincter. *Am J Physiol* 1989;257: G748–G759.

97. Kahrilas PJ, Dodds WJ, Dent J, et al. Upper esophageal sphincter function during deglutition. *Gastroenterology* 1988;95: 52–62.

98. Templeton FE. The cricopharyngeal sphincter: a roentgenologic study. *Laryngoscope* 1943;53:1.

99. Richter JE, Wu WC, Johns DN, et al. Esophageal manometry in 95 healthy adult volunteers. Variability of pressures with age and frequency of "abnormal" contractions. *Dig Dis Sci* 1987;32: 583–592.

100. Shi G, Pandolfino JE, Joehl RJ, et al. Distinct patterns of oesophageal shortening during primary peristalsis, secondary peristalsis and transient lower oesophageal sphincter relaxation. *Neurogastroenterol Motil* 2002;14:505–512.

101. Hollis JB, Castell DO. Esophageal function in elderly man. A new look at "presbyesophagus." *Ann Intern Med* 1974;80: 371–374.

102. Sears VW Jr, Castell JA, Castell DO. Comparison of effects of upright versus supine body position and liquid versus solid bolus on esophageal pressures in normal humans. *Dig Dis Sci* 1990;35:857–864.

103. Hollis JB, Castell DO. Effect of dry swallows and wet swallows of different volumes on esophageal peristalsis. *J Appl Physiol* 1975;38:1161–1164.

104. Janssens J, Valembois P, Hellemans J, et al. Studies on the necessity of a bolus for the progression of secondary peristalsis in the canine esophagus. *Gastroenterology* 1974;67:245–251.

105. Janssens J, Valembois P, Vantrappen G, et al. Is the primary peristaltic contraction of the canine esophagus bolus-dependent? *Gastroenterology* 1973;65:750–756.

106. El Ouazzani T, Mei N. Electrophysiologic properties and role of the vagal thermoreceptors of lower esophagus and stomach of cat. *Gastroenterology* 1982;83:995–1001.

107. Winship DH, Viegas dA Sr, Zboralske FF. Influence of bolus temperature on human esophageal motor function. *J Clin Invest* 1970;49:243–250.

108. Omari TI, Miki K, Fraser R, et al. Esophageal body and lower esophageal sphincter function in healthy premature infants. *Gastroenterology* 1995;109:1757–1764.

109. Paterson WG, Rattan S, Goyal RK. Esophageal responses to transient and sustained esophageal distension. *Am J Physiol* 1988;255:G587–G595.

110. Holloway RH. Esophageal body motor response to reflux events: secondary peristalsis. *Am J Med* 2000;108[Suppl 4a]:20S–26S.

111. Schoeman MN, Holloway RH. Stimulation and characteristics of secondary oesophageal peristalsis in normal subjects. *Gut* 1994;35:152–158.

112. Pai CG. Secondary oesophageal peristalsis in gastro-oesophageal reflux disease. *J Gastroenterol Hepatol* 2000;15:30–34.

113. Rydberg L, Ruth M, Lundell L. Characteristics of secondary oesophageal peristalsis in operated and non-operated patients with chronic gastro-oesophageal reflux disease. *Eur J Gastroenterol Hepatol* 2000;12:739–743.

114. Fleshler B. The characteristics and similarity of primary and secondary peristalsis in the esophagus. *J Clin Invest* 1959;38:110.

115. Paterson WG. Neuromuscular mechanisms of esophageal responses at and proximal to a distending balloon. *Am J Physiol* 1991;260:G148–G155.

116. Winship DH, Zboralske FF. The esophageal propulsive force: esophageal response to acute obstruction. *J Clin Invest* 1967;46: 1391–1401.

117. Williams D, Thompson DG, Heggie L, et al. Responses of the human esophagus to experimental intraluminal distension. *Am J Physiol* 1993;265:G196–G203.

118. Pouderoux P, Lin S, Kahrilas PJ. Timing, propagation, coordination, and effect of esophageal shortening during peristalsis. *Gastroenterology* 1997;112:1147–1154.

119. Paterson WG, Hynna-Liepert TT, Selucky M. Comparison of primary and secondary esophageal peristalsis in humans: effect of atropine. *Am J Physiol* 1991;260:G52–G57.

120. Ask P, Tibbling L. Effect of time interval between swallows on esophageal peristalsis. *Am J Physiol* 1980;238:G485–G490.

121. Meyer GW, Castell DO. Human esophageal response during chest pain induced by swallowing cold liquids. *JAMA* 1981; 246:2057–2059.

122. Siegel CI, Hendrix TR. Evidence for the central mediation of secondary peristalsis in the esophagus. *Bull Johns Hopkins Hosp* 1961;108:297.

123. Vanek AW, Diamant NE. Responses of the human esophagus to paired swallows. *Gastroenterology* 1987;92:643–650.

124. Mellow MH. Esophageal motility during food ingestion: a physiologic test of esophageal motor function. *Gastroenterology* 1983;85:570–577.

125. Mayrand S, Tremblay L, Diamant N. *In vivo* measurement of feline esophageal tone. *Am J Physiol* 1994;267:G914–G921.

126. Sifrim D, Janssens J. Secondary peristaltic contractions, like primary peristalsis, are preceded by inhibition in the human esophageal body. *Digestion* 1996;57:73–78.

127. Sifrim D, Janssens J, and Vantrappen G. A wave of inhibition precedes primary peristaltic contractions in the human esophagus *Gastroenterology* 1992;103:876-882.

128. Patapoutian A, Wold BJ, Wagner RA. Evidence for developmentally programmed transdifferentiation in mouse esophageal muscle. *Science* 1995;270:1818–1821.

129. Meyer GW, Austin RM, Brady CE III, et al. Muscle anatomy of the human esophagus. *J Clin Gastroenterol* 1986;8:131–134.

130. Toyama T, Yokoyama I, Nishi K. Effects of hexamethonium and other ganglionic blocking agents on electrical activity of the esophagus induced by vagal stimulation in the dog. *Eur J Pharmacol* 1975;31:63–71.

131. Neuhuber WL, Worl J, Berthoud HR, et al. NADPH-diaphorase-positive nerve fibers associated with motor endplates in the rat esophagus: new evidence for co-innervation of striated muscle by enteric neurons. *Cell Tissue Res* 1994;276:23–30.

132. Sang Q, Young HM. Development of nicotinic receptor clusters and innervation accompanying the change in muscle phenotype in the mouse esophagus. *J Comp Neurol* 1997;386:119–136.

133. Singaram C, Sengupta A, Sweet MA, et al. Nitrinergic and peptidergic innervation of the human oesophagus. *Gut* 1994;35:1690–1696.

134. Kuramoto H, Kawano H, Sakamoto H, et al. Motor innervation by enteric nerve fibers containing both nitric oxide synthase and galanin immunoreactivities in the striated muscle of the rat esophagus. *Cell Tissue Res* 1999;295:241–245.

135. Storr M, Geisler F, Neuhuber WL, et al. Characterization of vagal input to the rat esophageal muscle *Auton Neurosci* 2001; 91:1–9.

136. Janssens J, De W I, Vantrappen G, et al. Peristalsis in smooth muscle esophagus after transection and bolus deviation. *Gastroenterology* 1976;71:1004–1009.

137. Andrew BL. The nervous control of the cervical oesophagus of the rat during swallowing. *J Physiol* 1956;134:729–740.

138. Collman PI, Tremblay L, Diamant NE. The central vagal efferent supply to the esophagus and lower esophageal sphincter of the cat. *Gastroenterology* 1993;104:1430–1438.

139. Baumgarten HG, Lange W. Adrenergic innervation of the oesophagus in the cat (*Felis domestica*) and Rhesus monkey (*Macacus rhesus*). *Z Zellforsch Mikrosk Anat* 1969;95:529–545.

140. Jacobowitz D, Nemir P Jr. The autonomic innervation of the esophagus of the dog. *J Thorac Cardiovasc Surg* 1969;58:678–684.

141. Christensen J, Robison BA. Anatomy of the myenteric plexus of the opossum esophagus *Gastroenterology* 1982;83:1033–1042.

142. Sengupta A, Paterson WG, Goyal RK. Atypical localization of myenteric neurons in the opossum lower esophageal sphincter. *Am J Anat* 1987;180:342–348.

143. Seelig LL Jr, Doody P, Brainard L, et al. Acetylcholinesterase and choline acetyltransferase staining of neurons in the opossum esophagus. *Anat Rec* 1984;209:125–130.

144. Singaram C, Sengupta A, Sugarbaker DJ, et al. Peptidergic innervation of the human esophageal smooth muscle. *Gastroenterology* 1991;101:1256–1263.

145. Wattchow DA, Furness JB, Costa M. Distribution and coexistence of peptides in nerve fibers of the external muscle of the human gastrointestinal tract . *Gastroenterology* 1988;95:32–41.

146. Reynolds RP, El Sharkawy TY, Diamant NE. Lower esophageal sphincter function in the cat: role of central innervation assessed by transient vagal blockade. *Am J Physiol* 1984;246: G666–G674.

147. Ryan JP, Snape WJ Jr, Cohen S. Influence of vagal cooling on esophageal function. *Am J Physiol* 1977;232:E159–E164.

148. Tieffenbach L, Roman C. (The role of extrinsic vagal innervation in the motility of the smooth-muscled portion of the esophagus: electromyographic study in the cat and the baboon.) *J Physiol (Paris)* 1972;64:193–226.

149. Gidda JS, Cobb BW, Goyal RK. Modulation of esophageal peristalsis by vagal efferent stimulation in opossum. *J Clin Invest* 1981;68:1411–1419.

150. Gidda JS, Goyal RK. Influence of successive vagal stimulations on contractions in esophageal smooth muscle of opossum. *J Clin Invest* 1983;71:1095–1103.

151. Gidda JS, Goyal RK. Regional gradient of initial inhibition and refractoriness in esophageal smooth muscle. *Gastroenterology* 1985;89:843–851.

152. Rattan S, Gidda JS, Goyal RK. Membrane potential and mechanical responses of the opossum esophagus to vagal stimulation and swallowing. *Gastroenterology* 1983;85:922–928.

153. Weisbrodt NW, Christensen J. Gradients of contractions in the opossum esophagus. *Gastroenterology* 1972;62:1159–1166.

154. Yamato S, Saha JK, Goyal RK. Role of nitric oxide in lower esophageal sphincter relaxation to swallowing. *Life Sci* 1992;50: 1263–1272.

155. Diamant NE, El Sharkawy TY. Neural control of esophageal peristalsis. A conceptual analysis. *Gastroenterology* 1977;72: 546–556.

156. Dodds WJ, Christensen J, Dent J, et al. Pharmacologic investigation of primary peristalsis in smooth muscle portion of opossum esophagus. *Am J Physiol* 1979;237:E561–E566.

157. Gidda JS, Buyniski JP. Swallow-evoked peristalsis in opossum esophagus: role of cholinergic mechanisms. *Am J Physiol* 1986; 251:G779–G785.

158. Dodds WJ, Christensen J, Dent J, et al. Esophageal contractions induced by vagal stimulation in the opossum. *Am J Physiol* 1978;235:E392–E401.

159. Conklin JL, Du C, Murray JA, et al. Characterization and mediation of inhibitory junction potentials from opossum lower esophageal sphincter. *Gastroenterology* 1993;104: 1439–1444.

160. Murray J, Du C, Ledlow A, et al. Nitric oxide: mediator of nonadrenergic noncholinergic responses of opossum esophageal muscle. *Am J Physiol* 1991;261:G401–G406.

161. Yamato S, Spechler SJ, Goyal RK. Role of nitric oxide in esophageal peristalsis in the opossum. *Gastroenterology* 1992; 103:197–204.

162. Crist J, Surprenant A, Goyal RK. Intracellular studies of electrical membrane properties of opossum esophageal circular smooth muscle. *Gastroenterology* 1987;92:987–992.

163. Crist JR, Kauvar D, Goyal RK. Gradient of cholinergic innervation in opossum esophageal circular smooth muscle. *Gullet* 1991;1:92.

164. Crist J, Gidda JS, Goyal RK. Intramural mechanism of esophageal peristalsis: roles of cholinergic and noncholinergic nerves. *Proc Natl Acad Sci U S A* 1984;81:3595–3599.

165. Szymanski PT, Szymanska G, Goyal RK. Differences in calmodulin and calmodulin-binding proteins in phasic and tonic smooth muscles. *Am J Physiol Cell Physiol* 2002;282: C94–C104.

166. Szymanski PT, Chacko TK, Rovner AS, et al. Differences in contractile protein content and isoforms in phasic and tonic smooth muscles. *Am J Physiol* 1998;275:C684–C692.

167. Akbarali HI, Goyal RK. Effect of sodium nitroprusside on Ca2+ currents in opossum esophageal circular muscle cells. *Am J Physiol* 1994;266:G1036–G1042.

168. Akbarali HI, Hatakeyama N, Wang Q, et al. Transient outward current in opossum esophageal circular muscle. *Am J Physiol* 1995;268:G979–G987.

169. Wang Q, Akbarali HI, Hatakeyama N, et al. Caffeine- and carbachol-induced Cl- and cation currents in single opossum esophageal circular muscle cells. *Am J Physiol* 1996;271: C1725–C1734.

170. Salapatek AM, Ji J, Diamant NE. Ion channel diversity in the feline smooth muscle esophagus. *Am J Physiol Gastrointest Liver Physiol* 2002;282:G288–G299.

171. Muinuddin A, Xue S, Diamant NE. Regional differences in the response of feline esophageal smooth muscle to stretch and cholinergic stimulation. *Am J Physiol Gastrointest Liver Physiol* 2001;281:G1460–G1467.

172. Goyal RK, He XD. Evidence for NO$^\Sigma$ redox form of nitric oxide as nitrergic inhibitory neurotransmitter in gut. *Am J Physiol* 1998;275:G1185–G1192.

173. Crist JR, He XD, Goyal RK. Chloride-mediated inhibitory junction potentials in opossum esophageal circular smooth muscle. *Am J Physiol* 1991;261:G752–G762.

174. Zhang Y, Vogalis F, Goyal RK. Nitric oxide suppresses a Ca(2+)-stimulated Cl- current in smooth muscle cells of opossum esophagus. *Am J Physiol* 1998;274:G886–G890.

175. Zhang Y, Paterson WG. Nitric oxide contracts longitudinal smooth muscle of opossum oesophagus via excitation-contraction coupling. *J Physiol* 2001;536:133–140.

176. Jury J, Jager LP, Daniel EE. Unusual potassium channels mediate nonadrenergic noncholinergic nerve-mediated inhibition in opossum esophagus. *Can J Physiol Pharmacol* 1985;63: 107–112.

177. Hatakeyama N, Wang Q, Goyal RK, et al. Muscarinic suppression of ATP-sensitive K+ channel in rabbit esophageal smooth muscle. *Am J Physiol* 1995;268:C877–C885.

178. Hatakeyama N, Mukhopadhyay D, Goyal RK, et al. Tyrosine kinase-dependent modulation of calcium entry in rabbit colonic muscularis mucosae. *Am J Physiol* 1996;270: C1780–C1789.

179. Biancani P, Harnett KM, Sohn UD, et al. Differential signal transduction pathways in cat lower esophageal sphincter tone and response to ACh. *Am J Physiol* 1994;266:G767–G774.

180. Sohn UD, Kim DK, Bonventre JV, et al. Role of 100-kDa cytosolic PLA2 in ACh-induced contraction of cat esophageal circular muscle. *Am J Physiol* 1994;267:G433–G441.

181. Sohn UD, Cao W, Tang DC, et al. Myosin light chain kinase- and PKC-dependent contraction of LES and esophageal smooth muscle. *Am J Physiol Gastrointest Liver Physiol* 2001; 281:G467–G478.

182. Sohn UD, Hong YW, Choi HC, et al. Increase of (Ca(2+))i and release of arachidonic acid via activation of M2 receptor coupled to Gi and rho proteins in oesophageal muscle. *Cell Signal* 2000;12:215–222.

183. Sohn UD, Han B, Tashjian AH Jr, et al. Agonist-independent, muscle-type-specific signal transduction pathways in cat esophageal and lower esophageal sphincter circular smooth muscle. *J Pharmacol Exp Ther* 1995;273:482–491.

184. Sohn UD, Harnett KM, De Petris G, et al. Distinct muscarinic

185. receptors, G proteins and phospholipases in esophageal and lower esophageal sphincter circular muscle. *J Pharmacol Exp Ther* 1993;267:1205–1214.

185. Biancani P, Billett G, Hillemeier C, et al. Acute experimental esophagitis impairs signal transduction in cat lower esophageal sphincter circular muscle. *Gastroenterology* 1992;103: 1199–1206.

186. Xue S, Valdez D, Collman PI, et al. Effects of nitric oxide synthase blockade on esophageal peristalsis and the lower esophageal sphincter in the cat. *Can J Physiol Pharmacol* 1996; 74:1249–1257.

187. Chakder S, Rosenthal GJ, Rattan S. *In vivo* and *in vitro* influence of human recombinant hemoglobin on esophageal function. *Am J Physiol* 1995;268:G443–G450.

188. Conklin JL, Murray J, Ledlow A, et al. Effects of recombinant human hemoglobin on motor functions of the opossum esophagus. *J Pharmacol Exp Ther* 1995;273:762–767.

189. Kahrilas PJ, Wu S, Lin S, et al. Attenuation of esophageal shortening during peristalsis with hiatus hernia. *Gastroenterology* 1995;109:1818–1825.

190. Crist J, Gidda J, Goyal RK. Role of substance P nerves in longitudinal smooth muscle contractions of the esophagus. *Am J Physiol* 1986;250:G336–G343.

191. Hirano I, Kakkar R, Saha JK, et al. Tyrosine phosphorylation in contraction of opossum esophageal longitudinal muscle in response to SNP. *Am J Physiol* 1997;273:G247–G252.

192. Biancani P, Zabinski MP, Behar J. Pressure tension, and force of closure of the human lower esophageal sphincter and esophagus. *J Clin Invest* 1975;56:476–483.

193. Seelig LL Jr, Goyal RK. Morphological evaluation of opossum lower esophageal sphincter. *Gastroenterology* 1978;75:51–58.

194. Christensen J, Roberts RL. Differences between esophageal body and lower esophageal sphincter in mitochondria of smooth muscle in opossum. *Gastroenterology* 1983;85:650–656.

195. Behar J, Kerstein M, Biancani P. Neural control of the lower esophageal sphincter in the cat: studies on the excitatory pathways to the lower esophageal sphincter. *Gastroenterology* 1982; 82:680–688.

196. Christensen J, Rick GA, Soll DJ. Intramural nerves and interstitial cells revealed by the Champy-Maillet stain in the opossum esophagus. *J Auton Nerv Syst* 1987;19:137–151.

197. Daniel EE, Posey-Daniel V. Neuromuscular structures in opossum esophagus: role of interstitial cells of Cajal. *Am J Physiol* 1984;246:G305–G315.

198. Faussone-Pellegrini MS, Cortesini C. Ultrastructural features and localization of the interstitial cells of Cajal in the smooth muscle coat of human esophagus. *J Submicrosc Cytol* 1985;17: 187–197.

199. Stein HJ, Liebermann-Meffert D, DeMeester TR, et al. Three-dimensional pressure image and muscular structure of the human lower esophageal sphincter. *Surgery* 1995;117:692–698.

200. Richardson BJ, Welch RW. Differential effect of atropine on rightward and leftward lower esophageal sphincter pressure. *Gastroenterology* 1981;81:85–89.

201. Welch RW, Drake ST. Normal lower esophageal sphincter pressure: a comparison of rapid vs. slow pull-through techniques. *Gastroenterology* 1980;78:1446–1451.

202. Welch RW, Gray JE. Influence of respiration on recordings of lower esophageal sphincter pressure in humans. *Gastroenterology* 1982;83:590–594.

203. Boyle JT, Altschuler SM, Nixon TE, et al. Role of the diaphragm in the genesis of lower esophageal sphincter pressure in the cat. *Gastroenterology* 1985;88:723–730.

204. Heitmann P, Wolf BS, Sokol EM, et al. Simultaneous cineradiographic-manometric study of the distal esophagus: small hiatal hernias and rings. *Gastroenterology* 1966;50:737–753.

205. Lind JF, Cotton DJ, Blanchard R, et al. Effect of thoracic displacement and vagotomy on the canine gastroesophageal junctional zone. *Gastroenterology* 1969;56:1078–1085.

206. Dent J, Dodds WJ, Sekiguchi T, et al. Interdigestive phasic contractions of the human lower esophageal sphincter. *Gastroenterology* 1983;84:453–460.

207. Holloway RH, Blank E, Takahashi I, et al. Variability of lower esophageal sphincter pressure in the fasted unanesthetized opossum. *Am J Physiol* 1985;248:G398–G406.

208. Holloway RH, Blank E, Takahashi I, et al. Motilin: a mechanism incorporating the opossum lower esophageal sphincter into the migrating motor complex. *Gastroenterology* 1985;89:507–515.

209. Itoh Z, Aizawa I, Honda R, et al. Control of lower-esophageal-sphincter contractile activity by motilin in conscious dogs. *Am J Dig Dis* 1978;23:341–345.

210. Christensen J, Conklin JL, Freeman BW. Physiologic specialization at esophagogastric junction in three species. *Am J Physiol* 1973;225:1265–1270.

211. Papasova M, Milousheva E, Bonev A, et al. On the changes in the membrane potential and the contractile activity of the smooth muscle of the lower esophageal and ileo-caecal sphincters upon increased K in the nutrient solution. *Acta Physiol Pharmacol Bulg* 1980;6:41–49.

212. Zelcer E, Weisbrodt NW. Electrical and mechanical activity in the lower esophageal sphincter of the cat. *Am J Physiol* 1984;246:G243–G247.

213. Asoh R, Goyal RK. Electrical activity of the opossum lower esophageal sphincter *in vivo*. Its role in the basal sphincter pressure. *Gastroenterology* 1978;74:835–840.

214. Zhang Y, Miller DV, Paterson WG. Opposing roles of K(+) and Cl(-) channels in maintenance of opossum lower esophageal sphincter tone. *Am J Physiol Gastrointest Liver Physiol* 2000;279:G1226–G1234.

215. Reynolds JC, Ouyang A, Cohen S. A lower esophageal sphincter reflex involving substance P. *Am J Physiol* 1984;246:G346–G354.

216. Saha JK, Sengupta JN, Goyal RK. Role of chloride ions in lower esophageal sphincter tone and relaxation. *Am J Physiol* 1992;263:G115–G126.

217. Cao W, Harnett KM, Behar J, et al. PGF(2alpha)-induced contraction of cat esophageal and lower esophageal sphincter circular smooth muscle. *Am J Physiol Gastrointest Liver Physiol* 2002;283:G282–G291.

218. Cao W, Harnett KM, Behar J, et al. Group I secreted PLA2 in the maintenance of human lower esophageal sphincter tone. *Gastroenterology* 2000;119:1243–1252.

219. Hillemeier C, Bitar KN, Sohn U, et al. Protein kinase C mediates spontaneous tone in the cat lower esophageal sphincter. *J Pharmacol Exp Ther* 1996;277:144–149.

220. Kang HY, Lee TS, Lee YP, et al. Interaction of calmodulin- and PKC-dependent contractile pathways in cat lower esophageal sphincter (LES). *Arch Pharm Res* 2001;24:546–551.

221. Weisbrodt NW, Murphy RA. Myosin phosphorylation and contraction of feline esophageal smooth muscle. *Am J Physiol* 1985;249:C9–C14.

222. Christensen J. Oxygen dependence of contractions in esophageal and gastric pyloric and ileocecal muscle of opossums. *Proc Soc Exp Biol Med* 1982;170:194–202.

223. Schulze-Delrieu K, Crane SA. Oxygen uptake and mechanical tension in esophageal smooth muscle from opossums and cats. *Am J Physiol* 1982;242:G258–G262.

224. Robison BA, Percy WH, Christensen J. Differences in cytochrome c oxidase capacity in smooth muscle of opossum esophagus and lower esophageal sphincter. *Gastroenterology* 1984;87:1009–1013.

225. Biancani P, Goyal RK, Phillips A, et al. Mechanics of sphincter action. Studies on the lower esophageal sphincter. *J Clin Invest* 1973;52:2973–2978.

226. Goyal RK, Rattan S. Genesis of basal sphincter pressure: effect of tetrodotoxin on lower esophageal sphincter pressure in opossum in vivo. *Gastroenterology* 1976;71:62–67.

227. Barone FC, Lombardi DM, Ormsbee HS III. Effects of hindbrain stimulation on lower esophageal sphincter pressure in the cat. *Am J Physiol* 1984;247:G70–G78.

228. Paterson WG. Alteration of swallowing and oesophageal peristalsis by different initiators of deglutition. *Neurogastroenterol Motil* 1999;11:63–67.

229. Ward SM, Morris G, Reese L, et al. Interstitial cells of Cajal mediate enteric inhibitory neurotransmission in the lower esophageal and pyloric sphincters. *Gastroenterology* 1998;115:314–329.

230. Sivarao DV, Mashimo HL, Thatte HS, et al. Lower esophageal sphincter is achalasic in nNOS(-/-) and hypotensive in W/W(v) mutant mice. *Gastroenterology* 2001;121:34–42.

231. McNally AK, Chisolm GM III, Morel DW, et al. Activated human monocytes oxidize low-density lipoprotein by a lipoxygenase-dependent pathway. *J Immunol* 1990;145:254–259.

232. Smith CC, Brizzee KR. Cineradiographic analysis of vomiting in the cat. *Gastroenterology* 1960;40:654.

233. Wyman JB, Dent J, Heddle R, et al. Control of belching by the lower oesophageal sphincter. *Gut* 1990;31:639–646.

234. Mittal RK, McCallum RW. Characteristics of transient lower esophageal sphincter relaxation in humans. *Am J Physiol* 1987;252:G636–G641.

235. Mittal RK, Stewart WR, Schirmer BD. Effect of a catheter in the pharynx on the frequency of transient lower esophageal sphincter relaxations. *Gastroenterology* 1992;103:1236–1240.

236. Goyal RK, Rattan S. Nature of the vagal inhibitory innervation to the lower esophageal sphincter. *J Clin Invest* 1975;55:1119–1126.

237. Rattan S, Goyal RK. Neural control of the lower esophageal sphincter: influence of the vagus nerves. *J Clin Invest* 1974;54:899–906.

238. Rattan S, Goyal RK. Evidence of 5-HT participation in vagal inhibitory pathway to opossum LES. *Am J Physiol* 1978;234:E273–E276.

239. Rattan S, Goyal RK. Identification of M1 and M2 muscarinic receptor subtypes in the control of the lower esophageal sphincter in the opossum. *Trends Pharmacol Sci* 1984;[Suppl]:78.

240. Tottrup A, Forman A, Funch-Jensen P, et al. Effects of transmural field stimulation in isolated muscle strips from human esophagus. *Am J Physiol* 1990;258:G344–G351.

241. Tottrup A, Knudsen MA, Gregersen H. The role of the L-arginine-nitric oxide pathway in relaxation of the opossum lower oesophageal sphincter. *Br J Pharmacol* 1991;104:113–116.

242. Paterson WG, Anderson MA, Anand N. Pharmacological characterization of lower esophageal sphincter relaxation induced by swallowing, vagal efferent nerve stimulation, and esophageal distention. *Can J Physiol Pharmacol* 1992;70:1011–1015.

243. Goyal RK, Rattan S, Said SI. VIP as a possible neurotransmitter of non-cholinergic non-adrenergic inhibitory neurones. *Nature* 1980;288:378–380.

244. Szewczak SM, Behar J, Billett G, et al. VIP-induced alterations in cAMP and inositol phosphates in the lower esophageal sphincter. *Am J Physiol* 1990;259:G239–G244.

245. He XD, Goyal RK. Nitric oxide involvement in the peptide VIP-associated inhibitory junction potential in the guinea-pig ileum. *J Physiol* 1993;461:485–499.

246. Mao YK, Wang YF, Daniel EE. Distribution and characterization of vasoactive intestinal polypeptide binding in canine lower esophageal sphincter. *Gastroenterology* 1993;105:1370–1377.

247. Mashimo H, He XD, Huang PL, et al. Neuronal constitutive nitric oxide synthase is involved in murine enteric inhibitory neurotransmission. *J Clin Invest* 1996;98:8–13.

248. Miller CA, Barnette MS, Ormsbee HS III, et al. Cyclic nucleotide-dependent protein kinases in the lower esophageal sphincter. *Am J Physiol* 1986;251:G794–G803.

249. Rattan S, Moummi C. Influence of stimulators and inhibitors of cyclic nucleotides on lower esophageal sphincter. *J Pharmacol Exp Ther* 1989;248:703–709.

250. Torphy TJ, Fine CF, Burman M, et al. Lower esophageal sphincter relaxation is associated with increased cyclic nucleotide content. *Am J Physiol* 1986;251:G786–G793.

251. Lind JF, Warrian WG, Wankling WJ. Responses of the gastroesophageal junctional zone to increases in abdominal pressure. *Can J Surg* 1966;9:32–38.

252. Muller-Lissner SA, Blum AL. Fundic pressure rise lowers lower esophageal sphincter pressure in man. *Hepatogastroenterology* 1982;29:151–152.

253. Holloway RH, Blank EL, Takahashi I, et al. Electrical control activity of the lower esophageal sphincter in unanesthetized opossums. *Am J Physiol* 1987;252:G511–G521.

254. Biancani P, Sohn UD, Rich HG, et al. Signal transduction pathways in esophageal and lower esophageal sphincter circular muscle. *Am J Med* 1997;103:23S–28S.

255. Anand N, Paterson WG. Role of nitric oxide in esophageal peristalsis. *Am J Physiol* 1994;266:G123–G131.

256. Knudsen MA, Svane D, Tottrup A. Action profiles of nitric oxide, S-nitroso-L-cysteine, SNP, and NANC responses in opossum lower esophageal sphincter. *Am J Physiol* 1992;262:G840–G846.

257. Tottrup A, Svane D, Forman A. Nitric oxide mediating NANC inhibition in opossum lower esophageal sphincter. *Am J Physiol* 1991;260:G385–G389.

258. Gaumnitz EA, Bass P, Osinski MA, et al. Electrophysiological and pharmacological responses of chronically denervated lower esophageal sphincter of the opossum. *Gastroenterology* 1995;109:789–799.

259. Gilbert RJ, Dodds WJ. Effect of selective muscarinic antagonists on peristaltic contractions in opossum smooth muscle. *Am J Physiol* 1986;250:G50–G59.

260. Harris LD, Ashworkth WD, Ingelfinger FJ. Esophageal aperistalsis and achalasia produced in dogs by prolonged cholinesterase inhibition. *J Clin Invest* 1960;39:1744.

261. Dilawari JB, Newman A, Poleo J, et al. Response of the human cardia sphincter to circulating prostaglandins F2ALPHA and E2 and to antiinflammatory drugs. *Gut* 1975;16:137–143.

262. Terenghi G, Polak JM, Rodrigo J, et al. Calcitonin gene-related peptide-immunoreactive nerves in the tongue, epiglottis and pharynx of the rat: occurrence, distribution and origin. *Brain Res* 1986;365:1–14.

263. Thor K, Rokaeus A. Studies on the mechanisms by which (Gln4)-neurotensin reduces lower esophageal sphincter (LES) pressure in man. *Acta Physiol Scand* 1983;118:373–377.

264. Tuma SN, Mukhopadhyay A. The effect of parathyroid hormone on the esophageal smooth muscle of the opossum. *Am J Gastroenterol* 1980;74:415–418.

265. Gilbert R, Rattan S, Goyal RK. Pharmacologic identification, activation and antagonism of two muscarine receptor subtypes in the lower esophageal sphincter. *J Pharmacol Exp Ther* 1984;230:284–291.

266. Thorpe JA. Effect of propranolol on the lower oesophageal sphincter in man. *Curr Med Res Opin* 1980;7:91–95.

267. Biancani P, Beinfeld MC, Hillemeier C, et al. Role of peptide histidine isoleucine in relaxation of cat lower esophageal sphincter. *Gastroenterology* 1989;97:1083–1089.

268. Kim N, Sohn UD, Mangannan V, et al. Leukotrienes in acetyl-choline-induced contraction of esophageal circular smooth muscle in experimental esophagitis. *Gastroenterology* 1997;112:1548–1558.

269. Penagini R, Bianchi PA. Effect of morphine on gastroesophageal reflux and transient lower esophageal sphincter relaxation. *Gastroenterology* 1997;113:409–414.

270. Saha JK, Sengupta JN, Goyal RK. Effect of bradykinin on opossum esophageal longitudinal smooth muscle: evidence for novel bradykinin receptors. *J Pharmacol Exp Ther* 1990;252:1012–1020.

271. Saha JK, Sengupta JN, Goyal RK. Effects of bradykinin and bradykinin analogs on the opossum lower esophageal sphincter: characterization of an inhibitory bradykinin receptor. *J Pharmacol Exp Ther* 1991;259:265–273.

272. Kahrilas PJ, Gupta RR. Mechanisms of acid reflux associated with cigarette smoking. *Gut* 1990;31:4–10.

273. Wright LE, Castell DO. The adverse effect of chocolate on lower esophageal sphincter pressure. *Am J Dig Dis* 1975;20:703–707.

274. Mittal RK, Rochester DF, McCallum RW. Electrical and mechanical activity in the human lower esophageal sphincter during diaphragmatic contraction. *J Clin Invest* 1988;81:1182–1189.

275. Klein WA, Parkman HP, Dempsey DT, et al. Sphincterlike thoracoabdominal high pressure zone after esophagogastrectomy. *Gastroenterology* 1993;105:1362–1369.

276. Titchen DA. Diaphragmatic and oesophageal activity in regurgitation in sheep: an electromyographic study. *J Physiol* 1979;292:381–390.

277. Altschuler SM, Boyle JT, Nixon TE, et al. Simultaneous reflex inhibition of lower esophageal sphincter and crural diaphragm in cats. *Am J Physiol* 1985;249:G586–G591.

278. Mittal RK, Fisher MJ. Electrical and mechanical inhibition of the crural diaphragm during transient relaxation of the lower esophageal sphincter. *Gastroenterology* 1990;99:1265–1268.

279. De Troyer A, Rosso J. Reflex inhibition of the diaphragm by esophageal afferents. *Neurosci Lett* 1982;30:43–46.

280. Liu J, Yamamoto Y, Schirmer BD, et al. Evidence for a peripheral mechanism of esophagocrural diaphragm inhibitory reflex in cats. *Am J Physiol Gastrointest Liver Physiol* 2000;278:G281–G288.

281. Fryscak T, Zenker W, Kantner D. Afferent and efferent innervation of the rat esophagus. A tracing study with horseradish peroxidase and nuclear yellow. *Anat Embryol (Berl)* 1984;170:63–70.

282. Collman PI, Tremblay L, Diamant NE. The distribution of spinal and vagal sensory neurons that innervate the esophagus of the cat. *Gastroenterology* 1992;103:817–822.

283. Rodrigo J, de Felipe J, Robles-Chillida EM, et al. Sensory vagal nature and anatomical access paths to esophagus laminar nerve endings in myenteric ganglia. Determination by surgical degeneration methods. *Acta Anat (Basel)* 1982;112:47–57.

284. Rodrigo J, Hernandez CJ, Vidal MA, et al. Vegetative innervation of the esophagus. III. Intraepithelial endings. *Acta Anat (Basel)* 1975;92:242–258.

285. Rodrigo J, Hernandez J, Vidal MA, et al. Vegetative innervation of the esophagus. II. Intraganglionic laminar endings. *Acta Anat (Basel)* 1975;92:79–100.

286. Rodrigo J, Polak JM, Fernandez L, et al. Calcitonin gene-related peptide immunoreactive sensory and motor nerves of the rat, cat, and monkey esophagus. *Gastroenterology* 1985;88:444–451.

287. Rodrigo J, Robles Chillida EM, de Felipe J, et al. Sensorivagal nature of oesophageal submucous layer nerve endings. Determination of surgical degeneration methods. *Acta Anat (Basel)* 1980;108:540–550.

288. Clerc N, Mei N. Thoracic esophageal mechanoreceptors connected with fibers following sympathetic pathways. *Brain Res Bull* 1983;10:1–7.
289. Clerc N, Mei N. Vagal mechanoreceptors located in the lower oesophageal sphincter of the cat. *J Physiol* 1983;336:487–498.
290. Cervero F, Janig W. Visceral nociceptors: a new world order? *Trends Neurosci* 1992;15:374–378.
291. Sengupta JN, Kauvar D, Goyal RK. Characteristics of vagal esophageal tension-sensitive afferent fibers in the opossum. *J Neurophysiol* 1989;61:1001–1010.
292. Sengupta JN, Saha JK, Goyal RK. Stimulus-response function studies of esophageal mechanosensitive nociceptors in sympathetic afferents of opossum. *J Neurophysiol* 1990;64:796–812.
293. Sengupta JN, Saha JK, Goyal RK. Differential sensitivity to bradykinin of esophageal distension-sensitive mechanoreceptors in vagal and sympathetic afferents of the opossum. *J Neurophysiol* 1992;68:1053–1067.
294. DeVault KR, Beacham S, Castell DO, et al. Esophageal sensation in spinal cord-injured patients: balloon distension and cerebral evoked potential recording. *Am J Physiol* 1996;271:G937–G941.
295. Altschuler SM, Bao XM, Bieger D, et al. Viscerotopic representation of the upper alimentary tract in the rat: sensory ganglia and nuclei of the solitary and spinal trigeminal tracts. *J Comp Neurol* 1989;283:248–268.
296. Mehta AJ, De Caestecker JS, Camm AJ, et al. Sensitization to painful distention and abnormal sensory perception in the esophagus. *Gastroenterology* 1995;108:311–319.
297. Aziz Q, Andersson JL, Valind S, et al. Identification of human brain loci processing esophageal sensation using positron emission tomography. *Gastroenterology* 1997;113:50–59.
298. Frieling T, Enck P, Wienbeck M. Cerebral responses evoked by electrical stimulation of the esophagus in normal subjects. *Gastroenterology* 1989;97:475–478.
299. Hollerbach S, Kamath MV, Chen Y, et al. The magnitude of the central response to esophageal electrical stimulation is intensity dependent. *Gastroenterology* 1997;112:1137–1146.
300. Rathmann W, Enck P, Frieling T, et al. Visceral afferent neuropathy in diabetic gastroparesis. *Diabetes Care* 1991;14:1086–1089.

SYMPTOM OVERVIEW AND QUALITY OF LIFE

BRIAN T. JOHNSTON
DONALD O. CASTELL

In 1905, Lord Moynihan claimed that most patients who presented with dyspepsia could be diagnosed correctly by symptoms alone (1). Although the statement was made about 100 years ago, it remains relevant in this era of technology, emphasizing the importance of maintaining good history-taking skills. This chapter gives a brief overview of the sensory pathways from the esophagus and then concentrates on the discriminate value of different esophageal symptoms. The second part of the chapter, which addresses the impact that esophageal disease can have on quality of life (QoL) is summed up best by a quotation from Joseph Conrad's book, *Under Western Eyes*: "The joy of life depends on a sound stomach." Quantifying "the joy of life" is a function of QoL measures.

SENSORY PATHWAYS

Various receptors within the esophageal wall are responsible for esophageal sensation. Specific mechanical and thermal receptors have been identified, along with free nerve endings within the epithelium, which may respond to chemical or osmotic changes (2). Although some receptors are purely physiologic, many serve both physiologic and pain (nociceptive) functions (3). Different stimuli, such as acid and distention, can augment nociception (4).

Sensation from the esophagus travels along spinal (sympathetic) and vagal (parasympathetic) pathways (5). Physiologic sensation travels along both routes. Pain is conveyed via the third through eighth thoracic sympathetic nerves. This overlaps with the heart and pericardium, which are supplied by the first through fifth thoracic sympathetic nerves. Both organs give rise to deep-seated visceral pain felt retrosternally and in the epigastrium. Pain from both sites can radiate to the arm, the jaw, or the back. This overlap makes it impossible to discriminate with certainty between cardiac and esophageal pain solely on the characteristics of the pain.

Some symptoms do appear to be relatively specific to the esophagus, such as heartburn and retrosternal dysphagia. Other symptoms, such as chest pain, have a lower probability of arising from the esophagus. The next section of this chapter discusses these typical (high probability) and atypical (low probability) symptoms in greater detail (Table 2.1).

TYPICAL (HIGH PROBABILITY) SYMPTOMS
Esophageal Dysphagia (Chapters 11, 12, 13, 15, 28)

The word *dysphagia*, which is derived from the Greek *phagia* (to eat) and *dys* (with difficulty), is the symptom most specifically indicating an esophageal disorder. It refers to the sensation of ingested material being hindered in its normal passage down the esophagus. Patients with esophageal dysphagia most frequently complain that food "sticks" retrosternally, "hangs up," "gets caught," or "just won't go down right." They may occasionally note some associated pain, but the symptom of dysphagia should not be used interchangeably with odynophagia (see Odynophagia). Dysphagia is not uncommon, and 10% of people older than 50 years old report troublesome dysphagia (6). The importance of the clinical history in suggesting a specific etiology for the dysphagia cannot be overstated. When Schatzki described the lower esophageal ring that bears his name, he asserted that a careful history should give the physician a strong suspicion of the correct diagnosis in 80% to 85% of patients with dysphagia (7).

Esophageal dysphagia may be caused by obstruction to luminal flow (mechanical) or by altered motility in the esophageal wall (neuromuscular) (Table 2.2). Causes of obstruction include rings, strictures, carcinoma, and extrin-

D. O. Castell: Esophageal Disorders Program, Division of GI/Hepatology, Medical University of South Carolina, Charleston, South Carolina.
B.T. Johnston: Royal Victoria Hospital, Belfast, United Kingdom.

TABLE 2.1. SYMPTOMS OF ESOPHAGEAL ORIGIN

Typical (high probability)
1. Esophageal dysphagia
2. Heartburn and acid regurgitation
3. Odynophagia

Atypical (low probability)
1. Chest pain
2. Oropharyngeal dysphagia
3. Globus
4. Cough
5. Asthma
6. Hoarseness
7. Nonacid regurgitation
8. Waterbrash
9. Hiccups

sic masses. Causes of altered motility include failure of peristalsis (achalasia, scleroderma) or disruption of the normal peristaltic progression (diffuse esophageal spasm).

When approaching the patient with apparent esophageal dysphagia, three questions are crucial: (a) What kind of food (liquid or solid) produces the symptom (8)? (b) Is the dysphagia intermittent or progressive? (c) Is there associated heartburn? Based on the answers to these questions, it is often possible not only to identify the etiology as either a mechanical or a neuromuscular defect but also to postulate a specific diagnosis. An algorithm of the common causes of esophageal dysphagia based on the

TABLE 2.2. ETIOLOGIES OF ESOPHAGEAL DYSPHAGIA

Neuromuscular (motility) disorders
  Primary
  Achalasia
  Diffuse esophageal spasm
  Nutcracker esophagus (hypertensive peristalsis)
  Hypertensive lower esophagus
  Ineffective esophageal motility
  Secondary
  Scleroderma
  Other collagen disorders
  Chagas' disease
Mechanical lesions—intrinsic
  Most common
  Peptic stricture
  Lower esophageal (Schatzki's) ring
  Carcinoma
  Other
  Esophageal webs
  Esophageal diverticula
  Benign tumors
  Foreign bodies
  Medication-induced injury
Mechanical lesions—extrinsic
  Vascular compression
  Mediastinal abnormalities
  Cervical osteoarthritis

clinical history is shown in Figure 2.1. Additional helpful features to ascertain are onset (sudden or gradual), duration, associated pain, weight loss, associated coughing or choking, and drug history (especially use of nonsteroidal antiinflammatory drugs).

Patients with esophageal motility disorders usually complain of slowly progressive dysphagia for both liquids and solids from the onset. In *achalasia,* regurgitation of undigested food that had been eaten many hours previously is a common complaint, particularly at night, when it may result in aspiration and nocturnal coughing. Dysphagia in *progressive systemic sclerosis* is often associated with heartburn. Poor clearance of acid results in strictures in up to 40% of these patients (9). The dysphagia of *diffuse esophageal spasm* may occur with liquids or solid food. It is generally intermittent and nonprogressive and occasionally is associated with pain, features that separate it from the other motility disorders. Patients with diffuse esophageal spasm may report that a variety of factors precipitate dysphagia or chest pain, including ingestion of hot or cold foods or carbonated beverages, or being exposed to stress.

Conversely, patients with mechanical obstruction usually have dysphagia initially for solids only and more progressive symptoms, although the onset is occasionally sudden. The exception to this consistent, progressive dysphagia is in the case of the *lower esophageal ring,* in which intermittent dysphagia is the rule. If the solid food dysphagia is clearly progressive, then the major considerations in the differential diagnosis are peptic esophageal stricture and carcinoma. Patients with *peptic stricture* are usually middle aged or elderly and typically have a long antecedent history of heartburn and chronic antacid use. Peptic strictures can also occur in patients with learning difficulties whose gastroesophageal reflux disease (GERD) has been left untreated because they have been unable to adequately express their symptoms. Patients with *carcinoma* of the esophagus are more likely to present with a history of rapidly progressive dysphagia. They have anorexia and weight loss greater than the severity or duration of their dysphagia would support. Heavy alcohol and tobacco use is associated with squamous carcinoma.

Several *vascular anomalies* may produce dysphagia by compression of the esophagus. The dysphagia associated with these lesions (so-called dysphagia lusoria) usually begins early in childhood. Occasionally, symptoms may present in the adult, after increasing atherosclerosis or aneurysmal changes. The dysphagia is usually a constant, daily problem, described as a temporary arrest of a solid bolus beneath the manubrium. The compression may be caused by (a) a complete vascular ring (e.g., a double aortic arch), (b) an incomplete ring, such as a retroesophageal right aberrant subclavian artery (arteria lusoria), or (c) a massive thoracic aortic aneurysm or a rigid atherosclerotic aorta (dysphagia aortica).

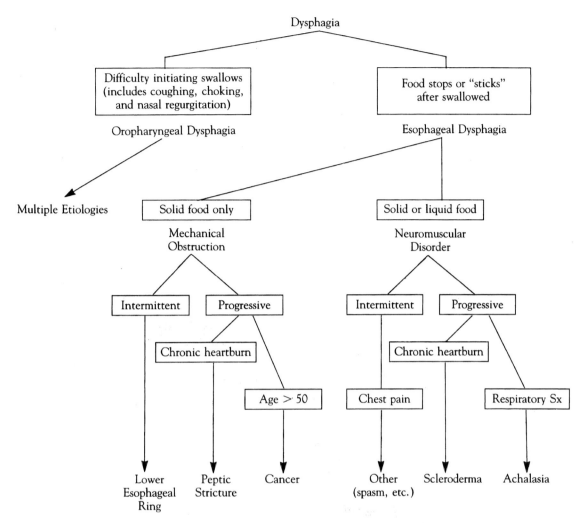

FIGURE 2.1. Algorithm for diagnostic symptom analysis of patients with dysphagia. Sx, symptoms.

The site at which the patient localizes his or her dysphagia is of limited value. Although dysphagia in the epigastric or retrosternal areas frequently corresponds to the site of obstruction, dysphagia localized by the patient to the neck is frequently referred from below. The term *cervical dysphagia* should be avoided because localization of the sensation in the suprasternal area can occur with either oropharyngeal or esophageal dysphagia. When the patient describes difficulty initiating a swallow and transferring food from the mouth to the esophagus, the dysphagia is oropharyngeal and not esophageal (see later text).

Physical examination is usually not revealing in patients with esophageal dysphagia, except in cases of scleroderma, in which other manifestations of CREST syndrome (*c*alcinosis, *R*aynaud's phenomenon, *e*sophagus, *s*clerodactyly, *t*elangiectasia) may be present. The two complementary tests for patients with dysphagia are a barium swallow and endoscopy. Because of the rapid sequence of pressure changes and movement of anatomic structures in the oropharynx, special radiologic techniques must be employed if there is an element of oropharyngeal dysphagia (Chapter 10). If the x-ray findings and endoscopy are negative or suggest a motility disorder, an esophageal and upper esophageal sphincter motility study should be performed (Chapter 5). These concepts are summarized in Figure 2.2.

Heartburn and Acid Regurgitation (Chapter 19)

Classic heartburn is a substernal burning sensation with a tendency to radiate toward the mouth. It may be associated with an acid or bitter taste, usually occurs within 30 minutes to 2 hours after meals, and is made worse when the patient lies down or bends over. It may awaken patients from sleep. A large meal, especially if it contains fat, chocolate, coffee, or alcohol, is particularly likely to precipitate heartburn. The discomfort often disappears quickly on drinking water or milk or after taking an antacid. If heartburn occurs fre-

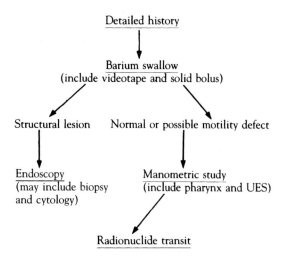

Detailed history

↓

Barium swallow
(include videotape and solid bolus)

Structural lesion   Normal or possible motility defect

↓   ↓

Endoscopy   Manometric study
(may include biopsy   (include pharynx and UES)
and cytology)

↓

Radionuclide transit

FIGURE 2.2. Suggested diagnostic testing sequence for the evaluation of patients with dysphagia. UES, upper esophageal sphincter.

quently, it can interfere with the patient's way of life, particularly work or pleasure involving lying or bending, including gardening and sexual intercourse. Sudden, unprecedented heartburn may indicate acute esophagitis or esophageal erosion caused by a corrosive, especially a drug.

Simply asking a patient whether he or she has experienced "heartburn" is insufficient. One study that excluded dyspeptic patients who admitted to "heartburn," still had 42% of patients whose predominant symptom was best described by the word picture "a burning feeling rising from your stomach or lower chest up towards your neck" (10). Using such a descriptive term improves diagnostic accuracy in documenting GERD.

Heartburn is often associated with the symptom of acid regurgitation, which is best described as the effortless appearance of an acid or bitter taste in the mouth. Regurgitation is particularly severe at night or when bending over. It can awaken patients from sleep because of coughing or choking and may occur with or independently from heartburn.

Heartburn and acid regurgitation can be regarded as the classic symptoms of reflux disease. In one study, pH monitoring showed a high specificity for excessive acid reflux (89% to 95%). Sensitivity, however, was poor (6% to 38%). No other symptom distinguished between patients with positive and negative esophageal pH testing (11). On the basis of this and other studies, it has been suggested that when either heartburn or acid regurgitation is present as the predominant symptom, a diagnosis of GERD can be made without further investigation (12). The importance of this has recently been emphasized in a primary care setting. A group of primary care physicians and gastroenterologists in Canada developed an algorithm for the management of uninvestigated dyspepsia (13). One step of this algorithm suggested a diagnosis of GERD be made and empirical treatment initiated on the basis of these symptoms being dominant. Diagnosis and treatment based on the most significant symptom is a more useful strategy than the previous approach of dividing dyspepsia on the basis of symptom clusters.

Acid perfusion studies and prolonged esophageal monitoring with recording of symptoms demonstrate a correlation between decreases in esophageal pH caused by acid reflux and the onset of a symptom (Fig. 2.3) This is called a *symptom index*. This index is not always 100% accurate for all patients with GERD (and other esophageal symptoms) (14). Patients differ in their sensitivity to the degree of acid-

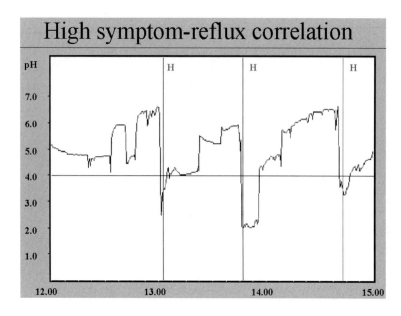

FIGURE 2.3. A tracing of esophageal pH monitoring demonstrating good symptom correlation with acid reflux (a high symptom index).

TABLE 2.3. FACTORS INFLUENCING SYMPTOM AWARENESS

Luminal factors
1. Nature of contents: pH, osmotic, ionic, temperature
2. Volume of contents and distention of lumen
3. Duration of exposure
4. Preceding sensitization

Mucosal factors
1. Pain threshold of nerve ending
2. Proximity of nerve ending to lumen
3. Inflammatory mediators

Central factors
1. Spinal modulation
2. Cerebral modulation
3. Psychological factors

ity (15), which may differ from day to day or throughout the day depending on preceding acid exposure (16), sensitization, and other factors (17) (Table 2.3). In particular, patients with Barrett's esophagus appear relatively insensitive to esophageal acidification (18).

Odynophagia (Chapters 34, 35, 36)

The term *odynophagia* is used to describe the symptom of pain associated with swallowing. This important symptom is highly indicative of a pharyngeal or esophageal problem. A sensation of burning or pain soon after swallowing hot, cold, spicy, or acidic food or drink is characteristic. It is common in erosive esophagitis whether it is acid-related, infective, or pill-induced, and it has been reported in 31% of acquired immunodeficiency syndrome patients (19). In corrosive esophagitis (particularly "pill"-induced injury), odynophagia may be severe enough to cause complete cessation of swallowing.

ATYPICAL (LOW PROBABILITY) SYMPTOMS

Chest Pain (Chapter 36)

Because of the overlapping sensory innervation described earlier, separating esophageal from cardiac chest pain is impossible based on the pain alone. If a cardiac cause has been excluded, esophageal pH monitoring and manometry can be used to demonstrate a temporal relationship between the pain and either a decrease in pH or motility changes. It seems increasingly likely that these individuals have abnormal visceral perception localized to the chest, with the "sensitive" viscus being the heart, esophagus, or other thoracic structure. The abnormality rendering them "sensitive" may be local nociceptors in the viscera, higher processing centers, cortical connections, or possibly other factors (including anxiety) (20–22).

Oropharyngeal Dysphagia (Chapter 10)

Oropharyngeal dysphagia is usually described as a problem with the initiation of swallowing and occurs before entry to the esophagus. It is a transfer problem, caused by impaired ability to transfer food from mouth to upper esophagus or by an impaired oral preparatory phase. These patients present with a variety of complaints, including food sticking in the throat, nasal regurgitation, and coughing during swallowing. They may also complain of dysarthria or display nasal speech because of associated muscle weakness. Many local, neurologic, and muscular diseases can produce oropharyngeal dysphagia. Usually, the dysphagia is only one of the manifestations of a relatively obvious disease and does not pose a diagnostic problem, but careful radiologic and manometric investigation may be required to make a specific diagnosis and to assist in planning therapy.

Globus (Chapter 10)

A generally accepted clinical truth is that dysphagia almost always indicates the presence of organic dysfunction. It is important, therefore, that one should not confuse dysphagia with globus sensation, the feeling of a lump, fullness, or "tickle" in the throat. Globus is usually a more constant symptom that does not interfere with swallowing and that may be relieved during deglutition. Globus has often been considered a symptom occurring in patients having hysterical personality traits, leading to the outdated term *globus hystericus*. This is not an appropriate name because psychological evaluations have revealed an increase in depression (23) and obsessive-compulsive tendencies (24) in patients with globus but little evidence of hysteria. Thus, the term *globus,* or *globus sensation,* is preferable. The diagnosis of globus should never be made without a thorough investigation for an otorhinolaryngeal lesion. In patients with this globus sensation in whom a physical cause in the pharynx, larynx, or neck has been excluded, a variety of esophageal associations have been made. Reports have linked the sensation to a hypertensive or poorly relaxing upper esophageal sphincter, altered visceral afferent sensation, or acid reflux (25–28) (Table 2.4).

TABLE 2.4. POTENTIAL ESOPHAGEAL ASSOCIATIONS WITH GLOBUS SENSATION

1. Hypertensive or poorly relaxing upper esophageal sphincter
2. Altered visceral afferent sensation
3. Gastroesophageal reflux
4. Esophageal dysmotility (e.g., achalasia, ineffective esophageal motility)
5. Esophageal webs and diverticula

Respiratory and Supraesophageal Symptoms (Chapters 29 and 30)

Certain *respiratory symptoms* are associated with and are possibly caused by gastroesophageal reflux and may be considered symptoms of esophageal disease. A higher than expected incidence of detectable reflux in patients with respiratory problems, such as asthma (29,30), bronchitis (31), and cough (32), has been repeatedly observed in recent years.

The suggestion that extraesophageal manifestations of chronic GERD may bring patients to various specialists is not a new concept. Otolaryngologists have been aware for many years that *hoarseness* can be a manifestation of GERD as a result of reflux laryngitis (33).

Nonacid Regurgitation

An esophageal problem alone does not cause true vomiting. Patients, however, may complain of "vomiting" when they are experiencing some form of *regurgitation*, that is, the effortless appearance of food or fluid in the mouth. When the contents of the regurgitation are tasteless or undigested food, a degree of esophageal obstruction is indicated as is often reported in achalasia. It can also be due to a pharyngeal pouch.

Water Brash

The term *water brash*, is frequently misused; it is intended to describe the sudden filling of the mouth with clear, slightly salty fluid. The fluid is not regurgitated gastric contents but, rather, secretions from the salivary glands occurring by reflex stimulation resulting from acid irritation in the distal esophagus (34). Although not a specific symptom on its own, water brash increases the certainty of a GERD diagnosis in patients who also report heartburn or acid regurgitation.

Hiccup

The easily recognized *hiccup* (hiccough, singultus) is caused by an abrupt, involuntary lowering of the diaphragm and closure of the glottis, producing a characteristic sound. Although most clinicians are aware that various systemic disorders, notably uremia, may cause hiccup, almost all sporadic hiccuping is of unclear origin (35). Esophageal disease can be a cause and the fact that sporadic hiccup particularly occurs after a large meal is compatible with the view that reflux is frequently the cause (36–38). Esophageal obstruction may also cause hiccup, sometimes without dysphagia, and has been reported by patients with achalasia or with benign or malignant strictures (36).

QUALITY OF LIFE

Definition

QoL has been defined by the World Health Organization not simply as absence of ill health but as a complete state of physical, psychological, and social health. Health-related QoL can be reduced by any illness or disease. However, until relatively recently, appropriate instruments to quantify this impact have not been available. Any global assessment of QoL must include measurement of the physical, social, and psychological consequences of the illness (39).

Three approaches can be adopted to assess QoL. First, a generic questionnaire such as the SF36 can be used. This approach allows QoL to be quantified and compared across a variety of illnesses. There are also normal values for the general population that facilitate comparison. Second, a disease-specific questionnaire acknowledges that there may be certain key aspects to a condition that merit particular assessment, for example, the psychological impact of receiving a diagnosis of esophageal cancer or the detrimental effect of chronic sleep disturbance from nocturnal reflux. The advantage of this approach is that it offers a sensitive measure of QoL for a specific disease and so may pick up more subtle effects of treatment options. It does not, however, facilitate comparison between different disease states unless it has been validated for each of them. The third approach is to use an individualized measure such as the Patient Generated Index (40). Just as the disease-specific measure seeks to pick up issues that are key to the impact of that disease on QoL, so the individualized measure seeks to determine issues that are of particular importance for the specific patient. It allows each patient to define the life domains that are important to him or her and that constitute their QoL. Although it is a sensitive method of quantifying QoL, this third approach requires greater expertise in its administration and interpretation.

Importance of Quality of Life

Relationship with Symptoms

There is a correlation between the severity of symptoms and the QoL score (41–43). It could therefore be argued that treating symptoms is sufficient without taking time to measure their impact on QoL. However, relying on symptoms alone is problematic. First, as highlighted earlier for heartburn, the patient's understanding of terms used for symptoms varies greatly. Second, the distress caused by a particular symptom differs between individuals. Third, treatment for symptoms alone may cease to be reimbursed by health care providers. For example, most patients with heartburn have no objective evidence of disease on esophagogastroduodenoscopy or esophageal pH monitoring. Do they have a disease, as suggested by the term *nonerosive reflux disease*, or are these symptoms physiologic and within normal limits? There is a danger that proton pump inhibitors could be classed as "lifestyle medications" for such individuals and not be funded by health care providers (44). Being able to quantify the effect such symptoms have on QoL is important in addressing this issue.

Evaluating Interventions

Increasingly, regulatory authorities are seeking evidence of cost effectiveness for new interventions before approving them. This is true of the Food and Drugs Administration in the United States and the National Institute for Clinical Excellence in the United Kingdom. QoL measures can be used to study the cost effectiveness of any treatment option.

Esophageal Cancer

QoL in esophageal carcinoma has been a neglected area. One review of 7,569 publications noted reference to QoL in only 44 studies (0.58%) (45). Furthermore, those studies that assessed QoL tended to be small, were based on postal surveys, or used nonstandardized, nonvalidated questionnaires. This defect has been addressed recently with the development of two validated questionnaires that incorporate both a general and a condition-specific component. These are the American FACT and the European Organization for Research and Treatment of Cancer (EORTC) questionnaire.

The FACT questionnaire contains four scales addressing physical, social, emotional, and functional well-being. The FACT-G has been widely used in many trials in oncology and an esophageal cancer module (FACT-E) is available. The EORTC questionnaire has a generic portion for patients with cancer (EORTC QLQ-C30) and a specific esophageal cancer module (EORTC QLQ-OES24). This site-specific module improves the sensitivity and specificity of the core instrument and has been tested in patients undergoing a variety of treatments for esophageal cancer (46).

For potentially operable patients, esophageal resection may offer the chance of cure. However, this may not be the best option for every patient. Improved information on postoperative QoL can help to guide patients appropriately. A recent study suggests that those patients who survived 2 years after esophagectomy regained preoperative levels of QoL 9 months after surgery. By contrast, those surviving less than 2 years never regained preoperative levels of QoL (47). In contrast, an earlier study suggested that even a palliative esophagectomy resulted in an overall improvement in QoL (48).

Those who survive 5 years after surgery have an equivalent QoL to that of an age-matched normal population (49). This is also true much sooner for patients who undergo limited resection for early esophageal cancer (50). This important information helps predict the effects of pro-

TABLE 2.5. KEY ELEMENTS OF A GOOD QoL AFTER ESOPHAGECTOMY

1. To eat adequately and enjoy it
2. To drink as desired, including alcohol
3. To eat and drink in a social setting
4. Weight stability
5. Sleep comfortably in a normal position
6. Free of pain
7. To earn one's living
8. To participate in sports and hobbies
9. Unimpaired libido

From Kirby JD. Quality of life after oesophagectomy: the patients' perspective. *Dis Esophagus* 1999;12:168–171.

phylactic esophagectomy for high-grade dysplasia in Barrett's esophagus (51). Patient groups are increasingly being asked to contribute to the debate regarding what constitutes a good QoL. One recent publication from a patient's perspective suggested nine parameters as representing a good QoL after esophagectomy (52) (Table 2.5).

For patients with inoperable esophageal cancer, QoL has been used effectively as a parameter to assess response to chemotherapy or radiotherapy. For example, a combination of epirubicin, cisplatin, and 5-fluorouracil offered better QoL results at 3 and 6 months compared with a different regimen (53). In another study, the addition of radiotherapy to endoscopic treatment in squamous carcinoma improved QoL over endoscopic treatment alone (54).

QoL assessment has been made of different palliative options in malignant dysphagia. One study demonstrated significant QoL benefits for metal stents over the traditional plastic Atkinson tubes (55). In another study, QoL deteriorated in those patients treated by stent insertion but not in patients treated by thermal tumor ablation (56).

Gastroesophageal Reflux Disease

Much of the information on QoL in GERD comes from tertiary referral centers treating esophagitis. It demonstrates an impairment in QoL comparable to that reported by patients with chronic heart failure (57,58) and it is persistent, being present at least 10 years after initial diagnosis (59) (Fig. 2.4). More recent studies have concentrated on nonerosive reflux disease. These studies have demonstrated an equal reduction in QoL compared to QoL in patients who do have erosive esophagitis (60,61). This is an important finding in light of the earlier discussion regarding whether reflux symptoms constitute a disease or are merely a lifestyle issue. Clearly, they are a significant factor in these individuals' lives. The impact of nocturnal reflux on QoL has recently been highlighted by an American Gastroenterological Association–sponsored Gallup telephone survey of 1,000 adults who admitted to having heartburn at least once per week (personal communication). Seventy-nine

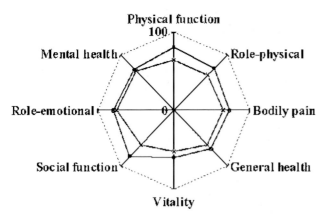

FIGURE 2.4. Impairment of quality of life in patients with chronic gastroesophageal reflux disease (—x—) compared with the normal population (—o—) as assessed by the SF36. (Adapted from McDougall NI, Johnston BT, Kee F, et al. Natural history of reflux oesophagitis: a 10 year follow up of its effect on patient symptomatology and quality of life. *Gut* 1996;38(4):481–486.)

percent reported nighttime symptoms and 63% of these individuals indicated their GERD-related symptoms interfered with sleep. Furthermore, 40% of them said that the nocturnal symptoms affected their performance the next day, emphasizing the effect of GERD on QoL through sleep deprivation. Data are also emerging of economic and productivity issues in a workforce in whom reflux symptoms have failed to be treated (44). The recently published "burden of digestive diseases" report documented that GERD was the third most common gastrointestinal disorder, following only infectious diarrheas and gallstones. The economic burden of GERD was greater than for any other gastrointestinal disease affecting 19 million individuals in the United States with an estimated cost of $9.3 billion dollars annually (in 1998 dollars) (62).

Proton pump inhibitors restore QoL levels to those of the normal population (60). Their QoL benefit is equivalent to that of antireflux surgery (63). They can improve QoL even when esophagitis has not been healed or reflux levels normalized (64). Histamine-2 receptor antagonists have also been shown to improve QoL in GERD (65).

What is lacking is information on the degree to which QoL is impaired in the vast number of patients who suffer reflux symptoms but who self-medicate or are contained within primary care. It is possible to hypothesize that their QoL is not markedly impaired if they choose not to consult (66).

Achalasia

There are limited data regarding the impact of achalasia on QoL and a virtual silence regarding the influence of other motility disorders. Only a few studies have been performed prospectively and they involved small numbers of patients. They indicate that QoL, as measured by the SF36,

improves with therapy (67,68). Two retrospective studies offer potentially conflicting results. The most recent, involving a laparoscopic or thoracoscopic approach, reported postoperative QoL levels that were equivalent to U.S. normal values on four subscales and significantly exceeded normal values on the other four (69).

The older study, which used a nonvalidated questionnaire but involved a follow-up period twice as long as that for Luketich and colleagues (69), reported restrictions in social and sporting activities in 8% to 15% of patients after therapy (70). In analyzing these results, one commentator has suggested that there is a tendency for QoL to deteriorate over time, even after initially successful therapy, and that these patients often fail to seek help (71).

CONCLUSION

Two points merit emphasizing regarding symptoms and QoL in esophageal disease. First, symptoms are subjective. Anxiety, fear of underlying malignancy, and somatization all potentially influence how patients perceive their symptoms, how they present, and how well they respond to treatment.

Second, patient outcome is influenced by what patients remember about their diagnosis. In a simple study from the pre-QoL era, chest pain patients with esophageal dysmotility who remembered being told their diagnosis had a better outcome than those who claimed that they had never been given a diagnosis (72).

These points emphasize the importance of communication between doctors and patients. This is true in the misunderstanding of esophageal symptoms and is equally applicable whether explaining a benign esophageal cause for chest pain or discussing the diagnosis of esophageal cancer. Good communication benefits the doctor diagnosing the symptoms and improves the QoL of the patient who is being informed and treated.

REFERENCES

1. Moynihan BGA. On duodenal ulcer: with notes of 52 operations. *Lancet* 1919;1:340–346.
2. Christensen J. Origin of sensation in the esophagus. *Am J Physiol* 1984;246:G221–G225
3. Sengupta JN, Saha JK, Goyal RK. Stimulus-response function studies of esophageal mechanosensitive nociceptors in sympathetic afferents of opossum. *J Neurophysiol* 1990;64(3):796–812.
4. De Caestecker JS, Heading RC. Esophageal pH monitoring. *Gastroenterol Clin North Am* 1990;19:645–670.
5. Cervero F. Sensory innervation of the viscera: peripheral basis of visceral pain. *Physiol Rev* 1994;74:95–138.
6. Lindgren S, Janzon L. Prevalence of swallowing complaints and clinical findings among 50–79-year-old men and women in an urban population. *Dysphagia* 1991;6(4):187–192.
7. Schatzki R. Panel discussion on diseases of the esophagus. *Am J Gastroenterol* 59 A.D.;31:117

8. Dakkak M, Bennett JR. A new dysphagia score with objective validation. *J Clin Gastroenterol* 1992;14(2):99–100.

9. Zamost BJ, Hirschberg J, Ippoliti AF, et al. Esophagitis in scleroderma. Prevalence and risk factors. *Gastroenterology* 1987;92(2):421–428.

10. Carlsson R, Dent J, Bolling-Sternevald E, et al. The usefulness of a structured questionnaire in the assessment of symptomatic gastroesophageal reflux disease. *Scand J Gastroenterol* 1998;33(10):1023–1029.

11. Klauser AG, Schindlbeck NE, Muller-Lissner SA. Symptoms in gastro-oesophageal reflux disease. *Lancet* 1990;335(8683):205–208.

12. Dent J. The role of the specialist in the diagnosis and short and long term care of patients with gastroesophageal reflux disease. *Am J Gastroenterol* 2001;96[Suppl 8]:S22–S26

13. Veldhuyzen vZS, Flook N, Chiba N, et al. An evidence-based approach to the management of uninvestigated dyspepsia in the era of *Helicobacter pylori*. Canadian Dyspepsia Working Group. *Can Med Assoc J* 2000;162[Suppl 12]:S3–23.

14. Johnston BT, McFarland RJ, Collins JS, et al. Symptom index as a marker of gastro-oesophageal reflux disease. *Br J Surg* 1992;79(10):1054–1055.

15. Smith JL, Opekun AR, Larkai E, Graham DY. Sensitivity of the esophageal mucosa to pH in gastroesophageal reflux disease. *Gastroenterology* 1989;96:683–689.

16. Siddiqui MA, Johnston BT, Leite LP, et al. Sensitization of esophageal mucosa by prior acid infusion: effect of decreasing intervals between infusions. *Am J Gastroenterol* 1996;91(9):1745–1748.

17. Johnston BT, Lewis SA, Love AH. Psychological factors in gastro-oesophageal reflux disease. *Gut* 1995;36(4):481–482.

18. Murphy PP, Johnston BT, Collins JSA. Mucosal sensitivity and salivary response to infused acid in patients with columnar-lined oesophagus. *Eur J Gastroenterol Hepatol* 1994;6:901–905.

19. Connolly GM, Hawkins D, Harcourt-Webster JN, et al. Oesophageal symptoms, their causes, treatment, and prognosis in patients with the acquired immunodeficiency syndrome. *Gut* 1989;30(8):1033–1039.

20. Bass C. Chest pain and breathlessness: relationship to psychiatric illness. *Am J Med* 1992;92(1A):12S–7S.

21. Barsky AJ. Palpitations, cardiac awareness, and panic disorder. *Am J Med* 1992;92(1A):31S–34S.

22. Lantinga LJ, Sprafkin RP, McCroskery JH, et al. One-year psychosocial follow-up of patients with chest pain and angiographically normal coronary arteries. *Am J Cardiol* 1988;62(4):209–213.

23. Pratt LW, Tobin WH, Gallagher RA. Globus hystericus—office evaluation by psychological testing with the MMPI. *Laryngoscope* 1976;86(10):1540–1551.

24. Puhakka H, Lehtinen V, Aalto T. Globus hystericus—a psychosomatic disease? *J Laryngol Otol* 1976;90(11):1021–1026.

25. Scharitzer M, Pokieser P, Schober E, et al. Morphological findings in dynamic swallowing studies of symptomatic patients. *Eur Radiol* 2002;12(5):1139–1144.

26. Moser G, Wenzel-Abatzi TA, Stelzeneder M, et al. Globus sensation: pharyngoesophageal function, psychometric and psychiatric findings, and follow-up in 88 patients. *Arch Intern Med* 1998;158(12):1365–1373.

27. Farkkila MA, Ertama L, Katila H, et al. Globus pharyngis, commonly associated with esophageal motility disorders. *Am J Gastroenterol* 1994;89(4):503–508.

28. Corso MJ, Pursnani KG, Mohiuddin MA, et al. Globus sensation is associated with hypertensive upper esophageal sphincter but not with gastroesophageal reflux. *Dig Dis Sci* 1998;43(7):1513–1517.

29. Harding SM. Gastroesophageal reflux, asthma, and mechanisms of interaction. *Am J Med* 2001;111[Suppl 8A]:8S–12S.

30. Sontag SJ, Schnell TG, Miller TQ, et al. Prevalence of oesophagitis in asthmatics. *Gut* 1992;33:872–876.

31. Ducolone A, Vandevenne A, Jouin H, et al. Gastroesophageal reflux in patients with asthma and chronic bronchitis. *Am Rev Respir Dis* 1987;135(2):327–332.

32. Irwin RS, French CT. Cough and gastroesophageal reflux: identifying cough and assessing the efficacy of cough-modifying agents. *Am J Med* 2001;111[Suppl 8A]:45S–50S.

33. Cherry J, Siegel CI, Margulies SI, et al. Pharyngeal localization of symptoms of gastroesophageal reflux. *Ann Otol Rhinol Laryngol* 1970;79(5):912–914.

34. Helm JF, Dodds WJ, Hogan WJ. Salivary response to esophageal acid in normal subjects and patients with reflux esophagitis. *Gastroenterology* 1987;93(6):1393–1397.

35. Kahrilas PJ, Shi G. Why do we hiccup? *Gut* 1997;41(5):712–713.

36. Fass R, Higa L, Kodner A, et al. Stimulus and site specific induction of hiccups in the oesophagus of normal subjects. *Gut* 1997;41(5):590–593.

37. Gluck M, Pope CE. Chronic hiccups and gastroesophageal reflux disease: the acid perfusion test as a provocative maneuver. *Ann Intern Med* 1986;105(2):219–220.

38. Shay SS, Myers RL, Johnson LF. Hiccups associated with reflux esophagitis. *Gastroenterology* 1984;87(1):204–207.

39. Wiklund I. Quality of life in patients with gastroesophageal reflux disease. *Am J Gastroenterol* 2001;96[8 Suppl]:S46–S53

40. Rutta D, Garrat A, Leng M, et al. A new approach to the measurement of quality of life: the Patient Generated Index. *Med Care* 1994;32:1109–1126.

41. Schuetz JA. Long-term outcomes following esophagectomy. *Chest Surg Clin North Am* 2000;10(3):639–48.

42. Glise H, Hallerback B, Wiklund I. Quality of life: a reflection of symptoms and concerns. *Scand J Gastroenterol Suppl* 1996;221:14–17.

43. Wiklund IK, Junghard O, Grace E, et al. Quality of Life in Reflux and Dyspepsia patients. Psychometric documentation of a new disease-specific questionnaire (QOLRAD). *Eur J Surg Suppl* 1998;(583):41–49.

44. Borchardt PJ. Employee productivity and gastroesophageal reflux disease: the payer's viewpoint. *Am J Gastroenterol* 2001;96[8 Suppl]:S62–S63

45. Gelfand GA, Finley RJ. Quality of life with carcinoma of the esophagus. *World J Surg* 1994;18(3):399–405.

46. Blazeby JM, Alderson D, Winstone K, et al. Development of an EORTC questionnaire module to be used in quality of life assessment for patients with oesophageal cancer. The EORTC Quality of Life Study Group. *Eur J Cancer* 1996;32A(11):1912–1917.

47. Blazeby JM, Farndon JR, Donovan J, et al. A prospective longitudinal study examining the quality of life of patients with esophageal carcinoma. *Cancer* 2000;88(8):1781–1787.

48. Branicki FJ, Law SY, Fok M, et al. Quality of life in patients with cancer of the esophagus and gastric cardia: a case for palliative resection. *Arch Surg* 1998;133(3):316–322.

49. McLarty AJ, Deschamps C, Trastek VF, et al. Esophageal resection for cancer of the esophagus: long-term function and quality of life. *Ann Thorac Surg* 1997;63(6):1568–1572.

50. Stein HJ, Feith M, Mueller J, et al. Limited resection for early adenocarcinoma in Barrett's esophagus. *Ann Surg* 2000;232(6):733–742.

51. Sonnenberg A, Soni A, Sampliner RE. Medical decision analysis of endoscopic surveillance of Barrett's oesophagus to prevent oesophageal adenocarcinoma. *Aliment Pharmacol Ther* 2002;16(1):41–50.

52. Kirby JD. Quality of life after oesophagectomy: the patients' perspective. *Dis Esophagus* 1999;12(3):168–171.

53. Ross P, Nicolson M, Cunningham D, et al. Prospective random-

ized trial comparing mitomycin, cisplatin, and protracted venous-infusion fluorouracil (PVI 5-FU) with epirubicin, cisplatin, and PVI 5-FU in advanced esophagogastric cancer. *J Clin Oncol* 2002;20(8):1996–2004.

54. Kharadi MY, Qadir A, Khan FA, et al. Comparative evaluation of therapeutic approaches in stage III and IV squamous cell carcinoma of the thoracic esophagus with conventional radiotherapy and endoscopic treatment in combination and endoscopic treatment alone: a randomized prospective trial. *Int J Radiat Oncol Biol Phys* 1997;39(2):309–320.

55. Nicholson DA, Haycox A, Kay CL, et al. The cost effectiveness of metal oesophageal stenting in malignant disease compared with conventional therapy. *Clin Radiol* 1999;54(4):212–215.

56. Dallal HJ, Smith GD, Grieve DC, et al. A randomized trial of thermal ablative therapy versus expandable metal stents in the palliative treatment of patients with esophageal carcinoma. *Gastrointest Endosc* 2001;54(5):549–557.

57. McDougall NI, Collins JS, McFarland RJ, et al. The effect of treating reflux oesophagitis with omeprazole on quality of life. *Eur J Gastroenterol Hepatol* 1998;10(6):459–464.

58. Hunter JG, Trus TL, Branum GD, et al. A physiologic approach to laparoscopic fundoplication for gastroesophageal reflux disease. *Ann Surg* 1996;223(6):673–685.

59. McDougall NI, Johnston BT, Kee F, et al. Natural history of reflux oesophagitis: a 10 year follow up of its effect on patient symptomatology and quality of life. *Gut* 1996;38(4):481–486.

60. Havelund T, Lind T, Wiklund I, et al. Quality of life in patients with heartburn but without esophagitis: effects of treatment with omeprazole. *Am J Gastroenterol* 1999;94(7):1782–1789.

61. Watson RG, Tham TC, Johnston BT, et al. Double blind crossover placebo controlled study of omeprazole in the treatment of patients with reflux symptoms and physiological levels of acid reflux—the "sensitive oesophagus." *Gut* 1997;40(5):587–590.

62. Sandler RS, Everhart JE, Donowitz M, et al. The burden of selected digestive diseases in the United States. *Gastroenterology* 2002;122(5):1500–1511.

63. Glise H, Hallerback B, Johansson B. Quality of life assessments in the evaluation of gastroesophageal reflux and peptic ulcer disease before, during and after treatment. *Scand J Gastroenterol Suppl* 1995;208:133–135.

64. Johnston BT. Gastroesophageal reflux disease and a HAPPI quality of life. *Am J Gastroenterol* 1999;94(7):1723–1724.

65. Chal KL, Stacey JH, Sacks GE. The effect of ranitidine on symptom relief and quality of life of patients with gastro-oesophageal reflux disease. *Br J Clin Pract* 1995;49(2):73–77.

66. Johnston BT, Gunning J, Lewis SA. Health care seeking by heartburn sufferers is associated with psychosocial factors. *Am J Gastroenterol* 1996;91(12):2500–2504.

67. Ben-Meir A, Urbach DR, Khajanchee YS, et al. Quality of life before and after laparoscopic Heller myotomy for achalasia. *Am J Surg* 2001;181(5):471–474.

68. Katilius M, Velanovich V. Heller myotomy for achalasia: quality of life comparison of laparoscopic and open approaches. *JSLS* 2001;5(3):227–231.

69. Luketich JD, Fernando HC, Christie NA, et al. Outcomes after minimally invasive esophagomyotomy. *Ann Thorac Surg* 2001;72(6):1909–1912.

70. Meshkinpour H, Haghighat P, Meshkinpour A. Quality of life among patients treated for achalasia. *Dig Dis Sci* 1996;41(2):352–356.

71. Massey BT. Management of idiopathic achalasia: short-term and long-term outcomes. *Curr Gastroenterol Rep* 2000;2(3):196–200.

72. Ward BW, Wu WC, Richter JE, et al. Long-term follow-up of symptomatic status of patients with noncardiac chest pain: is diagnosis of esophageal etiology helpful? *Am J Gastroenterol* 1987; 82(3):215–218.

3

RADIOLOGY OF THE PHARYNX AND ESOPHAGUS

MARC S. LEVINE
STEPHEN E. RUBESIN

As the population continues to age, pharyngeal disorders have become an increasingly common problem in modern medical practice. Many patients have swallowing dysfunction caused by neurologic conditions such as dementia or strokes, whereas others have morphologic lesions such as pharyngeal carcinoma or Zenker's diverticulum. The videofluoroscopic examination is a valuable technique for demonstrating a wide range of functional and structural lesions of the pharynx in these individuals. Esophagography (primarily double-contrast esophagography) is an equally valuable tool for detecting clinically significant disease of the esophagus in patients with gastroesophageal reflux disease, infectious esophagitis, esophageal carcinoma, or other structural lesions of the esophagus. Videofluoroscopic evaluation of the esophagus is also a useful technique for assessing esophageal motility and for detecting motility disorders such as achalasia and diffuse esophageal spasm. Thus, pharyngoesophagography has a major role in the evaluation of patients with pharyngeal or esophageal disease. This chapter reviews the various pathologic conditions involving the pharynx and esophagus and their associated findings on barium studies.

PHARYNX

Normal Pharyngeal Anatomy

The pharynx is a tube composed of skeletal muscle lined by squamous epithelium (1) (Fig. 3.1). The oropharynx (mesopharynx) is the portion of the pharynx associated with the oral cavity. The oropharynx extends craniocaudally from the soft palate to the pharyngoepiglottic fold. The base of the tongue forms the anterior wall of the oropharynx; the posterior wall of the oropharynx abuts the upper cervical spine. The laryngopharynx (hypopharynx) is the

portion of the pharynx associated with the larynx. The hypopharynx extends craniocaudally from the pharyngoepiglottic fold to the pharyngoesophageal segment (1). The nasopharynx is the part of the pharynx associated with the nasal cavity. It participates primarily in breathing and is not considered in this chapter. The anatomy and physiology of the oral and pharyngeal cavity are complex. Refer to references 1 through 12 for a detailed discussion of pharyngeal anatomy and physiology.

The anterior wall of the hypopharynx is shaped by the larynx; its epiglottic and arytenoid cartilages contribute to the anterior wall of the hypopharynx (2) (Figs. 3.2 and 3.3). The remainder of the anterior pharyngeal wall is formed by the piriform sinuses and surrounding thyroid cartilage. The posterior wall of the pharynx is bordered by the lower cervical spine. The junction of the pharynx and esophagus, the pharyngoesophageal segment, is lined by squamous epithelium and formed by the cricopharyngeus muscle. The pharyngoesophageal segment lies posterior to the cricoid cartilage.

The oropharynx and hypopharynx have four openings: superiorly, the velopharyngeal portal to the nasopharynx; anteriorly, the palatoglossal isthmus to the oral cavity; anteriorly, the laryngeal aditus to the larynx; and inferiorly, the pharyngoesophageal segment to the esophagus (1). Thus, the pharynx is the crossroads of speech, respiration, and swallowing.

The palatine fossae are bounded by the anterior and posterior tonsillar pillars, also known as the paired palatoglossal and palatopharyngeal folds. The vertical surface of the tongue is nodular because of the underlying circumvallate papillae and lingual tonsil (2). The valleculae are potential spaces created by a fold of tissue that extends posteriorly to the epiglottis (the median glossoepiglottic fold). The valleculae disappear when the epiglottis inverts during swallowing.

The piriform sinuses form the anterior portion of the lower hypopharynx. The piriform sinuses are pear-shaped spaces created by protrusion of the larynx into the pharynx (Fig. 3.4). These spaces are open posteriorly to the remain-

M. S. Levine, S. E. Rubesin: Department of Radiology, Hospital of the University of Pennsylvania, Philadelphia, Pennsylvania.

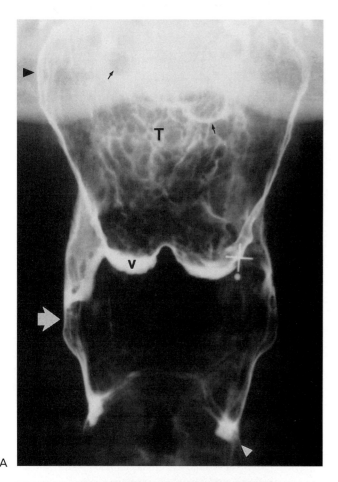

A

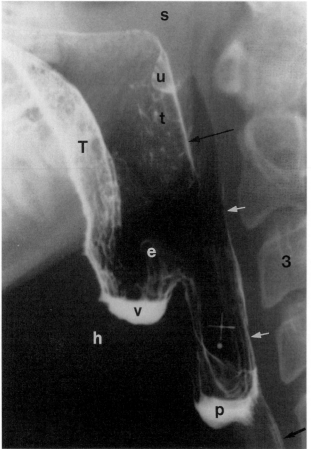

B

FIGURE 3.1. Normal pharynx. **A:** Frontal view of the pharynx. The surface of the tongue (*T*) has a reticular appearance due to underlying lingual tonsil. The right tonsillar fossa (*black arrowhead*), right vallecula (*V*), tip of the left piriform sinus (*white arrowhead*), and several of the circumvallate papillae (*black arrows*) are all identified. The right lateral wall of the hypopharynx is identified with a thick arrow. **B:** Lateral view of the pharynx during phonation. The soft palate (*s*) elevates to appose the posterior pharyngeal wall. The uvula (*u*) of the soft palate bows anteriorly. The palatopharyngeal fold (posterior tonsillar pillar) (*long black arrow*) overlies the palatopharyngeal muscle. The palatine tonsils (*t*) have barium trapped within their interstices. The vertical surface (base) of the tongue (*T*), epiglottic tip (*e*), valleculae (*v*), and tips of the piriform sinuses (*p*) are identified. The hyoid bone (*h*) is barely visible. The pharyngoesophageal segment (*short black arrow*) is closed. (From Rubesin SE, Jones B, Donner MW. Contrast pharyngography: the importance of phonation. *Am J Roentgenol* 1987;148:269–272, with permission.)

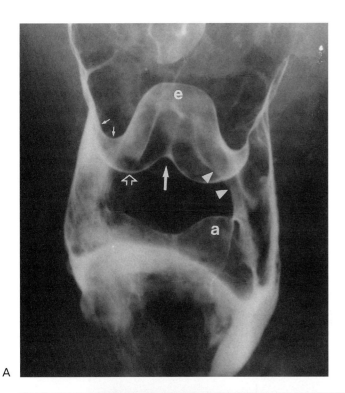

A

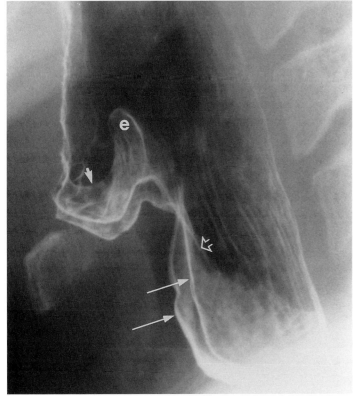

B

FIGURE 3.2. Folds of the epiglottis in a patient with radiation change. **A:** Frontal view of the pharynx. The median glossoepiglottic fold (*large arrow*) divides the space between the base of the tongue and tip of the epiglottis (e) into two halves. The pharyngoepiglottic folds overlying the paired stylopharyngeal muscles course from the lateral pharyngeal wall to the lateral edge of the epiglottis (right pharyngoepiglottic fold identified with *small arrows*, forming the posterior wall of the valleculae. The lateral wall of each vallecula is formed by the lateral glossoepiglottic fold. The lowest portion of the right vallecula is identified by an *open arrow*. The aryepiglottic folds course from the lateral edge of the epiglottis to the mucosa overlying the muscular processes of the arytenoid cartilages (left aryepiglottic fold identified by *arrowheads*; mucosa overlying left arytenoid cartilage identified by *a*). **B:** Lateral view of the pharynx demonstrates the median glossoepiglottic fold (*short arrow*), tip of epiglottis (e), aryepiglottic folds (*open arrow*), and anterior walls of the piriform sinuses (*long arrows*).

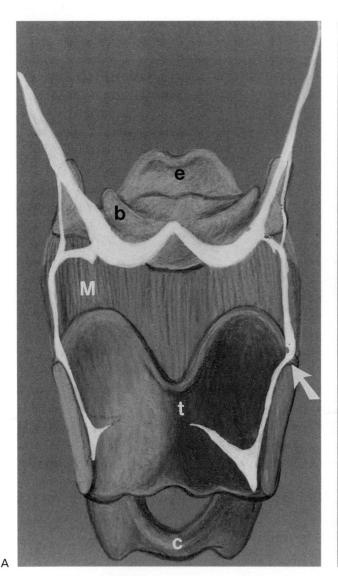

A

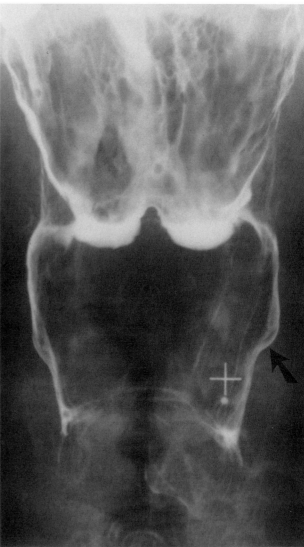

B

FIGURE 3.3. Relationship of the laryngeal cartilages to the pharynx. **A:** Line drawing in the frontal view demonstrates the tip of the epiglottic cartilage (*e*) above the level of the hyoid bone (*b*). The thyrohyoid membrane (*M*) connects the hyoid bone to the thyroid cartilage (*t*). The cricoid cartilage (*c*) is seen inferiorly. The white represents the barium-coated pharynx posterior to the larynx. **B:** Frontal view of the pharynx shows a notch in the lateral hypopharyngeal wall (*arrow* in both A and B) where the thyrohyoid membrane joins the thyroid cartilage. Inferiorly, the hypopharynx is confined anteriorly by the thyroid cartilage. (From Rubesin SE, Jesserun J, Robertson D, et al. Lines of the pharynx. *RadioGraphics* 1987;7:217–237, with permission.)

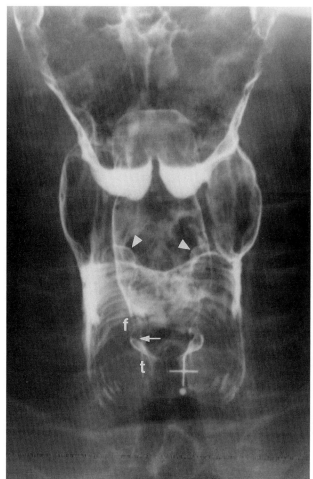

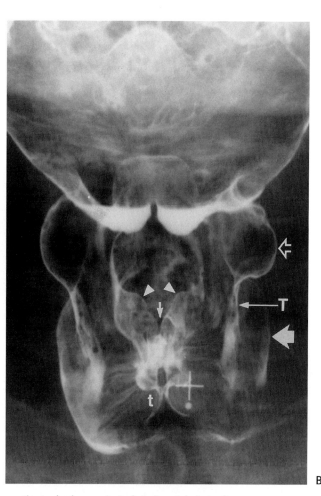

A

B

FIGURE 3.4. Relationship of larynx to pharynx in a patient who has aspirated. **A:** Frontal view of the pharynx during inspiration. The larynx is related to the lower hypopharynx, causing an extrinsic mass impression on the pharynx anteriorly. The true and false vocal cords are widely separated (the right true [*t*] and right false [*f*] vocal cords are identified). The laryngeal ventricle (*arrow*) is identified. The muscular processes of the arytenoids (*arrowheads*) are separated. **B:** Frontal view of the pharynx during a modified Valsalva maneuver demonstrates that the true vocal cords (right cord—*t*) are now apposed. The muscular processes of the arytenoids (*arrowheads*) close together. The space between them is the interarytenoid notch (*small arrow*). The pharynx is markedly distended in its posterior portion (*large arrow*), ballooning posterior to the confines of the thyroid cartilage (*arrow—T*). The pharynx also bulges at the thyrohyoid membrane (*open arrow*). (From Rubesin SE, Glick SN. The tailored double contrast pharyngogram. *CRC Crit Rev Diagn Imaging* 1988;28:133–179, with permission.)

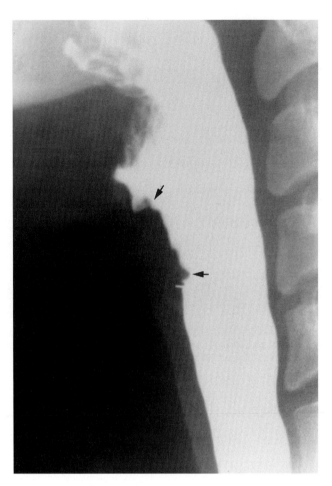

FIGURE 3.5. Postcricoid squamous mucosa. Just posterior to the cricoid cartilage, the anterior wall of the pharyngoesophageal segment has redundant mucosa that changes size and shape during swallowing. Note how the mucosa has a wavy appearance (*arrows*). When identified, this mucosa identifies the level of the cricoid cartilage and the level of the cricopharyngeus during pharyngography. (From Rubesin SE. Pharynx: normal anatomy and examination techniques. In: Gore RM, Levine MS, eds. *Textbook of gastrointestinal radiology*, second edition. Philadelphia: WB Saunders, 2000:190–211, with permission.)

der of the hypopharynx. The aryepiglottic folds and mucosa overlying the muscular process of the arytenoid cartilages form the medial boundaries of the piriform sinuses.

The anterior wall of the pharyngoesophageal segment abuts the cricoid cartilage (Fig. 3.5). The mucosa in this region contains abundant submucosal fat (2).

Normal Oral and Pharyngeal Motility

Swallowing is arbitrarily divided into four phases: (a) ingestion and bolus preparation, (b) the oral phase, (c) the pharyngeal phase, and (d) the esophageal phase. In reality, swallowing is a programmed sequence of skeletal, then smooth muscle contraction, altered by sensory input (13). There are no distinct phases of swallowing.

A bolus is selected and brought to the lips by volitional activity. A liquid is sucked or poured into the mouth. A solid is placed on top of the tongue. Liquids do not require much oral manipulation and are therefore easily transferred to the oropharynx. Solids must be chewed and mixed with saliva to achieve a satisfactory consistency for swallowing. During bolus preparation, the bolus is contained in the oral

cavity in young adults. Older "normal" adults frequently spill the bolus prematurely into the oropharynx before swallowing (12).

Once the bolus is prepared, the tongue collects and sizes the bolus and transfers it into the oropharynx. The tongue tip rises to appose the hard palate, and the midtongue forms an inclined plane directing the bolus into the oropharynx (10) (Fig. 3.6). The velopharyngeal portal is closed as the soft palate rises to appose the posterior pharyngeal wall and the superior constrictor muscle contracts to appose the soft palate (9).

The pharynx and larynx are elevated by the suprahyoid muscles and intrinsic elevators of the pharynx. Pharyngeal-laryngeal elevation participates in closure of the laryngeal aditus and vestibule, epiglottic tilt, and opening of the pharyngoesophageal segment (8). The epiglottis acts as a stream diverter, directing the bolus into the lateral swallowing channels. The tilting epiglottis also helps cover the laryngeal vestibule. The larynx closes in a retrograde fashion. The true vocal cords close at the beginning of the swallow, followed by the false vocal cords and the remainder of the laryngeal vestibule. Any portion of the bolus that has

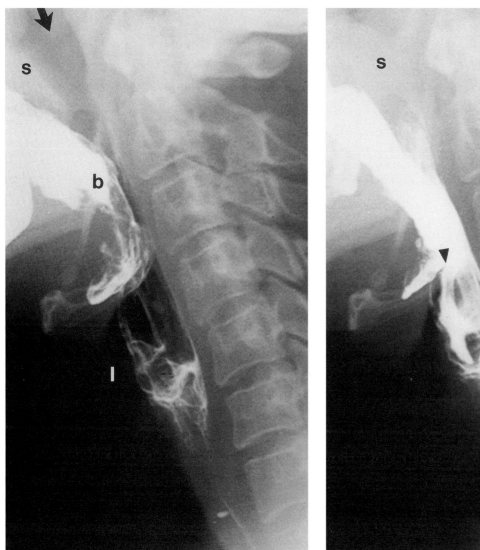

A   B

FIGURE 3.6. Representative frames from the pharyngeal phase of swallowing. **A:** The bolus (*b*) has just entered the oropharynx. The soft palate (*s*) is rising to appose the posterior pharyngeal wall, but the velopharyngeal portal (*arrow*) is still open. The epiglottic tip is just beginning to tilt posteriorly. The laryngeal vestibule (*l*) is still open. **B:** The bolus has just entered the hypopharynx. The soft palate (*s*) now apposes the posterior pharyngeal wall. The epiglottis (*arrowhead*) is partly obscured by the barium but is tilting. The pharyngoesophageal segment (*arrow*) remains closed.

penetrated the laryngeal vestibule therefore is pushed back into the hypopharynx by retrograde laryngeal closure.

The bolus flows through the pharynx by a combination of gravity, elevation of the pharynx over the bolus, tongue push, and sequential contraction of the constrictor muscles. Although the upper esophageal sphincter relaxes at the beginning of a swallow, the pharyngoesophageal segment does not open until the bolus reaches the lower hypopharynx. Elevation of the larynx and pharynx pulls the anterior wall of the pharyngoesophageal segment anteriorly. Tongue push, constrictor contraction, and gravity increase bolus pressure to open the pharyngoesophageal segment.

Neuromuscular Disorders

Most patients with swallowing dysfunction have neural or muscular disorders that alter timing of events or muscular contraction rather than causing oral or pharyngeal structural damage. Some diseases affect a patient's ability to self-feed

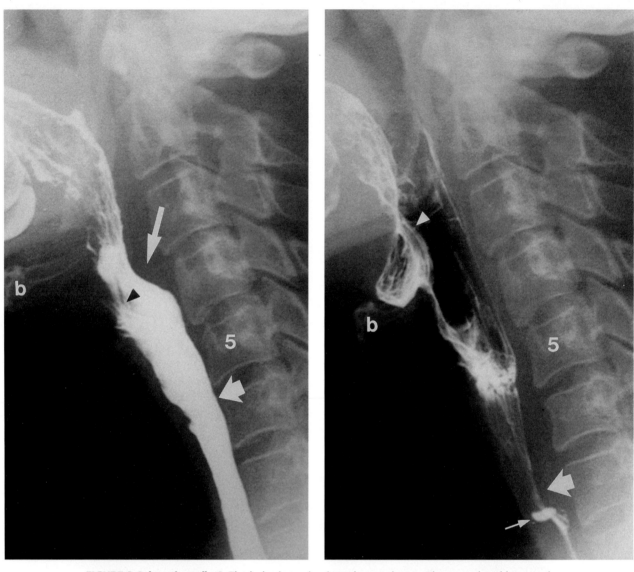

C

D

FIGURE 3.6 *(continued)*. C: The bolus is passing into the esophagus. Pharyngeal and laryngeal elevation is manifested by elevation of the hyoid bone (*b*) up underneath the mandible. The laryngeal vestibule is completely compressed and is no longer seen as an air-filled space. The epiglottis (*arrowhead*) has tilted to appose the anterior wall of the hypopharynx. The posterior pharyngeal contraction wave (*long arrow*) is in the thyropharyngeal muscle. The pharyngoesophageal segment (*short arrow*, identified by redundant postcricoid mucosa on the opposite wall) is open. The C5 vertebral body is labeled 5 to allow a direct comparison to D. **D:** The bolus has just passed through the pharynx. The pharynx and larynx have returned to their "resting" position. Compare the levels of the hyoid bone (*b*) and the pharyngoesophageal segment (*thick arrow*) on image C during swallowing and image D after swallowing. The epiglottic tip (*arrowhead*) has returned to its upright position. The soft palate now apposes the tongue and the laryngeal vestibule is open. A small Killian-Jamieson diverticulum (*thin arrow*) is present. The C5 vertebral body is labeled *5*.

despite normal swallowing. Other diseases affect both the ability to feed and to swallow. For example, patients with Parkinson's disease often have difficulty sitting and manipulating food as well as having abnormal bolus transfer (14).

About one fourth of cerebrovascular accidents cause dysphagia (14,15). In general, left-sided strokes alter the oral phase of swallowing, whereas right-sided strokes alter the pharyngeal phase (15,16). The corticobulbar pathways in the internal capsule can be damaged by large hemispheric strokes or small-vessel disease. Acute strokes or small-vessel disease resulting from hypertension, diabetes, or other causes can also affect the swallowing center in the pons and medulla (17).

Diseases that directly damage motor neurons in the swallowing center or cranial nerves in the skull base may result in bulbar palsy with oral and pharyngeal swallowing difficulties (18–22). Lower motor neural destruction occurs in amyotrophic lateral sclerosis and 10% to 15% of patients with acute poliomyelitis (19,20). Some patients with a history of poliomyelitis have progressive disintegration of axon terminals in surviving but overworked residual motor neurons, resulting in pharyngeal muscle weakness caused by "postpolio muscular atrophy" (21). Meningeal carcinomatosis may also result in dysphagia. Unilateral pharyngeal paresis is often caused by destruction of motor nerves at the skull base or in the neck as a result of tumor, trauma, or surgery (10). Abnormal transmission at the myoneural junction in myasthenia gravis may result in dysphagia that is initiated or exacerbated by prolonged swallowing.

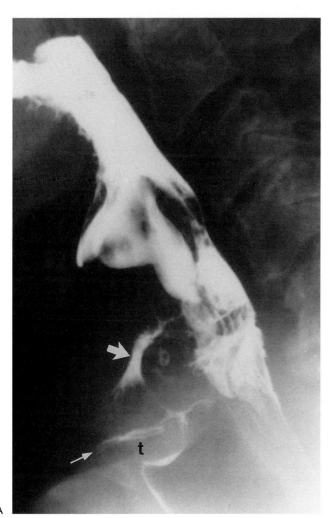
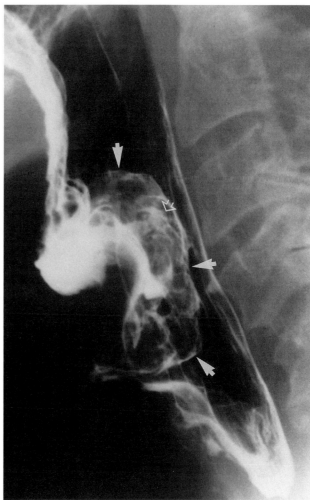

A

B

FIGURE 3.7. Laryngeal penetration. **A:** During drinking, barium enters the laryngeal vestibule (*thick arrow*). The anterior commissure (*thin arrow*) and true vocal cords (*t*) are identified. **B:** Spot radiograph during phonation shows a huge epiglottic mass (*arrows*) with nodular mucosa (*open arrow*) as the cause of the laryngeal penetration. (From Rubesin SE. Pharyngeal dysfunction. *Categorical course on gastrointestinal radiology.* Reston, VA: American College of Radiology, 1991:1–9, with permission.)

Dysphagia resulting from inflammatory or endocrine-related myopathies is potentially treatable (14). Dermatomyositis and polymyositis directly damage the intrinsic or extrinsic muscles of the pharynx. Pharyngeal muscle myopathy may be caused by a variety of endocrine disorders, including hyperthyroidism, hypothyroidism, and Cushing's syndrome (22).

The end result of these various neuromuscular disorders is poor timing of oral and pharyngeal events or abnormal movement of oral and pharyngeal structures. A bolus may be directed in a normal fashion, but because of poor timing, the bolus may enter the laryngeal vestibule or nasopharynx. Laryngeal penetration is defined as passage of the bolus into the laryngeal vestibule either just before the swallow or during swallowing (23,24). Abnormal tongue motion, pharyngeal contraction, or epiglottic tilt may also lead to laryngeal penetration (Figs. 3.7 and 3.8). Abnormal oral or pharyn-

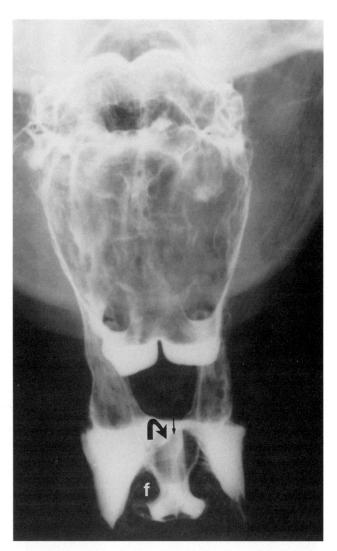

FIGURE 3.9. Overflow aspiration. This man had global pharyngeal weakness due to polymyositis and poor clearance of barium from the pharynx during swallowing with resultant stasis of barium in the piriform sinuses. Note that the barium level lies above the interarytenoid notch (*straight arrow*). After the swallow has passed, barium pours over and down into the larynx (*curved arrow*), outlining the false vocal cords (right cord—*f*) and laryngeal ventricle.

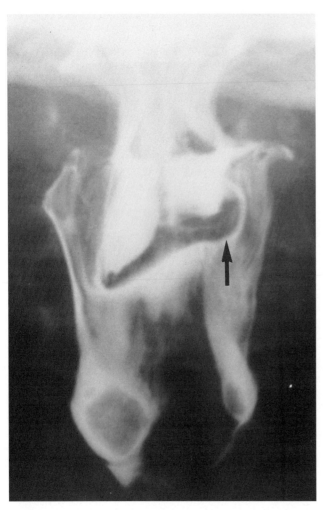

FIGURE 3.8. Asymmetric epiglottic tilt. There is diminished epiglottic tilt on its left side (*arrow*).

geal movement may result from a structural abnormality or neuromuscular disorder. Abnormal epiglottic tilt or pharyngeal muscular contraction may also lead to stasis in either the valleculae or piriform sinuses, respectively. Marked stasis in the piriform sinuses may cause the bolus to overflow into the larynx through the interarytenoid notch when the patient breathes or subsequently swallows a second time. Thus, overflow aspiration is defined as barium entering the laryngeal vestibule while the patient is breathing normally (23,24) (Fig. 3.9) or as barium entering the laryngeal vestibule as a result of poor timing when the patient swallows a second time, and there is moderate stasis in the valleculae and piriform sinuses. Aspiration may also result from regurgitation of esophageal contents into the pharynx.

Pouches and Diverticula

Zenker's Diverticulum

Zenker's diverticulum is an acquired mucosal herniation through an area of congenital muscle weakness in the cricopharyngeal muscle, known as Killian's dehiscence. This opening is found in about one third of people at autopsy and has been described as occurring between the thyropharyngeus and cricopharyngeus or between the oblique and horizontal fibers of the cricopharyngeus itself (25,26). The pathogenesis of Zenker's diverticulum is unknown. Mano-

metric studies have produced conflicting findings (27,28). Some of these studies have shown a normal tonic pressure in the upper esophageal sphincter (UES) and normal coordination between pharyngeal contraction and relaxation of the UES, whereas others have shown elevated UES pressure or abnormal relaxation of the UES. It also is unknown whether chronic gastroesophageal reflux predisposes patients with Killian's dehiscence to the development of a Zenker's diverticulum. Nevertheless, most patients with Zenker's diverticulum have a hiatal hernia and gastroesophageal reflux (29,30).

When detected on barium studies, Zenker's diverticulum appears on frontal views as a persistent, barium-filled sac in the midline below the tips of the piriform sinuses (Fig. 3.10). On lateral views during swallowing, the opening of the Zenker's diverticulum above the incompletely opened pharyngoesophageal segment is often surprisingly

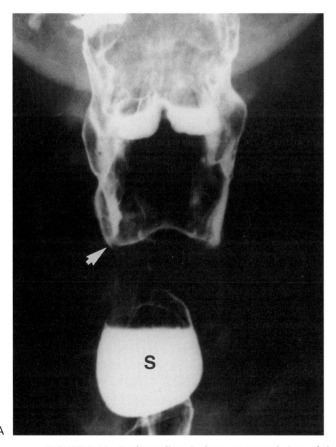 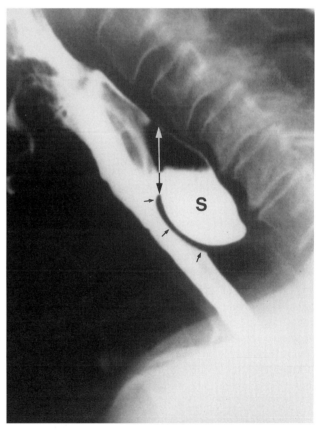

A   B

FIGURE 3.10. Zenker's diverticulum. **A:** Frontal view of the pharynx demonstrates a 3- × 2-cm sac (*S*) with an air/barium level. The sac lies in the midline below the tips of the piriform sinuses (right piriform sinus tip identified by *arrow*). **B:** Lateral view of the pharynx during drinking. The sac has a broad opening (*double arrow*). The sac (*S*) lies posterior to the pharyngoesophageal segment and proximal cervical esophagus (*small arrows*). (Laryngeal penetration resulted from abnormal timing between the oral and pharyngeal phases.) (**B:** from Rubesin SE. Pharyngeal dysfunction. *Categorical course on gastrointestinal radiology.* Reston, VA: American College of Radiology, 1991:1–9, with permission.)

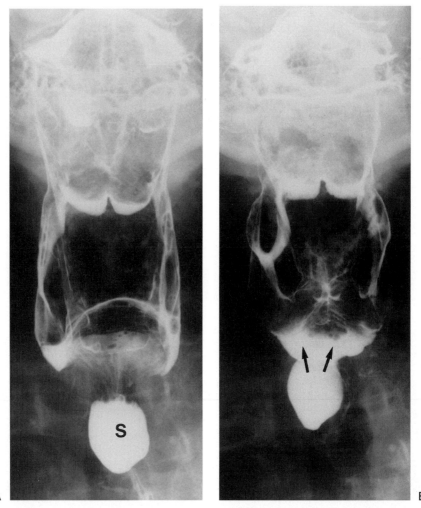

FIGURE 3.11. Pharyngeal regurgitation from Zenker's diverticulum. **A:** Frontal view of the pharynx shows a 2-cm sac (*S*) in the midline below the tips of the piriform sinuses. **B:** Frontal view of the pharynx as the patient begins a second swallow. Barium (*arrows*) has been regurgitated from the Zenker's diverticulum back into the lower hypopharynx.

broad (10,31). The sac then courses behind the pharyngoesophageal segment and proximal cervical esophagus. Barium within the diverticulum can be regurgitated back into the lower hypopharynx during breathing or additional swallowing (Fig. 3.11), but overflow aspiration is uncommon. Contour deformities in a Zenker's diverticulum may be caused by adherent debris, inflammation, or, rarely, carcinoma (32,33).

Barium trapped above a prematurely or incompletely opened cricopharyngeus may resemble a small Zenker's diverticulum, and has been termed a *pseudo-Zenker's diverticulum* (24) (Fig. 3.12). In such patients, no diverticulum is seen during swallowing. The saclike structure appears only when the cricopharyngeus closes early or when barium is trapped between the pharyngeal contrac-

tion wave and the incompletely opened cricopharyngeus. After a few moments, this barium enters the cervical esophagus, and the sac disappears. It is not known whether a pseudo-Zenker's diverticulum can progress to a true Zenker's diverticulum. Early closure and incomplete opening of the cricopharyngeus have also been associated with gastroesophageal reflux disease (34) (Figs. 3.13 and 3.14).

Killian-Jamieson Diverticulum

The Killian-Jamieson space is a triangular area of weakness in the upper anterolateral cervical esophagus, not to be confused with Killian's dehiscence. The Killian-Jamieson space is bounded superiorly by the inferior border of the

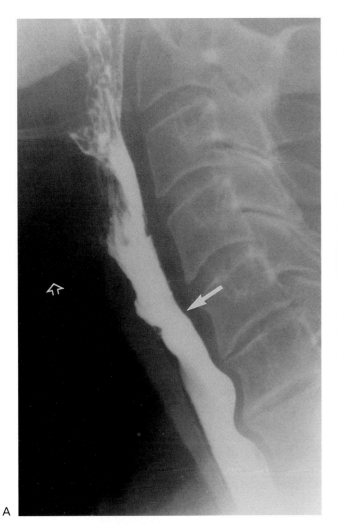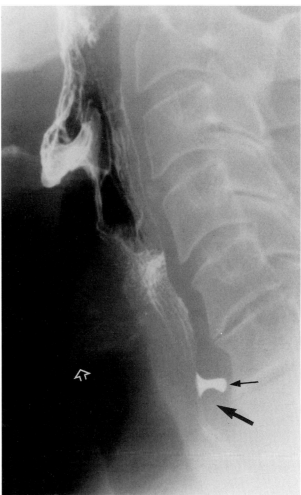

A

B

FIGURE 3.12. Pseudo-Zenker's diverticulum. **A:** Lateral view of the pharynx during drinking shows an open pharyngoesophageal segment (*arrow*) identified by redundant postcricoid mucosa. **B:** Lateral view of the pharynx just after the bolus passes shows how the pharynx is descending to its "resting" position. Barium is trapped (*thin arrow*) between the early closing pharyngoesophageal segment (*thick arrow*) and the posterior pharyngeal contraction wave that just passed. The transiently trapped barium entered the esophagus moments later. Note the difference in height of the pharyngoesophageal segment and the bottom of the vocal cords (*open arrows*) during and after swallowing.

cricopharyngeus, anteriorly by the cricoid cartilage, and inferomedially by the suspensory ligament of the esophagus (35). Transient protrusions through the Killian-Jamieson space are called *lateral proximal cervical esophageal pouches*, whereas persistent protrusions are called *lateral proximal cervical esophageal diverticula*. These structures are also known as Killian-Jamieson pouches and diverticula, respectively (36).

Killian-Jamieson diverticula, which are about one third as common as Zenker's diverticula, have a characteristic radiographic appearance (36). They are either unilateral,

usually on the left, or bilateral (6). The diverticula appear on barium studies as persistent 3- to 20-mm outpouchings with distinct necks (Fig. 3.15). The diverticula extend lateral to the cervical esophagus on frontal views and overlap the cervical esophagus on lateral views. In contrast, Zenker's diverticulum is in the midline on frontal views and posterior to the cervical esophagus on lateral views (Fig. 3.16). When barium is regurgitated from Killian-Jamieson diverticula, it enters the cervical esophagus because the diverticula are below the cricopharyngeal muscle. Thus, there is less risk of aspiration from Killian-Jamieson diverticula than

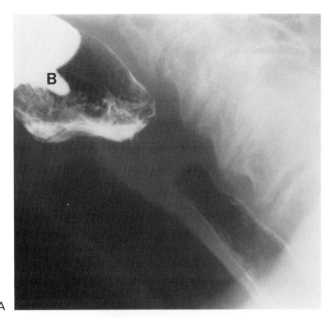
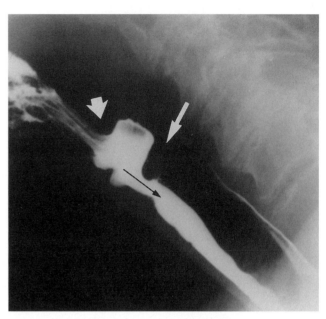

A

B

FIGURE 3.13. Incomplete opening of the cricopharyngeus. **A:** Lateral view of the pharynx obtained just as the bolus (*B*) is entering the hypopharynx. **B:** Lateral view of the pharynx at the end of bolus passage. The cricopharyngeus (*long white arrow*) is closing before the bolus has cleared the hypopharynx. The posterior pharyngeal contraction wave is identified (*thick white arrow*). A jet of barium (*black arrow*) spurts through the anterior wall of the cervical esophagus.

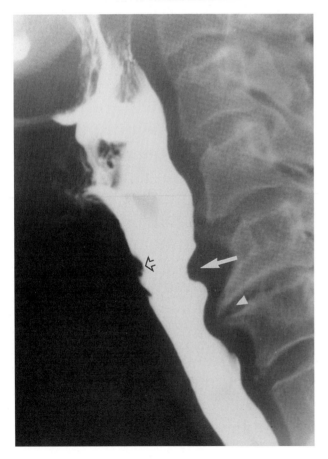

FIGURE 3.14. Extrinsic impressions during passage of bolus through the pharyngoesophageal segment. A smooth-surface hemispheric impression represents incomplete opening of the cricopharyngeus muscle (*white arrow*). Osteophytes impress the proximal cervical esophagus (*arrowhead*). Also note redundant postcricoid mucosa (*open arrow*) opposite the cricopharyngeal bar. (From Rubesin SE. Oral and pharyngeal dysphagia. *Gastroenterol Clin North Am* 1995;24:331–352, with permission.)

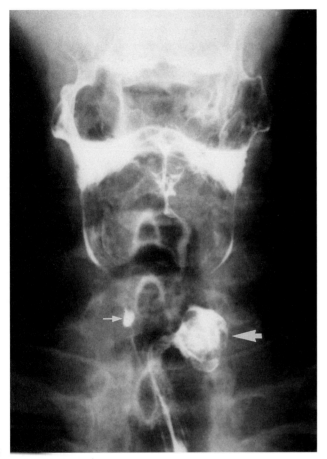

A

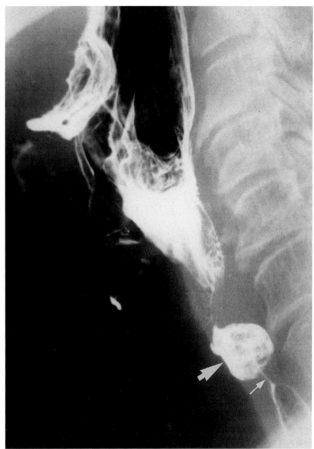

B

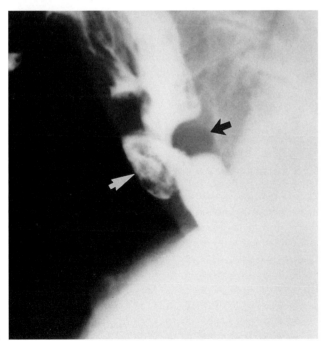

C

FIGURE 3.15. Killian-Jamieson diverticula. **A:** Frontal view of the pharynx demonstrates a 1.5-cm sac (*thick arrow*) just below the level of the cricopharyngeus. A tiny sac is also seen on the right (*thin arrow*). **B:** Lateral view of the pharynx shows that the 1.5-cm sac (*thick arrow*) extends anterior to the expected course of the cervical esophagus (*thin arrow*). **C:** Lateral view of the pharynx during bolus passage demonstrates that the Killian-Jamieson diverticulum (*white arrow*) lies below the level of an incompletely opening cricopharyngeus (*black arrow*). The sac arises from the anterolateral wall of the most proximal cervical esophagus. (From Rubesin SE, Levine MS. Killian-Jamieson diverticula: radiographic findings in 16 patients. *AJR Am J Roentgenol* 2001;177:85–89.)

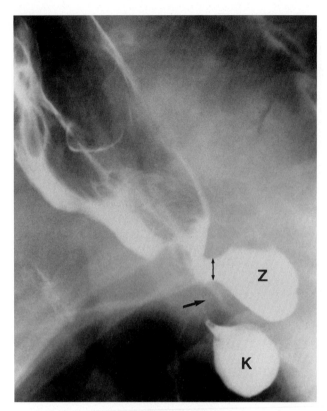

FIGURE 3.16. Synchronous Zenker's and Killian Jamieson diverticula. Oblique view of the pharynx shows a 2.5-cm Zenker's diverticulum (*Z*) with its opening (*double black arrow*) above the cricopharyngeal bar (*thick black arrow*). The Killian-Jamieson diverticulum (*K*) arises below the cricopharyngeal bar and a portion of the diverticulum extends anterior to the cervical esophagus. (From Rubesin SE. Structural abnormalities of the pharynx. In: Gore RM, Levine MS, eds. *Textbook of gastrointestinal radiology*, second edition. Philadelphia: WB Saunders, 2000:227–255, with permission.)

from Zenker's diverticula. Killian-Jamieson pouches appear as small, transient outpouchings just below the closing cricopharyngeus muscle and are only detected near the end of swallowing or after the bolus has passed through the cervical esophagus.

Lateral Pharyngeal Pouches and Diverticula

Lateral pharyngeal pouches are transient outpouchings of the proximal anterolateral hypopharyngeal wall, whereas lateral pharyngeal diverticula are persistent sacs through the same area of weakness in the pharyngeal wall (37). Lateral pharyngeal pouches protrude through an area bounded superiorly by the hyoid bone, anteriorly by the thyrohyoid muscle, inferiorly by the ala of the thyroid cartilage, and posteriorly by the superior cornu of the thyroid cartilage (37) (Fig. 3.17A).

Lateral pharyngeal pouches appear on barium studies as smooth-surfaced hemispheric outpouchings of the upper,

anterolateral hypopharyngeal wall just below the level of the hyoid bone (Fig. 3.17B and C). Barium enters the pouches and then spills into the ipsilateral piriform sinus, either late in the swallow or just after swallowing. Overflow aspiration is uncommon. In contrast, barium is retained in lateral pharyngeal diverticula long after the swallow has been completed (Fig. 3.18). Lateral pharyngeal pouches are usually bilateral, whereas lateral pharyngeal diverticula are usually unilateral (Fig. 3.18).

Lateral pharyngeal pouches are common and their incidence increases with age. Lateral pharyngeal diverticula are much less common, usually occurring in patients with elevated intrapharyngeal pressures. Most of these patients are asymptomatic, but about 5% with lateral pharyngeal pouches complain of a feeling of incomplete swallowing (38,39). Patients with lateral pharyngeal diverticula may also complain of dysphagia, choking, regurgitation of undigested food, or a painless neck mass.

Branchial Pouch Sinuses and Branchial Cleft Fistulae

In the 4-week embryo, paired grooves of ectodermal origin—the branchial clefts—appear on the sides of the neck. Four outpouchings of endodermal origin—the branchial pouches—grow to meet the branchial clefts (40). The second branchial cleft forms the middle ear, eustachian tube, and floor of the tonsillar fossa. The third and fourth branchial pouches form the piriform sinuses. Persistence of branchial clefts or pouches may lead to the development of sinus tracks (that end blindly beneath the skin), fistulae (that extend to the skin), or cysts. Branchial pouch sinus tracks arise from the tonsillar fossa (second pouch) (Fig. 3.19), the upper anterolateral piriform fossa (third pouch), or the lower anterolateral piriform sinus (fourth pouch).

Inflammatory Conditions

Although barium studies are of limited value in immunocompetent patients with an acute sore throat, they may be of value for demonstrating acute inflammatory lesions in the pharynx in immunocompromised patients with suspected *Candida* (Fig. 3.20) or herpes esophagitis. In patients with chronic sore throats, barium studies are primarily of value for assessing the presence and severity of gastroesophageal reflux disease.

Acute ulceration and chronic scarring of the pharynx may be caused by a variety of uncommon diseases, including Behçet's syndrome, bullous pemphigoid, benign mucous membrane pemphigoid, epidermolysis bullosa, erythema multiforme major (Stevens–Johnson syndrome), Reiter's syndrome, and Crohn's disease (41). Lye ingestion

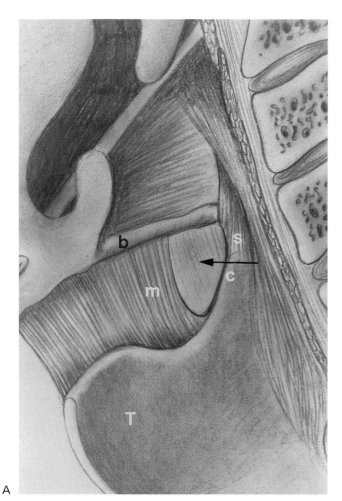

FIGURE 3.17. Lateral pharyngeal pouches. **A:** Line drawing of the pharynx in lateral view shows the area of weakness (*arrow*) that a lateral pharyngeal pouch protrudes through, bounded by the hyoid bone (*b*) superiorly, the posterior border of the thyrohyoid muscle (*m*) anteriorly, the superior cornu of the thyroid cartilage (*c*), and the insertion of the stylopharyngeal muscle (*s*) posteriorly. The ala of the thyroid cartilage (*T*) is identified. **B:** Frontal view of the pharynx just as the bolus reaches the valleculae shows no evidence of lateral pharyngeal pouches. **C:** Frontal view of the pharynx as the bolus passes through the pharyngoesophageal segment shows 1.5-cm and 1-cm barium-filled sacs (*arrows*) on the left and right pharyngeal walls, respectively. The tilting epiglottis is identified (*arrowhead*). (**A:** From Rubesin SE, Jesserun J, Robertson D, et al. Lines of the pharynx. *RadioGraphics* 1987;7:217–237, with permission.)

A

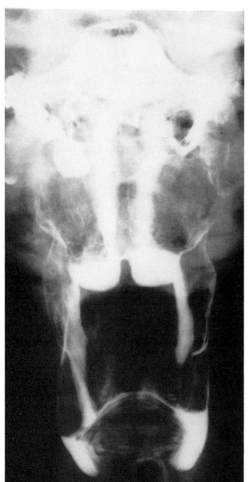

B

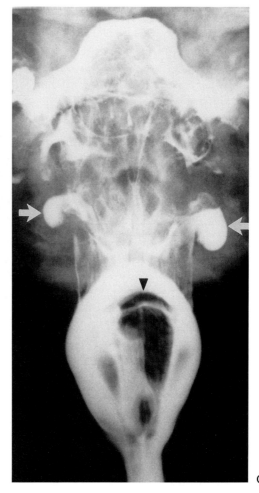

C

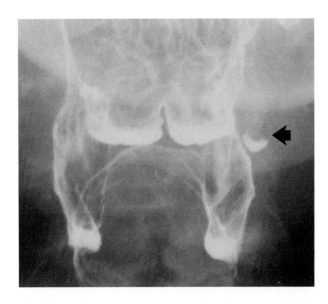

FIGURE 3.18. Lateral pharyngeal diverticulum. A 0.8-cm barium-filled sac (*arrow*) persists outside the left lateral wall of the pharynx after the bolus has passed.

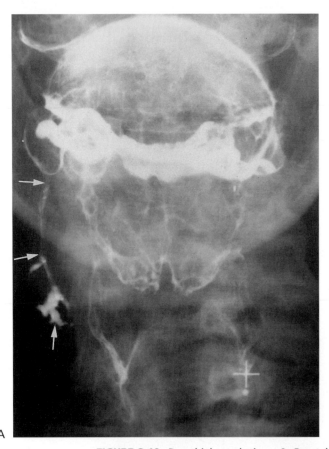

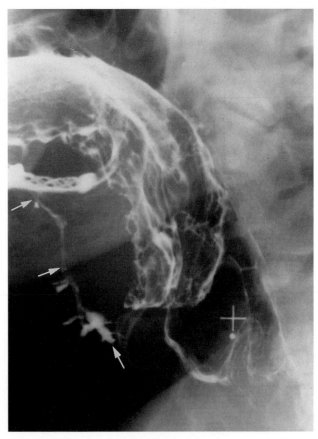

A   B

FIGURE 3.19. Branchial pouch sinus. **A:** Frontal view of the pharynx shows an 8-cm long track (*arrows*) that courses inferiorly from the floor of the mouth. **B:** Steep right posterior oblique view of the pharynx demonstrates the track (*arrows*) arising from the retromolar trigone/anterior portion of the tonsillar fossa. Dentures are in place. (From Rubesin SE, Glick SN. The tailored double contrast pharyngogram. *CRC Critical Rev Diagn Imaging* 1988;28:133–179.)

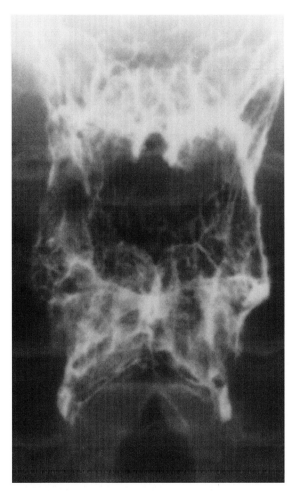

FIGURE 3.20. Candida pharyngitis. Innumerable nodules and plaquelike elevations have disrupted the normally smooth surface of the pharynx.

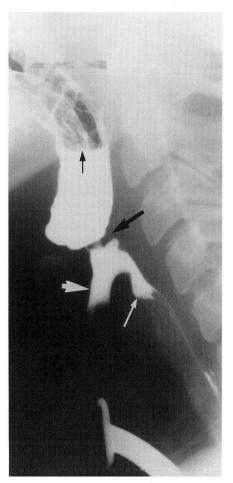

FIGURE 3.21. Scarring from corrosive ingestion. Lateral view of the pharynx shows a thick radiolucent band of soft tissue (*thick black arrow*) crossing the hypopharynx. Obstruction is implied by a large standing column of barium (*thin black arrow*) in the oropharynx. The hypopharynx is small and contracted (*thin white arrow*). Barium pours into the open laryngeal vestibule (*thick white arrow*). (From Rubesin SE. The pharynx: structural disorders. *Radiol Clin North Am* 1994;32:1083–1101, with permission.)

may cause marked ulceration with amputation of the epiglottis and severe scarring (Fig. 3.21).

Lymphoid Hyperplasia

Lymphoid hyperplasia is a nonspecific response to aging, allergies, and repeated infections, involving the palatine tonsils (Fig. 3.22) or base of the tongue (42). Lymphoid hyperplasia of the lingual tonsil may also occur as a compensatory response to prior tonsillectomy. Lymphoid hyperplasia may extend into the valleculae, vallecular surface of the epiglottis, or even the proximal hypopharynx. There are no radiographic criteria for differentiating lymphoid hyperplasia of the tongue base from the normal lingual tonsil. Lymphoid hyperplasia is characterized on barium studies by numerous 3- to 7-mm smooth-surfaced, ovoid nodules symmetrically distributed over the vertical surface of the tongue (42,43) (Fig. 3.23). These

nodules may protrude posteriorly into the oropharynx and valleculae. When lingual tonsil lymphoid hyperplasia is focal or masslike, it can mimic the appearance of tumor at the base of the tongue (42). Patients with asymmetric nodularity or mass lesions at the tongue base therefore should undergo further investigation to differentiated lymphoid hyperplasia of the lingual tonsil from malignant tumor.

Pharyngeal and Cervical Esophageal Webs

Webs are thin folds composed of mucosa and submucosa arising predominantly from the anterior wall of the

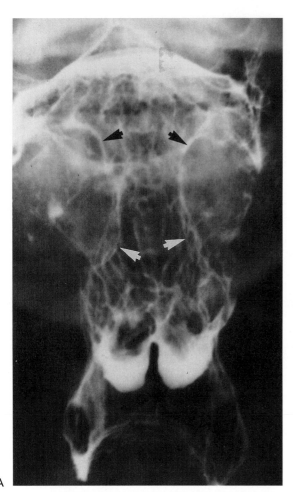
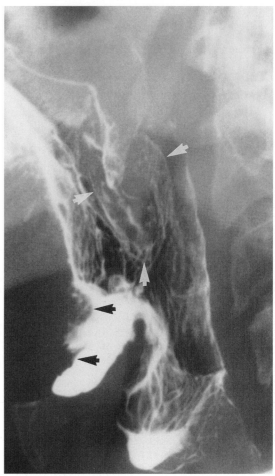

A

B

FIGURE 3.22. Lymphoid hyperplasia of the palatine tonsils and tongue base. **A:** A frontal view of the pharynx demonstrates that the left and right palatine tonsils (*arrows*) protrude deeply into the oropharynx. Ovoid nodules carpet the base of the tongue. **B:** Lateral view of the pharynx during phonation reveals a mass in the tonsillar fossae (*white arrows*) and nodules at the tongue base (*black arrows*). (From Rubesin SE. Structural abnormalities of the pharynx. In: Gore RM, Levine MS, eds. *Textbook of gastrointestinal radiology*, second edition. Philadelphia: WB Saunders, 2000:227–255.)

pharyngoesophageal segment and proximal cervical esophagus. Cervical esophageal webs are common findings, occurring in 3% to 8% of patients who undergo upper gastrointestinal barium studies and in 16% of patients at autopsy (44–47). The pathogenesis of these webs is uncertain. Some webs in the valleculae have been described as normal variants (48). Other webs result from diseases that cause chronic scarring. Many patients with cervical esophageal webs also have gastroesophageal reflux disease (31,49).

Webs are thin (1 to 2 mm in thickness) folds arising from the anterior wall of the pharyngoesophageal segment or proximal cervical esophagus. A web appears on barium studies as a radiolucent bar in the barium pool or as a thin structure etched in white by barium. Some webs extend circumferentially, with a deeper shelf on their anterior surface. Patients with dysphagia usually have circumferential cervical esophageal webs occluding greater than 50% of the luminal diameter (Fig. 3.24). Obstruction is implied by dilatation of the cervical esophagus proximal to the web or

FIGURE 3.24. Cervical esophageal web. Frontal **(A)** and lateral **(B)** views demonstrate a thin radiolucent band (*white arrows*) encircling the cervical esophagus. A jet of barium (*black arrow*) spurting through the opening in the web indicates that there is partial obstruction. Dilatation of the cervical esophagus (*E*) proximal to the web is also indicative of obstruction. (From Rubesin SE. Pharynx. In: Levine MS, Rubesin SE, Laufer I, eds. *Double contrast gastrointestinal radiology*, third edition. Philadelphia: WB Saunders, 2000:61–89, with permission.)

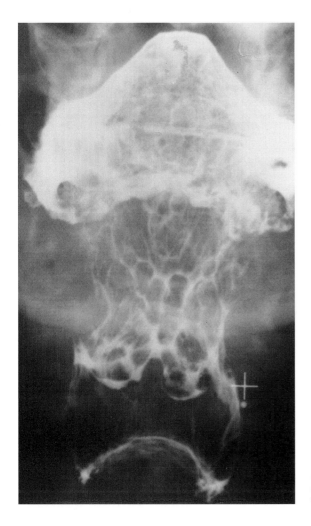

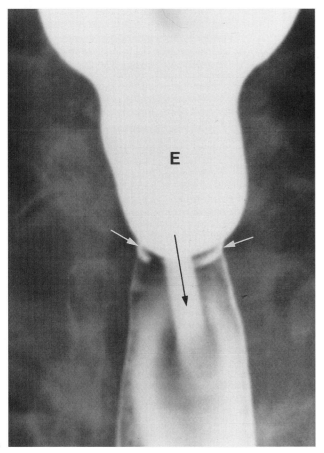

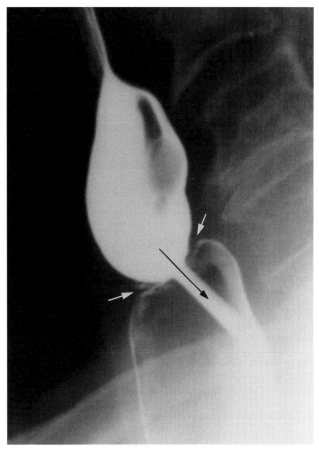

FIGURE 3.23. Lymphoid hyperplasia of the tongue base. Barium fills the grooves between smooth ovoid nodules symmetrically distributed on the vertical surface of the tongue.

A

B

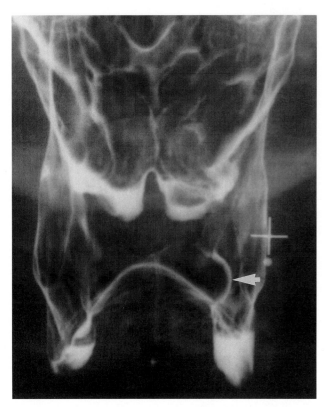

FIGURE 3.25. Retention cyst in medial left hypopharynx. A smooth-surfaced hemispheric line (*arrow*) protrudes into the left piriform sinus. (From Rubesin SE, Glick SN. The tailored double contrast pharyngogram. *CRC Crit Rev Diagn Imaging* 1988;28: 133–179, with permission.)

by a spurt of barium through the web (the so-called jet phenomenon) (50,51).

Tumors

Benign Tumors and Cysts

The most common benign lesions of the base of the tongue are retention cysts (43). Granular cell tumors as well as ectopic thyroid tissue and thyroglossal duct cysts also occur at the tongue base. The most common benign tumor-like lesions of the aryepiglottic folds are retention cysts and saccular cysts (43). Retention cysts are lined by squamous epithelium and are filled with desquamated debris. Saccular cysts are filled with mucus from glands of the appendix of the laryngeal ventricle (40) and are the mucus-filled variant

of internal laryngoceles. True soft tissue tumors are uncommon and include lipomas, neurofibromas, hamartomas, and oncocytomas, usually arising from the aryepiglottic folds or the mucosa overlying the muscular process of the arytenoid cartilages (40). Benign tumors arising from the mucoserous minor salivary glands are usually found in the soft palate or tongue base. Chondromas usually arise from the posterior lamina of the cricoid cartilage. Regardless of the specific histologic findings, benign pharyngeal tumors often appear on barium studies as smooth-surfaced hemispheric masses that protrude into the pharyngeal lumen (52) (Fig. 3.25).

Squamous Cell Carcinoma

In the United States, squamous cell carcinoma of the head and neck (tongue, pharynx, larynx) is five times more common than squamous cell carcinoma of the esophagus. More than 20% of patients with squamous cell carcinomas of the head and neck have synchronous or metachronous carcinomas of the oral cavity, pharynx, larynx, esophagus, or lungs (53). About 90% of malignant tumors in the oropharynx and hypopharynx are nonkeratinizing squamous cell carcinomas. Almost all of these tumors are detected in moderate or heavy abusers of alcohol, tobacco, or both.

The signs, symptoms, prognosis, and treatment of pharyngeal cancer depend on the location of the tumor. Most patients have symptoms of short duration (less than 4 months), including sore throat, hoarseness, dysphagia, and odynophagia. The overall 5-year survival rate for these patients is 20% to 40% (52–54).

The radiographic findings of squamous cell cancer are those of any mucosal tumor in the gastrointestinal tract (55–58). The normal contour of the involved structure is disrupted by a protrusion into the lumen or by an ulceration extending outside the expected luminal contour. Intraluminal tumor is manifested as an area of increased radiopacity replacing the normally air-filled lumen or as a radiolucent filling defect in the barium pool (55) (Fig. 3.26). The irregular mucosal surface of the tumor is manifested as a granular, nodular, ulcerated, or lobulated surface or as barium-etched lines in an unexpected configuration or location (57) (Fig. 3.26). The mobility or distensibility of the involved structure may be compromised (Fig. 3.27).

FIGURE 3.27. Infiltrative squamous cell carcinoma of right aryepiglottic fold. **A:** Frontal view of the pharynx during drinking shows diminished epiglottic tilt on the right (*arrow*). **B:** Spot radiograph after drinking demonstrates thickening of the right aryepiglottic fold (*short arrows*) and nodularity of the mucosa overlying the muscular process of the right arytenoid process (*open arrows*). (From Rubesin SE. *Pharyngeal dysfunction. Categorical course on gastrointestinal radiology.* Reston, VA: American College of Radiology, 1991:1–9, with permission.)

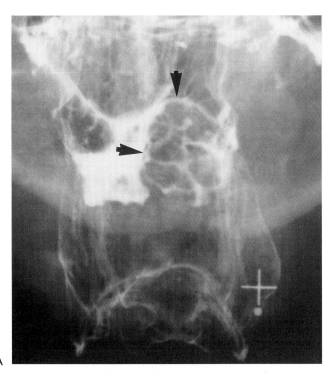

A

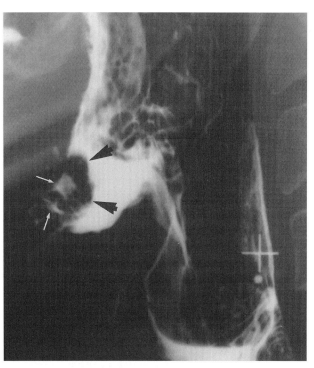

B

FIGURE 3.26. Polypoid squamous cell carcinoma of the base of the tongue. **A:** Frontal view of the pharynx demonstrates that the barium pool in the left vallecula is replaced by a 1.5-cm nodular mass (*arrows*) with barium in its interstices. **B:** Lateral view of the pharynx shows a 1.5 radiolucent filling defect (*black arrows*) in the barium pooling in the valleculae. Barium has entered the interstices of the tumor (*white arrows*) deep to the expected contour of the base of the tongue (From Rubesin SE, Glick SN. The tailored double contrast pharyngogram. *CRC Crit Rev Diagn Imaging* 1988;28:133–179, with permission.)

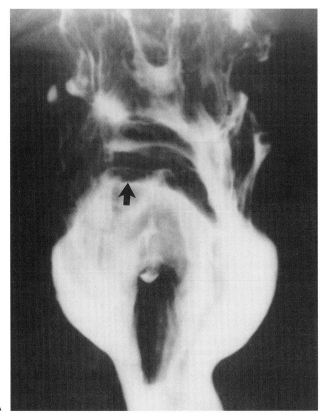

A

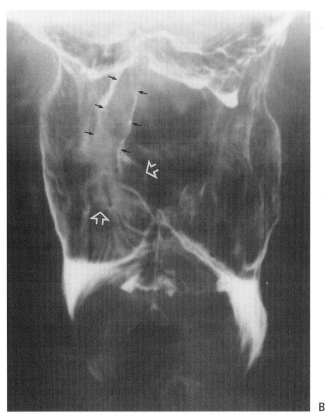

B

The palatine tonsil is the most common site of involvement of squamous cell carcinoma of the pharynx. Tonsillar tumors can spread to the posterior pharyngeal wall, soft palate, and base of the tongue. Lymph node metastases are seen in about one half of these patients (52,54). Squamous cell carcinomas of the tongue base are usually advanced tumors that already have spread deep into the intrinsic or extrinsic muscles of the tongue (59) (Fig. 3.26). These tumors can also invade the palatine tonsils, valleculae, or pharyngoepiglottic folds. Lymph node metastases are present in about 70% of cases at the time of presentation (52).

The supraglottic laryngeal structures (epiglottis, aryepiglottic folds, mucosa overlying the muscular process of the arytenoid cartilages, false vocal cords, and laryngeal ventricle) arise from pharyngobuccal anlage, forming a por-

tion of the anterior wall of the hypopharynx (1). Supraglottic cancers (Figs. 3.27 and 3.28) are often classified as a subsite of "laryngeal" rather than pharyngeal tumors. These lesions frequently cause coughing and choking (60). Hoarseness occurs in patients with supraglottic and laryngeal carcinomas as well as carcinomas of the medial piriform sinus infiltrating the arytenoid cartilage or cricoarytenoid joint (61). The supraglottic region has an extensive lymphatic bed; supraglottic cancers therefore tend to spread throughout the supraglottic region and into the preepiglottic space. Cervical lymphadenopathy is detected in one third to one half of these patients (52,54).

Squamous cell carcinomas of the piriform sinuses are usually bulky masses that already have spread to lymph nodes in 70% to 80% of patients at the time of presentation (52) (Fig. 3.29). Tumors of the medial piriform sinus

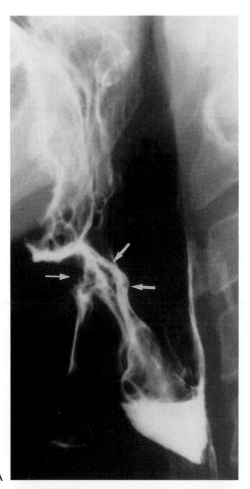 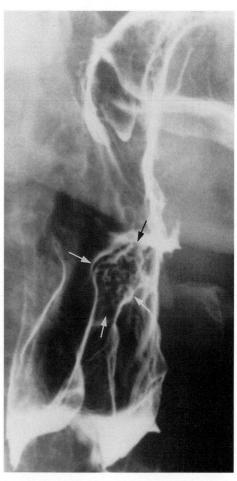

A   B

FIGURE 3.28. Ulcerative squamous cell carcinoma of the epiglottis. **A:** Lateral view of the pharynx shows that the epiglottic tip is missing. Fine mucosal nodularity is seen on the superior anterior wall of the laryngeal vestibule (*thin arrow*) and aryepiglottic folds (*thick arrows*). **B:** Left posterior oblique view of the pharynx demonstrates amputation of the epiglottic tip and nodularity of the mucosa (*arrows*). (From Rubesin SE. Structural abnormalities of the pharynx. In: Gore RM, Levine MS, eds. *Textbook of gastrointestinal radiology*, second edition. Philadelphia: WB Saunders, 2000:227–255, with permission.)

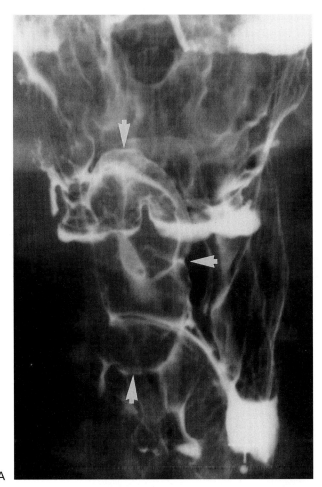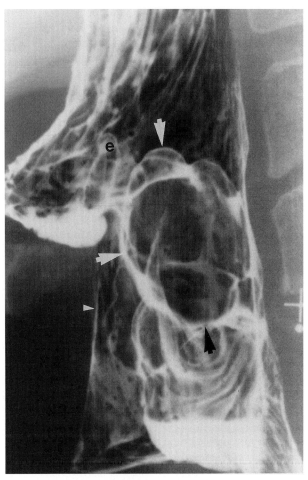

A   B

FIGURE 3.29. Polypoid squamous cell carcinoma of the right piriform sinus. **A:** Frontal view of the pharynx demonstrates loss of the normal contour of the right piriform sinus and a barium-etched mass (*arrows*) protruding into the lumen. The valleculae and epiglottic tip are spared. **B:** Lateral view of the pharynx demonstrates a large, lobulated barium-etched mass (*arrows*). The epiglottic tip (*e*) and laryngeal vestibule (*arrowhead*) are spared. (From Rubesin SE, Glick SN. The tailored double contrast pharyngogram. *CRC Crit Rev Diagn Imaging* 1988;28:133–179, with permission.)

wall may invade the ipsilateral aryepiglottic fold, arytenoid and cricoid cartilage, and paraglottic space, often resulting in hoarseness (61). Tumors of the lateral piriform sinus wall may invade the thyroid cartilage, thyrohyoid membrane, and neck, including the carotid sheath (52).

Squamous cell carcinomas of the posterior pharyngeal wall (Fig. 3.30) are large, bulky tumors that cause few symptoms, often presenting as painless neck masses resulting from metastases to cervical lymph nodes (62). More than half of these patients have lymph node metastases at the time of diagnosis. These exophytic tumors may spread superiorly or inferiorly into the nasopharynx or cervical esophagus and posteriorly into the retropharyngeal space. These tumors are the pharyngeal cancers most frequently associated with a synchronous or metachronous squamous

cell carcinoma of the oral cavity, pharynx, or esophagus (62).

Postcricoid carcinomas (Fig. 3.31) are an uncommon form of pharyngeal squamous cell carcinoma, except in Scandinavia. These tumors may also spread superiorly or inferiorly into the hypopharynx or cervical esophagus.

Lymphoma

About 10% of pharyngeal malignancies are non-Hodgkin's lymphomas arising in the abundant lymphoid tissue of Waldeyer's ring: the adenoids, palatine tonsils, and lingual tonsil (63). Hodgkin's disease involving the pharynx is uncommon, even though Hodgkin's disease is often first detected in cervical lymph nodes (64). Patients with pharyngeal lymphoma frequently present with a neck mass, and

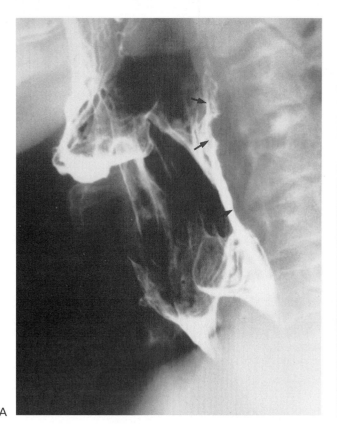
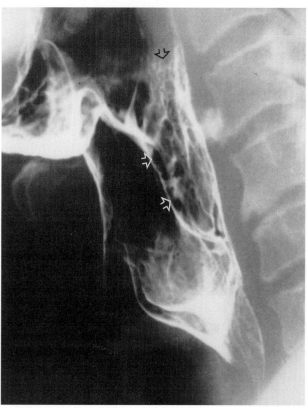

A

B

FIGURE 3.30. Plaquelike squamous cell carcinoma of the posterolateral pharyngeal wall. **A:** Steep oblique view of the pharynx demonstrates focal mucosal nodularity and plaquelike elevation (*arrows*) of the posterior pharyngeal wall. **B:** Lateral view of the pharynx demonstrates mucosal nodularity (*arrows*) *en face*.

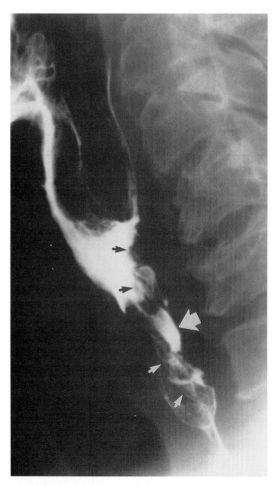

FIGURE 3.31. Ulcerated squamous cell carcinoma of the pharyngoesophageal segment. Lateral view of the pharynx shows a barium-filled ulcer (*large arrow*) at the pharyngoesophageal segment. The posterior pharyngeal wall is destroyed by tumor (*small arrows*) centered at the pharyngoesophageal segment but extending vertically into the distal hypopharynx and proximal cervical esophagus.

cervical lymph nodes are initially involved in 60% of cases (63). Other patients may present with nasal obstruction, sore throat, or dysphagia.

The palatine tonsil is the primary site of involvement by pharyngeal lymphoma in 40% to 60% of patients (Fig. 3.32), the nasopharynx in 18% to 28%, and the lingual tonsil in 10% (40,63). Multiple sites are involved in about 25% of patients, but the hypopharynx is rarely involved by this tumor. Pharyngeal lymphomas typically appear on barium studies as large, bulky, lobulated masses (Fig. 3.32). The mucosal surface may be smooth, however, because of the submucosal location of these tumors (31) (Fig. 3.33).

Other rare tumors involving the pharynx include Kaposi's sarcoma, carcinoma of the minor salivary glands, synovial sarcoma, and cartilaginous tumors of the larynx or cricoid cartilage.

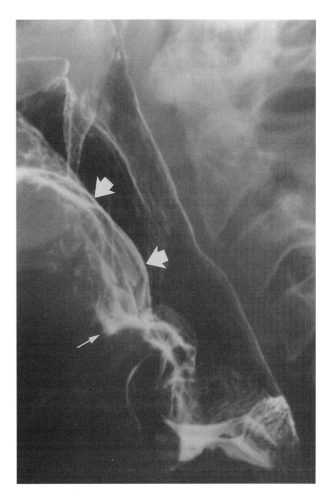

FIGURE 3.33. Lymphoma of the base of the tongue. Lateral view of the pharynx shows that the base of the tongue is enlarged (*thick arrows*) and protruding posteriorly. The valleculae are obliterated (*thin arrow*). (From Rubesin SE, Laufer I. Pictorial review: principles of double contrast pharyngography. *Dysphagia* 1991;6:170-178, Fig. 5B)

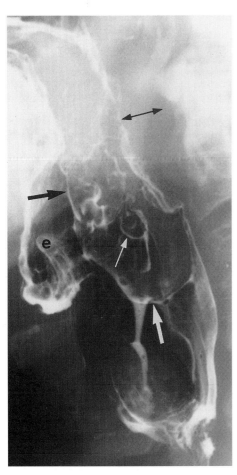

FIGURE 3.32. Lymphoma of the palatine tonsil. Lateral view of the pharynx after instillation of intranasal barium shows a large, smooth mass (*thick arrows*) filling the lateral hypopharynx. A barium-coated ring shadow (*thin arrow*) represents a central ulcer. The posterior pharyngeal wall is thickened (*double arrow*) and has a nodular surface. The epiglottic tip (e) is identified. (From Levine MS, Rubesin SE. Radiologic investigation of dysphagia. *AJR Am J Roentgenol* 1990;154:1157–1163, with permission)

Radiation Change

The pharynx is irradiated when patients undergo radiation therapy for squamous cell carcinoma of the larynx or pharynx, lymphoma of the pharynx or cervical lymph nodes, or metastases to the neck. Historically, the pharynx was included in the radiation portal in patients who also underwent radiation therapy for thyrotoxicosis and tuberculous lymphadenitis. Chronic radiation injury to the pharynx is characterized by vascular damage with mucosal atrophy and fibrosis of muscle and submucosal tissue. Edema caused by lymphatic and venous obstruction is most marked in the epiglottis and mucosa overlying the muscular processes of the arytenoid cartilages. Osteomyelitis and chondronecrosis are more severe complications.

Radiation edema and fibrosis is manifested on barium studies by smooth, bulbous enlargement of the epiglottis, smooth thickening of the aryepiglottic folds, and elevation

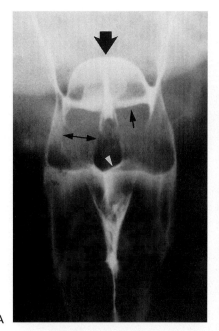
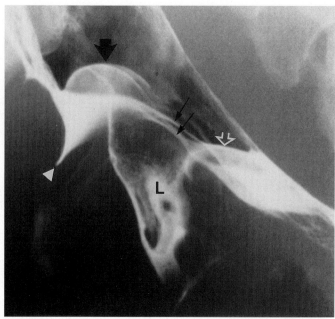

A

B

FIGURE 3.34. Diffuse radiation changes. **A:** Frontal view of the pharynx shows that epiglottis (*large arrow*) is enlarged and has a smooth bulbous contour. The valleculae are flattened (left valleculae identified with a *small arrow*). The aryepiglottic folds are markedly but smoothly enlarged (right aryepiglottic fold identified by *double arrow*). The mucosa overlying the muscular processes of the arytenoids is elevated (*white arrowhead* identifies mucosa overlying muscular process of the left arytenoid cartilage). **B:** Lateral view of the pharynx demonstrates a bulbous epiglottic tip (*black arrow*), elevated aryepiglottic folds (*thin arrows*), elevated mucosa overlying the muscular processes of the arytenoid cartilages (*open arrow*), and slitlike valleculae (*arrowhead*). Barium fills the laryngeal vestibule (*L*). (Reproduced with permission from Rubesin SE. Structural abnormalities of the pharynx. In: Gore RM, Levine MS, eds. *Textbook of gastrointestinal radiology*, second edition. Philadelphia: WB Saunders, 2000:227–255, with permission)

of the mucosa overlying the muscular processes of the arytenoid cartilages (31,40,65) (Fig. 3.34).Other findings include flattening of the valleculae and atrophy of the soft palate, if this structure is included in the radiation portal (3). Radiation fibrosis leads to diminished or absent epiglottic tilt and poor closure of the laryngeal vestibule with subsequent laryngeal penetration (66). Constrictor muscle paresis may result in poor clearance from the hypopharynx with stasis and overflow aspiration. Nodularity or focal ulceration of the mucosal surface should suggest the possibility of persistent or recurrent tumor (65).

ESOPHAGUS

Technique

Barium studies of the esophagus are usually performed as biphasic examinations that include both upright double-contrast views with a high-density barium suspension and prone single-contrast views with a low-density barium suspension (67). The patient first ingests an effervescent agent and then rapidly gulps the high-density barium in the upright, left posterior oblique (LPO) position in order to obtain double-contrast views of the esophagus. On such

views, the esophagus normally has a smooth, featureless appearance *en face* and a thin white etching where it is seen in profile (Fig. 3.35A). Occasionally, collapsed or partially collapsed views (also known as mucosal relief views) may show the normal longitudinal folds as thin, straight, delicate structures no more than 1 to 2 mm in width (Fig. 3.35B). The patient is then placed in a recumbent, right side down position for double-contrast views of the gastric cardia and fundus. The cardia can often be recognized by the presence of three or four stellate folds that radiate to a central point at the gastroesophageal junction, also known as the cardiac rosette (68) (Fig. 3.35C). In some patients with tumor involving the cardia, these lesions may be manifested by distortion, effacement, or obliteration of this cardiac rosette.

After the double-contrast phase of the examination is completed, the patient is placed in a prone, right anterior oblique (RAO) position and asked to take discrete swallows of a low-density barium suspension in order to evaluate esophageal motility. Esophageal dysmotility is considered to be present when abnormal peristalsis is detected on two or more of five separate swallows (69). The patient then rapidly gulps the low-density barium suspension to optimally distend the esophagus (particularly the distal esopha-

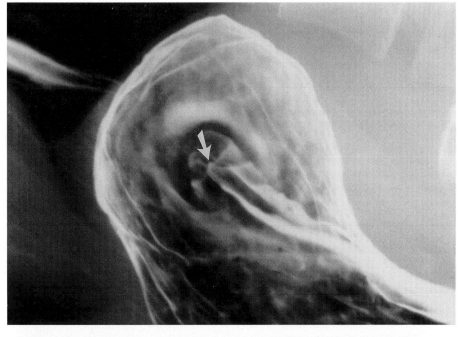

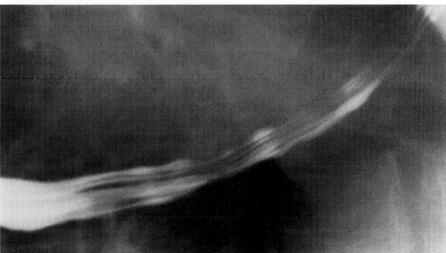

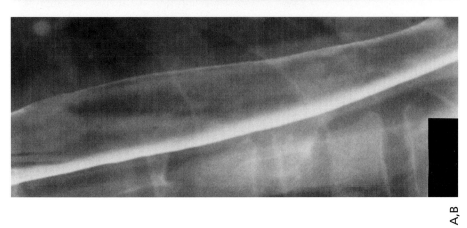

FIGURE 3.35. Normal esophagus and cardia. **A:** Double-contrast view of the esophagus shows how it normally has a smooth, featureless appearance *en face*. **B:** Mucosal relief view shows thin, straight longitudinal folds as a normal finding in the collapsed esophagus. **C:** Recumbent right lateral view of the gastric fundus shows stellate folds radiating to a central point (*arrow*) at the gastroesophageal junction, also known as the cardiac "rosette."

A,B

gus) to rule out rings or strictures that could be missed on the double-contrast phase of the examination. Finally, the patient is turned from a supine to a right lateral position to assess for spontaneous gastroesophageal reflux or for provoked reflux induced by a Valsalva maneuver.

In summary, the esophagram is ideally performed as a biphasic study. The double-contrast phase optimizes visualization of the mucosa for detection of subtle inflammatory or neoplastic disease that cannot be visualized on single-contrast images. Conversely, the single-contrast phase optimizes esophageal distention for detection of subtle esophageal rings or strictures that cannot be visualized on double-contrast images. The double- and single-contrast components of the biphasic esophagram therefore have complementary roles in the evaluation of patients with suspected esophageal disease.

Gastroesophageal Reflux Disease

The purpose of barium studies in patients with reflux symptoms is not simply to document the presence of a hiatal hernia or gastroesophageal reflux but rather to detect the morphologic sequelae of reflux, including reflux esophagitis, peptic strictures, Barrett's esophagus, and esophageal adenocarcinoma. These conditions are therefore considered separately in subsequent sections.

Reflux Esophagitis

Reflux esophagitis is by far the most common inflammatory disease involving the esophagus. This condition is characterized on single-contrast esophagrams by thickened folds, marginal ulceration, and decreased distensibility, but such findings are detected only in patients with advanced disease. In contrast, double-contrast esophagrams have a sensitivity approaching 90% for the diagnosis of reflux esophagitis because of the ability to detect superficial ulcers or other findings that cannot be visualized on single-contrast studies (70,71). Thus, double-contrast esophagography is the radiologic technique of choice for patients with suspected gastroesophageal reflux disease.

Early reflux esophagitis may be manifested on double-contrast studies by a finely nodular or granular appearance of the mucosa with poorly defined radiolucencies that fade peripherally as a result of mucosal edema and inflammation (72,73) (Fig. 3.36). In almost all cases, this nodularity or granularity extends proximally from the gastroesophageal junction as a continuous area of disease. With more advanced disease, barium studies may reveal shallow ulcers and erosions in the distal esophagus. The ulcers may have a punctate, linear, or stellate configuration and are frequently associated with surrounding halos of edematous mucosa, radiating folds, or sacculation of the adjacent esophageal wall (73) (Fig. 3.37A).Other patients may have a solitary ulcer at or near the gastroesophageal junction, often on the posterior wall of the

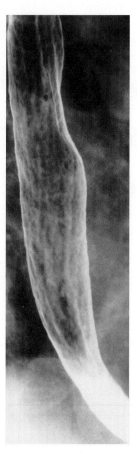

FIGURE 3.36. Reflux esophagitis with granular mucosa. Double-contrast view shows fine nodularity or granularity of the distal esophagus caused by edema and inflammation of the mucosa. Compare this image to the smooth, featureless appearance of the normal esophagus in Figure 3.35A.

distal esophagus (74) (Fig. 3.37B). It has been postulated that the location of these ulcers is related to prolonged exposure to refluxed acid that pools posteriorly when patients sleep in the supine position (74). Other patients may have widespread ulceration involving the distal third or even half of the thoracic esophagus. In such cases, however, the ulceration almost always extends distally to the region of the gastroesophageal junction. Thus, the presence of ulcers that are confined to the upper or midesophagus should suggest another cause for the patient's disease.

Reflux esophagitis may also be manifested on barium studies by thickened longitudinal folds as a result of edema and inflammation that extend into the submucosa (73) (Fig. 3.38). These folds may have a smooth or irregular contour, occasionally mimicking the appearance of esophageal varices (75). In general, thickened folds should be recognized as a nonspecific finding of esophagitis as a result of a host of causes. Other patients with chronic reflux esophagitis may have a single prominent fold that arises in the region of the gastric cardia and extends upward into the distal esophagus as a smooth, polypoid

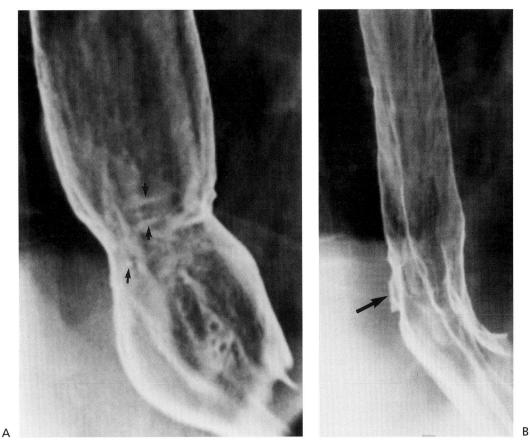

A

B

FIGURE 3.37. Reflux esophagitis with ulceration. **A:** Double-contrast view shows shallow linear and punctate ulcers (*arrows*) in the distal esophagus above a hiatal hernia. (From Levine MS. Gastroesophageal reflux disease. In: Gore RM, Levine MS, eds. *Textbook of gastrointestinal radiology*, second edition. Philadelphia: WB Saunders, 2000:329–349, with permission.) **B:** Double-contrast view in another patient shows a single flat ulcer (*arrow*) on the posterior wall of the distal esophagus. (From Levine MS. *Radiology of the esophagus*. Philadelphia: WB Saunders, 1989, with permission.)

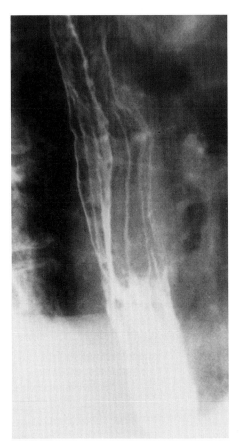

FIGURE 3.38. Reflux esophagitis with thickened folds. Double-contrast view shows considerably thickened folds in the esophagus caused by edema and inflammation extending into the submucosa. Compare this image to the normal appearance of the longitudinal folds in Figure 3.35B. (From Levine MS. *Radiology of the esophagus*. Philadelphia: WB Saunders, 1989, with permission.)

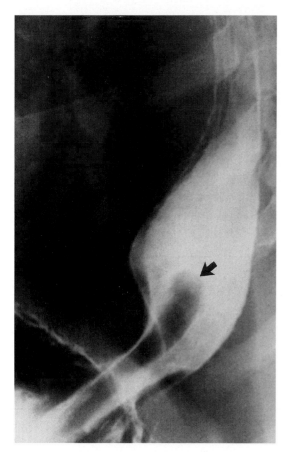

FIGURE 3.39. Reflux esophagitis with inflammatory esophagogastric polyp. Prone single-contrast view shows a prominent fold arising at the cardia that extends into the distal esophagus as a smooth polypoid protuberance (*arrow*). This appearance is characteristic of an inflammatory esophagogastric polyp.

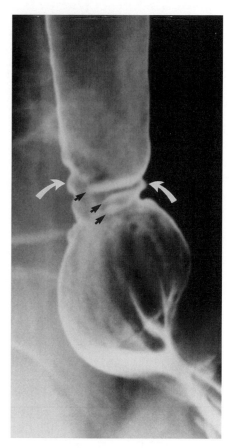

FIGURE 3.40. Scarring of distal esophagus with fixed transverse folds. Double-contrast view shows minimal narrowing of the distal esophagus above a hiatal hernia. Also note sacculation (*white arrows*) of the wall and pooling of barium between transverse folds (*black arrows*), producing a "stepladder" appearance. (From Levine MS, Laufer I. The upper gastrointestinal series at a crossroads. *AJR Am J Roentgenol* 1993;161:1131–1137, with permission.)

protuberance, also known as an inflammatory esophagogastric polyp (76,77) (Fig. 3.39). Because these lesions have no malignant potential, endoscopy is not warranted when barium studies reveal typical findings of an inflammatory polyp in the distal esophagus.

In advanced reflux esophagitis, extensive ulceration, edema, and spasm may cause the esophagus to have a grossly irregular contour with serrated or spiculated margins and loss of distensibility (73). Occasionally, the narrowing and deformity associated with severe esophagitis can mimic the appearance of an infiltrating esophageal carcinoma, so endoscopy and biopsy may be required for a definitive diagnosis.

Scarring and Strictures

As esophageal ulcers heal, localized scarring may be manifested on barium studies by flattening, puckering, or sacculation of the adjacent esophageal wall, often associated with the development of radiating folds (73) (Fig. 3.40).

Further scarring can lead to the development of circumferential strictures (also known as "peptic" strictures) in the distal esophagus, almost always above a hiatal hernia (73,78) (Fig. 3.41). These strictures often appear as concentric areas of smooth, tapered narrowing, but asymmetric scarring can lead to asymmetric narrowing with focal sacculation or ballooning of the esophageal wall between areas of fibrosis. When there is marked irregularity, flattening, or nodularity of one or more walls of the stricture, endoscopy and biopsy should be performed to rule out a malignant stricture as the cause of these findings. Scarring from reflux esophagitis can also lead to longitudinal shortening of the esophagus and the development of fixed transverse folds, producing a characteristic "stepladder" appearance caused by pooling of barium between the folds (79) (Fig. 3.40). These fixed transverse folds should be differentiated on barium studies from the thin transverse folds (also known as the "feline" esophagus) often seen in

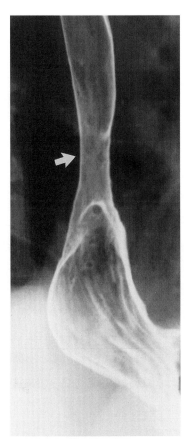

FIGURE 3.41. Peptic stricture. Double-contrast view shows a smooth, tapered area of concentric narrowing (*arrow*) in the distal esophagus above a hiatal hernia. (From Gilchrist AM, Levine MS, Carr RF, et al. Barrett's esophagus: diagnosis by double-contrast esophagography. *AJR Am J Roentgenol* 1988;150:97–102, with permission.)

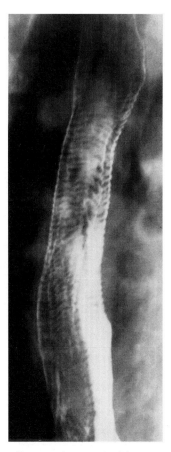

FIGURE 3.42. Feline esophagus. Double-contrast view shows delicate transverse folds as a transient finding in the esophagus. Compare this image to the fixed transverse folds in the distal esophagus in Figure 3.40.

patients with gastroesophageal reflux as a transient finding resulting from contraction of the longitudinally oriented muscularis mucosae (80,81) (Fig. 3.42).

Barrett's Esophagus

Barrett's esophagus is characterized by progressive columnar metaplasia of the distal esophagus caused by chronic gastroesophageal reflux and reflux esophagitis. The classic radiologic signs of Barrett's esophagus consist of a midesophageal stricture or ulcer occurring at a discrete distance from the gastroesophageal junction (82) (Fig. 3.43). In the presence of a hiatal hernia or gastroesophageal reflux, a midesophageal stricture or ulcer is thought to be highly suggestive, if not pathognomonic, of Barrett's esophagus. A distinctive reticular pattern of the mucosa has also been recognized as a relatively specific sign of Barrett's esophagus, particularly if adjacent to the distal aspect of a midesophageal stricture (83). This reticular pattern is characterized by tiny barium-filled

grooves or crevices resembling the areae gastricae on double-contrast studies of the stomach (Fig. 3.44). However, the classic radiologic signs of Barrett's esophagus (a midesophageal stricture or ulcer or a reticular mucosal pattern) are seen in only 5% to 10% of all patients with Barrett's esophagus (83,84). Other more common findings in Barrett's esophagus, such as reflux esophagitis and peptic strictures, are often present in patients with uncomplicated reflux disease who do not have Barrett's esophagus. Thus, those radiographic findings that are more specific for Barrett's esophagus are not sensitive, and those findings that are more sensitive are not specific. As a result, many investigators have traditionally believed that esophagography has limited value in diagnosing Barrett's esophagus.

Even so, other investigators have shown that double-contrast esophagography can be a useful imaging test for Barrett's esophagus in patients with reflux symptoms when these individuals are classified as being either at high, moderate, or low risk for Barrett's esophagus based on specific radiologic criteria (85). Patients who are clas-

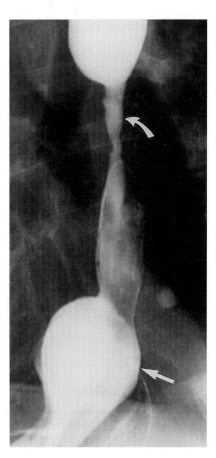

FIGURE 3.43. Barrett's esophagus with midesophageal stricture. Prone single-contrast view shows a large hiatal hernia (*straight arrow*) and a moderately long stricture (*curved arrow*) in the midesophagus a considerable distance from the hernia. In the proper clinical setting, the presence of a midesophageal stricture should be highly suggestive of Barrett's esophagus, but this finding is seen on barium studies in only a small percentage of patients.

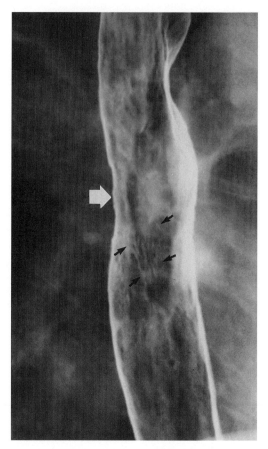

FIGURE 3.44. Barrett's esophagus with reticular pattern. Double-contrast view shows the earliest stage of a stricture in the midesophagus with slight flattening of one wall (*white arrow*). Also note a distinctive reticular pattern of the mucosa (*black arrows*) just below the level of the stricture. This radiographic finding is thought to be highly suggestive of Barrett's esophagus. (From Levine MS, Kressel HY, Caroline DF, et al. Barrett esophagus: reticular pattern of the mucosa. *Radiology* 1983;147: 663–667, with permission.)

sified at high risk for Barrett's esophagus because of a midesophageal stricture or ulcer or a reticular pattern are almost always found to have this condition, so endoscopy and biopsy should be performed for a definitive diagnosis. A larger group of patients are at moderate risk for Barrett's esophagus because of esophagitis or peptic strictures in the distal esophagus, so the decision for endoscopy should be based on the severity of symptoms, age, and overall health of the patient. However, most patients are at low risk for Barrett's esophagus because of the absence of esophagitis or strictures, and the risk of Barrett's esophagus is so small in this group that these individuals can be treated empirically for their reflux symptoms without need for endoscopy. Thus, double-contrast esophagography can be used to separate patients into various risk groups for Barrett's esophagus to deter-

mine the relative need for endoscopy and biopsy in these patients.

Infectious Esophagitis

Candida Esophagitis

Candida albicans is the most common cause of infectious esophagitis. It usually occurs as an opportunistic infection in immunocompromised patients, particularly those with acquired immunodeficiency syndrome (AIDS), but *Candida* esophagitis may also result from local esophageal stasis caused by severe esophageal motility disorders such as achalasia and scleroderma (86). In some patients with these motility disorders, a "foamy" esophagus may develop with innumerable tiny bubbles layering out in the barium column; this phenomenon presumably results from esophageal infection by the yeast form of the organism (87). Only about 50% of patients with *Candida* esophagitis have oropharyngeal candidiasis (i.e., thrush), so the absence of oropharyngeal disease in no way excludes this diagnosis. Single-contrast barium studies have limited value in detecting *Candida* esophagitis because of the superficial nature of the disease. In contrast, double-contrast barium studies have a sensitivity of about 90% in diagnosing *Candida* esophagitis in relation to endoscopy (88,89), primarily because of the ability to demonstrate mucosal plaques with this technique.

Candida esophagitis is usually manifested on double-contrast studies by discrete plaquelike lesions corresponding to the white plaques seen on endoscopy (88). The plaques may appear as linear or irregular filling defects that are often oriented longitudinally in relation to the long axis of the esophagus and are separated by segments

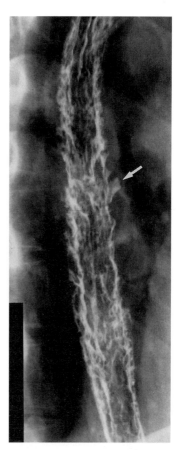

FIGURE 3.46. Advanced *Candida* esophagitis with "shaggy" esophagus. Double-contrast view shows a grossly irregular or shaggy esophagus caused by innumerable coalescent plaques and pseudomembranes with trapping of barium between the lesions. Also note a superimposed ulcer (*arrow*) due to sloughing of diseased mucosa. This patient had acquired immunodeficiency syndrome. (From Levine MS, Woldenberg R, Herlinger H, et al. Opportunistic esophagitis in AIDS: radiographic diagnosis. *Radiology* 1987;165:815–820, with permission.)

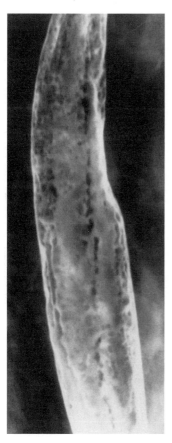

FIGURE 3.45. *Candida* esophagitis with plaques. Double-contrast view shows multiple discrete plaquelike lesions in the esophagus. Note how the plaques have a linear configuration and are separated by segments of normal intervening mucosa. This appearance is characteristic of *Candida* esophagitis. (From Levine MS, Macones AJ, Laufer I. *Candida* esophagitis: accuracy of radiographic diagnosis. *Radiology* 1985;154:581–587.)

of normal intervening mucosa (88) (Fig. 3.45). During the past 2 decades, a much more fulminant form of candidiasis has been encountered in patients with AIDS, who may present with a grossly irregular or "shaggy" esophagus caused by innumerable coalescent plaques and pseudomembranes with trapping of barium between the lesions (90) (Fig. 3.46). Some of these plaques may eventually slough, producing one or more deep ulcers superimposed on a background of diffuse plaque formation (Fig. 3.46). Occasionally, AIDS patients may present with the shaggy esophagus of candidiasis as the initial manifestation of their disease, so the radiologist performing the examination may be the first to suggest that the patient has AIDS. When typical findings of *Candida* esophagitis are encountered on double-contrast esophagography, these patients can be treated with antifungal agents such as fluconazole without need for endoscopic evaluation.

Herpes Esophagitis

The herpes simplex virus is another frequent cause of infectious esophagitis. Most patients with this condition are immunocompromised, but herpes esophagitis may occasionally develop as an acute, self-limited disease in otherwise healthy patients who have no underlying immunologic problems (91). Herpes esophagitis is initially manifested by small esophageal vesicles that subsequently rupture to form discrete, punched-out ulcers on the mucosa. Although some patients have associated herpetic lesions in the oropharynx, most do not have oropharyngeal disease, and others with herpetic infection of the oropharynx have *Candida* esophagitis.

Herpes esophagitis may be manifested on double-contrast studies by small, discrete ulcers on a normal background mucosa (92,93). The ulcers can have a punctate, stellate, or volcano-like appearance and are often surrounded by radiolucent mounds of edema (Fig. 3.47). Multiple discrete ulcers are found on double-contrast esophagography in about 50% of patients with herpes esophagitis (93). In the appropriate clinical setting, the presence of small, discrete ulcers without plaques should be highly suggestive of herpes esophagitis on barium studies, because ulceration in candidiasis almost always occurs on a background of diffuse plaque formation. As the disease progresses, however, herpes esophagitis may be manifested by a combination of ulcers and plaques, mimicking the appearance of *Candida* esophagitis. Occasionally, herpes esophagitis in otherwise healthy patients may be manifested by innumerable tiny ulcers that tend to be clustered together in the midesophagus below the level of the left main

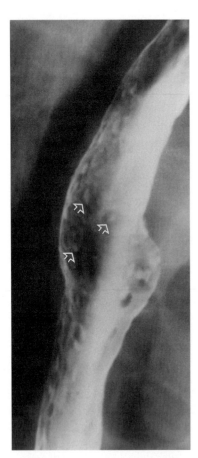

FIGURE 3.47. Herpes esophagitis. Double-contrast view shows multiple tiny ulcers (*arrows*) with surrounding mounds of edema in the midesophagus. In an immunocompromised patient with odynophagia, this finding should be highly suggestive of herpes esophagitis. (From Levine MS, Rubesin SE, Laufer I, eds. *Double contrast gastrointestinal radiology*, third edition. Philadelphia: WB Saunders, 2000, with permission.)

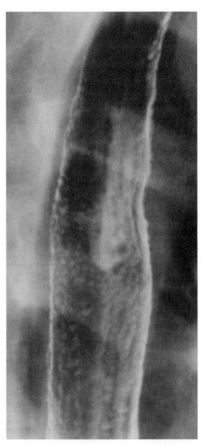

FIGURE 3.48. Herpes esophagitis in an otherwise healthy patient. Double-contrast view shows innumerable punctate ulcers clustered together in the midesophagus below the level of the left main bronchus. (From DeGaeta L, Levine MS, Guglielmi GE, et al. Herpes esophagitis in an otherwise healthy patient. *AJR Am J Roentgenol* 1985;244:1205–1206, with permission.)

bronchus (91) (Fig. 3.48). The ulcers are even smaller than those in immunocompromised patients with herpes esophagitis, presumably because these individuals have an intact immune system that can prevent the ulcers from enlarging.

Cytomegalovirus Esophagitis

Cytomegalovirus (CMV) is another cause of infectious esophagitis that occurs primarily in patients with AIDS. CMV esophagitis may be manifested on double-contrast studies by the development of one or more giant, flat ulcers that are several centimeters or more in length (94) (Fig. 3.49). The ulcers may have an ovoid or diamond-shaped configuration and are often surrounded by a radi-

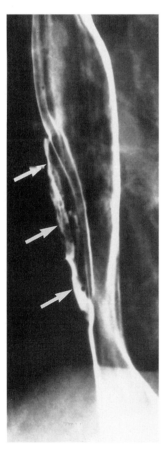

FIGURE 3.49. Cytomegalovirus (CMV) esophagitis in an acquired immunodeficiency syndrome (AIDS) patient. Double-contrast view shows a giant, flat ulcer (*arrows*) in the distal esophagus. Note the thin rim of edema abutting the ulcer. Because herpetic ulcers rarely become this large, the presence of one or more giant ulcers should be highly suggestive of CMV esophagitis in patients with AIDS. (From Laufer I, Levine MS, eds. *Double contrast gastrointestinal radiology*, second edition. Philadelphia: WB Saunders, 1992, with permission.)

olucent rim of edematous mucosa. Because herpetic ulcers rarely become this large, the presence of one or more giant ulcers should suggest the possibility of CMV esophagitis in patients with AIDS. However, the differential diagnosis also includes giant HIV ulcers in the esophagus (see next section). Less commonly, CMV esophagitis may be manifested by small, superficial ulcers indistinguishable from those in herpes esophagitis (94). Because CMV esophagitis is treated with relatively potent antiviral agents such as ganciclovir, which has associated bone marrow toxicity, endoscopy (with biopsy specimens, brushings, or cultures from the esophagus) is required to confirm the presence of CMV infection before treating these patients.

Human Immunodeficiency Virus Esophagitis

Human immunodeficiency virus (HIV) infection of the esophagus can lead to the development of giant esophageal ulcers indistinguishable from those caused by CMV esophagitis. Double-contrast esophagrams typically reveal one or more large, ovoid or diamond-shaped ulcers surrounded by a radiolucent rim of edema, sometimes associated with a cluster of small satellite ulcers (95,96) (Fig. 3.50). The diagnosis is established by obtaining endoscopic biopsy specimens, brushings, or cultures from the esophagus to rule out CMV esophagitis as the cause of the ulcers. Unlike CMV ulcers, HIV-related esophageal ulcers usually heal dramatically on treatment with oral steroids (95,96). Thus, endoscopy is required in HIV-positive patients with giant esophageal ulcers to differentiate esophagitis caused by HIV and CMV, so appropriate therapy can be instituted in these patients.

Drug-Induced Esophagitis

Tetracycline and its derivative, doxycycline, are two of the agents most commonly responsible for drug-induced esophagitis in the United States, but other offending medications include potassium chloride, quinidine, aspirin or other nonsteroidal antiinflammatory drugs (NSAIDs), and alendronate (97–99). Affected individuals typically ingest the medications with little or no water immediately before going to bed. The pills or capsules tend to become lodged in the upper or midesophagus where it is compressed by the adjacent aortic arch or left main bronchus. Prolonged contact of the esophageal mucosa with the pills presumably causes an irritant contact esophagitis. These patients may present with severe odynophagia, but there is often marked clinical improvement after withdrawal of the offending agent.

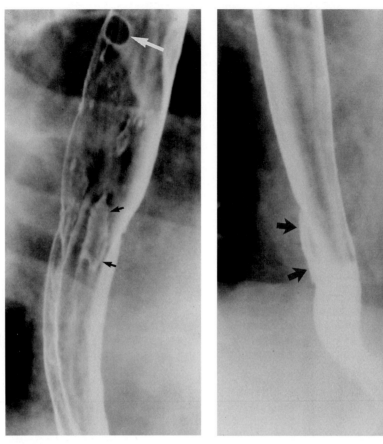

FIGURE 3.50. Human immunodeficiency virus (HIV) esophagitis in patients with acquired immunodeficiency syndrome (AIDS). **A:** Double-contrast view shows a large diamond-shaped ulcer (*black arrows*) with a cluster of small satellite ulcers in the midesophagus. The rounded filling defect (*white arrow*) proximally is an air bubble. **B:** Double-contrast view in another patient shows a large, flat ulcer (*arrows*) in profile in the distal esophagus. HIV ulcers are impossible to differentiate from cytomegalovirus ulcers on the basis of the radiographic findings, so endoscopy is required for a definitive diagnosis before treating these patients. (**A:** From Levine MS, Loercher G, Katzka DA, et al. Giant, human immunodeficiency virus-related ulcers in the esophagus. *Radiology* 1991;180:320–323, with permission.)

The radiographic findings in drug-induced esophagitis depend on the nature of the offending medication. Tetracycline and doxycycline are associated with the development of small, superficial ulcers in the upper or midesophagus indistinguishable from those in herpes esophagitis (100,101) (Fig. 3.51). Because of the superficial nature of the disease, these ulcers almost always heal without associated scarring or stricture formation. In contrast, potassium chloride, quinidine, and NSAIDs may cause more severe esophageal injury, sometimes leading to the development of much larger ulcers and subsequent strictures (102–104) (Fig. 3.52). Alendronate may also cause a severe form of esophagitis with extensive ulceration and strictures, but these strictures are usually confined to the distal esophagus (105). When drug-induced esophagitis is detected on barium studies, a repeat esophagram may be performed to doc-

ument ulcer healing after withdrawal of the offending medication.

Radiation Esophagitis

A radiation dose of 5,000 cGy or more to the mediastinum may cause severe injury to the esophagus. Acute radiation esophagitis usually occurs 2 to 4 weeks after the initiation of radiation therapy (106). This condition may be manifested by ulceration or by a granular appearance of the mucosa and decreased distensibility resulting from edema and inflammation of the irradiated segment (106) (Fig. 3.53A). In all cases, the extent of disease conforms to the margins of the radiation portal. Most cases of acute radiation esophagitis are self limited, but some patients may have progressive dysphagia as a result of the development of radi-

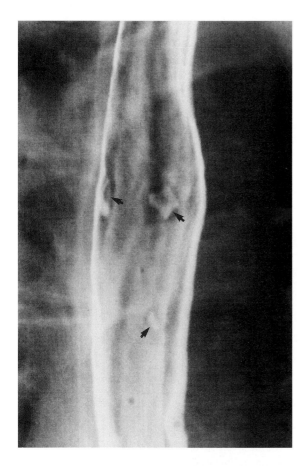

FIGURE 3.51. Drug-induced esophagitis. Double-contrast view shows several small, discrete ulcers (*arrows*) in the midesophagus. This patient developed odynophagia after taking tetracycline. Herpes esophagitis could produce similar findings. (From Levine MS. *Radiology of the esophagus.* Philadelphia: WB Saunders, 1989, with permission.)

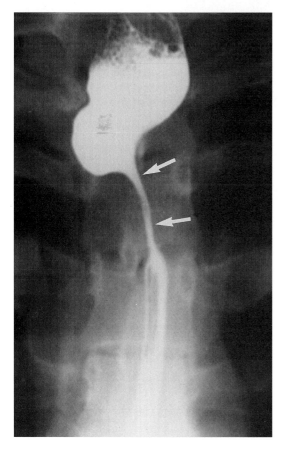

FIGURE 3.52. Drug-induced stricture. Double-contrast view shows a smooth, tapered stricture (*arrows*) in the upper thoracic esophagus caused by previous potassium chloride ingestion.

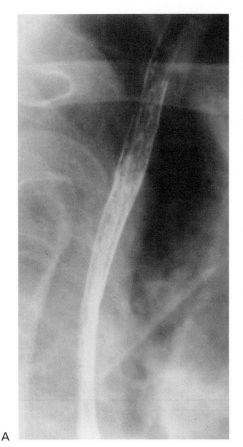
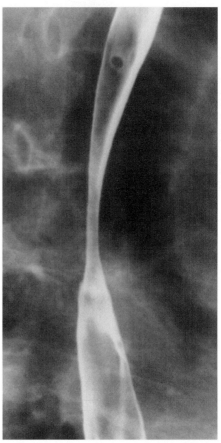

A

B

FIGURE 3.53. Radiation injury to the esophagus. **A:** Double-contrast view shows decreased distensibility of the midesophagus and a granular appearance of the mucosa caused by acute radiation esophagitis. **B:** Double-contrast view from a follow-up study 6 months later shows a smooth, tapered area of narrowing in the midesophagus due to the development of a radiation stricture. (From Levine MS. Other esophagitides. In: Gore RM, Levine MS, eds. *Textbook of gastrointestinal radiology*, second edition. Philadelphia: WB Saunders, 2000;364–386, with permission.)

ation strictures 4 to 8 months after completion of radiation therapy (107). These strictures typically appear as smooth, tapered areas of concentric narrowing within a preexisting radiation portal (Fig. 3.53B). Fistula formation is another uncommon complication of chronic radiation injury to the esophagus.

Caustic Esophagitis

Whether accidental or intentional, ingestion of lye or other caustic agents can lead to a severe form of esophageal injury characterized by marked esophagitis and stricture formation. When esophagography is performed after a patient ingests a caustic agent, water-soluble contrast media should be used because of the risk of esophageal perforation. Such studies may reveal marked edema, spasm, and ulceration of the affected esophagus, and in some cases, esophageal dis-

ruption (108) (Fig. 3.54). As the esophagitis heals, follow-up studies may reveal marked stricture formation, typically involving a long segment of the thoracic esophagus (108) (Fig. 3.55). Patients with chronic lye strictures also have an increased risk of developing squamous cell carcinoma of the esophagus (109), so a new area of mucosal irregularity or nodularity within a preexisting lye stricture on barium studies should raise concern about the possibility of a superimposed carcinoma.

Other Esophagitides

Alkaline reflux esophagitis is caused by reflux of bile or pancreatic secretions into the esophagus after partial or total gastrectomy (110). The esophagitis is characterized on barium studies by mucosal nodularity or ulceration, or, in severe disease, by the development of distal esophageal stric-

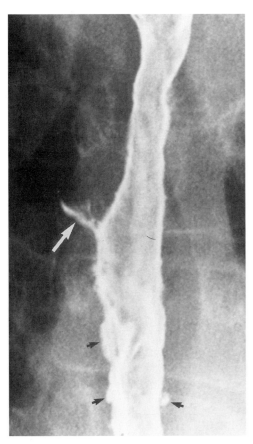

FIGURE 3.54. Acute caustic esophagitis. View of the esophagus with water soluble contrast agent shows multiple ulcers (*black arrows*) and a sealed-off perforation with a small tract (*white arrow*) extending into the mediastinum. This patient ingested lye 2 days earlier.

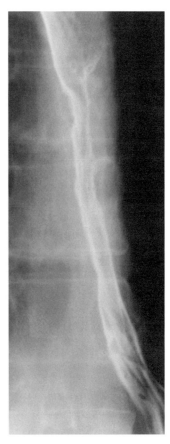

FIGURE 3.55. Chronic lye stricture. Double-contrast view shows a long stricture in the mid and distal esophagus caused by extensive scarring and fibrosis from lye ingestion many years earlier.

tures that can progress rapidly in length and severity over a short period of time (110). The risk of developing alkaline reflux esophagitis can be decreased by performing a roux-en-Y type of reconstruction to prevent or minimize reflux of bile or pancreatic secretions into the esophagus after partial or total gastrectomy.

Nasogastric intubation is an uncommon cause of esophagitis and stricture formation in the distal esophagus (108). Most strictures develop after prolonged nasogastric intubation, but some patients have developed strictures from nasogastric tubes that were in place for as little as 48 hours (108). It has been postulated that these strictures result from severe reflux esophagitis caused by constant reflux of acid around the tube into the distal esophagus. In affected individuals, marked esophageal strictures sometimes develop that can progress rapidly in length and severity on follow-up barium studies (108).

Other uncommon causes of esophagitis include Crohn's disease, eosinophilic esophagitis, acute alcohol-induced esophagitis, chronic graft-versus-host disease, Behçet's dis-

ease, and, rarely, skin disorders involving the esophagus, such as epidermolysis bullosa dystrophica and benign mucous membrane pemphigoid (108).

Benign Tumors

Papilloma

Squamous papillomas are uncommon benign mucosal tumors in the esophagus. These lesions consist histologically of a central fibrovascular core with multiple digit-like projections covered by hyperplastic squamous epithelium. Papillomas usually appear on double-contrast esophagography as small, sessile polyps with a smooth or slightly lobulated contour (111). Occasionally, papillomas are difficult to distinguish from small esophageal cancer on the basis of the radiographic findings (Fig. 3.56), so biopsy or resection of the lesions may be required. Some patients can have innumerable papillomas in the esophagus, a rare entity known as *esophageal papillomatosis* (112).

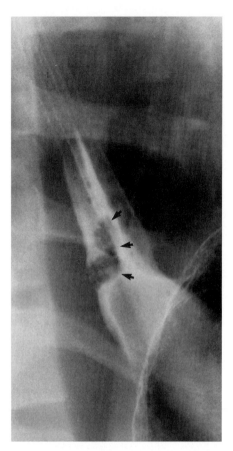

FIGURE 3.56. Squamous papilloma. Single-contrast view shows a small, lobulated mass (*arrows*) in the distal esophagus. A small esophageal cancer could produce similar findings.

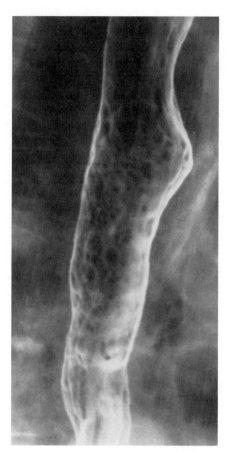

FIGURE 3.57. Glycogenic acanthosis. Double-contrast view shows multiple small, rounded plaques and nodules in the midesophagus. Although *Candida* esophagitis could produce similar findings, this elderly patient was not immunocompromised and had no esophageal symptoms. The clinical history therefore is extremely helpful for differentiating these conditions. (From Levine MS. *Radiology of the esophagus.* Philadelphia: WB Saunders, 1989, with permission.)

Adenoma

Esophageal adenomas are rare benign lesions that usually arise in metaplastic columnar epithelium associated with Barrett's esophagus (112). Because these lesions have the same potential for malignant degeneration as colonic adenomas, endoscopic or surgical resection is warranted. Adenomas typically appear on barium studies as sessile or pedunculated polyps in the distal esophagus at or near the gastroesophageal junction (112). Adenomatous polyps should be differentiated from inflammatory esophagogastric polyps, benign lesions in the distal esophagus that have no malignant potential (see Reflux Esophagitis).

Glycogenic Acanthosis

Glycogenic acanthosis is a benign condition in which there is accumulation of cytoplasmic glycogen in the squamous epithelial cells lining the esophagus, causing focal, plaque-like thickening of the mucosa (113). It is a benign, degenerative condition, occurring primarily in elderly individu-

als. Glycogenic acanthosis can often be recognized on double-contrast studies by the presence of multiple small, rounded nodules or plaques in the mid or, less commonly, distal esophagus (114) (Fig. 3.57). The major consideration in the differential diagnosis is *Candida* esophagitis. However, the plaques of candidiasis tend to have a more linear configuration and typically occur in immunocompromised patients with odynophagia, whereas glycogenic acanthosis typically occurs in older individuals who are not immunocompromised and have no esophageal symptoms. Thus, it is usually possible to differentiate these conditions on the basis of the clinical and radiographic findings.

Leiomyoma

Leiomyomas (also known as gastrointestinal stromal tumors) are by far the most common benign submucosal tumors in the esophagus. Unlike gastrointestinal stromal tumors elsewhere, esophageal leiomyomas almost never undergo sarcomatous degeneration and, unlike gastrointestinal stromal tumors in the stomach, they are almost never ulcerated (112). Patients with esophageal leiomyomas are usually asymptomatic but occasionally may present with dysphagia, depending on the size of the tumor and how much it encroaches on the lumen.

When esophageal leiomyomas grow exophytically into the mediastinum, they can sometimes be recognized on chest radiographs by the presence of a mass in the right superior mediastinum, occasionally containing punctate calcifications (112). Esophageal leiomyomas are usually manifested on esophagography by a smooth submucosal mass, etched in white, that forms right angles or slightly obtuse angles with the adjacent esophageal wall when viewed in profile (112) (Fig. 3.58). These lesions therefore may be indistinguishable on barium studies from other mesenchymal tumors such as granular cell tumors, lipomas, hemangiomas, fibromas, and neurofibromas, except that

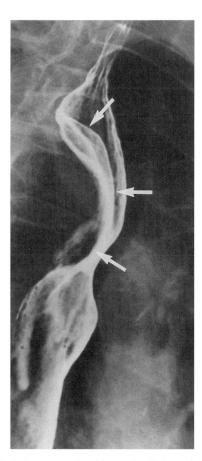

FIGURE 3.58. Leiomyoma. Double-contrast view shows a submucosal mass (*arrows*) in the upper thoracic esophagus. Note how the lesion has a smooth surface and forms slightly obtuse angles with the adjacent esophageal wall. These features are characteristic of a submucosal mass.

leiomyomas are more likely on empirical grounds. Occasionally, computed tomography (CT) may be helpful for differentiating submucosal esophageal masses from extrinsic tumors or lymphadenopathy in the mediastinum compressing the esophagus.

Fibrovascular Polyp

Fibrovascular polyps are rare benign mesenchymal tumors characterized by the development of a pedunculated intraluminal mass that can grow to enormous sizes in the esophagus (115). These lesions consist histologically of varying amounts of fibrovascular and adipose tissue covered by normal squamous epithelium. Fibrovascular polyps are almost always thought to arise near the level of the cricopharyngeus, gradually elongating over a period of years as they are dragged inferiorly by esophageal peristalsis. Some of these polyps can become so large that they cause dysphagia or wheezing as a result of extrinsic compression of the trachea by the polyp (115). Rarely, these patients have a spectacular clinical presentation with regurgitation of a fleshy mass into the pharynx or mouth or even asphyxia and sudden death if the regurgitated polyp occludes the larynx (116).

Fibrovascular polyps usually appear on esophagography as smooth, expansile, sausage-shaped masses that expand the lumen of the upper or upper and midesophagus (115) (Fig. 3.59A). Occasionally, a discrete pedicle can be seen originating near the level of the cricopharyngeus. Fibrovascular polyps that contain a considerable amount of adipose tissue may appear as fat-density lesions on CT scan (Fig. 3.59B), whereas fibrovascular polyps that contain varying amounts of fibrovascular and adipose tissue may have a heterogeneous appearance with areas of fat juxtaposed with areas of soft tissue density (115). Thus, fibrovascular polyps may be manifested by a spectrum of findings on CT, depending on their predominant histologic components.

Granular Cell Tumor

Granular cell tumors arise from Schwann cells of the peripheral nervous system. About 7% of granular cell tumors involve the gastrointestinal tract, and one third of these lesions occur in the esophagus (112). Granular cell tumors usually appear on esophagography as one or more small, round or ovoid submucosal masses that are often mistaken for leiomyomas on the basis of the radiographic findings (117) (Fig. 3.60). Most patients with granular cell tumors are asymptomatic, so these lesions are usually detected as incidental findings. However, large granular cell tumors that cause dysphagia may require local excision.

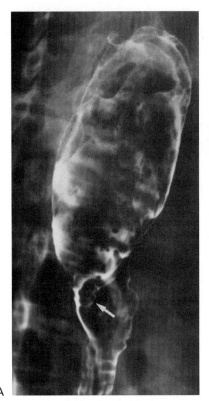

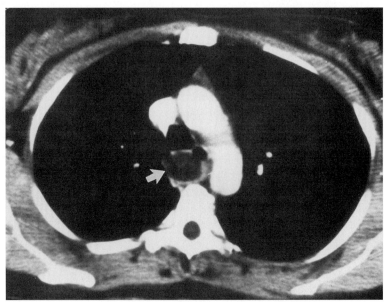

A   B

FIGURE 3.59. Giant fibrovascular polyp. **A:** Double-contrast view shows a smooth, expansile, sausage-shaped mass in the upper thoracic esophagus (*arrow* denotes tip of polyp). **B:** Computed tomography (CT) scan also shows an expansile mass (*arrow*) in the esophagus, with a thin rim of contrast surrounding the lesion, confirming its intraluminal location. Also note the predominantly fat density of the polyp. This CT finding is characteristic of fibrovascular polyps containing abundant adipose tissue. (From Levine MS, Buck JL, Pantongrag-Brown L, et al. Fibrovascular polyps of the esophagus: clinical, radiographic, and pathologic findings in 16 patients. *AJR Am J Roentgenol* 1996;166:781–787, with permission.)

Duplication Cyst

Duplication cysts are not true neoplasms, but they may also appear on esophagography as submucosal masses. Esophageal duplications cysts comprise about 20% of all duplication cysts in the gastrointestinal tract (112). The cysts are development anomalies in which nests of cells are sequestered from the primitive foregut. Duplication cysts contain multiple layers of the bowel, including a mucosa, submucosa, and muscularis propria. Affected individuals are usually asymptomatic, but symptoms may occasionally be caused by bleeding or infection of the cyst. The cysts generally do not communicate with the esophageal lumen (so-called noncommunicating cysts) and tend to be located in the right lower mediastinum. As a result, they can sometimes be recognized on frontal chest radiographs by the presence of a mass in the right lower mediastinum (112). The cysts typically appear on barium studies as smooth submucosal masses indistinguishable from esophageal leiomyomas (112). When duplication cysts do communicate with the

esophageal lumen, they occasionally may be recognized as tubular, branching outpouchings from the esophagus that fill with barium (112) (Fig. 3.61). These fluid-filled cysts usually appear as homogeneous low-attenuation structures on CT and as high-signal intensity structures on T2-weighted magnetic resonance imaging (MRI) (118).

Malignant Tumors

Esophageal Carcinoma

Esophageal carcinoma comprises about 1% of all cancers in the United States and 7% of all gastrointestinal tumors (119). Patients with esophageal carcinoma usually present with dysphagia, but this is a late finding that usually develops only after the tumor has invaded periesophageal lymphatics or other mediastinal structures. As a result, most patients have advanced, unresectable lesions at the time of diagnosis, with overall 5-year survival rates of less than 10% (119). Histologically, 50% to 70% of these tumors are

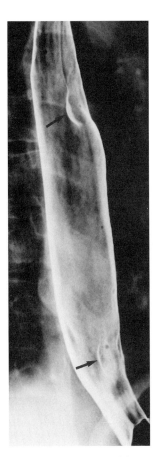

FIGURE 3.60. Granular cell tumors. Double-contrast view shows two discrete submucosal masses (*arrows*) in the mid and distal esophagus. Both of these lesions were granular cell tumors. (From Levine MS. *Radiology of the esophagus.* Philadelphia: WB Saunders, 1989, with permission.)

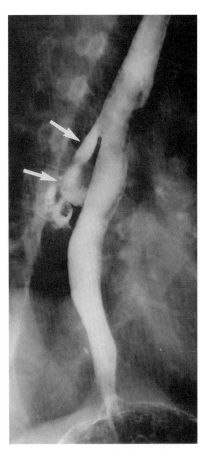

FIGURE 3.61. Communicating esophageal duplication cyst. Single-contrast view shows a branching, tubular outpouching (*arrows*) from the midesophagus. This is a rare type of esophageal duplication cyst. (From Levine MS. Benign tumors of the esophagus. In: Gore RM, Levine MS, eds. *Textbook of gastrointestinal radiology*, second edition. Philadelphia: WB Saunders, 2000:387–402, with permission.)

squamous cell carcinomas and the remaining 30% to 50% are adenocarcinomas (119).

Tobacco and alcohol are the two major risk factors that predispose to the development of squamous cell carcinoma of the esophagus, but other premalignant conditions associated with an increased risk of developing esophageal carcinoma include achalasia, lye strictures, head and neck tumors, celiac disease, Plummer-Vinson syndrome, and tylosis (119). Some authors advocate periodic screening of patients with these conditions in the hope of detecting a developing carcinoma at the earliest possible stage.

Unlike squamous cell carcinomas of the esophagus, adenocarcinomas virtually always arise on a background of Barrett's mucosa in the esophagus. The reported prevalence of adenocarcinoma in patients with Barrett's esophagus is about 10% (119). Studies using incidence rather than prevalence data indicate that the relative risk of adenocarcinoma developing in patients with Barrett's esophagus may be 30 to 40 times greater than that in the general population (120).

Early esophageal cancer is defined histologically as cancer limited to the mucosa or submucosa without lymph node metastases. Unlike advanced carcinoma, early esophageal cancer is a readily curable lesion with 5-year survival rates of about 90% (119). As mentioned previously, early diagnosis of esophageal cancer is usually limited by the late onset of symptoms in patients with this disease. However, in a minority of patients, dysphagia or upper gastrointestinal bleeding develops while the tumor is still at an early stage. Patients with early adenocarcinoma arising in Barrett's mucosa may also seek medical attention because of their underlying reflux disease, so some early esophageal cancers may be detected fortuitously in patients with reflux symptoms (119).

Double-contrast esophagography has a sensitivity of greater than 95% in detecting esophageal cancer (121), a figure comparable to the reported endoscopic sensitivity of 95% to 100% when multiple brushings and biopsy specimens are obtained (119). Early esophageal cancers

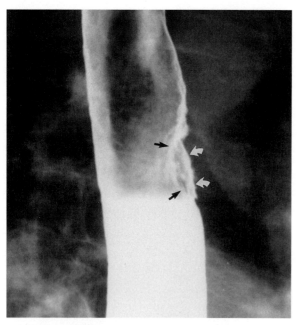

FIGURE 3.62. Early esophageal carcinoma. Double-contrast view shows a plaquelike lesion (*black arrows*) in the midesophagus with a flat, central ulcer (*white arrows*).

are usually small, protruded lesions less than 3.5 cm in diameter. These tumors may be manifested on double-contrast studies by plaquelike lesions (often containing a flat central ulcer) (Fig. 3.62), by sessile polyps with a smooth or slightly lobulated contour, or by focal irregularity of the esophageal wall (119, 122). Early adenocarcinomas in Barrett's esophagus may also be manifested by a localized area of wall flattening or irregularity within a preexisting peptic stricture (119) (Fig. 3.63). Superficial spreading carcinoma is another form of early esophageal cancer characterized on double-contrast studies by a confluent area of poorly defined mucosal nodules or plaques that merge with one another (119,122) (Fig. 3.64). Although these lesions can sometimes be confused with focal *Candida* esophagitis, the plaques in candidiasis tend to be discrete lesions with normal intervening mucosa, whereas the nodules in superficial spreading carcinoma tend to coalesce, producing a continuous area of disease.

Advanced esophageal carcinomas usually appear on barium studies as infiltrating, polypoid, ulcerative, or, less

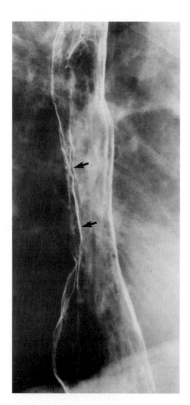

FIGURE 3.63. Early adenocarcinoma in Barrett's esophagus. Double-contrast view shows a long peptic stricture in the distal esophagus above a hiatal hernia. Also note irregular flattening (*arrows*) of one wall of the stricture. Endoscopic and surgical biopsy specimens revealed an early adenocarcinoma arising in Barrett's esophagus. (From Levine MS, Caroline D, Thompson JJ, et al. Adenocarcinoma of the esophagus: relationship to Barrett mucosa. *Radiology* 1984;150:305–309.)

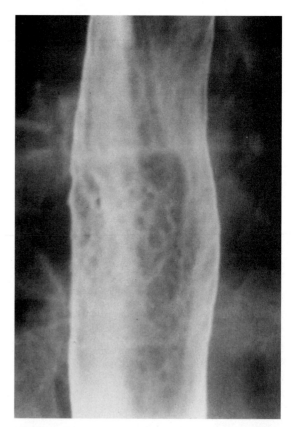

FIGURE 3.64. Superficial spreading carcinoma. Double-contrast view shows focal nodularity of the mucosa in the midesophagus. Note how the nodules are poorly defined, producing a confluent area of disease. This appearance should be highly suspicious for a superficial spreading carcinoma. (From Levine MS. *Radiology of the esophagus*. Philadelphia: WB Saunders, 1989, with permission.)

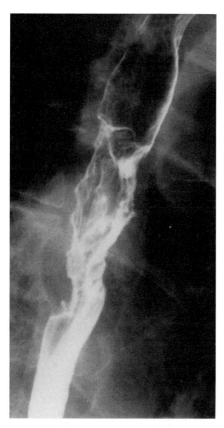

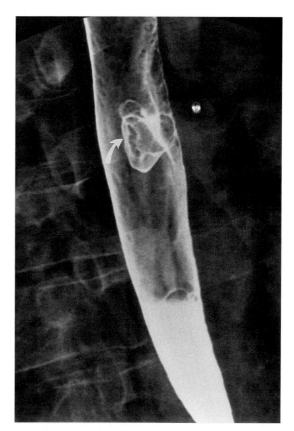

FIGURE 3.65. Infiltrating squamous cell carcinoma. Double-contrast view shows an irregular area of narrowing in the midesophagus with nodularity and ulceration of the narrowed segment. Also note the abrupt, shelflike margins of the lesion.

FIGURE 3.66. Polypoid squamous cell carcinoma. Double-contrast view shows a polypoid mass (*arrow*) in the midesophagus.

commonly, varicoid lesions (119). Infiltrating carcinomas are manifested by irregular luminal narrowing with mucosal nodularity or ulceration and abrupt, often shelflike borders (Fig. 3.65). Polypoid carcinomas appear as lobulated intraluminal masses (Fig. 3.66). Primary ulcerative carcinomas are manifested by a giant, meniscoid ulcer surrounded by a radiolucent rind of tumor (123) (Fig. 3.67). Finally, varicoid carcinomas are those in which submucosal spread of tumor produces thickened, tortuous longitudinal defects, mimicking the appearance of varices (124). However, varicoid tumors have a fixed configuration, whereas varices tend to change in size and shape at fluoroscopy. Also, varices rarely cause dysphagia because they are soft and compressible. Thus, it is usually possible to differentiate varices from varicoid tumors on the basis of the clinical and radiographic findings.

Squamous cell carcinomas and adenocarcinomas of the esophagus cannot be reliably differentiated on esophagography. Nevertheless, squamous cell carcinomas tend to involve the upper or midesophagus, whereas adenocarcinomas are located predominantly in the distal esophagus (Fig. 3.68). Unlike squamous carcinomas, esophageal adenocarcinomas also have a marked tendency to invade the gastric cardia or fundus, comprising as many as 50% of all malignant tumors involving the gastroesophageal junction (125,126).

Esophageal carcinomas tend to metastasize to other parts of the esophagus by way of a rich network of submucosal lymphatic channels. These lymphatic metastases may appear as polypoid, plaquelike, or ulcerated lesions separated from the primary lesion by normal intervening mucosa (119). Tumor may also spread subdiaphragmatically to the proximal portion of the stomach by way of submucosal esophageal lymphatic vessels. These metastases to the gastric cardia and fundus may appear as large submucosal masses, often containing central areas of ulceration (127).

Appropriate treatment strategies for esophageal carcinoma depend on accurate staging of the tumor. Various imaging techniques such as CT, MRI, and endoscopic sonography are used for staging esophageal carcinoma (119). The tumor stage is assessed by evaluating the depth of esophageal wall invasion and the presence or absence of lymphatic or distant metastases.

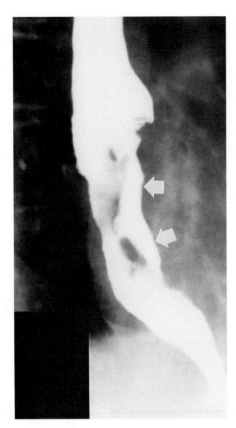

FIGURE 3.67. Primary ulcerative squamous cell carcinoma. Double-contrast view shows a large, meniscoid ulcer (*arrows*) surrounded by a thin rind of tumor in the distal esophagus. (From Levine MS. *Radiology of the esophagus.* Philadelphia: WB Saunders, 1989, with permission.)

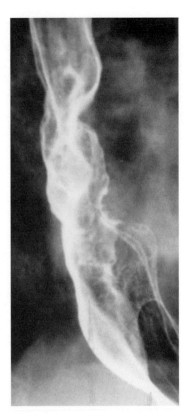

FIGURE 3.68. Infiltrating adenocarcinoma. Double-contrast view shows an irregular area of narrowing in the distal esophagus. Note how lesion extends into proximal edge of hiatal hernia. This patient had an adenocarcinoma arising in Barrett's esophagus. (From Levine MS. *Radiology of the esophagus.* Philadelphia: WB Saunders, 1989, with permission.)

Other Malignant Tumors

Non-Hodgkin's lymphoma and, rarely, Hodgkin's lymphoma may involve the esophagus. Esophageal lymphoma may be manifested on barium studies by submucosal masses, polypoid lesions, enlarged folds, or strictures (128). Spindle cell carcinoma is another rare tumor characterized by a bulky, polypoid intraluminal mass that expands the lumen of the esophagus without causing obstruction (129). Other rare malignant tumors involving the esophagus include leiomyosarcoma, malignant melanoma, and Kaposi's sarcoma (128).

Lower Esophageal Rings

Lower esophageal rings are a common finding on esophagography, but only a small percentage of patients are symptomatic. The term *Schatzki ring* should be reserved for those patients with symptomatic lower esophageal rings who present with dysphagia. These rings almost always occur at the gastroesophageal junction. Histologically, the superior surface of the ring is lined by stratified squamous epithelium

and the inferior surface by columnar epithelium. The exact pathogenesis of Schatzki rings is uncertain, but some rings are thought to develop as a result of scarring from reflux esophagitis.

Symptomatic lower esophageal rings typically appear on barium studies as 2- to 3-mm high, symmetric, weblike constrictions (usually less than 13 mm in diameter) at the gastroesophageal junction above a hiatal hernia (Fig. 3.69). The rings can be missed if the distal esophagus is not adequately distended at fluoroscopy (Fig. 3.69A), so it is important to obtain prone views of the esophagus during continuous drinking of a low-density barium suspension in order to visualize these structures (Fig. 3.69B). Studies have shown that biphasic esophagography is a sensitive technique for the diagnosis of symptomatic lower esophageal rings, occasionally detecting rings that are missed on endoscopy (130).

Diverticula

Esophageal diverticula may be classified as *pulsion* or *traction* diverticula. The more common pulsion diverticula

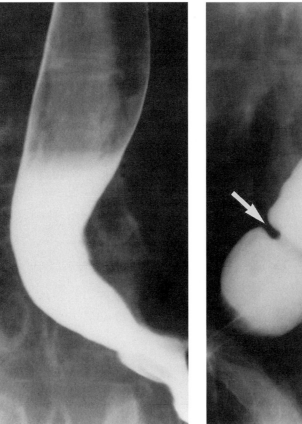

FIGURE 3.69. Schatzki ring. **A:** Double-contrast view shows no evidence of a ring in the distal esophagus, but the region abutting the gastroesophageal junction is not optimally distended. **B:** Prone single-contrast view from the same examination shows a smooth, symmetric ringlike constriction (*arrow*) at the gastroesophageal junction above a hiatal hernia. This Schatzki ring caused intermittent dysphagia for solids.

result from esophageal dysmotility with increased intraluminal pressures in the esophagus, whereas traction diverticula are caused by scarring in the soft tissues surrounding the esophagus. Diverticula most commonly occur in the region of the pharyngoesophageal junction (i.e., Zenker's diverticulum), midesophagus, and distal esophagus above the gastroesophageal junction (i.e., epiphrenic diverticulum). Other patients may develop tiny outpouchings from the esophagus known as esophageal intramural pseudodiverticula.

Pulsion Diverticula

Pulsion diverticula tend to be located in the distal esophagus and are often associated with fluoroscopic or manometric evidence of esophageal dysmotility. The diverticula are usually detected as incidental findings in patients who have no esophageal symptoms. However, a large epiphrenic diverticulum adjacent to the gastroesophageal junction may fill with debris, causing dysphagia, regurgi-

tation, or aspiration (Fig. 3.70). Pulsion diverticula appear on barium studies as rounded outpouchings from the esophageal lumen that have wide necks. They often do not empty completely when the esophagus collapses and may be associated with other radiologic findings of esophageal motor dysfunction.

Traction Diverticula

Traction diverticula occur in the midesophagus and are usually caused by scarring from tuberculosis or histoplasmosis involving perihilar or subcarinal lymph nodes. Traction diverticula are true diverticula containing all layers of the esophageal wall and therefore maintain their elastic recoil. As a result, they tend to empty their contents when the esophagus collapses at fluoroscopy. Traction diverticula often have a triangular or tented appearance resulting from traction on the diverticulum by the fibrotic process in the adjacent mediastinum (Fig. 3.71). Thus, it is often possible to distinguish traction divertic-

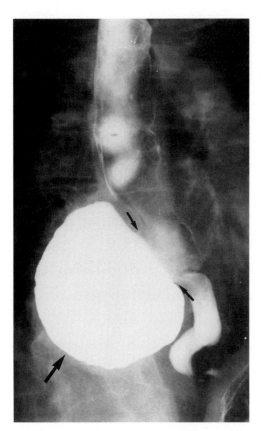

FIGURE 3.70. Giant epiphrenic diverticulum. Single-contrast view shows a large epiphrenic diverticulum (*large arrow*) arising from the right lateral wall of the distal esophagus. Note the wide neck (*small arrows*) of the diverticulum.

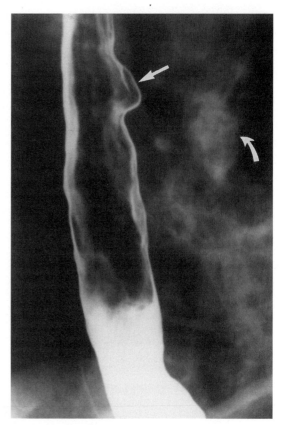

FIGURE 3.71. Traction diverticulum. Double-contrast view shows a triangular outpouching (*straight arrow*) from the left lateral wall of the midesophagus. Also note a clump of calcified lymph nodes (*curved arrow*) in the adjacent pulmonary hilum. This traction diverticulum presumably was caused by scarring from old tuberculous disease in the mediastinum.

ula from pulsion diverticula on the basis of the radiographic findings.

Esophageal Intramural Pseudodiverticula

Esophageal intramural pseudodiverticula consist pathologically of dilated excretory ducts of deep mucous glands in the esophagus. The pseudodiverticula typically appear on esophagography as flask-shaped outpouchings in longitudinal rows parallel to the long axis of the esophagus (131) (Fig. 3.72A). The pseudodiverticula classically have a diffuse distribution in the esophagus and are sometimes associated with strictures in the upper or midesophagus (131) (Fig. 3.72A). However, it is more common to have an isolated cluster of pseudodiverticula in the distal esophagus in the region of a peptic stricture (131) (Fig. 3.72B). In such cases, the pseudodiverticula probably occur as a sequela of scarring from reflux esophagitis.

When viewed *en face* on double-contrast esophagrams, esophageal intramural pseudodiverticula can sometimes be mistaken for tiny ulcers. When viewed in profile, however, they often appear to be "floating" or "levitating" outside the wall of the esophagus without any apparent communication with the lumen (131) (Fig. 3.72B), whereas true esophageal ulcers are almost always seen to communicate directly with the lumen. This sign is extremely helpful for differentiating esophageal intramural pseudodiverticula from ulcers.

Congenital Esophageal Stenosis

A severe form of congenital esophageal stenosis occurs in newborns or infants who generally require surgery. However, a milder form of congenital esophageal stenosis may occasionally be encountered in young or even middle-aged adults, typically men with a lifelong history of mild "compensated" dysphagia and recurrent food impactions (132). The stenotic segment may appear on barium studies as a midesophageal stricture with distinctive ringlike indentations resembling tracheal rings (132) Fig. 3.73). These ring-

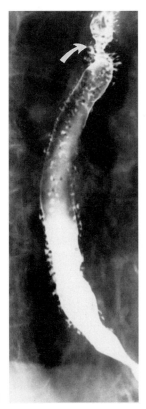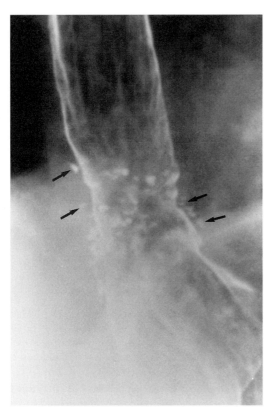

A,B

FIGURE 3.72. Esophageal intramural pseudodiverticulosis. **A:** Double-contrast view shows multiple flask-shaped outpouchings throughout the esophagus in a patient with diffuse esophageal intramural pseudodiverticulosis. Also note a focal stricture (*arrow*) in the upper thoracic esophagus. **B:** Double-contrast view in another patient shows a mild peptic stricture in the distal esophagus with multiple pseudodiverticula clustered together in the region of the stricture. When viewed *en face*, the pseudodiverticula could be mistaken for tiny ulcers. When viewed in profile, however, these structures (*arrows*) appear to be "floating" outside the esophagus without communicating with the lumen. This feature is characteristic of pseudodiverticula. (From Levine MS. *Radiology of the esophagus.* Philadelphia: WB Saunders, 1989, with permission.)

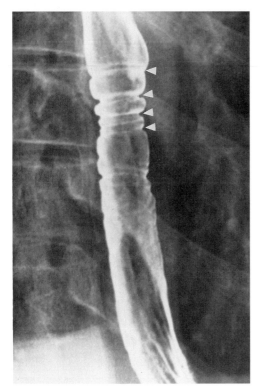

FIGURE 3.73. Congenital esophageal stenosis. Double-contrast view shows a mild stricture in the midesophagus with distinctive ringlike indentations (*arrows*) in the region of the stricture. This finding may be related to the presence of cartilaginous rings in the esophageal wall. (From Katzka DA, Levine MS, Ginsberg GG, et al. Congenital esophageal stenosis in adults. *Am J Gastroenterol* 2000;95:32–36, with permission.)

like indentations may result from cartilaginous rings in the wall of the esophagus. Whatever the explanation, the presence of a midesophageal stricture with multiple ringlike indentations should suggest the diagnosis of congenital esophageal stenosis in the appropriate clinical setting.

Esophageal Motility Disorders

Achalasia

Achalasia can be classified as primary when it occurs as an idiopathic condition involving the myenteric plexus of the esophagus or as secondary when it is caused by other underlying conditions, most commonly malignant tumor involving the gastroesophageal junction (especially carcinoma of the gastric cardia and fundus). Primary achalasia is characterized by absent primary peristalsis in the body of the esophagus and incomplete relaxation of the lower esophageal sphincter, manifested on barium studies by tapered, beaklike narrowing of the distal esophagus directly adjacent to the gastroesophageal junction (133) (Fig. 3.74). In advanced disease, the esophagus can become massively

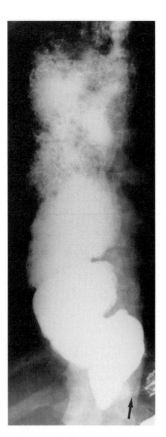

FIGURE 3.74. Primary achalasia. Single-contrast esophagram shows a markedly dilated esophagus filled with debris. Also note beaklike narrowing (*arrow*) of the distal esophagus near the gastroesophageal junction in this patient with longstanding achalasia.

dilated and tortuous distally (also known as a *sigmoid* esophagus). Because of the slow, insidious progression of symptoms, affected individuals typically have longstanding dysphagia when they seek medical attention.

In contrast, secondary achalasia usually results from tumor at the gastroesophageal junction that simulates the findings of primary achalasia because of destruction of ganglion cells in the distal esophagus. As a result, secondary achalasia is also characterized by absent peristalsis in the body of the esophagus and beaklike narrowing near the gastroesophageal junction. In secondary achalasia, however, the length of the narrowed segment is often considerably greater than that in primary achalasia because of spread of tumor into the distal esophagus (134) (Fig. 3.75). The narrowed segment also may be asymmetric, nodular, or ulcerated because of underlying tumor in this region. In some cases, barium studies may reveal other signs of malignancy in the region of the gastric cardia and fundus. The clinical history also is extremely helpful, in that patients with primary achalasia almost always have longstanding dysphagia, whereas patients with secondary achalasia are usually older individuals (older than age 60 years) with recent onset of dysphagia (less than 6 months) and weight loss (134). Thus, it is often possible to differentiate these conditions on the basis of the clinical and radiographic findings.

Other Motility Disorders

Symptomatic diffuse esophageal spasm may occasionally be manifested on barium studies by intermittent weakening or absence of primary peristalsis and severe, repetitive, lumen-obliterating nonperistaltic contractions, producing a classic "corkscrew" appearance (133). More commonly, older patients have intermittent weakening of primary peristalsis and multiple nonperistaltic contractions in the absence of esophageal symptoms, a relatively common manifestation of aging known as *presbyesophagus* (133) (Fig. 3.76). In other normal patients, there may be splitting of the barium column at or near the level of the aortic arch with retrograde flow of a portion of the bolus because of weakening of the amplitude of primary peristalsis at the transition zone between the striated and smooth muscle portions of the esophagus, a clinically trivial phenomenon known as *proximal escape* (133).

Varices

Esophageal varices can be classified as *uphill* or *downhill*. Uphill varices are caused by portal hypertension with increased pressure in the portal venous system transmitted upward via dilated esophageal collaterals to the superior vena cava. In contrast, downhill varices are caused by superior vena cava obstruction with downward flow via dilated

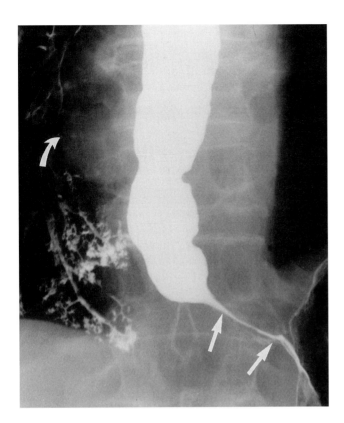

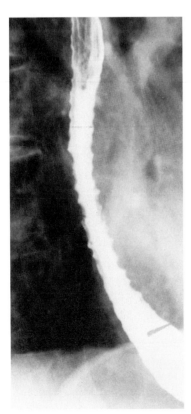

FIGURE 3.75. Secondary achalasia caused by bronchogenic carcinoma. Double-contrast view shows a mildly dilated esophagus with beaklike distal narrowing (*straight arrows*). Unlike the patient with primary achalasia in Figure 3.74, however, the narrowed segment extends 4 to 5 cm above the gastroesophageal junction. Also note the large mass (*curved arrow*) abutting the right side of the mediastinum in a patient with bronchogenic carcinoma that had metastasized to the gastroesophageal junction. (Aspirated barium is seen in the right lung.) (From Levine MS. *Radiology of the esophagus.* Philadelphia: WB Saunders, 1989, with permission.)

FIGURE 3.76. Presbyesophagus. Double-contrast view shows multiple nonperistaltic contractions in the distal esophagus. This elderly patient had no esophageal symptoms.

esophageal collaterals to the portal venous system and inferior vena cava. Uphill varices are much more common than downhill varices. Whether uphill or downhill, varices are important because of the risk of upper gastrointestinal bleeding.

Uphill Varices

Uphill esophageal varices develop as a result of portal hypertension or other causes of portal venous obstruction. Varices appear on barium studies as serpiginous or tortuous longitudinal filling defects in the distal half of the thoracic esophagus (135) (Fig. 3.77). They are best seen on mucosal relief views of the collapsed or partially collapsed esophagus using a high-density barium suspension to increase mucosal adherence (135). The differential diagnosis for varices includes submucosally infiltrating esophageal carcinomas (so-called varicoid carcinomas) and esophagitis with thickened folds caused by submucosal edema and inflammation.

Esophageal varices are characterized on CT scan by a thickened, lobulated esophageal wall containing tubular structures that enhance markedly after intravenous administration of contrast material (135). Additional varices may be seen elsewhere in the abdomen at other sites of communication between the portal and systemic venous circulations. Angiography of the celiac or superior mesenteric arteries can be used to confirm the presence of

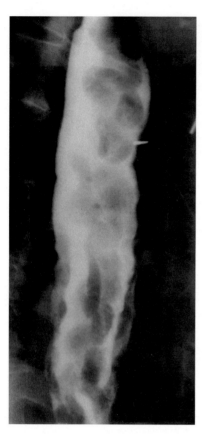

FIGURE 3.77. Esophageal varices. Single-contrast view shows multiple large serpiginous defects in the lower third of the esophagus in a patient with portal hypertension and uphill esophageal varices.

varices in and around the distal esophagus. However, the need for portal venography for presurgical planning of portosystemic shunts has decreased with the widespread use of transjugular intrahepatic portosystemic shunting procedures.

Downhill Varices

The most common cause of downhill varices is bronchogenic carcinoma with mediastinal metastases and superior vena cava obstruction (135). Additional causes include other primary or metastatic tumors involving the mediastinum, mediastinal irradiation, sclerosing mediastinitis, substernal goiter, and central catheter-related thrombosis of the superior vena cava. Most patients with downhill varices present clinically with superior vena cava syndrome.

Downhill varices typically appear as serpiginous longitudinal filling defects, which, unlike uphill esophageal varices, are confined to the upper or midesophagus (135). Venography may be performed to confirm the presence of superior vena cava obstruction, and chest radiographs or CT may be performed to determine the underlying cause.

Foreign Body Impactions

In adults, esophageal foreign body impactions most commonly are caused by inadequately chewed pieces of meat. Most of these foreign bodies pass spontaneously into the stomach, but 10% to 20% require some form of therapeutic intervention (136). The risk of perforation is less than 1% during the first 24 hours, but this risk increases substantially after 24 hours because of schemia and pressure necrosis at the site of impaction (136). Affected individuals typically present with acute onset of dysphagia and substernal chest pain.

Contrast studies are often performed in patients with suspected food impaction to confirm the presence of obstruction, to determine its level, and to rule out esophageal perforation. An impacted food bolus typically appears as a polypoid defect with an irregular meniscus superiorly (136) (Fig. 3.78A). Because of the degree of obstruction, it may be difficult to assess the underlying esophagus at the time of impaction. It is prudent, therefore, to perform a follow-up barium study after the impaction has been relieved to determine whether the impaction was caused by a pathologic area of narrowing (Fig. 3.78B). The most common causes are Schatzki rings and peptic strictures (136).

Intravenous glucagon may be used to relax the lower esophageal sphincter and facilitate passage of an impacted bolus from the distal esophagus into the stomach (137). Effervescent agents may also help to distend the esophagus, promoting passage of the bolus (137). Over time, however, pressure necrosis may develop at the site of impaction, so gas-forming agents should be avoided if the obstruction has been present more than 24 hours because of an increased risk of perforation. Combination therapy with intravenous glucagon, an effervescent agent, and water has a success rate of 70% in relieving esophageal food impactions without need for endoscopic intervention (137).

Fistulae

Esophageal-airway fistulae most commonly result from direct invasion of the tracheobronchial tree by advanced esophageal carcinoma (Fig. 3.79). Such fistulae have been reported in 5% to 10% of all patients with esophageal cancer, often occurring after treatment with radiation therapy (136). Other causes of esophageal-airway fistulae include esophageal instrumentation, trauma, foreign bodies, and surgery. Affected individuals typically present with violent episodes of coughing and choking during deglutition. When an esophageal-airway fistula is suspected on clinical grounds, barium should be used instead of water-soluble contrast agents, because these hyperosmolar agents may cause severe pulmonary edema if a fistula is present (136).

Esophagopleural fistulae may be caused by esophageal carcinoma, radiation therapy, surgery, or instrumentation (136).

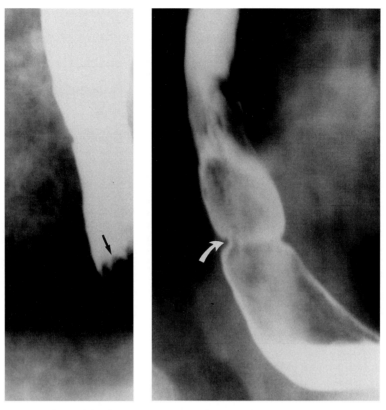

FIGURE 3.78. Esophageal food impaction. **A:** On the initial barium study, an impacted bolus of meat in the distal esophagus appears as a polypoid defect (*arrows*) with complete obstruction at this level. **B:** A repeat study 10 days after endoscopic removal of the bolus reveals a lower esophageal ring (*arrow*) as the cause of the impaction.

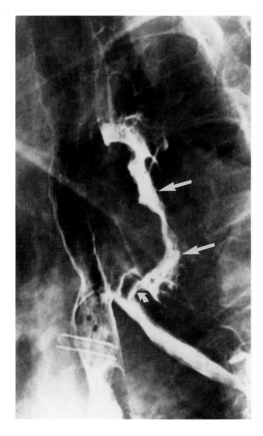

FIGURE 3.79. Esophageal carcinoma with esophagobronchial fistula. A barium study shows an advanced infiltrating squamous cell carcinoma of the midesophagus (*straight arrows*) with an esophagobronchial fistula (*curved arrow*).

Such patients may present with a pleural effusion, pneumothorax, or hydropneumothorax. When an esophagopleural fistula is suspected, the presence and location of the fistula can be confirmed by a study with water-soluble contrast media.

Aortoesophageal fistulae are extremely rare but are associated with a high mortality rate. Such fistulae may be caused by a ruptured aortic aneurysm, aortic dissection, infected aortic graft, swallowed foreign body, or esophageal carcinoma (138). Patients with aortoesophageal fistulae may present with an initial episode of arterial hematemesis followed by a variable latent period, before experiencing massive hematemesis, exsanguination, and death (138). Oral studies with water-soluble contrast agents are unlikely to show the fistula because of high aortic pressures, whereas contrast aortography may fail to show the fistula because of occlusion of the fistulous tract by thrombus (138).

Perforation

If untreated, perforation of the esophagus is associated with a mortality rate of nearly 100% because of a fulminant mediastinitis that occurs in these patients (136). Early diagnosis is critical. Endoscopy is the most common cause of esophageal perforation, accounting for up to 75% of cases (136). Other causes include foreign bodies, food impactions, penetrating and blunt trauma, and spontaneous esophageal perforation resulting from a sudden, rapid increase in intraluminal esophageal pressure (Boerhaave's syndrome).

Cervical esophageal perforation may be manifested on plain films by subcutaneous emphysema, retropharyngeal air, and pneumomediastinum (136). Lateral films of the neck may also show widening of the prevertebral space or a retropharyngeal abscess containing loculated gas or air-fluid levels. In contrast, thoracic esophageal perforation may be associated with pneumomediastinum, mediastinal widening, and a pleural effusion or hydropneumothorax (136). In the proper setting, the presence of mediastinal gas on CT should be highly suggestive of esophageal perforation, whereas other findings such as pleural effusion or mediastinal fluid are less specific (136). However, CT is unreliable for determining the site of perforation.

Esophagography is often performed on patients with suspected esophageal perforation. Some patients may have free leaks into the mediastinum (Fig. 3.80),whereas others may have small, sealed-off leaks. Although barium is the most sensitive contrast agent for detecting small leaks, it can potentially cause a granulomatous reaction in the mediastinum. In contrast, water-soluble agents do not incite a mediastinal reaction and are readily absorbed from the mediastinum if a leak is present. However, water-soluble contrast agents are less radiopaque than barium and can miss a substantial percentage of esophageal perforations (136). It is therefore recommended that the examination be

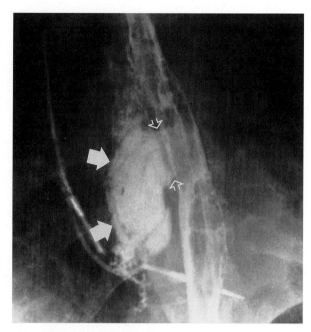

FIGURE 3.80. Esophageal perforation after traumatic endoscopy. A study with a water-soluble contrast agent shows focal extravasation of contrast from the right lateral wall of the midesophagus (*open arrows*) into the right side of the mediastinum (*closed arrows*).

repeated with barium to detect subtle leaks if the initial study with water-soluble contrast media shows no evidence of perforation (136).

REFERENCES

1. DuBrul EL. *Sicher's Oral Anatomy,* seventh edition. St. Louis: CV Mosby, 1980:319–350.
2. Rubesin SE, Jesserun J, Robertson D, et al. Lines of the pharynx. *RadioGraphics* 1987;7:217–237.
3. Rubesin SE, Rabischong P, Bilaniuk LT, et al. Contrast examination of the soft palate with cross-sectional correlation. *RadioGraphics* 1988;4:641–665.
4. Pitman RG, Fraser GM. The post-cricoid impression of the esophagus. *Clin Radiol* 1965;16:34–39.
5. Donner MW, Bosma JF, Robertson DL. Anatomy and physiology of the pharynx. *Gastrointest Radiol* 1985;10:196–212.
6. Rubesin SE. Pharynx: normal anatomy and techniques. In: Gore RM, Levine MS, Laufer I, eds. *Textbook of gastrointestinal radiology.* Philadelphia: WB Saunders, 1994:202–225.
7. Dodds WJ. The physiology of swallowing. *Dysphagia* 1989;3: 171–178.
8. Dodds WJ, Stewart ET, Logemann JA. Physiology and radiology of the normal oral and pharyngeal phases of swallowing. *AJR Am J Roentgenol* 1990;154:953–963.
9. Rubesin SE, Stiles TD. Principles of performing a "modified barium swallow" examination. In: Balfe DM, Levine MS, eds. *Categorical course in diagnostic radiology: gastrointestinal.* Oak Brook, IL: RSNA Publications, 1997:7–20.
10. Rubesin SE. Pharyngeal dysfunction. In: Gore R, ed. *Syllabus for categorical course on gastrointestinal radiology.* Reston, VA: American College of Radiology, 1991:1–9.

11. Dodds WJ, Taylor AJ, Stewart ET, et al. Tipper and dipper types of oral swallows. *AJR Am J Roentgenol* 1989;153:1197–1199.

12. Logemann JA. Effects of aging on the swallowing mechanism. *Otolaryngol Clin North Am* 1990;23:1045–1056.

13. Doty RW, Bosma JF. An electromyographic analysis of reflex deglutition. *J Neurophysiol* 1956;19:44–60.

14. Buchholz DW. Neurologic causes of dysphagia. *Dysphagia* 1987;1:152–156.

15. Buchholz DW. Dysphagia associated with neurological disorders. *Acta Otorhinolaryngol Belg* 1994;48:143–155.

16. Robbins J, Levine RL. Swallowing after unilateral stroke of the cerebral cortex; preliminary evidence. *Dysphagia* 1988;3:11–17.

17. Buchholz DW. Clinically-probable brainstem stroke presenting primarily as dysphagia and non-visualized by MRI. *Dysphagia* 1993;8:235–238.

18. Leopold NA, Kagel MC. Pharyngo-esophageal dysphagia in Parkinson's disease. *Dysphagia* 1997;12:11–18.

19. Bosma JF, Brodie DR. Disabilities of the pharynx in ALS demonstrated by cineradiography. *Radiology* 1969;92:97–103.

20. Bosma JF. Studies of disability of the pharynx resultant from poliomyelitis. *Ann Otol Rhinol Laryngol* 1953;62:529–547.

21. Buchholz D, Jones B. Dysphagia occurring after polio. *Dysphagia* 1991;6:165–169.

22. Branski D, Levy J, Globus M, et al. Dysphagia as a primary manifestation of hyperthyroidism. *J Clin Gastroenterol* 1984;6:437–440.

23. Rubesin SE, Glick SN. The tailored double-contrast pharyngogram. *Crit Rev Diagn Imaging* 1988;28:133–179.

24. Rubesin SE. Pharynx. In: Laufer I, Levine MS, eds. *Double contrast gastrointestinal radiology*, second edition. Philadelphia: WB Saunders, 1992;73–105.

25. Zaino C, Jacobson HG, Lepow H, et al. The pharyngoesophageal sphincter. *Radiology* 1967;89:639–645.

26. Zaino C, Jacobson HG, Lepow H, et al. *The pharyngoesophageal sphincter*. Springfield, IL: Charles C. Thomas, 1970.

27. Frieling T, Berges W, Lubke HJ, et al. Upper esophageal sphincter function in patients with Zenker's diverticulum. *Dysphagia* 1988;3:90–92.

28. Knuff TE, Benjamin SB, Castell DO. Pharyngoesophageal (Zenker's) diverticulum: a reappraisal. *Gastroenterology* 1982;82:734–736.

29. Smiley TB, Caves PK, Porter DC. Relationship between posterior pharyngeal pouch and hiatus hernia. *Thorax* 1970;25:725–731.

30. Delahunty JE, Margulies SE, Alonso UA, et al. The relationship of reflux esophagitis to pharyngeal pouch (Zenker's diverticulum). *Laryngoscope* 1971;81:570–577.

31. Rubesin SE. Structural abnormalities of the pharynx. In: Gore RM, Levine MS, eds. *Textbook of gastrointestinal radiology*, second edition. Philadelphia: WB Saunders, 2000:227–255.

32. Shirazi KK, Daffner RH, Gaede JT. Ulcer occurring in Zenker's diverticulum. *Gastrointest Radiol* 1977;2:117–118.

33. Wychulis AR, Gunnulaugsson GH, Clagett OT. Carcinoma arising in pharyngoesophageal diverticulum. *Surgery* 1969;66:976–979.

34. Brady AP, Stevenson GW, Somers S, et al. Premature contraction of the cricopharyngeus: new sign of gastroesophageal reflux disease. *Abdom Imaging* 1995;20:225–228.

35. Ekberg O, Nylander G. Lateral diverticula from the pharyngoesophageal junction area. *Radiology* 1983;146:117–122.

36. Rubesin SE, Levine MS. Killian-Jamieson diverticula: radiographic findings in 16 patients. *AJR Am J Roentgenol* 2001;177:85–89.

37. Bachman AL, Seaman WB, Macken KL. Lateral pharyngeal diverticula. *Radiology* 1968;91:774–782.

38. Curtis DJ, Cruess DF, Crain M, et al. Lateral pharyngeal outpouchings: a comparison of dysphagic and asymptomatic patients. *Dysphagia* 1988;2:156–161.

39. Lindbichler F, Raith J, Uggowitzer M, et al. Aspiration resulting from lateral hypopharyngeal pouches. *AJR Am J Roentgenol* 1998;170:129–132.

40. Hyams VJ, Batsakis JG, Michaels L. Tumors of the upper respiratory tract and ear. In: *Atlas of tumor pathology*, second series, fascicle 25. Bethesda: Armed Forces Institute of Pathology, 1988.

41. Bosma JF, Gravkowski EA, Tryostad CW. Chronic ulcerative pharyngitis. *Arch Otolaryngol* 1968;87:85–96.

42. Gromet M, Homer MJ, Carter BL. Lymphoid hyperplasia at the base of the tongue. *Radiology* 1982;144:825–828.

43. Bachman AL. Benign, non-neoplastic conditions of the larynx and pharynx. *Radiol Clin North Am* 1978;16:273–290.

44. Clements JL, Cox GW, Torres WE, et al. Cervical esophageal webs—a roentgen-anatomic correlation. *AJR Am J Roentgenol* 1974;121:221–231.

45. Nosher JL, Campbell WL, Seaman WB. The clinical significance of cervical esophageal and hypopharyngeal webs. *Radiology* 1975;117:45–47.

46. Seaman WB. The significance of webs in the hypopharynx and upper esophagus. *Radiology* 1967;89:32–38.

47. Ekberg O. Cervical oesophageal webs in patients with dysphagia. *Clin Radiol* 1981;32:633–641.

48. Ekberg O, Nylander G. Webs and web-like formations in the pharynx and cervical esophagus. *Diagn Imaging* 1983;52:10–18.

49. Gordon AR, Levine MS, Redfern RO, et al. Cervical esophageal webs: association with gastroesophageal reflux. *Abdom Imaging* 2001;26:574–577.

50. Shauffer IA, Phillips HE, Sequeira J. The jet phenomenon: a manifestation of esophageal web. *AJR Am J Roentgenol* 1977;129:747–748.

51. Taylor AJ, Stewart ET, Dodds WJ. The esophageal jet phenomenon revisited. *AJR Am J Roentgenol* 1990;155:289–290.

52. Balfe DM, Heiken JP. Contrast evaluation of structural lesions of the pharynx. *Curr Probl Diagn Radiol* 1986;15:73–160.

53. Goldstein HM, Zornoza J. Association of squamous cell carcinoma of the head and neck with cancer of the esophagus. *AJR Am J Roentgenol* 1978;131:791–794.

54. Kirchner JA, Owen JR. Five hundred cancers of the larynx and piriform sinus: results of treatment by radiation and surgery. *Laryngoscope* 1977;87:1288–1303.

55. Seaman WB. Contrast radiography in neoplastic disease of the larynx and pharynx. *Semin Roentgenol* 1974;9:301–309.

56. Ekberg O, Nylander G. Double contrast examination of the pharynx. *Gastrointest Radiol* 1985;10:263–271.

57. Rubesin SE, Laufer I. Pictorial review: principles of double contrast pharyngography. *Dysphagia* 1991;6:170–178.

58. Jing BS. Roentgen examination of the larynx and hypopharynx. *Radiol Clin North Am* 1970;8:361–386.

59. Apter AJ, Levine MS, Glick SN. Carcinomas of the base of the tongue: diagnosis using double-contrast radiography of the pharynx. *Radiology* 1984;151:123–126.

60. Mong A, Levine MS, Rubesin SE, et al. Epiglottic carcinoma as a cause of laryngeal penetration and aspiration. *AJR Am J Roentgenol* 2003;180:207–211.

61. Carpenter RJ III, DeSanto LW, Devine KD, et al. Cancer of the hypopharynx. *Arch Otolaryngol* 1976;102:716–721.

62. Cunningham MP, Catlin D. Cancer of the pharyngeal wall. *Cancer* 1967;20:1859–1866.

63. Banfi A, Bonadonna G, Carnevali G, et al. Lymphoreticular sarcomas with primary involvement of Waldeyer's ring. *Cancer* 1970;26:341–351.

64. Todd GB, Michaels L. Hodgkin's disease involving Waldeyer's lymphoid ring. *Cancer* 1974;34:1769–1778.

65. Quillen SP, Balfe DM, Glick SN. Pharyngography after head and neck irradiation: differentiation of postirradiation edema from recurrent tumor. *AJR Am J Roentgenol* 1993;161:1205–1208.

66. Ekberg O, Nylander G. Pharyngeal dysfunction after treatment for pharyngeal cancer with surgery and radiotherapy. *Gastrointest Radiol* 1983;8:97–104.

67. Levine MS, Rubesin SE, Herlinger H, et al. Double-contrast upper gastrointestinal examination: technique and interpretation. *Radiology* 1988;168:593–602.

68. Herlinger H, Grossman R, Laufer I, et al. The gastric cardia in double-contrast study: its dynamic image. *AJR Am J Roentgenol* 1980;135:21–29.

69. Ott DJ, Chen YM, Hewson EG, et al. Esophageal motility: assessment with synchronous video tape fluoroscopy and manometry. *Radiology* 1989;173:419–422.

70. Koehler RE, Weyman PJ, Oakley HF. Single- and double-contrast techniques in esophagitis. *AJR Am J Roentgenol* 1980;135:15–19.

71. Creteur V, Thoeni RF, Federle MP, et al. The role of single- and double-contrast radiography in the diagnosis of reflux esophagitis. *Radiology* 1983;147:71–75.

72. Graziani L, Bearzi I, Romagnoli A, et al. Significance of diffuse granularity and nodularity of the esophageal mucosa at double-contrast radiography. *Gastrointest Radiol* 1985;10:1–6.

73. Levine MS. Gastroesophageal reflux disease. In: Gore RM, Levine MS, eds. *Textbook of gastrointestinal radiology*, second edition. Philadelphia: WB Saunders, 2000:329–349.

74. Hu C, Levine MS, Laufer I. Solitary ulcers in reflux esophagitis: radiographic findings. *Abdom Imaging* 1997;22:5–7.

75. Rabin M, Schmaman IB. Reflux oesophagitis resembling varices. *S Afr Med J* 1979;55:293–295.

76. Bleshman MH, Banner MP, Johnson RC, et al. The inflammatory esophagogastric polyp and fold. *Radiology* 1978;128:589–593.

77. Styles RA, Gibb SP, Tarshis A, et al. Esophagogastric polyps: radiographic and endoscopic findings. *Radiology* 1985;154:307–311.

78. Ho CS, Rodrigues PR. Lower esophageal strictures, benign or malignant? *J Can Assoc Radiol* 1980;31:110–113.

79. Levine MS, Goldstein HM. Fixed transverse folds in the esophagus: a sign of reflux esophagitis. *AJR Am J Roentgenol* 1984;143:275–278.

80. Gohel VK, Edell SI, Laufer I, et al. Transverse folds in the human esophagus. *Radiology* 1978;128:303–308.

81. Furth EE, Rubesin SE, Rose D. Feline esophagus. *AJR Am J Roentgenol* 1995;164:900.

82. Robbins AH, Hermos JA, Schimmel EM, et al. The columnar-lined esophagus: analysis of 26 cases. *Radiology* 1977;123:1–7.

83. Levine MS, Kressel HY, Caroline DF, et al. Barrett esophagus: reticular pattern of the mucosa. *Radiology* 1983;147:663–667.

84. Chen YM, Gelfand DW, Ott DJ, et al. Barrett esophagus as an extension of severe esophagitis: analysis of radiologic signs in 29 cases. *AJR Am J Roentgenol* 1985;145:275–281.

85. Gilchrist AM, Levine MS, Carr RF, et al. Barrett's esophagus: diagnosis by double-contrast esophagography. *AJR Am J Roentgenol* 1988;150:97–102.

86. Gefter WB, Laufer I, Edell S, et al. Candidiasis in the obstructed esophagus. *Radiology* 1981;138:25-28.

87. Sam JW, Levine MS, Rubesin SE, et al. The "foamy" esophagus: a radiographic sign of *Candida* esophagitis. *AJR Am J Roentgenol* 2000;174:999–1002.

88. Levine MS, Macones AJ, Laufer I. *Candida* esophagitis: accuracy of radiographic diagnosis. *Radiology* 1985;154:581–587.

89. Vahey TN, Maglinte DDT, Chernish SM. State-of-the-art barium examination in opportunistic esophagitis. *Dig Dis Sci* 1986;31:1192–1195.

90. Levine MS, Woldenberg R, Herlinger H, et al. Opportunistic esophagitis in AIDS: radiographic diagnosis. *Radiology* 1987;165:815–820.

91. Shortsleeve MJ, Levine MS. Herpes esophagitis in otherwise healthy patients: clinical and radiographic findings. *Radiology* 1992;182:859–861.

92. Levine MS, Laufer I, Kressel HY, et al. Herpes esophagitis. *AJR Am J Roentgenol* 1981;136:863–866.

93. Levine MS, Loevner LA, Saul SH, et al. Herpes esophagitis: sensitivity of double-contrast esophagography. *AJR Am J Roentgenol* 1988;151:57–62.

94. Balthazar EM, Megibow AJ, Hulnick D, et al. Cytomegalovirus esophagitis in AIDS: radiographic features in 16 patients. *AJR Am J Roentgenol* 1987;149:919–923.

95. Levine MS, Loercher G, Katzka DA, et al. Giant, human immunodeficiency virus-related ulcers in the esophagus. *Radiology* 1991;180:320–323.

96. Sor S, Levine MS, Kowalski TE, et al. Giant ulcers of the esophagus in patients with human immunodeficiency virus: clinical, radiographic, and pathologic findings. *Radiology* 1995;194:447–451.

97. Kikendall JW, Friedman AC, Oyewole MA, et al. Pill-induced esophageal injury: case reports and review of the medical literature. *Dig Dis Sci* 1983;28:174–182.

98. Coates AG, Nostrand TT, Wilson JAP, et al. Esophagitis caused by nonsteroidal antiinflammatory medication. *South Med J* 1986;79:1094–1097.

99. de Groen PC, Lubbe DF, Hirsch LJ, et al. Esophagitis associated with the use of alendronate. *N Engl J Med* 1996;335:1016–1021.

100. Creteur V, Laufer I, Kressel HY, et al. Drug-induced esophagitis detected by double contrast radiography. *Radiology* 1983;147:365–368.

101. Bova JG, Dutton NE, Goldstein HM, et al. Medication-induced esophagitis: diagnosis by double-contrast esophagography. *AJR Am J Roentgenol* 1987;148:731–732.

102. Teplick JG, Teplick SK, Ominsky SH, et al. Esophagitis caused by oral medication. *Radiology* 1980;134:23–25.

103. Levine MS, Rothstein RD, Laufer I. Giant esophageal ulcer due to Clinoril. *AJR Am J Roentgenol* 1991;156:955–956.

104. Levine MS, Borislow SM, Rubesin SE, et al. Esophageal stricture caused by a Motrin tablet (ibuprofen). *Abdom Imaging* 1994;19:6–7.

105. Ryan JM, Kelsey P, Ryan BM, et al. Alendronate-induced esophagitis: case report of a recently recognized form of severe esophagitis with esophageal stricture—radiographic features. *AJR Am J Roentgenol* 1998;206:389–391.

106. Collazzo LA, Levine MS, Rubesin SE, et al. Acute radiation esophagitis: radiographic findings. *AJR Am J Roentgenol* 1997;169:1067–1070.

107. Lepke RA, Libshitz HI. Radiation-induced injury of the esophagus. *Radiology* 1983;148:375–378.

108. Levine MS. Other esophagitides. In: Gore RM, Levine MS, eds. *Textbook of gastrointestinal radiology*, second edition. Philadelphia: WB Saunders, 2000:364–386.

109. Appleqvist P, Salmo M. Lye corrosion carcinoma of the esophagus: a review of 63 cases. *Cancer* 1980;45:2655–2658.

110. Levine MS, Fisher AR, Rubesin SE, et al. Complications after total gastrectomy and esophagojejunostomy: radiologic evaluation. *AJR Am J Roentgenol* 1991;157:1189–1194.

111. Montesi A, Alessandro P, Graziani L, et al. Small benign tumors of the esophagus: radiological diagnosis with double-contrast examination. *Gastrointest Radiol* 1983;8:207–212.

112. Levine MS. Benign tumors of the esophagus. In: Gore RM, Levine MS, eds. *Textbook of gastrointestinal radiology*, second edition. Philadelphia: WB Saunders, 2000:387–402.

113. Rose D, Furth EE, Rubesin SE. Glycogenic acanthosis. *AJR Am J Roentgenol* 1995;164:96.

114. Glick SN, Teplick SK, Goldstein J, et al. Glycogenic acanthosis of the esophagus. *AJR Am J Roentgenol* 1982;139:683–688.

115. Levine MS, Buck JL, Pantongrag-Brown L, et al. Fibrovascular polyps of the esophagus: clinical, radiographic, and pathologic findings in 16 patients. *AJR Am J Roentgenol* 1996;166:781–787.

116. Cochet B, Hohl P, Sans M, et al. Asphyxia caused by laryngeal impaction of an esophageal polyp. *Arch Otolaryngol* 1980;106:176–178.

117. Rubesin SE, Herlinger H, Sigal H. Granular cell tumors of the esophagus. *Gastrointest Radiol* 1985;10:11-15.

118. Rafal RB, Markisz JA. Magnetic resonance imaging of an esophageal duplication cyst. *Am J Gastroenterol* 1991;86:1809–1811.

119. Levine MS, Halvorsen RA. Carcinoma of the esophagus. In: Gore RM, Levine MS, eds. *Textbook of gastrointestinal radiology*, second edition. Philadelphia: WB Saunders, 2000:403–433.

120. Cameron AJ, Ott BJ, Payne WS. The incidence of adenocarcinoma in the columnar-lined (Barrett's) esophagus. *N Engl J Med* 1985;313:857–859.

121. Levine MS, Chu P, Furth EE, et al. Carcinoma of the esophagus and esophagogastric junction: sensitivity of radiographic diagnosis. *AJR Am J Roentgenol* 1997;168:1423–1426.

122. Levine MS, Dillon EC, Saul SH, et al. Early esophageal cancer. *AJR Am J Roentgenol* 1986;146:507–512.

123. Gloyna RE, Zornoza J, Goldstein HM. Primary ulcerative carcinoma of the esophagus. *AJR Am J Roentgenol* 1977;129:599–600.

124. Yates CW, LeVine MA, Jensen KM. Varicoid carcinoma of the esophagus. *Radiology* 1977;122:605–608.

125. Levine MS, Caroline D, Thompson JJ, et al. Adenocarcinoma of the esophagus: relationship to Barrett mucosa. *Radiology* 1984;150:305–309.

126. Keen SJ, Dodd GD, Smith JL. Adenocarcinoma arising in Barrett's esophagus: pathologic and radiologic features. *Mt Sinai J Med* 1984;51:442–450.

127. Glick SN, Teplick SK, Levine MS, et al. Gastric cardia metastasis in esophageal carcinoma. *Radiology* 1986;160:627–630.

128. Levine MS. Other malignant tumors of the esophagus. In: Gore RM, Levine MS, eds. *Textbook of gastrointestinal radiology*, second edition. Philadelphia: WB Saunders, 2000:435–451.

129. Agha FP, Keren DF. Spindle-cell squamous carcinoma of the esophagus: a tumor with biphasic morphology. *AJR Am J Roentgenol* 1985;145:541–545.

130. Ott DJ, Chen YM, Wu WC, et al. Radiographic and endoscopic sensitivity in detecting lower esophageal mucosal ring. *AJR Am J Roentgenol* 1986;147:261–265.

131. Levine MS, Moolten DN, Herlinger H, et al. Esophageal intramural pseudodiverticulosis: a reevaluation. *AJR Am J Roentgenol* 1986;147:1165–1170.

132. Oh CH, Levine MS, Katzka DA, et al. Congenital esophageal stenosis in adults: clinical and radiographic findings in seven patients. *AJR Am J Roentgenol* 2001;176:1179–1182.

133. Ott DJ. Motility disorders of the esophagus. In: Gore RM, Levine MS, eds. *Textbook of gastrointestinal radiology*, second edition. Philadelphia: WB Saunders, 2000:316–328.

134. Woodfield CA, Levine MS, Rubesin SE, et al. Diagnosis of primary versus secondary achalasia: reassessment of clinical and radiographic criteria. *AJR Am J Roentgenol* 2000;175:727–731.

135. Levine MS. Varices. In: Gore RM, Levine MS, eds. *Textbook of gastrointestinal radiology*, second edition. Philadelphia: WB Saunders, 2000:452–463.

136. Levine MS. Miscellaneous abnormalities of the esophagus. In: Gore RM, Levine MS, eds. *Textbook of gastrointestinal radiology*, second edition. Philadelphia: WB Saunders, 2000:465–483.

137. Robbins MI, Shortsleeve MJ. Treatment of acute esophageal food impaction with glucagon, an effervescent agent, and water. *AJR Am J Roentgenol* 1994;162:325–328.

138. Baron RL, Koehler RE, Gutierrez FR, et al. Clinical and radiographic manifestations of aortoesophageal fistulas. *Radiology* 1981;141:599–605.

SPECIAL ENDOSCOPIC IMAGING AND OPTICAL TECHNIQUES

MICHAEL B. WALLACE

Endoscopy has played a critical role in advancing the knowledge and management of esophageal disease. It is difficult to imagine management of esophageal diseases such as gastroesophageal reflux disease (GERD), esophageal cancer, and strictures without endoscopy. Endoscopy has expanded the ability to understand the mechanisms of esophageal disease through imaging of mucosa, endoscopic ultrasound imaging of the deeper layers, and endoscopic therapy such as mucosal ablation and antireflux procedures. In the past 5 years, several major endoscopic advances have been made in relation to esophageal disease. Major advances in diagnostic and imaging technologies include the development of new methods of analyzing the interaction of light and tissue called *spectroscopy*, particularly in the area of detecting dysplasia; improvements in mucosal staining techniques and increasingly powerful magnification endoscopy; and continued improvement in endoscopic ultrasound imaging of a variety of esophageal disorders. There is a continuing convergence of endoscopic therapy with minimally invasive surgery to develop techniques for endoscopic treatment of GERD, Zenker's diverticula, and Barrett's esophagus. This chapter reviews the role of special diagnostic techniques for esophageal diseases, focusing on optical and ultrasound methods. The role of endoscopy in specific diseases is discussed in each of relevant chapters.

HISTORY OF ENDOSCOPY OF THE ESOPHAGUS

The evolution of modern endoscopy has been the cumulative result of the work of many innovative individuals who have furthered endoscopic development over the past 150 years. Their combined efforts are described in historical works that delineate the development of the modern videoendoscope since the steel tube that was first intro-

duced in 1868 to visualize the esophagus and stomach by Kussmaul. Modern flexible endoscopy began with the development of optical fibers in 1954 by Hopkins and Kapany (1) and their adaptation to medical endoscopy by Hirschowitz in 1957 (2). Advances since then include the development of charged couple devices (CCD) and videoendoscopy in 1983 by the Welch Allyn Corporation, endoscopic ultrasound by Hisanaga (3) and DiMagno (4) in 1980, and a variety of spectroscopic technologies that expanded endoscopy beyond the visible wavelength. At the same time, the standard video endoscope became increasing smaller, more maneuverable, and equipped with high-resolution video images (Fig. 4.1). These changes allow for improved diagnostic abilities, more extensive options for image documentation and transmission, and easier delivery of endoscopic therapies. In addition, endoscopes and endoscopic accessories, such as band ligation, and mucosal resection devices opened the door to therapeutic procedures in the esophagus. This door has swung wide open with the development of techniques for treatment of GERD (5,6).

The history of endoscopic technology is distinct from most scientific advances in gastroenterology. Major advances have occurred at the boundary between medicine, optical physics, and engineering. This has demanded a new breed of physician-endoscopists who can serve as translators between clinical medicine, biomedical research, and optical engineering.

TECHNIQUES FOR ENDOSCOPY OF THE ESOPHAGUS

The technique of diagnostic upper endoscopy has not changed significantly in the past decade. Most patients can easily undergo upper endoscopy with minimal effort and preparation. Relative contraindications to upper endoscopy are listed in Table 4.1. Even though patient preparation, facilities, and certain aspects of endoscopy may vary by region, the procedure is essentially performed in the same manner at all locations. Instruments vary slightly in design

M. B. Wallace: Department of Gastroenterology and Biometry, Medical University of South Carolina, Charleston, South Carolina.

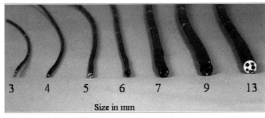

	3	4	5	6	7	9	13

Size in mm

Biopsy: No No Yes ⟶

Image: Fiber Fiber CCD ⟶

Air/H2O: Yes ⟶

Sedation: No No Maybe ⟶Yes ⟶

Nasal: Yes Yes Maybe ⟶No ⟶

FIGURE 4.1. Range of diameter and capabilities of endoscopes. *Biopsy* refers to the availability of an accessory channel for biopsy forceps. *Air/H20* refers to the availability of external air and water installation. *Sedation* refers to the ability to tolerably perform endoscopy without sedation. *Nasal* refers to the ability to pass the endoscope transnasally.

and characteristics. In general, they appear to be well suited for diagnostic upper endoscopy (which is described in detail in references 7 and 8).

Examination of the esophagus by endoscopy begins with insertion of the endoscope into the posterior pharynx. The posterior pharynx and larynx are examined for abnormalities (see Chapter 29). The endoscope is advanced under direct vision into the upper esophageal sphincter, and the patient is instructed to swallow. With relaxation of the sphincter, the endoscope is advanced into the upper esophagus and the mucosa is carefully examined. The esophageal mucosa is continuously examined for abnormalities as the endoscope is slowly advanced. Extrinsic compression of the esophagus by the aortic arch, left atrium, or left ventricle may be noted. The area of the gastroesophageal junction is carefully examined to document the location of the squamocolumnar junction and the gastroesophageal junction. Delineation of these two locations is critical for the diagnosis of Barrett's esophagus. In the presence of a hiatus hernia, it is important to avoid overinflation with air that can flatten the proximal gastric folds and give a false impression of columnar lined mucosa in the distal esophagus. The endoscope should then be advanced into the stomach and the cardia examined in retroflexion to visualize a hiatus hernia or other abnormality of the cardia.

TABLE 4.1. RELATIVE CONTRAINDICATIONS TO UPPER ENDOSCOPY

Medically unstable patient (i.e., marked hypotension, acute myocardial infarction, respiratory distress)
Unstable cervical spine
Coagulopathy, unresponsive to therapy
Known or suspected perforation of the gastrointestinal tract

Several situations require special consideration when endoscopy is used to evaluate patients with suspected specific esophageal disorders. Patients with suspected achalasia should have a prolonged fast preceded by a clear liquid diet for 24 to 48 hours to allow any food matter to pass into the stomach before endoscopy (see Chapter 11). Large-bore tube lavage may be required to remove semisolid material that does not pass spontaneously into the stomach. The staff assisting with the endoscopy should be prepared to suction the oropharynx and prevent aspiration. Similar precautions should be used in patients with significant dysphagia. They may have structural abnormalities of the upper esophagus that could increase the risk of perforation or aspiration. If a recent barium study is not available, caution should be used in passing the endoscope. If patients have severe dysphagia for solids, it may be advantageous to schedule the procedure with the availability of fluoroscopy to assist in dilatation if a significant stricture is encountered. Patients with a known or suspected Zenker's diverticulum should also undergo endoscopy with caution because the lumen of the esophagus may be difficult to identify and follow. Forceful manipulation of the endoscope inside the diverticulum could lead to perforation (see Chapter 16).

DIAGNOSTIC UPPER ENDOSCOPY AND TISSUE SAMPLING

Imaging the esophageal mucosa during endoscopy is extremely useful in clarifying symptoms. High-resolution video images allow the endoscopist and others in the endoscopy suite to view mucosal irregularities with great convenience and excellent image quality. Even though some abnormalities appear unique enough to lead to a specific diagnosis, most abnormalities require histologic or cytologic confirmation. This can be easily accomplished with standard biopsy techniques, brush cytology, or endoscopic mucosal resection.

Biopsy forceps are used to obtain tissue at endoscopy. Forceps vary by size, style, and design. Adequate mucosal sampling can be obtained with most standard biopsy forceps. Certain endoscopic maneuvers, such as the "turn and suction" technique (9), may be used to increase the biopsy size. This technique involves pulling an open-jawed forceps until it is flush with the end of the endoscopy, turning the entire endoscope into the tissues, suctioning air from the lumen to allow esophageal mucosa to collapse into the open forceps, and then closing the forceps. Jumbo, or large-capacity, forceps have a very low risk of complication. Jumbo forceps require an endoscope with at least a 3.2-mm diameter biopsy channel. These accessories allow the endoscopist to obtain larger samples of mucosa and submucosa for histologic evaluation (10), although current data suggest that this may not reduce the sampling error inherent in small mucosal biopsies (11). Endoscopic mucosal resection is both a diagnostic and a therapeutic technique that can remove larger sections (>1 cm^2) of tissue. A variety of techniques have been described (12,13), although all involve separating the mucosa from deeper layers by injection of fluid into the submucosa, followed by mucosal resection with specially developed snaring devices.

Brush cytology is routinely performed in all areas of the gastrointestinal tract with specially designed disposable brushes (14). The sheathed cytology brush is advanced through the biopsy channel of the endoscope and placed in contact with the mucosa to be examined. Vigorous motion of the brush against the mucosa allows cells to be captured on the bristles of the brush. The brush is then retracted into its sheath and removed from the endoscope. The brush is then placed in contact with a glass slide, and the captured cells are transferred to its surface. The slide is treated with a fixative and submitted to the cytologist for staining. Malignancy (14), infections, dysplasia, and even *Helicobacter pylori* (15) can be detected by brush cytology.

Endoscopic Ultrasound

Endoscopic ultrasound (EUS) is a valuable tool for imaging the entire depth of the esophagus, and periesophageal structures. The main applications of EUS in the esophagus are staging of cancer of the esophagus (16), imaging submucosal lesions (17,18), and evaluation of esophageal varices (19,20). Transesophageal EUS is also a safe and effective method for imaging the mediastinum in patients with mediastinal masses or lung cancer (21).

The principal advantage of EUS over other imaging modalities is the ability to image from directly adjacent to or within the lesion of interest. This eliminates the problem of intervening structures (bone, bowel gas) and allows the use of higher ultrasound frequencies (5.0 to 30 MHz), which provide higher resolution images. Another major advance in EUS is the ability to perform image-guided fine needle aspiration (FNA) and core biopsy, which have substantially improved the accuracy, especially in assessing lymph nodes for tumor spread (22).

Currently available ultrasound technologies include dedicated radial and linear endoscope systems and through-the-scope miniprobes (Fig. 4.2). These devices are attached to an ultrasound processor that includes a control panel to manipulate the ultrasound image on a high-resolution monitor. The most commonly used system for the evaluation of esophageal disease is the Olympus (Tokyo, Japan) 360-degree radial-scanning instrument operating at 5.0 to 20 MHz. These devices also have standard video optics for endoscopic evaluation. The outer diameter of echoendoscopes (12 to 13 mm) is larger than for standard endoscopes. In patients with esophageal cancer, approximately one third require dilation to perform a complete EUS examination, although this procedure is safe when performed using standard dilation methods (23,24). A narrow-

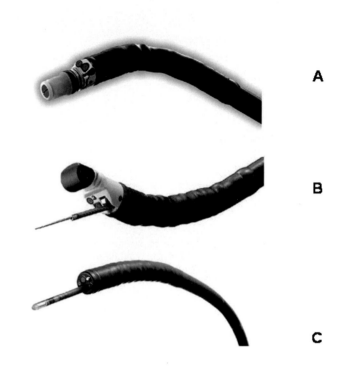

FIGURE 4.2. A: Radial echoendoscope. **B:** Linear echoendoscope with fine needle aspiration device. **C:** Endoscopic ultrasound miniprobe within the accessory channel of a standard gastroscope (all from Olympus, Melville, NY).

diameter, non-optical EUS device can be passed over a guidewire and does not require dilation of esophageal strictures (25).

EUS miniprobes are particularly useful in evaluation of superficial lesions of the esophagus. These catheter-type systems can be passed through the accessory channel of standard endoscopes and provide 360-degree imaging at 12, 20, and 30 MHz. Miniprobes provide excellent resolution of the esophageal wall (Fig. 4.3) but have a limited depth of penetration (26). They are best used for imaging mucosal and small submucosal abnormalities involving the esophageal wall. Special water-filled balloons or condoms are useful for obtaining good acoustic coupling and reducing aspiration risk in the esophagus (27). One novel application of EUS miniprobes is the investigation of noncardiac chest pain through ambulatory imaging of longitudinal esophageal muscle contractions (and thus thickening of the muscle layer) (28).

Two dedicated endoscope systems (Pentax and Olympus) have curved linear array transducers. Both devices are designed primarily for ultrasound guidance during FNA procedures such as sampling celiac lymph nodes in patients with esophageal cancer (29) or transesophageal FNA of mediastinal lesions (21). These devices also have Doppler

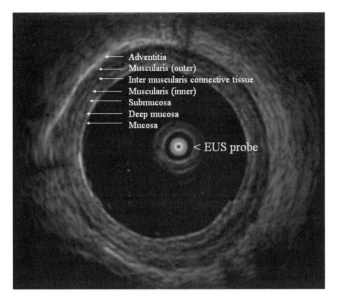

FIGURE 4.3. Endoscopic ultrasound image of the esophagus using a high-frequency (20 MHz) miniprobe. The anatomic layers of the esophagus wall, including the inner and outer muscularis propria, are identified as alternating bright and dark bands.

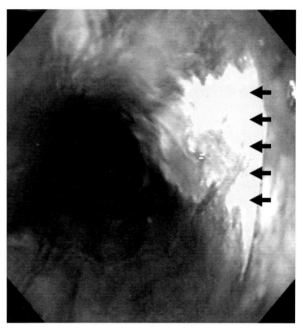

FIGURE 4.4. Lugol's iodine chromoendoscopy of patient with superficial squamous cell carcinoma. Note the focal area of non-staining (*arrows*) in the region of carcinoma compared to the rich brown-green staining of normal squamous epithelium.

ultrasound capability and have been applied to the evaluation of portal hypertension (20), flow within the thoracic duct (30), identification of aberrant vascular anatomy as a cause of dysphagia lusoria (31), and characterization and guiding resection of esophageal submucosal tumors (17,32).

Chromoendoscopy

Chromoendoscopy refers to methods in which dyes are applied to enhance specific mucosal details followed by endoscopic inspection. The two most commonly used dyes are Lugol's iodine and methylene blue. In general, Lugol's iodine is most useful for evaluation of the squamous mucosa of the esophagus, and methylene blue is most useful for evaluation of Barrett's and other columnar epithelium of the esophagus.

Lugol's solution stains the glycogen-containing normal esophageal mucosa a dark green-brown. Any abnormality of the squamous epithelium that does not contain glycogen (carcinoma, intestinal metaplasia, and inflammation) appears unstained when the dye is sprayed throughout the mucosa (33) (Fig. 4.4). Up to 50 mL of a 1% solution can be sprayed onto the mucosa during endoscopy to detect subtle areas of abnormality and to direct biopsy. Lugol's iodine has been used to detect early carcinoma of the esophagus and areas of dysplasia in patients at high risk of squamous cell cancer (see Chapter 13). A population study in a region of China with a high incidence of squamous cell cancer found that Lugol's staining significantly improved the sensitivity for detection of dysplasia and early cancer (34).

Other potential high-risk populations who may benefit from Lugol's chromoendoscopy include patients with head and neck cancers (35), and heavy users of alcohol and tobacco (36,37).

Although generally safe, Lugol's iodine can cause local irritation to the esophagus, and retrosternal pain. One study suggests that application of sodium thiosulfate following the procedure reduced this symptom (38). Lugol's should be avoided in patients with known allergy to iodine.

Methylene blue is another stain that is taken up into the cytoplasm of actively absorbing epithelial cells such as normal small intestine, colon, and specialized intestinal metaplasia (SIM) of the esophagus. The technique involves application of a mucolytic agent, typically 10% *N*-acetylcysteine (Mucomyst), followed by methylene blue 0.5% to 1.0%, then washing the excess dye with water. In theory, methylene blue should improve the ability to detect SIM and dysplasia of the esophagus. However, results of published trials have been highly variable, with some studies suggesting it is useful (39–42) and other studies finding it did not detect SIM or dysplasia more than random biopsy (43,44). At least one study has suggested methylene blue increases complications (primarily vomiting) and procedure duration (44). Reasons for the variable results include variation in the application technique and study design (45). Until better standardization and consistent results are available, methylene blue should be considered investigational.

Magnification Endoscopy

Magnification endoscopy uses endoscopes capable of viewing mucosal detail at high magnification (35- to 100-fold) in conjunction with chromoendoscopy techniques to enhance mucosal architecture and biochemical staining patterns. This technique has been used in Barrett's esophagus, to improve detection of SIM and dysplasia with encouraging early results. Guelrud and colleagues (46) used a 35× magnification endoscope (GIF-200z, Olympus America, Melville, NY) and 10% acetic acid, which causes reversible denaturation of intracellular cytoplasmic proteins and enhances mucosal details in Barrett's esophagus and the uterine cervix. They classified the mucosal pattern into four distinct patterns based on the pattern of "pits" in the mucosa (Color Plate 4.5). SIM was seen in 100% of pattern IV, 87% of pattern III, 11% of pattern II, and 0% of pattern I.

Endo and co-workers found similar results using a 100× magnification endoscope (GIF Q240z, Olympus, Japan) and methylene blue staining. They classified the pattern slightly differently, but found that mucosa with irregular, villiform or nonlinear sulci was highly associated with SIM, intestinal type mucins, and a high proliferation index as measured by antibody staining to Ki-67.

As with early results of chromoendoscopy, further study is needed to confirm the value of magnification endoscopy. A further limitation of magnification endoscopy is the inherent focus on small regions of tissue. Methods to survey large areas rapidly and then focus down on potentially abnormal regions are still needed.

Tissue Spectroscopy

In the gastrointestinal tract, spectroscopy is largely applied to the detection of dysplasia. By quantifying the color and brightness of light, spectroscopy can detect a variety of properties relevant to esophageal diseases, including biochemical changes within the cell, extracellular matrix, and nuclear size and density. Because of this ability, many spectroscopic techniques have been referred to as *optical biopsy*, although this term is misleading in that spectroscopy does not require excisional biopsy and provides both qualitative and quantitative information about tissues.

Although spectroscopy is unlikely to replace tissue biopsy, many aspects of spectroscopy offer advantages over standard biopsy. A major problem of current gastrointestinal pathology is the significant variability in the diagnosis of dysplasia. This is especially true in Barrett's esophagus (48). One reason for such variation is the subjective nature of determining dysplastic characteristics such as increased nuclear size, nuclear crowding, and architectural disorganization. By providing a more quantitative measure of features such as nuclear size and number, or changes in collagen and porphyrin concentrations, spectroscopic methods

may enhance the current qualitative measures used in pathologic diagnosis.

Endoscopic biopsy is also limited by the time delay between endoscopy and the histologic results. Spectroscopic methods are capable of rendering a diagnosis in "real time," thus allowing spectroscopy-directed biopsy of patients with dysplasia and avoiding unnecessary biopsy in patients without dysplasia.

A third limitation of endoscopic biopsy is the inherent "sampling error." This is exemplified by the fact that 30% to 50% of Barrett's patients with the diagnosis of high-grade dysplasia on random biopsy have invasive cancer at the time of esophagectomy (49–58). Spectroscopy has the potential to overcome many of these problems by providing objective, real-time information over large areas of tissue.

Types of Spectroscopy

Several types of spectroscopy have been applied to diseases of the esophagus, including laser-induced fluorescence (LIF), light scattering (LSS), and reflectance spectroscopy. LIF relies on the principle that many biologic molecules (called *fluorophores*) give off "fluorescence" when stimulated by light (Table 4.2). Fluorescence is cause by absorption of light energy and elevation of electrons to higher energy states. When the electrons fall back to a lower (but not the original) energy state, light energy of a different (longer) wavelength is emitted. Because diseased tissue contains different concentrations and different structures of these fluorophores, the pattern of light that they give off provides a "fingerprint" of the tissue that can be used to diagnose whether it is normal or diseased.

Laser-Induced Fluorescence

LIF requires the use of monochromatic or narrowband light to induce fluorescence. This can be accomplished with laser devices or filtered white light sources. One advantage of filtered white light is the lower cost and smaller size of the light source, thus making these more adaptable to current endoscope systems. Fluorescence from the tissue is detected using optical probes, which are passed through the endo-

TABLE 4.2. IMPORTANT FLUOROPHORES USED IN LASER INDUCED FLUORESCENCE

Fluorophore	Maximum Excitation Wavelength	Maximum Emission Wavelength
Collagen	335 nm	390 nm
NADH	340 nm	460 nm
FAD	460 nm	520 nm
Porphyrins 390 nm	390 nm	630–680 nm

FAD, flavin adenine dinucleotide; NADH, nicotinamide adenine dinucleotide.

scope channel, or analysis of images from specialized, highly sensitive CCD video cameras. LIF used alone is accurate for the detection of high-grade dysplasia in Barrett's esophagus but has poor sensitivity for low-grade dysplasia (59,60).

One of the fluorophores that characterizes dysplastic epithelium is protoporphyrin IX (PPIX) which accumulates in dysplastic and malignant cells as a result of relative deficiencies of ferrochelatase, the enzyme that metabolizes PPIX (61). One of the limitations of LIF (and all spectroscopy methods) is that the weak signal often requires highly sensitive optical probes in direct contact with the tissue. This limits the amount of mucosa that can be examined similar to the way biopsy is limited to the site in contact with the biopsy forceps. One method to enhance the LIF effect is to apply an exogenous precursor to PPIX, such as aminolevulinic acid. This technique, commonly termed "photodynamic diagnosis," increases the relative fluorescence signal in dysplastic tissue, allows imaging of broad areas of mucosa with specially adapted endoscopic instruments, and appears capable of detecting dysplasia in Barrett's mucosa (62).

Light Scattering Spectroscopy

LSS measures the extent to which photons of light are elastically (without loss of energy) scattered by the structures they encounter. Three factors that determine how light scatters are the size of the structures, the number of structures, and the color of light used to illuminate the structure. We have exploited this phenomenon by measuring the number and the size of nuclei in patients with Barrett's esophagus as a measure of dysplasia (63–65). Dysplasia in Barrett's esophagus is characterized by an increased population of enlarged and more optically dense nuclei, likely due to the increased ploidy of tightly wound DNA in the replicating cell (Fig. 4.6). As with LIF, LSS has also been applied to broad area imaging *ex vivo* (66) and instruments are in development for *in vivo* broad area imaging.

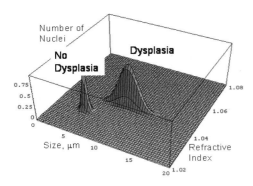

FIGURE 4.6. Light-scattering spectroscopy (LSS) plot of Barrett's epithelium with and without dysplasia. LSS determines the size and population density of nuclei in the superficial esophageal layer and classifies dysplasia when an increased number and size of nuclei are found.

Reflectance Spectroscopy

Reflectance spectroscopy measures the color and intensity of light that is either absorbed or reflected from tissues. The wavelength (color) of light is not altered; however, if one uses a white light, which contains many colors of the spectrum, some of those colors are absorbed and some reflected. Thus, if white light is used to illuminate an inflamed colon, it appears red because the blue light is absorbed by hemoglobin and the red is reflected back. By analyzing the exact amount of blue light that is absorbed, the concentration of hemoglobin, a measure of blood flow, can be precisely determined.

Summary

Each type of spectroscopy measures independent and complementary information about the tissue. By combining these three forms (LIF, LSS, reflectance), the detection of dysplasia in Barrett's is improved compared to any single technique (67).

Spectroscopic techniques, like many fundamental scientific developments, are slow in transitioning from the laboratory to clinical applications. None of the current methods is currently suitable for routine use in surveillance of patients with Barrett's esophagus but all are being investigated. As the techniques become more sensitive, rapid, and capable of imaging broad areas of esophagus, they will likely become an important adjunct to routine endoscopic inspection and biopsy.

Optical Coherence Tomography

Optical coherence tomography (OCT), like EUS, provides two-dimensional cross-sectional images of the GI tract and is capable of resolving the four layers of the intestine (mucosa, submucosa, muscularis, and serosa or adventitia). Instead of using ultrasound, OCT uses light waves. This increases the resolution up to tenfold greater than high-frequency EUS and approaches that of light microscopy.

Tearney and colleagues (68) reported the first use of OCT to image the human esophagus and colon in postmortem specimens. For this study, tissues were excised and imaged in saline (although OCT images, unlike ultrasound, can be obtained through air) and compared with histologic specimens. Newer OCT systems have substantially improved the optical resolution and applied OCT to the imaging of Barrett's mucosa and early carcinoma (69–74).

OCT has many advantages over currently available imaging modalities and tissue biopsy. In comparison to histology, OCT does not require excision of tissue with all of its associated complications, cost, and time delay. Thus, large regions of tissue can be surveyed for pathology and biopsy reserved to confirm abnormalities seen on imaging. OCT is readily adaptable to current endoscopic instruments. The system can be engineered to approximately the size of a personal computer, and the optical probes are easily passed through small-diameter endoscope channels. In comparison to high-frequency ultrasound, the tenfold increase in image resolution may overcome several limitations of EUS, namely identification of high-grade dysplasia (75) and poor accuracy of distinguishing tumor invasion of muscularis propria (76). In comparison to spectroscopy methods, the primary advantage of OCT is the quality of anatomic images obtained, which are critical to tumor differentiation and staging.

CONCLUSION

Just as the invention of fiberoptics allowed major advances in our understanding of the esophagus, advanced imaging methods will further expand our knowledge and clinical options. Advanced optical methods will likely play a valuable role in gastrointestinal imaging, giving the endoscopist a window into intracellular anatomy and function. They will also provide a unique method of monitoring disease *in vivo* and overcoming many of the limitations of endoscopic biopsy.

ACKNOWLEDGMENTS

I thank Steve Edmundowicz for his contribution to this chapter in the third edition of the textbook and for materials adapted to this edition. I also thank Mrs. Sylvia Holmes for editorial assistance.

REFERENCES

1. Hopkins H, Kapany N. A flexible fiberscope using static scanning. *Nature* 1954;173:39–41.
2. Hirschowitz B. A personal history of the fiberscope. *Gastroenterology* 1979;76:864–869.
3. Hisanaga K, Hisanaga A, Nagata K, et al. High speed rotating scanner for transgastric sonography. *AJR Am J Roentgenol* 1980; 135:627–639.
4. DiMagno EP, Buxton JL, Regan PT, et al. Ultrasonic endoscope. *Lancet* 1980;22:629–631.
5. Triadafilopoulos G, Utley DS. Temperature-controlled radiofrequency energy delivery for gastroesophageal reflux disease: the Stretta procedure. *J Laparoendosc Adv Surg Tech A* 2001;11(6): 333–339.
6. Filipi CJ, Lehman GA, Rothstein RI, et al. Transoral, flexible endoscopic suturing for treatment of GERD: a multicenter trial. *Gastrointest Endosc* 2001;53(4):416–422.
7. Cotton PB, Williams CB, eds. *Practical gastrointestinal endoscopy*, third ed. Cambridge: Blackwell Science, 1990.
8. Baillie J. *Gastrointestinal endoscopy: basic principles and practice.* Boston: Butterworth-Heinemann, 1992.
9. Levine DS, Reid BJ. Endoscopic biopsy technique for acquiring larger mucosal samples. *Gastrointest Endosc* 1991;37(3):332–337.
10. Bernstein DE, Barkin JS, Reiner DK, et al. Standard biopsy forceps versus large-capacity forceps with and without needle. *Gastrointest Endosc* 1995;41(6):573–576.
11. Falk GW, Rice TW, Goldblum JR, et al. Jumbo biopsy forceps protocol still misses unsuspected cancer in Barrett's esophagus with high-grade dysplasia. *Gastrointest Endosc* 1999;49(2): 170–176.
12. Inoue H, Takeshita K, Hori H, et al. Endoscopic mucosal resection with a cap-fitted panendoscope for esophagus, stomach, and colon mucosal lesions [see comments]. *Gastrointest Endosc* 1993; 39(1):58–62.
13. Matsuda K. Introduction to endoscopic mucosal resection. *Gastrointest Endosc Clin North Am* 2001;11(3):439–443.
14. Camp R, Rutkowski MA, Atkison K, et al. A prospective, randomized, blinded trial of cytological yield with disposable cytology brushes in upper gastrointestinal tract lesions. *Am J Gastroenterol* 1992;87(10):1439–1442.
15. Mendoza ML, Martin-Rabadan P, Carrion I, et al. *Helicobacter pylori* infection. Rapid diagnosis with brush cytology. *Acta Cytol* 1993;37(2):181–185.
16. Mallery S, Van Dam J. EUS in the evaluation of esophageal carcinoma. *Gastrointest Endosc* 2000;52[Suppl 6]:S6–S11.
17. Waxman I, Saitoh Y, Raju GS, et al. High-frequency probe EUS-assisted endoscopic mucosal resection: a therapeutic strategy for submucosal tumors of the GI tract. *Gastrointest Endosc* 2002;55 (1):44–49.
18. Takada N, Higashino M, Osugi H, et al. Utility of endoscopic ultrasonography in assessing the indications for endoscopic surgery of submucosal esophageal tumors. *Surg Endosc* 1999;13 (3):228–230.
19. Hino S, Kakutani H, Ikeda K, et al. Hemodynamic assessment of the left gastric vein in patients with esophageal varices with color Doppler EUS: factors affecting development of esophageal varices. *Gastrointest Endosc* 2002;55(4):512–517.
20. Miller LS. Endoscopic ultrasound in the evaluation of portal hypertension. *Gastrointest Endosc Clin North Am* 1999;9(2): 271–285.
21. Wallace MB, Silvestri GA, Sahai AV, et al. Endoscopic ultrasound-guided fine needle aspiration for staging patients with carcinoma of the lung. *Ann Thorac Surg* 2001;72(6):1861–1867.
22. Vazquez-Sequeiros E, Norton ID, Clain JE, et al. Impact of EUS-guided fine-needle aspiration on lymph node staging in patients with esophageal carcinoma. *Gastrointest Endosc* 2001;53(7): 751–757.
23. Wallace MB, Hawes RH, Sahai AV, et al. Dilation of malignant esophageal stenosis to allow EUS guided fine-needle aspiration: safety and effect on patient management. *Gastrointest Endosc* 2000;51(3):309–313.
24. Pfau PR, Ginsberg GG, Lew RJ, et al. Esophageal dilation for endosonographic evaluation of malignant esophageal strictures is safe and effective. *Am J Gastroenterol* 2000;95(10): 2813–2815.
25. Mallery S, Van Dam J. Increased rate of complete EUS staging of patients with esophageal cancer using the nonoptical, wire-guided echoendoscope. *Gastrointest Endosc* 1999;50(1):53–57.
26. Chak A, Canto M, Stevens PD, et al. Clinical applications of a new through-the-scope ultrasound probe: prospective comparison with an ultrasound endoscope. *Gastrointest Endosc* 1997;45 (3):291–295.
27. Wallace MB, Hoffman BJ, Sahai AS, et al. Imaging of esophageal tumors with a water-filled condom and a catheter US probe. *Gastrointest Endosc* 2000;51(5):597–600.
28. Pehlivanov N, Liu J, Mittal RK. Sustained esophageal contraction: a motor correlate of heartburn symptom. *Am J Physiol Gastrointest Liver Physiol* 2001;281(3):G743–G751.
29. Eloubeidi MA, Wallace MB, Reed CE, et al. The utility of EUS and EUS-guided fine needle aspiration in detecting celiac lymph

node metastasis in patients with esophageal cancer: a single-center experience. *Gastrointest Endosc* 2001;54(6):714–719.

30. Parasher VK, Meroni E, Malesci A, et al. Observation of thoracic duct morphology in portal hypertension by endoscopic ultrasound. *Gastrointest Endosc* 1998;48(6):588–592.

31. De Luca L, Bergman JJ, Tytgat GN, et al. EUS imaging of the arteria lusoria: case series and review. *Gastrointest Endosc* 2000; 52(5):670–673.

32. Sun S, Wang M. Use of endoscopic ultrasound-guided injection in endoscopic resection of solid submucosal tumors. *Endoscopy* 2002;34(1):82–85.

33. Fennerty MB. Tissue staining. *Gastrointest Endosc Clin North Am* 1994;4(2):297–311.

34. Dawsey SM, Fleischer DE, Wang GQ, et al. Mucosal iodine staining improves endoscopic visualization of squamous dysplasia and squamous cell carcinoma of the esophagus in Linxian, China. *Cancer* 1998;83(2):220–231.

35. Tincani AJ, Brandalise N, Altemani A, et al. Diagnosis of superficial esophageal cancer and dysplasia using endoscopic screening with a 2% Lugol dye solution in patients with head and neck cancer. *Head Neck* 2000;22(2):170–174.

36. Fagundes RB, de Barros SG, Putten AC, et al. Occult dysplasia is disclosed by Lugol chromoendoscopy in alcoholics at high risk for squamous cell carcinoma of the esophagus. *Endoscopy* 1999;31(4):281–285.

37. Meyer V, Burtin P, Bour B, et al. Endoscopic detection of early esophageal cancer in a high-risk population: does Lugol staining improve videoendoscopy? *Gastrointest Endosc* 1997;45(6): 480–484.

38. Kondo H, Fukuda H, Ono H, et al. Sodium thiosulfate solution spray for relief of irritation caused by Lugol's stain in chromoendoscopy. *Gastrointest Endosc* 2001;53(2):199–202.

39. Canto MI, Setrakian S, Petras RE, et al. Methylene blue selectively stains intestinal metaplasia in Barrett's esophagus. *Gastrointest Endosc* 1996;44(1):1–7.

40. Canto MI, Setrakian S, Willis J, et al. Methylene blue-directed biopsies improve detection of intestinal metaplasia and dysplasia in Barrett's esophagus. *Gastrointest Endosc* 2000;51(5):560–568.

41. Sharma P, Topalovski M, Mayo MS, et al. Methylene blue chromoendoscopy for detection of short-segment Barrett's esophagus. *Gastrointest Endosc* 2001;54(3):289–293.

42. Kiesslich R, Hahn M, Herrmann G, et al. Screening for specialized columnar epithelium with methylene blue: chromoendoscopy in patients with Barrett's esophagus and a normal control group. *Gastrointest Endosc* 2001;53(1):47–52.

43. Wo JM, Ray MB, Mayfield-Stokes S, et al. Comparison of methylene blue-directed biopsies and conventional biopsies in the detection of intestinal metaplasia and dysplasia in Barrett's esophagus: a preliminary study. *Gastrointest Endosc* 2001;54(3): 294–301.

44. Dave U, Shousha S, Westaby D. Methylene blue staining: Is it really useful in Barrett's esophagus? *Gastrointest Endosc* 2001;53 (3):333–335.

45. Wong RK, Horwhat JD, Maydonovitch CL. Sky blue or murky waters: the diagnostic utility of methylene blue. *Gastrointest Endosc* 2001;54(3):409–413.

46. Guelrud M, Herrera I, Essenfeld H, et al. Enhanced magnification endoscopy: a new technique to identify specialized intestinal metaplasia in Barrett's esophagus. *Gastrointest Endosc* 2001;53 (6):559–565.

47. Endo T, Awakawa T, Takahashi H, et al. Classification of Barrett's epithelium by magnifying endoscopy. *Gastrointestinal Endoscopy* 2002;55(6):641–647.

48. Reid BJ, Haggitt RC, Rubin CE, et al. Observer variation in the diagnosis of dysplasia in Barrett's esophagus. *Hum Pathol* 1988; 19(2):166–178.

49. Reid BJ, Weinstein WM, Lewin KJ, et al. Endoscopic biopsy can detect high-grade dysplasia or early adenocarcinoma in Barrett's esophagus without grossly recognizable neoplastic lesions. *Gastroenterology* 1988;94(1):81–90.

50. DeMeester TR, Attwood SE, Smyrk TC, et al. Surgical therapy in Barrett's esophagus. *Ann Surg* 1990;212(4):528–540; discussion 540–542.

51. Altorki NK, Skinner DB, Segalin A, et al. Indications for esophagectomy in nonmalignant Barrett's esophagus: a 10- year experience [see comments]. *Ann Thorac Surg* 1990;49(5): 724–726; discussion 727.

52. Pera M, Trastek VF, Carpenter HA, et al. Barrett's esophagus with high-grade dysplasia: an indication for esophagectomy? *Ann Thorac Surg* 1992;54(2):199–204.

53. Rice TW, Falk GW, Achkar E, et al. Surgical management of high-grade dysplasia in Barrett's esophagus [see comments]. *Am J Gastroenterol* 1993;88(11):1832–1836.

54. Rusch VW, Levine DS, Haggitt R, et al. The management of high grade dysplasia and early cancer in Barrett's esophagus. A multidisciplinary problem. *Cancer* 1994;74(4):1225–1229.

55. Cameron AJ, Carpenter HA. Barrett's esophagus, high-grade dysplasia, and early adenocarcinoma: a pathological study. *Am J Gastroenterol* 1997;92(4):586–591.

56. Ferguson MK, Naunheim KS. Resection for Barrett's mucosa with high-grade dysplasia: implications for prophylactic photodynamic therapy. *J Thorac Cardiovasc Surg* 1997;114(5): 824–829.

57. Heitmiller RF, Redmond M, Hamilton SR. Barrett's esophagus with high-grade dysplasia. An indication for prophylactic esophagectomy. *Ann Surg* 1996;224(1):66–71.

58. Edwards MJ, Gable DR, Lentsch AB, et al. The rationale for esophagectomy as the optimal therapy for Barrett's esophagus with high-grade dysplasia. *Ann Surg* 1996;223(5):585–589; discussion 589–591.

59. Mayinger B, Horner P, Jordan M, et al. Light-induced autofluorescence spectroscopy for the endoscopic detection of esophageal cancer. *Gastrointest Endosc* 2001;54(2):195–201.

60. Panjehpour M, Overholt BF, Vo-Dinh T, et al. Endoscopic fluorescence detection of high-grade dysplasia in Barrett's esophagus. *Gastroenterology* 1996;111(1):93–101.

61. Grant WE, Hopper C, MacRobert AJ, et al. Photodynamic therapy of oral cancer: photosensitisation with systemic aminolaevulinic acid. *Lancet* 1993;342(8864):147–148.

62. Messmann H, Knuchel R, Baumler W, et al. Endoscopic fluorescence detection of dysplasia in patients with Barrett's esophagus, ulcerative colitis, or adenomatous polyps after 5-aminolevulinic acid-induced protoporphyrin IX sensitization [see comments]. *Gastrointest Endosc* 1999;49(1):97–101.

63. Wallace M, Shields S, Perelman LT, et al. Fiber-optic detection of low-grade dysplasia in patients with Barrett's esophagus using reflectance spectroscopy [abstract]. *Gastroenterology* 1998;114: A1336.

64. Perelman LT, Backman V, Wallace MB, et al. Observation of periodic fine structure in reflectance from biological tissue: a new technique for measuring nuclear size distribution. *Phys Rev Let* 1998;80(3):627–630.

65. Backman V, Wallace MB, Perelman LT, et al. Detection of preinvasive cancer cells. *Nature* 2000;406(6791):35–36.

66. Gurjar RS, Backman V, Perelman LT, et al. Imaging human epithelial properties with polarized light-scattering spectroscopy. *Nat Med* 2001;7(11):1245–1248.

67. Georgakoudi I, Jacobson BC, Van Dam J, et al. Fluorescence, reflectance, and light-scattering spectroscopy for evaluating dysplasia in patients with Barrett's esophagus. *Gastroenterology* 2001; 120(7):1620–1629.

68. Tearney GJ, Brezinski ME, Southern JF, et al. Optical biopsy in

human gastrointestinal tissue using optical coherence tomography. *Am J Gastroenterol* 1997;92(10):1800–1804.

69. Kobayashi K, Izatt JA, Kulkarni MD, et al. High-resolution cross-sectional imaging of the gastrointestinal tract using optical coherence tomography: preliminary results. *Gastrointest Endosc* 1998;47(6):515–523.

70. Pitris C, Jesser C, Boppart SA, et al. Feasibility of optical coherence tomography for high-resolution imaging of human gastrointestinal tract malignancies. *J Gastroenterol* 2000;35(2): 87–92.

71. Sivak MV Jr, Kobayashi K, Izatt JA, et al. High-resolution endoscopic imaging of the GI tract using optical coherence tomography. *Gastrointest Endosc* 2000;51(4 Pt 1):474–479.

72. Bouma BE, Tearney GJ, Compton CC, et al. High-resolution imaging of the human esophagus and stomach *in vivo* using optical coherence tomography. *Gastrointest Endosc* 2000;51(4 Pt 1):467–474.

73. Jackle S, Gladkova N, Feldchtein F, et al. *In vivo* endoscopic optical coherence tomography of esophagitis, Barrett's esophagus, and adenocarcinoma of the esophagus. *Endoscopy* 2000;32(10): 750–755.

74. Li XD, Boppart SA, Van Dam J, et al. Optical coherence tomography: advanced technology for the endoscopic imaging of Barrett's esophagus. *Endoscopy* 2000;32(12):921–930.

75. Falk GW, Catalano MF, Sivak MV Jr, et al. Endosonography in the evaluation of patients with Barrett's esophagus and high-grade dysplasia. *Gastrointest Endosc* 1994;40(2 Pt 1):207–212.

76. Brugge WR, Lee MJ, Carey RW, et al. Endoscopic ultrasound staging criteria for esophageal cancer. *Gastrointest Endosc* 1997;45 (2):147–152.

ESOPHAGEAL MANOMETRY

JANICE FREEMAN
AMINE HILA
DONALD O. CASTELL

During the past 2 decades, there has been increased interest in studies of esophageal function, stimulated primarily by the growing use of laparoscopic antireflux surgery. Improvements in methodology providing accurate measurement of intraluminal pressures began this reawakening, with studies of the lower esophageal sphincter (LES), continuing through the refinements in the measurement of esophageal peristaltic pressures and, finally, upper esophageal sphincter (UES) evaluation. In addition, initial studies showing that large amounts of gastrin could increase LES pressure opened the door to a whole series of investigations of the effects of hormones and the effects of a variety of other possible pharmacologic agents on esophageal function.

Esophageal manometry is a diagnostic test that measures intraluminal pressures and coordination of pressure activity of the muscles of the esophagus (Fig. 5.1). It provides both qualitative and quantitative assessment of the esophageal pressures, coordination, and motility. Manometric studies are used in the assessment of patients with symptoms suggestive of esophageal origin such as dysphagia, odynophagia, noncardiac chest pain, and chronic cough. A manometric study is also indicated before antireflux surgery and assessment of possible esophageal involvement in systemic disorders such as scleroderma and chronic idiopathic pseudoobstruction (Table 5.1).

MATERIALS AND EQUIPMENT

The equipment and materials required to perform esophageal motility testing can be divided into a primary equipment group and a secondary materials group. The primary group consists of relatively expensive, interconnected electronic equipment that make up the permanent part of the motility system. The secondary group is made up of relatively inexpensive and generally consumable materials required to assist in the performance of the motility study.

There are two types of esophageal motility systems within the primary equipment group: water perfusion and solid-state. Both systems use esophageal motility catheters, series of measuring instruments (transducers), and a recording and analysis device (physiograph or computer). In addition, a water perfusion pump is required for the former. Both systems measure strength and assess the coordination of the muscles of the esophagus and its sphincters, and they both transmit and convert this information into a permanent record that is easy to read and interpret. However, each system performs this function differently.

Primary Equipment

The function of the primary equipment is to sense the pressure activity of the esophagus and to transmit and convert this to a permanent record that is easily read, measured, and stored. This equipment includes the manometry catheter system, transducers, and the physiograph or computer.

The motility catheter is inserted into the esophagus and measures the pressures of the esophageal contractions. It is a specially designed long, flexible tube. There are two main types of manometry catheter systems. The water infusion system consists of a catheter made up of small capillary tubes that make up the manometry catheter, have an internal diameter of approximately 0.8 mm, and have an opening or port at a known point along the length of the catheter. One commonly used catheter has eight capillary tubes around a larger central tube with an overall diameter of 4.5 mm (Fig. 5.2). The eight orifices, or ports, of this catheter are arranged so that the four distal ports have a radial orientation of 90

J. Freeman, A. Hila, D.O. Castell: Medical University of South Carolina, Charleston, South Carolina.

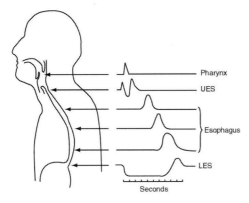

FIGURE 5.1. Schematic representation of the pressure sequence of a normal primary peristaltic wave. At the onset of the swallow, both the upper and lower esophageal sphincters relax. A peristaltic contraction begins at the pharynx and continues through the esophagus.

degrees and are either 1 cm apart or at the same level. The four proximal ports are 5 cm apart and are also radially oriented (Fig. 5.3). Each lumen is connected to an external transducer. The infusion pump perfuses the capillary tubes with water at a rate of 0.5 mL/min. When a catheter port is occluded (e.g., by a muscular contraction), the water pressure builds within the catheter exerting a force, which is transmitted to the external transducer.

The solid-state esophageal motility catheter is a soft, flexible tube with microtransducers contained within the catheter. These microtransducers measure esophageal contractions directly from the esophageal or sphincter wall (Fig. 5.4). Type of transducer (circumferential or unidirectional) and number and placement of transducers are variable (Fig. 5.5).

The diameter of the catheter used in our laboratory is 4.6 mm, although transducer number, spacing, and size

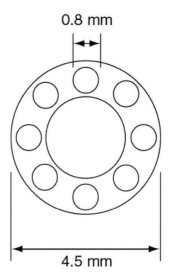

FIGURE 5.2. Cross section of an eight-lumen water-perfused esophageal manometry catheter showing the internal diameter of individual catheters and the diameter of the entire catheter.

(length and diameter) vary among manufacturers. Catheters or transducers of different diameter (water perfusion or solid-state) measure different pressures, both in the two sphincters (LES and UES), and the esophageal body (1,2). Small catheter diameter or transducer diameter yields lower pressures. Conversely, large diameter or larger transducer diameter yields higher pressures. When using catheters with smaller diameter, this should be an important consideration in the determination of normal values for minimum and maximum pressures.

TABLE 5.1. SUGGESTED CLINICAL INDICATIONS FOR MANOMETRIC TESTING

Evaluation of patients with dysphagia
   Pharyngeal and upper esophageal sphincter abnormalities
   Primary esophageal motility disorders (e.g., achalasia)
   Secondary esophageal motility disorders (e.g., scleroderma)
Evaluation of patients with possible gastroesophageal reflux
   disease
   Assist in placement of pH probe
   Evaluate lower esophageal sphincter pressure (e.g., poor
    treatment response)
   Evaluate defective peristalsis (particularly before fundoplication)
Evaluation of patients with noncardiac chest pain
   Primary esophageal motility disorders
   Pain response to provocative testing
Exclude generalized gastrointestinal tract disease
   Scleroderma
   Chronic idiopathic intestinal pseudoobstruction
Exclude esophageal etiology for suspected anorexia nervosa

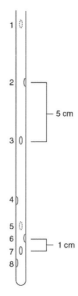

FIGURE 5.3. Distal end of an eight-lumen catheter showing placement and radial orientation of recording orifices.

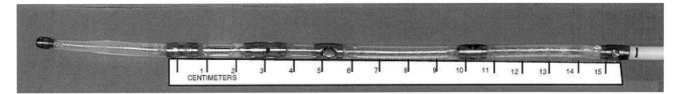

FIGURE 5.4. Esophageal motility catheter (solid-state) alongside a centimeter ruler showing centimeter marks on catheter aligned with catheter marks on the ruler. Catheters are measured to distal transducer.

Solid-state catheters have the advantage that intraluminal pressures are measured directly and, unlike the water perfusion system, are unrelated to the relative position of the patient and the equipment; therefore, studies may be performed with the subject in the upright position. This, and the fact that no continuous source of water is required, has made the development of special equipment for studies such as long-term ambulatory monitoring possible. In addition, the response time of solid-state catheters is much faster than that of the water-perfused system, making possible more accurate measurements of the cricopharyngeal region where the pressure rise rate exceeds the response time of water-perfused external transducers.

Development of a specialized solid-state transducer that senses pressures circumferentially over 360 degrees has simplified measurement of sphincter pressures (Fig. 5.6). This is accomplished through the use of a polymeric silicone (silastic) circumferential anulus filled with a viscous fluid, (USP grade castor oil), which surrounds a single miniature titanium strain gauge. The oil-filled chamber surrounding the transducer produces an extremely noncompliant system. Studies by the manufacturer (Konigsberg Instruments, Inc., Pasadena, CA) reveal low hysteresis (0.40% of full scale) and low volumetric compliance (7×10^6 mm^3/mm Hg). This transducer has a pressure rise rate greater than 2,000 mm Hg/sec. The pressure-sensing portion of this transducer has an active length of 3.1 mm and a diameter range between 4.65 mm and 5.2 mm. The pressure-sensing diaphragm of the transducer is exposed to the fluid-filled anulus, whose silicone rubber membrane makes direct contact with the sphincter wall. The pressure exerted by the sphincter is transmitted through the contained fluid to the strain gauge within the transducer. This transducer assembly provides a measure of circumferential squeeze, which is especially useful for pressure measurements in areas where pressure is not exerted symmetrically, such as the UES and LES (3–5).

Secondary Equipment

In addition to the primary equipment, there are pieces of smaller equipment and consumable supplies that are needed for esophageal manometry. A mercury manometer attached to a calibration chamber (stoppered flask or test tube) should be available to calibrate the equipment. Miscellaneous equipment includes a stretcher or bed, pillow, sheets, towels, patient gowns, and an intravenous pole. Necessary materials includes viscous lidocaine, lubricating jelly, tissue, tape, an emesis basin, 20-mL syringe, 8-oz disposable cup, straw and a container of room temperature water, and cotton swab for applying lidocaine to the nares. A pen-

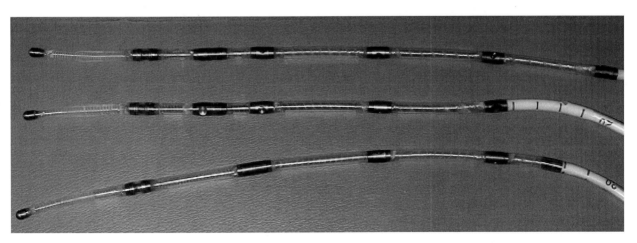

FIGURE 5.5. Examples of three catheter designs containing solid-state transducers.

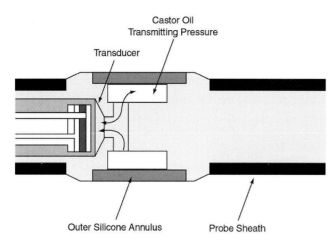

Castor Oil
Transmitting Pressure

Transducer

Outer Silicone Annulus

Probe Sheath

FIGURE 5.6. Schematic drawing of the circumferential pressure-sensing sphincter transducer showing the strain gauge surrounded by a fluid-filled chamber (USP grade castor oil) through which the pressure is transmitted.

light and a tongue blade may be helpful for insertion of the tube. During the study, we use the 20-mL syringe to give swallows of water (5 mL each).

Secondary materials used for special provocative testing are also needed. The Bernstein test requires three 60-mL syringes and 0.1N HCL and 0.9% saline solutions. A Harvard infusing pump can aid in the constant infusions of the solutions. Alternatively, intravenous bags and Y- tubing may be used. The edrophonium test requires 1-mL tuberculin syringes, alcohol swabs, injectable saline, edrophonium chloride, and atropine (the antidote to edrophonium).

Finally, a word on cleanup after the motility study: A ready-to-use surface disinfectant is used to wipe down the wheeled cart and associated equipment. In our laboratory, motility catheters are washed with soap and water, dried, and then immersed in Cidex (glutaraldehyde) for approximately 20 minutes. *Caution:* Do not immerse the connectors in the cleaning solutions. Follow the manufacturer's recommendations and the hospital's policy for proper cleaning and care.

STUDY TECHNIQUE

Careful attention to detail is essential for a successful manometric study. The esophageal manometry is performed while the patient is awake, alert, and in a supine position. Therefore, the cooperation and comfort of the patient are important for a good study outcome.

Patient Preparation

The patient should have fasted for at least 6 hours. Medications that might alter normal esophageal function should be discontinued at least 24 hours before the study. These include

nitrates, calcium channel blockers, anticholinergics, promotility agents, and sedatives. Patients who must take one or more of these medications for a serious, chronic medical condition may be studied while on the medication. All medications prescribed "as needed," or PRN, should be discontinued.

Intubation and Patient Calibration

Intubation is the most uncomfortable part of the study for the patient and can be the most intimidating part for the clinician. It is important not to rush this part of the study. The patient should be informed of what to expect and how important cooperation is to the success of the study. The patient should be in a comfortable seated position. Have the patient remove his or her glasses and any plates or dentures that are not strongly secured. Ask whether the patient has a preference as to which side of the nose to use. Explain that it is best to intubate through the nose instead of the mouth, because the tube has a tendency to make patients gag if inserted through the mouth. Also explain that the patient will be able to breathe with the tube in place. Gagging is a normal reflex. In patients with nasal congestion, a nasal spray used 30 minutes before intubation may open up the nasal passages. Passing a motility catheter is much like placing a nasal gastric tube.

The tip of the catheter is lubricated with 2% viscous Xylocaine. If the patient feels the intubation is too uncomfortable, 0.5 mL of Xylocaine can be injected in the nose and sniffed back into the nasal passage or a cotton swab moistened with Xylocaine may be used to apply the Xylocaine to the nasal passage.

Intubation through the nasal route may be a little more uncomfortable than through the mouth, but it is much better tolerated during the procedure. With nasal insertion, the catheter runs down the posterior pharynx away from the teeth and tongue. With oral insertion, the catheter lies across the tongue and teeth, causing the patient discomfort and a tendency to gag. An emesis basin should be close by; some patients have a sensitive gag reflex and may vomit. The tip of the catheter is placed into the nose and advanced slowly straight back. There is some resistance as the tip of the catheter reaches the back of the nose and begins to make the bend into the throat. At this point, the patient should tip his or her chin down toward the chest to help the catheter slip into the esophagus. Instruct the patient to sip water through the straw and advance the catheter as the patient swallows. Once through the UES, the catheter may be advanced fairly rapidly as the patient continues to swallow. Advance the catheter to a probe depth of 60 cm. If the patient coughs repeatedly and is unable to speak, the catheter may have slipped into the trachea instead of the esophagus. Withdraw the catheter and attempt to reinsert it. Reassure the patient throughout the intubation process. Once the catheter is down, having the patient take some deep breaths helps calm him or her. Secure the catheter in place with tape. At this point with most patients, the recording sites are in the stomach. The patient is then placed in the supine position and a "patient calibration" is performed. This procedure sets to zero all recording sites regardless of the pressure exerted against them. This allows gastric pressure to be used as a zero baseline when measuring LES pressures. The patient remains supine (head elevated no more than 30 degrees) during evaluation of the LES and esophageal body for two reasons: first, most published normal values for stationary manometry were obtained in the supine position; second, gravity is removed as a compounding factor. Once in the supine position, the patient should be reminded that it is important to be relaxed and to hold swallows until requested. In our laboratory, we use music to aid in patient relaxation.

Gastric Baseline

In our laboratory, we begin the study by placing the two distal pressure transducers (the circumferential transducers) in the stomach. It is important to start the manometric study by measuring gastric pressure through a series of quiet respirations. A relatively flat, smooth tracing with small pressure changes with inspiration indicates proper gastric placement (Fig. 5.7). Appropriate placement can be confirmed by having the patient take a deep breath and noting a rise in pressure with full inspiration. The gastric baseline pressure becomes the zero set for the subsequent LES pressure measurement. Thus, the LES pressure value is not an absolute pressure but is a relative pressure related to the gastric baseline pressure. The study of the LES and the esophageal body are traditionally done with the patient in the supine position.

Lower Esophageal Sphincter

The LES is composed of tonically contracted smooth muscle, which relaxes with a swallow. The aim of the manometric assessment of the LES is to measure its resting pressure and to assess its relaxation during swallowing. The LES resting pressure (LESP) is measured at the point of highest pressure. Assessment of the LES is best performed with a catheter containing distal averaging or circumferential sensors. This is important because of the asymmetric nature of the LES. With this type of catheters, the sensor is positioned in the high pressure zone (HPZ) of the LES, and LES relaxation is assessed by giving the patient a series of 5

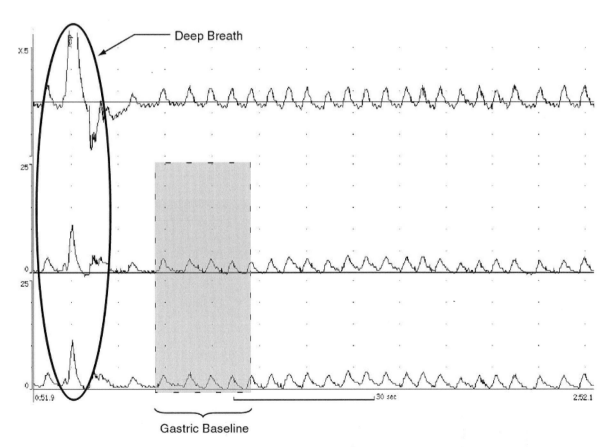

FIGURE 5.7. This tracing shows respiratory recording above and recordings from two transducers located in the stomach below. Note the increase in intragastric pressure with the deep inspiration. The gastric baseline pressure is obtained during a period of quiet respiration.

mL water swallows. It is important to use water that is at room temperature. If the catheter contains directional sensors or water ports, the LES pressure must be measured with each port or sensor and the results averaged to get an accurate measurement of the LESP. Assessment of LES function is composed of two steps: profiling the LES and evaluation of sphincter relaxation.

Profiling the Lower Esophageal Sphincter

The station pullthrough technique for determining LES pressure involves a slow, stepwise withdrawal of the catheter through the LES. The catheter is moved in 0.5-cm increments and should remain at each position or "station" long enough to register a stable LESP. This usually requires waiting for a period of three to five respiratory cycles. This pullthrough technique allows the identification of the LES distal border, the HPZ, the pressure inversion point (PIP) or point of respiratory reversal, and the proximal border of the LES.

The LES is first identified by increased respiratory pressure changes in the channel displaying waveforms from the proximal circumferential sensor, located directly above the distal sensor. This sensor is sometimes referred to as the *scout*, because it is used to identify the different landmarks in the LES. The increased respiratory pressure changes are followed by the rising of the bottom of the

pressure tracing above the baseline (Fig. 5.8). As the catheter is withdrawn, the pressure increases, and at the point where the transducer moves from the abdominal portion of the sphincter to the thoracic portion, the tracing shows a marked change in configuration, with a fall in pressure during inspiration instead of a rise in pressure. This is the PIP (Fig. 5.8). The PIP is not the end of the sphincter, but rather a landmark within the sphincter that is used to calculate intraabdominal LES length, because the PIP identifies the location of the diaphragm. The abdominal length of the LES is calculated by subtracting the probe depth where the PIP is located from the probe depth where the distal LES border is located (Fig. 5.9). This measurement and total LES length are used as important parameters in the assessment of the LES as a competent reflux barrier in some laboratories (6,7). As the catheter is further withdrawn, the pressure tracing drops and flattens. When the transducer leaves the LES, the pressure drops below gastric baseline pressure, indicating that the transducer is then measuring esophageal baseline pressure. The proximal border of the LES is located at the probe depth where the pressure falls to or below the gastric baseline pressure (Fig. 5.8). Subtracting this probe depth from that obtained for the distal border gives the total length of the LES (Fig. 5.9).

Measurement of the LESP must take into account the changes in pressure resulting from respiration. As noted ear-

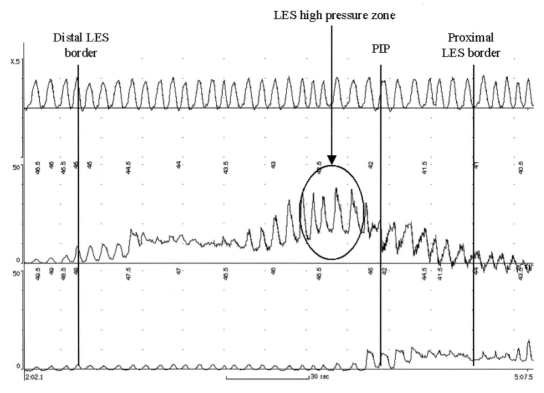

FIGURE 5.8. Pressure profile of the LES obtained by a station pull-through of a transducer from the stomach across the sphincter to the esophagus (*middle tracing*).

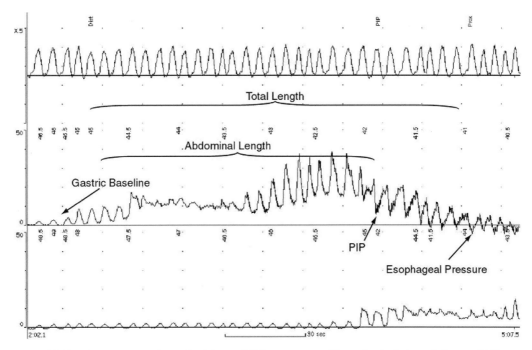

FIGURE 5.9. Lower esophageal sphincter (LES) pressure profile and calculation of the total LES length and the length of its abdominal portion.

lier, the LESP is not an absolute pressure but is a relative pressure related to the gastric baseline pressure. This is why LESP is always calculated as a pressure differential between the gastric baseline pressure and the highest LES pressure. There are two popular ways to measure LESP: from the gastric baseline to either the midrespiratory or the end-expira-

tory pressure at the station with the highest overall pressure, that is, the HPZ (Fig. 5.10). There is some controversy concerning which of these methods is most accurate, but it is important to know which method was used when comparing results from different laboratories. One study suggested that end-expiratory pressures are more indicative of the true

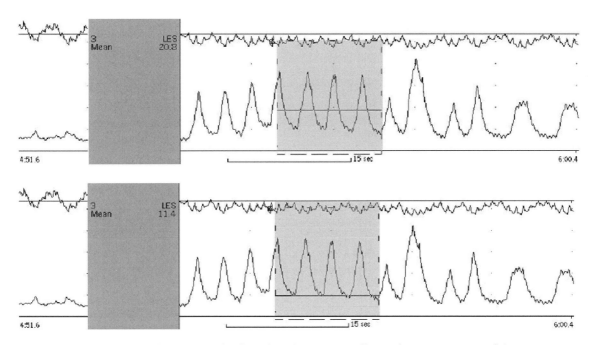

FIGURE 5.10. Midrespiratory (*top*) and end expiratory (*bottom*) measurements of lower esophageal sphincter pressure.

LESP, because it is at this point in the respiratory cycle that the diaphragmatic contribution to the observed pressure is at a minimum (8). Other investigators have shown that the midrespiratory pressure provides an LESP measurement that most reliably distinguishes patients with normal amounts of gastroesophageal reflux from those with abnormal reflux (9). Thus, the pressure contributed by the diaphragm during respiration is an important component of the antireflux mechanism of the LES and should be included in the assessment of LESP.

The LESP measurement should include three or four respiratory cycles of level, even amplitude obtained at a fixed location (Fig. 5.10). High pressure spikes are usually artifact and not a true representation of LESP; these should be disregarded. Also, pressure measurements should not be obtained after a swallow-induced relaxation because the pressure is often elevated for a while. In general, the highest pressure in the LES occurs on the abdominal side of the LES just distal to the PIP.

The results of any method must be compared with normal values obtained from using the same technique to test a cohort of age-matched normal subjects. The most comprehensive study of normal esophageal manometric parameters (10) established the following normal values (relative to gastric baseline pressure) in 95 healthy adult volunteers (mean age 43 years): end inspiration, 39.7 ± 13.2 mm Hg; midrespiration, 24.4 ± 10.1 mm Hg; end expiration, 15.2 ± 10.7 mm Hg. All values are expressed as the mean ± 1 standard deviation.

Evaluation of Sphincter Relaxation

After the LES pullthrough with the proximal transducer, the clinician continues to pull the catheter in 0.5-cm increments until the distal transducer is located in the HPZ of the LES. (Fig. 5.11). This placement allows evaluation of sphincter relaxation during swallowing. The catheter is taped in place and the LESP is recorded. Dry swallows often do not induce complete LES relaxation. Thus, in our laboratory, we give the patient a 5-mL bolus of room temperature water. After a swallow, the LES pressure should drop to approximately the level of the gastric baseline. We observe the relaxation as the pressure falls, allowing the sphincter to open, and then the pressure returns to or exceeds the LESP as the sphincter contracts following the passage of the bolus. During the LES relaxation, the parameters that are usually evaluated are the duration of the relaxation and either the percent relaxation or the residual pressure. The residual pressure is defined as the difference between the lowest pressure achieved during relaxation and the gastric baseline pressure. This residual pressure is a better indicator of LES function than percent relaxation because it is independent of the resting LES baseline pressure (11) (Fig. 12). A normal residual pressure should be 8 mm Hg or less.

Once the relaxation is complete, a 20- to 30-second interval passes before another water swallow is given. Five to ten relaxations should be repeated in this manner. Once the water swallows are completed, the catheter is pulled in 0.5-cm increments until the sensor exits the LES.

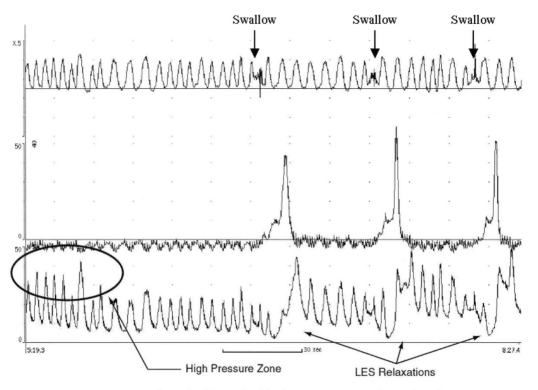

FIGURE 5.11. Lower esophageal sphincter (LES) high-pressure zone and LES relaxations.

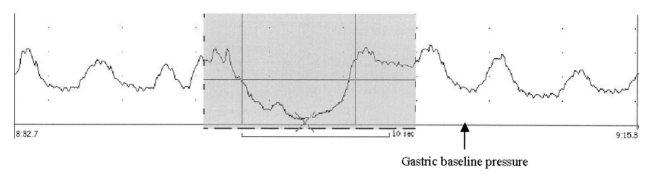

FIGURE 5.12. Normal swallow-induced lower esophageal sphincter relaxation showing measurement of residual pressure at the *X*.

If using a catheter with directional sensors only, it is important that the sensors be rotated around the axis of the catheter so that the pressure in all four quadrants of the sphincter can be measured and averaged to produce an accurate measure of the resting pressures and relaxation. The foregoing procedure should be performed for each sensor, pulling it through the sphincter, assessing resting pressure and relaxation. The results for all sensors should be averaged. If a catheter with only a distal circumferential sensor is used, the directional sensor just proximal to the distal sensor may be used to profile the LES; it should not be used to assess resting pressure because of the asymmetry of the LES.

Manual interpretation of LES parameters, particularly the relaxation parameters, is highly subjective and qualitative. Attempts to provide a more objective and quantitative measure of these parameters have resulted in computer algorithms for an automated analysis (11,12). It is imperative, however, that the user review and adjust, if necessary, the analysis provided by the computer (Fig. 5.13). Most of these computer algorithms for LES evaluation have been adapted by manufacturers of motility equipment.

Body of the Esophagus

The study of the body of the esophagus evaluates the esophageal body response to a water swallow. The muscle normally contracts beginning from the proximal (top) portion of the esophagus and progresses in an orderly sequence to the distal (bottom) portion of the esophagus. This organized progression of the esophageal contractions represents a peristaltic wave. In the esophageal body, manometry measures amplitude, duration, and velocity of the esophageal contractions, allowing an assessment of the peristaltic activity and detection of possible motility abnormalities. A complete evaluation should include measurements of both the smooth muscle of the distal esophagus and the striated muscle of the distal esophagus. Special attention is directed to measurements made at 3 and 8 cm above the LES, because esophageal motil-

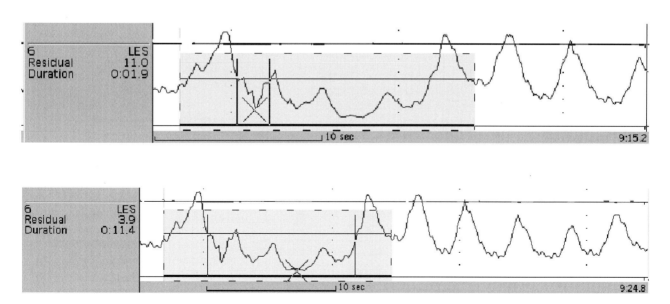

FIGURE 5.13. Incorrect computer generated analysis of lower esophageal sphincter (LES) relaxation (*top*) and user-corrected analysis (*bottom*).

ity abnormalities occur more frequently in the distal segment of the esophagus comprised exclusively of smooth muscle. Dry swallows or double swallows are not measured.

When using catheters with two distal circumferential sensors, the distal sensor is usually placed in the HPZ of the LES. The sensors are 5 cm apart, thus censors are at 5, 10, 15, and 20 cm above the HPZ of the LES. This positioning allows simultaneous evaluation of the LES relaxation and the esophageal body contractions. Placing the distal sensor 3 cm above the proximal border of the LES is also a frequent positioning method. Most catheters have sensors or ports positioned 5 cm apart to allow assessment of the esophageal peristalsis. Usually, catheters have three to five sensors, with the most frequent spacing at 5 cm.

Once the catheter has been properly positioned and taped in place, a period of 10 to 15 seconds is allowed to elapse to establish the esophageal resting pressure as a baseline or reference point for assessing body contractions. The patient is then given a series of 5-mL boluses of room temperature water with a 20- to 30-second interval between swallows (Fig. 5.14). This allows time for the smooth muscle to repolarize. Each swallow should be annotated using the computer keys designated for swallow. If a strip chart is used, swallows should be marked on the graph to distinguish the water swallow from a dry swallow.

Usually, ten wet swallows are assessed and parameters are based on the mean values. A study from our laboratory evaluated the reproducibility of swallow parameters and concluded that the mean values from five to eight swallows reli-

ably characterize an individual's esophageal peristalsis (13). Analysis of these parameters, especially those involving the identification of the onset of the peristaltic wave, can be subjective and time consuming. To obtain more objective and quantitative data, most laboratories use computer systems that collect, digitize, and analyze esophageal body pressure data (12,14,15). Most manufacturers of manometric equipment have adapted and improved upon these programs for general use and they are commercially available.

In evaluating the esophageal body, we measure, at least, the following peristaltic parameters: amplitude, duration, and velocity. Amplitude is a measurement of how tightly the muscles of the esophagus are squeezing during a contraction and is expressed in mm Hg. The baseline (0 mm Hg) is the pressure in the body of the esophagus between swallows. Contraction amplitude is measured from the baseline to the peak of the pressure wave (Fig. 5.15). The reported amplitude of each sensor location within the esophageal body is the mean value of the amplitude of ten contractions in response to wet swallows. Mean values from the two most distal transducers can be averaged to obtain the distal esophageal amplitude, for which normal values of ten swallows are 99 ± 49 (mean ± SD) mm Hg.

Duration is a measurement of how long, in seconds, the muscles of the esophagus are squeezing during a contraction. The measurement is made from the onset of the major upstroke of the contraction to the point where the downstroke of the contraction returns to the baseline (Fig. 5.16).

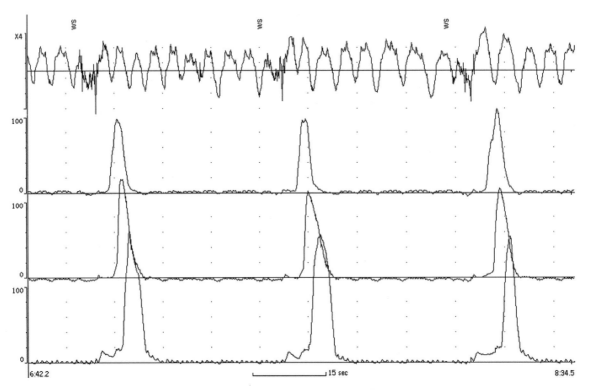

FIGURE 5.14. Esophageal body contractions.

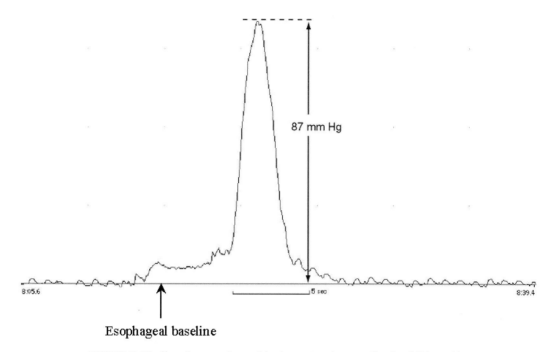

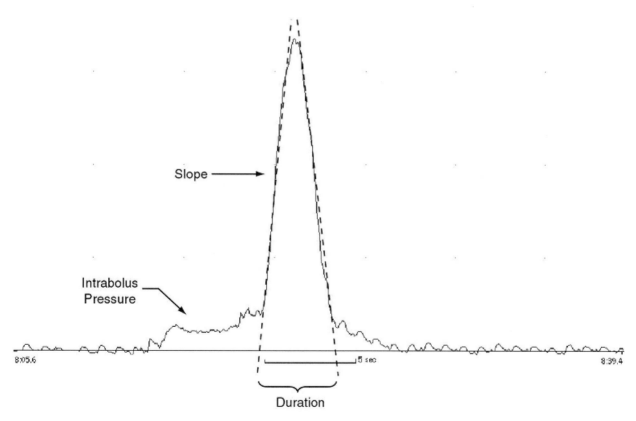

FIGURE 5.15. Showing esophageal body contraction amplitude of 87 mm Hg.

FIGURE 5.16. Esophageal body contraction showing the intrabolus pressure, slope of the pressure wave, and duration of the contraction.

The esophageal baseline sometimes rises slightly before the actual contraction: this is called the *intrabolus pressure* and is due to the presence of the ingested water bolus (Fig. 5.16). Normal duration values are 3.9 ± 0.9 seconds.

Velocity is the rate (cm/sec) of progression of the contraction down the esophagus. It can be obtained between any two sites in the esophagus. The measurement is made by determining the time between the beginning of the upstroke of the contractions and dividing it by the centimeters separating the sensors. Normal values should be less than 8 cm/sec (Fig. 5.17).

Normal peristalsis in the distal esophagus is an orderly, sequential contraction down the esophagus, with amplitude, duration, and velocity in the normal range (Fig. 5.14). In the striated muscle segment of the esophagus, the contractions are usually sharper than in the smooth muscle areas, with a shorter duration. If a transducer is placed in the transition zone between the striated and smooth muscle portions of the esophagus (usually around 6 cm below the UES), absent or very low amplitude contractions may be seen ("pressure trough"). The presence of a midesophageal pressure trough was confirmed by Clouse and co-workers (16–18), who recorded esophageal pressures at 1-cm intervals and generated isobaric contour plots for a detailed analysis of intraesophageal pressures. They also showed a difference in shape and peristaltic velocity between the distal and proximal esophagus. However, a study by Peghini and colleagues (19) determined that the striated muscle of the esophagus has manometric characteristics much closer to those of the smooth muscle portion than to those of the striated muscle in the pharynx. They also confirmed the presence of a pressure trough in the middle esophagus, although they found it in less than one third of the subjects studied.

TABLE 5.2. NORMAL ESOPHAGEAL PRESSURE DATA FROM 95 HEALTHY VOLUNTEERS

Parameter Measured at Given Recording Site	Value
Amplitude (mm Hg)	
At 18 cm above lower esophageal sphincter (LES)	62 ± 29
At 13 cm above LES	70 ± 32
At 8 cm above LES	90 ± 41
At 3 cm above LES	109 ± 45
Distal esophageal amplitude duration (sec)	99 ± 40
At 18 cm above LES	2.8 ± 0.8
At 13 cm above LES	3.5 ± 0.7
At 8 cm above LES	3.9 ± 0.9
At 3 cm above LES	4.0 ± 1.1
Distal esophageal duration velocity (cm/sec)	3.9 ± 0.9
Proximal	3.0 ± 0.6
Distal	3.5 ± 0.9

The definition of normal range comes from measurements of the contraction parameters in a large number of normal volunteers. The largest such study is the one by Richter and colleagues (10). This study established normal values in 95 healthy volunteers. Table 5.2 gives the values from that study. When comparing studies done in patients with this or any other group of normal values, it is necessary to remember that these measurements are affected by the age of the subject, body position, size of the bolus, size of the catheter, and location of the transducer.

Peristaltic contractions that have two pressure peaks are called double-peaked contractions and are considered a variant of normal. Each separate peak should be at least 10% of the overall wave amplitude and 1 second in duration (Fig. 5.18). Contraction amplitude should be measured from the higher peak. Duration is measured from the upstroke of the first peak to the downstroke of the last. Triple peaked or more (Fig. 5.19), peristaltic contractions are considered abnormal and usually indicate distal esophageal spasm.

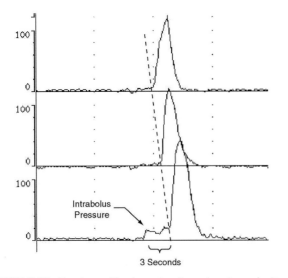

FIGURE 5.17. Esophageal body contractions showing velocity of the peristaltic wave.

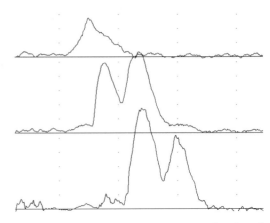

FIGURE 5.18. Esophageal body contractions showing double-peaked contraction waves.

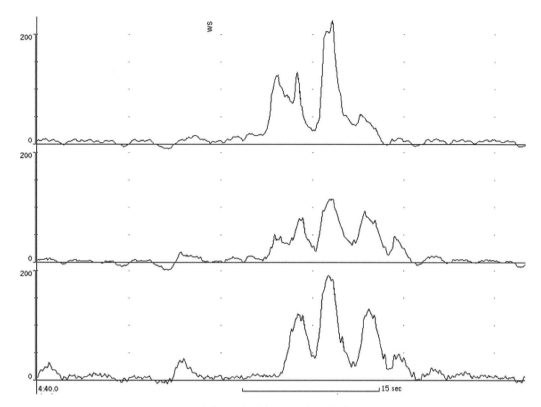

FIGURE 5.19. Triple-peaked (or more) peristaltic contractions.

The occurrence of a nonperistaltic contraction following a wet swallow is abnormal. Simultaneous and retrograde contractions constitute nonperistaltic contractions. Contractions are considered simultaneous when their velocity is more than 8 cm/sec. A simultaneous contraction indicates that large portions of the esophagus are contracting at the same time, instead of in the normal, peristaltic sequence (Fig. 5.20). In some cases, the entire esophagus contracts together, whereas in other cases, only the mid or distal esophagus contracts simultaneously. Greater than 10% simultaneous contractions during water swallows is abnormal. Retrograde contractions occur

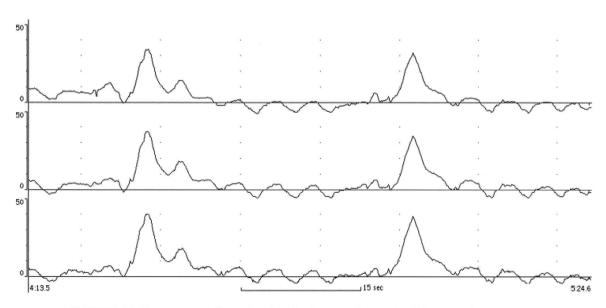

FIGURE 5.20. Two water swallows showing simultaneous (nonperistaltic) contractions.

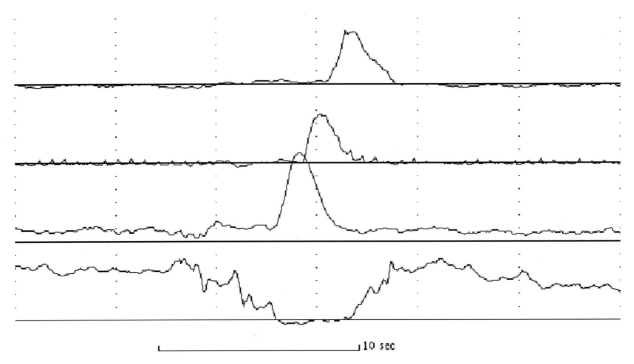

FIGURE 5.21. A water swallow showing a retrograde contraction.

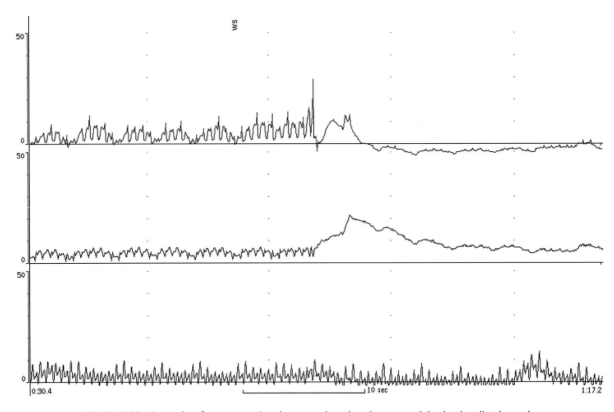

FIGURE 5.22. Example of nontransmitted contraction showing no activity in the distal esophagus.

when the distal esophagus contracts before the proximal esophagus (Fig. 5.21).

Sometimes, a wet swallow is followed by no activity in the distal esophagus (Fig. 5.22) or a contraction failing to reach an amplitude of 30 mm Hg (Fig. 5.23). These are both examples of ineffective motility (20,21). The former is known as a nontransmitted wave. A measurement of more than 20% ineffective waves after wet swallows is considered abnormal. Simultaneous comparisons of manometry with radiography (22) and scintigraphy (23) have shown that contractions with an amplitude of less than 30 mm Hg may lack the necessary force to move a bolus through the esophagus. However, the recent introduction of multichannel intraluminal impedance technology (see Chapter 7), which allows measurement of bolus transit simultaneously with pressure, suggests that a lower threshold than 30 mm Hg may be needed because there appears to be frequent bolus transit with pressures between 25 and 30 mm Hg.

In patients with a skeletal muscular disorder (including scleroderma), it may be desirable to assess striated muscle function. To do this, the catheter is pulled orad until a pressure rise is noted in the proximal channel, indicating the sensor is entering the UES. The sensor is repositioned 1 cm lower, placing the sensor 1 cm below the distal border of the UES (Fig. 5.24) to ensure that the proximal sensor is in striated muscle. Ten to 15 seconds of resting pressure establishes an esophageal baseline or reference point for the body contractions resulting from the water swallows. The patient is given five to ten water swallows. It is not necessary to wait the 20 to 30 seconds required for assessing smooth muscle, because striated muscle does not require as long a recovery time.

Provocative Testing

Provocative testing is an optional part of the esophageal manometry study. It elicits or reproduces symptoms that might be esophageal in origin. Interpretation is based on the patient's subjective complaints rather than on specific manometric change. Because of this subjective factor, the provocative tests must have a blinded placebo phase. It is important not to draw any special attention to this part of the test.

Bernstein Test

The Bernstein test assesses esophageal sensitivity to acid. Saline and 0.1N HCL are alternately infused through the Bernstein port of the catheter. The patient reports any discomfort. This discomfort must duplicate the patient's symptoms to be considered positive. If a patient complains

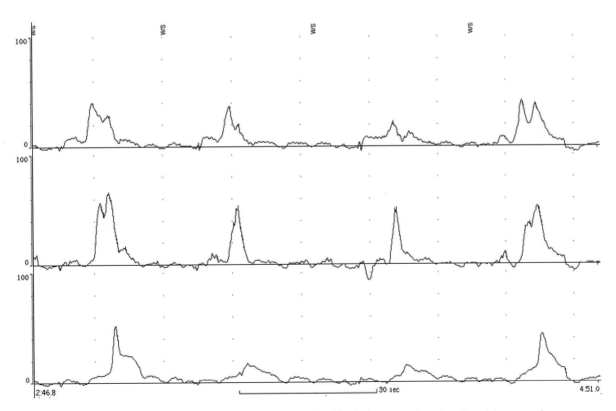

FIGURE 5.23. Example of two low-amplitude (ineffective) contractions bracketed by normal peristaltic waves.

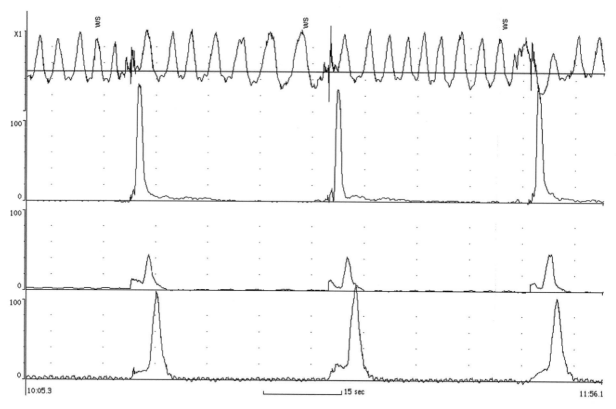

FIGURE 5.24. Upper esophageal body contractions.

of burning but the original symptoms were of chest pain, then the test is negative. The test is conducted as follows:

1. Infuse normal saline for 3 to 5 minutes.
2. Switch to the dilute HCL (without the patient being aware) at a rate of 10 mL/min. Infuse the HCL for 10 minutes or until the patient experiences symptoms.
3. Switch back to saline. The symptoms should subside in patients exhibiting a response to the acid.
4. Repeat the process to ensure the acid is the cause of the symptoms.

If the patient did not experience symptoms or if the symptoms are not those that the patient normally experiences, the test is negative. The symptoms should subside with infusion of saline and return with the second infusion of acid.

Edrophonium (Tensilon) Test

The patient is given two injections: one of 0.9% normal saline (placebo) and one of edrophonium chloride. Tensilon is a short-acting cholinesterase inhibitor that increases the amplitude and duration of esophageal contraction. The patient is instructed to report any symptoms. The test is conducted as follows:

1. Begin with an injection of 0.2 mL 0.9% normal saline either intravenously or subcutaneously.

2. Give the patient water swallows (every 30 seconds) and record the presence of any symptoms.
3. Give an intravenous injection of edrophonium (10 mg or less as determined by patient weight). If the patient experiences burning at the injection site, the medication is not being administered in a vein.
4. Give the patient ten swallows of water.

If the patient complains of typical chest pain after the injection, the test is considered positive. There should be an association between the patient's symptoms and high-amplitude esophageal contractions, although change in manometry without symptoms is not indicative of a positive test. The chest pain is usually mild to moderate in intensity. *Do not use more than 1.0 mL (10 mg) of edrophonium,* even if the patient's weight warrants it. Some patients may complain of side effects from the edrophonium such as watery eyes, dizziness, and abdominal cramping. These usually pass quickly. We do not give edrophonium to patients with asthma, chronic obstructive lung disease, or cardiac arrhythmia. Atropine is the antidote and should be kept close at hand; it is rarely needed.

Upper Esophageal Sphincter

The final portion of the study involves assessment of the UES, which includes a determination of the resting pressure of the UES, the relaxation of the UES, pharyngeal contraction and peristalsis, and an assessment of the coordination between UES relaxation and the pharyngeal contraction (24). This study is best performed with the patient in a sitting position.

Like the LES, the UES is a sphincter that is tonically contracted and relaxes with swallowing. The UES and pharyngeal region differ from the body of the esophagus in several ways that markedly affect the manner in which manometry must be performed. First, the UES and pharynx are composed of striated muscle; therefore, the muscular contractions and responses are much more rapid than those in the smooth muscle distal esophagus. The more rapid rate of contraction of the striated muscle far exceeds the response time of low-compliance infusion systems, which substantially misrecord pharyngeal waveforms (25). In addition to limitations imposed by the response of the transducer system, an analog recording system has a recording frequency that impacts the interpretation of the signal from the transducers. The mechanical recording pens of the polygraph generally record faithfully only to a frequency of 20 to 40 Hz (26). A computerized manometry system allows more flexibility in recording frequencies. Although it is possible to collect data at much higher rates, practical considerations of memory and disk space utilization have kept those computer systems currently in use to a recording frequency of 100 to 128 Hz (8), which allows for a resolution of ±10 msec.

The second difference that affects UES and pharyngeal manometry is inherent in the anatomy of the UES. The asymmetry of the UES pressure profile has been confirmed in humans by the use of an eight-lumen perfused manometry catheter in which the orientation of each orifice was known (27,28). The highest pressures are recorded from the anterior and posterior directions, and the lowest from the lateral direction. One possible solution to this dilemma is to use an oval catheter that ensures proper orientation within the sphincter and records only maximum and minimum pressures (29,30). Use of such a catheter instead of the round tube routinely used for esophageal manometry would present some practical problems. Green and colleagues (31) reported on a comparison between a round and an oval catheter, each with

four orifices spaced radially at 90 degrees. They found that mean values for the oval and round catheters were not significantly different. Therefore, the recording of average sphincter pressures greater than 360 degrees is independent of catheter shape. Thus, the development of a circumferential sphincter transducer has allowed for accurate sphincter measurements without the need to control catheter orientation (32).

The assessment of the UES begins by establishing a baseline or reference point in the body of the esophagus. The HPZ of the UES is usually found by the slow or station pullthrough method. The UES is reactive to catheter movement, so it is necessary to allow the recording device to remain in the HPZ for 15 to 20 seconds before measuring the pressure (Fig. 5.25).

In addition to measuring the resting UES pressure, a manometric evaluation must also include an analysis of UES relaxation during swallowing. This analysis has been confounded by swallow-related movements of the sphincter (13). Kahrilas and co-workers (33) have shown that a measuring device positioned in the HPZ of the UES records a duration of UES relaxation considerably longer than the period of UES opening observed radiographically. They concluded that this is an artifact caused by the sensor falling distal to the sphincter (i.e., into the body of the esophagus) as the UES moves orad.

If the sensor is positioned in the HPZ for the swallow, the pressure tracing produces what appears to be a prolonged relaxation (i.e., a relaxation without the elevation spike). This is due to the UES moving completely off the sensor as it moves orad with the swallow. The sensor actually drops into the body of the esophagus. When the UES returns to resting pressure, it moves back onto the sensor, giving the appearance that the UES has closed (Fig. 5.26). A prolonged relaxation of more than 0.5 second (500 msec) should be an indication that the sensor may not be correctly positioned.

To properly assess UES relaxation, it is necessary to position the sensor above or proximal to the HPZ of the UES. If the sensor is properly positioned, the tracing seen during a swallow appears as an M-configuration (Fig. 5.27). Initially, the pressure is well below that of the UES HPZ. However, as the UES moves orad with the initiation of the swallow, the pressure increases, corresponding to

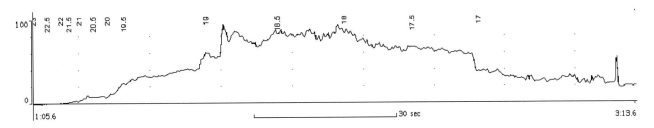

FIGURE 5.25. Upper esophageal sphincter pull-through localizing the high-pressure zone.

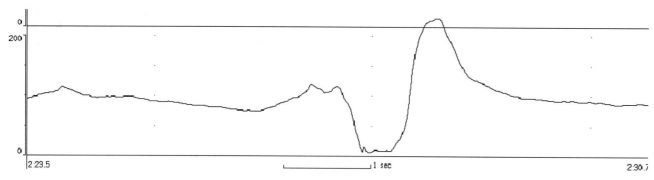

FIGURE 5.26. Artifactual apparent relaxation of upper esophageal sphincter with sensor improperly positioned within the high-pressure zone.

the movement of the HPZ onto the sensor. The pressure then drops and again increases as the sphincter relaxes and regains its resting tone. There is finally a slow drop in pressure as the HPZ returns to its original position distal to the sensor.

Once the sensor is properly positioned, it is possible to study both the UES function during swallowing and the coordination between the relaxation of the UES and the contraction of the pharynx. The pharynx, like the UES, is asymmetric with the highest pressures recorded in the anterior and posterior direction, and the lower pressures laterally. A study using a special catheter with four solid-state

transducers separated by 3 cm and oriented circumferentially at 90 degrees measured pharyngeal pressures in four directions from the proximal edge of the UES through the hypopharynx and oropharynx (5). There was statistically significant asymmetry in both the longitudinal and radial directions. Pressures varied from 365 ± 29 to 86 ± 13 mm Hg (mean ± 1 standard error).

To properly assess UES and pharyngeal contraction coordination, the catheter should contain three pressure sensors within a 5-cm total spacing. The best catheter configuration has two circumferential sensors spaced 3 cm apart, with a third unidirectional sensor positioned 2

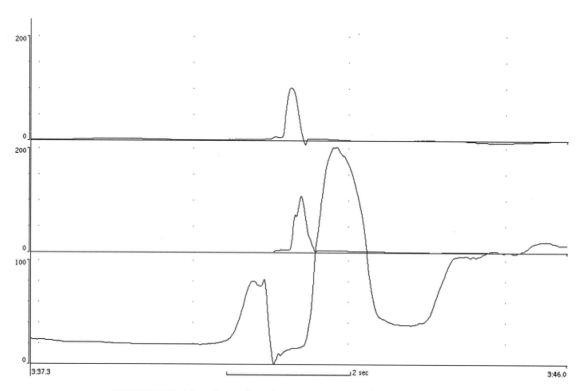

FIGURE 5.27. M configuration of upper esophageal sphincter relaxation.

cm above the secondary or proximal circumferential sensor. This configuration allows evaluation of the pharyngeal contractions with the two proximal sensors (one circumferential, one directional) while assessing UES relaxation with the distal circumferential sensor, as shown in Figure 5.27. There is no reason to wait between the swallows because the area being assessed is in striated muscle which has rapid repolarization. Once a swallow is completed, the next one may be given as soon as the patient is ready.

The accurate evaluation of pharyngeal peristalsis and UES-pharyngeal coordination requires computer analysis. The sequence of events is so rapid (usually less than 1 second) that the higher resolution of computer-recorded data is necessary.

CONCLUSION

It has been generally believed that the barium examination is the only useful technique for assessing patients with pharyngeal dysphagia, because it provides the opportunity to assess actual bolus transfer and the possible presence of aspiration. However, using the technology described, manometric studies can also provide important information on the swallowing mechanism of the pharynx and the UES. In particular, such studies can provide details of the force of the pharyngeal contraction and specific timing of this contraction and the relaxation of the UES. A manometric evaluation allows quantitation of the forces of the pharyngeal propulsive wave, the squeezing tone of the UES, and the timing of the coordination between the pharyngeal contraction and the UES relaxation to an accuracy of 1/100th of a second. We believe that this information will augment that provided by the barium swallow and allow for a more complete assessment of the patient with dysphagia.

REFERENCES

1. Cardoso, et al. The effect of catheter diameter on upper esophageal sphincter measurements in normal subjects. *Gullet* 1992;2:145–149.
2. Lydon SB, et al. The effect of manometric assembly diameter on intraluminal esophageal pressure recording. *Dig Dis Sci* 1975; 20:968.
3. Castell JA, Dalton CB, Castell DO. Pharyngeal and upper esophageal sphincter manometry in humans. *Am J Physiol* 1990; 258:G173.
4. Pursnani KG, Oeffner C, Gideon RM, et al. Comparison of lower oesophageal sphincter pressure measurement using circumferential vs unidirectional transducers. *Neurogastroenterol Motil* 1997;9:177.
5. Sears VW, Castell JA, Castell DO. Radial and longitudinal asymmetry of the human pharynx. *Gastroenterology* 1991;101:1559.
6. Bonavina L, Evander A, Demeester TR. Length of the distal esophageal sphincter and competency of the cardia. *Am J Surg* 1986;151:25.
7. O'Sullivan, GC, Demeester TR, Joelsson BE. Interaction of lower esophageal sphincter pressure and length of sphincter in the abdomen and determinants of gastroesophageal competence. *Am J Surg* 1982;143:40.
8. Castell JA, Castell DO. Modern solid state computerized manometry of the pharyngoesophageal segment. *Dysphagia* 1993;8:270.
9. Kraus BB, Wu WC, Castell DO. Comparison of lower esophageal sphincter manometries and gastroesophageal reflux measured by 24-hour pH recording. *Am J Gastroenterol* 1990;85:692.
10. Richter JE, et al. Esophageal manometry in 95 healthy adult volunteers. *Dig Dis Sci* 1987;32:583.
11. Castell JA, Dalton CB, Castell DO. On-line computer analysis of human lower esophageal sphincter relaxation. *Am J Physiol* 1988;255:G794.
12. Castell JA, Castell DO. Computer analysis of human esophageal peristalsis and lower esophageal sphincter pressure. II. An interactive system for on-line data collection and analysis. *Dig Dis Sci* 1986;31:1211.
13. De Vault K, Castell JA, Castell DO. How many swallows are required to establish reliable esophageal peristaltic parameters in normal subjects? An on-line computer analysis. *Am J Gastroenterol* 1987;82:754.
14. Tijskens G, et al. Validation of a fully automated analysis of esophageal body contractility and lower esophageal sphincter function: a study on the effect of the PGE, analogue rioprostil on human esophageal motility. *J Gastrointentest Motil* 1989;1:21.
15. Wilson JA, et al. Computerized manometric recording: an evaluation. *Gullet* 1991;1:87.
16. Clouse RE, Staiano A. Topography of normal and high-amplitude esophageal peristalsis. *Am J Physiol* 1993;268:G1098.
17. Clouse RE, Staiano A. Topography of the esophageal peristaltic pressure wave. *Am J Physiol* 1991;261:G677.
18. Clouse RE, et al. Characteristics of the propagating pressure wave in the esophagus. *Dig Dis Sci* 1996;41:2369.
19. Peghini PL, et al. Proximal and distal esophageal contractions have similar manometric features. *Am J Physiol* 1998;37:G325.
20. Kahrilas PJ, Dodds WJ, Hogan WJ. Effect of peristaltic dysfunction on esophageal volume clearance. *Gastroenterology* 1988;94: 73.
21. Leite LP, et al. Ineffective esophageal motility (IEM): the primary finding in patients with non-specific esophageal motility disorder. *Dig Dis Sci* 1997;42:1853.
22. Hogan WJ, Doodds WJ, Stewart ET. Comparison of roentgenology and intraluminal manometry for evaluating oesophageal peristalsis. *Rend Gastroenterol* 1973:5:28.
23. Richter JE, et al. Relationship of radionuclide liquid bolus transport and esophageal manometry. *J Lab Clin Med* 1987; 109:217.
24. Castell JA, Castell DO. Stationary esophageal manometry. In: Scarpignato C, Galiche JP, eds. *Functional investigation in esophageal disease*, first ed. Basel: Karger, 1994:109–129.
25. Dodds WJ, et al. Considerations about pharyngeal manometry. *Dysphagia* 1987;1:209.
26. Stef JJ, et al. Intraluminal esophageal manometry :an analysis of variables affecting recording fidelity of peristaltic pressures. *Gastroenterology* 1974:67:221.
27. Welch RW, et al. Manometry of the normal upper esophageal sphincter and its alteration in laryngectomy. *J Clin Invest* 1979; 63:1036.
28. Winans CS. The pharyngoesophageal closure mechanism. A manometric study. *Gastroenterology* 1972;63:1036.

29. Gergardt DC, et al. Esophageal dysfunction in esophagopharyngeal regurgitation. *Gastroenterology* 1980;78:893.

30. Knuff TE, Benjamin SB, Castell DO. Pharyngoesophageal (Zenker's) diverticulum, a reappraisal. *Gastroenterology* 1982; 82:734.

31. Green WER, Castell JA, Castell DO. Upper esophageal sphincter pressure recording: is an oval manometry catheter necessary? *Dysphagia* 1988;2:162.

32. Castell JA, Dalton CB, Castell DO. Effects of body position and bolus consistency on the manometric parameters and coordination of the upper esophageal sphincter and pharynx. *Dysphagia* 1990;5:179.

33. Deleted in press.

34. Boyle JT, et al. Role of the diaphragm in the genesis of lower esophageal sphincter pressure in the cat. *Gastroenterology* 1985; 88:723.

6

AMBULATORY MONITORING OF ESOPHAGEAL PH AND PRESSURE

BAS L.A.M. WEUSTEN
ANDRÉ J.P.M. SMOUT

During the last two decades, both researchers and clinicians have learned to appreciate the relevance of prolonged recording of esophageal functions in ambulatory subjects. The first report on prolonged recording of esophageal pH dates from 1969 (1). This pioneering work was done with stationary equipment in hospitalized patients. Esophageal pH monitoring in truly ambulatory subjects was first described in 1980 (2). The first report on ambulatory 24-hour esophageal pressure recording dates from 1982 (3). Since the early 1980s, the development in this field has been rapid, and numerous reports on ambulatory monitoring of esophageal function have been published. In this chapter, information on ambulatory esophageal pH and pressure monitoring in health and disease is reviewed. Because ambulatory pH recording has found and will find more widespread clinical application than ambulatory pressure recording, emphasis is placed on the former technique.

pH RECORDING

Recording Techniques and Conditions

Some of the technical details of intraesophageal pH recording greatly influence the outcome of the procedure and are thus relevant to the clinician. In this chapter, technical details are discussed only when considered of clinical relevance.

pH Electrodes

There are several types of small pH electrodes suitable for intraesophageal use. Important differences exist between monopolar electrodes that require an external reference electrode and combination electrodes with a built-in reference. The former recording technique is more susceptible to artifacts than the latter. The cutaneous reference electrode may be the source of totally unreadable tracings caused by loose contact, and inaccurate readings may be caused by perspiration-induced changes of the ionic composition of the electrolyte solution surrounding the electrode (4–6). Until recently, pH electrodes with built-in reference were available only as glass electrodes. Bipolar glass electrodes have a larger diameter (up to 4.5 mm) than monopolar electrodes, making transnasal insertion somewhat more difficult. Currently, antimony electrodes with a built-in reference are commercially available, but these appear to be vulnerable and less reliable than their glass equivalent.

Monocrystalline antimony electrodes are less expensive than glass electrodes but have a much shorter life. Furthermore, their performance is clearly inferior to that of glass electrodes. *In vitro* studies have shown that antimony electrodes respond more slowly to sudden pH changes, drift more, and have a far less linear response than glass electrodes (5,6). In addition, the response curves of antimony electrodes show considerable hysteresis. From the standpoint of a basic scientist, these shortcomings of antimony electrodes render them inadequate for accurate measurement of intraesophageal pH. In clinical esophageal pH studies, however, both types of electrodes appear to provide similar results (5,7).

Several years ago, the ion-sensitive field effect (ISFET) pH electrode was developed. ISFET pH sensors appear to be comparable to glass electrodes with respect to linearity and drift, but they respond more rapidly to sudden pH changes (8,9). They offer the advantage of miniaturization, which makes it feasible to incorporate up to six sensors into one catheter. ISFET pH electrodes are no longer commercially available.

Recently, a new wireless esophageal pH recording device was introduced. It consists of a pH-sensitive cap-

B.L.A.M. Weusten: Department of Gastroenterology, St. Antonius Ziekenhuis, Nieuwegein, The Netherlands.

A.J.P.M. Smout: Gastrointestinal Research Unit, Departments of Gastroenterology and Surgery, University Hospital Utrecht, Utrecht, The Netherlands.

sule to be attached to the esophageal mucosa. Data are sent from the capsule to a receiver/data logger by means of radio transmission. The absence of a transnasal catheter is more comfortable to the patient, and patients may find it easier to maintain normal daily activities (10). However, a recent study in 100 consecutive patients undergoing 24-hour pH monitoring showed that presence of a conventional transnasal pH probe led to only minimal lifestyle alteration during the recording period (i.e., habits of eating, drinking, posture, and physical activity) (11). The wireless pH capsule must be placed endoscopically, which may be a major drawback.

Before each 24-hour pH study, a two-point calibration of the pH electrode must be performed using a neutral buffer and an acidic buffer. At return of the patient after the 24-hour recording period, the calibration should be repeated to rule out pH electrode failure and to allow for correction for slow pH drift. When glass electrodes are used, any type of pH buffer suffices. With antimony electrodes, only the buffer solutions provided by the manufacturer should be used, because antimony electrodes are also sensitive to agents other than the hydrogen ion.

Data Loggers

Various types of portable data loggers are commercially available. The analog recording systems initially used have generally been replaced by digital data loggers. A sampling rate of eight per minute and a resolution of 0.1 pH unit are sufficient for clinical purposes (4), but defection of short-lived reflux events my require a sampling rate of 1 Hz. All available systems contain one or more event markers that allow the patient to indicate when symptoms occur. At first, the availability of a larger number of event markers seems to be advantageous, but most users of this equipment have become disappointed by the capability of the average patient to use these multiple event markers appropriately. An example of an overview plot of a 24-hour esophageal pH recording is shown in Figure 6.1.

Electrode Positioning

Global consensus has been reached that the pH electrode should be positioned at 5 cm above the upper border of the lower esophageal sphincter. For accurate positioning, an esophageal manometric study should be performed before the 24-hour pH study to determine the distance from the lower sphincter to the nares. Because esophageal manometry is not as widely available as 24-hour pH recording, other techniques for electrode placement have been used. Measurement based on the pH profile recorded on withdrawal of the electrode from the stomach has been found to be inferior to placement on manometric guidance (12). Measurement of the distance from the sphincter to the mouth at endoscopic examination, fluoroscopic placement, and use of certain formulas in which body height is used to calculate sphincter depth are other alternatives, but they have disadvantages. Fluoroscopic placement carries the risk that the pH electrode will be inadvertently positioned in a hiatal hernia. The endoscopic measurement technique suffers from the disadvantage that the differences between sphincter-to-mouth and sphincter-to-nose distance varies from patient to patient.

Food Intake and Exercise Level

The acidity and buffering capacity of meals and beverages consumed during the 24-hour study period can vary considerably. Therefore, standardization of food intake during pH monitoring has been recommended. Acidic foods, such as carbonated beverages, fruit-based products, pickles, and yogurt, are usually forbidden. However, the intake of these products has a short-lived effect on esophageal pH, so the quantitative effect of their consumption on reflux variables is minimal. Hence, the use of acid-restricted or nonacidic diets probably is not required for a routine clinical study. Exclusion of the actual eating period from the overall analysis eliminates the artifact introduced by meal constituents having pH less than 4.0 (coffee, tea, citrus, carbonated drinks) and improves the separation of normal and abnormal total times for which pH is less than 4 (13,14). In some

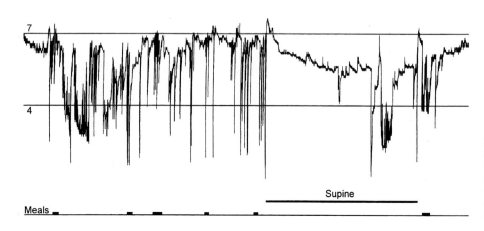

FIGURE 6.1. Twenty-four–hour overview plot of esophageal pH recorded in an ambulatory subject with gastroesophageal reflux disease. Periods of eating and drinking are indicated by *horizontal bars*. Supine position is indicated by *horizontal line*.

institutions, the use of coffee or cigarettes is routinely prohibited to patients undergoing 24-hour pH monitoring. Not only is it doubtful that all patients will adhere to these regulations but also the evidence for a substantial influence of these factors on esophageal acid exposure is poor. Alcohol and chocolate consumption have a significant reflux-promoting effect (15,16). It is likely that other food constituents also have demonstrable effects on gastroesophageal reflux. The ideal pH study for research is one during which the patient ingests standardized meals at standardized times (17). In clinical practice, however, such an approach is unfeasible and perhaps even undesirable, because information on esophageal pH profile and symptoms during a period in which the patient adheres to his or her own dietary habits is probably more relevant. Other factors of considerable influence are the level of physical exercise displayed by the patient during 24-hour recording (18) and the time spent in a supine position (19).

Data Reproducibility

The intrasubject reproducibility of 24-hour recording of esophageal pH was studied by several groups of investigators. In some studies, subjects (patients and healthy control subjects) underwent two ambulatory pH studies on separate days (20,21). In another, reflux patients were studied for 48 hours, that is, during 2 consecutive days (22). Consecutive-day testing was also performed in infants and children (23). Reproducibility was found to be most consistent for the parameters of percent of time with a pH of less than 4. Total percent of time with a pH of less than 4 showed 85% reproducibility (i.e., 85% of the tested subjects retained a normal or abnormal test result on both study days) (24). The degree of concordance for this parameter was 77% (22). Whereas most groups concluded that the reproducibility was "good" or "satisfactory" (20,22,23), others stressed the fact that the total percent of time with a pH of less than 4 may vary between tests by a factor of 3.2-fold (218% higher to 69% lower) (21). In a recent Scandinavian study, 22 adult patients were investigated twice, 6 weeks apart, under identical in-hospital conditions (25). Although no significant differences in reflux parameters were found between the two test occasions, six patients had normal total reflux time on one test occasion but pathologic results on the other. In another study, two antimony pH electrodes were positioned at the same level in the esophagus. Discrepancies between the readings from the two electrodes were such that a change in clinical diagnosis (normal versus abnormal) occurred for two of the ten patients studied (26).

Duration of pH Monitoring

There has been some debate on the optimal duration of a prolonged ambulatory pH monitoring study. Some investigators have made a case for short-term postprandial recording rather than a 24-hour study (27,28). However, evidence for the superiority of 24-hour over shorter interval pH monitoring as been produced; the sensitivity of a 24-hour test is significantly higher than that of a 12-hour test (29). Furthermore, in outpatients, a 24-hour recording period usually is more practical than a shorter test and the reproducibility of 24-hour recordings is significantly better than that of 4- or 8-hour recordings (22). Although 24-hour recording is the method of choice, a 16-hour study from 4:00 p.m. to 8:00 a.m. can provide accurate information and improve patient tolerance (30).

INTERPRETATION

Criteria for Reflux

In the analysis of esophageal pH recordings, pH decreases to less than 4 are usually taken as evidence of acid gastroesophageal reflux. The cutoff limit of pH 4 has been chosen arbitrarily, but there seems to be some rationale for this choice. First, the proteolytic enzyme pepsin is inactive at more than pH 4.0; second, patients with symptomatic reflux usually report heartburn at an intraesophageal pH of less than 4 (31). Different cutoff limits have been formally compared in a number of studies. In an early study in nonambulatory subjects, the discriminatory power of pH cutoff levels 3, 4, and 5 was calculated and the best discrimination between healthy control subjects and patients with reflux symptoms was found to be obtained with pH 5 (32). Others compared cutoff levels of pH 3, 4, 5, and 6 using an ambulatory technique. The best discrimination between healthy subjects and reflux patients occurred within the full range from pH 3 to 6 rather than at any single pH (33). Yet another group reported cutoff limits of pH 3, 4, and 5 to be superior to pH 2 with respect to the discrimination of patients with endoscopic evidence of grade II or III esophagitis from normal subjects (34). A combination of cutoff limits was not found to be superior in the latter group's data. Consequently, the authors suggested that pH 4 should be used to define reflux episodes (34).

In a study in which we used pH distribution curves to identify the point of separation between "reflux" and "nonreflux" pH values, optimal pH thresholds from 5.0 to 6.4 (upright) and from 4.5 to 5.7 (supine) were found (24). On the basis of the results, it can be concluded that use of the conventional threshold of pH 4 leads to underestimation of the severity of gastroesophageal reflux. Nevertheless, given the widespread acceptance of the pH 4 threshold, it would be unwise to advocate the use of any other threshold in clinical practice. In the analysis of the association between symptoms and reflux, however, we advocate taking rapid pH decreases of more than 1 pH unit into account, even when the threshold of 4 is not reached (see Association between Symptoms and Reflux).

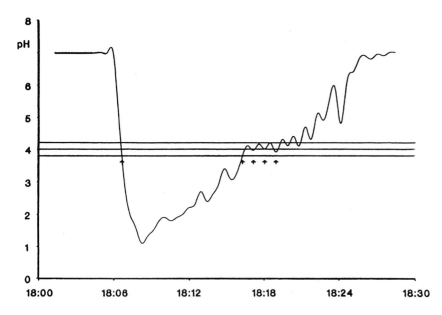

FIGURE 6.2. Figure illustrating that the number of reflux episodes counted in a 24-hour esophageal pH study depends on the algorithm used for determination of onset and end of a reflux episode. Small oscillations around the threshold level of pH 4 may lead to a spuriously high number of reflux episodes. (From Hopert R, Emde C, Riecken EO. Recommendations for long-term oesophageal pH monitoring. *Neth J Med* 1989;34:S55–S61, with permission.)

The proportion of time that the pH is below the cutoff level of 4, called *reflux time* or *acid exposure time,* is the most widely used reflux variable. It can be expressed either in minutes or in percentage of time. It has the often underestimated advantage that its calculation is straightforward. In contrast, the number of reflux episodes counted during a 24-hour study period depends highly on the algorithm used for identification of a reflux episode. With some algorithms, oscillations of the pH around the threshold value lead to a spuriously high number of reflux episodes counted (4,35) (Fig. 6.2). The results from different centers cannot be compared as far as the numbers of reflux episodes are concerned. The number of reflux episodes shows a much poorer correlation with the grade of esophagitis than does reflux time. In addition, the parameter of number of episodes was less reproducible than the parameter of percent of time with a pH less than 4 (21). These limitations of the number-of-episodes parameter have made some investigators abandon its use completely.

The mean duration of a reflux episode can be calculated by dividing the reflux time by the number of reflux episodes. The variable has been called the *acid clearance time* because it is dependent on the clearance capacity of the esophagus. This variable is as algorithm dependent as is the number of reflux episodes.

The number of reflux episodes longer than 5 minutes, a variable introduced in 1974 (36), is still popular to use. Whereas one should be aware that the choice of a 5-minute period is arbitrary, many clinicians have learned to appreciate this variable as a measure of esophageal clearance capacity. Three or more reflux episodes longer than 5 minutes occurring in a 24-hour study is considered abnormal.

Mean and median pH in certain time intervals have been used as variables by some investigators in this field, but have not gained much popularity.

More complex reflux parameters composed of a number of different variables have been advocated by some users of the 24-hour recording technique. The frequency–duration index (FDI), for example, is defined as the mean number of reflux episodes per hour multiplied by the mean cumulative duration of reflux episodes per hour (37). Johnson and DeMeester (36,38) advocated the use of a pH score that takes into account the six different variables listed in Table 6.1. It is questionable whether such composite scores have sufficient advantages over simpler variables. Studies that compared composite scores with reflux time (time with a pH less than 4) showed that the latter discriminates at least as well as the former between health and disease (34,39). Calculation of the area less than pH 4 has recently been advocated as an alternative to reflux time or acid exposure

TABLE 6.1. NORMAL VALUES IN 24-HOUR ESOPHAGEAL pH RECORDING

Variable	Normal Value
Percent of time pH <4	
Total period	<4.2%
Upright period	<6.3%
Supine period	<1.2%
Number of episodes	
Total	<50
Longer than 5 min	<3
Duration of longest episode	<9.2 min

From Johnson LF, DeMeester TR. Twenty-four-hour pH monitoring of the distal esophagus. *Am J Gastroenterol* 1974;62:323–332, with permission.

time. In this parameter, the duration as well as the depth of pH decreases are taken into account. Although the sensitivity for the diagnosis of gastroesophageal reflux disease was found to be superior to that of the conventional percent of time with pH less than 4 in two studies (40,41), the technique has not yet found widespread clinical application.

The patterns of reflux in healthy subjects are very different during the day and during the night. At night, reflux episodes are rare, although their incidence increases with age (42–44). When nighttime gastroesophageal reflux occurs, it appears to be related to the interdigestive migrating motor complex (42). During the day, up to 50 reflux episodes may be observed in health. These observations necessitate the separate analysis of daytime (upright) and nighttime (supine) portions of the recordings.

DeMeester and colleagues (19) described three patterns of abnormal gastroesophageal reflux: reflux in the upright position only, in the supine position only, and in both positions. Of the 100 symptomatic patients studied, nine were upright refluxers, 37 were supine refluxers, and 54 were combined refluxers. In patients with an upright reflux pattern, reflux occurred predominantly in the postprandial period. Supine refluxers differed from upright refluxers by having a higher incidence of esophagitis. Combined refluxers had an even higher incidence of esophagitis than supine refluxers (19). Others were unable to confirm that three distinct patterns of reflux occur (45). Also, acid exposure during the 3 hours following the evening meal was more closely correlated with esophagitis than was nighttime exposure (45). Others reported that although the increase in nighttime reflux in esophagitis patients was proportionally greater than the increase in postprandial reflux, the latter still formed the greatest contribution to the acid contact time (43).

Reflux of alkaline duodenal contents into the esophagus has been put forward as a putative factor in the pathogenesis of reflux esophagitis, and it has been claimed that episodes of alkaline gastroesophageal reflux can be detected as increases of esophageal pH in excess of 7. However, in a patient with an intact and acid-secreting stomach, most episodes of esophageal alkalinization are associated with gastric pH of less than 7. Esophageal pH values of greater than 7 may also occur as a result of increased secretion of saliva (46). Furthermore, the esophageal mucosa can also be a source of bicarbonate in the esophageal lumen (47). Using an esophageal aspiration technique, Mittal and colleagues found that, in patients with gastroesophageal reflux disease, bile acids do not reflux into the esophagus in potentially harmful quantities (48). In a study using a bilirubin-sensitive probe, significant correlations were found between esophageal acid and bilirubin exposure values, but not between alkaline and bilirubin exposures. This observation suggests that bilirubin exposure of the esophagus mainly runs parallel with acid exposure and that duodenogastroe-

sophageal reflux cannot be recorded reliably by esophageal pH monitoring (49). Therefore there is no rationale for quantifying the number of episodes or percentages of time with an esophageal pH greater than 7 in a clinical 24-hour esophageal pH study.

Normal Values

A prerequisite for any diagnostic test aimed at detecting disease is that the limits of normal for that test have been well defined. This is usually done by subjecting a sufficiently large group of healthy subjects to the test. When the values found in these normal subjects are normally distributed, the mean plus or minus 2 standard deviations can be used to determine the upper and lower limits of normal. Many investigators have indeed used the mean plus or minus 2 standard deviations in calculating the upper limit of normal of ambulatory esophageal pH variables. It has been shown, however, that most variables measured in ambulatory 24-hour esophageal recording do not fit the assumption of gaussian distribution (34,50). Nonparametric methods, such as estimation of the fifth and ninety-fifth percentiles (or the 2.5th and 97.5th percentiles), must therefore be used in the determination of normal values in ambulatory 24-hour esophageal pH recording. Another approach is to study a group of healthy control subjects and a group of patients with reflux disease and to determine the values that provide optimal separation between the groups. This can be done with discriminant analysis or with receiver-operating characteristics analysis (39). The threshold values found with such an approach should be evaluated prospectively in a new group of patients and control subjects before statements about the sensitivity and specificity of the test are made.

As shown in Table 6.2, the normal values for ambulatory esophageal pH recording in adults reported in the literature vary widely (5,7,33,34,39,44,45,51–53) because of differences in the age distribution of the control subjects studied and in the algorithms used for calculation of the parameters, and because of the method used for determination of the upper limit of normal.

Controversial data have been published on the relation between age and pH variables in normal subjects. Whereas some investigators found no significant relation with age (54), others reported an increase in some reflux variables with age (50,53).

In a study of 285 infants, the esophageal exposure time was found to be relatively low in the first months of life (1.20% ± 0.91% to 2.52% ± 2.25%) (31). At 4 months, the reflux index had increased significantly (to 4.18% ± 2.6%). At 15 months, the reflux index had decreased again, to 2.65% ± 1.90%. The low values of the reflux variables found in newborns have been attributed to a low level of body movements and the hyposecretion of gastric acid.

TABLE 6.2. REPORTED LIMITS OF NORMAL VALUES AS FOUND IN AMBULATORY ESOPHAGEAL pH RECORDING IN ADULTS

| Study | Ref. | Percent of Time Esophageal pH < 4 | | Analytic Method Used |
		Upright	Supine	
Johnson and DeMeester 1974	36	6.3	1.2	Mean ± 2 SD
Weiser et al. 1982	44	5.9	2.1	Mean ± 2 SD
Vitale et al. 1985	33	5.9	4.6	Mean ± 2 SD
Ward et al. 1986	7	5.9	1.8	Mean ± 2 SD
Bonavina et al. 1986	51	6.3	4.6	Mean ± 2 SD
De Caestecker 1989	45	9.1	11.2	95th percentile
Gignoux et al. 1987	5	14.2	3.6	Mean ± 2 SD
Schindlbeck et al. 1987	39	10.5	6.0	ROC
Johnsson et al. 1987	34	4.6	3.2	95th percentile
Smout et al. 1989	50			
<45 yr		7.3	3.6	95th percentile
>45 yr		16.0	6.7	95th percentile
Richter et al. 1992	53	8.15	3.45	95th percentile

ROC, receiver-operating characteristic analysis; SD, standard deviation.

Association between Symptoms and Reflux

As discussed in more detail later, the importance of determining whether a patient's reflux is pathologic or is still within physiologic limits is probably overstressed. Rather, the most important piece of information to be obtained from a 24-hour pH study is whether and to what extent the symptoms reported by the patient are related to gastroesophageal reflux. The temporal correlation between symptoms and reflux can be convincing on inspection of the pH–time curves (Fig. 6.3), but a quantitative measure of such a relationship is desirable. In the (automated) analysis of the relationship between symptoms and reflux, a 2-minute time window beginning at 2 minutes before the onset of the symptoms appears to be optimal (55).

In 1988, Wiener and colleagues (56) proposed a parameter to express the relationship between symptoms and reflux episodes, which they labeled the *symptom index* (SI). It is defined as the percentage of the symptom episodes that are related to reflux:

$$\frac{\text{Number of reflux-related symptom episodes}}{\text{Total number of symptom episodes}} \times 100\%$$

There is evidence, based on receiver-operating characteristic analysis, that 50% is the optimal threshold for the SI (57).

The distribution of SIs in a population of patients with reflux disease is bimodal (i.e., high and low values occur more often than intermediate values) (Fig. 6. 4). The correlation between the severity of esophageal acid exposure and the SI is poor (Fig. 6.4), indicating that acid exposure and acid sensitivity are different phenomena.

The disadvantage of the SI is that it does not take into account the number of reflux episodes. The significance of an SI of 100% in a patient with only a single reflux episode per 24 hours is different from that in a patient with more than 100 reflux episodes per 24 hours. For this reason, Breumelhof and colleagues proposed the additional use of another index, which they called the *symptom sensitivity index* (SSI) (58), defined as

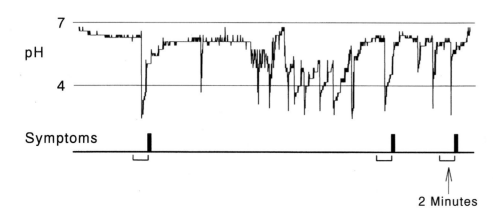

FIGURE 6.3. Association between reflux symptoms and esophageal pH decreases in a patient with pyrosis and regurgitation, but without esophagitis. The three *vertical bars* mark the onset of reflux symptoms, as indicated by the patient by pressing the symptom marker button on the pH recorder. Each of the three symptom episodes is preceded by reflux.

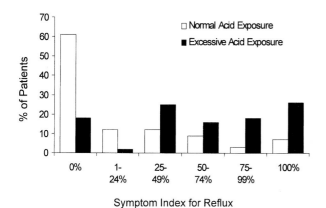

FIGURE 6.4. Distribution of symptom indices (SI) for the symptom heartburn or chest pain in 125 patients who experienced one or more symptom episodes during a 24-hour esophageal pH study. Note that many patients with a low SI have excessive esophageal acid exposure and that some patients with a high SI have normal acid exposure. (From Weusten BLAM, Akkermans LMA, van Berge Henegouwen GP, Smout AJPM. Ambulatory combined oesophageal pressure and pH monitoring: relationships between pathological reflux, oesophageal dysmotility and symptoms of oesophageal dysfunction. *Eur J Gastroenterol Hepatol* 1993;5:1055–1060, with permission.)

$$\frac{\text{Number of symptom-associated reflux episodes}}{\text{Total number of reflux episodes}} \times 100\%$$

SSI values of 10% or higher are considered to be positive (58). Calculation of both SI and SSI for one and the same pH monitoring test may yield discordant results. From discordant test results, conclusions can be drawn as to the cause of the patient's symptoms. A high SSI and a low SI, for example, would indicate that the patient's esophagus is sensitive to reflux but that other causes than acid reflux are likely to contribute to the symptoms as well.

Both the SI and the SSI suffer from the disadvantage that they do not integrate all factors determining the relationship between symptoms and reflux. Weusten and colleagues therefore developed another parameter that expresses the likelihood that a patient's symptoms are related to reflux (59). This parameter, labeled the *symptom association probability* (SAP), is calculated by dividing the 24-hour pH data into 2-minute segments. Then, for each of these 2-minute segments, it is determined whether reflux occurred in it and whether a symptom was reported. A 2 × 2 contingency table is then made in which the number of 2-minute segments with and without reflux and with and without symptoms are tabulated. A modified chi-squared test is used to calculate the probability that the observed distribution could have been brought about by chance. The SAP is calculated as $(1-P) \times 100\%$. By statistical convention, SAP values greater than 95% are positive.

In the analysis of the association between symptoms and reflux, rigorous adherence to the criterion that a threshold of pH 4 should be passed may lead to underestimation of the reflux-related origin of the symptoms. In patients using acid secretion inhibitors, in patients with atrophic gastritis, and during postprandial periods, the intragastric pH may be greater than 4. In our laboratory, any decrease in pH of more than 1 pH unit that occurs within 8 seconds is considered indicative of gastroesophageal reflux. These episodes may be responsible for up to one third of reflux-related symptom episodes (60).

Clinical Relevance of Ambulatory pH Recording

pH Monitoring in Patients with Reflux Esophagitis

It will come as no surprise to learn that patients with reflux esophagitis have more reflux episodes and a higher esophageal acid exposure time than do normal control subjects (43,61–64) and that the severity of reflux esophagitis is significantly correlated with the extent of gastroesophageal reflux, or reflux time (62) (Fig. 6.5). Even though the diagnosis of reflux esophagitis can be made endoscopically with accuracy, much effort has been made to determine the sensitivity and specificity of 24-hour pH recording in making this diagnosis. Sensitivities between 84% and 96% and specificities ranging from 91% to 98% have been reported (29,33,34,39,61,65). The gold standard in the aforementioned reports was variable; hence, the results of the various studies cannot be compared directly. Furthermore, the design of some of the studies was insufficient in that determination of the optimally discriminating pH values and the calculation of specificity and sensitivity were done in the same patient group and control group. This may result in spuriously high sensitivity and specificity values. More importantly, it is incorrect to view esophageal pH monitoring as an alternative to endoscopy in the diagnosis of reflux esophagitis; therefore, calculation of sensitivity and specificity with esophagitis as the gold standard is useless.

Once the diagnosis of reflux has been made endoscopically, there is generally no indication for 24-hour monitoring. Only when the esophagitis fails to respond to medical treatment should 24-hour pH recording be considered. Ideally, the pH study should then be performed repetitively with the patient using increasingly high doses of an acid secretion–inhibiting drug. With this approach, one should be able to find the dose that adequately reduces esophageal acid exposure. It has been argued, however, that the large intrasubject variability in 24-hour acid exposure may limit the usefulness of this test as a measurement of therapeutic improvement (21). Dual pH monitoring with one electrode in the esophagus and one in the stomach may be helpful in the management of these therapy-resistant patients (66).

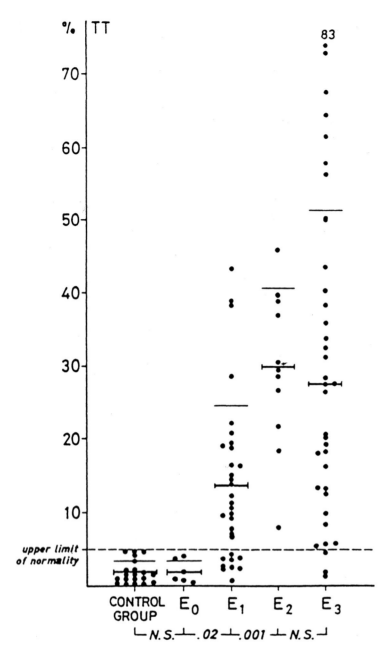

FIGURE 6.5. Relationship between percent total time (%TT) with esophageal pH of less than 4 and grade of esophagitis. E_0, no esophagitis; E_1, microscopic esophagitis; E_2, nonconfluent erosions; E_3, confluent erosions, ulcer, stenosis, or Barrett's esophagus; N.S., not significant. (From Mattioli S, Pilotti V, Spangaro M, et al. Reliability of 24-hour home esophageal pH monitoring in diagnosis of gastroesophageal reflux. *Dig Dis Sci* 1989;34:71–78, with permission.)

pH Monitoring in Patients with Reflux Symptoms

The symptoms of heartburn and regurgitation are commonly held to be reliable indicators of gastroesophageal reflux. However, heartburn may also be the principal complaint of patients with peptic ulcer disease, cholelithiasis, and nonulcer dyspepsia. On the other hand, patients with severe reflux disease (resulting in severe esophagitis) may deny all typical reflux symptoms. Not infrequently, atypical symptoms—in particular, angina-like chest pain and pulmonary symptoms—are the only manifestations of reflux disease. Therefore, ambulatory pH monitoring is the preferred method to document abnormal reflux and its associ-

ation with specific symptoms. The correlation between typical reflux symptoms and 24-hour esophageal acid exposure, as measured by 24-hour monitoring, is weak (59,62) (Fig. 6.6). This finding should not be interpreted as indicative of a limited value of 24-hour esophageal pH monitoring, but rather as a result of the large individual variability in the perception of reflux. Esophageal pH monitoring is the most appropriate technique to prove (or disprove) that the symptoms (typical or not) are reflux related (67). For quantitative analysis of the temporal relation between symptoms and reflux, the SI, the SSI, and the SAP can be used (56,58,68), as discussed previously. The indications for ambulatory 24-hour esophageal pH recording are summarized in Table 6.3.

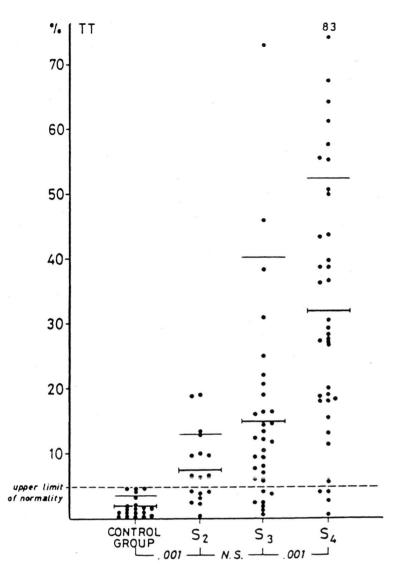

FIGURE 6.6. Relationship between percent of total time (%TT) with esophageal pH of less than 4 and severity of reflux symptoms. S₂, Postural heartburn or pain once or twice daily; S₃, postural or spontaneous heartburn or pain up to four times daily; S₄, spontaneous or postural heartburn or pain more than four times per day; N.S., not significant. (From Mattioli S, Pilotti V, Spangaro M, et al. Reliability of 24-hour home esophageal pH monitoring in diagnosis of gastroesophageal reflux. *Dig Dis Sci* 1989;34:71–78, with permission.)

PRESSURE RECORDING

Recording Technique

Since the early 1980s, esophageal pressure signals have been recorded in ambulatory subjects, using intraesophageal microtransducers. All groups that have evaluated 24-hour esophageal pressure recording have combined this technique with 24-hour esophageal pH recording. The pioneering work in this field was done with analog recording systems, using Holter types of tape recorders and audiocassettes (52,67,69–72). With the advent of digital recording systems with large memory capacity, many of the technical problems of ambulatory esophageal pressure recording have been overcome (73–75). One of the advantages of digital recording is that the digitized data can easily be displayed graphically at any desired time base and amplitude scale, without excessive paper consumption. When a digital system is used to store 24-hour esophageal pressure data, the

---

TABLE 6.3. INDICATIONS FOR AMBULATORY 24-HOUR ESOPHAGEAL pH RECORDING

Assessment of relationships between symptoms and (acid) reflux
   Typical reflux symptoms in the absence of esophagitis
   Atypical symptoms with or without esophagitis
   When antireflux surgery is considered
Evaluation of the effect of symptomatically or endoscopically unsuccessful treatment (medical or surgical) on esophageal acid exposure

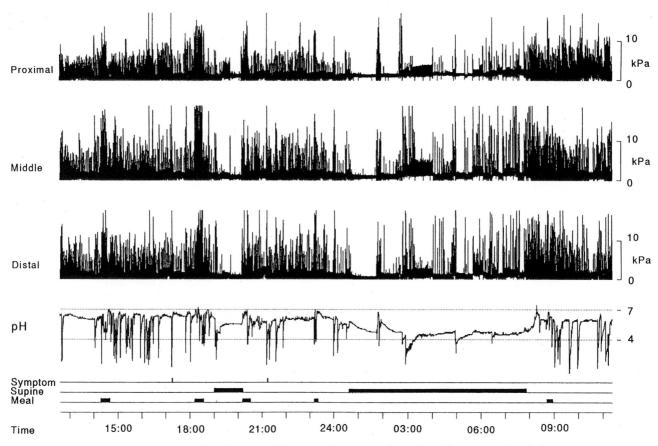

FIGURE 6.7. Twenty-four–hour overview plot of esophageal pH signal (lower panel) and three esophageal pressure signals (*upper three panels*) recorded in an ambulatory patient with chest pain. The proximal, middle, and distal pressure transducers were positioned 15, 10, and 5 cm proximal to the upper border of the lower esophageal sphincter, respectively. 10 kPa = 75 mm Hg.

sampling rate must be 4 Hz or higher to prevent unacceptable waveform distortion and underestimation of contraction amplitude.

Since esophageal contractile activity is different during meals and between meals and different during sleep and during the day (Fig. 6.7), it is imperative that records be kept of these activities. These records must be precise to the minute. Use of a marker button to indicate accurately the beginning and end of a meal and supine episodes is helpful.

At present, 24-hour recording of esophageal pH and pressure no longer is a research technique. Clinical application of this technique in the noncardiac chest pain syndrome is worthwhile (52,69,71,76). However, standardization of recording and analysis techniques has not yet been achieved.

Analysis Techniques

The problems encountered in the analysis of 24-hour esophageal pressure data are far more complex than those encountered in the analysis of 24-hour pH data. As mentioned earlier, esophageal motility and its relation to symptoms cannot be adequately assessed by simply looking at a 24-hour plot. It can be estimated that complete manual analysis of a 24-hour pressure recording, comprising categorization of each contraction and measurement of its amplitude, duration, and propagation velocity, would take one person approximately 2 weeks. Even in a research environment, this is an unacceptable investment of time and money. Solutions to this problem are to just browse through the data and analyze only certain proportions (e.g., the episodes during which the patient reported presence of a symptom) or to rely on computer algorithms for fully automated analysis of the data. Even when commercially developed computer software can be used, the clinician relying on it must be sure that he or she fully understands what the program does. Ambulatory esophageal pressure recording is certainly an area in medicine in which there is a danger of incorrect decisions being made based on insufficiently understood computer-generated figures.

In the automated analysis of ambulatorily recorded esophageal pressure, criteria have been developed to differentiate contractions from artifacts (e.g., respiration artifacts) and to categorize contractions as peristaltic, simultaneous, or nontransmitted (nonpropagated). Most contractions recorded in a 24-hour study are not initiated by wet swallows and these have a considerably lower amplitude than those recorded in a conventional manometric study. Even in healthy control subjects, the smallest esophageal contractions are indistinguishable from respiratory pressure variations and other artifacts. A threshold of approximately 15 mm Hg above baseline is usually used to distinguish contractions from artifacts (73,75). The criteria to differentiate peristaltic contractions from simultaneous and nontransmitted contractions are summarized in Table 6.4 (73,75,50). Results of automated pressure data analysis have been validated by comparing the results of computer analysis with those of manual analysis by a panel of experts (50,74).

In a study in 32 healthy volunteers ranging in age from 20 to 73 years, it was found that contractions recorded during meal consumption (perprandial contractions) had a significantly ($p < .001$) higher amplitude (66 ± 5.3 mm Hg) than the interprandial contractions recorded at daytime (49.6 ± 3.8 mm Hg). Only $50.9\% \pm 2.0\%$ of the $2,141 \pm 163$ contractions recorded in the 24-hour period were peristaltic, $10.4\% \pm 1.2\%$ were simultaneous, and the remaining portion was nontransmitted (segmental). Repetitive contractions, defined as having more than two peaks, were rare (50). Upper and lower limits of normal are listed in Table 6.5.

As in the analysis of pH data, the analysis of the temporal association between symptoms and abnormalities in tracings is of more importance than the overall analysis. This symptom-oriented analysis is complex, because the pressure tracings must be analyzed for abnormal contraction amplitude, abnormal contraction duration, abnormal contraction configuration (repetitive contractions), and abnormal contraction type (increased number of simultaneous waves). The optimal approach appears to be to use the patient as his or her own control (i.e., to use the motor activity in symptom-free episodes to determine what is normal for that patient). Analysis that uses asymptomatic baseline periods throughout the entire 24-hour period leads to more reliable results than analysis in which only 10-minute periods before each chest pain episode are used (77). Algorithms for fully automated computer analysis according to this principle have been developed and applied, and are now commercially available (77). In this symptom association analysis, different time windows have been used arbitrarily by various groups. A recent study has indicated, however, that a window beginning at 2 minutes before the onset of pain and ending at the onset of pain yields optimal results (55). This is the same window that is also optimal for the analysis of reflux-related symptoms.

Clinical Relevance of Ambulatory Pressure Recording

The development of systems for ambulatory recording of esophageal motor activity was prompted by the frequency with which diagnostic problems are encountered in patients with noncardiac chest pain. Because some of the esophageal motor abnormalities that may lead to esophageal chest pain occur intermittently, they can easily be missed during a brief conventional study. The aim of 24-hour pressure monitoring is to increase the chance of catching these abnormalities. Second, the demonstration of a continuously present esophageal motor abnormality, such as the nutcracker esophagus, does not yet prove that the patient's intermittent symptoms are caused by that abnormality. Much more convincing evidence of the causal role of such an abnormality is obtained when a temporal relationship between symptoms and abnormal motor events is found.

Although 24-hour esophageal pressure monitoring may yield valuable information on the pathophysiology of esophageal dysmotility (78), it is not likely that the technique will prove to be very useful in the diagnosis of continuously present (i.e., nonintermittent) esophageal motor disorders. It may be argued that prolonged monitoring is slightly more sensitive and specific in the diagnosis of nutcracker esophagus, because the diagnosis of this condition depends on the quantitative evaluation of contraction amplitude, but it is doubtful whether this diagnostic yield

TABLE 6.4. PROPAGATION VELOCITIES USED AS CRITERIA IN COMPUTERIZED CLASSIFICATION OF ESOPHAGEAL CONTRACTIONS IN AMBULATORY 24-HOUR STUDIES

	Velocity (cm/sec)	
Contraction Type	Breedijk et al. 1989 (73)[a] Smout et al. 1989 (50)[a]	Emde et al. 1990 (75)[b]
Peristaltic	≥1.8 and ≤12.5	>1 and <10
Simultaneous	>12.5 or <−25.0	>10
Nontransmitted	<1.8 and ≥−25.0	<1

[a]Reference point: passing of 15-mm Hg threshold.
[b]Reference point: maximal slope during upstroke.

TABLE 6.5. NORMAL VALUES IN 24-HOUR AMBULATORY ESOPHAGEAL MANOMETRY (2.5TH AND 97.5TH PERCENTILES) AS DERIVED FROM A STUDY IN 32 HEALTHY SUBJECTS[a]

	15 cm from LES	5 cm from LES
Mean amplitude (kPa)		
Peristaltic contractions		
Interprandial, daytime	3.71–9.31	3.84–10.39
Interprandial, nighttime	3.38–12.63	3.26–13.97
Perprandial	3.50–11.42	3.60–15.09
Simultaneous contractions		
Interprandial, daytime	3.63–7.65	3.84–8.13
Interprandial, nighttime	3.11–9.73	3.68–15.41
Perprandial	3.43–7.59	3.48–7.51
Nontransmitted contractions		
Interprandial, daytime	3.43–7.24	3.56–6.86
Interprandial, nighttime	2.91–6.93	3.59–8.08
Perprandial	3.60–9.29	3.54–10.85
Mean duration (sec)		
Peristaltic contractions		
Interprandial, daytime	1.3–2.9	1.3–3.5
Interprandial, nighttime	1.3–3.7	1.8–4.9
Perprandial	1.5–3.7	1.4–3.7
Simultaneous contractions		
Interprandial, daytime	1.0–2.2	1.2–2.9
Interprandial, nighttime	1.2–3.3	1.4–6.3
Perprandial	0.9–2.4	1.1–2.8
Nontransmitted contractions		
Interprandial, daytime	1.1–2.2	1.1–2.4
Interprandial, nighttime	1.2–2.3	1.4–3.4
Perprandial	1.2–4.0	1.2–2.9
Percent peristaltic contractions	30.4–71.1	
Percent simultaneous contractions	2.65–29.8	
Percent nontransmitted contractions	19.6–59.4	

LES, Lower esophageal sphincter.
[a]1 kPa = 7.5 mm Hg.
From Smout AJPM, Breedijk M, Van der Zouw C, et al. Physiological gastroesophageal reflux and esophageal motor activity studied with a new system for 24-hour recording and automated analysis. *Dig Dis Sci* 1989;34:372–378, with permission.

outweighs the costs and efforts associated with ambulatory pressure monitoring.

The first report on 24-hour ambulatory pressure monitoring in noncardiac chest pain was published in 1986 (52). In that year, the Louvain group reported that, in a group of 60 patients with chest pain of unexplained origin, combined 24-hour monitoring of esophageal pH and pressure increased from 16 to 29 the number of patients in whom an esophageal origin of the pain could be proved (52). The authors described their findings in a positive way, by stating that the combination of all conventional examinations and the 24-hour test made an esophageal origin of the pain likely in 48% of the patients (29 of 60 patients) (61). However, a correlation between chest pain and abnormal motility alone was demonstrated in only 8 of 60 patients, six of whom also showed abnormalities during the conventional manometric study. Therefore, the most pessimistic interpretation of the data would be that in only 2 of 60 patients studied did the ambulatory pressure study provide new evidence of the esophageal origin of the symptoms.

One year later, the same group of investigators described a group of 33 patients with angina-like chest pain in whom a positive correlation between chest pain and reflux or an esophageal motor disorder was found on 24-hour monitoring (72). An intriguing finding was that in ten of these patients, some of the episodes of chest pain were associated with reflux and other episodes with motor abnormalities. The increased tendency to perceive esophageal stimuli of various types as pain was designated *irritable esophagus*.

In a U.S. study in 24 patients with daily noncardiac chest pain in which quantitative criteria were used to determine whether a patient's esophageal motility was (more) abnormal during symptom episodes than during asymptomatic periods, the majority of the symptom episodes (64%) had no associations with abnormal motility or reflux, 20% were reflux related, 18% were dysmotility related, and 4% of the episodes were related to both abnormalities (69).

Overall, 13 patients (59%) had at least one chest pain episode correlating with abnormal motility or pH. The authors concluded that ambulatory monitoring of esophageal motility and pH is useful in the evaluation of noncardiac chest pain. However, their individual patient data show that some association between chest pain and abnormal motility alone was found in only four patients (14%), only one of whom had an SI higher than 50% (for motor abnormality).

In a study from the United Kingdom of 20 patients with noncardiac chest pain, ambulatory pH and pressure recording were reported to have a low diagnostic yield. The ambulatory pH study helped to establish the esophagus as the likely source of pain in one patient, and the ambulatory pressure recording did the same in another (71).

Our first experiences with 24-hour pH and pressure monitoring in unexplained chest pain were published in 1990 (7). Breumelhof and colleagues studied 44 consecutive tertiary referral patients with daily chest pain without making a selection of the basis of the frequency of their pain attacks. Nineteen of the patients did not experience chest pain during the 24-hour study period. Using computerized analysis of the association between chest pain and reflux or abnormal motility and using the rather stringent criterion of SI greater than 75%, proof of an esophageal origin of the symptoms was found in eight of the remaining 25 patients (reflux in two, dysmotility in two, both reflux and dysmotility in four patients). Thus, it was concluded that combined esophageal monitoring provided a diagnosis in 8 of 44 patients (18%) only.

Later we learned that the yield of ambulatory 24-hour pH and pressure monitoring in noncardiac chest pain depends largely on patient selection. Whereas the test was positive in only 18% of tertiary referral patients, much higher yields were found in patients acutely referred to a general hospital. Lam and colleagues studied 41 patients admitted to the coronary care unit as soon as it was considered unlikely that their pain was of cardiac origin (76). Using the same techniques for recording and data analysis as in Breumelhof's study (79), they found pain episodes to be related to reflux in 14 patients (34%) and to abnormal motility in 12 patients (29%) (76). In another general hospital, a 24-hour monitoring study was carried out in 28 patients who were newly referred to a cardiac outpatient clinic because of chest pain. Symptomatic gastroesophageal reflux disease was identified as the cause of the pain in 36% of the patients. In none of the patients was evidence of a esophageal motility disorder found (80).

Hewson and colleagues compared the yield of conventional tests, such as short-term esophageal manometry, the acid perfusion test, and the edrophonium test, with that of 24-hour pH and pressure monitoring in 45 patients with noncardiac chest pain (67). All patients experienced chest pain during ambulatory monitoring. Patients with normal manometry were significantly more likely to have acid reflux chest pain than were nutcracker esophagus patients. A positive result on the acid perfusion test was significantly associated with abnormal motility during pain, whereas a positive result on the edrophonium test predicted acid reflux-associated pain. The authors concluded that conventional tests may point to the esophagus as the likely source of the chest pain but that ambulatory monitoring is required to prove the association between symptoms and reflux or dysmotility. However, an association between pain and abnormal motility alone (i.e., in the absence of an association with reflux) occurred in only 4 of 45 patients (9%) (67).

The general conclusion to be drawn from these studies is that, in tertiary referral patients, the addition of 24-hour pressure recording to 24-hour pH recording does not lead to a substantial increase in the number of cases in which evidence for an esophageal origin of the symptoms can be obtained. On the basis of currently available information, it can be estimated that the additional diagnostic yield in these patients is less than 10%. One of the problems encountered is that only a minority of the noncardiac chest pain patients have pain every day. The diagnostic yield of the technique appears to be higher, however, when it is applied to patients in an early phase of the diagnostic workup or to patients with frequent pain attacks.

However, even though the yield of combined pH and pressure monitoring in unselected patients with chest pain is limited, we consider it worthwhile to perform the test because a positive result may greatly influence the patient's quality of life. It has been reported that an affirmative diagnosis of esophageal chest pain reduces the number of coronary care unit admissions, the consumption of drugs, and even the incidence of chest pain episodes (81).

Ambulatory Lower Esophageal Sphincter Pressure Monitoring

Recent technologic developments have made it possible to record lower esophageal sphincter (LES) pressure during prolonged periods of time in ambulatory subjects. Basically, two types of devices can be used to measure LES pressure continuously. Both employ a sensor of several centimeters' length that is positioned across the LES. With such a sensor, small longitudinal movements of the sphincter with respect to the sensor (caused by respiration, body movements, or swallowing) do not influence the LES pressure readings. One of these devices is a so-called sphinctometer, consisting of a nonperfused chamber filled with a viscous fluid (82). The other is a modification of the water-perfused sleeve sensor, requiring a portable perfusion pump and transducer assembly (83). A disadvantage of the latter system is that it is rather bulky and heavy. These technical obstacles, as well as the fact that the additional value of LES pressure monitoring for clinical decision making has not yet been established, presently limit

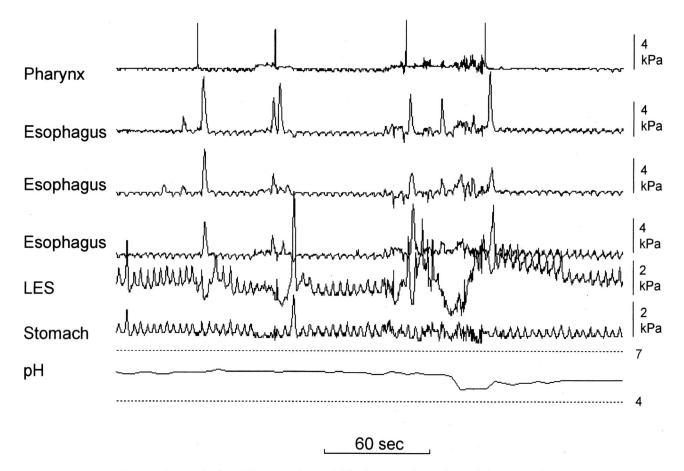

FIGURE 6.8. Detail of a 24-hour study in which pharyngeal, esophageal, lower esophageal sphincter (LES), and gastric pressures were recorded in a patient with (endoscopy-negative) reflux disease. A reflux episode can be seen during which the esophageal pH decreases from 5.8 to 4.7. This reflux episode is caused by a transient LES relaxation.

the application of the technique to the research domain. New observations on the mechanisms of gastroesophageal reflux and achalasia have been made with this technique (83–85). In particular, the important role of transient LES relaxations in the pathogenesis of gastroesophageal reflux has been elucidated with the aid of ambulatory LES pressure monitoring (Fig. 6.8).

REFERENCES

1. Spencer J. Prolonged pH recording in the study of gastro-oesophageal reflux. *Br J Surg* 1969;56:912–914.
2. Falor WH, Hansell JR, Chang B, et al. Outpatient 24-hour esophageal monitoring by pH telemetry. *Gastroenterology* 1980; 78:1163–1168.
3. Vantrappen G, Servaes J, Janssens J, et al. Twenty-four hour esophageal pH- and pressure recording in outpatients. In: Wienbeck M, ed. *Motility of the digestive tract.* New York: Raven Press, 1982:293–297.
4. Emde C, Garner A, Blum A. Technical aspects of intraluminal pH-metry in man: current status and recommendations. *Gut* 1987;28:1177–1188.
5. Gignoux C, Bonnet-Eymard DO, Holstein J, et al. Enregistrement ambulatoire du pH oesophagien pendant 24 heures dans une population de 27 témoins: analyse des facteurs techniques et methodologiques influençant les resultats. *Gastroenterol Clin Biol* 1987;11:17–23.
6. McLauchlan G, Rawlings JM, Lucas ML, et al. Electrodes for 24-hour pH monitoring: a comparative study. *Gut* 1987;28:935–939.
7. Ward BW, Wu WC, Richter JE, et al. Ambulatory 24-hour esophageal pH monitoring: technology searching for a clinical application. *J Clin Gastroenterol* 1986;8:59–67.
8. Duroux P, Emde C, Bauerfeind P, et al. The ion sensitive field effect transistor (ISFFT) pH electrode: a new sensor for long term ambulatory pH monitoring. *Gut* 1991;32:240–245.
9. Kuit JA, Schepel SJ, Bijleveld CMA, et al. Evaluation of a new catheter for esophageal pH monitoring. *Hepatogastroenterology* 1991;38:78–80.
10. Ours P, Richter J. Bravo pH vs ambulatory 24 hour catheter pH monitoring: a prospective assessment of patient satisfaction, discomfort and impairment of daily activities. *Gastroenterology* 2002;122[Suppl]:A580.
11. Lim PL, Gibbons MJ, Crawford EJ, et al. The effect of lifestyle changes on results of 24-h ambulatory oesophageal pH monitoring. *Eur J Gastroenterol Hepatol* 2000;12:655–656.
12. Mattox HE, Richter JE, Sinclair JW, et al. Gastroesophageal pH

step-up inaccurately locates proximal border of lower esophageal sphincter. *Dig Dis Sci* 1992;37:1185–1195.

13. Ter RB, Johnston BT, Castell DO. Exclusion of the meal period improves the clinical reliability of esophageal pH monitoring. *J Clin Gastroenterol* 1997;25:314–316.

14. Wo JM, Castell DO. Exclusion of meal periods from ambulatory pH monitoring may improve diagnosis of esophageal acid reflux. *Dig Dis Sci* 1994;39:1601–1607.

15. Murphy DW, Castell DO. Chocolate and heartburn: evidence of increased esophageal acid exposure after chocolate ingestion. *Am J Gastroenterol* 1988;83:633–636.

16. Vitale GC, Cheddle WG, Patel B, et al. The effect of alcohol on nocturnal gastroesophageal reflux. *JAMA* 1987;258:2077–2079.

17. Rodriquez S, Miner P, Robinson M, et al. Meal type affects heartburn severity. *Dig Dis Sci* 1998;43:485-490.

18. Clark CS, Kraus BB, Sinclair J, et al. Gastroesophageal reflux induced by exercise in healthy *volunteers. JAMA* 1989;261:3599–3601.

19. DeMeester TR, Johnson LF, Joseph GJ, et al. Patterns of gastroesophageal reflux in health and disease. *Ann Surg* 1976;184:459–469.

20. Wang H, Beck IT, Paterson WG. Reproducibility and physiological characteristics of 24-hour ambulatory esophageal manometry/pH-metry. *Am J Gastroenterol* 1996;91:492–497.

21. Wiener GJ, Morgan TM, Copper JB, et al. Ambulatory 24-hour esophageal pH monitoring. Reproducibility and variability of pH parameters. *Dig Dis Sci* 1988;33:1127–1133.

22. Johnsson F, Joelsson B. Reproducibility of ambulatory oesophageal pH monitoring in the diagnosis of gastroesophageal pH monitoring. *Gut* 1988;29:886–889.

23. Vandenplas Y, Helven R, Goyvaerts H, Sacré L. Reproducibility of continuous 24 hour oesophageal pH monitoring in infants and children. *Gut* 1990;31:374–377.

24. Weusten BL, Roelofs JM, Akkermans LM, et al. Objective determination of pH thresholds in the analysis of 24 h ambulatory oesophageal pH monitoring. *Eur J Clin Invest* 1996;26:151–158.

25. Franzen T, Grahn LT. Reliability of 24-hour oesophageal pH monitoring under standardized conditions. *Scand J Gastroenterol* 2002;37:6–8.

26. Murphy DW, Yuan Y, Castell DO. Does the intraesophageal pH probe accurately detect acid reflux? Simultaneous recording with two pH probes in humans. *Dig Dis Sci* 1989;34:649–656.

27. Grande L, Pujol A, Ros E, et al. Intraesophageal pH monitoring after breakfast and lunch in gastroesophageal reflux. *J Clin Gastroenterol* 1988;10:373–376.

28. Jörgensen F, Elsborg L, Hesse B. The diagnostic value of computerized short term esophageal pH monitoring in suspected gastroesophageal reflux. *Scand J Gastroenterol* 1988;23:363–367.

29. Bianchi Porro G, Pace F. Comparison of three methods of intraesophageal pH recording in the diagnosis of gastroesophageal reflux. *Scand J Gastroenterol* 1988;23:743–750.

30. Dobhan R, Castell DO. Prolonged intraesophageal pH monitoring with 16-hour overnight recording. *Dig Dis Sci* 1992;37:857–864.

31. Tuttle SG, Rufin F, Bettarello A. The physiology of heartburn. *Ann Intern Med* 1961;55:292–300.

32. Stanciu R, Hoarc RC, Bennett JR. Correlations between manometric and pH tests for gastro-oesophageal reflux. *Gut* 1977;18:536–540.

33. Vitale GC, Sadek S, Tulley FM, et al. Computerized 24-hour ambulatory esophageal pH monitoring and esophagogastroduodenoscopy in the reflux patient. *J Lab Clin Med* 1985;105:686–693.

34. Johnsson F, Joelsson B, Isberg PE. Ambulatory 24 hour intraesophageal pH monitoring in the diagnosis of gastroesophageal reflux disease. *Gut* 1987;28:1145–1150.

35. Hopert R, Emde C, Riecken EO. Recommendations for long-term oesophageal pH monitoring. *Neth J Med* 1989;34:S55–S61.

36. Johnson LF, DeMeester TR. Twenty-four-hour pH monitoring of the distal esophagus. *Am J Gastroenterol* 1974;62:323–332.

37. Branicki FJ, Evans DF, Jones JA, et al. A frequency-duration index (FDI) for the evaluation of ambulatory recordings of gastro-oesophageal reflux. *Br J Surg* 1984;71:425–430.

38. Johnson LF, DeMeester TR. Development of the 24-hour intraesophageal pH monitoring composite scoring system. *J Clin Gastroenterol* 1986;8[Suppl 1]:52–58.

39. Schindlbeck NE, Heinrich C, König A, et al. Optimal thresholds, sensitivity, and specificity of long-term pH-metry for the detection of gastroesophageal reflux disease. *Gastroenterology* 1987;93:85–90.

40. Dinelli, M, Passaretti S, Di Francia I, et al. Area under pH 4: a more sensitive parameter for the quantitative analysis of esophageal acid exposure in adults. *Am J Gastroenterol* 1999;94:3139–3144.

41. Rebecchi F, Di FI, Giaccone C, et al. Improving the analysis of esophageal acid exposure by a new parameter: area under H+. *Am J Gastroenterol* 2002;97:568–574.

42. Gill RC, Kellow JE, Wingate DI. Gastro-oesophageal reflux and the migrating motor complex. *Gut* 1987;28:929–934.

43. Kruse-Andersen S, Wallin L, Madsen T. Acid gastro-oesophageal reflux and oesophageal pressure activity during postprandial and nocturnal periods. *Scand J Gastroenterol* 1987;22:926–930.

44. Weiser HF, Pace F, Lepsien C, et al. Gastroösophagealer Reflux—was ist physiologisch? *Dtsch Med Wochenschr* 1982;107:366–370.

45. De Caestecker JS. Twenty-four-hour oesophageal pH monitoring: advances and controversies. *Neth J Med* 1989;34:S20–S39.

46. Singh S, Bradley LA, Richter JE. Determinants of oesophageal "alkaline" pH environment in controls and patients with gastro-oesophageal reflux disease. *Gut* 1993;34:309–316.

47. Meyers RL, Orlando RC. *In vivo* bicarbonate secretion by the human esophagus. *Gastroenterology* 1992;103:1174–1178.

48. Mittal RK, Reuben A, Whitney JO, et al. Do bile acids reflux into the esophagus? *Gastroenterology* 1987;92:371–375.

49. Champion G, Richter JE, Vaezi MF, et al. Duodenogastroesophageal reflux: relationship to pH and importance in Barrett's esophagus. *Gastroenterology* 1994;107:747–754.

50. Smout AJPM, Breedijk M, Van der Zouw C, et al. Physiological gastroesophageal reflux and esophageal motor activity studied with a new system for 24-hour recording and automated analysis. *Dig Dis Sci* 1989;34:372–378.

51. Bonavina L, DeMeester TR. Prolonged esophageal pH monitoring. In: Sigel B, ed, *Diagnostic patient studies in surgery*. Philadelphia: Lea & Febiger, 1986:353–363.

52. Janssens J, Vantrappen G, Ghillebert G. 24-Hour recording of esophageal pressure and pH in patients with noncardiac chest pain. *Gastroenterology* 1986;90:1978–1984.

53. Richter JE, Bradley LA, DeMeester TR, et al. Normal 24-hour ambulatory esophageal pH values. Influences of study center, pH electrode, age and gender. *Dig Dis Sci* 1992;37:849–856.

54. Sponce RAJ, Collins BJ, Parks TG, et al. Does age influence normal gastroesophageal reflux? *Gut* 1985;26:799–801.

55. Lam HGT, Breumelhof R, Roelofs JMM, et al. What is the optimal time window in symptom analysis of 24-hour esophageal pressure and pH data? *Dig Dis Sci* 1994;39:402–409.

56. Wiener GJ, Richter JE, Copper JB, et al. The symptom index: a clinically important parameter of ambulatory 24-hour esophageal pH monitoring. *Am J Gastroenterol* 1988;83:358–361.

57. Singh S, Richter JE, Bradley LA, et al. The symptom index. Differential usefulness in suspected acid-related complaints of heartburn and chest pain. *Dig Dis Sci* 1993;38:1402–1408.

58. Breumelhof R, Smout AJPM. The symptom sensitivity index: a

valuable additional parameter in 24-hour esophageal pH recording. *Am J Gastroenterol* 1991;86:160–164.

59. Weusten BLAM, Akkermans LMA, van Berge Henegouwen GP, et al. Ambulatory combined oesophageal pressure and pH monitoring: relationships between pathological reflux, oesophageal dysmotility and symptoms of oesophageal dysfunction. *Eur J Gastroenterol Hepatol* 1993;5:1055–1060.

60. Klauser AG, Schindlbeck HC, Müller-Lissner SA. Is long-term esophageal pH monitoring of clinical value? *Am J Gastroenterol* 1989;84:362–366.

61. Fuchs KH, DeMeester TR, Albertucci M. Specificity and sensitivity of objective diagnosis of gastroesophageal reflux disease. *Surgery* 1987;102:575–580.

62. Mattioli S, Pilotti V, Spangaro M, et al. Reliability of 24-hour home esophageal pH monitoring in diagnosis of gastroesophageal reflux. *Dig Dis Sci* 1989;34:71–78.

63. Pujol A, Grande L, Ros F, et al. Utility of inpatient 24-hour intraesophageal pH monitoring in diagnosis of gastroesophageal reflux. *Dig Dis Sci* 1988;33:1134–1140.

64. Rokkas T, Sladen GE. Ambulatory esophageal pH recording in gastroesophageal reflux. Relevance to the development of esophagitis. *Am J Gastroenterol* 1988;83:629–632.

65. Schlesinger PK, Donahue PE, Schmid B, et al. Limitations of 24-hour intraesophageal pH monitoring in the hospital setting. *Gastroenterology* 1985;98:797–804.

66. Katzka DA, Paoletti V, Lelte L, et al. Prolonged ambulatory pH monitoring in patients with persistent gastroesophageal reflux symptoms: testing while on therapy identifies the need for more aggressive anti-reflux therapy. *Am J Gastroenterol* 1996;91:2110–2113.

67. Hewson LG, Dalton CB, Richter JE. Comparison of esophageal manometry, provocative testing, and ambulatory monitoring in patients with unexplained chest pain. *Dig Dis Sci* 1990;35:302–309.

68. Weusten BLAM, Roelofs JMM, Akkermans LMA, et al. The symptom association probability: an improved method for symptom analysis of 24-hour esophageal pH data. *Gastroenterology* 1994;107:1741–1745.

69. Peters L, Maas L, Petty D, et al. Spontaneous noncardiac chest pain. *Gastroenterology* 1988;94:878–886.

70. Pfister CJ, Harrison MA, Hamilton JW, et al. Development of a three-channel, 24-h ambulatory esophageal pressure monitor. *IEEE Trans Biomed Eng* 1989;36:487–490.

71. Soffer EE, Scalabrini P, Wingate DL. Spontaneous noncardiac chest pain: value of ambulatory esophageal pH and motility monitoring. *Dig Dis Sci* 1989;34:1651–1655.

72. Vantrappen G, Janssens J, Ghillebert G. The irritable oesopha-

gus: a frequent cause of angina-like pain. *Lancet* 1987;2:1232–1234.

73. Breedijk M, Smout AJPM, Van der Zouw C, et al. Microcomputer based system for 24-hour recording of oesophageal motility and pH profile with automated analysis. *Med Biol Eng Comput* 1989;27:41–46.

74. Bumm R, Emde C, Armstrong D, et al. Ambulatory esophageal manometry: comparison of expert and computer-aided manometry analyses. *J Gastrointest Motil* 1990;2:216–223.

75. Emde C, Armstrong D, Bumm R, et al. Twenty-four-hour continuous ambulatory measurement of oesophageal pH and pressure: a digital recording system and computer-aided manometry analysis. *J Ambul Monit* 1990;3:47–62.

76. Lam HGT, Dekker W, Kan G, et al. Acute noncardiac chest pain in a coronary care unit: evaluation by 24-hour pressure and pH monitoring of the esophagus. *Gastroenterology* 1992;102:453–460.

77. Richter JF, Castell DO. 24-Hour ambulatory oesophageal motility monitoring: how should motility data be analyzed? *Gut* 1989;30:1040–1047.

78. Barham CP, Gotley DC, Mills A, et al. Oesophageal acid clearance in patients with severe reflux oesophagitis. *Br J Surg* 1995;82:333–337.

79. Breumelhof R, Nadorp JHSM, Akkermans LMA, et al. Analysis of 24-hour esophageal pressure and pH data in unselected patients with noncardiac chest pain. *Gastroenterology* 1990;99:1257–1264.

80. Voskuil JH, Cramer MJ, Breumelhof R, et al. Prevalence of esophageal disorders in patients with chest pain newly referred to the cardiologist. *Chest* 1996;109:1210–1214.

81. Ward BW, Wallace C, Wu WC, et al. Longterm follow-up of symptomatic status of patients with noncardiac chest pain: is diagnosis of esophageal etiology helpful? *Am J Gastroenterol* 1987;82:215–218.

82. Trudgill NJ, Riley SA. Monitoring the lower oesophageal sphincter: sphinctometer or sleeve? *Neurogastroenterol Motil* 1999;11:173–178.

83. Schoeman MN, Tippett M, Akkermans LMA, et al. Mechanisms of gastroesophageal reflux in ambulant healthy human subjects. *Gastroenterology* 1995;108:83–91.

84. Van Herwaarden MA, Samsom M, Smout AJPM. Excess gastroesophageal reflux in patients with hiatus hernia is caused by mechanisms other than transient LES relaxations. *Gastroenterology* 2000;119:1439–1446.

85. Van Herwaarden MA, Samsom M, Smout AJPM. Prolonged manometric recordings of oesophagus and lower oesophageal sphincter in achalasia patients. *Gut* 2001;49:813–821.

7

ESOPHAGEAL FUNCTION TESTING AND GASTROESOPHAGEAL REFLUX TESTING USING MULTICHANNEL INTRALUMINAL IMPEDANCE

RADU TUTUIAN
MARCELO F. VELA
STEVEN S. SHAY

Multichannel intraluminal impedance (MII) is a new technique for evaluating esophageal function. This chapter reviews the current status in the development of this new method in esophageal function testing (EFT) and gastroesophageal reflux (GER) testing. EFT is an important step in evaluating patients with possible esophageal symptoms. This is currently performed using a combination of esophageal manometry and barium or radioisotope esophagram. Approximately a decade ago, Silny and coworkers (1) first described this new technique of assessing intraluminal bolus movement.

BASIC PRINCIPLES

The principle of this technique depends on changes in resistance to alternating current (i.e., impedance) between two metal electrodes (i.e., impedance measuring segment) produced by the presence of bolus inside the esophageal lumen. Electric conductivity (the opposite of resistance or impedance) is directly related to the ionic concentration of the intraluminal content. Intraluminal content with high ionic concentrations (i.e. refluxate, food, saliva) have a relative low resistance (high conductivity) compared to the esophageal lining or air.

Combined video-impedance measurements have validated changes observed with bolus entry, presence, and clearing in the impedance-measuring segment (1,2) (Fig. 7.1). In the absence of bolus, impedance is determined by the electrical conductivity of the esophageal lining. Upon arrival of bolus between the electrodes, impedance may increase abruptly as a result of the presence of a pocket of air in front of the head of the bolus. Intraluminal impedance then rapidly decreases as high ionic content of the bolus provides good electrical conductivity. While the bolus is present in the impedance measuring segment, intraluminal impedance remains low. Esophageal contractions clearing the intraluminal content increase the impedance with a slight "overshoot" caused by a decrease in esophageal cross section during contraction before returning to baseline.

Multiple impedance measuring segments within the esophagus allow determination of direction of bolus movement within the esophagus, or MII (Fig. 7.2). Antegrade (i.e., swallows) bolus movement (Fig. 7.3) is detected by impedance changes of bolus presence progressing proximal to distal. Retrograde (i.e., reflux) bolus movement is detected by changes in impedance progressing distal to proximal followed by proximal to distal clearance of bolus by either a primary or a secondary contraction wave (Fig. 7.4).

By mounting MII on classic manometry or pH catheters allows MII to complement traditional manometry or pH testing. Combined MII and manometry (MII-EM) provides simultaneous information on intraluminal pressure changes and bolus movement, whereas combined MII and pH (MII-pH) allows detection of pH episodes regardless of their pH values (i.e., acid and nonacid reflux).

R. Tutuian: Division of GI/Hepatology, Medical University of South Carolina, Charleston, South Carolina.
M. F. Vela, S. S. Shay: Department of Gastroenterology, The Cleveland Clinic Foundation, Cleveland, Ohio.

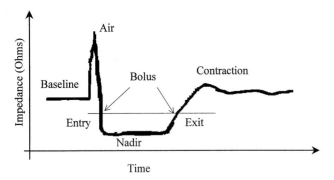

FIGURE 7.1. Impedance changes observed during bolus transit over a single pair of measurement rings separated by 2 cm. A rapid increase in resistance is noted when air traveling in front of the bolus head reaches the impedance measuring segment followed by a decrease in impedance once higher conductive bolus material passes the measuring site. Bolus entry is considered at the 50% decrease in impedance from baseline relative to nadir, and bolus exit is considered at the 50% recovery point from nadir to baseline. Lumen narrowing produced by the contraction transiently increases the impedance above baseline.

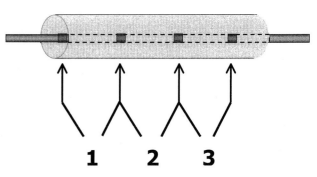

FIGURE 7.2. Multiple impedance measuring segments within the esophagus allow determination of direction of bolus movement within the esophagus; that is, multichannel intraluminal impedance, or MII.

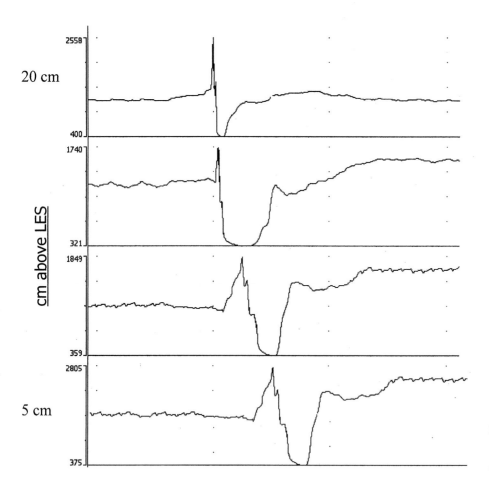

FIGURE 7.3. Antegrade (i.e., swallows) bolus movement detected by impedance changes of bolus presence progressing proximal to distal.

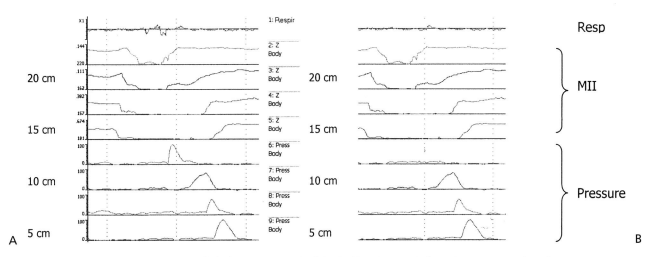

FIGURE 7.4. Retrograde bolus movement is detected by changes in impedance progressing distal to proximal followed by proximal to distal clearance of bolus by either a primary **(A)** or a secondary contraction wave **(B)**. Primary contraction identified by swallowing activity shown in the respiratory channel (*Respir*) not shown with secondary contractions.

ESOPHAGEAL FUNCTION TESTING USING COMBINED MULTICHANNEL INTRALUMINAL IMPEDANCE AND MANOMETRY

MII-EM is a new technique using two complementary methods of EFT: (a) Esophageal manometry provides information about intraluminal pressures generated during swallowing, and (b) MII assesses bolus movement during swallowing. Although it does not provide the anatomic details offered by radiographic barium swallow, MII has the advantage of not requiring radiation exposure in evaluating bolus movement. Furthermore, bolus transit and pressures are obtained during a single test procedure.

The indications for combined MII-EM are the same as for esophageal manometry: evaluation of dysphagia, noncardiac chest pain, and GERD, including preoperative evaluation before antireflux surgery or endoscopic antireflux procedures.

Initial studies performed in our laboratory on normal subjects indicated that MII could detect presence of small volumes of swallowed liquid (i.e., 1 mL) and confirmed known pharmacologic effects of cholinergic medication on esophageal peristalsis and bolus movement (3).

Materials and Equipment

The EFT catheter is a specially designed, flexible tube incorporating pressure sensors and impedance measuring rings. The nine-channel EFT catheter (Konigsberg Instruments, Pasadena, CA; Sandhill Scientific, Inc., Highlands Ranch, CO) incorporates five pressure (two circumferential and three unidirectional) sensors and four impedance measuring segments (Fig. 7.5). The two circumferential

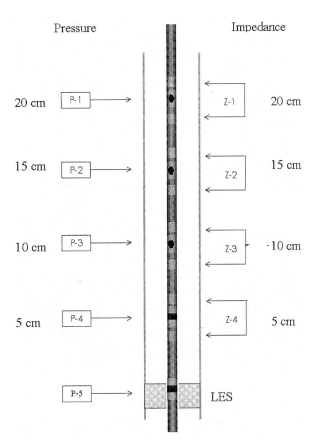

FIGURE 7.5. Nine-channel combined multichannel intraluminal impedance (MII) and manometry (EM) catheter. Circumferential solid-state pressure sensors located in lower esophageal sphincter (LES) high-pressure zone (P5) and 5 cm above it (P4); unidirectional solid-state pressure sensors located 10 cm (P3), 15 cm (P2), and 20 cm (P1) above LES. Impedance measuring segments centered at 5 cm (Z4), 10 cm (Z3), 15 cm (Z2), and 20 cm (Z1) above LES.

solid-state pressure sensors are located at 5 and 10 cm from the tip, and three unidirectional pressure sensors are at 15, 20, and 25 cm. Impedance measuring segments consist of pairs of metal rings placed 2 cm apart, centered at 10, 15, 20, and 25 cm from the tip, thus straddling the four proximal pressure transducers. The signal from the catheter is transferred to an amplifying and digitizing interface (SensorPAC-Z, Sandhill Scientific, Inc., Highlands Ranch, CO) and is then recorded and stored using dedicated software (Insight Acquisition, Sandhill Scientific, Inc., Highlands Ranch, CO). Upon completion of data acquisition, tracings are edited and analyzed using a second dedicated software program (BioView Analysis, Sandhill Scientific, Inc., Highlands Ranch, CO). The analysis software reports manometric (contraction amplitude, duration and velocity, LES resting and residual pressure) and impedance (bolus presence time, bolus head advance time, total and segmental bolus transit times) parameters. Based on predefined criteria, the software determines bolus entry, presence, and clearing parameters that assess completion of bolus transit. The summary reports percent of manometric normal peristaltic, ineffective, and simultaneous contractions, and percent of swallows with complete and incomplete bolus transit.

Study Procedure

The study procedure is similar to standard esophageal manometry with some modulation determined by the design of the catheter. The EFT catheter is inserted transnasally into the stomach. The lower esophageal sphincter (LES) is identified using a stationary pullthrough technique, and the most distal sensor is placed in the high-pressure zone of the LES. The remaining intraesophageal pressure sensors and impedance measuring segments are thus located at 5, 10, 15, and 20 cm above LES. In the supine position, subjects are given ten swallows of 5 mL liquid (normal saline solution 0.9%) and ten swallows of 5 mL EFT viscous solution (Sandhill Scientific, Inc., Highlands Ranch, CO), which has the consistency of applesauce. The use of standard normal saline 0.9% solution is preferred over the use of water because it has higher ionic content, which increases the ability of the impedance circuit to identify bolus presence. Also, the impedance of bottled or tap water varies with brand or geographic location.

During data acquisition, it is important to allow at least 20 seconds between individual swallows so the esophageal body and LES have time to recover. Findings from double swallows should be discarded and the swallow repeated because of deglutitive inhibition produced by closely spaced swallows. Completion of the LES pullthrough using the most distal circumferential pressure sensor after the administration of both sets of ten liquid and viscous swallows ends

the procedure. The entire procedure can be completed in approximately 25 to 30 minutes.

Data Analysis

Lower Esophageal Sphincter

The location of the LES and its pressure profile are evaluated in the standard manner (see Chapter 5). The circumferential sensor in the LES measures LES relaxation duration and residual pressure during swallowing.

Esophageal Body

Combined MII-EM offers simultaneous evaluation of both esophageal contraction characteristics and bolus transit. Manometric parameters of amplitude, duration, and velocity are measured as per standard manometry (see Chapter 5).

Bolus entry at a specific level measured by impedance is considered to occur at the 50% point between 3 seconds before swallow impedance baseline and impedance nadir during bolus presence. Bolus exit is determined as return to this 50% point on the impedance recovery curve (Fig. 7.1). These relationships have been validated by simultaneous MII and barium swallow (1,2). Calculated impedance parameters are shown in Figure 7.6: (a) total bolus transit time as time elapsed between bolus entry at 20 cm above LES and bolus exit at 5 cm above LES, (b) bolus head advance time as time elapsed between bolus entry at 20 cm above LES and bolus entry at 15, 10, and 5 cm above LES, (c) bolus presence time as time elapsed between bolus entry and bolus exit at each impedance measuring site (5, 10, 15, and 20 cm above LES), and (d) segmental transit times as time elapsed between bolus entry at a given level above LES and bolus exit at the next lower level.

Swallows are manometrically classified (4) as (a) normal, if contraction amplitudes at 5 and 10 cm above the LES are each greater than or equal to 30 mm Hg and distal onset velocity is less than 8 cm/sec; (b) ineffective, if either of the contraction amplitudes at 5 and 10 cm above the LES is less than 30 mm Hg; (c) simultaneous, if contraction amplitudes at 5 and 10 cm above the LES are each greater than or equal to 30 mm Hg and distal onset velocity is greater than 8 cm/sec. These criteria are based on studies in normal volunteers (5) and simultaneous videofluoromanometry (6).

Swallows are classified by MII as showing (a) complete bolus transit (Fig. 7.7A), if bolus entry is seen at the most proximal site (20 cm above LES) and bolus exit points are recorded in all three distal impedance-measuring sites (i.e., 15, 10, and 5 cm above the LES) and (b) incomplete bolus transit (Fig. 7.7B) if bolus exit is not identified at any of the three distal impedance measuring sites.

Total bolus transit time (TBTT)

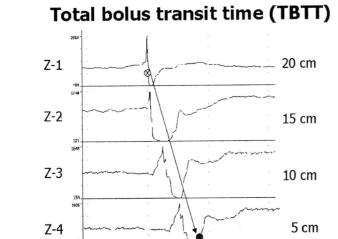

Bolus head advance time (BHAT)

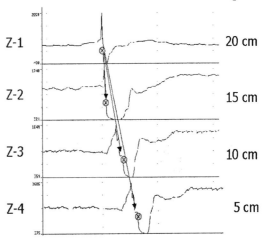

A

B

Bolus Presence Time (BPT)

Segment Transit Time (STT)

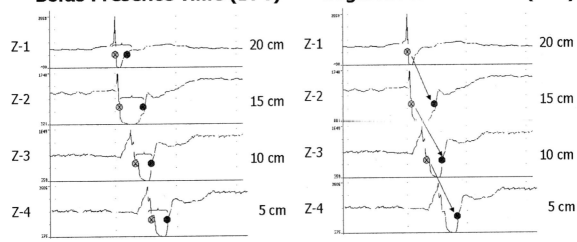
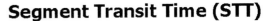

C

D

FIGURE 7.6. Definitions of impedance parameters. **A:** Total bolus transit time (TBTT) as time elapsed between bolus entry at 20 cm above lower esophageal sphincter (LES) and bolus exit at 5 cm above LES. **B:** Bolus head advance time as time elapsed between bolus entry at 20 cm above LES and bolus entry at 15, 10, and 5 cm above LES. **C:** Bolus presence time (BPT) as time elapsed between bolus entry and bolus exit at each impedance measuring site (5, 10, 15, and 20 cm above LES). **D:** Segment transit times (STT) as time elapsed between bolus entry at a given level above LES and bolus exit at the next lower level.

Study Interpretation

Previously published studies in normal volunteers established normal values for classic esophageal manometry (Chapter 5). Normal EFT parameters (Tables 7.1 and 7.2) have been recently determined in a multicenter study (7). Normal values for impedance parameters were proposed based on the 95 percentile in healthy volunteers (Table 7.3).

Manometric parameters define a study as being normal if it does not contain more than 20% ineffective and 10% simultaneous liquid swallows (4).

Impedance parameters define a study as normal if at least 80% of liquid and at least 70% of viscous swallows showed complete MII-detected bolus transit (7). When using viscous testing substances, a study is considered normal if it does not contain more than 20% ineffective and 10% simultaneous swallows (7).

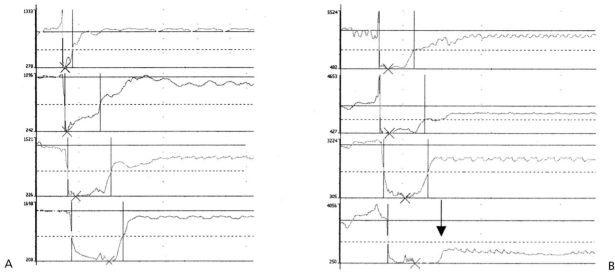

FIGURE 7.7. Classification of swallows by MII criteria. **A:** Complete bolus transit if bolus entry is seen at the most proximal site (20 cm above lower esophageal sphincter [LES]) and bolus exit points are recorded in all three distal impedance-measuring sites (i.e., 15, 10, and 5 cm above the LES). **B:** Incomplete bolus transit if bolus exit is not identified at any one of the three distal impedance measuring sites.

Classification of manometric abnormal swallows is presented in Chapter 12. Studies using MII-EM in patients with manometrically defined motility abnormalities are in progress. These studies should provide a better understanding of bolus transit of various categories of motility abnormalities. Preliminary observations in our laboratory suggest that more than half of patients with manometrically defined distal esophageal spasm (DES) or ineffective esophageal motility (IEM) have complete bolus transit measured by MII. Patients with nutcracker esophagus or isolated LES abnormalities (i.e., hypertensive or hypotensive LES, poorly relaxing LES) have complete bolus transit during swallowing, whereas patients with achalasia or scleroderma have incomplete bolus transit during swallowing (Fig. 7.8).

MII-EM studies in healthy volunteers and patients with various manometric abnormalities suggest a new classifica-

TABLE 7.1. NORMATIVE DATA OF MANOMETRIC PARAMETERS (AMPLITUDE, DURATION, AND ONSET VELOCITY OF CONTRACTIONS) OF ESOPHAGEAL FUNCTION TESTING FOR LIQUID AND VISCOUS SWALLOWS

	Liquid (N = 429) Percentile				Viscous (N = 425) Percentile			
	Median	25th	75th	95th	Median	25th	75th	95th
Amplitude of contractions (mm Hg)								
at 15 cm	57.1	41.3	88.7	125.8	71.7	51.3	93.4	136.8
at 10 cm	86.4	64.7	120.6	185.9	87.5	64.6	123.9	173.4
at 5 cm	118.1	92.9	146.1	239.6	125.8	88.6	170.1	246.6
Distal esophageal amplitude (mean of 5 and 10 cm)	104.6	81.3	132.5	195.1	109.8	80.0	141.3	197.7
Duration of contraction (sec)								
at 15 cm	2.7	2.2	3.3	4.5	3.2	2.7	3.8	5.1
at 10 cm	3.0	2.4	3.8	5.1	3.1	2.6	4.2	5.9
at 5 cm	3.4	2.7	4.2	6.2	3.5	2.8	4.5	6.6
Onset velocity of contractions (cm/sec)								
15–5 cm	3.5	2.9	4.4	5.5	3.0	2.4	3.6	5.3
10–5 cm	3.9	2.7	5.2	7.4	3.1	2.3	4.0	6.5

95th Percentile values should define upper limit of normal for given parameters.
N, total number of swallows in 43 healthy volunteers.
Data from Tutuian R, Vela MF, Balaji N, et al. Esophageal function testing using combined multichannel intraluminal impedance and manometry. Multicenter Study in healthy volunteers. *Clin Gastroenterol Hepatol* 2003 (*in press*).

TABLE 7.2. NORMATIVE DATA OF IMPEDANCE PARAMETERS OF ESOPHAGEAL FUNCTION TESTING FOR TEN LIQUID AND TEN VISCOUS SWALLOWS IN 43 HEALTHY VOLUNTEERS

	Liquid (N = 429) Percentile				Viscous (N = 425) Percentile			
	Median	25th	75th	5th–95th	Median	25th	75th	5th–95th
Bolus head advance time (sec)								
20–15 cm	0.2	0.1	0.3	0.0–0.7	1.0	0.6	1.5	0.2–2.5
20–10 cm	0.6	0.4	0.9	0.1–1.7	3.3	2.4	4.0	0.9–5.1
20–5 cm	1.3	0.8	2.2	0.5–5.0	4.9	4.3	5.6	2.8–7.4
Bolus presence time (sec)								
at 20 cm	1.7	1.1	2.7	0.6–5.9	1.9	1.2	2.9	0.8–5.0
at 15 cm	4.1	3.0	5.1	1.4–8.8	3.5	2.8	4.1	1.9–5.9
at 10 cm	5.3	4.5	6.3	3.5–9.9	3.4	2.6	4.3	1.9–7.6
at 5 cm	5.8	4.6	6.7	2.3–9.3	3.1	2.3	4.1	1.5–6.3
Segment transit time (sec)								
20–15 cm	4.4	3.3	5.4	1.6–9.0	4.6	4.0	5.3	2.8–7.3
15–10 cm	5.7	5.0	6.7	3.9–10.5	5.3	4.5	6.3	3.8–10.1
10–5 cm	6.6	5.8	7.6	4.5–10.6	4.9	3.9	6.0	3.0–8.3
Total bolus transit time (sec)	7.2	6.6	8.2	5.2–11.9	7.9	7.0	9.0	5.9–12.4

95th Percentile values can be considered upper limit of normal for given parameters.
Data from Tutvian R, Vela MF, Balaji N, et al. Esophageal function testing using combined multichannel intraluminal impedance and manometry. Multicenter Study in healthy volunteers. *Clin Gastroenterol Hepatol* 2003 (*in press*).

TABLE 7.3. PROPOSED NORMAL VALUES (BASED ON 95TH PERCENTILE) FOR MII PARAMETERS FOR LIQUID AND VISCOUS SWALLOWS

	Liquid	Viscous
Total bolus head advance time 20–5 cm (sec)	5.0	7.5
Total bolus transit time (sec)	12.5	12.5
Smooth muscle transit time 10–5 cm (sec)	10.5	8.5
Percent complete bolus transit	≥80%	≥70%

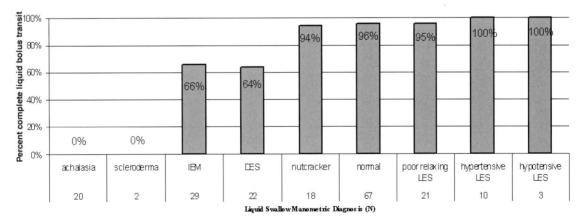

FIGURE 7.8. Preliminary data on bolus transit in various manometric diagnoses. Whereas all patients with achalasia and scleroderma have incomplete bolus transit, more than half of patients with distal esophageal spasm and ineffective esophageal motility have complete bolus transit. Almost all patients with nutcracker esophagus, normal esophageal manometry, and isolated lower esophageal sphincter abnormalities have complete bolus transit for liquid.

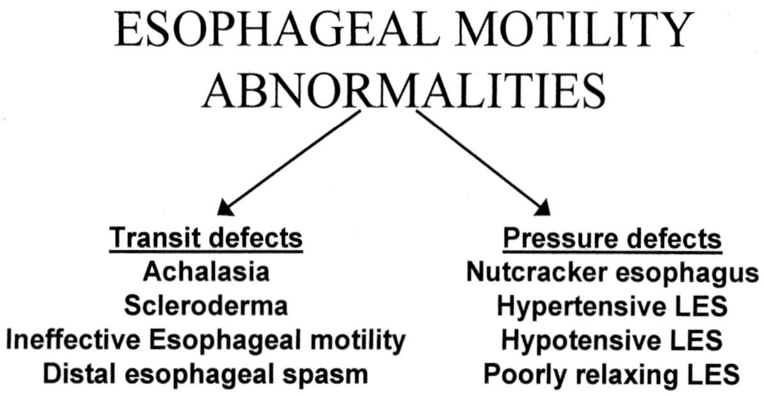

ESOPHAGEAL MOTILITY ABNORMALITIES

Transit defects
Achalasia
Scleroderma
Ineffective Esophageal motility
Distal esophageal spasm

Pressure defects
Nutcracker esophagus
Hypertensive LES
Hypotensive LES
Poorly relaxing LES

FIGURE 7.9. New separation of esophageal motility abnormalities into bolus transit defects and pressure defects based on multichannel intraluminal impedance and manometry findings.

tion for esophageal motility abnormalities into bolus transit defects (i.e., achalasia, scleroderma, IEM, and DES) and pressure defects (i.e., nutcracker esophagus, hypertensive LES, hypotensive LES, and poorly relaxing LES) as shown in Figure 7.9.

MII-EM provides a more detailed evaluation of both aspects of esophageal function: esophageal contractility and bolus transit. Given differences in transit pattern of liquid and viscous bolus transit identified by MII-EM, we recommend using both testing substances for a more refined characterization of esophageal function.

COMBINED MULTICHANNEL INTRALUMINAL IMPEDANCE AND PH FOR DETECTION OF ACID AND NONACID GASTROESOPHAGEAL REFLUX

The pathophysiologic role of acid in GERD has been well established by a number of studies in both animals and humans (8). The accepted gold standard for the assessment of GER is distal esophageal pH recording (9), which bases detection of reflux of acidic material into the esophagus on changes in hydrogen ion concentration. In a number of patients, reflux symptoms persist despite treatment with medications that decrease gastric acid secretion; it has been suggested that these symptoms may be due to reflux having pH greater than 4 (i.e., nonacid reflux) (10). When the contents of the stomach are buffered, such as in the postprandial period, or during treatment with potent acid-suppressing medications, such as proton pump inhibitors, a significant proportion of GER is nonacid and therefore hard to detect by conventional pH recording (11–14). This limitation of pH-metry has created the need for a method that can accurately measure nonacid reflux.

Currently available techniques for the study of nonacid or alkaline reflux include aspiration, scintigraphy, ambulatory pH monitoring, and bilirubin monitor-

ing (Bilitec) (15–19), all of which have certain limitations. Aspiration studies allow for only short analysis periods, and the accuracy of enzymatic determination of the contents of the aspirates has been questioned (8,18,20). Scintigraphic studies are expensive, involve radiation exposure, and are usually limited to short monitoring periods (8,16,18,20). Ambulatory pH monitoring uses pH of 7 or greater as the definition of "alkaline" reflux, but increased saliva production or bicarbonate secreted by esophageal submucosal glands confounds measurements by increasing esophageal pH in the absence of reflux (8,18,20,21). Some authors propose that reflux can be detected by pH-metry even when intraesophageal pH remains greater than 4.0 through measurement of pH decreases greater than 1 unit (22). However, pH-metry is unable to detect nonacid reflux that occurs in the absence of pH changes or with small pH changes (less than 1 unit). Monitoring with the Bilitec probe is based on the presence of bilirubin and is therefore incapable of measuring bile-free nonacid reflux; furthermore, simultaneous determination of bile and pH in the stomach has been shown to correlate poorly (23). Additionally, bilirubin monitoring requires a special diet to avoid false-positive readings (8,18).

Multichannel intraluminal impedance used in combination with pH-metry (MII-pH) accurately records GER at all pH levels and is emerging as a useful tool to study both acid and nonacid reflux (11,12). The technique has been validated fluoroscopically and manometrically to detect bolus movement in the esophagus, both in the oral and aboral direction (24), thus enabling measurement of and distinction between swallows and reflux. Because MII records retrograde flow of gastric contents into the esophagus in a pH-independent fashion, combining the technique with pH-metry enables detection of nonacid as well as acid reflux. Additionally, MII-pH provides detailed characterization of the reflux episode, including determination of the composition (gas, liquid, mixed) and the height reached by the refluxate (11,12,25).

PRINCIPLES OF MEASUREMENT OF ACID AND NONACID REFLUX THROUGH COMBINED MULTICHANNEL INTRALUMINAL IMPEDANCE AND PH

Measurement of Reflux

As discussed earlier, by placing a series of conducting rings throughout the length of the esophagus, changes in intraluminal impedance can be recorded in response to the movement of intraluminal material in either an oral or aboral direction. As shown in Figures 7.3 and 7.4, this means that a swallow can be clearly distinguished from retrograde movement of gastric contents into the esophagus. Furthermore, clearance of the refluxate (volume clearance) can be established at the point where impedance returns to baseline in the most distal recording segment.

Acid Reflux, Nonacid Reflux, and Re-reflux

Simultaneous MII and pH measurements are achievable through catheters that combine several impedance measuring segments with one or more pH electrodes. An

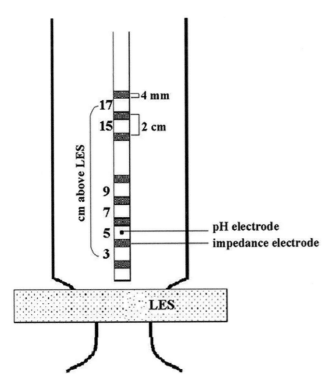

FIGURE 7.10. Schematic representation of the 2-mm diameter multichannel intraluminal impedance pH catheter with impedance electrodes (4 mm in length) set in pairs at 2-cm intervals, allowing for six impedance measuring segments as well as one pH electrode. Once properly positioned, this catheter allows recording of pH at 5 cm above the LES and impedance in six measuring segments, with their centers at 3, 5, 7, 9, 15, and 17 cm above the LES.

example of such a catheter that allows for recordings in six impedance recording sites and one pH site is shown in Figure 7.10.

When MII is combined with pH, a distinction between acid and nonacid reflux can be made because MII detects the presence of the refluxate, whereas pH simply determines the acid or nonacid nature of the refluxate. Furthermore, MII-pH enables the measurement of additional reflux episodes during an ongoing acid reflux episode, so-called re-reflux. Examples of GER of three types (acid, nonacid, and re-reflux) recorded with a six-impedance/one-pH catheter are shown in Figure 7.11.

Determination of Reflux Composition and Height

Assisted by the observation that air and gastric contents each produce a different change in impedance, reflux episodes can be characterized as containing gas, liquid, or both. Air conducts electricity poorly and therefore has high impedance, whereas liquid gastric contents have a low impedance. As illustrated in Figure 7.12, gas produces increases in intraluminal impedance, and liquid gastric contents result in decreased impedance.

In summary, MII-pH enables refined characterization of the reflux episode. Because it measures both volume presence (through MII) as well as changes in acidity (through pH), it enables detection of reflux of all types—acid, nonacid, and re-reflux—while providing details about the volume and acid clearance as well as information on the composition and height reached by the refluxate.

Ambulatory MII-pH

All of the initial studies using MII-pH were done with stationary setups and over relatively short periods of time (2- to 3-hour recording sessions). More recently, equipment to perform ambulatory MII-pH studies over prolonged periods of time has become available (Sleuth, Sandhill Scientific, Inc., Highlands Ranch, CO) (31). The equipment is similar to that used in clinical pH-metry: the 2-mm flexible catheter (2 mm in diameter) is placed transnasally and is connected to a data logger that the patient carries for 24 hours (Fig. 7.13).

APPLICATION OF MULTICHANNEL INTRALUMINAL IMPEDANCE AND PH IN GASTROESOPHAGEAL REFLUX DISEASE

Pediatric Applications

In the first published study describing the use of MII-pH as a means of assessing acid and nonacid reflux, Skopnik and colleagues (26) reported on 17 infants with GERD who underwent MII-pH measurements in the postprandial

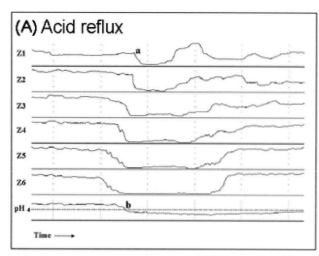

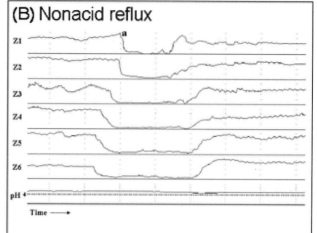

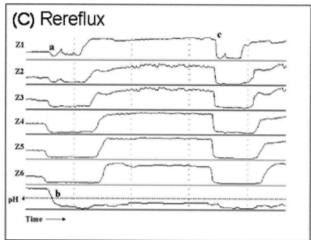

FIGURE 7.11. Impedance changes in ohms during three episodes of reflux. The six impedance measuring segments (Z1 to Z6) and pH changes are shown in the Y-axis. The *dotted line* marks a pH of 4.0. **A:** Point *a* indicates the proximal extent of the reflux event. It is preceded by a sequential drop in impedance starting at the most distal measuring segment that proceeds toward the proximal esophagus. Arrival of the refluxate into the distal esophagus causes a decrease in pH to less than 4.0, an acid reflux episode. **B:** The proximal extent is indicated by point *a*. This is not accompanied by a decrease in pH to less than 4.0 and is thus considered an episode of nonacid reflux. **C:** Reflux detected by multichannel intraluminal impedance (MII) (*a*) causes a decrease in pH to less than 4.0 (*b*). A second MII-detected reflux episode (re-reflux, *c*) occurs before pH returns to 4.0.

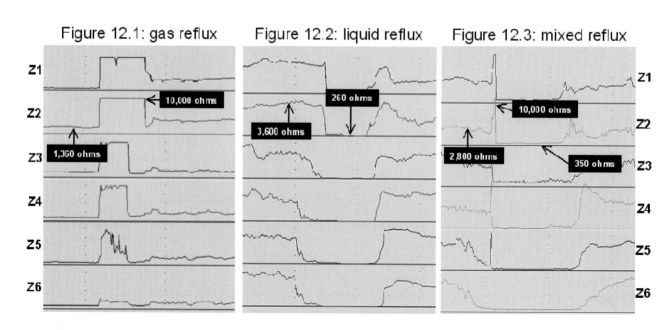

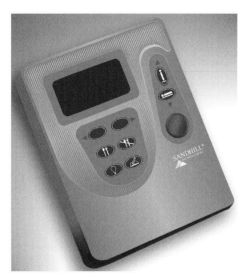

FIGURE 7.13. The ambulatory multichannel intraluminal impedance pH logger.

period. They found that the technique allowed detection of a large number of nonacid reflux episodes that would otherwise be undetectable by conventional pH-metry. Further reports in the pediatric literature have described the use of MII-pH to study the relationship between reflux, both acid and nonacid, and apnea in infants and premature babies (27,28).

Adult Applications

Several studies have examined different patterns of reflux using MII-pH in stationary conditions and over short periods of time.

Sifrim and colleagues (29) used the technique with concurrent manometry to study patterns of gas and liquid reflux during transient LES relaxations (TLESRs) in 11 normal volunteers in the postprandial period; their findings showed that, in upright normal subjects, although belching can precipitate acid reflux, most acid reflux occurs as a primary event (29). In a subsequent study (9), this group of investigators evaluated the composition of postprandial refluxate in 16 patients with GERD and 15 healthy control subjects and found that, in the postprandial period,

TLESRs and reflux of gastric contents are similarly frequent in patients with GERD and control subjects; however, GERD patients showed more acid reflux and less nonacid reflux. They postulated that differences in the air-liquid composition of the refluxate may contribute to a higher rate of acid reflux in the patient group.

More recently, Shay and colleagues (25) used MII-pH in combination with manometry in ten GERD patients and ten normal volunteers to evaluate the accuracy of MII in detecting individual reflux events identified by pH probe and manometry. The subjects were studied fasting in both the left and right lateral decubitus. Overall, patients had 30-fold more reflux episodes than normal volunteers; MII detected 95% of all reflux events identified by pH metry or manometry alone and showed that liquid reflux predominates in the right recumbent posture, with gas reflux being more common in the left recumbent position.

Two studies have used MII-pH to assess acid and nonacid reflux and their associated symptoms after pharmacologic manipulation. Vela and co-workers (11) reported in a group of subjects with frequent heartburn studied in the postprandial period that treatment with omeprazole resulted in a significant decrease in the number of acid reflux episodes; however, nonacid reflux continued to occur and was responsible for some symptoms. Thus, acid suppression did not result in a decrease in reflux episodes but rather in a shift from acid to nonacid reflux in the immediate postprandial period. This study also showed that taking all reflux episodes into account both acid and nonacid reflux—results in a higher calculated symptom index. In a subsequent study of patients with heartburn, these investigators studied the effect of baclofen, a γ-aminobutyric acid B agonist, on acid and nonacid reflux and their associated symptoms (30). By inhibiting TLESRs, this medication decreased acid and nonacid reflux as well as their associated symptoms in the postprandial period.

All of the aforementioned studies were performed in stationary setups and over short periods of time (3 hours or less). The findings described by these investigators await confirmation in ambulatory conditions and over prolonged periods of time.

In the only published study using 24-hour ambulatory MII-pH, Sifrim and colleagues (29) described acid, nonacid, and gas reflux in 30 patients with symptomatic

FIGURE 7.12. Impedance changes in ohms during reflux of gas, liquid, and mixed contents, obtained with a catheter incorporating six impedance measuring segments (Z1 to Z6), which are shown in the Y-axis. Impedance values for the second measuring segment (Z2) are shown for the three reflux episodes. **A:** Reflux of gas is characterized by sharp increases in impedance beginning in the most distal recording segment and rapidly progressing upward toward the proximal esophagus. In Z2 impedance rises from a baseline of 1,360 ohms to a peak of 10,000 ohms. **B:** Reflux of liquid is characterized by sequential impedance decreases starting in the distal esophagus and moving upward toward the mouth. In Z2, impedance decreases from a baseline of 3,600 ohms to a trough of 260 ohms. **C:** Reflux of gas mixed with liquid. In Z2, impedance increases from a baseline of 2,860 ohms to a peak of 10,000 ohms; this is followed by an impedance decrease to a trough of 350 ohms.

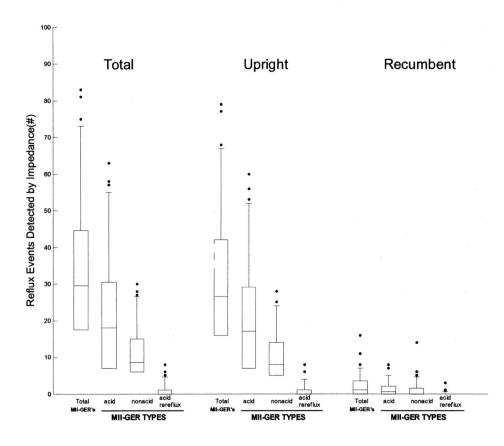

FIGURE 7.14. Number of gastroesophageal reflux (GER) events detected by multichannel intraluminal impedance 5 cm above the lower esophageal sphincter. Data are expressed as median with interquartile ranges (*box*: 25% to 75%; *bar*: 95% value) per subject, and individual values greater than 95% are shown.

GERD and erosive esophagitis and 28 healthy controls. Interestingly, they found that the total rate of reflux episodes was similar in the patients and the healthy controls. However, GERD patients had a higher proportion of acid reflux. One third of the reflux episodes were nonacid in both groups. In terms of reflux composition, mixed reflux (liquid and gas) was most frequent in both groups,

and GERD patients had more pure liquid reflux than the normal control subjects.

Shay and colleagues (31) recently defined normal values for acid and nonacid reflux in 24-hour ambulatory MII-pH based on studies in 60 normal volunteers (Fig. 7.14 and Table 7.4) and have suggested abnormal parameters based on 95 percentile values in the normal volunteers.

TABLE 7.4. TWENTY-FOUR-HOUR MII-pH VALUES 5 cm ABOVE THE LES IN 60 NORMAL VOLUNTEERS

| | MII Parameters | | | | | | | |
| | MII-GER | | MII-GER Type and Frequency[a] | | | | pH Parameters | |
	Total	Duration (sec)	Acid	Nonacid	Acid Re-reflux	% Bolus Exposure	pH-Only GER[c]	% Acid Exposure
Total 24-hr:								
Median (25th, 75th)	30 (18,45)	10 (6,16)	18 (7,31)	9 (6,15)	0 (0,1)	0.5 (0.3,0.9)	0 (0,1)	1.2 (0.3,2.5)
95th percentile	73	*	55	26	4	1.4	3	6.3
Upright:								
Median (25th, 75th)	27 (16,42)	10 (6,16)	17 (7,29)	8 (5,14)	0 (0,1)	0.7 (0.4,1.3)	0 (0,1)	1.3 (0.4,3.3)
95th percentile	67	*	52	24	4	2.1	3	9.7
Recumbent:								
Median (25th, 75th)	1 (0,4)	7 (4,14)	0 (0,2)	0 (0,2)	0.04 (0.0,0.12)	0 (0,5)	0.0 (0.0,0.3)	
95th percentile	7	*	5	4	0	0.7	0	2.1

GER, gastroesophageal reflux; MII, multichannel intraluminal impedance.
[a]MII-GER types are based on pH probe findings. Acid MII-GER and pH-GER: pH fall above to below 4; nonacid: MII-GER while pH > 4; acid re-reflux: MII-GER while pH < 4.
[b]% Bolus exposure: duration of all MII-GERs/time monitored.
[c]pH-Only GERs: GERs detected by the pH probe, but not by MII.

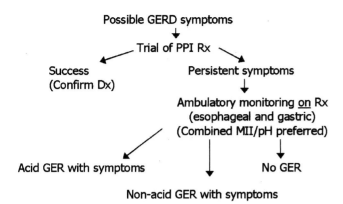

FIGURE 7.15. Proposed gastroesophageal reflux disease diagnostic algorithm.

Preliminary data from a multicenter study involving the Medical University of South Carolina, Cleveland Clinic, and Catholic University in Leuven, Belgium, suggest that only 20% of patients with persistent symptoms on proton pump inhibitor therapy have symptoms associated with acid reflux. MII-pH was able to evaluate association of persistent symptoms in the remaining 80% of patients, finding that half of patients had symptoms associated with nonacid reflux while the other half of patients had neither acid nor nonacid preceding their symptoms. Based on this observation, we propose using the algorithm in Figure 7.15 for a more complete diagnosis of GERD.

Summary

In summary, MII-pH testing brings a shift in GER testing paradigm. In MII-pH studies reflux events are no longer detected by pH. Refluxate presence, distribution, and clearing is primarily detected by MII and characterized as acid versus nonacid based on pH change and as liquid, gas, or mixed based on MII. MII determines refluxate clearance time, whereas pH measures acid clearance time. MII-pH shows promise to become an important clinical tool, particularly to assess GER in the postprandial period and in patients with persistent symptoms on therapy and with atypical symptoms.

REFERENCES

1. Silny J. Intraluminal multiple electric impedance procedure for measurement of gastrointestinal motility. *J Gastrointest Motil* 1991;3:151–162.
2. Blom D, Mason RJ, Balaji NS, et al. Esophageal bolus transport identified by simultaneous multichannel intraluminal impedance and manofluoroscopy. *Gastroenterology* 2001;120:P103.
3. Srinivasan R, Vela MF, Katz PO, et al. Esophageal function testing using multichannel intraluminal impedance. *Am J Physiol Gastrointest Liver Physiol* 2001;280:G457–G462.
4. Spechler SJ, Castell DO. Classification of oesophageal motility abnormalities. *Gut* 2001;49:145–151.
5. Richter JE, Wu WC, Johns DN, et al. Esophageal manometry in 95 healthy adult volunteers. *Dig Dis Sci* 1987;32:583–592.
6. Kahrilas PJ, Doods WJ, Hogan WJ. Effect of peristaltic dysfunction on esophageal volume clearance. *Gastroenterology* 1988;94:73–80.
7. Tutuian R, Vela MF, Balaji N, et al. Esophageal function testing using combined multichannel intraluminal impedance and manometry. Multicenter study in healthy volunteers. *Clin Gastroenterol Hepatol* 2003;1:174–182.
8. Vaezi MF, Singh S, Richter JE. Role of acid and duodenogastric reflux in esophageal mucosal injury: a review of animal and human studies. *Gastroenterology* 1995;108:1897–1907.
9. DeVault KR, Castell DO. Updated guidelines for the diagnosis and treatment of gastroesophageal reflux disease. *Am J Gastroenterol* 1999;94:1434–1442.
10. Navaratnam RM, Winslet MC. Gastro-oesophageal reflux: the disease of the millennium. *Hosp Med* 1998;59:646–649.
11. Vela MF, Camacho-Lobato L, Srinivasan R, et al. Intraesophageal impedance and pH measurement of acid and nonacid reflux: effect of omeprazole. *Gastroenterology* 2001;120:1599–1606
12. Sifrim D, Holloway RH, Silny J, et al. Composition of the postprandial refluxate in patients with gastroesophageal reflux disease. *Am J Gastroenterol* 2001;96:647–655.
13. Washington N, Steele RJC, Jackson SJ, et al. Patterns of food and acid reflux with low-grade esophagitis—the role of an anti-reflux agent. *Aliment Pharmacol Ther* 1998;12:53–58.
14. Shay SS, Egli D, Johnson LF. Simultaneous esophageal pH monitoring and scintigraphy during the postprandial period in patients with severe reflux esophagitis. *Dig Dis Sci* 1991;36:558–564.
15. Stein HJ, Feussner H, Kauer W, et al. Alkaline gastroesophageal reflux: assessment by ambulatory esophageal aspiration and pH monitoring. *Am J Surg* 1994;167:163–168.
16. Velasco N, Pope CE, Gannan RM, et al. Measurement of esophageal reflux by scintigraphy. *Dig Dis Sci* 1984;29:977–982.
17. Iftikhar SY, Ledingham S, Evans DF, et al. Alkaline gastro-oesophageal reflux: dual probe pH monitoring. *Gut* 1995;37: 465–470.
18. Vaezi MF, Richter JE. Importance of duodeno-gastro-esophageal reflux in the medical outpatient practice. *Hepatogastroenterology* 1999;46:40–47.
19. Stein HJ, Kauer WKH, Feussner H, et al. Bile acids as components of the duodenogastric refluxate: detection, relationship to bilirubin, mechanism of injury, and clinical relevance. *Hepatogastroenterology* 1999;46:66–73.
20. Girelli CM, Cuvello P, Limido E, et al. Duodenogastric reflux: an update. *Am J Gastroenterol* 1996;91:648–653.
21. DeVault KR, Georgeson S, Castell DO. Salivary stimulation mimics esophageal exposure to refluxed duodenal contents. *Am J Gastroenterol* 1993;88:1040–1043.
22. Smout AJPM. Ambulatory monitoring of esophageal pH and pressure. In: Castell DO, Richter JE, eds. *The esophagus*, third ed. Philadelphia: Lippincott Williams & Wilkins, 1999:119–133.
23. Just RJ, Leite LP, Castell DO. Changes in overnight fasting intragastric pH show poor correlation with duodenogastric bile reflux in normal subjects. *Am J Gastroenterol* 1996;91:1567–1570.
24. Silny J, Knigge KP, Fass J, et al. Verification of the intraluminal multiple electrical impedance measurement for the recording of gastrointestinal motility. *J Gastrointest Motil* 1993;5:107–122.
25. Shay S, Bomeli S, Richter J. Multichannel intraluminal impedance accurately detects fasting, recumbent reflux events and their clearing. *Am J Physiol Gastrointest Liver Physiol* 2002;283: G376–G383.
26. Skopnik H, Silny J, Heiber O, et al. Gastroesophageal reflux in infants: evaluation of a new intraluminal technique. *J Pediatr Gastroenterol Nutr* 1996;22:591–598.
27. Wenzl T, Schenke S, Peschgens T, et al. Association of apnea and nonacid gastroesophageal reflux in infants: investigations with

the intraluminal impedance technique. *Pediatr Pulmonol* 2001; 31:144–149.

28. Peter C, Prodowski N, Bonhorst B, et al. Gastroesophageal reflux and apnea of prematurity: no temporal relationship. *Pediatrics* 2002;109:8–11.

29. Sifrim D, Silny J, Holloway R, et al. Patterns of gas and liquid reflux during transient lower oesophageal sphincter relaxation: a study using intraluminal electrical impedance. *Gut* 1999;44:47–54.

30. Vela MF, Tutuian R, Katz P, et al. Baclofen reduces acid and nonacid postprandial gastroesophageal reflux measured by combined multichannel intraluminal impedance and pH. *Aliment Pharmacol Ther* 2003;17:243–251.

31. Shay SS, Vela MF, Tutuian R, et al. Twenty-four hour ambulatory multichannel intraluminal impedance and pH (24h MII-pH): a multicenter report of normal values from 45 healthy volunteers. *Gastroenterology* 2002;122[Suppl 1]:A577.

8

PROVOCATIVE TESTS FOR PAIN OF ESOPHAGEAL ORIGIN

RONNIE FASS

Noncardiac chest pain (NCCP), or unexplained chest pain, is a highly prevalent disorder that affects up to 23% of the general population (1). Predominance in women has been primarily reported by tertiary referral centers, but community-based studies revealed no gender predilection (1). The prevalence of NCCP in various ethnic groups remains to be elucidated. Tendency to report symptoms and seek medical attention may vary amongst the different ethnic groups.

It is well recognized that many individuals with NCCP who seek medical attention become avid and sometimes relentless users of the health care system (2–4). These patients are more likely to see a physician repeatedly or multiple physicians for their chest pain (5). A significant number of patients report poor quality of life and admit taking cardiac medications despite lack of evidence for a cardiac cause. Only a small fraction of patients feel reassured. This disease-related behavior results in a considerable toll on the health care system. In one study, the health care cost for NCCP was estimated at more than $315 million annually, primarily because of multiple clinic visits, emergency department visits, hospitalizations, and prescription medications (4). This cost estimate does not include indirect costs such as lost days of work (absenteeism) or intangible cost, such as the impact of symptoms on the patient's quality of life, which have been demonstrated to be considerable when evaluating the economic burden of functional bowel disorders. In Australia, the annual costs associated with NCCP presentations to the Nepean Hospital amount to approximately $1.4 million (2). The researchers extrapolated these costs to the Australian health care system and conservatively estimated that NCCP accounts for at least $30 million of the health care budget annually.

Gastroesophageal reflux is the most common cause of NCCP. An association with gastroesophageal reflux disease (GERD) has been demonstrated by abnormal 24-hour esophageal pH monitoring or upper endoscopy in up to 60% of patients with NCCP (6–9).

Various esophageal motility abnormalities may present with chest pain only or with other esophageal-related symptoms (such as dysphagia). The motility abnormalities include diffuse esophageal spasm, nutcracker esophagus, achalasia, long-duration contractions, multipeaked waves, and hypertensive lower esophageal sphincter (LES) (10). However, esophageal manometry appears to have a relatively poor sensitivity in evaluating patients with NCCP. When evaluated by esophageal manometry, most patients with NCCP demonstrate normal esophageal motor function. In different studies, only one third of the patients with NCCP have some type of esophageal dysmotility (11,12). Furthermore, patients rarely experienced chest pain during esophageal manometry, regardless of whether esophageal dysmotility was documented (13). Some authorities suggest that motility abnormalities in NCCP should be used as a marker of an underlying esophageal motor disorder that may be responsible for patient's symptoms (14).

Patients with NCCP who lack any evidence of pathologic gastroesophageal reflux or motility disorder with a recognized pathologic basis have been defined by the Rome II committee as having functional chest pain of presumed esophageal origin (15). It is postulated that altered perception of sensations that arise from the esophagus is the mechanism responsible for symptoms of chest pain in these patients.

The introduction of various provocative tests was prompted by lack of demonstration of esophageal pathology with the currently available esophageal physiologic tests in a significant number of NCCP patients. The hope was to improve the diagnostic yield of esophageal testing.

PHYSIOLOGY OF ESOPHAGEAL PAIN

The esophagus, like the rest of the viscera, receives dual sensory innervation, traditionally referred to as parasympathetic

R. Fass: Department of Medicine, University of Arizona, and Director of GI Motility Laboratories, Southern Arizona VA Health Care System and University of Arizona Health Sciences Center, Tucson, Arizona.

and sympathetic, but more properly based on the actual nerves, vagal and spinal (16) (Fig. 8.1). The vagal afferent neurons compose 80% of the vagal trunk and have cell bodies in the nodose ganglia (17). Vagal afferents whose receptive fields are located in the esophageal smooth muscle layer are sensitive to mechanical distention, whereas polymodal (responding to multiple modalities of stimuli) vagal afferents with receptive fields in the mucosa are sensitive to a variety of chemical or mechanical intraluminal stimuli, which, under normal circumstances, are not associated with conscious perception (18). In general, vagal afferents do not play a direct role in visceral pain transmission at the level of the gut, except for certain types of vagal afferents that appear to have a pain modulatory effect (19). Recent reports suggest that vagal afferents may also play a role in perception of esophageal distention (19,20). In contrast, spinal afferents, which have their cell bodies in the dorsal root ganglia, are primarily acting as nociceptors and are central to the perception of discomfort and pain (21). Spinal afferents with receptive fields in the muscle layer and serosa are primarily mechanosensitive. The intraepithelial nerve endings of spinal afferent are likely to be involved in mediating acid-induced pain during topical exposure to intraluminal acid (22,23). Many of the afferents contain calcitonin gene-related peptide and substance P, which are neurotransmitters that are important in mediating visceral nociception (17).

Data regarding cortical loci involved in processing of esophageal sensation in humans are relatively scarce (24). Nonpainful esophageal balloon distentions elicit bilateral activation along the central sulcus, the insular cortex, and the frontal and parietal operculum (25). In contrast, painful esophageal balloon distentions result in intense activation of the same areas and additional activation of the right anterior insular cortex (important in affective processing) and anterior cingulate gyrus (important in pain processing and generating an affective and cognitive response to pain) (26–28). Nonpainful infusions of 0.1N hydrochloric acid resulted in cerebral cortical activity that was concentrated in the posterior cingulate and the parietal and anteromesial frontal lobes (29). The superior frontal lobe regions activated corresponded to Brodmann's areas 32, the insula, the operculum, and the anterior cingulate.

Chest pain symptoms may represent an activation of a common pathway in response to different intraesophageal stimuli. Different intraesophageal stimuli (e.g., acid, balloon distention) may elicit similar symptoms in different patients or different symptoms in the same patient (22,30). Thus, esophageal symptoms such as heartburn or chest pain are not stimulus specific.

A recent study demonstrated that chest pain and heartburn may be provoked in normal subjects during esophageal balloon distention either in the proximal or dis-

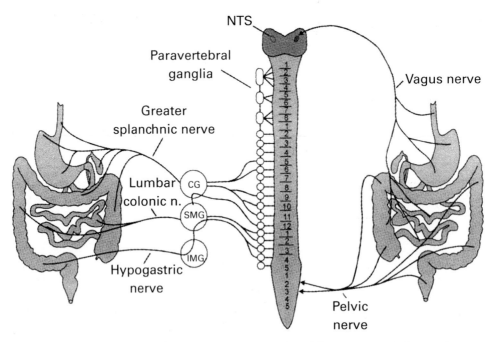

FIGURE 8.1. Representation of visceral sensory innervation of the gastrointestinal tract. The sensory innervation that anatomically exists in association with the sympathetic nervous system is shown on the left. These spinal visceral sensory fibers traverse both prevertebral and paravertebral ganglia en route to the spinal cord. Pelvic and vagus nerve innervation to the sacral spinal cord and brainstem, respectively, is shown on the right. *CG,* celiac ganglion; *IMG,* inferior mesenteric ganglion; *SMG,* superior mesenteric ganglion. (Adapted from Gebhart GF. Visceral pain—peripheral sensitisation. *Gut* 2000;47[Suppl 4]:iv54–iv55.)

tal portion of the esophagus (22). Volume thresholds for heartburn and chest pain in both esophageal locations were similar, suggesting that, for a specific volume, some patients develop chest pain and others heartburn. Furthermore, volume thresholds for both chest pain and heartburn did not differ significantly at each esophageal location and between locations. In this study, esophageal balloon distention reproduced typical heartburn symptoms in some patients with documented GERD and chest pain in others. This study clearly demonstrates that balloon distention may result in different types of esophageal symptoms.

The mechanism by which an esophageal stimulus causes heartburn in some patients and chest pain in others remains poorly understood. Balaban and colleagues (31) have recently demonstrated a temporal correlation between sustained contractions of the esophageal longitudinal muscle and both spontaneous and provoked esophageal chest pain. In a subsequent study that assessed the temporal relationship between sustained esophageal longitudinal muscle contractions and heartburn (32), the investigators suggested that shorter duration of the sustained esophageal contraction was associated with heartburn and longer duration with chest pain.

Perception of intraesophageal events, either physiologic or pathologic, is a complicated process that involves central and peripheral mechanisms. Several studies have shown that most intraesophageal stimuli are not perceived by subjects (33). For example, less than 20% of all acid reflux events result in GERD symptoms, regardless of whether mucosal injury is present (33). It is yet to be elucidated what factors determine perception of an intraesophageal event, leading to symptom generation. In GERD, is it a specific acid reflux event, the actual hydrogen ion concentration (H^+) of the refluxate, the summation of several short reflux events, the distribution of acid along the esophagus, or the increased number or duration of acid reflux events (24)? Several recent studies have demonstrated that fat and other nutrients can modulate perception of intraluminal events that are mediated by gut neurotransmitters, hormones, or enzymes. Meyer and colleagues have recently shown that intraduodenal fat significantly shortened latency to onset of heartburn and intensified the perception of acid-induced heartburn in subjects with GERD who underwent intraesophageal acid perfusion (34).

Central neural mechanisms appear to have an important role in modulating esophageal perception as well (35). Psychological comorbidity (e.g., anxiety, depression) can modulate esophageal perception and cause subjects to perceive low-intensity esophageal stimuli (pathologic or physiologic) as being painful (36). Another important factor is stress that appears to enhance perception of intraesophageal stimuli by reducing perception thresholds for pain (37). Stress has recently emerged as an important factor in symptom generation and exacerbation of both functional and organic gastrointestinal disorders (38). Traditionally, stress is consid-

ered a domain of psychology, and, thus, commonly lumped together with the role of psychiatric comorbidity (39). However, recent developments in the understanding of brain–gut interactions in functional bowel disorders resulted in reassessment of the role of chronic stress in the pathophysiology and management of gastrointestinal disorders such as NCCP. Certain stressful life events have been associated with the onset or symptom exacerbation of functional bowel disorders. In addition, daily experiences of stress appear to have an important modulating effect on perception of intraluminal events (Fig. 8.2).

Other central factors, such as sleep quality, may also alter perception of intraesophageal events. Further research is needed to better define the brain–gut (or gut–brain) relationship as it is related to symptom generation in esophageal disorders.

ESOPHAGEAL PROVOCATION TESTS

Acid Perfusion Test (Bernstein Test)

Bernstein and Baker (40) introduced the acid perfusion test as an objective method to identify esophageal chemosensitivity to acid. A nasogastric tube was passed through the nares of a fasting, sitting subject and into the stomach (40,41). After the gastric content was aspirated, the tube was withdrawn until it measured 30 cm from the nares to the tip (41). This maneuver assumed that the solution would be delivered at a level near the junction of the upper and middle thirds of the esophagus. The tube was connected to an intravenous bottle. A control administration of 0.9% NaCl was perfused for 10 to 15 minutes at a rate of 6 to 7.5 mL per minute. This was followed by administration of 0.1N HCl acid, at a similar rate, for 30 minutes or until discomfort was induced (41). If symptoms appeared, the test was discontinued and saline solution was given.

The acid perfusion test was originally devised to distinguish between chest pain of cardiac and esophageal origin. However, since the initial description, many modifications have been made to the original Bernstein test. Although the basic principal of the test remained similar, many investigators have tried different acid perfusion rates, concentrations, and durations in the hope of increasing the sensitivity of the test (42–49). Furthermore, some have even suggested the addition of bile salts to the acid solution (50). Others required that, for a result to be positive, the acid-induced symptoms should quickly disappear by the reinfusion of saline or bicarbonate (51).

Many attempts were made to change the test from a qualitative to a quantitative tool. Time to onset of symptoms during acid perfusion was used to compare the extent of chemosensitivity to acid between GERD and Barrett's patients (52). Fass and colleagues (22) placed a manometry catheter 10 cm above the upper border of the LES to ensure sufficient exposure of the esophageal mucosa to acid. Saline

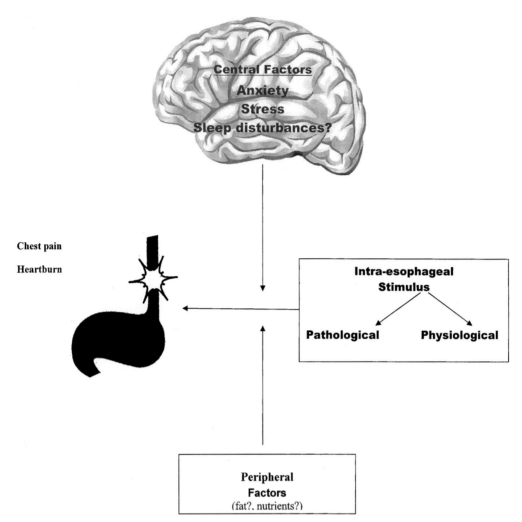

FIGURE 8.2. Proposed conceptual model for esophageal symptom generation. This model suggests that central (through brain–gut interactions) and peripheral mechanisms are essential for intraesophageal stimuli (either physiologic or pathologic) to reach the conscious level and thus be perceived. (Adapted from Fass R, Tougas G. Functional heartburn—the stimulus, the pain and the brain. *Gut* 2002;51:885–892.)

was infused initially for 2 minutes and then without the patient's knowledge 0.1N HCl acid was infused for 10 minutes at a rate of 10 mL per minute. Patients were instructed to report whenever their typical symptoms were reproduced. Esophageal chemosensitivity was assessed by both the duration until typical symptom perception was induced (expressed in seconds) and the total sensory intensity rating reported by the subject at the end of acid perfusion by using a verbal descriptor scale. The scale consisted of a 20-cm vertical bar flanked by descriptors of increasing intensity (no sensation, faint, very weak, weak, very mild, mild, moderate, barely strong, slightly intense, strong, intense, very intense, and extremely intense). Placement of words along each scale was determined from their relative log intensity rating in a normative study (53). The validity of these scales for assessing the perceived intensity of visceral sensations has been confirmed (54).

An acid perfusion test intensity score (cm × sec) was then calculated as follows:

$$\frac{I \times T}{100}$$

where I is the total intensity rating at the end of acid perfusion and T is the duration of report of typical symptom perception during the test. For convenience, the score was divided by 100.

Although the test appears to be highly specific (55), its sensitivity is relatively low, with figures ranging from 6% to almost 60% (56–62). A negative test result has little clinical value and does not exclude an esophageal origin of the chest pain. Patients with Barrett's esophagus have been reported to demonstrate a decrease in esophageal chemosensitivity to acid, resulting in even more false-negative results (52). However, this alteration in pain perception disappeared after esophageal ablation resulted in complete Barrett's reversal (63).

It has been debated whether the contact of acid with the mucosa on its own, or acid-induced motility disorder (64,65), or a combination of both are involved in the pain production. Smith and colleagues (66) showed that symptom production is clearly pH dependent, which strongly suggests that acid and not the associated motility disorder is responsible for the symptoms.

Presently, the acid perfusion test is rarely performed in clinical practice because of its limited diagnostic value in NCCP and other esophageal disorders. Because of the low sensitivity and the emergence of noninvasive and highly sensitive modalities, such as the proton pump inhibitor (PPI) test and empirical therapy with a PPI, many authors have considered the acid perfusion test to be obsolete (42,67,68).

Edrophonium (Tensilon) Test

Edrophonium is an anticholinesterase that increases cholinergic activity at muscarinic receptors (69). A short-acting drug, edrophonium pharmacologic action is manifested within 30 to 60 seconds after injection and lasts an average of 10 minutes. The aim of the edrophonium test is to induce greater esophageal body amplitude contractions in the hope of provoking the patient's typical chest pain (70). The test is performed by injecting either 80 mg/kg or 10 mg edrophonium intravenously, immediately followed by five to ten swallows of 5 to 10 mL of water over a period of 5 to 10 minutes (71–75). The pain occurs on swallowing, within 5 minutes after the administration of the drug, and disappears quickly as the drug is rapidly metabolized.

Edrophonium has shown no effect on coronary artery diameter and actually decreases cardiac workload (71). Overall, the side effects are minimal and the antidote atropine is almost never required. Side effects are chiefly due to excessive cholinergic stimulation and may include increased salivation, nausea, vomiting, and abdominal cramps.

The sensitivity of the edrophonium test is relatively low and has varied from as high as 55% to as low as 0% (56,57,59–62). The correct sensitivity is unknown because of the lack of a gold standard. Although edrophonium is known to increase esophageal contraction amplitude and duration as well as the number of repetitive contractions after a swallow, some studies showed that this increase is not greater in chest pain patients with a positive (pain) response than patients in whom the test did not induce pain. The changes in contraction observed in chest pain patients after administration of edrophonium are similar to those in healthy control subjects who never experience pain during the test (76). This indicates that the mechanism by which edrophonium induces chest pain in NCCP patients is

unclear, but may be related to hypersensitivity to augmented esophageal motor activity (13).

Overall, it appears that if the edrophonium test is positive, then the esophagus is the likely origin of chest pain. However, due to lack of differences in esophageal contractile activity after the edrophonium test between NCCP patients and normal healthy subjects, several authorities have suggested to perform the test without concomitant esophageal manometric studies (4,71).

Other Provocative Tests

The bethanechol test is presently rarely performed in clinical practice because of its questionable diagnostic value and frequent side effects. Bethanechol chloride, a cholinergic agonist, is a synthetic ester that is structurally and pharmacologically related to acetylcholine. Doses of 40 to 50 mg/kg have been administered subcutaneously, inducing chest pain in 12% to 33% of NCCP patients (51,77,78). Improved sensitivity was achieved when the dose of bethanechol was increased to two injections of 50 μg/kg, with an interval of 15 minutes. As many as 77% of the patients had their chest pain reproduced, but at the cost of severe side effects (78). Side effects reported after the bethanechol test included symptomatic bradycardia requiring atropine treatment, hypotension, headache, increased salivation, sweating, and nervousness, among others (70). Presence of other medical problems, such as asthma, epilepsy, cardiac or vascular disorders, hypotension, and Parkinson's disease should be elicited and, if present, the test should be avoided.

The intravenous ergonovine stimulation test has been demonstrated to induce augmentation of esophageal contractions and chest pain in many NCCP patients (4). Ergonovine is a sympathomimetic agent of the ergoalkaloid group and is used by cardiologists to diagnose vasospastic angina in chest pain patients with normal coronary arteries. The drug reportedly is as sensitive as edrophonium in the provocation of esophageal chest pain in patients without changes in the ST-T segment on electrocardiogram (ECG) or coronary artery spasm on angiography (69,79–81). However, because side effects are common and serious cardiac effects and even death have been reported, the test should not be used for standard esophageal testing (82).

Pentagastrin directly stimulates esophageal smooth muscle, especially in patients with primary esophageal dysmotility. Its sensitivity to induce pain in patients with NCCP is low and the drug is no longer used for a provocation test.

Proton Pump Inhibitor Test

GERD is the most common esophageal cause for NCCP. Studies have demonstrated that GERD is prevalent in up to 60% of the patients with NCCP (6–9). The frequency of reports of NCCP increases in patients who report more frequent typical GERD symptoms (1). The prevalence of erosive esophagitis in patients with GERD-related NCCP has been reported to be as low as 10% and as high as 70% (7–9). The wide range is likely to be related to the different patient populations that were studied. The extent of esophageal mucosal involvement in community-based patients with GERD-related NCCP remains to be elucidated. Abnormal esophageal acid exposure, using ambulatory 24-hour esophageal pH monitoring, has been recorded in up to 60% of the patients presented with NCCP (7,83).

The presence of abnormal acid exposure or esophageal mucosal injury may suggest an association with GERD, but not necessarily causality. However, studies have shown that approximately 80% of the NCCP patients with either abnormal upper endoscopy or pH testing responded to potent antireflux treatment (84–86). These data suggest that, in most NCCP patients with evidence of GERD, the latter is the likely cause of their symptoms.

The mechanism by which acid reflux causes heartburn in some patients and chest pain in others remains poorly understood. This is compounded by the fact that a large subset of patients with NCCP report heartburn in addition to their chest pain symptom.

The different diagnostic tests that are currently available to detect GERD in patients with NCCP include barium esophagram, upper endoscopy, and ambulatory 24-hour esophageal pH monitoring. Due to lack of gold standard for the diagnosis of GERD, assessment of sensitivity and specificity of these modalities is relatively limited. In addition, these tests are invasive, costly, not readily available, and demonstrate inherent limitations in their diagnostic capabilities, all of which significantly limit their usefulness.

The PPI test is a very attractive alternative to the aforementioned diagnostic tests for GERD-related NCCP. The test uses a short course of high-dose PPI to diagnose patients with GERD-related NCCP. The PPI test is a simple and clinically practical diagnostic tool that is at the disposal of primary care physicians as well as subspecialists (87). The PPI test can be used in the other atypical and extraesophageal manifestations of GERD as well (88). The main requirement of the PPI test is to achieve a significant symptomatic improvement from as many patients as possible within a relatively short period of drug administration (89).

PPIs are the preferred agents for testing in NCCP because of their profound acid inhibition and relatively consistent effect (90–92).

In two early studies that assessed the diagnostic accuracy of the PPI test in NCCP patients, a single dose of 80 mg omeprazole resulted in variable sensitivity (69% vs. 90%) (91,92). Patients were randomized to placebo or a single-dose omeprazole on day 1 and then crossed over to the opposite arm after a washout period of 2 to 5 days. However, no attempt to ensure lack of carryover effect was made

in these two studies. In a double-blind, placebo-controlled trial, 37 patients with NCCP were randomized to either placebo or high-dose omeprazole (40 mg in the morning plus 20 mg in the evening for 7 days) (7). Diagnosis of GERD was established by an upper endoscopy or by 24-hour esophageal pH monitoring. After a washout period and repeated baseline symptom assessment, patients crossed over to the opposite arm. The calculated sensitivity of the test was 78.3% (95% CI, 61.4 to 95.1); specificity of 85.7% (95% CI, 67.4 to 100) and the positive predictive value 90% (95% CI, 74.4 to 100). Results of this study have been recently replicated in a more diverse group of patients that included mostly women and a small number of subjects with erosive esophagitis on endoscopy (93). Recent usage of lansoprazole, 60 mg in the morning and 30 mg in the evening, over a period of 7 days demonstrated similar sensitivity and specificity (78% and 82%, respectively) (94). Moreover, the investigators discovered that the lansoprazole test was able to diagnose most of the responders within the first 48 hours and, thus, suggested that a shorter duration of therapy can be used in selected patients. Rabeprazole, 20 mg twice daily given over a period of 7 days, demonstrated an 83% sensitivity and 75% specificity (95) in diagnosing GERD in patients with NCCP. By day 3, all GERD-related NCCP responders had either complete or almost complete symptom resolution.

The use of PPI test is highly dependent on the frequency of chest pain symptoms. The test may be extended to 2 weeks or even longer if symptoms occur less than once a week.

When using the PPI test, there was a significant correlation between the extent of esophageal acid exposure as determined by ambulatory 24-hour esophageal pH monitoring and the change in symptom intensity score after treatment (96). This suggests that the higher the esophageal acid exposure, the greater the response to the PPI test in patients with GERD-related NCCP.

Studies have also demonstrated that the PPI test is cost effective. In patients with NCCP, the potential impact of implementing a strategy of the PPI test rather than a conventional diagnostic strategy (1: upper endoscopy; 2: pH test; 3: esophageal manometry) was estimated in a cost-minimization analysis (7). The PPI test saved $573 (US) per average patient with NCCP. The test was also associated with 79% reduction in the use of ambulatory 24-hour esophageal pH monitoring and 81% reduction in the number of upper endoscopies. This reduction in the use of diagnostic tests was attributed to the high positive predictive value of the PPI test for GERD in NCCP.

When a decision analytic model using bayesian analysis was developed to compare the costs and outcomes of alternative diagnostic strategies for NCCP, noninvasive strategies using the PPI test as the initial step resulted in significant cost savings compared with invasive strategies (97). These cost savings resulted from the reduced use of invasive diagnostic tests that are of unproven utility in the diagnosis and subsequent management of patients with NCCP (98).

If the PPI test is used initially and is inconclusive, then a pH test should be performed when the patient is off therapy. However, a recent study revealed that the PPI test, using omeprazole 40 mg in the morning and 20 mg in the evening for 7 days, was at least as sensitive as ambulatory 24-hour esophageal pH monitoring in diagnosing GERD (99). Furthermore, none of the patients with a negative PPI test had an abnormal pH test.

Electrical Stimulation

Electrical stimulation of the esophagus has been used by several research groups to study visceral perception as well as cortical responses to different intensities of intraesophageal stimuli. The technique has yet to be standardized and published protocols are difficult to compare.

Electrical stimulation of the esophageal mucosa is performed by using a 5-mm stainless steel electrode attached to a standard manometric catheter assembly (76). The electrode is made from fine stainless steel wire wrapped around the end of the catheter and fixed with surgical silk (100). The electrodes are connected to an electrical stimulator. The catheter assembly is then passed through the nostril and the electrode is placed in the esophagus. Electrical stimuli are applied repeatedly in series of 24 stimuli (duration 200 μs at 0.2 Hz). A reference electrode is placed on the abdominal wall, 5 cm below the xiphoid process. Electrical stimulation of the upper and lower esophagus can be achieved by two pairs of silver/silver chloride bipolar ring electrodes located at 5 and 20 cm proximal to the tip of the catheter (101).

The ascending stimulus paradigm includes stimuli that are delivered at a frequency of 0.2 Hz at intensities between 0 and 100 mA (101). Severity and qualitative perceptual responses are usually assessed by a verbal descriptor (102). Descriptors are used in ascending order of severity. Sensory threshold is the intensity (measured in mA) at which the participant reports faint sensation, and pain threshold is the intensity at which the participant reports an intense sensation (101). A somewhat different stimulus paradigm is used in patients who undergo recording of cerebral evoked responses to esophageal electrical stimulation (103).

Impedance Planimetry

Originally, impedance planimetry was developed to measure the cross-sectional area of the ureter (104,105). Over the years, the technique was further perfected and was recently used to describe the biomechanical characteristics of the human esophagus (106–108). The sensing system includes a thin latex balloon, which was used by some investigators to assess esophageal sensory thresholds. Balloon pressure was increased stepwise by 5 cm H_2O incre-

ments from 0 to determine sensory thresholds for pain in several studies (19,107,110). After each inflation, the balloon was completely deflated for a rest period of 3 minutes. Balloon distentions were maintained each for 3 to 5 minutes. In this protocol, at each level of distention, the cross-sectional area was measured and sensory response was determined using verbal descriptor. Grade 1 was considered a sensation of fullness, grade 2 was considered moderate discomfort, and grade 3 was considered severe pain. In validating this technique, the authors found that the threshold pressure required to induce a sensation of fullness varied between 20 and 50 cm H_2O (107).

Multichannel intraluminal impedance (see Chapter 7).

Recent introduction of improved impedance probes with integrated pH sensors allowed further assessment of refluxate composition and its relationship to symptoms (111,112). Because the electrical conductivity of the esophageal muscular wall, air, and any given bolus is different, the presence of different substances in the esophageal lumen provides a different impedance pattern (112). With a highly conductive bolus (e.g., saliva), the impedance decreases; with poorly conductive material (e.g., air) the impedance increases (113,114).

The combination of an impedance catheter and a pH probe provides a unique opportunity to study physiologic events within the esophagus and their relationship to symptoms. In addition, the recording assembly can disclose the characteristics of the gastric refluxate (acid, nonacid, gas, and mixed gas and liquid). The value of such technique has been demonstrated by recent studies that demonstrated that nonacid reflux is not uncommon in GERD patients and may lead to classic heartburn symptoms as well (111,112).

It is apparent that the esophageal impedance technique needs to be standardized and further studies are required to determine its proper clinical utility. However, future usage of this unique technique may further expand our understanding of symptom generation in patients with esophageal disorders.

Intraluminal Ultrasonography

High-frequency intraluminal ultrasonography has been recently introduced as a novel modality to study the relationship between esophageal motor events and symptoms. The technique has been a useful tool for evaluating smooth muscle contractions (115) (Fig. 8.3). Esophageal ultrasonography can be performed continuously using a catheter-based probe, which allows direct visualization of changes in smooth muscle conformation (31). The capability of intraluminal ultrasonography to evaluate changes in the thickness of the longitudinal muscle of the esophagus has been used to determine the relationship between esophageal symptoms and motor changes of the esophageal wall. Although the technique is yet to be standardized, investigators have used an esophageal catheter assembly that

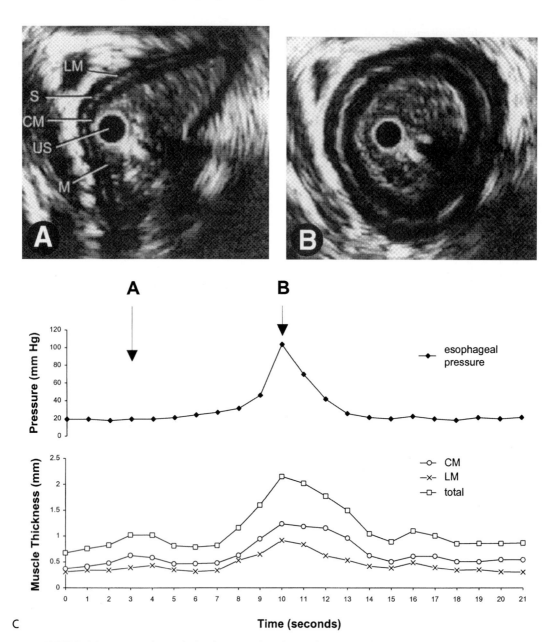

FIGURE 8.3. Temporal correlation between intraluminal pressure change and ultrasonographic muscle thickness during a swallow-induced contraction. Ultrasound images, esophageal pressure, and muscle thickness during a 5-mL water swallow are shown. Before the swallow (image **A**, time *A*), the esophageal muscle is thin and the cross-sectional configuration is oblong. During contraction (image **B**, time *B*), there is thickening of the muscular wall. The increase in intraluminal pressure is associated with an increase in thickness of both the circular and longitudinal muscles. *LM*, longitudinal muscle; *S*, intermuscular septum; *CM*, circular muscle; *US*, ultrasound probe; *M*, mucosa. (Adapted from Balaban DH, Yamamoto Y, Liu J, et al. Sustained esophageal contraction: a marker of esophageal chest pain identified by intraluminal ultrasonography. *Gastroenterology* 1999;116[1]:29–37.)

included a 12.5-MHz ultrasound transducer, solid-state pressure catheter, and monocrystant antimony pH catheter (31). The ultrasound transducer was placed 5 cm above the LES. The 24-hour recordings were analyzed every 2 seconds for a period of 2 minutes before and 30 seconds after the onset of the studied symptom. Rules for image analysis remain at the discretion of the investigator. Because of the limited number of centers that are proficient with this technique, image analysis is primarily operator dependent and interobserver and intraobserver agreements have yet to be determined.

Using intraluminal ultrasonography, Balaban and colleagues demonstrated that most chest pain episodes in patients with NCCP were preceded by sustained thickening of the esophageal smooth muscle wall due to longitudinal muscle contraction that was not detected by esophageal manometry catheter (31). The same muscular changes were noted after edrophonium-induced chest pain. The authors suggested that the duration rather than the magnitude of the longitudinal muscle contraction is the determining factor for generating esophageal pain. In this study, swallow-associated longitudinal muscle contractions lasted an average of 6.4 seconds, whereas contractions associated with chest pain persisted for a mean of 68.0 seconds. Similar studies in patients with GERD revealed that the mean duration of sustained longitudinal muscle contractions during heartburn was 44.9 seconds (32). The motor changes were also observed in patients who reported heartburn that was unrelated to acid reflux events, further supporting the investigator's hypothesis that this sustained esophageal muscle contraction is responsible for generation of esophageal symptoms, such as chest pain and heartburn.

Even though high-frequency intraluminal ultrasonography has been a valuable research tool to assess the biomechanics of the human esophagus, its exact role in evaluating esophageal related symptoms has not been fully elucidated (116). Initial studies provided intriguing data, but other investigators have yet to replicate these findings. Additionally, sustained contractions of the esophageal longitudinal muscle may represent an epiphenomenon that occurs with symptoms, rather than being the trigger for symptoms.

Balloon Distention

Balloon distention has been used primarily for research purposes to determine perception thresholds for pain. This modality has been used extensively in studies of various functional bowel disorders, most notably, irritable bowel syndrome, functional dyspepsia, and NCCP (117–119).

More than 40 years ago, intraesophageal balloon distention in humans was reported to produce pain referred to the chest (120). Early data indicated that, in patients with documented ischemic heart disease, balloon distention of the esophagus produced pain indistinguishable from anginal pain, but without ECG changes (121). This may be explained by convergence of sensory pathways at the level of spinal cord or in the midbrain. Despite this similarity in pain, it appears that esophageal balloon distention itself has no effect on coronary function or blood flow (122).

Several painful clinical syndromes are associated with esophageal distention. These include esophageal dilation and aperistalsis induced by the ingestion of cold liquids (123), acute food impaction, the drinking of carbonated beverages (124), and dysfunction of the belch reflex (125). It has also been suggested that esophageal pain is, at times, due to esophageal dilation secondary to a lack of coordination between the esophageal body and the LES (126).

Balloon distention was reintroduced during the mid-1980s in a seminal study that evaluated perception thresholds for pain in patients with NCCP (117). The latex balloon was attached to a manometric catheter and filled with air. The balloon was positioned 10 cm above the LES and distended in a stepwise fashion using a handheld syringe. When air was injected (within 2 second) in 1-mL increments to a maximum of 10 mL into the balloon attached to a manometry catheter, patients with NCCP were more likely to experience pain (18 of 30) than were normal control subjects (6 of 30) (117). Concurrent ECG monitoring showed no ischemic changes. In this study the intraesophageal volume at the onset of pain also distinguished patients from control subjects, with chest pain patients experiencing pain at balloon volumes of less than 8 mL and the few control subjects experiencing pain at volumes of 9 mL or more. A second report evaluating 50 patients with NCCP found that 28 (56%) had their "typical" chest pain during balloon inflation. Again, most of these patients (24 of 28) had their pain at volumes less than 8 mL (127). Abnormal motility did not predict a positive test result. When intraballoon pressures were used as a measure of esophageal wall tone, no difference between control subjects and NCCP patients was noted. The response appears to be fairly specific in that only one patient had a negative response on the balloon study and a positive result on the edrophonium test and no patient had a negative response on the balloon study and a positive result on the acid perfusion test.

A further development in the balloon distention technique was the introduction of a pump that was powered by compressed air (128). The pump ensured inflations at a predetermined rate, which was difficult to achieve with a handheld syringe. However, neither system was able to provide concomitant pressure measurements that could have been helpful to determine whether the balloon remained within the esophageal lumen during each inflation. This was particularly critical in protocols that inflated balloons within the distal portion of the esophagus. Fass and colleagues (22) demonstrated that balloon distention in the esophagus resulted in phasic esophageal contractions that increased with increase in balloon volume (Fig. 8.4). These powerful contractions in association with shortening of the esophagus may propel the balloon into the stomach without being recognized by the subject or the investigator. Concomitant pressure measurements would have been helpful to detect the migration of the balloon into the gastric fundus by demonstrating a sudden decrease in intraluminal pressure despite continued increase in the balloon's volume.

The introduction of the electronic barostat, a computer-driven volume-displacement device has helped to ensure proper location of the balloon, regardless of inflation paradigm that was used (129). The basic principal of the barostat is to maintain a constant pressure within the balloon/bag in the lumen despite muscular contractions and relaxations (129,130). To maintain a constant pressure, the barostat aspirates air with contractions and injects air with

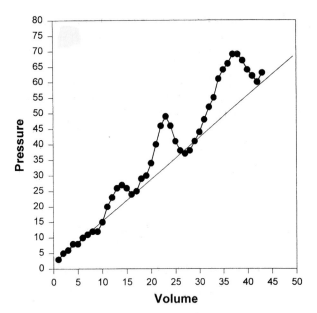

FIGURE 8.4. Pressure-volume relationship during ramp distention of the esophagus. Each *dot* indicates 1-mL volume increment. Increase in volume results in progressively high phasic esophageal contraction amplitude superimposed on the linear pressure volume relationship (*straight line*). Compliance is expressed as dV/dp. (Adapted from Fass R, Naliboff B, Higa L, et al. Differential effect of long-term esophageal acid exposure on mechanosensitivity and chemosensitivity in humans. *Gastroenterology* 1998;115[6]:1363–1373.)

relaxations. Presently, many prefer the use of a polyethylene bag to that of a latex balloon. Bags are infinitely compliant and show no increase in intrabag pressure until about 90% of the maximum bag volume is achieved (129,131). In contrast, latex balloons resist inflation and thus show a rapid increase in intraballoon pressure with small volumes of distention (22,129,132). When the pressure increases above the elastance threshold, the balloon becomes plastic and accommodates large volumes of air with very little change in pressure (129,131). For tubular organs in the gastrointestinal tract, such as the esophagus, experts recommend the use of a cylindrical bag (rather than spherical) with a fixed length (22,129).

Barostat has been used extensively in studies evaluating rectosigmoid and gastric perception thresholds for pain. However, this technique has been rarely used to assess esophageal mechanosensitivity in humans. Unlike the rectum and the stomach, the esophagus does not serve as a storage organ but rather as a conduit. Consequently, intraesophageal distentions do not mimic a normal, physiologic stimulus and thus perceptual responses to such a stimulus may have no scientific merit. This factor, in addition to the patient's difficulties in tolerating balloon distention, which commonly results in poor recruitment rates as well as the potential for esophageal perforation, have made esophageal balloon distentions by a barostat a less attractive research tool.

Various distention protocols have been used in different studies. Like any other technique that assesses esophageal sensation, balloon distention has yet to be standardized. Slow ramp distention is an ascending method that involves slow (rate varies from one study to another) increase in volume or pressure of the balloon usually until the desired perceptual response has been reported by the subject (22,133, 134). In contrast, phasic distentions are rapid inflations of the balloon that can be delivered in random sequence or double random staircase (22,133). The latter includes two series of distention stimuli (staircases), and the computer alternates between the two staircases on a random basis (22,129,134). With the tracking method (Fig. 8.5), the barostat is programmed to deliver a series of intermittent phasic stimuli separated by interpulse rest period within an interactive stimulus tracking procedure (22,135,136). If subject indicates a sensation below the tracked intensity then the following stimulus will increase in pressure. If the subject reports the desired sensation, then the following pressure step is randomized to stay the same or decrease. The random element is placed to mask the relationship between ratings and subsequent stimulus change, and, therefore, decrease potential scaling bias (137).

Quantification of perceptual responses depends on the characteristics of the mechanoreceptors in a specific region of the gastrointestinal tract. Volume or pressure distention can be considered the most physiologic stimuli (119,138).

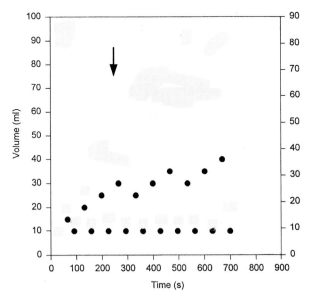

FIGURE 8.5. Discomfort threshold tracking during a 700-second trial using volume. *Arrow* indicates the time point when subject first indicated discomfort and barostat switched into tracking mode. Tracking based on intrabag volume gives more reliable and stable thresholds. Symbols around 10 mL (baseline volume) indicate that subject could differentiate well between stimulus and interstimulus interval. (Adapted from Fass R, et al. Differential effect of long-term esophageal acid exposure on mechanosensitivity and chemosensitivity in humans. *Gastroenterology* 1998;115[6]:1363–1373.)

As can be shown for a representative subject in Figure 8.4, the most reliable reports of sensory thresholds were obtained during volume distention. Although the overall pressure-volume curve is linear, the pressure at any given volume may vary as a result of the presence or absence of a superimposed esophageal phasic contraction (22) (Fig. 8.5). Despite this physiologic phenomenon, other investigators rely primarily on pressure when performing balloon studies in the esophagus.

Commonly, qualitative and quantitative perceptual responses are evaluated during balloon distention studies. Qualitative perceptual responses include symptom reports in response to balloon distention, such as chest pain, heartburn, bloating, and fullness, among others (22,139). Heartburn is a common sensation that occurs during balloon distention and may mimic the patient's typical heartburn symptom (139). Quantitative perceptual responses are commonly obtained during slow-ramp distention and include the minimal distention volume or pressure at which the individual first reports moderate sensation (innocuous sensation), discomfort, and pain (aversive sensation) (22). Discomfort threshold is commonly defined as the first unpleasant esophageal sensation, and pain threshold is defined as the first sensation of pain (22).

Pitfalls that may modify perceptual responses to balloon distention are listed in Table 8.1. Increased rate of balloon distention results in reported perception at lower volumes or pressures (140). Longer durations of balloon distention are more likely to elicit sensation than shorter durations (140). Elderly subjects demonstrate diminished visceral pain perception and female patients appear to have lower perception thresholds for pain compared to male patients (141–143). The proximal esophagus has been suggested to be more sensitive to chemical and mechanical stimuli than the distal esophagus (22,144). Additionally, reduced sensitivity to intraluminal stimuli has been demonstrated in specific patient populations, such as those with Barrett's mucosa or esophageal stricture (52,145,146). A recent study demonstrated the development of secondary allodynia (visceral hypersensitivity to innocuous stimulus in normal tissue that is in proximity to site of tissue injury) in the adjacent portion of the esophagus that was not sensitized by a chemical stimulus (acid) (147).

Esophageal balloon distention has been shown to produce increased motility proximal to the balloon and inhibition distally and to initiate secondary peristalsis in normal subjects (148,149). Sustained balloon distention produces a strong, proximal, aboral contraction force referred to as the *duration response*, or the *esophageal propulsive force* (150). In the opossum, this contraction proximal to a distending balloon is abolished with cervical vagotomy, whereas contractions distal to the balloon are retained and believed to be mediated by an intramural nonadrenergic noncholinergic system (151). Human studies showed that atropine inhibits proximal contraction when balloon distention is carried out in the distal, but not proximal, esophagus, indirectly indicating some difference in the innervation of these two regions (152). In addition to the aforementioned effects in the body of the esophagus, balloon distention produces increases in upper esophageal sphincter and decreases in LES pressure (153). In studies performed on a group of dysphagia patients, both patients and control subjects experi-

TABLE 8.1. FACTORS THAT MODULATE ESOPHAGEAL SENSATION

Factors	Effect on Sensory Response
Rate of balloon inflation	
Increase	Reduce perception threshold for pain
Decrease	Increase perception threshold for pain
Duration of balloon distention	
Longer	Increase sensation
Shorter	Reduce sensation
Gender	
Female	Reduce perception threshold for pain
Male	Increase perception threshold for pain
Age	
Elderly	Increase perception threshold for pain
Younger	Reduce perception threshold for pain
Esophageal region	
Proximal	Reduce perception threshold for pain
	Secondary allodynia in distal portion
Distal	Increase perception threshold for pain
	Secondary allodynia in proximal portion
Patient population	
Barrett's esophagus	Increase perception threshold for pain
Peptic stricture	Increase perception threshold for pain

Functional heartburn decreases perception thresholds for pain.

enced a sustained increase in pressure proximal to the balloon. In 21 (70%) of 30 patients, but in no control subjects, there was evidence of repeated simultaneous contractions (spasm) distal to the balloon (154). Similar findings of distal esophageal "spasm" with balloon distention were noted in 38 (61%) of 62 chest pain patients but in no control subjects (155).

Balloon studies are primarily designed to assess the presence of visceral hyperalgesia in various esophageal disorders. Early studies demonstrated that pain develops with balloon distention more frequently in NCCP patients than in normal control subjects and that their pain occurs at smaller volumes (117,127,156). Short-term sensitization of mechanosensitive afferent pathways by transient exposure to irritants has been shown in both humans and animal models of visceral hyperalgesia (157,158). Human studies that evaluated the effect of esophageal acid perfusion on perception of esophageal distention in healthy control subjects and patients with gastroesophageal reflux disease had varying results (157,159–161).

Mehta and colleagues (157) reported that perfusion of the esophagus with 0.1N HCl acid for 30 minutes resulted in enhanced sensitivity to esophageal balloon distention. Similarly, Sarkar and colleagues (161) reported that acid perfusion into the distal esophagus was associated with the development of mechanical hyperalgesia in the proximal esophagus, which had not been exposed to acid, suggesting the development of secondary visceral hyperalgesia. Peghini and co-workers (159) found a lowering of the pain threshold to distention only in those individuals who were symptomatic during acid perfusion (160). In contrast, DeVault (160) reported that a 15-minute acid perfusion had no significant effect on pain perception during esophageal distention. The mechanisms underlying the sensitizing effect of acute tissue irritation on visceral afferent pathways have been well characterized in the form of peripheral and central sensitization (21). Such sensitization manifests as increased background activity of sensory neurons, the lowering of nociceptive thresholds, changes in stimulus response curves, and enlargement of receptive fields. During a noxious event, a series of counterregulatory mechanisms are activated that are aimed at containing the development of both the acute and any long-lasting sensitization (21).

Studies evaluating balloon distentions in patients with chronic acid exposure or esophageal mucosal injury are scarce. Fass and colleagues demonstrated that mild to moderate chronic tissue injury in GERD differentially affects mechanosensitive and chemosensitive afferent pathways (22). GERD patients showed enhanced perception of acid perfusion but not of esophageal distention. Chemosensitivity but not mechanosensitivity was correlated with reflux symptoms and with the degree of endoscopically shown tissue injury at baseline. Trimble and co-workers evaluated patients with heartburn and excess reflux defined by abnor-

mal upper endoscopy or 24-hour esophageal pH monitoring and compared them with patients with heartburn and a normal 24-hour pH test. The results demonstrated that the latter group had lower volume thresholds for perception of esophageal balloon distention and discomfort (36). This study suggests that patients with typical heartburn who lack any evidence of excess acid are highly sensitive to mechanical stimuli.

The use of balloon distention as a tool to test the pharmacologic response to various agents being considered for use in patients with chest pain is evolving. Imipramine has been demonstrated to improve symptoms in patients with NCCP (162) and it has been shown to increase perception threshold for pain during balloon distention in a group of normal control subjects (163). Octreotide was found to improve both sensory and pain thresholds in a group of chest pain patients (164). Nifedipine has been studied using both standard balloon distention and with barostat testing and has not been found to change reliably sensory thresholds or esophageal wall tone (165,166).

Esophageal Evoked Potentials

Cerebral evoked potentials are recorded as a reflection of the electrical activity of the brain in response to stimuli applied in the periphery (Fig. 8.6). Visual evoked potentials (secondary to a flashing light) and auditory evoked potentials (secondary to repetitive clicks) have found clinical applicability. In addition, somatosensory evoked potentials (secondary to repetitive electrical stimulation) have been used to evaluate peripheral nerves. The recording of cerebral evoked potentials in response to visceral stimulation has

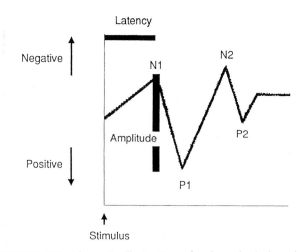

FIGURE 8.6. Schematic illustration of a hypothetical evoked potential. By convention, negative is up and positive is down. The peaks are numbered consecutively as negative (N1, N2) or positive (P1, P2). Amplitude is expressed on the vertical axis as a difference between peaks (N1 to P1, P1 to N2). Latency is on the horizontal axis and is measured from the stimulus to a given peak.

Color Plates

Color Plates

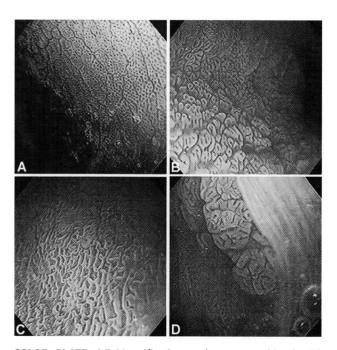

COLOR PLATE 4.5 Magnification endoscopy combined with acetic acid. **A:** Pattern I: round pits with a characteristic pattern of regular and orderly arranged circular dots. **B:** Pattern II: reticular. Pits were circular or oval and were regular in shape and arrangement. **C:** Pattern III: villous. No pits were present but there was a fine villiform appearance with regular shape and arrangement. **D:** Pattern IV: ridged. No pits were present but there was a thick villous convoluted shape with a cerebriform appearance with regular shape and arrangement. Specialized intestinal metaplasia is predominantly found in patterns III and IV.

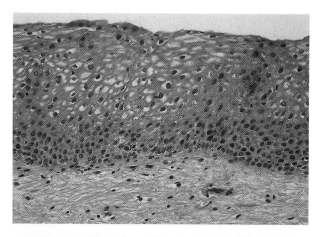

A

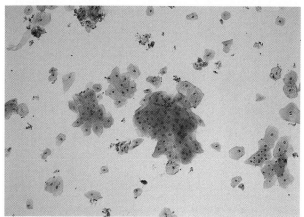

B

COLOR PLATE 9.1. A: Normal esophageal squamous mucosa with a thin basal epithelial zone and lamina propria papillae that are less than about 20% of the total epithelial thickness. **B:** Normal esophageal brushing composed predominantly of mature squamous epithelial cells and rare benign glandular cells. (Papanicolaou stain; courtesy of Dr. Jennifer Brainard.)

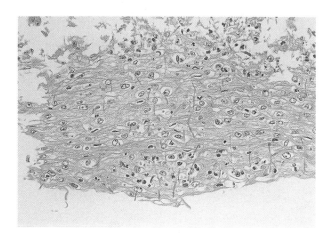

COLOR PLATE 9.2. Candida esophagitis. Pseudohyphal organisms are identified perpendicular to the squamous mucosa. Acute inflammatory cells are prominent within the mucosa. (Courtesy of Dr. Joel Greenson.)

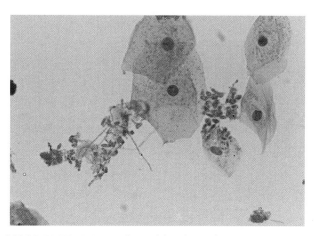

COLOR PLATE 9.3. Esophageal brush cytology specimen with squamous epithelial cells and pseudohyphae consistent with candida esophagitis.

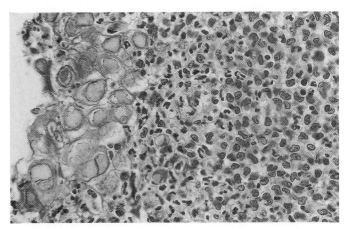

COLOR PLATE 9.4. Herpes esophagitis. Squamous epithelial cells with ground-glass nuclei are prominent. A sheet of macrophages is seen beneath the infected cells. (Courtesy of Dr. Joel Greenson.)

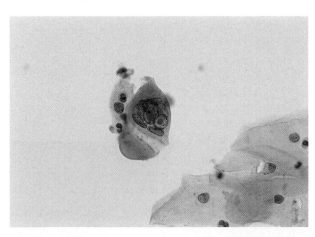

COLOR PLATE 9.5. Esophageal brush cytology specimen showing multinucleated squamous epithelial cells diagnostic of herpes esophagitis.

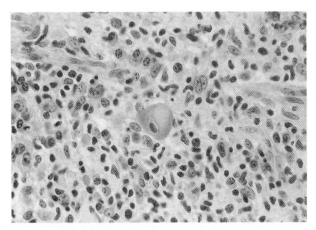

COLOR PLATE 9.6. Cytomegalovirus (CMV) esophagitis. In the center of the field, there is an enlarged CMV-infected cell with a prominent intranuclear eosinophilic inclusion and smaller granular cytoplasmic inclusions. This likely represents an infected mesenchymal cell. (Courtesy of Dr. Joel Greenson.)

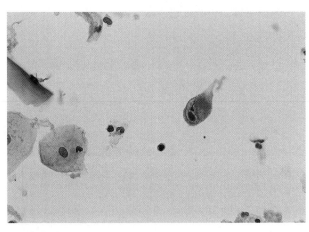

COLOR PLATE 9.7. Esophageal brush cytology specimen showing an intranuclear inclusion diagnostic of cytomegalovirus esophagitis.

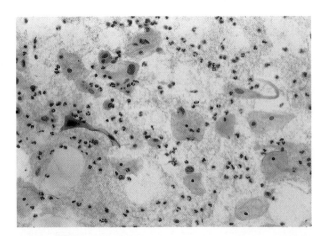

COLOR PLATE 9.8. Atypical squamous epithelial cells and inflammatory exudate following radiation therapy. Residual neoplasm is not identified.

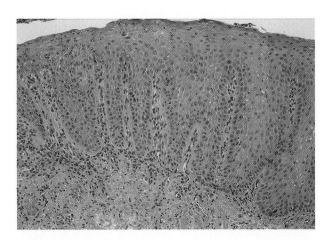

COLOR PLATE 9.9. Squamous hyperplasia with papillomatosis. The lamina propria papillae extend more than two thirds of the full thickness of the esophageal mucosa. These changes are not specific but are frequently seen in patients with gastroesophageal reflux disease.

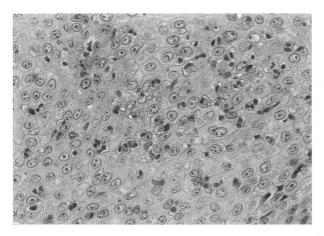

COLOR PLATE 9.10. Marked intraepithelial eosinophilia in a patient with gastroesophageal reflux disease.

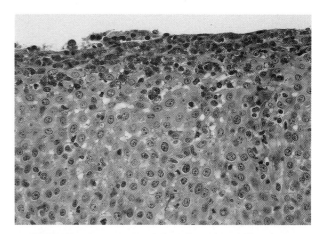

COLOR PLATE 9.11. Eosinophilic (allergic) esophagitis characterized by numerous itraepithelial eosinophils with a clustering of eosinophils near the surface of the squamous mucosa. This pattern of intraepithelial eosinophilia is characteristic of allergic esophagitis.

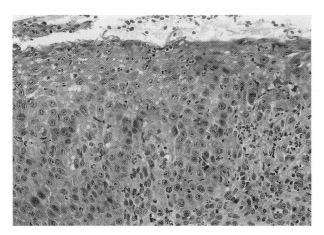

COLOR PLATE 9.12. Intraepithelial neutrophils in a patient with gastroesophageal reflux disease.

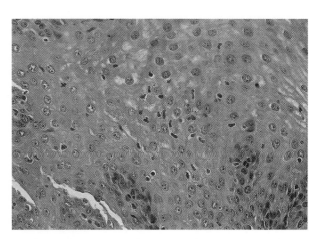

COLOR PLATE 9.13. Lymphocytic esophagitis in a patient with gastroesophageal reflux disease.

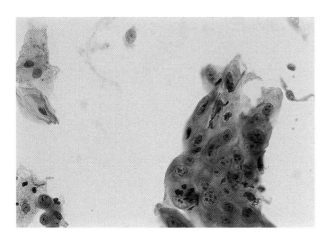

COLOR PLATE 9.14. Epithelial repair characterized by cohesive cell clusters with prominent nucleoli and intraepithelial acute inflammatory cells.

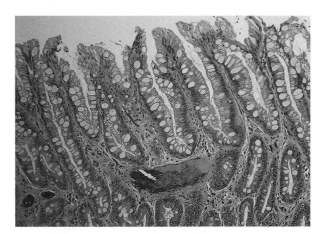

COLOR PLATE 9.15. Low-magnification view of Barrett's esophagus. Goblet cells are easily identified. The base of the mucosa shows nuclear stratification, a feature that is characteristically found in the basal portion of Barrett's mucosa.

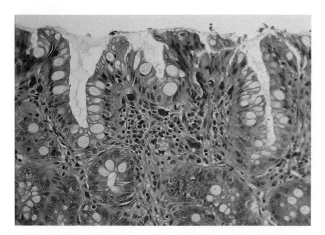

COLOR PLATE 9.16. Higher magnification view of Barrett's mucosa, characterized by acid mucin-containing goblet cells.

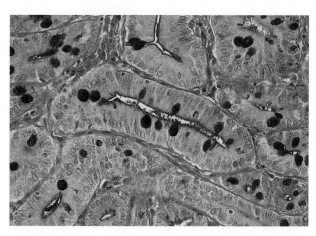

COLOR PLATE 9.17. Barrett's esophagus with complete intestinal metaplasia. The Alcian blue portion of this combined Alcian blue and periodic acid–Schiff (PAS) stain highlights the goblet cells. The PAS portion of the stain highlights the luminal aspect of the glands, suggesting a primitive brush border.

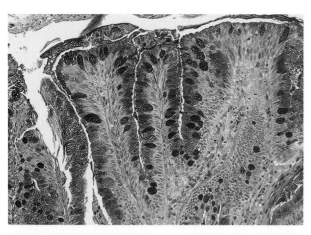

COLOR PLATE 9.18. Alcian blue and periodic acid–Schiff (PAS) stain highlighting incomplete intestinal metaplasia in Barrett's esophagus. The Alcian blue portion of the stain highlights the goblet cells. The cells between the goblet cells are stained by PAS, indicating that they are filled with neutrophil mucins reminiscent of foveolar-type cells.

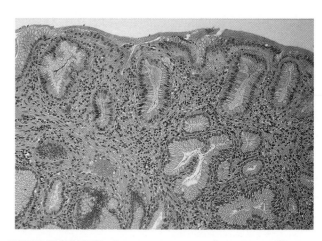

COLOR PLATE 9.19. Squamous mucosa adjacent to cardiac-type mucosa in a biopsy obtained from the distal esophagus. Because goblet cells are not present, this would not be diagnostic of Barrett's esophagus.

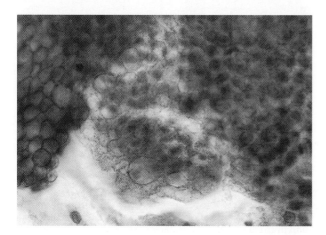

COLOR PLATE 9.20. Brush cytology specimen from nondysplastic Barrett's esophagus showing cohesive cell fragments with a "honeycomb" architecture and goblet cells.

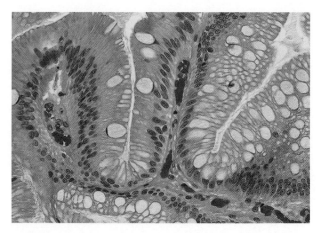

COLOR PLATE 9.21. Intestinal metaplasia in a biopsy specimen obtained near the esophagogastric junction. Although this could represent short-segment Barrett's esophagus, it could just as easily represent intestinal metaplasia of the gastric cardia.

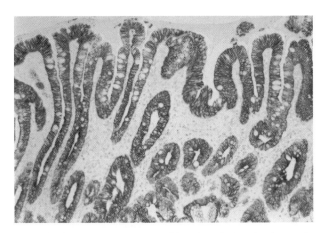

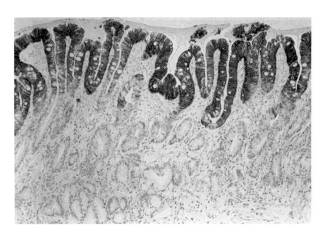

COLOR PLATE 9.22. Immunohistochemical-stained section using an antibody to cytokeratin 7 from a resection specimen with long-segment Barrett's esophagus. The antibody stains the superficial and deep portion of the intestinalized mucosa. (From Goldblum JR. Inflammation and intestinal metaplasia of the gastric cardia: *Helicobacter pylori*, gastroesophageal reflux disease, or both (review). *Dig Dis* 2000;18[1]:14–19, with permission.)

COLOR PLATE 9.23. Immunohistochemical-stained section using an antibody to cytokeratin 20 from a resection specimen with long-segment Barrett's esophagus. There is superficial band-like staining of the intestinalized mucosa. This pattern of cytokeratin 7 and 20 immunoreactivity (including Fig. 9.22) is characteristic of Barrett's esophagus. (From Goldblum JR. Inflammation and intestinal metaplasia of the gastric cardia: *Helicobacter pylori*, gastroesophageal reflux disease, or both (review). *Dig Dis* 2000;18[1]:14–19, with permission.)

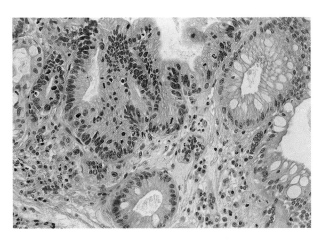

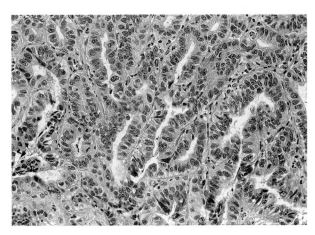

COLOR PLATE 9.24. Barrett's esophagus with low-grade dysplasia. The glands on the left show nuclear hyperchromasia and loss of polarity, which are not identified in the nondysplastic Barrett's epithelium to the right.

COLOR PLATE 9.25. High-grade dysplasia in Barrett's esophagus. There is marked cytologic atypia and architectural complexity that exceeds that seen in low-grade dysplasia.

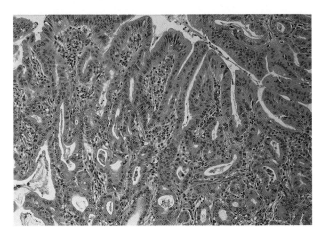

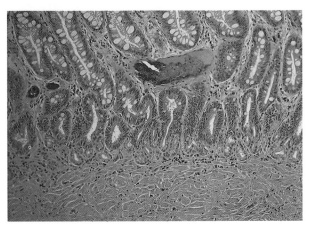

COLOR PLATE 9.26. Intramucosal adenocarcinoma arising in Barrett's esophagus. There is a complex glandular architectural pattern with apparent infiltration of glands into the lamina propria.

COLOR PLATE 9.27. Nondysplastic Barrett's esophagus. The base of the mucosa shows glands with hyperchromasia and slight nuclear stratification. However, this is the "baseline atypia" characteristic of Barrett's esophagus. There is cellular maturation toward the surface.

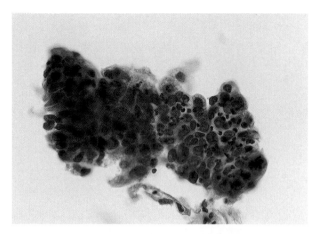

COLOR PLATE 9.28. Brush cytology specimen of Barrett's esophagus with high-grade dysplasia. Nuclear pleomorphism and hyperchromasia are present in cohesive cell aggregates.

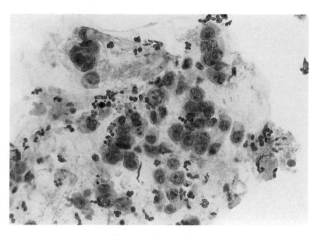

COLOR PLATE 9.29. Adenocarcinoma arising in Barrett's esophagus, characterized by atypical and discohesive tumor cells.

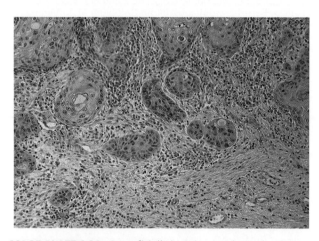

COLOR PLATE 9.30. Superficially invasive esophageal squamous cell carcinoma. Small nests of infiltrating cells with obvious squamous differentiation are seen.

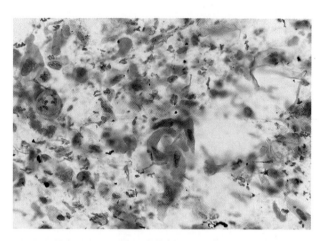

COLOR PLATE 9.31. Well-differentiated squamous cell carcinoma. The cells show dense organophilic cytoplasm indicative of keratin production.

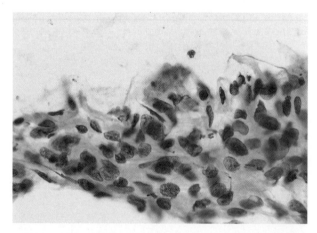

COLOR PLATE 9.32. Brush cytology specimen of a poorly differentiated squamous cell carcinoma. The neoplastic cells show a spindled morphology without evidence of squamous differentiation.

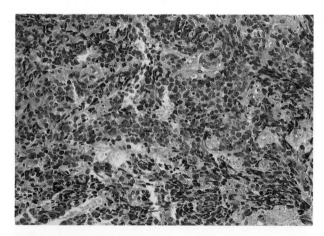

COLOR PLATE 9.33. Esophageal small cell carcinoma. At low magnification, the cells are markedly hyperchromatic, and there is significant crush artifact.

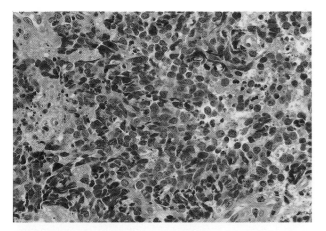

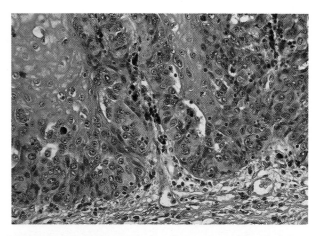

COLOR PLATE 9.34. High-magnification view of an esophageal small cell carcinoma. Many of the cells show crush artifact. Single-cell necrosis is also prominent. Nuclear molding and a finely granular chromatin pattern suggest neuroendocrine differentiation.

COLOR PLATE 9.35. Atypical melanocytic proliferation in an esophageal melanoma. The presence of atypical junctional melanocytic activity is strong evidence that the underlying melanoma (not pictured) is primary to this site

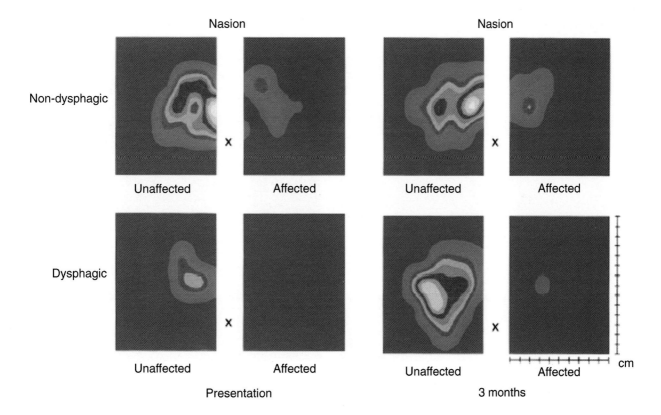

COLOR PLATE 10.5. Topographic maps of the pharynx in two patients who were studied at presentation and 3 months after a right hemisphere stroke. The maps represent areas of relative cortical representation of the pharynx determined by pharyngeal electromyographic responses to transcranial magnetic stimulation of each cortex. The top panel maps are from a patient who had normal swallowing throughout. The bottom panel maps are from a patient who had dysphagia at presentation, but who recovered normal swallowing by 3 months. Note that the dysphagic patient has a smaller area of pharyngeal representation on the unaffected hemisphere than the nondysphagic patient at presentation, but by 3 months it has enlarged to an area comparable to that of the nondysphagic patient. In contrast, in the affected hemisphere of both patients, the area of pharyngeal representation is small and remains unchanged with time. Hemispheric asymmetry of topographic representation determines whether a hemispheric stroke will cause dysphagia, and cortical plasticity in the unaffected hemisphere is a determinant of recovery of swallowing following stroke. (From Hamdy S, Aziz Q, Rothwell JC, et al. The cortical topography of human swallowing musculature in health and disease [see comments]. *Nat Med* 1996;2[11]: 1217–1224, with permission.)

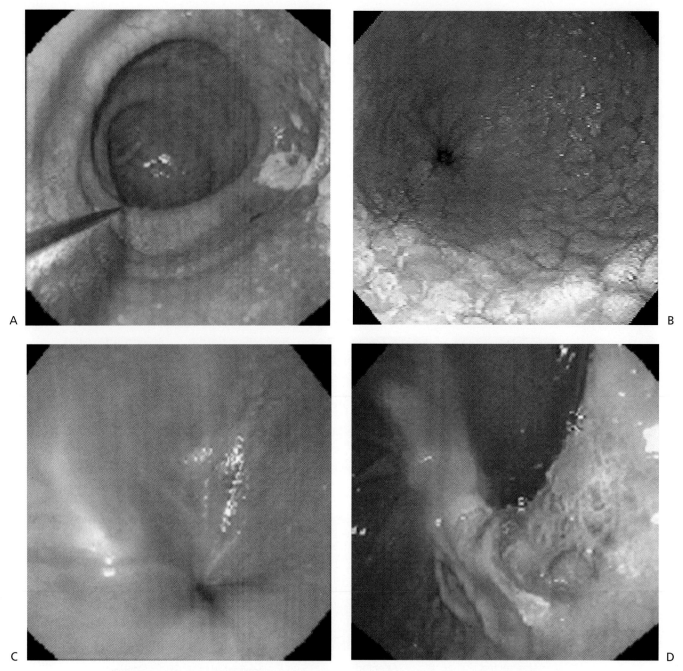

COLOR PLATE 11.7. Endoscopic findings in achalasia. **A:** Dilated atonic esophagus with normal appearing mucosa. Savary wire has been placed in the stomach to aid in esophageal manometry catheter placement. **B:** Reddened, friable, thickened, and cracked mucosa in a patient with megaesophagus from longstanding achalasia. **C:** Puckered esophagogastric junction, which remains closed with air insufflation but opens easily, sometimes with a "pop," with gentle pressure from the endoscope. **D:** Pseudoachalasia from an adenocarcinoma of the gastric cardia noted at retroflexion of the endoscope.

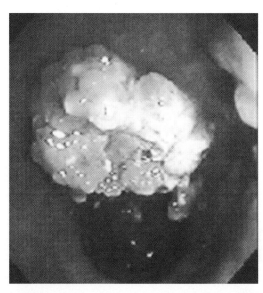

COLOR PLATE 13.1. A large squamous papilloma leading to dysphagia. The lesion was treated with laser therapy to palliate the dysphagia.

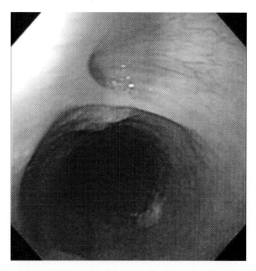

COLOR PLATE 13.2. Extrinsic compression of the esophagus from a large foregut cyst. The overlying mucosa is normal. Note the small traction diverticulum caused by the cyst.

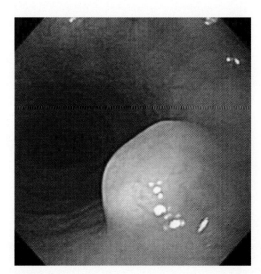

COLOR PLATE 13.4. An esophageal granular cell tumor. These are firm to touch, but can be diagnosed with precise forceps biopsy.

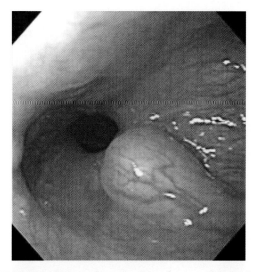

COLOR PLATE 13.5. Endoscopic view of an esophageal leiomyoma. The overlying mucosa is normal.

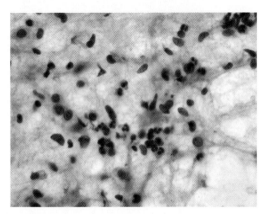

COLOR PLATE 13.8. High magnification view fine needle aspirate shows malignant spindled gastrointestinal stromal tumor cells admixed with occasional small lymphocytes.

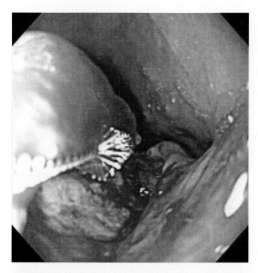

COLOR PLATE 13.9. Brush cytology of an esophageal adenocarcinoma.

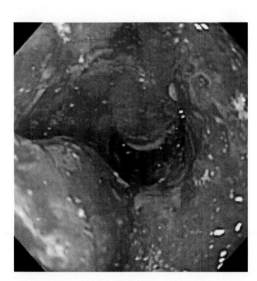

COLOR PLATE 13.10. A long cancer stricture in a patient with adenocarcinoma. On histopathologic evaluation, the cancer is poorly differentiated. It is highly likely that this lesion extends beyond the esophageal wall.

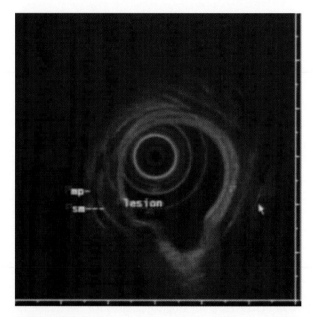

COLOR PLATE 13.11. Endoscopic ultrasound image of a T1 cancer, extending to but not through the submucosal layer of the esophageal wall.

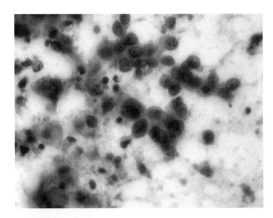

COLOR PLATE 13.14. Fine needle aspirate reveals large malignant adenocarcinoma cells with scattered lymphocytes.

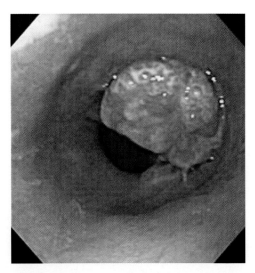

COLOR PLATE 13.15. An exophytic adenocarcinoma prior to chemoradiotherapy.

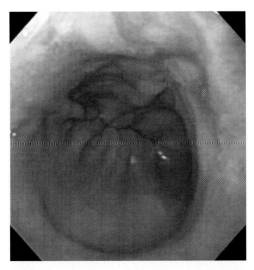

COLOR PLATE 13.16. After chemoradiotherapy, there is no visible tumor at endoscopy. This does not always predict pathologic T0.

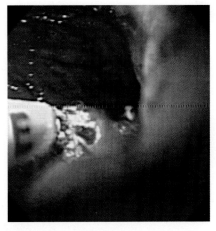

COLOR PLATE 13.18. Argon plasma coagulation of an exophytic tumor for palliation of malignant dysphagia.

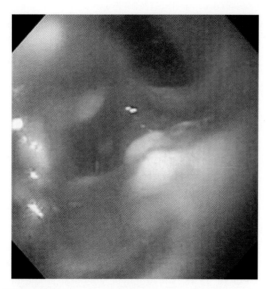

COLOR PLATE 13.19. A tracheoesophageal fistula in a patient with proximal squamous cell cancer.

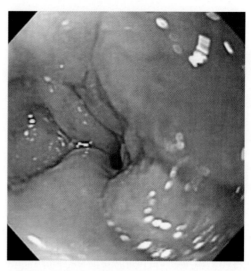

COLOR PLATE 13.20. A tight stricture caused by adenocarcinoma of the distal esophagus. The patient received subsequent dilation and laser therapy for palliation of malignant dysphagia.

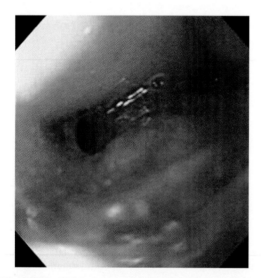

COLOR PLATE 13.21. Several hours after the procedure, the patient returned with fever and chest pain. Chest radiograph revealed the presence of free air consistent with perforation. The perforation is identified at endoscopy.

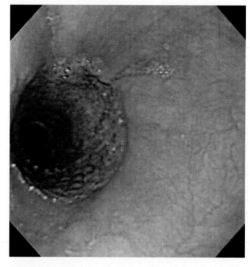

COLOR PLATE 13.22. Emergency placement of a covered stent in the same patient. With parenteral antibiotics and supportive care, the patient left the hospital in 48 hours.

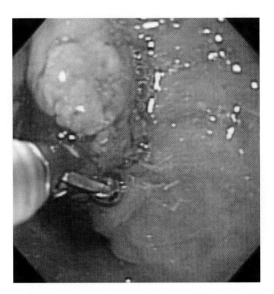

COLOR PLATE 14.1. Esophagoscopy and biopsy, following brush cytology, of a malignant esophageal stricture.

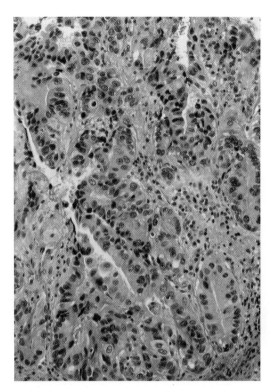

COLOR PLATE 14.4. Intramucosal adenocarcinoma: neoplastic glands infiltrate into the lamina propria but do not invade below muscularis mucosa.

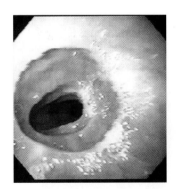

COLOR PLATE 15.3. Endoscopic photograph of ringed esophagus.

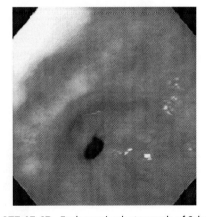

COLOR PLATE 15.4B. Endoscopic photograph of Schatzki's ring.

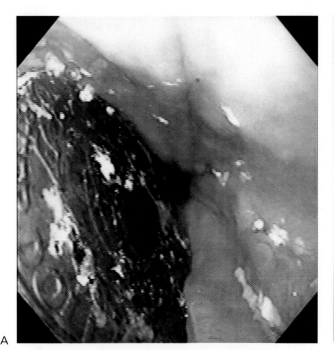

A

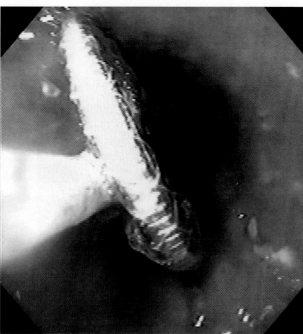

B

COLOR PLATE 17.3. Endoscopic views of a "quarter" lodged in the distal esophagus that was successfully removed with a Roth retrieval net.

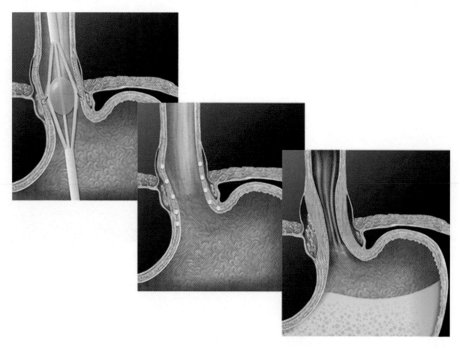

COLOR PLATE 26.2. Sequential steps of the Stretta procedure. **Left:** Balloon inflation and needle deployment at the level of the gastroesophageal junction (GEJ). **Right:** Upon completion of Stretta, radiofrequency energy (*white dots*) has been applied across the GEJ. **Right:** Tightening of the GEJ prevents reflux.

been used in the past decade to objectively assess central responses to provocation of visceral pain.

Evoked potential recording after electrical stimulation of the esophagus demonstrated a clear relationship between stimulus frequency and amplitude of cerebral evoked responses (76). With increasing stimulus frequency, a significant and progressive decrease of evoked potential amplitudes were observed (between frequencies of 0.2 and 1.0 Hz), suggesting rapid attenuation of the cerebral autonomic neural responses with increased electrical stimulation frequency. Additionally, there is a clear dose-response relationship in the brain response with increasing stimulus intensities, which probably reflects increased recruitment of afferent fibers (167). Although investigators have recently defined optimal parameters for recording esophageal cerebral evoked potentials to mechanical and electrical stimulation, it is yet to be determined which technique is better (168,169). Balloon distention is considered a relatively more physiologic stimulus than electrical stimulation. Additionally, the use of large electrical currents and the potential current flow to neighboring tissue result in the uncertainty about the structures and receptors activated (168). However, experienced investigators report that electrical stimulation produces good quality cerebral evoked potentials as a result of abrupt and easily controlled stimulation.

Evoked potential recording after mechanical distention of a visceral organ was first reported for the rectum (170). This led to initial studies of cerebral potentials evoked by esophageal balloon distention (164). In this study, a latex balloon was placed in the distal esophagus and inflated repeatedly at the level of pain threshold by a mechanical pump that also triggered the evoked potential recorder. A characteristic triphasic evoked potential was obtained (Fig. 8.7). Considerable intersubject, but minimal intrasubject variability was noted. In a follow-up study, Smout and colleagues (128) clarified this response. A rapid inflation rate (170 mL/min) was found to be superior to a slower rate (30 mL/min) in the production of evoked potentials. Perhaps most importantly, evoked potential quality and amplitude were found to be dependent on the level of sensation provided by the stimulus. The specificity and reproducibility of esophageal evoked potential recordings have been confirmed (171). Balloon distention with cerebral evoked potential recording was sequentially carried out in the distal and proximal esophageal body. The latencies were significantly shorter with balloon distention in the proximal esophagus. This change in latency is similar whether electrical or mechanical stimulation is used (172).

Evoked potential recording has been performed in patients with esophageal disease (173). Ten patients with NCCP having either nutcracker esophagus or diffuse esophageal spasm experienced chest pain at lower balloon volumes than did control subjects. Both amplitude and quality of the evoked potentials increased with increasing

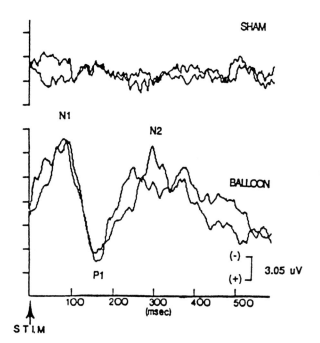

FIGURE 8.7. Evoked potential recorded after esophageal balloon distention (50 repetitions). Amplitude is expressed in microvolts on the vertical axis, while latency from stimulus (Stim) to peak in milliseconds is on the horizontal axis. The typical configuration of two negative peaks (N1, N2) and one positive peak (P1) is demonstrated. Note the close similarity of the two studies in this subject and the lack of evoked potential with sham distention.

sensation while the latencies remained stable. Interestingly, the amplitude and quality of the evoked potentials were lower in patients than in control subjects, with similar levels of sensation produced by lower balloon volumes in the patients. The authors concluded that these data suggest an abnormality in central processing of visceral sensory information in NCCP patients and not an abnormality at the peripheral receptor. An interesting correlate to this was provided by a report of increased evoked potentials produced with auditory stimulation in patients with somatization disorder, which may indicate an increase in general central nervous system sensitivity (174), and by the finding of abnormal pain thresholds in multiple areas in patients with nonulcer dyspepsia and irritable bowel syndrome (175).

Esophageal balloon distention and cerebral evoked potential recording may help define the pathway and type of nerves involved in esophageal nociception in the human. In one report, both esophageal pain perception and esophageal evoked potentials were found to be normal in patients with C5 to C6 sensory spinal cord lesions (176). Two comparisons of evoked potentials obtained with balloon and electrical stimulation concluded that sensation evoked by balloon distention was carried by unmyelinated C fibers, whereas electrical stimulation more likely activated myelinated A delta fibers (177,178). Conversely, Aziz and co-workers (179) found a decrease in evoked potential amplitude but an increase in sensation with increasing frequency of stimulation. They suggested that the evoked potential may therefore be dependent on slowly adapting fibers, although an alternative explanation would hold that their higher frequency stimulation may have initiated motor or other activity too diffuse to be measured with evoked potential recording. The above studies emphasize the potential utility of esophageal evoked potential recording in examining the innervation of the human esophagus.

Evoked potential recording has been also used to provide evidence that specific portions of the brain are responsible for esophageal pain. A small study used source modeling to suggest that the scalp evoked potential was coming from cortical sources located in the cingulate gyri and insular cortex (180). An additional study supported the role of the insular cortex and suggested that there was some evidence for hemispheric dominance that was independent of handedness (181).

Brain Imaging

In addition to cortical evoked potentials, other techniques have been increasingly used to evaluate brain-gut relationship in patients with esophageal disorders. These techniques include positron emission tomography (PET) and functional magnetic resonance imaging (fMRI). The gastrointestinal tract is intricately connected to the central nervous system by pathways that are continuously sampling and modulating gut function (182).

PET scanning is an established method to study the functional neuroanatomy of the human brain (183,184). Radiolabeled compounds allow the study of biochemical and physiologic processes involved in cerebral metabolism (182). Tomographic images represent spatial distribution of radioisotopes in the brain. Regional cerebral blood flow is studied with labeled water ($H_2^{15}O$) and glucose metabolism with ^{18}Fl-labeled fluorodeoxyglucose. Unlike PET, fMRI does not require radioisotopes and hence is considered a safer imaging technique. fMRI detects increases in oxygen concentration in areas of heightened neuronal activity (173,184,185). This imaging technique is best suited for locating the site but not the sequence or duration of neuronal activity. Overall, fMRI provides both anatomic and functional information.

Thus far, only a few studies have attempted to assess the cortical process of esophageal sensation in humans. Aziz and colleagues examined the human brain loci involved in the process of esophageal sensation using PET and distal esophageal balloon distention in eight healthy volunteers (25). Nonpainful stimuli elicited bilateral activation along the central sulcus, insular cortex, and the frontal and parietal operculum. Painful stimuli resulted in intense activation of the same areas and additional activation of right anterior insular cortex and anterior cingulate gyrus. The former is important in affective processing while the latter

in pain processing and generating an affective and cognitive response to pain (26–28). In another study, Kern and colleagues evaluated activation of cerebral cortical responses to esophageal mucosal acid exposure by using an fMRI (29). Ten healthy subjects underwent intraesophageal perfusion of 0.1N hydrochloric acid over 10 minutes. None of the study subjects reported GERD symptoms during acid perfusion. Cerebral cortical activity was concentrated in the posterior cingulate, parietal, and anteromesial frontal lobes. The superior frontal lobe regions activated in this study corresponded to Brodmann's area 32, the insula, the operculum, and the anterior cingulate.

Further studies are needed to assess cerebral activation in patients with different esophageal disorders. In addition, it would be of great interest to determine whether there are differences in central processing of an intraesophageal stimulus in patients with NCCP, nonerosive reflux disease, or functional heartburn. It is also important to begin to examine the role of psychophysiologic states such as stress, anxiety, and depression, and their effects on central nuclei involved with perception of esophageal stimuli. Moving forward will require going from purely topographical and phenomenologic studies to more mechanistic studies designed to address the pathways and neurotransmitters involved in these symptoms (24). Even though the technology is there (e.g., PET and fMRI,) it is essential that the right questions be asked for the necessary progress to take place.

REFERENCES

1. Locke GR 3rd, Talley NJ, Fett SL, et al. Prevalence and clinical spectrum of gastroesophageal reflux: a population-based study in Olmstead County, Minnesota. *Gastroenterology* 1997;112 (5):1448–1456.
2. Eslick GD, Talley NJ. Non-cardiac chest pain: squeezing the life out of the Australian healthcare system? *Med J Aust* 2000; 173(5):233–234.
3. Wielgosz AT, Fletcher RH, McCants CB, et al. Unimproved chest pain in patients with minimal or no coronary disease: a behavioral phenomenon. *Am Heart J* 1984;108(1):67–72.
4. Richter JE, Bradley LA, Castell DO. Esophageal chest pain: current controversies in pathogenesis, diagnosis, and therapy. *Ann Intern Med* 1989;110(1):66–78.
5. Fass R. Chest pain of esophageal origin. *Curr Opin Gastroenterol* 2002;18:464–470.
6. Cherian P, Smith LF, Bardhan KD, et al. Esophageal tests in the evaluation of non-cardiac chest pain. *Dis Esophagus* 1995;8:129.
7. Fass R, Fennerty MB, Ofman JJ, et al. The clinical and economic value of a short course of omeprazole in patients with noncardiac chest pain. *Gastroenterology* 1998;115(1):42–49.
8. Hsia PC, Maher KA, Lewis JH, et al. Utility of upper endoscopy in the evaluation of noncardiac chest pain. *Gastrointest Endosc* 1991;37(1):22–26.
9. Frobert O, Funch-Jensen P, Jacobsen NO, et al. Upper endoscopy in patients with angina and normal coronary angiograms. *Endoscopy* 1995;27(5):365–370.
10. Kahrilas PJ, Clouse RE, Hogan WJ. American Gastroenterolog-

ical Association technical review on the clinical use of esophageal manometry. *Gastroenterology* 1994;107(6):1865–1884.

11. Fass R, Pulliam G, Hayden CW. Patients with non-cardiac chest pain (NCCP) receiving an empirical trial of high dose lansoprazole, demonstrate early symptom response—a double blind, placebo-controlled trial. *Gastroenterology* 2001;120[5, Suppl 1]:A221, #1162.

12. Katon W, Hall ML, Russo J, et al. Chest pain: relationship of psychiatric illness to coronary arteriographic results. *Am J Med* 1988;84(1):1–9.

13. DiMarino AJJ, Allen ML, Lynn RB, et al. Clinical value of esophageal motility testing. *Dig Dis* 1998;16(4):198–204.

14. Chauhan A, Petch MC, Schofield PM. Cardio-oesophageal reflex in humans as a mechanism for "linked angina." *Eur Heart J* 1996;17(3):407–413.

15. Drossman DA, Corazziari R, Talley NJ, et al, and the Rome II Multinational Work Teams. In: Drossman DA, ed. *Rome II The functional gastrointestinal disorders*, second ed. Lawrence, KS: Allen Press, 2000.

16. Gebhart GF. Visceral pain-peripheral sensitisation. *Gut* 2000; 47[Suppl 4]:iv54–iv55; discussion iv58.

17. Goyal RK, Hirano I. The enteric nervous system. *N Engl J Med* 1996;334(17):1106–1115.

18. Grundy D, Scratcherd T. Sensory afferents from the gastrointestinal tract. In: Schultz SG, Wood JD, Rauner BB, eds. *Handbook of physiology*. New York: Oxford University, 1989: 593–620.

19. Randich A. Visceral nerve stimulation and pain modulation. In: Josh LR, ed. *Physiology of the gastrointestinal tract*, third ed. Amsterdam: Elsevier, 1993:126–139.

20. Tougas G, Kamath MV, Garnett S, et al. Mapping of cerebral response to vagal and esophageal stimulation using positron emission tomography (PET) and topographic EEG in humans. *Gastroenterology* 1994;106(4, part 2):A846.

21. Mayer EA, Gebhart GF. Basic and clinical aspects of visceral hyperalgesia. *Gastroenterology* 1994;107(1):271–293.

22. Fass R, Naliboff B, Higa L, et al. Differential effect of long-term esophageal acid exposure on mechanosensitivity and chemosensitivity in humans. *Gastroenterology* 1998;115(6):1363–1373.

23. Rodrigo J, Hernandez CJ, Vidal MA, et al. Vegetative innervation of the esophagus. III. Intraepithelial endings. *Acta Anat* (Basel) 1975;92(2):242–258.

24. Fass R, Tougas G. Functional heartburn—the stimulus, the pain and the brain. *Gut* 2002 *(in press)*.

25. Aziz Q, Andersson JL, Valind S, et al. Identification of human brain loci processing esophageal sensation using positron emission tomography. *Gastroenterology* 1997;113(1):50–59.

26. Minshohima S, Morrow TJ, Koeppe RA. Involvement of insular cortex in central autonomic regulation during painful thermal stimulation. *J Cereb Blood Flow Metab* 1995;15[Suppl 1]:1355–1358.

27. Talbot JD, Marrett S, Evans AC, et al. Multiple representations of pain in human cerebral cortex. *Science* 1991; 251(4999):1355–1358.

28. Vogt BA, Sikes RW, Vogt LJ. anterior cingulate cortex and the medial pain system. In: Vogt BA, Gabriel M, eds. *Neurobiology of cingulate cortex and limbic thalamus*. Boston: Birkhauser; 1994:313–344.

29. Kern MK, Birn RM, Jaradeh S, et al. Identification and characterization of cerebral cortical response to esophageal mucosal acid exposure and distention. *Gastroenterology* 1998;115(6): 1353–1362.

30. Takeda T, Liu J, Gui A, et al. Heartburn not chest pain, is the most common symptoms in response to esophageal distension in normal subjects. *Gastroenterology* 2001;120[5 Suppl 1]:A-222, #1167.

31. Balaban DH, Yamamoto Y, Liu J, et al. Sustained esophageal contraction: a marker of esophageal chest pain identified by intraluminal ultrasonography. *Gastroenterology* 1999;116(1):29–37.

32. Pehlivanov N, Liu J, Mittal RK. Sustained esophageal contraction: a motor correlate of heartburn symptom. *Am J Physiol Gastrointest Liver Physiol* 2001;281(3):G743–G751.

33. Baldi F, Ferrarini F, Longanesi A, et al. Acid gastroesophageal reflux and symptom occurrence. Analysis of some factors influencing their association. *Dig Dis Sci* 1989;34(12):1890–1893.

34. Meyer JH, Lembo A, Elashoff JD, et al. Duodenal fat intensifies the perception of heartburn. *Gut* 2001;49(5):624–628.

35. Fass R. Focused clinical review—nonerosive reflux disease. *Medscape Gastroenterol* 2001;3(1):1–13.

36. Trimble KC, Pryde A, Heading RC. Lowered oesophageal sensory thresholds in patients with symptomatic but not excess gastro-oesophageal reflux: evidence for a spectrum of visceral sensitivity in GORD. *Gut* 1995;37(1):7–12.

37. Fass R, Malagon I, Naliboff B, et al. Effect of psychologically induced stress on symptom perception and autonomic nervous system response of patients (PTS) with erosive esophagitis (EE) and non-erosive reflux disease (NERD). *Gastroenterology* 2000;118(4):A637, #3250.

38. Fass R, Malagon I, Pulliam G, et al. Gender differences in perceptual and emotional ratings of intra-esophageal stimuli in GERD patients undergoing auditory-induced stress. *Gastroenterology* 2002;122[4, Suppl 1]:A-187, #S1228.

39. Mayer EA. The neurobiology of stress and gastrointestinal disease. *Gut* 2000;47(6):861–869.

40. Bernstein LM, Baker LA. A clinical test for esophagitis. *Gastroenterology* 1958;347:760.

41. Bernot R, Norton RA. The esophageal acid perfusion test. *Lahey Clin Found Bull* 1965;14(2):58–63.

42. Richter JE, Hewson EG, Sinclair JW, et al. Acid perfusion test and 24-hour esophageal pH monitoring with symptom index. Comparison of tests for esophageal acid sensitivity. *Dig Dis Sci* 1991;36(5):565–571.

43. Price SF, Smithson KW, Castell DO. Food sensitivity in reflux esophagitis. *Gastroenterology* 1978;75(2):240–243.

44. Kaul B, Petersen H, Grette K, et al. The acid perfusion test in gastroesophageal reflux disease. *Scand J Gastroenterol* 1986; 21(1):93–96.

45. Howard PJ, Maher L, Pryde A, et al. Symptomatic gastro-oesophageal reflux, abnormal oesophageal acid exposure, and mucosal acid sensitivity are three separate, though related, aspects of gastro-oesophageal reflux disease. *Gut* 1991;32(2): 128–132.

46. Battle WS, Nyhus LM, Bombeck CT. Gastroesophageal reflux: diagnosis and treatment. *Ann Surg* 1973;177(5):560–565.

47. Behar J, Biancani P, Sheahan DG. Evaluation of esophageal tests in the diagnosis of reflux esophagitis. *Gastroenterology* 1976; 71(1):9–15.

48. Breen KJ, Whelan G. The diagnosis of reflux oesophagitis: an evaluation of five investigative procedures. *Aust N Z J Surg* 1978;48(2):156–161.

49. Fisher RS, Cohen S. Gastroesophageal reflux. *Med Clin North Am* 1978;62(1):3–20.

50. Bachir GS, Leigh-Collis J, Wilson P, et al. Diagnosis of incipient reflux esophagitis: a new test. *South Med J* 1981;74(9): 1072–1074.

51. Benjamin SB, Richter JE, Cordova CM, et al. Prospective manometric evaluation with pharmacologic provocation of patients with suspected esophageal motility dysfunction. *Gastroenterology* 1983;84(5, part 1):893–901.

52. Johnson DA, Winters C, Spurling TJ, et al. Esophageal acid sensitivity in Barrett's esophagus. *J Clin Gastroenterol* 1987;9 (1):23–27.

53. Gracely RH, McGrath F, Dubner R. Ratio scales of sensory and affective verbal pain descriptors. *Pain* 1978;5(1):5–18.

54. Silverman DH, Munakata JA, Ennes H, et al. Regional cerebral activity in normal and pathological perception of visceral pain. *Gastroenterology* 1997;112(1):64–72.

55. Richter JE. Provocative tests in esophageal diseases. In: Scarpignato C, Galmiche JP, eds. *Functional evaluation in esophageal disease.* Basel: Karger; 1994.

56. De Caestecker JS, Pryde A, Heading RC. Comparison of intravenous edrophonium and oesophageal acid perfusion during oesophageal manometry in patients with non-cardiac chest pain. *Gut* 1988;29(8):1029–1034.

57. Ghillebert G, Janssens J, Vantrappen G, et al. Ambulatory 24 hour intraoesophageal pH and pressure recordings v provocation tests in the diagnosis of chest pain of oesophageal origin. *Gut* 1990;31(7):738–744.

58. Hewson EG, Dalton CB, Richter JE. Comparison of esophageal manometry, provocative testing, and ambulatory monitoring in patients with unexplained chest pain. *Dig Dis Sci* 1990;35(3):302–309.

59. Nevens F, Janssens J, Piessens J, et al. Prospective study on prevalence of esophageal chest pain in patients referred on an elective basis to a cardiac unit for suspected myocardial schemia. *Dig Dis Sci* 1991;36(2):229–235.

60. Peters L, Maas L, Petty D, et al. Spontaneous noncardiac chest pain. Evaluation of 24-hour ambulatory esophageal motility and pH monitoring. *Gastroenterology* 1988;94(4):878–886.

61. Soffer EE, Scalabrini P, Wingate DL. Spontaneous noncardiac chest pain: value of ambulatory esophageal pH and motility monitoring. *Dig Dis Sci* 1989;34(11):1651–1655.

62. Vantrappen G, Janssens J, Ghillebert G. The irritable oesophagus—a frequent cause of angina-like pain. *Lancet* 1987;1 (85444):1232–1234.

63. Fass R, Yalam JM, Camargo L, et al. Increased esophageal chemoreceptor sensitivity to acid in patients after successful reversal of Barrett's esophagus. *Dig Dis Sci* 1997;42(9):1853–1858.

64. Burns TW, Venturatos SG. Esophageal motor function and response to acid perfusion in patients with symptomatic reflux esophagitis. *Dig Dis Sci* 1985;30(6):529–535.

65. Richter JE, Johns DN, Wu WC, et al. Are esophageal motility abnormalities produced during the intraesophageal acid perfusion test? *JAMA* 1985;253(13):1914–1917.

66. Smith JL, Opekun AR, Larkai E, et al. Sensitivity of the esophageal mucosa to pH in gastroesophageal reflux disease. *Gastroenterology* 1989;96(3):683–689.

67. Hewson EG, Sinclair JW, Dalton CB, et al. Acid perfusion test: does it have a role in the assessment of non cardiac chest pain. *Gut* 1989;30(3):305–310.

68. Eslick GD, Fass R. Non-cardiac chest pain: evaluation and treatment. *Gastroenterol Clin North Am* 2002 *(in press)*.

69. London RL, Ouyang A, Snape WJJ, et al. Provocation of esophageal pain by ergonovine or edrophonium. *Gastroenterology* 1981;81(1):10–14.

70. Nostrant TT. Provocation testing in noncardiac chest pain. *Am J Med* 1992;92:565–645.

71. Richter JE, Hackshaw BT, Wu WC, et al. Edrophonium: a useful provocative test for oesophageal chest pain. *Ann Intern Med* 1985;103(1):14–21.

72. Frobert O, Funch-Jensen P, Bagger JP. Diagnostic value of esophageal studies in patients with angina-like chest pain and normal coronary angiograms. *Ann Intern Med* 1996;124 (11):959–969.

73. Katz PO, Dalton CB, Richter JE, et al. Esophageal testing of patients with noncardiac chest pain or dysphagia. *Ann Intern Med* 1987;106(4):593–597.

74. Cooke RA, Anggiansah A, Chambers JB, et al. A prospective study of oesophageal function in patients with normal coronary angiograms and controls with angina. *Gut* 1998;42(3):323–329.

75. Dalton CB, Hewson EG, Castell DO, et al.. Edrophonium provocative test in noncardiac chest pain. Evaluation of testing techniques. *Dig Dis Sci* 1990;35(12):1445–1451.

76. Hollerbach S, Kamath MV, Fitzpatrick D, et al. The cerebral response to electrical stimuli in the oesophagus is altered by increasing stimulus frequencies. *Neurogastroenterol Motil* 1997;9 (2):129–139.

77. Mellow M. Symptomatic diffuse esophageal spasm. Manometric follow-up and response to cholinergic stimulating and cholinesterase inhibition. *Gastroenterology* 1977;73(2):237–240.

78. Nostrant TT, Sams J, Huber T. Bethanechol increases the diagnostic yield in patients with esophageal chest pain. *Gastroenterology* 1986;91(5):1141–1146.

79. Davies HA, Kaye MD, Rhodes J, et al. Diagnosis of oesophageal spasm by ergometrine provocation. *Gut* 1982;23:89–97.

80. Eastwood GL, Weiner BH, Dickerson WJ II, et al. Use of ergonovine to identify esophageal spasm in patients with chest pain. *Ann Intern Med* 1981;94(6):768–771.

81. Koch KL, Curry RC, Feldman RL, et al. Ergonovine-induced esophageal spasm in patients with chest pain resembling angina pectoris. *Dig Dis Sci* 1982;27(12):1073–1080.

82. Buxton A, Goldberg S, Hirshfeld JW, et al. Refractory ergonovine-induced coronary vasospasm: importance of intracoronary nitroglycerin. *Am J Cardiol* 1980;46(2):329–334.

83. Hewson EG, Sinclair JW, Dalton CB, et al. Twenty-four-hour esophageal pH monitoring: the most useful test for evaluating noncardiac chest pain. *Am J Med* 1991;90(5):576–583.

84. Achem SR, Kolts BE, MacMath T, et al. Effects of omeprazole versus placebo in treatment of noncardiac chest pain and gastroesophageal reflux. *Dig Dis Sci* 1997;42(10):2138–2145.

85. Fass R, Fennerty MB, Vakil N. Nonerosive reflux disease - current concepts and dilemmas. *Am J Gastroenterol* 2001;96(2):303–314.

86. Fass R, Winters GF. Evaluation of the patient with noncardiac chest pain: is gastroesophageal reflux disease or an esophageal motility disorder the cause? *Medscape Gastroenterol* 2001;3(6):1–7.

87. Euler AR, Byrne WJ. Twenty-four-hour esophageal intraluminal pH probe testing: comparative analysis. *Gastroenterology* 1981;80(5 part 1):957–961.

88. Fass R. Empirical trials in treatment of gastroesophageal reflux disease. *Dig Dis* 2000;18(1):20–26.

89. Fass R. Testing of diagnosis with a therapeutic trial: concept and requirements for a therapeutic trial. *Eur J Gastroenterol Hepatol* 2001;13[suppl 3]:S49–S50.

90. Schenk BE, Kuipers EJ, Klinkenberg-Knol EC, et al. Omeprazole as a diagnostic tool in gastroesophageal reflux disease. *Am J Gastroenterol* 1997;92(11):1997–2000.

91. Squillace SJ, Young MF, Sanowski RA. Single dose omeprazole as a test for noncardiac chest pain. *Gastroenterology* 1993;104:A197.

92. Young MF, Sanowski RA, Talbert GA, et al. Omeprazole administration as a test for gastroesophageal reflux. *Gastroenterology* 1992;102:192.

93. Pandak WM, Arezo S, Everett S, et al. Short course of omeprazole. A better first diagnostic approach to noncardiac chest pain than endoscopy, manometry, or 24-hour esophageal pH monitoring. *J Clin Gastroenterol* 2002;35(4):307–314.

94. Deleted in proofs.

95. Fass R, Fullerton H, Hayden CW, et al. Patients with noncardiac chest pain (NCCP) receiving an empirical trial of high dose rabeprazole, demonstrate early symptom response—a double

blind, placebo-controlled trial. *Gastroenterology* 2002;122[4 Suppl 1]:A580–A581, #W1175.

96. Fass R, Fennerty MB, Johnson C, et al. Correlation of ambulatory 24-hour esophageal pH monitoring results with symptom improvement in patients with noncardiac chest pain due to gastroesophageal reflux disease. *J Clin Gastroenterol* 1999;28(1): 36–39.

97. Ofman J, Gralnek I, Udani J, et al. The cost-effectiveness of the omeprazole test in noncardiac chest pain (NCCP). *Gastroenterology* 1998;114(4 part 2):A-31, #G0127.

98. Ofman JJ, Gralnek IM, Udani J, et al. The cost-effectiveness of the omeprazole test in patients with noncardiac chest pain. *Am J Med* 1999;107(3):288–289.

99. Fass R, Ofman JJ, Sampliner RE, et al. The omeprazole test is as sensitive as 24-h oesophageal pH monitoring in diagnosing gastro-oesophageal reflux disease in symptomatic patients with erosive esophagitis. *Aliment Pharmacol Ther* 2000;14(4): 389–396.

100. Tougas G, Hudoba P, Fitzpatrick D, et al. Cerebral-evoked potential responses following direct vagal and esophageal electrical stimulation in humans. *Am J Physiol* 1993;264(3 part 1):G486–G491.

101. Sarkar S, Aziz Q, Woolf CJ, et al. Contribution of central sensitisation to the development of noncardiac chest pain. *Lancet* 2000;356(9236):1154–1159.

102. Heft MW, Parker SR. An experimental basis for revising the graphic rating scale for pain. *Pain* 1984;19(2):153–161.

103. Hollerbach S, Bulat R, May A, et al. Abnormal cerebral processing of oesophageal stimuli in patients with noncardiac chest pain (NCCP). *Neurogastroenterol Motil* 2000;12(6):555–565.

104. Harris JH, Therkelsen EE, Zinner NR. Electrical measurement of urethral flow. In: Boyarsky S, Tanagho EA, Gottschalf CW, et al, eds. *Urodynamics*. London: Academic Press, 1971:465–472.

105. Rask-Andersen H, Djurhuus JC. Development of a probe for endoureteral investigation of peristalsis by flow velocity and cross section area measurement. *Acta Chir Scand Suppl* 1976;472:59–65.

106. Silny J, Knigge KP, Fass J, et al. Verification of the intraluminal multiple electrical impedance measurement for the recording of gastrointestinal motility. *J Gastrointest Motil* 1993;5:107–122.

107. Rao SSC, Hayek B, Summers RW. Impedance planimetry: an integrated approach for assessing sensory, active, and passive biomechanical properties of the human esophagus. *Am J Gastroenterol* 1995;90(3):431–438.

108. Orvar KB, Gregersen H, Christensen J. Biomechanical characteristics of the human esophagus. *Dig Dis Sci* 1993;38(2):197–205.

109. Rao SS, Gregersen H, Hayek B, et al. Unexplained chest pain: the hypersensitive, hyperreactive, and poorly compliant esophagus. *Ann Intern Med* 1996;124(11):950–958.

110. Rao SSC, Hayek B, Summers RW. Functional chest pain of esophageal origin: hyperalgesia or motor dysfunction. *Am J Gastroenterol* 2001;96(9):2584–2589.

111. Sifrim D, Holloway R, Silny J, et al. Acid, nonacid, and gas reflux in patients with gastroesophageal reflux disease during ambulatory 24-hour pH-impedance recordings. *Gastroenterology* 2001;120(7):1588–1598.

112. Vela MF, Camacho-Lobato L, Srinivasan R, et al. Simultaneous intraesophageal impedance and pH measurement of acid and nonacid gastroesophageal reflux: effect of omeprazole. *Gastroenterology* 2001;120(7):1599–1606.

113. Silny J. Intraluminal multiple electric impedance procedure for measurement of gastrointestinal motility. *J Gastrointest Motil* 1991;3:151–162.

114. Fass J, Silny J, Braun J, et al. Measuring esophageal motility with a new intraluminal impedance device. First clinical results in reflux patients. *Scand J Gastroenterol* 1994;29(8):693–702.

115. Nguyen HN, Silny J, Matern S. Multiple intraluminal electrical impedancometry for recording of upper gastrointestinal motility: current results and further implications. *Am J Gastroenterol* 1999;94(2):306–317.

116. Takeda T, Kassab G, Liu J, et al. A novel ultrasound technique to study the biomechanics of the human esophagus *in vivo*. *Am J Physiol Gastrointest Liver Physiol* 2002;282(5):G785–G793.

117. Richter JE, Barish CF, Castell DO. Abnormal sensory perception in patients with esophageal chest pain. *Gastroenterology* 1986;91(4):845–852.

118. Ritchie J. Pain from distension of the pelvic colon by inflating a balloon in the irritable colon syndrome. *Gut* 1973;14(2): 125–132.

119. Mertz H, Walsh JH, Sytnik B, et al. The effect of octreotide on human gastric compliance and sensory perception. *Neurogastroenterol Motil* 1995;7(3):175–185.

120. Kramer P, Hollander W. Comparison of experimental esophageal pain with clinical pain of angina pectoris and esophageal disease. *Gastroenterology* 1955;29:719.

121. Lipkin M, Sleisenger MH. Studies of visceral pain: measurements of stimulus intensity and duration associated with the onset of pain in esophagus, ileum and colon. *J Clin Invest* 1958; 37:28.

122. Yakshe PN, et al. Does provocative esophageal testing influence coronary blood flow or coronary flow reserve? Preliminary results of concurrent esophageal and cardiac testing. *Gastroenterology* 1993;104:A227.

123. Meyer GW, Castell DO. Human esophageal response during chest pain induced by swallowing cold liquids. *JAMA* 1981;246(18):2057–2059.

124. Kaye MD, Kilby AE, Harper PC. Changes in distal esophageal function in response to cooling. *Dig Dis Sci* 1987;32(1):22–27.

125. Kahrilas PJ, Dodds WJ, Hogan WJ. Dysfunction of the belch reflex. A cause of incapacitating chest pain. *Gastroenterology* 1987;93(4):818–822.

126. Kaye MD. Anomalies of peristalsis in idiopathic diffuse oesophageal spasm. *Gut* 1981;22(3):217–222.

127. Barish CF, Castell DO, Richter JE. Graded esophageal balloon distention. A new provocative test for noncardiac chest pain. *Dig Dis Sci* 1986;31(12):1292–1298.

128. Smout AJ, DeVore MS, Castell DO. Cerebral potentials evoked by esophageal distension in human. *Am J Physiol* 1990;259(6 part 1):G955–G959.

129. Whitehead WE, Delvaux M. The Working Team. Standardization of barostat procedures for testing smooth muscle tone and sensory thresholds in the gastrointestinal tract. *Dig Dis Sci* 1997;42(2):223–241.

130. Azpiroz F, Malagelada JR. Physiological variations in canine gastric tone measured by an electronic barostat. *Am J Physiol* 1985;248:G229–G237.

131. Toma TD, Zighelboim J, Phillips SF, et al. Methods for studying intestinal sensitivity and compliance: *in vitro* studies of balloons and a barostat. *Neurogastroenterol Motil* 1996;8(1):19–28.

132. Khan MI, Feinle C, Read NW. Investigating gastric and sensory response to distention: comparative studies using flaccid bags and latex balloons. *Second United European Gastroenterology Meeting* 1992;13(A):175.

133. Hu WHC, Martin CJ, Talley NJ. Intraesophageal acid perfusion sensitizes the esophagus to mechanical distension: a barostat study. *Am J Gastroenterol* 2000;95(9):2189–2194.

134. Sun WM, Read NW, Prior A, et al. Sensory and motor responses to rectal distention vary according to rate and pattern of balloon inflation. *Gastroenterology* 1990;99(4):1008–1015.

135. Munakata J, Naliboff B, Harraf F, et al. Repetitive sigmoid stimulation induces rectal hyperalgesia in patients with irritable bowel syndrome. *Gastroenterology* 1997;112(1):55–63.

136. Whitehead WE, Crowell MD, Shone D, et al. Sensitivity to rectal distension: validation of a measurement system. *Gastroenterology* 1993;104:A600.

137. Cornsweet TN. The staircase-method in psychophysics. *Am J Psychol* 1996;75:485–491.

138. Lembo T, Niazi N, Mayer EA. Do mucosal mechanoreceptors contribute to rectal hyperalgesia in IBS patients? *Gastroenterology* 1993;104:A540.

139. Pehlivanov N, Liu J, Mittal R. Sustained esophageal contraction: a motor correlate of heartburn symptom. *Gastroenterology* 1999;116(4):A1062, #G4613.

140. Nguyen P, Castell DO. Stimulation of esophageal mechanoreceptors is dependent on rate and duration of distension. *Am J Physiol* 1994;267(1 part 1):G115–G118.

141. Lasch H, Castell DO, Castell JA. Evidence of diminished visceral pain with aging: studies using graded intraesophageal balloon distension. *Am J Physiol* 1997;272(1 part 1):G1–G3.

142. Fass R, Pulliam G, Johnson C, et al. Symptom severity and oesophageal chemosensitivity to acid in older and young patients with gastro-oesophageal reflux. *Age Ageing* 2000;29 (2):125–130.

143. Nguyen P, Lee SD, Castell DO. Evidence of gender differences in esophageal pain threshold. *Am J Gastroenterol* 1995;90 (6):901–905.

144. Niemantsverdriet EC, Timmer R, Breumelhof R, et al. Regional differences in esophageal acid sensitivity studied with pH-controlled segmental acid perfusion. *Gastroenterology* 1997;112(4):A237.

145. Winwood PJ, Mavrogiannis CC, Smith CL. Reduced sensitivity to intra-oesophageal acid in patients with reflux-induced strictures. *Scand J Gastroenterol* 1993;28(2):109–112.

146. Grade A, Pulliam G, Johnson C, et al. Reduced chemoreceptor sensitivity in patients with Barrett's esophagus may be related to age and not to the presence of Barrett's epithelium. *Am J Gastroenterol* 1997;92(11):2040–2043.

147. Sarkar S, Aziz Q, Woolf CJ, et al. Contribution of central sensitisation to the development of non-cardiac chest pain. *Lancet* 2000;356(9236):1154–1159.

148. Creamer B, Schlegel J. Motor responses of the esophagus to distention. *J Appl Physiol* 1957;100:498.

149. Enzmann DR, Harell GS, Zboralske FF. Upper esophageal responses to intraluminal distention in man. *Gastroenterology* 1977;72(6):1292–1298.

150. Winship DH, Zboralske FF. The esophageal propulsive force: esophageal response to acute obstruction. *J Clin Invest* 1967; 46(9):1391–1401.

151. Paterson WG. Neuromuscular mechanisms of esophageal responses at and proximal to a distending balloon. *Am J Physiol* 1991;260(1 part 1):G148–G155.

152. Paterson WG, Selucky M, Hynna-Liepert TT. Effect of intraesophageal location and muscarinic blockade on balloon distension-induced chest pain. *Dig Dis Sci* 1991;36(3):282–288.

153. Andreollo NA, Thompson DG, Kendall GP, et al. Functional relationships between cricopharyngeal sphincter and oesophageal body in response to graded intraluminal distension. *Gut* 1988;29(2):161–166.

154. Deschner WK, Maher KA, Cattau EL Jr, et al. Manometric responses to balloon distention in patients with nonobstructive dysphagia. *Gastroenterology* 1989;97(5):1181–1185.

155. Deschner WK, Maher KA, Cattau EL Jr, et al. Intraesophageal balloon distention versus drug provocation in the evaluation of noncardiac chest pain. *Am J Gastroenterol* 1990;85(8):938–943.

156. Clouse RE, McCord GS, Lustman PJ, et al. Clinical correlates of abnormal sensitivity to intraesophageal balloon distension. *Dig Dis Sci* 1991;36(8):1040–1045.

157. Mehta AJ, De Caestecker JS, Camm AJ, et al. Sensitization to painful distention and abnormal sensory perception in the esophagus. *Gastroenterology* 1995;108(2):311–319.

158. Garrison DW, Chandler MJ, Foreman RD. Viscerosomatic convergence onto feline spinal neurons from esophagus, heart and somatic fields: effects of inflammation. *Pain* 1992;49(3):373–382.

159. Peghini PL, Johnston BT, Leite LP, et al. Mucosal acid exposure sensitizes a subset of normal subjects to intra-oesophageal balloon distension. *Eur J Gastroenterol Hepatol* 1996;8(10):979–983.

160. DeVault KR. Acid infusion does not affect intraesophageal balloon distention-induced sensory and pain thresholds. *Am J Gastroenterol* 1997;92(6):947–949.

161. Sarkar S, Woolf CJ, Aziz Q, et al. Secondary hyperalgesia is induced by acid in the healthy human oesophagus. *Gut* 1997; 41[Suppl 3]:A26.

162. Cannon RO 3rd, Quyyumi AA, Mincemoyer R, et al. Imipramine in patients with chest pain despite normal coronary angiograms. *N Engl J Med* 1994;330(20):1411–1417.

163. Peghini PL, Katz PO, Castell DO. Imipramine decreases oesophageal pain perception in human male volunteers. *Gut* 1998;42(6):807–813.

164. Castell DO, Wood JD, Frieling T, et al. Cerebral electrical potentials evoked by balloon distention of the human esophagus. *Gastroenterology* 1990;98(3):662–666.

165. DeVault KR. Nifedipine does not alter barostat determined esophageal smooth muscle tone. *Gastroenterology* 1995;108(4):A591.

166. Smout AJ, DeVore MS, Dalton CB, et al. Effects of nifedipine on esophageal tone and perception of esophageal distension. *Dig Dis Sci* 1992;37(4):598–602.

167. Hollerbach S, Kamath MV, Chen Y, et al. The magnitude of the central response to esophageal electrical stimulation is intensity dependent. *Gastroenterology* 1997;112(4):1137–1146.

168. Hobson AR, Sarkar S, Furlong PL, et al. Identification of the optimal parameters for recording cortical potentials evoked by mechanical stimulation of the human oesophagus. *Neurogastroenterol Motil* 2000;12(2):163–171.

169. Hobson AR, Aziz Q, Furlong PL, et al.. Identification of the optimal parameters for recording cortical evoked potentials to human oesophageal electrical stimulation. *Neurogastroenterol Motil* 1998;10(5):421–430.

170. Collett L, Meunier P, Duclaux R, et al. Cerebral evoked potentials after endorectal mechanical stimulation in humans. *Am J Physiol* 1988;254(4 part 1):G477–G482.

171. DeVault KR, Beacham S, Streletz LJ, et al. Cerebral evoked potentials. A method of quantification of central nervous system response to esophageal pain. *Dig Dis Sci* 1993;38(12):2241–2246.

172. Frieling T, Enck P, Wienbeck M. Cerebral responses evoked by electrical stimulation of rectosigmoid in normal subjects. *Dig Dis Sci* 1989;34(2):202–205.

173. Smout AJPM, DeVore MS, Dalton CB, et al. Cerebral potentials evoked by oesophageal distension in patients with non-cardiac chest pain. *Gut* 1992;33(3):298–302.

174. James L, Gordon E, Kraiuhin C, et al. Augmentation of auditory evoked potentials in somatization disorder. *J Psychiatr Res* 1990;24(2):155–163.

175. Trimble KC, Farouk R, Pryde A, et al. Heightened visceral sensation in functional gastrointestinal disease is not site-specific. Evidence for a generalized disorder of gut sensitivity. *Dig Dis Sci* 1995;40(8):1607–1613.

176. DeVault KR, Beacham S, Castell DO, et al. Esophageal sensation in spinal cord-injured patients: balloon distension and cerebral evoked potential recording. *Am J Physiol* 1996;271(6 part 1):G937–G941.

177. Sollenbohmer C, Enck P, Haussinger D, et al. Electrically evoked cerebral potentials during esophageal distension at perception and pain threshold. *Am J Gastroenterol* 1996;91(5): 970–975.

178. Tougas G, Fitzpatrick D, Upton ARM, et al. The cortical evoked responses produced by balloon distention and electrical stimulation of the esophagus involve different vagal fibers. *Gastroenterology* 1993;104(A592).

179. Aziz Q, et al. Effect of stimulation frequency on sensory perception and cortical evoked potentials in the human esophagus. *Gastroenterology* 1993;104:A810.

180. Franssen H, Weusten BL, Wieneke GH, et al. Source modeling of message evoked potentials. *Electroencephalogr Clin Neurophysiol* 1996;100(2):85–95.

181. Aziz Q, Furlong PL, Barlow J, et al. Topographic mapping of cortical potentials evoked by distension of the human proximal and distal oesophagus. *Electroencephalogr Clin Neurophysiol* 1995;96(3):219–228.

182. Aziz Q, Thompson DG. Brain-gut axis in health and disease. *Gastroenterology* 1998;114(3):559–578.

183. Hartshorne MF. Positron emission tomography. In: Orrison WW, Lewine JD, Sanders JA, et al, eds. *Functional brain imaging*. St. Louis: Mosby—Year Book, 1995:187–212.

184. Aine CJ. A conceptual overview and critique of functional neuroimaging techniques in humans: I. MRI/FMRI and PET. *Crit Rev Neurobiol* 1995;9(2-3):229–309.

185. Sanders JA, Orrison WW. Functional magnetic resonance imaging. In: Orrison WW, Lewine JD, Sanders JA, et al, eds. *Functional brain imaging*. St. Louis: Mosby—Year Book, 1995: 239–326.

ROLE OF HISTOLOGY AND CYTOLOGY IN ESOPHAGEAL DISEASES

JOHN R. GOLDBLUM
TERRY L. GRAMLICH

In some patients with esophageal diseases, morphologic confirmation of the clinical and endoscopic picture is required, thereby necessitating the procurement of endoscopic biopsy specimens or cytologic brushings. In such cases, morphologic assessment of these specimens can provide a specific diagnosis, or at least help to narrow the diagnostic considerations. We believe that the histologic evaluation of biopsy specimens and cytologic brushings is diagnostically complementary (1,2) for both neoplastic and nonneoplastic conditions.

The benefits of cytologic evaluation of esophageal specimens are not generally well appreciated. Cytology may provide a definitive diagnosis of carcinoma when a biopsy specimen is inconclusive. Cytology has the advantage of greater accessibility over biopsy for stenotic or obstructive lesions. The distinction between carcinoma and lymphoma in some cases can be made with greater ease in cytologic specimens than in biopsy specimens. Cytology may cost less and decrease sampling error when large areas of the esophageal mucosa (e.g., Barrett's esophagus [BE]) must be evaluated. Finally, cytology can provide a faster turnaround time from endoscopy to diagnosis than can standard tissue processing.

Nonendoscopic, exfoliative cytology can be used to screen for squamous cell carcinoma in patients living in high-risk regions of the world (3–7), for screening and surveillance of BE (8), to detect metachronous and recurrent neoplasms in the follow-up of patients with previously treated carcinomas of the ear, nose, and throat (9), and to identify infectious agents (10). Endoscopically directed brushing is the method of choice for the diagnosis of visible mucosal lesions; however, balloon, sponge, mesh, or a combination of these has been used in screening and surveillance programs (11). Once the specimen has been obtained, the cells may be prepared in a variety of ways including direct smear, cytospin, and cell block preparations (12).

One alternative uses a liquid-based method to prepare a slide that contains a representative sample of the obtained cells. This alternative technique has provided superior results in recent years and allows additional slides to be prepared for special studies including immunohistochemistry and *in situ* hybridization (13,14). Finally, endoscopic fine needle aspiration can provide diagnostic material from lesions arising from the mucosa, esophageal intramural masses, or periesophageal lymph nodes.

NORMAL HISTOLOGY AND CYTOLOGY

Like other gastrointestinal tract organs, the esophagus has four concentric layers: the mucosa, submucosa, muscularis propria, and adventitia. The esophageal mucosa is lined by nonkeratinized, stratified squamous epithelium with basal, intermediate, and superficial cell layers. The basal cell compartment comprises less than 15% of the thickness of the mucosa and is usually composed of no more than two to three cell layers (15). Mitotic figures are restricted to the basal cell zone under normal circumstances. The cells above the basal cell zone have more cytoplasm with a decrease in the nuclear-to-cytoplasmic ratio. A basement membrane separates the epithelium from the lamina propria, which itself is composed of loose fibrovascular tissue (Color Plate 9.1A). Unlike the colon, lymphatic channels are found within the esophageal mucosa. Lamina propria papillae cause infoldings of the esophageal squamous mucosa and are generally evenly spaced and project less than two thirds of the way through the epithelium. The muscularis mucosae separate the mucosa from the submucosa and are composed of slips of smooth muscle cells. This structure is often markedly thickened in BE. The submucosa is composed of dense collagenous and elastic connective tissue containing nerves, lymphatic channels, and blood vessels. The composition of the muscularis propria changes throughout the esophagus, because it is composed of skele-

J.R. Goldblum, T.L. Gramlich: Department of Anatomic Pathology, Cleveland Clinic Foundation, Cleveland, Ohio.

tal muscle in the upper one third, smooth muscle in the lower one third, and a mixture of skeletal and smooth muscle in the middle one third. The myenteric plexus is found between the inner and outer layers of the muscularis propria and is composed of nerves, ganglion cells, and scattered inflammatory cells. The adventitia is composed of loose connective tissue.

Cytologic preparations obtained from a histologically normal esophagus typically result in a cellular sample of squamous epithelial cells that are similar to those designated as "intermediate" and "superficial" in the cervical (Papanicolaou) smear (Color Plate 9.1B). Both intermediate and superficial squamous cells contain abundant cytoplasm with small, round, regular nuclei, resulting in cells with low nuclear-to-cytoplasmic ratios. Intermediate nuclei contain finely granular chromatin with inconspicuous nucleoli. In contrast, the superficial nuclei are dense and pyknotic without discernible chromatic structure. Both cell types occur as individual cells, loosely cohesive cell aggregates, or large sheets. Glandular epithelial cells may represent a normal finding if the esophagogastric junction is sampled (discussed later). These glandular cells occur as single cells or cohesive tissue fragments. The individual cells have a columnar appearance with a small basally located nucleus with small nucleoli. These tissue fragments appear as either flat, "honeycomb" sheets if viewed *en face* or as columnar cells if oriented on edge. Slight pseudostratification of the nuclei can be seen and does not necessarily indicate a dysplastic phenomenon. The specimen may be contaminated by cells originating from the oral cavity, pharynx, or respiratory tract. Thus, ciliated columnar cells, pulmonary macrophages, or squamous cells with adherent bacterial or fungal colonies are often present.

ESOPHAGITIS

Inflammation of the esophageal mucosa is common, and a variety of insults may result in a similar histologic pattern of injury. Thus, although clinical and radiologic findings may suggest a specific etiology, the histologic and cytologic alterations present in these specimens are often not specific. However, in some types of infectious esophagitis, histologic or cytologic evaluation can offer a specific diagnosis (16).

Candida Esophagitis

Candida albicans is the most frequent cause of clinically significant infectious esophagitis, often occurring in patients who are immunosuppressed. Esophageal obstructions secondary to neoplasm, benign stricture, or even achalasia also predispose to infection by this organism (17,18).

Grossly, *candida* esophagitis usually results in slightly raised, white plaques arising in a background of erythematous squamous mucosa. Histologically, a pseudomembrane

composed of a mixture of pseudohyphae, necrotic squamous cells, and fibrinopurulent exudate are often adherent to the underlying squamous mucosa, which often shows marked regenerative epithelial changes and intramucosal neutrophils (19) (Color Plate 9.2).

Cytologically, fungal pseudohyphae and yeast are readily identified as red or pink structures within Papanicolaou-stained material (Color Plate 9.3). The organism may be more readily identified in cytologic brushings than in biopsy specimens (20). The presence of normal squamous epithelial cells with adherent yeast raises the possibility of oral contamination, whereas the presence of organisms admixed with acute inflammatory cells and reparative epithelial changes provides more convincing evidence of a true pathologic infection. These reparative changes may be so profound as to be easily confused with squamous dysplasia. Features that support a nonneoplastic process include an even distribution of nuclear chromatin and the absence of nuclear pleomorphism. The atypical cells of repair frequently occur as cohesive sheets of cells with streaming nuclei containing acute inflammatory cells. Normal polarity is retained in these cell groupings. In contrast, dysplastic cells are discohesive, showing greater degrees of chromatin abnormalities and nuclear pleomorphism, as well as loss of polarity. Equivocal cases can result in suspicious but not diagnostic findings (21).

Herpes Esophagitis

Herpes simplex virus (HSV) is the most commonly recognized cause of viral esophagitis. Mucosal trauma, cancer, chemotherapy, radiation therapy, immunosuppressive therapy, and other immunodeficiency states (especially infection with human immunodeficiency virus) predispose to herpes esophagitis (22–24). In addition, this form of esophagitis can occur in immunocompetent patients (25).

Many patients with herpes esophagitis are asymptomatic, and thus the true incidence of this infection is unknown. The endoscopic appearance is that of multiple shallow, small ulcers with sharply delineated borders that most commonly affect the distal one third of the esophagus (26). Given that the characteristic morphologic findings are present in the squamous mucosa adjacent to the ulcer, it is important for the endoscopist to be aware of where the optimal site of biopsy should be. The virus affects the squamous mucosa and results in two types of viral cytopathic alterations. Cowdry's type A inclusion bodies are round, densely eosinophilic structures that are separated from a thickened nuclear membrane by a clear halo. So-called ground-glass nuclei result in a homogeneous, faintly basophilic chromatin pattern (Color Plate 9.4). In both types of virocytes, the nuclei and the cytoplasm are increased in volume. Multinucleated squamous cells are also characteristic (27). Other squamous mucosal alterations are also present in herpes esophagitis. Frequently, the mucosa adjacent to the characteristic inclusions is ulcerated, and the ulcer base is composed of necrotic cellular debris, acute inflammatory cells, granulation tissue, and sheets of macrophages (28). As mentioned previously, the characteristic virocytes are present in the squamous mucosa adjacent to the ulcer.

Because herpes infects the squamous epithelial cells, their identification is possible by brush cytology. The infected squamous cells show similar nuclear changes to those described earlier, including ground-glass nuclei, nuclei with Cowdry's type A inclusions, and multinucleated squamous cells with nuclear molding (Color Plate 9.5). The characteristic chromatin changes are more difficult to appreciate in poorly preserved, air-dried smears. Multinucleated glandular cells, a feature found in reactive glandular cells, may mimic infection with herpes. The nature of the chromatin with the characteristic inclusion distinguishes HSV infection from reactive changes.

Cytomegalovirus Esophagitis

Cytomegalovirus infection (CMV) is the second most common cause of viral esophagitis. Like infection with HSV, CMV tends to affect immunocompromised patients (29–31). Infection of the esophagus is less common than infection of the stomach or small intestine.

Endoscopically, the alterations in CMV esophagitis lack specificity. Unlike HSV infection in which the characteristic alterations are found in the squamous mucosa, CMV tends to infect cells in the ulcer base, including fibroblasts and capillary endothelial cells. Thus, the endoscopist is more likely to find these diagnostic features if the ulcer bed is biopsied.

Histologically, cells that are infected by CMV show marked nuclear and cytoplasmic enlargement. There is a characteristic homogeneous, basophilic inclusion within the enlarged nucleus that is separated from a thickened nuclear membrane by a clear halo (Color Plate 9.6). In addition, although not always identified, some infected cells contain small eosinophilic cytoplasmic inclusions. As with HSV infection, sheets of macrophages are often seen at the base of the ulcer bed (32). When the inclusions are not classic, ancillary tests including immunohistochemistry or *in situ* hybridization are useful in confirming CMV infection (33).

As discussed earlier, CMV does not typically infect the squamous epithelial cells, thereby making the diagnosis by cytology less likely. A cytologic diagnosis is more likely if the ulcer base is vigorously brushed to produce a sample of the underlying connective tissue. CMV inclusions are readily identified by the Papanicolaou stain (Color Plate 9.7). The intranuclear inclusions can be confused with prominent nucleoli seen with repair or carcinoma. Esophageal brushing smears also show a background of reparative epithelial cells, acute inflammation, necrotic debris, and granulation tissue (1,34).

Other Infections of the Esophagus

Other less common infectious types of esophagitis are rarely encountered. Bacterial esophagitis is an uncommon clinical problem and typically affects immunocompromised patients or patients who have been subjected to prolonged antibiotic therapy (35,36). Bacterial esophagitis may result in esophageal ulcers or pseudomembranes or a less severe inflammatory process. The bacterial organisms can be detected by Gram stain. In cytologic specimens, bacterial colonies are often admixed with acute inflammatory cells, reactive epithelial cells, and necrotic debris. However, it can be difficult to determine whether the bacterial colonies are contributing to the esophagitis or simply a superinfection. Even less common than bacterial esophagitis, rare cases of esophagitis secondary to *Aspergillus, Mucor, Histoplasma,* and *Cryptococcus* have been described (37–40).

Radiation and Chemotherapy-Associated Esophagitis

Many chemotherapeutic agents as well as external beam radiotherapy can induce severe esophageal mucosal injury. Radiation therapy for neoplasms of the chest and mediastinum frequently induce esophagitis, and the severity of injury appears to be related to the total radiation dose, the fraction delivered per treatment, and the time period over which the radiation is given (41,42). The threshold for esophageal mucosal injury appears to be lower in patients who are treated with both chemotherapy and radiation than with either therapy alone (43–45). Endoscopic abnormalities associated with chemotherapy or radiation-induced esophagitis include erythema, mucosal friability, erosions, and ulcers. In severe cases, there may be mucosal sloughing with upper gastrointestinal bleeding that can be life threatening. Esophageal mural fibrosis can be a long-term complication of either chemotherapy or radiation.

Histologically, as with radiation-induced injury to other tissues, radiation esophagitis is characterized by atypical mesenchymal cells and prominent vascular changes with intimal fibrosis or foam cells. The atypical mesenchymal cells have enlarged irregularly shaped nuclei with a "smudgy" chromatin pattern. Squamous epithelial cells may also be bizarre-appearing and are characterized by atypical nuclei associated with a commensurate increase in the cytoplasm such that the nuclear-to-cytoplasmic ratio is not significantly increased. Multinucleated squamous cells, as well as prominent mitotic activity, including atypical mitotic figures, may be seen. Nonspecific alterations of the squamous mucosa that are similar to those seen in other causes of esophagitis are often present. All of the aforementioned changes may also be seen in chemotherapy-induced esophagitis.

In cytologic preparations, highly atypical epithelial cells are characteristic of radiation or chemotherapy-induced esophagitis (1,43) (Color Plate 9.8). The cells, however, have an increased amount of cytoplasm that is frequently vacuolated. Multinucleated squamous epithelial cells are also seen and are easily distinguished from HSV virocytes by their significantly different nuclear features. Obviously, knowledge of treatment with chemotherapeutic agents or radiotherapy is the key to the diagnosis, although in patients with esophageal carcinoma who are treated with such therapies, it may be difficult to distinguish these alterations. In such cases, histologic evaluation of biopsy specimens is often more useful in distinguishing radiation or chemotherapy-induced esophagitis from esophageal carcinoma.

Reflux Esophagitis

Reflux esophagitis is caused by reflux of gastric or duodenal contents into the esophagus with resultant esophageal mucosal injury. Although the etiology is multifactorial, the presence of a hiatal hernia plays a major role (46,47). There is not complete correlation between clinical, endoscopic, and histologic findings in that up to 60% of patients with symptomatic gastroesophageal reflux disease (GERD) with other objective parameters suggesting reflux have normal or minimally hyperemic esophageal mucosa at endoscopy (48). In contrast, esophageal mucosa with histologic esophagitis may occur in asymptomatic patients or in patients with normal or minimally abnormal endoscopic findings (49). In symptomatic patients, esophageal mucosal biopsy is warranted not only to document the presence of esophagitis but also to exclude other diagnostic considerations including infectious esophagitis, BE, and neoplasm.

There are several important caveats with respect to the histologic documentation of esophagitis in patients with GERD. Reflux esophagitis may affect the mucosa in a patchy fashion, and, as such, multiple biopsies are warranted to document histologic abnormalities (50). Physiologic gastroesophageal reflux may cause minor histologic alterations in the most distal 2 to 3 cm of the esophageal mucosa. Therefore, biopsies of the most distal esophagus are of limited diagnostic value because it may not be possible to distinguish physiologic from pathologic alterations. Often, biopsies of this region are more useful in identifying other causes of esophagitis, BE, or neoplasm than for making a definitive diagnosis of reflux esophagitis.

No single or group of histologic features is entirely specific for GERD-related esophagitis. Numerous etiologies can result in a similar histologic picture. Thus, reflux esophagitis is a clinicopathologic/endoscopic diagnosis. The major histologic components of reflux esophagitis include squamous hyperplasia and its attendant alterations and esophageal inflammation. It has been suggested that squamous hyperplasia is among the earliest histologic manifestations of reflux-induced esophageal injury (51). Under normal circumstances, the lamina propria papillae only extend approximately one third into the thickness of the esophageal mucosa, and the basal zone occupies less than 15% of the mucosal thickness. In squamous hyperplasia, the lamina propria papillae typically exceed two thirds, and the basal zone occupies more than 15% of the mucosal thickness (Color Plate 9.9). Johnson and colleagues have shown a strong correlation between length of lamina propria papillae and severity of GERD as measured by the 24-hour pH score (52).

Intraepithelial inflammatory cells are also an important component of reflux esophagitis. In adult patients, scattered intraepithelial eosinophils are considered to be normal. Thus, intraepithelial eosinophils are only considered to be significant when there are more than six eosinophils present in a biopsy section (53–55) (Color Plate 9.10). Because intraepithelial eosinophils are not normally present in the esophageal mucosa of pediatric patients, recognition of any degree of eosinophilia is considered to be pathologic (56–58). However, intraepithelial eosinophils are not specific for reflux esophagitis (59). Recently, Walsh and colleagues reported that marked intraepithelial eosinophilia (near 30 eosinophils per high-power field) with collections of eosinophils in the superficial layers is more suggestive of eosinophilic (allergic) esophagitis than reflux esophagitis in pediatric patients (60) (Color Plate 9.11). Other diagnostic considerations when intraepithelial eosinophils are seen include pill-induced esophagitis, eosinophilic gastroenteritis, and drug reactions (Stevens-Johnson syndrome) (61).

Intraepithelial neutrophils are also identified in patients with reflux esophagitis, although this histologic feature lacks sensitivity because neutrophils are present in less than one third of patients with GERD (Color Plate 9.12). Furthermore, anything that causes an erosion or ulcer of the adjacent squamous mucosa can result in the presence of intraepithelial neutrophils; thus, this feature lacks specificity as well. The presence of intraepithelial neutrophils should prompt the pathologist to exclude candida infection.

Although scattered lymphocytes, particularly T lymphocytes, are normal within the esophageal squamous mucosa, an increased number of lymphocytes are frequently seen in patients with reflux esophagitis (62,63) (Color Plate 9.13). These lymphocytes typically have irregular nuclear contours and often appear to be squeezed between squamous cells. As such, they can be easily mistaken for neutrophils. Other histologic features can be seen in reflux esophagitis, but these features also lack sensitivity and specificity. For example, marked dilatation of capillaries within the lamina propria is often seen (64), but similar histologic findings may be seen as a biopsy artifact in normal patients (65). Cytoplasmic ballooning of squamous cells, presumably secondary to injury to cell membranes and influx of fluid, is a frequent accompaniment of reflux esophagitis. Erosions and ulcers associated with granulation tissue may also be seen but lack specificity.

Cytology specimens provide limited information in the evaluation of reflux esophagitis in the absence of BE. The cytologic abnormalities resulting from GERD are similar to those noted with any inflammatory process involving the esophagus. Specifically, basal cell hyperplasia results in numerous cells with a high nuclear-to-cytoplasmic ratio in cytologic preparations. An inflammatory background containing neutrophils or eosinophils and degenerating squamous cells are present when frank ulcers are found. Care must be taken not to overinterpret reparative epithelial changes as dysplastic or neoplastic. There is considerable overlap in the cytologic features between repair and carcinoma; reparative epithelial cells are characterized by vesicular nuclei with single large nucleoli and delicate uniform nuclear membranes (Color Plate 9.14). An absence of diffuse nuclear hyperchromasia and marked nuclear membrane abnormalities are typically seen in squamous dysplasia.

Barrett's Esophagus

BE is a complication of chronic gastroesophageal reflux and results in the replacement of the normal stratified squamous epithelium of the esophagus with columnar epithelium of various types (66), particularly specialized columnar epithelium. The importance of diagnosing this condition is related to its association with the development of esophageal adenocarcinoma (67), the frequency of which has rapidly increased over the past several decades (68,69). Although the definition of BE has been modified numerous times over the past decade, the American College of Gastroenterology and its Practice Parameters Committee recently provided a definition of BE as "a change in the esophageal epithelium of any length that can be recognized at endoscopy and is confirmed to have intestinal metaplasia by biopsy" (70,71). Thus, the identification of acid mucin-containing goblet cells (specialized columnar epithelium) is the histologic *sine qua non* for making this diagnosis, regardless of the precise site of the biopsy within the tubular esophagus (Color Plates 9.15 and 9.16). Cytologically, goblet cells have distended, mucin-filled cytoplasm and a barrel-shaped configuration. These cells contain both sialo- and sulfated mucin that stains positively with Alcian blue at pH 2.5. The columnar cells between the goblet cells may resemble either intestinal absorptive cells (complete intestinal metaplasia) (Color Plate 9.17) or gastric foveolar cells (incomplete intestinal metaplasia) (Color Plate 9.18). The columnar cells between the goblet cells may also contain some Alcian blue-positive acid mucin (so-called columnar blue cells), although the intensity of staining is not as great as is seen in the goblet cells (72). The identification of such cells is not sufficient to render a definitive diagnosis of BE.

In 1976, it was recognized that both cardiac-type and fundic-type epithelia may be seen in a segment of BE (73). However, if only cardiac-type or fundic-type mucosa is identified in a biopsy specimen in the absence of intestinal metaplasia, the biopsy specimen would not be considered sufficient evidence for a diagnosis of BE (Color Plate 9.19). However, this problem is exceedingly rare. Weinstein and Ippoliti found nonintestinal tongues of columnar epithelium extending more than 2 cm into the lower esophagus in less than 1% of 250 cases of BE (74). Thus, the longer the segment of columnar epithelium, the higher the likelihood of identifying goblet cells such that virtually all columnar-lined segments of 3 cm or more have goblet cells (if adequately sampled) and are diagnostic of BE.

Endoscopic brushings of nondysplastic BE containing specialized columnar epithelium produce a cellular sample of columnar epithelial cells. The cells typically occur as cohesive sheets with occasional single cells being present (Color Plate 9.20). These sheets of cells have evenly distributed nuclei with distinct cell borders, producing a "honeycomb" arrangement when viewed *en face*. The individual tissue fragments exhibit sharp, defined smooth edges. Large villiform structures as well as small acini and rosette formations can also be encountered. Nondysplastic nuclei have an oval configuration with smooth external contours of uniform thickness and only mild variation in size. The chromatin is fine and evenly distributed and is associated with small or inconspicuous nucleoli. Nucleolar prominence is a finding associated with ongoing inflammation and reactive epithelial changes. The columnar nature of the individual epithelial cells is more apparent when the tissue fragments are viewed on edge. In this profile, the nuclei are basally located with apical cytoplasmic mucin. Goblet cells contain a single, large apical mucin vacuole that displaces the nucleus, resulting in a crescent rather than a round/oval configuration. Goblet cell differentiation results in a "Swiss cheese" appearance of the tissue fragments when viewed *en face*. In an attempt to apply more objective criteria, Wang and colleagues defined the cells as definite goblet cells when the mucin vacuole was at least three times the width of a normal columnar cell and probable goblet cells when the cell width was increased but less than three times that of the columnar cell (75). This cytologic description of goblet cells fails to address the recognized histologic pitfall whereby gastric foveolar-type cells contain distended cytoplasmic mucin vacuoles that mimic goblet cells but are Alcian blue negative. Atypical squamous epithelial cells are commonly associated with the columnar epithelial cells. Such cells represent reparative squamous cells secondary to ongoing reflux esophagitis.

There are problems with equating intestinal metaplasia to BE in all cases because one may occasionally encounter a biopsy specimen obtained near the esophagogastric junction with intestinal metaplasia (76,77). In such cases, it can be difficult to distinguish short-segment BE from intestinal metaplasia of the gastric cardia (Color Plate 9.21). Histologically, intestinal metaplasia of the upper stomach and distal esophagus can be difficult to distinguish from one another. Furthermore, given the difficulties in accurately and reproducibly recognizing the anatomic landmarks of the esophagogastric junction, it may not be possible to be sure whether the biopsy specimen came from above or below the esophagogastric junction. Beginning with the classic study by Spechler and co-workers (78), which first recognized the relatively high frequency of intestinal metaplasia in biopsy specimens obtained near the esophagogastric junction, there has been intense interest in identifying the etiology of intestinal metaplasia as well as the clinical significance with respect to progression to dysplasia and carcinoma. In fact, the prevalence of intestinal metaplasia near the esophagogastric junction in various studies has ranged from 9% to as high as 36% (79–81). The data on the relative roles of *Helicobacter pylori* infection and gastroesophageal reflux disease in the development of intestinal metaplasia near the esophagogastric junction are conflicting. Although some investigators have found intestinal metaplasia in this location to be more strongly associated with GERD (82), others have found it to be more closely associated with *H. pylori* infection and intestinal metaplasia in other parts of the stomach (83–86).

Although the data are relatively sparse, several studies have suggested a much lower risk of progression to dysplasia and carcinoma of intestinal metaplasia of the cardia when compared with either short- or long-segment BE (87,88). If these risks are truly different, as the evidence would suggest, then it would be important to distinguish intestinal metaplasia of esophageal from proximal gastric origin. As such, immunohistochemical stains for cytokeratin (CK) subsets may be useful in this regard. Several studies have shown that there is a characteristic CK 7/20 immunoreactivity pattern in long- and short-segment BE (89–91) (Color Plates 9.22 and 9.23). In virtually all cases, there is superficial and deep CK7 staining in the intestinalized mucosa with only superficial CK20 staining in the areas of intestinal metaplasia. In contrast, intestinal metaplasia of gastric origin, including the proximal stomach, virtually never has a Barrett's CK 7/20 immunoreactivity pattern (89,91).

Barrett's Esophagus-Related Dysplasia

Although all patients with BE are at an increased risk for developing adenocarcinoma, some patients are at higher risk than others (92,93). From an epidemiologic standpoint, most patients with BE-associated adenocarcinoma are elderly white men (66). Only patients with intestinal metaplasia (as opposed to those with cardiac-type and fundic-type mucosa) are at increased risk of progression, and, as such, the presence of this type of epithelium has become the histologic diagnostic criterion of BE. Epithelial dysplasia, particularly high-grade dysplasia, is a risk factor for synchronous or metachronous adenocarcinoma (94–96). In addition, most studies have found an increased

risk of progression with increasing lengths of intestinalized mucosa (83).

Dysplasia can be defined as the presence of neoplastic epithelium that is confined within the basement membrane of the gland from which it arises (97). Both cytologic and architectural alterations are components in making this diagnosis (98,99). Unlike inflammatory bowel disease-related dysplasia, dysplastic lesions in BE do not resemble colorectal adenomas. In every biopsy with BE, a comment should be made as to the presence or absence of dysplasia using the following classification scheme: negative for dysplasia; BE with dysplasia, low-grade (LGD); BE with dysplasia, high-grade (HGD); BE with changes indefinite for dysplasia.

In LGD, there is preservation or only minimal distortion of crypt architecture (Color Plate 9.24). Cytologically, the nuclei tend to be basally located and show variable nuclear hyperchromasia and irregular nuclear contours. Dystrophic goblet cells are often present. HGD shows more severe cytologic atypia and architectural complexity than LGD, although in some cases, this distinction is difficult and somewhat arbitrary. In HGD, the cells show more nuclear pleomorphism and hyperchromasia, and there is usually nuclear stratification with prominent mitotic figures, including atypical mitotic figures (Color Plate 9.25). There is usually more crypt architectural complexity, and a villiform mucosal configuration is common. Branched and cribriform glands can be seen. Intramucosal adenocarcinoma (IMC), defined as the presence of neoplastic cells that have penetrated through the basement membrane into the lamina propria or muscularis mucosae, but not below, can be difficult to distinguish from HGD. Given the presence of lymphatic channels within the esophageal mucosa, there is a small but definite risk of regional lymph node metastasis in patients with IMC alone (100). Given that architectural changes are the only way to separate HGD from IMC, it is not surprising that this distinction is exceedingly difficult in some cases, particularly in poorly oriented biopsy specimens, even among experienced gastrointestinal pathologists (101) (Color Plate 9.26).

A diagnosis of "indefinite for dysplasia" is a legitimate histologic diagnosis because, in some cases, it may be difficult to distinguish regenerative changes from dysplasia, particularly in biopsies with significant background inflammation.

The mucosa in BE always displays a certain degree of "baseline atypia" (99), which is most pronounced at the base of the mucosa and does not involve the surface epithelium (Color Plate 9.27). In well-oriented biopsy specimens, it is usually easy to determine whether the cytologic alterations involve the surface epithelium, an important criterion for making a definitive diagnosis of dysplasia. However, in tangentially sectioned biopsy specimens, this evaluation may be challenging, and in such cases a diagnosis of "indefinite for dysplasia" may be rendered. In addition, one should be cautious in making a definitive diagnosis of dysplasia in the face of active inflammation.

Prospective and retrospective studies correlating histology with endoscopic brush cytology have characterized the cytologic abnormalities that correspond to the histologic stages of this neoplastic progression (102–105). In endoscopic brush cytology specimens with dysplasia, the cell groups tend to be smaller when compared with benign BE cells. These smaller epithelial groups frequently occur as three-dimensional clusters, although flat sheets, acini, and isolated single cells may be found. Dysplastic cells typically form cohesive cell aggregates, but the edges of the aggregates are frayed, resulting in the appearance of cells falling away from the group. The individual cells show indistinct cell borders, loss of nuclear polarity with crowding, and nuclear overlap. Dysplastic nuclei have an increased nuclear-to-cytoplasmic ratio when compared with benign BE cells. Alterations in the nuclear membranes such as thickening, notching, and irregular contours are likewise noted in dysplasia. The distinction between LGD and HGD may be subtle, with the latter showing greater degrees of abnormalities (Color Plates 9.28 and 9.29). Large numbers of atypical aggregates and single atypical cells as well as giant nuclei have been reported as features favoring the diagnosis of adenocarcinoma (102).

Investigators have attempted to determine the correlation between cytology and histology in the diagnosis of BE and BE-related dysplasia and adenocarcinoma. Robey and colleagues claimed a sensitivity of 82% in the cytologic detection of specialized columnar epithelium in their retrospective study (106), whereas Geisinger and co-workers identified BE in all 65 cytology specimens studied (103). In a prospective study, Falk and colleagues identified columnar cells in 97% of their patients undergoing surveillance for BE by endoscopic brushing (8). Specialized columnar epithelium diagnostic of BE was noted in 47 of these 59 patients. Wang and colleagues showed a poor correlation between the detection of goblet cells by brush cytology and histologic findings, especially in those individuals without endoscopic evidence of columnar epithelium in the esophagus (75).

Several groups have investigated the ability of brush cytology to detect dysplastic or neoplastic cells in comparison to tissue biopsy. Geisinger and co-workers reported an agreement of 72% between the brush cytology diagnosis and that of histology in 65 patients undergoing endoscopy for BE (103). Interestingly, endoscopic brushings revealed a higher grade lesion than the histologic diagnosis in 13 cases, thereby suggesting the combined techniques would detect a greater number of significant lesions versus histology alone. Falk and colleagues prospectively analyzed 66 patients undergoing surveillance endoscopy for BE (8). The columnar epithelium was classified as follows: no abnormal cells (negative for dysplasia) or abnormal cells present (indefinite for dysplasia, high-grade dysplasia/adenocarcinoma, or ade-

nocarcinoma). The cytologic diagnosis was compared with a histologic diagnosis as follows: negative for dysplasia, low-grade or indefinite dysplasia, high-grade dysplasia, or intramucosal/submucosal adenocarcinoma. Abnormal cells were detected by brush cytology in all 11 cases with a histologic diagnosis of HGD or adenocarcinoma, but in only 22% (two of nine) with LGD. Wang and co-workers, however, detected both LGD and HGD by cytology in their study (75). In addition, one of two patients with a cytologic diagnosis of LGD but negative histology was subsequently found to have LGD on follow-up biopsy. These studies suggest that endoscopic brush cytology is a valuable and complementary technique to endoscopic biopsy.

Nonendoscopic cytologic techniques have also been evaluated in the context of BE. In the study by Fennerty and co-workers (107), balloon cytology identified columnar epithelial cells in eight of ten patients with specialized columnar epithelium on concurrent biopsy. Falk and colleagues studied a much larger group of patients using nonendoscopic balloon cytology, endoscopic brush cytology, and tissue biopsy (8). Columnar epithelium was detected in 52 of 63 (83%) patients by balloon cytology with only 15 of these having recognizable goblet cells diagnostic of BE. Balloon cytology obtained abnormal cells in six of eight patients with adenocarcinoma, two of two patients with HGD, but only two of eight patients with LGD. Two of 39 patients without dysplasia on biopsy had abnormal cells by balloon cytology. Rader and colleagues (12) used a different approach in 11 BE patients undergoing endoscopic surveillance. A flexible mesh catheter was used to obtain the cytologic material, which was then processed into a cell block, resulting in slides that were stained by hematoxylin and eosin and Alcian blue, rather than using the standard smear technique followed by Papanicolaou staining. Glandular cells were identified in 8 of 11 (73%) patients. Seven of these eight patients had goblet cells diagnostic of BE.

Squamous Cell Carcinoma

Although the incidence of squamous cell carcinoma has been steadily decreasing in Western countries, including the United States, and is now far surpassed by Barrett's-related adenocarcinoma, squamous cell carcinoma still comprises the vast majority of esophageal cancers worldwide. Most patients present at an advanced stage of disease, and prognosis is generally poor (108).

Histologically, esophageal squamous cell carcinoma resembles squamous cell carcinomas that arise in other anatomic sites (Color Plate 9.30). Most arise from an identifiable *in situ* component that can be seen in the adjacent mucosa. These tumors may be keratinizing or nonkeratinizing and are classified as well, moderately, or poorly differentiated neoplasms. Well-differentiated squamous cell carcinoma is characterized by infiltrative nests of cells that are generally surrounded by a desmoplastic stroma. On occasion, tumor may invade as nests of cells with an expanding as opposed to infiltrative growth pattern. Cytoplasmic keratinization and keratin pearls as well as intercellular bridges (desmosomes) are easily identified. As the degree of tumor differentiation decreases, it becomes more difficult to immediately recognize the neoplastic cells as squamous in origin. As such, poorly differentiated squamous cell carcinomas typically lack easily identifiable features of squamous differentiation, and thus keratin pearls and desmosomes are difficult to identify. In such tumors, the cells show considerable nuclear pleomorphism and easily identifiable mitotic figures, including atypical forms. The histologic grade of the neoplasm should be based on the most poorly differentiated portion of the neoplasm, even if it only comprises a small component of the tumor. In addition, the relationship of tumor to the surgical resection margins should be noted, because the risk of local recurrence is significantly increased with positive surgical margins with a consequent dismal prognosis. Tumor stage is also a major prognostic factor. Early squamous cell carcinomas are defined as those in which invasion is limited to the mucosa or submucosa (109). Most tumors, however, are more deeply invasive at the time of esophagectomy. Vascular invasion may also be present and should be specifically noted.

The cytologic features of esophageal squamous cell carcinoma are dependent on the degree of tumor differentiation (Color Plates 9.31 and 9.32). Poorly differentiated tumors are composed of cells with classic malignant cytologic features but without obvious squamous differentiation. The malignant cells show increased nuclear-to-cytoplasmic ratios with nuclei containing coarse, clumped chromatin and often prominent nucleoli. The malignant cells may occur as cohesive tissue fragments or as individual neoplastic cells. Poorly differentiated squamous cell carcinoma may be difficult to distinguish from poorly differentiated adenocarcinoma, lymphoma, or melanoma, and special studies, particularly immunohistochemical studies, are often required to make a definitive diagnosis.

Well-differentiated squamous cell carcinomas are clearly squamous in nature and produce numerous individual atypical keratinizing cells. The production of keratin causes the cytoplasm to be dense, refractile, and orange with a Papanicolaou stain. Difficulties may arise in distinguishing carcinoma from a hyperkeratotic reactive process. Biopsy may be required to document stromal invasion because, in some cases, this may be the only feature that allows the distinction of carcinoma from a reactive process. Verrucous carcinoma, an uncommon form of squamous cell carcinoma, by definition does not exhibit malignant cytologic features but shows a pushing infiltrating border into the underlying stroma (110–112). Spindled or sarcomatoid squamous cell carcinomas yield spindle-shaped tumor cells with sarcomatous features as well as more conventional keratinizing or nonkeratinizing polygonal cells. Basaloid squamous cell carcinoma, a distinctive variant that is more commonly found in the head and neck region, must be distinguished cytologically from small cell carcinoma (described later). Basaloid squamous cell carcinoma contains cohesive clusters of small cells that are hyperchromatic with irregularly distributed coarse chromatin. Immunohistochemistry may be required to distinguish this variant from small cell carcinoma, because the latter typically marks with neuroendocrine antigens including neuron-specific enolase, synaptophysin, and chromogranin.

Preinvasive lesions of the squamous mucosa result in a spectrum of cytologic abnormalities. Two general classification schemes have been devised over the years to describe these findings. The Chinese have developed a system based on their experience with esophageal balloon cytology and corresponding histology. In contrast, Western pathologists have applied the classification scheme commonly used in the cervix as a result of the relative lack of experience with esophageal cytology specimens. The Chinese classification scheme includes categories of hyperplasia, dysplasia 1, dysplasia 2, and near-cancer (7). In contrast, Roth and colleagues (113) devised a modification of the Bethesda system used for the evaluation of cervical cytology. This classification scheme uses categories such as atypical squamous cells of undetermined significance, low-grade dysplasia, and high-grade dysplasia.

The use of cytology to screen for esophageal squamous cell carcinoma in high-risk regions of the world has been attempted. Esophageal balloon cytology has been used in China for many years with the hopes of identifying patients with early stage disease or preinvasive lesions (3–7,113). Lesions identified in such screening programs are frequently *in situ* or minimally invasive carcinomas, providing the potential for improved long-term survival over that typically seen in other parts of the world without screening programs. Although cytology is highly sensitive in detecting carcinoma in symptomatic patients, the ability to detect significant lesions in asymptomatic patients has been less impressive (113). For example, in a study of 439 asymptomatic patients from China, Roth and colleagues found that balloon cytology had a sensitivity and specificity of 44% and 99%, respectively, for the detection of biopsy-proven squamous cell carcinoma (113). In the same study, a sponge device yielded results of 18% sensitivity and 100% specificity for carcinoma, highlighting the importance of optimizing the device used to obtain the cells.

Small Cell Carcinoma

Esophageal small cell carcinoma is an exceedingly rare neoplasm and accounts for far less than 5% of all esophageal malignancies (114). Interestingly, unlike other portions of the gastrointestinal tract, well-differentiated neuroendocrine neoplasms (carcinoid tumors) are exceedingly rare, and small cell carcinoma is by far the most common esophageal neuroendocrine tumor. Similar to other anatomic sites, this tumor typically occurs in middle-aged or elderly patients and usually arises in the middle or distal portion of the esophagus (115–117). Histologically, esophageal small cell carcinoma is identical to that seen in other sites and is composed of varying sized nests of small, highly malignant cells and exhibiting nuclear molding and significant crush artifact (Color Plates 9.33 and 9.34). These tumors are typically deeply invasive at the time of their discovery (118).

The cytologic features of small cell carcinoma are identical to that of the more common small cell carcinoma of the lung (119). The tumor is composed of cells with prominent nuclear molding and nuclei with finely stippled chromatin without prominent nucleoli. The high nuclear-to-cytoplasmic ratio is reminiscent of lymphocytes when the cells are scattered individually. A necrotic background is frequently conspicuous.

The histologic and cytologic differential diagnosis of esophageal small cell carcinoma includes metastatic small cell carcinoma from another site, poorly differentiated squamous cell carcinoma, and lymphoma. Given the rarity of primary esophageal small cell carcinoma, the possibility of a pulmonary metastasis should always be excluded. On occasion, it may be difficult to distinguish small cell carcinoma from poorly differentiated squamous cell carcinoma, and, in such cases, immunohistochemical findings of neuroendocrine differentiation are useful. However, mixed carcinomas with areas of both squamous and small cell differentiation may be seen. In addition, a panel of lymphoid and neuroendocrine markers may be useful in distinguishing small cell carcinoma from lymphoma.

Malignant Melanoma

Primary or metastatic melanoma of the esophagus is exceedingly rare (120–123). Melanocytes are normally scattered within the esophageal squamous mucosa, and, as such, primary esophageal malignant melanoma does occur and characteristically exhibits an exophytic growth pattern producing an intraluminal polypoid mass. The presence of atypical junctional melanocytic activity is useful in distinguishing primary from metastatic melanoma (Color Plate 9.35). This finding is often only observed at the tumor periphery because the esophageal mucosa is often ulcerated overlying the neoplasm. The submucosal portion of the tumor is composed of nests of loosely cohesive, large epithelioid to spindle-shaped cells with abundant granular cytoplasm and eccentric vesicular nuclei with macronucleoli. Obvious finely granular cytoplasmic pigmentation may or may not be found. Scattered multinucleated cells and intranuclear cytoplasmic inclusions are also seen.

In cytologic specimens, highly cellular specimens composed of large obviously malignant cells with vesicular nuclei, macronucleoli, and abundant granular cytoplasm

are seen. Cytoplasmic melanin appears as finely dispersed dark brown granules. Nuclei are typically eccentrically located and may have intranuclear cytoplasmic inclusions. The cells may be in loosely cohesive aggregates or they may occur singly in the specimen. In difficult cases, immunohistochemical stains for S-100 protein and melanocytic antigens (HMB-45 and MART-1) are useful in distinguishing melanoma from other malignant spindled or epithelioid neoplasms.

REFERENCES

1. Geisinger KR. Endoscopic biopsies and cytologic brushings of the esophagus are diagnostically complimentary. *Am J Clin Pathol* 1995;103:295–299.
2. Geisinger KR. Alimentary tract (esophagus, stomach, small intestine, colon, rectum, anus, biliary tract). In: Bibbo M, ed. *Comprehensive cytopathology*, second ed. Philadelphia: WB Saunders, 1997:413–444.
3. Shu Y-J. Cytopathology of the esophagus: an overview of esophageal cytopathology in China. *Acta Cytol* 1983;27:7–16.
4. Shen Q, Liu SF, Dawsey SM, et al. Cytologic screening for esophageal cancer: results from 12,877 subjects from a high-risk population in China. *Int J Cancer* 1993;54:185–188.
5. Dawsey SM, Yu Y, Taylor PR, et al. Esophageal cytology and subsequent risk of esophageal cancer: a prospective follow-up study from Linxian, China. *Acta Cytol* 1994;38:183–192.
6. Liu Sf, Shen Q, Dawsey SM, et al. Esophageal balloon cytology and subsequent risk of esophageal and gastric-cardia cancer in a high-risk Chinese population. *Int J Cancer* 1994;57:775–780.
7. Dawsey SM, Shen Q, Nieberg RK, et al. Studies of esophageal balloon cytology in Linxian, China. *Cancer Epid Biomark Prev* 1997;6:121–130.
8. Falk GW, Chittajallu R, Goldblum JR, et al. Surveillance of patients with Barrett's esophagus for dysplasia and cancer with balloon cytology. *Gastroenterology* 1999;112:1787–1797.
9. Leoni-Parvex S, Mihaescu A, Pellanda A, et al. Esophageal cytology in the follow-up of patients with treated upper aerodigestive tract malignancies. *Cancer Cytopathol* 2000;90:10–16.
10. Brandt LJ, Coman E, Schwartz E, et al. Use of a new cytology balloon for diagnosis of symptomatic esophageal disease in acquired immunodeficiency syndrome. *Gastrointest Endosc* 1993;39:559–561.
11. Sepehr A, Razavi P, Saidi F, et al. Esophageal exfoliative cytology samplers: a comparison of three types. *Acta Cytol* 2000;44:797–804.
12. Rader AE, Faigel DO, Ditomasso J, et al. Cytological screening for Barrett's esophagus using a prototype flexible mesh catheter. *Dig Dis Sci* 2001;46:2681–2686.
13. Fischler DF, Toddy SM. Non-gynecologic cytology utilizing the ThinPrep processor. *Acta Cytol* 1996;40(4):669—675.
14. Wang HH, Sovie S, Trawinski G, et al. ThinPrep processing of endoscopic brushing specimens. *Am J Clin Pathol* 1996;105:163–167.
15. DeNardi FG, Riddell RH. The normal esophagus. *Am J Surg Pathol* 1991;15:296–309.
16. Baehr PH, McDonald GB. Esophageal infections: risk factors, presentation, diagnosis and treatment. *Gastroenterology* 1994;106:509–532.
17. Gefter WB, Laufer I, Edell S, et al. Candidiasis in the obstructed esophagus. *Radiology* 1981;138:25–28.
18. Kodsi BE, Wickremeisinghe PC, Kozinn PJ, et al. Candida

esophagitis. A prospective study of 27 cases. *Gastroenterology* 1976;71:715–719.

19. Mathieson R, Dutta SK. Candida esophagitis. *Dig Dis Sci* 1983;28:365–370.

20. Wang HH, Jonasson JG, Ducatman BS. Brushing cytology of the upper gastrointestinal tract: obsolete or not? *Acta Cytol* 1991;35:195–198.

21. Hoover L, Berman JJ. Epithelial repair versus carcinoma in esophageal brush cytology. *Diagn Cytopathol* 1988;4:217–223.

22. Buss DH, Scharyj M. Herpes virus infection of the esophagus and other visceral organs in adults. Incidence and clinical significance. *Am J Med* 1979;66:457–462.

23. McDonald GB, Sharma P, Hackman RC, et al. Esophageal infections in immunosuppressed patients after marrow transplantation. *Gastroenterology* 1985;88:1111–1117.

24. McBane RD, Gross JB. Herpes esophagitis: clinical syndrome, endoscopic appearance and diagnosis in 23 patients. *Gastrointest Endosc* 1991;37:600–603.

25. Kirsch M. Herpes esophagitis in an immunocompetent host. *Am Fam Phys* 1998;57:1778.

26. Amaro R, Poniecka AW, Goldberg RI. Herpes esophagitis. *Gastrointest Endosc* 2000;51:68.

27. Singh SP, Odze RD. Multinucleated epithelial giant cell changes in esophagitis: a clinicopathologic study of 14 cases. *Am J Surg Pathol* 1998;22:93–99.

28. Greenson JK, Beschorner WE, Boitnott JK, et al. Prominent mononuclear cell infiltrate is characteristic of herpes esophagitis. *Hum Pathol* 1991;22:541–549.

29. Chetty R, Roskell DE. Cytomegalovirus infection in the gastrointestinal tract. *J Clin Pathol* 1994;47:968–972.

30. Wilcox CM, Straub RF, Schwartz DA. Prospective endoscopic characterization of cytomegalovirus esophagitis in AIDS. *Gastrointest Endosc* 1994;40:481–484.

31. Hackman RC, Wolford JL, Cleaves CA, et al. Recognition and rapid diagnosis of upper gastrointestinal cytomegalovirus infection in bone marrow transplant recipients. *Transplantation* 1994;57:231–237.

32. Greenson JK. Macrophage aggregates in cytomegalovirus esophagitis. *Hum Pathol* 1997;28:375–378.

33. Schwartz DA, Wilcox CM. Atypical cytomegaloviral inclusions in gastrointestinal biopsy specimens from patients with the acquired immunodeficiency syndrome: diagnostic role of in situ nucleic acid hybridization. *Hum Pathol* 1992;23:1019–1026.

34. Teot LA, Ducatman BS, Geisinger KR. Cytologic diagnosis of cytomegaloviral esophagitis. A report of three acquired immunodeficiency syndrome-related cases. *Acta Cytol* 1993;37:93–96.

35. Walsh TJ, Belitsos NJ, Hamilton SR. Bacterial esophagitis in immunocompromised patients. *Arch Intern Med* 1986;146:1345–1348.

36. McManus JPA, Webb JN. A yeast-like infection of the esophagus caused by *Lactobacillus acidophilus*. *Gastroenterology* 1975;68:583–586.

37. Jacobs DH, Macher AM, Handler R, et al. Esophageal cryptococcosis in a patient with hyperimmunoglobulin E-recurrent infection (Job's syndrome). *Gastroenterology* 1984;87:201–203.

38. Jenkins DW, Fisk DE, Byrd RB. Mediastinal Histoplasmosis with esophageal abscess. *Gastroenterology* 1976;70:109–111.

39. Lamps LW, Molina CP, West AB, et al. The pathologic spectrum of gastrointestinal and hepatic Histoplasmosis. *Am J Clin Pathol* 2000;113:64–72.

40. Mineur PH, Ferrant A, Walton J, et al. Bronchoesophageal fistula caused by pulmonary Aspergillosis. *Eur J Respir Dis* 1985;66:360–366.

41. Berthrong M, Fajardo LE. Radiation injury in surgical pathology: II. Alimentary tract. *Am J Surg Pathol* 1981;5:153–178.

42. Novak JM, Collins JT, Donowitz M, et al. Effects of radiation on the human gastrointestinal tract. *J Clin Gastroenterol* 1979;1:9–39.

43. O'Morchoe PJ, Lee DC, Korak CA. Esophageal cytology in patients receiving Cytoxan drug therapy. *Acta Cytol* 1983;27:630–634.

44. Greco FA, Brereton HD, Kent H, et al. Adriamycin and enhanced radiation reaction in normal esophagus and skin. *Ann Intern Med* 1976;85:294–298.

45. Phillips TL, Fu K. Quantification of combined radiation therapy and chemotherapy effects on critical normal tissues. *Cancer* 1976;37:1186–1200.

46. Vaezi MF, Richter JR. Role of acid and duodenogastroesophageal reflux in gastroesophageal reflux disease. *Gastroenterology* 1996;111:1192–1199.

47. Pope CE. Acid-reflux disorders. *N Engl J Med* 1994;331:656–660.

48. Knuff TE, Benjamin SB, Worsham GF, et al. Histologic evaluation of chronic gastroesophageal reflux: an evaluation of biopsy methods and diagnostic criteria. *Dig Dis Sci* 1984;29:194–201.

49. Frierson HF. Histology in the diagnosis of reflux esophagitis. *Gastroenterol Clin N Am* 1990;19:631–644.

50. Weinstein WM, Bogoch ER, Bowes KL. The normal human esophageal mucosa: a histological reappraisal. *Gastroenterology* 1975;68:40–44.

51. Ismail-Beigi F, Horton PF, Pope CE, et al. The histological consequences of gastroesophageal reflux in man. *Gastroenterology* 1970;58:163–174.

52. Johnson LF, DeMeester TR, Haggitt RC. Esophageal epithelial response to gastroesophageal reflux: a quantitative study. *Am J Dig Dis* 1978;23:498–509.

53. Haggitt RC. Histopathology of reflux-induced esophageal and supraesophageal injuries. *Am J Med* 2000;108[Suppl 4A]:109 S–111S.

54. Brown LF, Goldman H, Antonioli DA. Intraepithelial eosinophils in endoscopic biopsies of adults with reflux esophagitis. *Am J Surg Pathol* 1984;8:899–905.

55. Tummala V, Barwick KW, Sontag SJ, et al. The significance of intraepithelial eosinophils in the histologic diagnosis of gastroesophageal reflux. *Am J Clin Pathol* 1987;87:43–48.

56. Orenstein SR. Gastroesophageal reflux. *Curr Probl Pediatr* 1991;21:193–241.

57. Black DD, Haggitt RC, Orenstein SR, et al. Esophagitis in infants: morphometric histological diagnosis and correlation with measures of gastroesophageal reflux. *Gastroenterology* 1990;98:1408–1414.

58. Winter HS, Madara JL, Stafford RJ, et al. Intraepithelial eosinophils: a new diagnostic criterion for reflux esophagitis. *Gastroenterology* 1982;83:818–823.

59. Kelley KJ, Lazenby AJ, Rowe PC, et al. Eosinophilic esophagitis attributed to gastroesophageal reflux: improvement with an amino acid-based formula. *Gastroenterology* 1995;109:1503–1512.

60. Walsh SV, Antonioli DA, Goldman H, et al. Allergic esophagitis in children: a clinicopathologic entity. *Am J Surg Pathol* 1999;23:390–396.

61. Lee RG. Marked eosinophilia in esophageal biopsies. *Am J Surg Pathol* 1985;9:475–479.

62. Mangano MM, Antonioli DA, Schnitt SJ, et al. Nature and significance of cells with irregular nuclear contours in esophageal mucosal biopsies. *Mod Pathol* 1992;5:191–196.

63. Wang HH, Mangano MM, Antonioli DA. Evaluation of T-lymphocytes in esophageal mucosal biopsies. *Mod Pathol* 1994;7:55–58.

64. Geboes K, Desmet V, Vantrappen G, et al. Vascular changes in the esophageal mucosa. An early histologic sign of esophagitis. *Gastrointest Endosc* 1980;26:29–32.

65. Collins BJ, Elliott H, Cloan JM, et al. Oesophageal histology in reflux esophagitis. *J Clin Pathol* 1985;38:1265–1272.

66. Spechler SJ, Goyal RK. Barrett's esophagus. *N Engl J Med* 1986;315:362–371.

67. Haggitt RC, Tryzelaar J, Ellis FH, et al. Adenocarcinoma complicated columnar epithelial-lined (Barrett's) esophagus. *Am J Clin Pathol* 1978;7:1–5.

68. Haggitt RC. Adenocarcinoma in Barrett's esophagus: a new epidemic? *Hum Pathol* 1992;23:475–476.

69. Blot WJ. Esophageal cancer trends and risk factors. *Semin Oncol* 1994;21:403–410.

70. Sampliner RE. Practice guidelines on the diagnosis, surveillance and therapy of Barrett's esophagus. *Am J Gastroenterol* 1998;93:1028–1031.

71. Sampliner RE. Updated guidelines for the diagnosis, surveillance and therapy of Barrett's esophagus. *Am J Gastroenterol* 2002;97:1888–1895.

72. Offner FA, Lewin KJ, Weinstein WM. Metaplastic columnar cells in Barrett's esophagus: a common and neglected cell type. *Hum Pathol* 1996;27:885–889.

73. Paull A, Trier JS, Dalton MD, et al. The histologic spectrum of Barrett's esophagus. *N Engl J Med* 1976;295:476–480.

74. Weinstein WM, Ippoliti AF. The diagnosis of Barrett's esophagus. Goblets, goblets, goblets. *Gastrointest Endosc* 1996;44:91–94.

75. Wang HH, Sovie S, Zeroogian JM, et al. Value of cytology detecting intestinal metaplasia and associated dysplasia at the gastroesophageal junction. *Hum Pathol* 1997;28:465–471.

76. Goldblum JR. Gastric cardia: controversial topics. *Pathol Case Rev* 2002;7:12–18.

77. Goldblum JR. The significance and etiology of intestinal metaplasia of the esophagogastric junction. *Ann Diagn Pathol* 2002;6:67–73.

78. Spechler SJ, Zeroogian JM, Antonioli DA, et al. Prevalence of metaplasia of the gastroesophageal junction. *Lancet* 1994;344:1533–1536.

79. Johnston MH, Hammond AS, Laskin W, et al. The prevalence and clinical characteristics of short segments of specialized intestinal metaplasia in the distal esophagus on routine endoscopy. *Am J Gastroenterol* 1996;91:1507–1511.

80. Nandukar S, Talley MJ, Martin CJ, et al. Short segment Barrett's esophagus: prevalence, diagnosis and associations. *Gut* 1997;40:710–715.

81. Trudgill MJ, Suvarna SK, Kapur KC, et al. Intestinal metaplasia of the squamocolumnar junction in patients attending for diagnostic gastroscopy. *Gut* 1997;41:585–589.

82. Oberg S, Peters JH, DeMeester TR, et al. Inflammation and specialized intestinal metaplasia of cardiac mucosa is a manifestation of gastroesophageal reflux disease. *Ann Surg* 1997;26:522–532.

83. Hirota WK, Loughney TN, Lazas DJ, et al. Specialized intestinal metaplasia, dysplasia and cancer of the esophagus and esophagogastric junction: prevalence and clinical data. *Gastroenterology* 1999;116:277–285.

84. Morales TG, Sampliner RE, Bhattacharyya A. Intestinal metaplasia of the gastric cardia. *Am J Gastroenterol* 1997;92:414–418.

85. Hackelsberger A, Gunther T, Schultze V, et al. Intestinal metaplasia of the gastroesophageal junction: *Helicobacter pylori* gastritis or gastro-esophageal reflux disease? *Gut* 1998;43:17–21.

86. Goldblum JR, Vicari JJ, Falk GW, et al. Inflammation and intestinal metaplasia of the gastric cardia: the role of gastroesophageal reflux and *H. pylori* infection. *Gastroenterology* 1998;114:633–639.

87. Sharma P, Weston AP, Morales T, et al. Relative risk of dysplasia for patients with intestinal metaplasia in the distal oesophagus and in the gastric cardia. *Gut* 2000;46:9–13.

88. Morales TG, Camargo E, Bhattacharyya A, et al. Long-term follow-up of intestinal metaplasia of the gastric cardia. *Am J Gastroenterol* 2000;95:1677–1680.

89. Ormsby AH, Goldblum JR, Rice TW, et al. Cytokeratin subsets can reliably distinguish Barrett's esophagus from intestinal metaplasia of the stomach. *Hum Pathol* 1999;30:288–294.

90. Ormsby AH, Vaezi MF, Richter JE, et al. Cytokeratin immunoreactivity patterns in the diagnosis of short-segment Barrett's esophagus. *Gastroenterology* 2000;119:682–690.

91. Couvelard A, Cauvin J-M, Goldfain D, et al. Cytokeratin immunoreactivity of intestinal metaplasia of the normal oesophagogastric junction indicates its aetiology. *Gut* 2001;49:761–766.

92. Sampliner RE. Appearance and prognosis of dysplasia in Barrett's esophagus. *Chest Surg Clin N Am* 2002;12:69–76.

93. Haggitt RC. Barrett's esophagus, dysplasia and adenocarcinoma. *Hum Pathol* 1994;25:982–993.

94. Reid BJ, Weinstein WM, Lewin KJ, et al. Endoscopic biopsies diagnose high-grade dysplasia or early operative adenocarcinoma in Barrett's esophagus without grossly recognizable neoplastic lesions. *Gastroenterology* 1988;94:81–90.

95. Schmidt HG, Riddell RH, Walther B, et al. Dysplasia in Barrett's esophagus. *J Cancer Res Clin Oncol* 1985;110:145–152.

96. Smith RRL, Hamilton SR, Boitnoit JK, et al. The spectrum of carcinoma arising in Barrett's esophagus: a clinicopathologic study of 26 patients. *Am J Surg Pathol* 1984;8:562–573.

97. Riddell RH, Goldman H, Ransohoff DF, et al. Dysplasia in inflammatory bowel disease: standardized classification with provisional clinical applications. *Hum Pathol* 1983;14:931–968.

98. Montgomery E, Bronner MP, Goldblum JR, et al. Reproducibility of the diagnosis of dysplasia in Barrett esophagus: a reaffirmation. *Hum Pathol* 2001;32:368–378.

99. Goldblum JR, Lauwers GY. Dysplasia arising in Barrett's esophagus: diagnostic pitfalls and natural history. *Semin Diagn Pathol* 2002;19:12–19.

100. Sabik JF, Rice TW, Goldblum JR, et al. Superficial esophageal carcinoma. *Ann Thorac Surg* 1995;60:896–902.

101. Ormsby AH, Petras RE, Henricks WH, et al. Observer variation in the diagnosis of superficial esophageal adenocarcinoma. *Gut* 2002;51:671–676.

102. Shurbaji M, Erozan YS. The cytopathologic diagnosis of esophageal adenocarcinoma. *Acta Cytol* 1991;35:189–194.

103. Geisinger KR, Teot LA, Richter JE. A comparative cytopathologic and histologic study of atypia, dysplasia and adenocarcinoma in Barrett's esophagus. *Cancer* 1992;69:8–16.

104. Wang HH, Ducatman BS, Thibault S. Cytologic features of premalignant glandular lesions in the upper gastrointestinal tract. *Acta Cytol* 1991;35:199–203.

105. Wang HH, Doria MI, Purohit-Buch S, et al. Barrett's esophagus: the cytology of dysplasia and comparison to benign and malignant lesions. *Acta Cytol* 1992;36:60–64.

106. Robey SS, Hamilton SR, Gupta P, et al. Diagnostic value of cytopathology in Barrett esophagus and associated adenocarcinoma. *Am J Clin Pathol* 1988;89:493–498.

107. Fennerty MB, Ditomasso J, Morales T, et al. Screening for Barrett's esophagus by balloon cytology. *Am J Gastroenterol* 1995;90:1230–1232.

108. Adelstein DJ, Forman WB, Beavers B. Esophageal carcinoma: a 6-year review of the Cleveland Veterans' Administration Hospital experience. *Cancer* 1984;54:918–923.

109. Ohno S, Mori M, Tsutsui S, et al. Growth patterns and prognosis of submucosal carcinoma of the esophagus. A pathologic study. *Cancer* 1991;68:335–340.

110. Ereno C, Lopez JI, Loizate A, et al. Verrucous carcinoma of the esophagus. *Endoscopy* 2001;33:297.

111. Tajiri H, Muto M, Boku N, et al. Verrucous carcinoma of the esophagus completely resected by endoscopy. *Am J Gastroenterol* 2000;95:1076–1077.

112. Malik AB, Bidani JA, Rich HG, et al. Long-term survival in a patient with verrucous carcinoma of the esophagus. *Am J Gastroenterol* 1996;91:1031–1033.

113. Roth MJ, Liu SF, Dawsey SM, et al. Cytologic detection of esophageal squamous cell carcinoma and precursor lesions using balloon and sponge samplers in asymptomatic adults in Linxian, China. *Cancer* 1997;84:2047–2059.

114. Briggs JC, Ibrahim NBN. Oat cell carcinoma of the esophagus: a clinicopathologic study of 23 cases. *Histopathology* 1983;7: 261–277.

115. Madroszyk A, Egreteau J, Martin L, et al. Small-cell carcinoma of the esophagus: report of three cases and review of the literature with emphasis on therapy. *Ann Oncol* 2001;12:1321–1325.

116. Yashida S, Matsushita K, Usuki H, et al. Long-term survival after resection for small cell carcinoma of the esophagus. *Ann Thorac Surg* 2001;72:596–597.

117. Bennouna J, Bardet E, Deguiral P, et al. Small cell carcinoma of the esophagus: analysis of 10 cases and review of the published data. *Am J Clin Oncol* 2000;23:455–459.

118. Nemoto K, Zhao HJ, Goto T, et al. Radiation therapy for limited-stage small-cell esophageal cancer. *Am J Clin Oncol* 2002; 25:404–407.

119. Chen KTK. Cytology in small-cell carcinoma arising in Barrett's esophagus. *Diagn Cytopathol* 2000;23:180–182.

120. Holck S, Siemsen M, Jensen DB, et al. Endoscopic ultrasonography-guided fine needle aspiration biopsy for staging malignant melanoma of the esophagus. A case report. *Acta Cytol* 2002;46:744–748.

121. Boni L, Benevento A, Cabrini L, et al. Primary melanoma of the esophagus. *J Am Coll Surg* 2002;194:840.

122. Matsutani T, Onda M, Miyashita M, et al. Primary malignant melanoma of the esophagus treated by esophagectomy and systemic chemotherapy. *Dis Esoph* 2001;14:241–244.

123. Archer HA, Owen WJ. Primary malignant melanoma of the esophagus. *Dis Esoph* 2000;13:320–323.

DISORDERS CAUSING OROPHARYNGEAL DYSPHAGIA

IAN J. COOK

Pharyngeal dysphagia most commonly arises from neurogenic or myogenic diseases in which dysphagia is frequently a part of a wider neurologic syndrome, making it necessary for the clinician to consider a wide range of diagnostic possibilities and appropriate investigations. Oropharyngeal dysphagia, the most common cause of which is stroke, carries a high morbidity, mortality, and cost. Oropharyngeal dysphagia occurs in one third of all stroke patients (1,2). Other special populations such as those with head injuries, Parkinson's disease, or Alzheimer's have a 20% to 40% prevalence of oropharyngeal dysphagia (1,3–6). In our aging population, oropharyngeal dysphagia is a large and growing problem, the consequences of which can be severe: malnutrition, aspiration, choking, pneumonia, and death. It is common in the chronic care setting, with up to 60% of nursing home occupants having feeding difficulties (7,8), of whom a substantial proportion have dysphagia. The cost implications are significant and it is recognized that the resulting complications significantly increase the chance of institutionalization and hospital readmission following stroke (9,10). Responsiveness to currently available treatments is extremely variable and unpredictable in many instances with response being dependent upon on several factors, including the underlying cause of the dysphagia, the severity and nature of the mechanical dysfunction, the degree of cognitive dysfunction, and the prognosis of the underlying disease (11). Finally, pharyngeal dysphagia, more so than esophageal dysphagia, is a problem that frequently demands a multidisciplinary management approach, which may involve the radiologist, gastroenterologist, gerontologist, neurologist, speech-language pathologist, otolaryngologist, dietitian, and, sometimes, the palliative care physician.

PRESENTATION AND CLINICAL ASSESSMENT OF OROPHARYNGEAL DYSPHAGIA

It is a common mistake for the clinician, confronted with a patient reporting bolus holdup in the neck, to assume that patient has pharyngeal dysphagia. If dysfunction does relate to the oral or pharyngeal region, the patient can localize accurately the site of such dysfunction, which correlates well with radiologic localization of the problem (12). However, distal esophageal obstruction can give rise to a sensation of the bolus catching either in the retrosternal region or in the cervical region in 15% to 30% of cases (13–15). Hence, a perception by the patient of apparent bolus holdup in the neck has low diagnostic specificity and cervical localization per se does not help the clinician distinguish pharyngeal from esophageal causes of dysphagia. Nonetheless, a careful history can reliably distinguish esophageal from pharyngeal dysphagia in most cases. The clinician may mistake the purely sensory symptom of globus for pharyngeal dysphagia. Globus is a common, nonpainful sensation of a lump, fullness, or tightness in the throat of unknown etiology in which deglutitive food bolus transport is unimpaired (16,17). Indeed, globus sensation is usually most apparent to the patient between meals, is not necessarily related to the act of swallowing, and is usually alleviated by eating. The minority of affected patients who do report associated dysphagia may have associated esophageal dysmotility (18). A number of pharyngeal and esophageal radiologic appearances have been described in association with globus but none have been proven to have a causative relationship with the symptom (19). The patient with pure globus sensation without pain, dysphagia, or weight loss generally only requires otolaryngologic evaluation to exclude local inflammatory or infiltrative disorders followed by explanation and reassurance.

Because of the complexity of functions served by the upper aerodigestive tract, oropharyngeal dysphagia should be considered to be one component of a multidimensional symptom complex. The patient with oropharyngeal dysphagia my have oral or pharyngeal dysfunction, or both. Typical symptoms of oral dysfunction might include drooling from the mouth or spillage of food as a result of poor labial and facial muscle function; sialorrhea or xerostomia; difficulty with swallow initiation; piecemeal swallows; and dysarthria. Typical symptoms of pharyngeal dysfunction

I. J. Cook: Department of Gastroenterology, St. George Hospital, Kogarah, Sydney, Australia.

include the following: an immediate sense of bolus holdup localized to the neck; postnasal regurgitation; the need to swallow repeatedly to clear food or fluid from the pharynx; coughing or choking during meals, suggesting aspiration; and dysphonia. Pain on swallowing or persistent sore throat may indicate malignancy. Immediate expectoration of an offending bolus is indicative of bolus retention in the hypopharyngeal or cricopharyngeal region. Delayed regurgitation of old food is typical of a large pharyngeal diverticulum. Dysphagia solely for solids is indicative of a structural lesion such as a stenosis, web, or tumor. However, distinction between dysphagia for liquids and solids is of little diagnostic value in distinguishing oropharyngeal dysphagia from esophageal dysphagia because it is the specific type of mechanical pharyngeal dysfunction rather than the presence of pharyngeal dysfunction that dictates which bolus type generates most symptoms.

The circumstances of symptom onset, duration, and progression of dysphagia provide useful diagnostic information. For example, malignant dysphagia usually presents with a relatively short history of progressive dysphagia and is frequently associated with weight loss. A sudden onset of dysphagia, often in association with other neurologic symptoms or signs, usually indicates a cerebrovascular cause such as stroke. A subacute or more insidious onset is more consistent with disorders such as inflammatory myopathy, myasthenia, or amyotrophic lateral sclerosis. Oropharyngeal dysphagia usually has a neurologic basis. A prior history of stroke may be obtained. Symptoms of bulbar muscle dysfunction or other brainstem symptoms (e.g., vertigo, nausea, vomiting, hiccup, tinnitus, diplopia, and drop attacks) should be sought. More widespread neuromuscular symptoms such as dysarthria, diplopia, limb weakness, or fatigability are variably present in motor neuron disease, myasthenia, and myopathy. The patient may report tremor, ataxia, or unsteadiness, which might indicate an underlying movement disorder such as Parkinson's disease (Table 10.1).

TABLE 10.1. ETIOLOGY OF OROPHARYNGEAL DYSPHAGIA

Central nervous system
  Stroke
  Extrapyramidal syndromes (Parkinson's, Huntington's chorea, Wilson's disease)
  Head trauma
  Brainstem tumors
  Alzheimer's disease
  Multiple sclerosis
  Cerebral palsy
  Amyotrophic lateral sclerosis
  Drugs (phenothiazines, benzodiazepines)
Peripheral nervous system
  Spinal muscular atrophy
  Guillain-Barré syndrome
  Poliomyelitis
  Postpolio syndrome
  Diphtheria
  Drugs (botulinum toxin, procainamide, cytotoxics)
Myogenic
  Myasthenia gravis
  Botulism
  Dermatomyositis
  Polymyositis
  Mixed connective tissue disease
  Sarcoidosis
  Thryotoxic myopathy
  Paraneoplastic syndromes
  Myotonic dystrophy
  Oculopharyngeal muscular dystrophy
  Drugs (amiodarone, alcohol, cholesterol-lowering drugs)
Structural disorders
  Posterior (Zenker's) pharyngeal diverticulum
  Lateral pharyngeal diverticulum
  Cricopharyngeal bar
  Cricopharyngeal stenosis
  Cervical web
  Oropharyngeal tumors
  Head and neck surgery
  Radiotherapy
  Cervical osteophytes

Xerostomia is frequently accompanied by dysphagia and is a common symptom in the elderly, being present in 16% of men and 25% of women (20). Dysphagia is attributed to the loss of the lubricating qualities of saliva. Dry mouth may be accompanied by dry eyes, inflammatory arthropathy (e.g., rheumatoid arthritis, Sjögren's syndrome), a prior history of head and neck radiotherapy, or concurrent medications displaying anticholinergic side effects. A detailed drug history is also important because a number of centrally acting drugs can impair oral-pharyngeal dysfunction and can cause tardive dyskinesia with masticatory and swallowing difficulties (Table 10.2).

The aims of the physical examination in the dysphagic patient are to (a) identify features of underlying systemic or metabolic disease when present, (b) localize where possible the neuroanatomic level and severity of a causative neurologic lesion when present, and (c) detect adverse sequelae such as pulmonary sepsis or nutritional deficiency, which are important indicators of the severity of dysphagia. In addition to the diagnostic assessment, an assessment by a speech language pathologist provides further information about language, cognitive and behavioral dysfunction, and the strength and range of movement of the muscles involved in speech and swallowing. This information directly influences decisions as to the patient's suitability for swallow therapy and the type of therapy adopted.

A careful neurologic examination is important unless a certain cause of dysphagia is apparent. However, examination, even when combined with magnetic resonance imaging (MRI), is frequently unremarkable despite videoradiographic demonstration of severe impairment of the pharyngeal swallow (21) and the absence of neurologic signs does not preclude significant pharyngeal neuromuscular dysfunction. When present, physical findings in affected patients might include cranial nerve dysfunction, cerebellar dysfunction, or signs of movement disorder or muscle disease. The clinician should remember that the gag reflex is absent in 20% to 40% of healthy adults (22) and in the patient is neither predictive of pharyngeal swallow efficiency, the severity of swallow dysfunction, nor adequacy of deglutitive airway protection (23,24). Nasal speech is indicative of soft palatal dysfunction, which commonly results in deglutitive postnasal regurgitation. Tremor and gait disturbances may reflect an extrapyramidal movement disorder, the most common cause of which is Parkinson's disease (25,26). Muscle fasciculation, wasting and weakness or fatigability should be sought to detect underlying motor neuron disease, myopathy, or myasthenia.

The examiner should palpate the neck for masses, lymph nodes, or a goiter. Sometimes a pharyngeal pouch can be felt, nearly always on the left, and may be com-

TABLE 10.2. DRUGS ASSOCIATED WITH OROPHARYNGEAL DYSPHAGIA

Centrally acting drugs
Phenothiazines[a]
Metoclopramide[a]
Benzodiazepines[a] (nitrazepam, clonazepam)
Antihistamines[a]

Drugs acting at neuromuscular junction
Botulinum A toxin[a]
Procainamide[a]
Penicillamine
Erythromycin
Aminoglycosides

Drugs toxic to muscle
Amiodarone[a]
Alcohol[a]
HMG-CoA reductase inhibitors[a]
Cyclosporin
Penicillamine
Other (colchicine, L-tryptophan, emetine, chloroquine, steroids, cimetidine, ipecac)

Miscellaneous, mechanism presumed neuromyopathic
Digoxin[a]
Trichloroethylene[a]
Vincristine[a]

Drugs influencing salivation
Inhibit salivation[a] (anticholinergics, antidepressants, antipsychotics, antihistamines, antiparkinsonian drugs, antihypertensives, diuretics)
Enhance salivation[a] (anticholinesterase, nitrazepam, clonazepam, clozapine)

[a]Indicates that specific reports of drug-related dysphagia exist.

pressed causing regurgitation of a small amount of food residue into the pharynx with an audible "gurgle." Signs of prior surgery, tracheostomy, and radiotherapy are usually obvious when present. The oral cavity including natural dentition or dentures, tongue, and oropharynx should be inspected.

Examination of the eyes and ocular movements is relevant. Bilateral ptosis might indicate a myopathy or myasthenia, and unilateral ptosis, if associated with Horner's syndrome (descending sympathetic tract), is typical of lateral medullary infarction causing dysphagia. Eye signs, sweating, tremor, and tachycardia of thyrotoxicosis may be present in patients with thyrotoxic myopathy causing pharyngeal dysfunction. The typical features of thyrotoxicosis, however, may not be present in elderly patients or in individuals taking β-adrenergic antagonists and dysphagia may be the only presenting symptom of thyrotoxicosis (27). With the index and middle fingers resting lightly on the hyoid and laryngeal cartilages, respectively, axial motion of the larynx and hyoid bone should be noted while the patient swallows a mouthful of water. Inadequate laryngeal ascent is frequently seen in neurogenic dysphagia and also impairs airway protection during the swallow and can be associated with aspiration. Aspiration often causes coughing or choking during the swallow. Radiologic studies have shown that aspiration is underestimated by roughly 50% on the basis of clinical assessment alone (28,29). A video barium swallow therefore is vital to confidently establish the risk of significant aspiration in most cases (30).

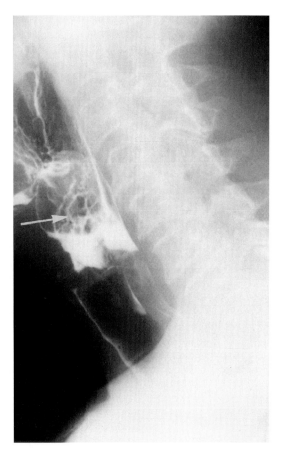

FIGURE 10.1. Hypopharyngeal carcinoma (*arrow*) arising from the aryepiglottic fold and presenting with pharyngeal dysphagia and aspiration during meals.

EVALUATION OF THE ORAL-PHARYNGEAL SWALLOW

Videofluoroscopy

Static films of the oropharynx obtained during a standard barium swallow can readily identify structural causes of dysphagia, such as diverticula, webs, stenoses, or cancers (Figs. 10.1 and 10.2). However, static films frequently detect various anomalies, such as osteophytes or a cricopharyngeal bar, which may or may not be linked causatively with the patient's dysphagia. These entities must be interpreted with caution because they are usually not the cause of the patient's dysphagia (see later discussion). Static films may also provide important clues to oral or pharyngeal dysfunction such as barium pooling in the valleculae or piriform sinuses or aspiration of contrast, but because of the rapidity and complexity of the oropharyngeal swallow, static films are inadequate to define any disturbance of the mechanics of the swallow. The most commonly used radiographic method to achieve this is the videofluoroscopic swallow study, frequently referred to as a modified barium swallow (31). This test acquires dedicated lateral and anteroposterior views of the oral and pharyngeal phases of the swallow and permits standard and slow motion replay of the swallow to define the mechanisms and severity of dysfunction and, if desired, the influence of modifications to bolus consistency, postures, and other swallow maneuvers on bolus flow and clearance. Videofluoroscopy is a sensitive means of confirming oral-pharyngeal dysfunction if its presence is uncertain on the basis of history. This technique provides information on the presence and severity of the major categories of dysfunction such as an absent or delayed pharyngeal swallow response, timing of aspiration if present, velopharyngeal competence, and impaired pharyngeal clearance of contrast (Table 10.3). One of the most important pieces of information provided by videofluoroscopy is the presence, timing, and severity of aspiration, which is frequently silent. Identification of these mechanisms assist the therapist in deciding on specific swallow therapies. On the other hand, videofluoroscopy does not permit quantification of pharyngeal contractile forces or intrabolus pressure, or the detection of incomplete upper esophageal sphincter (UES) relaxation, which can occur despite normal UES opening (32).

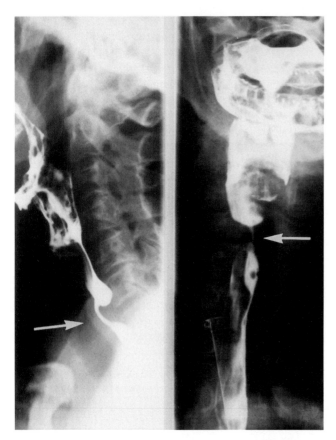

FIGURE 10.2. Radiograph of a woman with longstanding dysphagia caused by cricopharyngeal stenosis. Note that the reduction in sphincter lumen is circumferential, indicating that this lesion is not a simple cricopharyngeal bar. The lateral view (*left*) also demonstrates the early formation of a pouch above the stenosed cricopharyngeus. The patient had significant benefit from cricopharyngeal myotomy, and histopathology of the resected muscle showed hypertrophy only without fibrosis. (From Cook IJ. Cricopharyngeal function and dysfunction. *Dysphagia* 1993;8[3]:244–251, with permission).

Nasoendoscopy

Fiberoptic nasoendoscopy is the optimal method for identifying and biopsying mucosal abnormalities and is mandatory in all cases in which malignancy is suspected. Frequently in the workup of the patient with dysphagia, the gastroenterologist examines the laryngopharynx during routine fiberoptic esophagogastroduodenoscopy. However, the standard gastroscope passed per oral route is frequently unreliable in the detection of glottic and pharyngeal cancers (33). If there is any doubt about a possible malignancy, fiberoptic nasoendoscopy or even examination under anesthesia is recommended. Nasoendoscopy, frequently referred to as *fiberoptic endoscopic examination of swallowing* (FEES), is less well suited to the assessment of swallow mechanics than videofluoroscopy but can detect the absence of or profound delay in initiating the pharyngeal swallow response and can provide indirect evidence of aspiration (34,35).

Manometry

Intraluminal manometry can quantify pharyngeal deglutitive forces, detect failure of UES relaxation, and the relative coordination of pharyngeal contraction with UES relaxation (36–39). Pharyngeal manometry is technically more demanding and more complex than esophageal manometry because of transducer requirements for high-fidelity recording, extreme longitudinal and radial asymmetry of intraluminal pressures recorded from within the pharynx during swallow, and unpredictable structural movements during the pharyngeal swallow response, which have the effect of displacing the pressure sensor from its preswallow position (40–43). Age effects on manometric parameters are also recognized and dictate the need for comparison with appro-

TABLE 10.3. MECHANISMS OF OROPHARYNGEAL DYSPHAGIA

Dysfunction	Mechanism	Etiology
Oral phase		
Drooling	Poor lip closure	Facial muscle weakness
Poor oral clearance	Lingual dysfunction	Central lesion, myopathy
	Delayed swallow initiation	Afferent or central lesion
Premature bolus spill	Incompetent glossopalatal closure	Myopathy, palatal surgery
Pharyngeal phase		
Postnasal regurgitation	Velopharyngeal incompetence	Central, tenth cranial nerve myopathy
Laryngeal penetration/aspiration	Reduced laryngeal elevation	Suprahyoid muscle dysfunction
	Incomplete epiglottal closure	Suprahyoid muscle dysfunction tumor
	Impaired closure vocal cords	Medullary or tenth cranial nerve lesion
	Impaired pharyngeal clearance	Central lesion, myopathy
Impaired pharyngeal propulsion	Absent or delayed pharyngeal response	Central lesion
	Impaired tongue base motion	Central lesion, myopathy
	Impaired constrictor muscle action	Central lesion, myopathy
Increased outflow resistance	Failed upper esophageal sphincter (UES) relaxation	Medullary lesion
	Loss of UES compliance	Cricopharyngeal fibrosis
	Impaired hyoid traction	Suprahyoid muscle dysfunction

priate normative values (44–46). Manometry has been combined with videofluoroscopy by some investigators. This permits determination of precise catheter position relative to the UES and facilitates correlation of motion of anatomic structures with the resulting intraluminal pressures (38,47–49). This technique permits identification of intrabolus pressure, which is an indirect measure of UES compliance (50,51). Impaired UES opening can also be distinguished from impaired sphincter relaxation, and weak propulsive pharyngeal forces can be distinguished from increased outflow resistance as manifest by high intrabolus pressure (32). Failure of UES relaxation, detected manometrically, is frequently indicative of a rostral medullary lesion or Parkinson's disease (32,39,52). Identification of certain manometric abnormalities, particularly failed UES relaxation or elevated intrabolus pressure, may help in diagnosis and may influence management decisions, particularly relating to the advisability of cricopharyngeal myotomy or dilatation (37–39,53–55). However, it remains to be proven that such intervention in this context influences clinical outcome. The precise role of UES-pharyngeal manometry in the dysphagic patient, therefore, remains controversial (56); for example, when routinely added to standard esophageal manometry, it does pick up more UES abnormalities in a dysphagic population than in those undergoing esophageal manometry for chest pain (57). However, the clinical implications of many of the more nonspecific findings (e.g., hypertonic UES, short relaxation duration) remain unclear. Furthermore, unexpected pharyngeal manometric findings in one study made little impact on management decisions or treatment (58). Further prospective evaluation of the impact on diagnosis and on treatment outcomes in appropriately selected patients with oropharyngeal dysphagia are required to clarify the future role of manometry in this context.

NORMAL AND ABNORMAL SWALLOW

Voluntary initiation of the oral-pharyngeal swallow requires synthesis of sensory queues from the oropharynx into both the cerebral cortex and the medulla (59). The interneuronal pool within the medulla, the so-called medullary swallow center, then orchestrates the entire sequence of motor responses, predominantly via the lower cranial nerves, that constitute the oral-pharyngeal swallow. The pharyngeal swallow is a rapid sequence of responses involving propulsive forces coordinated with valving functions. These valving functions regulate antegrade and retrograde flow to and from the esophagus through the UES, control bolus exit from the oral cavity (glossopalatal closure mechanism), and prevent laryngeal penetration and nasopharyngeal regurgitation (velopharyngeal closure mechanism). Sequential contact of the tongue against the palate propels the bolus into the pharynx. As the bolus passes the tonsillar arches, the pharyngeal swallow response is initiated and involves velopharyngeal closure, hyolaryngeal elevation with laryngeal closure, and relaxation and then opening of the UES (48,49,60). Tongue pulsion combined with pharyngeal constrictor action then propels the bolus through the UES into the esophagus, and the progressive pharyngeal contraction clears the pharynx of any residue (61,62).

Oropharyngeal dysphagia results from disturbances in one or more of these functions and can manifest in several ways (Table 10.3). Swallow initiation may be delayed or absent. Aspiration may manifest as coughing or choking. Nasopharyngeal regurgitation may be reported. Excessive postswallow residue commonly necessitates repeated swallows to effect clearance or the patient may describe the bolus holding up in the neck. It is usual for several of these dysfunctions to manifest simultaneously in the dysphagic patient. Furthermore, none of these phenomena are specific for any particular disease process. Therefore while it is convenient to categorize neurogenic oropharyngeal dysphagia according to the underlying disease, it is more useful in the evaluation and management of individual patients to conceptualize the disorder in functional terms. With several important exceptions (see later discussion), management is based more on these mechanisms of dysfunction than on the underlying disease causing the dysphagia (Table 10.3).

STRUCTURAL CAUSES OF OROPHARYNGEAL DYSPHAGIA

Tumors, Head and Neck Surgery, Radiotherapy

Intrinsic tumors of the tongue, palate, pharynx, tonsil, and glottis may present with dysphagia (Fig. 10.1). Radiology and nasoendoscopy are imperative for diagnosis (33). Much less commonly, extrinsic tumors of the head and neck, particularly of the thyroid, can also cause dysphagia if they reach a substantial size (63,64). Surgical resection of head and neck cancer commonly causes oropharyngeal dysphagia. The impact of head and neck cancer surgery on swallowing varies markedly among individuals and depends on many factors, including extent of surgical resection; whether flap reconstruction is required; which muscular, boney, or cartilaginous structures are removed or deranged; whether surgery causes collateral damage to neural innervation; and whether surgery is accompanied by radiotherapy, which damages both muscles and nerves (65). Because tongue base motion is important in the generation of pharyngeal propulsive forces, both the extent of oral tongue and tongue base resection is the most important variable determining dysphagia severity in those undergoing surgery for oral cancer (66,67). Mandibular resection and oropharyngeal flap reconstructions, for example, seem to have a lesser impact on swallow function than does lingual resection. The degree of preservation of tongue base motion is also an important predictor of recovery of swallow function following laryngeal surgery (68).

Laryngectomy with or without radiotherapy can cause dysphagia as a result of a combination of anatomic derangements and pharyngeal muscular dysfunction (68,69). Following laryngectomy, the middle and inferior constrictors are reconstituted anteriorly with their opposite number and with the tongue base in a T-configuration. Partial breakdown of this repair gives rise to a pseudodiverticulum or a pouchlike defect anterior to the pharyngeal chamber at the tongue base in which food boluses become trapped, thereby impairing pharyngeal clearance. After removal of the cricoid cartilage, the free margins of the cricopharyngeus muscle are approximated anteriorly, converting the sphincter lumen from an oval to a smaller ringlike structure (70). This alteration in its configuration and diameter significantly reduces the extent of UES opening and increases outflow resistance. Pharyngeal stenosis at the superior surgical closure site is also common (69). Intrinsic pharyngeal muscle and nerve damage from the surgery and frequently exacerbated by radiotherapy, may impair pharyngeal propulsive forces. Although less common, dysphagia can complicate head and neck surgery performed for benign disease. For example, dysphagia has been reported following anterior cervical fusion, carotid endarterectomy and ventral rhizotomy for spasmodic torticollis (71,72).

Radiotherapy is well recognized to cause structural and functional damage to oral and pharyngeal structures. Careful videofluoroscopic or manometric studies demonstrate a range of disturbances, including pharyngeal dysmotility, muscular weakness, and incoordination to account for dysfunction in both oral and pharyngeal phases (73–75). The cricopharyngeus seems particularly susceptible to radiation damage. Cricopharyngeal stenosis is commonly seen in these cases and often responds well to simple dilation (Cook, unpublished observations, 2002). It is not uncommon for radiation-induced dysphagia to manifest clinically more than 10 years after administration of the radiotherapy (76). Radiation-induced xerostomia is an important contributor to swallow dysfunction in the cancer patient because the salivary glands are extremely radiosensitive.

Postcricoid Web, Stenosis, and the Cricopharyngeal Bar

A postcricoid web is a thin, shelflike, usually eccentric but sometimes circumferential constriction that occurs in the proximal few centimeters of the esophagus and is comprised of a thin layer of mucosa and submucosa. Webs typically present with dysphagia for solids, but, because of their proximal location, deglutitive aspiration may occur. One consecutive series of 1,134 videofluoroscopic examinations reported a cervical esophageal web in 7.5% of cases investigated for dysphagia and were twice as common in women as in men (77). The web has been associated with iron deficiency anemia, in which case, the terms *Patterson-Brown-Kelly* or *Plummer-Vinson syndromes* have been applied (78). The incidence of this syndrome appears to have declined markedly in recent decades and webs occur in the absence of iron deficiency (79). Squamous carcinoma is a recognized complication of this syndrome (80). Webs are frequently more readily appreciated on barium swallow than they are endoscopically. Indeed, inadvertent disruption of the lesion at endoscopy and a somewhat retrospective appreciation of its existence is common. The lesion is often only visible transiently on standard barium swallow and is usually better visualized on videofluoroscopy or cine fluoroscopy.

A cricopharyngeal bar is a common incidental radiologic finding, the clinical significance of which is controversial. There is no universally accepted term used to describe the cricopharyngeal bar. Frequently adopted but erroneous terminology includes achalasia, spasm, and hypertrophy. The former two manometric terms have been inappropriately applied to radiologic appearances. Careful manometric evaluation of a group of patients with cricopharyngeal bars confirmed normal resting UES pressure and complete deglutitive UES relaxation (50). The term *hypertrophy* is only applicable when histopathologic examination of the cricopharyngeus muscle confirms hypertrophy because the radiologic appearance of fibrotic and hypertrophic stenoses can be indistinguishable (Fig. 10.2). A cricopharyngeal bar has been reported in 5% to 19% of patients undergoing pharyngeal cineradiography or videoradiography (81–85), and, in patients undergoing videofluoroscopy, dysphagia is no more prevalent in those individuals found to have a cricopharyngeal bar (13%) than it is in those without one (84). Inevitably, the cricopharyngeal bar will turn up in the investigation of many patients with dysphagia but it causes dysphagia in the minority. In one series of 124 patients, a cricopharyngeal bar was identified in 24 (19%) but esophageal pathology that could have accounted for dysphagia was found in all but one of these; in at least eight patients (33%), the esophageal lesions almost certainly accounted for the dysphagia (85). Pharyngeal motor dysfunction may coexist with a cricopharyngeal bar and, in this context, the accompanying neurogenic pharyngeal dysfunction is the dominant mechanism of the dysphagia (Fig. 10.3). Notwithstanding, the argument that the cricopharyngeal bar might cause holdup of the swallowed bolus is plausible. Careful radiologic and manometric measurements of the sphincter zone in these patients demonstrate normal manometric UES relaxation but restricted UES opening and increased resistance to bolus flow across the sphincter (50,86). In some cases, however, the postcricoid narrowing may only be apparent, being accounted for by widening of the gullet above and below the cricopharyngeus (87). Histologic examination of the cricopharyngeus muscle retrieved from patients undergoing myotomy for a cricopharyngeal bar has shown muscle fiber degeneration and interstitial fibrosis in some cases (88–90), similar to

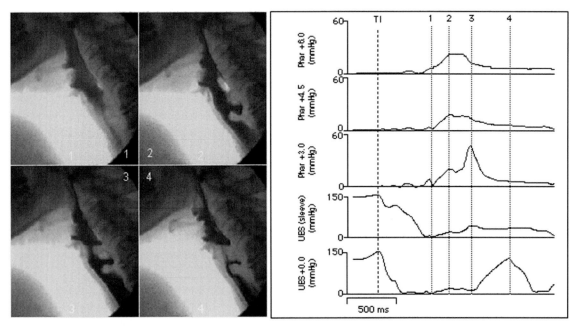

FIGURE 10.3. Videoradiographic sequence (*left*) and corresponding manometry in a patient with myositis, a cricopharyngeal bar, and early diverticulum. Note the poor pharyngeal bolus clearance from a combination of pharyngeal weakness and restrictive defect at the upper esophageal sphincter. Each vertical dashed line represents the time corresponding to the numbered radiographic frame on the left. Note that the sphincter relaxes completely and there is a pharyngeal swallow response detected both radiographically and manometrically. Although the pharyngeal stripping wave is apparent, it is of low amplitude. Hypopharyngeal intrabolus pressure (*frame 2, channel 3*) is increased as a result of the marked restriction in sphincter opening. TI refers to onset of swallow indicated by initial tongue tip motion at the maxillary incisors. (From Williams RB, Grehan MJ, Hersch M, et al. Biomechanics, diagnosis, and treatment outcome in inflammatory myopathy presenting as oropharyngeal dysphagia. *Gut* 2002;52:471–478, with permission.)

that found in the cricopharyngeus retrieved from Zenker's patients at surgery (91). Recent histopathologic studies also report inflammatory myopathic changes with muscle fiber necrosis and phagocytosis and that these pathologic changes appeared to be confined to the cricopharyngeus muscle (92–94). Furthermore, there appears to be an increased prevalence of a cricopharyngeal bar and stenosis with or without Zenker's diverticulum in patients with dysphagia resulting from polymyositis or dermatomyositis (95,96). These observations suggest that some cases of cricopharyngeal bar or cricopharyngeal stenosis might be secondary to a focal or more generalized myopathy.

The functional significance of cricopharyngeal bars is variable. The constriction causes symptoms under the following circumstances:

1. If the constriction is circumferential (i.e., visible on both anteroposterior and lateral radiographs) and if additional esophageal or pharyngeal abnormalities have been ruled out by appropriate radiologic, manometric, and endoscopic investigation. In this situation, the author believes that the descriptor *cricopharyngeal stenosis* is a term to apply to such a circumferential lesion because the term makes no unsubstantiated assumptions about the underlying pathogenesis and could be applicable to

a fibrotic, hypertrophic, or other histopathologic process (Fig. 10.2).
2. If a posterior hypopharyngeal (Zenker's) diverticulum is present.
3. If coexistent pharyngeal neuromuscular dysfunction is identified, the functional significance of the combined abnormalities is likely to be greater than that of the CP bar in isolation (Fig. 10.3).

These structural lesions, when considered the cause of symptoms, are treated by mechanical disruption, either by cricopharyngeal myotomy or dilatation. Cricopharyngeal myotomy reduces resting sphincter tone by approximately 50% (53,97,98). The fact that myotomy does not abolish tone suggests that therapeutic benefit is derived from the increased capacity for sphincter opening and decreased resistance to transsphincteric flow (51,98). Myotomy is most efficacious when applied to patients with structural disorders that limit opening the cricopharyngeus in association with preserved pharyngeal contractility as seen in webs and stenoses (99,100). Data supporting efficacy of either dilatation or myotomy for cervical esophageal webs and postcricoid stenosis are also consistently favorable, albeit uncontrolled (99,101–103). However, repeated dilations over many years seem to be required in at least 40%

of such patients and, in one study, 20% eventually required myotomy (101,102).

Lateral Pharyngeal Diverticula

Pharyngeal diverticula are most conveniently classified according to anatomic site. Broadly speaking, these anatomic structures can be lateral or posterior. Lateral pharyngeal diverticula or pharyngoceles are frequently bilateral, are more common in the elderly, and occur at the level of the vallecula in an area of relative weakness through the thyrohyoid membrane at a site that is relatively poorly supported by cartilage or muscle. Because this anomaly is a common incidental radiologic finding, symptoms may be erroneously attributed to it and the clinician should carefully consider alternative causes of dysphagia or regurgitation in these patients. Lateral diverticula protrude from the lateral wall of the midpharynx and should not be confused with the typical posterior, hypopharyngeal (Zenker's) diverticulum that arises just above the proximal margin of the cricopharyngeus. Lateral diverticula may be congenital or, more commonly, acquired. Congenital lateral pouches are true branchial cleft cysts representing an embryologic remnant of the third pharyngeal pouch corresponding to the thyrohyoid membrane (104). The area of relative weakness is bounded by the hyoid bone superiorly, at a site where there is incomplete overlap of the thyrohyoid muscle anteriorly and the inferior constrictor muscle inferiorly (105). At this site, the thyrohyoid membrane is also perforated by the superior laryngeal artery and the internal laryngeal branch of the superior laryngeal nerve. Lateral diverticula rarely cause symptoms and they are a common incidental finding. However, there are sporadic case reports of successful alleviation of dysphagia after surgical ligation or removal of the diverticulum (106,107).

Zenker's Diverticulum

The posterior hypopharyngeal pouch, Zenker's diverticulum, arises in the posterior hypopharyngeal wall through an area of relative muscular weakness (Killian's dehiscence) just proximal to the upper margin of the cricopharyngeus muscle. Patients are usually elderly with the median age at presentation being in the eighth decade (51). Presenting symptoms include dysphagia combined with varying degrees of regurgitation depending on the size of the pouch. Regurgitation of food particles ingested many hours earlier is often reported. Aspiration symptoms and recurrent chest infections are common features. Audible gurgling during the swallow may be present.

Since Zenker and Ziemssen first hypothesized in 1878 that herniation of the pouch was due to increased hypopharyngeal pressures (108), there has been much debate about its pathogenesis. Initially it was believed that UES incoordination, specifically premature sphincter closure, in some cases combined with early UES relaxation, was the cause of the proposed elevated hypopharyngeal pressure (109–111). The validity of those early observations is questionable, however, because UES relaxation profiles were recorded with a discrete sidehole positioned within the sphincter without appreciation of its deglutitive axial mobility (40). Other theories proposed include UES spasm (112), failure of UES relaxation (113), and a second swallow against a closed sphincter (110,114). There has been no consistent demonstration of any of these phenomena and a number of subsequent carefully conducted manometric studies reported normal or low basal sphincter tone and normal pharyngosphincteric coordination (51,115).

More recently, opening of the UES has been shown to be restricted by an intrinsic cricopharyngeal muscle disease (91). Simultaneous videofluorography and manometry confirmed normal pharyngosphincteric coordination, normal UES tone, and complete UES relaxation but that UES opening is restricted during the swallow (51) (Fig. 10.4). That study showed that inadequate UES opening markedly increases hypopharyngeal intrabolus pressure during transsphincteric bolus flow. It is possible that such an increase in hypopharyngeal pressure just proximal to the sphincter might contribute to pouch herniation. The cause of inadequate sphincter opening is muscle fiber degeneration and fibroadipose tissue replacement confined to the cricopharyngeus muscle (91). These combined observations suggest that Zenker's diverticulum is due to a poorly compliant but normally relaxing UES that cannot fully distend during the process of sphincter opening. Further evidence supporting this concept lies in the finding that cricopharyngeal myotomy, effectively a curative surgical procedure, normalizes both the extent of UES opening and hypopharyngeal intrabolus pressure (98).

Treatment is cricopharyngeal myotomy, either alone or in combination with pouch resection or suspension (100). The early observation that cricopharyngeal dilatation by bougienage gave temporary relief of dysphagia (116) prompted the introduction of cricopharyngeal myotomy (117). Simple dilatation can afford symptomatic benefit of variable duration (116,118,119). Cricopharyngeal myotomy is the key element for successful long-term relief of dysphagia and it has been established that resection of the pouch alone is inadequate treatment and that myotomy is the essential element in treatment of this condition (120–126). Indeed, excellent symptomatic results can be achieved from myotomy alone (100,124). Regression of the intact pouch can be observed following myotomy (127, 128), and radiologic recurrence of the pouch is reduced after myotomy (111). No controlled trials of the efficacy of

NORMAL **ZENKERS**

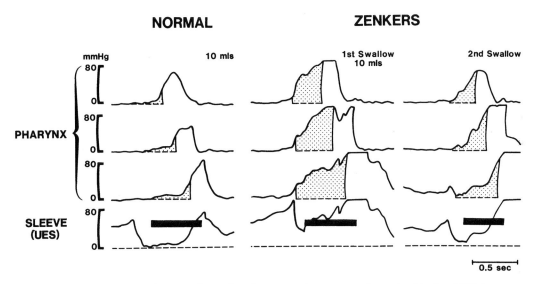

FIGURE 10.4. Manometric traces from the pharynx and upper esophageal sphincter (UES) in a patient with a hypopharyngeal (Zenker's) diverticulum (*right*) compared with that of a healthy subject (*left*). Recordings were synchronized with concurrent videofluoroscopy to permit identification of UES opening and bolus flow across the sphincter (*black horizontal bar*). Resting UES tone, recorded by a perfused sleeve sensor, is normal and UES relaxation is complete in response to a "dry" swallow (2nd swallow on right). Note also the marked increase in hypopharyngeal intrabolus pressure (*stippled*) compared with that in the control subject. (From Cook IJ, Gabb M, Panagopoulos V, et al. Pharyngeal [Zenker's] diverticulum is a disorder of upper esophageal sphincter opening. *Gastroenterology* 1992;103:1229–1235, with permission).

surgical treatment for Zenker's diverticulum exist. However, the consistency of published response rates of between 80% and 100% is in keeping with the strong clinical impression that surgery is nearly always curative in this disorder (97–99,129–132).

Transoral treatment of the pouch, either by endosurgical stapling or laser, has gained wide acceptance in the past 10 years. The technique was first described in 1960 (133). If the pouch is deep enough (>2 cm), it is possible to straddle the cricopharyngeal bridge with a diverticuloscope and incise and staple the cricopharyngeus. This removes the "common wall" between cervical esophagus and the diverticulum, thereby achieving a cricopharyngeal myotomy and facilitating drainage of the pouch without removing it. Limited numbers of this technique have also been performed using the flexible endoscope (134). No controlled efficacy data exist for these endosurgical approaches. Uncontrolled series consistently report success rates of 81% to 96%; complication rates of up to 6% (mediastinitis, hemorrhage, aspiration) have been reported with an estimated mortality rate after combining published studies of around 0.5% (135–140). These figures are comparable to those for open surgical approaches, but patients are generally fed sooner and incur shorter hospital stays. Endosurgical stapling is the treatment of choice for the elderly or high-risk patient and is rapidly gaining acceptance as first line therapy for average risk cases with favorable anatomy.

Cervical Osteophytes

Cervical osteophytes are a common incidental finding in the dysphagic patient, occurring in 6% to 30% of the elderly (141,142). On the other hand, only 0.7% of patients with cervical disc disease report dysphagia (143). Hence, the finding of prominent osteophytes should prompt a careful search for an alternative cause of dysphagia, which is found in the majority of patients. Nonetheless, if prominent, osteophytes can cause dysphagia, which is correctable by surgical removal of the bony spur (144–146). The major mechanism of dysphagia is mechanical compression of the posterior pharyngeal wall, but associated periesophageal inflammation induced by pharyngoesophageal motion over the cervical exostoses (predominantly over the C3-6 vertebrae) might contribute as well (147,148). Development of osteophytes may be related to DISH (diffuse idiopathic skeletal hyperostosis ankylosing spondylosis), infectious spondylosis, previous surgical fusion of the cervical vertebrae, or local trauma, or it may be of idiopathic origin (71,149). Surgical treatment of cervical osteophytes remains controversial, and appropriate objective criteria have not been consistently used to assess results. Complications of surgical excision include vocal fold paresis, vertebral disc prolapse, fistula, hematoma, infection, aspiration, and Horner's syndrome (150). In view of these limitations, most researchers feel surgery should be performed only for those patients with severe dysphagia in whom conservative treatment has failed (149).

NEUROGENIC CAUSES OF OROPHARYNGEAL DYSPHAGIA

Stroke

Stroke is the most common cause of oropharyngeal dysphagia. Oropharyngeal dysphagia affects one third of all stroke patients at presentation (1,2). Although much more common and more severe in bilateral or brainstem stroke, dysphagia affects 25% to 40% of patients in the acute phase of a unilateral hemisphere stroke (3,4,151–153).

The anterolateral frontal cortex and caudolateral precentral cortex are known to be involved in cortical control of swallowing (154,155). Recent studies on the cortical topographic representation of swallow musculature in health and following hemispheric stroke have implicated hemispheric asymmetry as a determinant of dysphagia after unilateral hemisphere stroke (156). By stimulating the cortex using transcutaneous magnetic stimulation, the size and location of cortical areas involved in swallowing can be determined by inference from the magnitude of the resulting peripheral electromyographic (EMG) response recorded from the swallowing muscles. Such studies show that the swallowing musculature is somatotopically organized on the human motor and premotor cortex, with consistent cortical lateralization of both pharynx and esophagus to one or other hemisphere, which is independent of handedness (156). Whether or not an individual develops dysphagia following stroke seems to be determined by the size of pharyngeal representation within the affected cortex. When compared with nondysphagic stroke patients, those with dysphagia demonstrated smaller areas of cortical representation in the intact hemisphere and stimulation of the unaffected hemisphere also evoked smaller pharyngeal EMG responses (157). Furthermore, the degree of natural recovery of swallowing following stroke parallels the increase in size of cortical representation in the intact hemisphere (Color Plate 10.5). Hence, recovery of swallow function after stroke depends on the presence of intact projections from the undamaged hemisphere, which, by the process of "plasticity," can develop increased control over brainstem swallow centers with time.

Of stroke patients with dysphagia, 45% to 68% are dead within 6 months, largely due to dysphagia-related nutritional and pulmonary complications (3,158). In addition to a higher mortality rate, dysphagia infers a higher risk of infection, poor nutrition, longer hospital stay, and institutionalization (2,4,9). The most prevalent complication of stroke-related pharyngeal dysphagia is aspiration pneumonia, occurring in one third of all patients and in 67% of those with brainstem stroke (1,2).

Hence, determination of the risk of aspiration in this population is a fundamental aim of management. However, the risk of developing pneumonia cannot be predicted accurately from any single clinical sign or symptom at the bedside (159). Furthermore, bedside evaluation underestimates the prevalence of deglutitive aspiration. Radiography detects aspiration not evident at the time of bedside assessment in 42% to 60% of patients (1,28,151, 160,161). This may represent a laryngopharyngeal sensory deficit as regional mucosal sensory thresholds have been found to be increased in stroke cases when compared with control subjects (162). In addition, an absent or depressed gag reflex does not have predictive value for aspiration, in that only 60% of aspirators have an impaired gag reflex (1). Similarly, whereas dysphonia has a 91% sensitivity for aspiration, it has a positive predictive value of only 58%. Radiographic demonstration of a markedly delayed or absent pharyngeal swallow response, combined with a poor pharyngeal contraction, carries the highest risk of aspiration (1,151,163). These facts underpin the importance of videofluoroscopy as being the only certain way of detecting aspiration and, if such gross features of pharyngeal dysfunction are demonstrated along with aspiration, immediate introduction of nonoral feeding is indicated. Typical videofluoroscopic findings are as follows: difficulty in initiating the swallow, delayed or absent pharyngeal swallow response, pharyngeal weakness with poor pharyngeal clearance and postswallow pooling in vallecula and piriform sinuses, and aspiration. In hemispheric stroke, the lesion location seems to be more critical than hemisphere or size of lesion in predicting the risk of aspiration. Lesions in anterior locations and subcortical periventricular white matter may carry a higher risk of aspiration than do posterior lesions and involvement in subcortical gray matter (164). Does systematic evaluation of the stroke patient with dysphagia reduce the risk of pneumonia and influence outcome? There are no randomized controlled studies that address this question. Although the level of evidence is weak, reports of pneumonia rates from centers with dysphagia programs compared with historical data from centers without formal programs suggest that systematic evaluation by videofluoroscopy or nasoendoscopy coupled with a structured treatment program may reduce pneumonia rates (165, 166).

Parkinson's Disease

Dysphagia in Parkinson's disease is common and is associated with considerable morbidity from nutritional and pulmonary sequelae (25,167–169). Dysphagia is also common in related parkinsonian disorders such as dementia with Lewy bodies, corticobasal degeneration, multiple system atrophy, and progressive supranuclear palsy (170). The median survival time from onset of dysphagia to death in these disorders is short, ranging from 15 to 24 months (170). The true prevalence of dysphagia in Parkinson's is uncertain but may be as high as 52% (25,171,172). Drooling of saliva is even more common than dysphagia being reported in up to 78% of patients (25,173). Although symptoms are referable to the oropharynx in most patients, esophageal dysfunction is also common in Parkinson's disease (174,175). Most investigators who have examined the relationships among symptoms, severity of disease, and dysphagia found that the duration of the disease, the severity of underlying disease, and the specific cardinal parkinsonian features did not correlate with severity or mechanism of dysphagia (39,167,174,176). However, latency from disease onset to onset of dysphagia correlates positively with overall long-term survival (170).

Preparatory and oral phase dysfunction is common in Parkinson's disease. Impaired preparatory lingual movements and mastication, piecemeal swallows, increased oral residue, preswallow spill, and swallow hesitancy are common radiologic observations (39,177). Lingual tremor appears to be specific for extrapyramidal movement disorders (39,167,174). All Parkinson's patients with dysphagia and many without dysphagia demonstrate one or more radiologic indicators of pharyngeal dysfunction, such as postswallow contrast coating of pharyngeal wall, vallecula and piriform sinus pooling, abnormal pharyngeal wall motion, and impaired UES opening (26,39). Intraswallow or postswallow aspiration occurs in one third of those with dysphagia, and silent aspiration has been reported in up to 15% of those reporting neither dysphagia nor symptoms of aspiration (39,167,176,178).

Manometric studies may demonstrate diminished pharyngeal contraction pressures, pharyngosphincteric incoordination, or synchronous pressure waves, and failure of UES relaxation is common, occurring in up to 25% of cases (39,113,179). Failed UES relaxation, although relatively common, is not the major determinant of dysphagia in Parkinson's disease, in that its presence correlates neither with the severity of the associated motor disorder nor the severity of dysphagia (39). Impaired pharyngeal bolus transport is the major determinant of dysphagia in Parkinson's disease.

Cricopharyngeal myotomy seems to be a logical treatment in view of the high prevalence of failed UES relaxation. A favorable response to myotomy has been reported in a small series of patients, many of whom had additional structural abnormalities, but more data are required before surgery could be recommended (180). Similarly, there has been little systematic evaluation of the responsiveness of dysphagia to antiparkinsonian medication. The acute effect of central dopaminergic stimulation on pharyngeal mechanics is controversial. An early study assessed swallow function cineradiographically and reported no difference in swallow function following acute administration of oral levodopa compared with placebo (181). A

subsequent study using videofluoroscopy found that central dopaminergic stimulation by apomorphine improved pharyngeal bolus clearance acutely in roughly 50% of patients with mild disease (182). Bushmann and colleagues (167) studied the acute effects of levodopa using videofluoroscopy and a clinical rating. Whereas they found general improvement in parkinsonian motor features, such improvement was not an indicator of improved swallow function. In that study, 15% of those with abnormal videofluoroscopic studies demonstrated acute improvement following oral administration of levodopa (167). Hunter and co-workers (183) studied subjective dysphagia symptoms and videofluoroscopic parameters before and after acute administration of oral levodopa and apomorphine. Despite an unequivocal motor response to both drugs, there was no or minimal detectable change in oral-pharyngeal swallow function. These findings strongly suggest that parkinsonian dysphagia is not solely related to nigrostriatal dopamine deficiency (183).

The longer term effects of drug therapy on swallow function also remain unclear. It has been the experience of the author that the dysphagia is relatively unresponsive to antiparkinsonian drug therapy. Nevertheless, evidence for a good clinical response to drug therapy exists in isolated case reports (184), and optimal pharmacotherapy generally improves the patients' ability to feed themselves by minimizing hand tremor and bradykinesia; treatment of mood disturbance, when present, may also improve feeding behavior and appetite. Appropriate timing of medication, 1 hour before meals, would seem logical and was found to be beneficial in at least one case report (185). There are no controlled studies of swallow rehabilitation in Parkinson's disease. One uncontrolled study found that a combination of levodopa and swallow therapy improved swallow function, but it is uncertain to what extent improvement could be attributed to pharmacotherapy (167). A recent systematic review concluded that there are no controlled data at all upon which to base firm treatment guidelines in this disease (186,187). However, the general principles of swallow rehabilitation that are applicable after stroke are generally adopted in Parkinson's disease (see later discussion).

Motor Neuron Disease

Oropharyngeal dysphagia commonly complicates motor neuron disease, affecting the majority of affected patients at some stage in their disease (188). In the most common variant of this disease, amyotrophic lateral sclerosis (ALS), there is degeneration of motor neurons in the cortex, brainstem, and the spinal cord, leading to both upper and lower motor neuronal weakness. Bulbar involvement with dysarthria and dysphagia is a primary manifestation in 25% to 30% of cases of ALS (189). The onset of the disease is insidious. Early symptoms include coughing or choking during liquid swallows, followed by progressive dysphagia and weight loss. The sequence of involvement of bulbar musculature is relatively predictable, in that the tongue is generally involved early and nearly always before the pharyngeal muscles. Aspiration pneumonia is a common complication, and when coupled with diminished respiratory muscle reserve, is the most common cause of death (190,191).

Videofluoroscopic findings are variable and depend on the stage of disease (192). By the time dysphagia is a significant problem, lingual dysfunction is almost invariably present and manifests as repetitive tongue movements, premature retrolingual bolus spill, and significant retention of barium in the oral sulci, requiring several swallows for clearance. The pharyngeal swallow response may be delayed and is eventually lost with markedly impaired bolus clearance from the pharynx and intraswallow and postswallow aspiration of contrast. There have been few systematic manometric studies of these patients. Although UES relaxation appears to be complete and sphincter spasm is not a feature (32,193), an EMG study found unexpected bursts of cricopharyngeal muscle motor activity during the phase of sphincter opening and that the duration of UES opening is shortened (194).

Management of these patients is difficult and necessitates involvement of the palliative care team along with institution of swallow therapy (see later discussion), appropriately timed introduction of PEG feeding, and control of troublesome drooling (195). Although the disease is inexorably progressive and leads to death with a median survival of 3 years (191), the rate of disease progression is variable (196). One study has shown a close temporal correlation among speech, swallowing, and lung vital capacity and noted a rapid deterioration in swallowing with the onset of compromised speech intelligibility (196). These findings suggest that monitoring of vital capacity and speech are useful prognostic indicators that guide the clinician as to the timing of intervention with swallow therapy and consideration of nonoral feeding. In the absence of adequately controlled studies, no clear, evidence-based guidelines exist for the optimal timing of PEG tube insertion. Whether or not early PEG placement results in increased survival or improved outcomes has not yet been demonstrated convincingly (197,198). The decision is made on clinical grounds considering a range of factors, including nutritional and hydration status, aspiration risk, and patient attitude to dietary modification and the feeding process (199). Excessive drooling can be a major management problem. Drugs such as glycopyrrolate, hyoscine dermal patches, amitriptyline, atropine/benztropine, or clonidine can be helpful. More recently, intraparotid injection of botulinum toxin has been reported in the treatment of sialorrhea in ALS as well as in Parkinson's disease and muscular sclerosis (200). Reports of success are currently anecdotal and systematic efficacy studies are awaited. Complications have included worsening of dysphagia and impaired oral and jaw function (201,202).

Poliomyelitis and Postpolio Syndrome

Although less common than the spinal involvement in this disease, bulbar poliomyelitis carries a much greater mortality rate, primarily from depression of respiratory muscles associated with an inability to clear pharyngeal secretions. Pharyngeal involvement with dysphagia probably occurs in about 60% of cases of bulbar poliomyelitis (203). Dysphagia, when present, involves the neurons of the nucleus ambiguus in the medulla with variable involvement of the adjacent reticular formation. Furthermore, the rostrocaudal level of involvement in poliomyelitis determines the likelihood of dysphagia occurring because involvement of the rostral nucleus ambiguus has a much stronger correlation with dysphagia than involvement of the mid or distal medulla (204). Cineradiographic swallow studies in affected patients commonly show velopharyngeal incompetence affecting speech and causing deglutitive, postnasal regurgitation. Abnormal pharyngeal wall motion reflecting constrictor muscle and suprahyoid muscle dysfunction is commonly seen and results in impaired pharyngeal bolus clearance (205).

Since the widespread introduction of vaccination, acute poliomyelitis is rarely seen. However, a late onset and very slowly progressive muscular weakness, the postpolio syndrome, is now recognized in some patients who have partially or totally recovered from acute poliomyelitis many years before (206). Typically, the postpolio syndrome manifests 25 to 35 years after the original attack of poliomyelitis. Patients report an insidious onset of new fatigability, muscle wasting, weakness, and sometimes muscle pain. These symptoms are generally most prominent in previously affected muscles, and regions not previously involved with the original attack may be affected. Only 50% of those with postpolio dysphagia experienced dysphagia at the time of their acute poliomyelitis (207,208). One survey determined the prevalence of dysphagia in a polio survivors support group to be 18% (209). The videofluoroscopic features are not specific for this syndrome and may include those described in poliomyelitis such as velopharyngeal incompetence, pharyngeal weakness, and silent aspiration. Silent aspiration is reported in up to 50% of these patients (207). Additionally, whereas pharyngeal dysfunction is the most common deficit, oromotor dysfunction is also common, affecting about half of these patients (209–212). It is now appreciated that, in people affected by postpolio syndrome, motor neurons continue to undergo damage, and slowly progressive deterioration of swallow function can occur once the syndrome is apparent (210).

MYOGENIC CAUSES OF OROPHARYNGEAL DYSPHAGIA

Myasthenia Gravis

Myasthenia usually has an insidious onset and protean manifestations. Muscles most frequently involved include the facial, laryngeal, pharyngeal, and respiratory groups, but limb muscles are usually affected also. Facial and pharyngeal weakness is present in 70%, and dysphagia affects 30% to 60% of cases (213,214). Dysphagia is present at diagnosis in around 20% of cases (213,215), and dysphagia may dominate the clinical picture, being the sole presenting symptom in 6% to 17% of affected individuals (216,217). The so-called fatigable flaccid dysarthria is manifested by hypernasal speech (velopharyngeal incompetence), imprecise articulation and breathiness reflects bulbar dysfunction and is usually prominent in those with dysphagia, and progressive difficulty chewing and swallowing during the course of a long meal may also be reported (214,218). The ocular features of palpebral ptosis and diplopia are usually but not invariably present. Atrophy of the tongue may be prominent also (219). Diagnosis may be apparent from typical clinical signs, including fatigability, but should be considered in any dysphagic patient, even though typical ocular signs may be absent.

Diagnosis is confirmed by detecting AChR antibodies, which are present in 85% of cases overall (220). The finding of AChR antibodies is highly specific and virtually diagnostic, but antibodies may be absent in up to 50% of patients without typical ocular signs. The Tensilon (edrophonium) stimulation test may be positive. The diagnosis may also be made electromyographically using repetitive nerve stimulation; even more sensitive is single-fiber EMG recordings, which are the most sensitive diagnostic tests (214,220,221). Pharyngeal pressure recordings during Tensilon test may be useful to quantify the response, particularly if response as judged by other muscle groups is equivocal (Cook, unpublished data, 1999). Videoradiographic examination reveals obvious features of virtually all the muscle groups involved, including both oral and pharyngeal phases and the suprahyoid muscles responsible for hyolaryngeal ascent (218,222). Poor oral delivery with incomplete oral clearance, premature bolus spill, deglutitive velopharyngeal incompetence, abnormal pharyngeal wall motion with aspiration, and vallecula and piriform sinus pooling are characteristic features. Subnormal hyolaryngeal ascent results in incomplete epiglottal inversion, further predisposing to aspiration.

The response of pharyngeal swallow dysfunction to medical therapy (acetylcholinesterase inhibitor and immunosuppressive drugs) is variable and may respond at a different rate and less satisfactorily than other muscle groups. For example, the dysphagia in only three of eight elderly men whose primary symptoms of myasthenia gravis were dysarthria and dysphagia responded satisfactorily; the remaining five required long-term enteral feeding tubes (218). Some have reported dramatic improvement in hypopharyngeal bolus clearance in response to edrophonium (215), but this is not a consistent observation. Even in those with a satisfactory clinical response, the videofluoroscopic improvement following therapy may be marginal, which casts doubt on the use of videofluoroscopy in assessing progress of these patients (218). Notwithstanding the frequently disappointing response to medical therapy, establishing the diagnosis does influence management because it always warrants drug therapy, a search for thymoma, and avoidance of risk factors for myasthenic crisis, to which the dysphagic patient is frequently exposed, including respiratory tract infections, anesthesia, and surgery.

Inflammatory Myopathies

Dysphagia is a frequent and sometimes the only presenting symptom, occurring in 30% to 60% of cases of inflammatory myopathy (214,223). The inflammatory myopathies comprise three distinct groups: polymyositis, dermatomyositis, and inclusion body myositis (223). Pharyngeal dysphagia can occur in the mixed connective tissue disease overlap syndrome in up to 20% of cases (224,225). In this syndrome, patients may display the clinical features of polymyositis with those of lupus, Sjögren's, or scleroderma, and antibodies to extractable nuclear antigen are detectable. The clinical features of inflammatory myopathy generally include a subacute or chronic and progressive symmetrical, proximal muscular weakness. However, one third of those affected who have dysphagia as their only presenting symptom have no clinically apparent extrabulbar muscular weakness (96).

Diagnosis maybe confirmed by abnormalities on one or more of muscle enzymes, EMG, or muscle biopsy. Serum creatine phosphokinase (CPK) is the most sensitive enzyme but alanine transaminase, aspartate aminostransferase, lactate dehydrogenase, and aldolase are also sensitive indicators of muscle injury. Whereas CPK levels generally parallel disease activity, the CPK is frequently normal even in active disease (223,224). Specifically in those with dysphagia as the presenting complaint, CPK is normal in 25% (96). Elevated erythrocyte sedimentation rate or positive antinuclear antibodies (ANA) may be found in 30% to 50% of those presenting with dysphagia but have low diagnostic sensitivity and specificity in this population (96). A positive ANA is much more likely to be present (85% to 90%) if the myositis occurs as part of an overlap syndrome (224). Needle electromyography is useful in excluding neurogenic disorders and demonstrates features consistent with inflammatory myositis in 85% to 90% (224). Muscle biopsy is required for definitive diagnosis and to distinguish among dermatomyositis, polymyositis, and inclusion body myositis. Notwithstanding, muscle biopsy is diagnostic in only 80%, emphasizing that diagnosis of myositis can be elusive and that there is a need for complete clinical, biochemical, and laboratory evaluation in all suspected cases (96,224). Selection of the site for muscle biopsy is important and attempts should be made to sample muscles that are affected but that are not yet atrophic, either clinically or electromyographically. The inflammatory process my be patchy and is occasionally confined to the pharyngeal musculature (92–94). If cricopharyngeal myotomy is undertaken in suspected cases without prior confirmation of the diagnosis by the aforementioned techniques, fresh muscle samples should be obtained from the cricopharyngeus and other neck muscles (e.g., omohyoid, sternomastoid) for histologic examination.

The videofluoroscopic features are variable. Pharyngeal dysfunction is almost universal in radiologic studies of patients with dysphagia resulting from inflammatory myopathy, and radiographic evidence of aspiration is seen in 60% (96,113,226). Restrictive cricopharyngeal disorders (cricopharyngeal bar, cricopharyngeal stenosis, and Zenker's) are more commonly seen in inflammatory myopathy presenting with dysphagia than they are in neurogenic dysphagia (96,113,227,228). For example, in one controlled series of patients, cricopharyngeal bar or circumferential stenosis (three of whom also had Zenker's diverticula) was found in 69% of patients with myositis and dysphagia, which was a significantly higher percentage than that observed (5%) in controls with neurogenic dysphagia (96). Combined videoradiographic and manometric evaluation of this population showed normal sphincter relaxation, restricted sphincter opening, and raised hypopharyngeal intrabolus pressures (Fig. 10.3). These observations indicate that the limitation of UES opening is not fully explained by the associated diminished pharyngeal propulsive force during the swallow, but that the intrinsic distensibility of the cricopharyngeus muscle is reduced in this disease. Indeed, histologic examination of cricopharyngeus muscle in affected patients has demonstrated necrosis, inflammatory infiltration, and fibrosis (227,229). Interestingly, focal inflammation and fibrosis can affect the cricopharyngeus without the usual biochemical, electromyographic, or histologic evidence of muscle involvement elsewhere (92,93).

Manometric studies in this population demonstrate that basal UES pressure is either normal or low when compared with aged healthy controls, but that sphincter relaxation is preserved. Manometric studies in this population demonstrate normal or low resting UES pressure with normal deglutitive relaxation and reduced peak pharyngeal contraction pressures (96,230,231).

The mainstay of treatment for inflammatory myopathies is immunosuppressive therapy with steroids in the first instance, with azathioprine or methotrexate as second line or steroid-sparing agents. Despite the lack of controlled efficacy trials, significant number of patients respond favorably to these agents. High-dose intravenous immunoglobulin has been shown to be of clear benefit in a controlled trial for those with polymyositis and dermatomyositis (232). Inclusion body myositis is generally resistant to standard therapies (233), although high-dose intravenous immunoglobulin may be helpful in this variant also (234). Reports of response of swallowing function in response to drug therapy are anecdotal but generally favorable. Given the high prevalence of upper esophageal restriction in this population, one might expect cricopharyngeal disruption might be beneficial. Although no controlled efficacy data exist, either cricopharyngeal dilation or myotomy carries a 50% (short term) response rate (227,228,235). Prognosis in those with significant dysphagia is poor, with one third dying within 12 months of diagnosis, generally from pulmonary complications (96).

Toxic and Metabolic Myopathies

Hyperthyroidism is a well-recognized cause of myopathy, which is believed to be due to mitochondrial dysfunction (236). Muscle weakness affects 80% of thyrotoxic patients and men are affected more commonly than women (236). The myopathy of thyrotoxicosis can cause pharyngeal dysphagia, which is generally slowly progressive and which may be the presenting feature of this endocrinopathy (27,237). Although uncommon, this condition should always be considered, particularly in the elderly when the more classic thyrotoxic features may be absent, because it is a reversible cause of dysphagia (27,238). Serum CPK is not increased in contrast to the myopathy of myxedema in which CPK is usually increased but in which weakness is uncommon (239). The response of limb muscle function to specific treatment of thyrotoxicosis is usually excellent. Although published data are limited, there are case reports of resolution of pharyngeal dysphagia with return to the euthyroid state (27); this has also been the anecdotal experience of the author. A number of drugs capable of causing toxic or inflammatory myopathy should be considered in the assessment of the patient with dysphagia because removal of the drug generally reverses the dysphagia (Table 10.2).

Oculopharyngeal Muscular Dystrophy

Taylor, who was first to describe this rare syndrome in 1915, originally postulated that the disorder was a neuropathy 1915 (240). Oculopharyngeal muscular dystrophy has subsequently been shown to be a myopathy affecting nearly exclusively the bulbar muscles and the levator muscles of the eyes (241). The disease usually presents between the ages of 40 and 70 years, most often initially with bilateral ptosis followed some years later by dysphagia. The ptosis usually develops before, or sometimes simultaneously with, the dysphagia but it is unusual for the dysphagia to develop first. The disease is slowly progressive. Variable but mild facial weakness may develop, as may a minor degree of ophthalmoplegia, and limb muscle weakness is occasionally present. However, the pharyngeal and levator palpebral involvement always dominate the clinical picture. The disorder is inherited in an autosomal dominant fashion. There is a high incidence of this disorder in French Canadians. However, the disorder has been well documented in many other racial groups including the Italian, Spanish, English, Armenian, Australian, Norwegian, and Japanese populations (242–244).

Dystrophic changes in muscle biopsy have been demonstrated by light and electron microscopy on levator, pharyngeal, and vastus lateralis muscles (242–247). Although the findings are variable, a number of investigators report histologic and ultrastructural features, suggesting that this disorder is a heterogeneous syndrome and that it may be a manifestation of mitochondrial myopathy (242,246,247). Histopathologic findings in cricopharyngeus muscle specimens must be interpreted with caution, however, because the normal cricopharyngeus muscle demonstrates features, which if identified in limb muscle, would be consistent with a mitochondrial myopathy (91). Nonetheless, the reported changes of cricopharyngeal muscle fiber degeneration and fibrosis are definitely pathologic (242), and such changes in the cricopharyngeus would be expected to impair sphincter opening and compliance and might account for the reported favorable response to cricopharyngeal myotomy in this disease (53,248). Elevated IgG and IgA levels are frequently found in the serum of these patients (247). The major differential diagnoses are myasthenia gravis and mitochondrial myopathies.

Videoradiographic findings include relative preservation of oral function, incomplete UES opening, pharyngeal weakness with impaired pharyngeal bolus clearance, variable aspiration, and postnasal regurgitation. Manometric recordings have generally shown a normally relaxing UES, which is sometimes hypotensive, and markedly reduced pharyngeal pressure wave amplitudes (53,113,249–251). Although the syndrome is a disease of striated muscle, manometric abnormalities have also been described in the esophagus. A high prevalence of nonpropulsive, simultaneous pressure waves and failed peristalsis is reported (242,251,252), which is associated with delayed esophageal isotope clearance (53,252).

Because of its late onset and slow progression, the prognosis of oculopharyngeal muscular dystrophy is generally good and the disease in many cases does not adversely influence life expectancy. This syndrome is one homogenous condition in which the results of cricopharyngeal myotomy appear to be fairly consistently favorable (53,253). Despite the lack of controlled trials of efficacy of myotomy, this procedure appears to be appropriate in cases with severe dysphagia.

DRUGS CAUSING OROPHARYNGEAL DYSPHAGIA

It is important for the clinician to obtain a detailed drug history from the patient who has oropharyngeal dysphagia because a range of drugs can act either centrally or peripherally to impair neural function, neuromuscular transmission, muscle function, or salivary secretion and thereby cause dysphagia (Table 10.2). Drugs can impair swallow function indirectly by either inhibiting or enhancing salivary flow.

Centrally acting drugs with dopamine antagonist action, such as phenothiazines and metoclopramide, can cause extrapyramidal movement disorders such as dystonia and dyskinesia, resulting in dysphagia. Phenothiazines in particular can cause tardive dyskinesia in which choreoathetoid movements of the tongue can severely impair swallowing (254–256). This syndrome, which is frequently irreversible, is characterized by repetitive, involuntary tongue movements that render the masticatory process and oral delivery ineffective. These centrally acting drugs may also impair pharyngeal propulsive and clearance functions by causing a clinical picture similar to Parkinson's disease (257,258). The benzodiazepines nitrazepam (259,260) and clonazepam (261) have been documented to cause oropharyngeal dysphagia. Nitrazepam, a drug frequently used to treat myoclonic epilepsy, has been associated with fatalities in children, probably as a result of a combination of excessive salivation, poor pharyngeal clearance, and bronchospasm resulting in fatal respiratory distress (259,260).

A number of drugs can produce a myasthenic syndrome. Botulinum A toxin (Botox), when injected into the neck muscles to treat spasmodic torticollis, may cause pharyngeal dysphagia, presumably because of regional spread of the toxin to adjacent muscles (262–264). Other drugs capable of causing a myasthenic syndrome include penicillamine (265), large doses of aminoglycosides (214), and procainamide (266). In some cases, anti-AChR antibodies are detectable (265). The myasthenia and dysphagia, if present, are reversible on cessation of the offending drug. Erythromycin may aggravate neuromuscular function in existing myasthenia gravis and should be avoided in this condition (267).

Drugs are a relatively common cause of myopathy, which may be complicated by oropharyngeal dysphagia. A drug can cause either an inflammatory or a toxic myopathy (Table 10.2). Penicillamine (268) and zidovudine (269), for example, can cause an endomysial inflammation similar to that observed in polymyositis, although recent evidence shows that zidovudine is primarily toxic to muscle mitochondria (270). A number of drugs capable of causing a reversible toxic myopathy should also be considered because some of these have been linked specifically with dysphagia. Amiodarone-induced thyroid myopathy may present as dysphagia (271). The cholesterol-lowering HMG-CoA reductase inhibitors (e.g., lovastatin, simvastatin) are a relatively common cause of toxic myopathy (270,272) and may cause reversible oropharyngeal dysphagia associated with elevated CPK levels (Cook, unpublished observations, 1999).

MANAGEMENT OF OROPHARYNGEAL DYSPHAGIA

Management Principles

Because oropharyngeal dysphagia can be the presenting or accompanying manifestation of one of many systemic diseases (Table 10.1), a multidisciplinary strategy is usually necessary to make a diagnosis and optimize management. Furthermore, the accompanying neurologic impairment by limiting the patient's cognitive and physical competence can compromise his or her ability to understand and cooperate with the process of investigation and therapy. Broadly speaking, the aims of management are to identify and treat an underlying primary disease when possible and then try to compensate or circumvent the specific mechanical disturbances responsible for the dysphagia (11). Hence, there is no single strategy appropriate for all cases nor indeed for dysphagia caused by a single disease process because the mechanical disturbances are generally neither homogeneous nor specific for a particular disease. However, there are logical, generic management principles that are widely applicable, whereas specific surgical or rehabilitative swallow therapies should be tailored to individual cases:

1. Confirm that oropharyngeal dysphagia is a problem and attempt to identify the underlying cause. A careful history generally distinguishes oropharyngeal dysphagia from globus, xerostomia, and esophageal dysphagia. History and physical examination may provide clues of a treatable systemic, metabolic, or drug-related disorder. It also identifies the pulmonary and nutritional sequelae of dysphagia. Based on this information, the clinician can prioritize subsequent investigations, including laboratory tests and imaging techniques, to verify a systemic, metabolic, or neuromyogenic disease. Laboratory tests should aim to detect treatable metabolic diseases (e.g., thyrotoxicosis, Cushing's disease, drug-related disease), inflammatory myopathies, and myasthenia.

2. Identify the structural or neuromyogenic mechanisms of oropharyngeal dysfunction. Structural disorders are generally readily detected by radiographic or endoscopic evaluation. Identification of a neoplasm or a Zenker's diverticulum dictate the need for surgery. A cervical web or a cricopharyngeal stenosis prompts dilatation or, in some cases, cricopharyngeal myotomy. Identification of a cricopharyngeal bar or cervical osteophytes should prompt a careful search for a coexistent or alternative explanation for dysphagia but may, in some circumstances, warrant dilatation or surgery (see earlier discus-

sion). The evidence supporting the efficacy of mechanical disruption (usually surgical) for structural disorders is consistently favorable (11). Nasoendoscopic examination of the laryngopharynx is mandatory if neoplasm is suspected. Nasoendoscopy may also provide useful indirect information about some aspects of pharyngeal dysfunction and aspiration (34). In some instances, particularly in the assessment of disorders with a high prevalence of failed UES relaxation, such as Parkinson's disease and medullary lesions (Fig. 10.6), pharyngeal manometry with or without concurrent videofluoroscopy may allow further delineation of the underlying mechanism of dysfunction (36,39,52). In some instances, manometry is able to identify abnormalities that are not apparent on videofluoroscopy (38,39), but whether such decisions based on manometric findings can influence outcome remains unproven (54).

3. Determine the risk of aspiration pneumonia, which is the primary factor in the decision as to whether and when nonoral feeding should be instituted. The risk of aspiration is determined by videofluoroscopic examination because clinical estimation of aspiration underestimates this risk by about 50% (28). The decision on the advisability of gastrostomy feeding is also influenced by (a) the likelihood that therapeutic maneuvers, which may be tested during videofluoroscopy, will reduce or eliminate aspiration, (b) the natural history of the underlying disease, and (c) the patient's cognitive ability (9,10,158).

4. After exclusion of structural lesions and underlying treatable diseases, and having established the safety of oral feeding, consider specific "local" therapy. The therapeutic options are dietary modification, swallow therapy, surgery, or a combination of all three.

Surgical Options

Although the data supporting the efficacy of cricopharyngeal myotomy for structural cricopharyngeal disorders is strong, the outcome following myotomy for neuromyogenic dysphagia is far less certain. There are no controlled trials of cricopharyngeal myotomy in neurogenic dysphagia, but the available evidence suggests an overall response rate of approximately 60% with an operative mortality rate of 1% to 2% (53,273). Indicators that may predict a favorable outcome from myotomy include intact swallow initiation, "adequate" lingual and pharyngeal propulsive forces, radiographic or manometric evidence of increased outflow resistance at the UES, and a relatively good prognosis for the underlying neurologic disease (54,274). However, myotomy has not been proven conclusively to influence outcome in neurogenic dysphagia nor have any preoperative variables been proven to predict response to myotomy. Hence, the decision to undertake myotomy remains largely empirical at present.

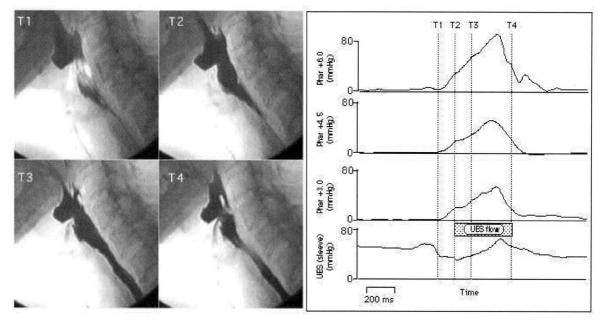

FIGURE 10.6. Failed upper esophageal sphincter (UES) relaxation demonstrated by simultaneous videoradiographs and manometry traces in a patient with moderately severe dysphagia due to Parkinson's disease. UES opening is present but extent of sphincter opening is subnormal. Some bolus flow across the sphincter is seen (*black horizontal bar*) between T2 and T4. Pressure within the UES, measured by a sleeve sensor (*bottom trace*), does not go below 35 mm Hg during the swallow. The pharyngeal pressure waves are synchronous in onset as a result of a lack of pharyngeal wall closure; the radiographic correlate of which is an absence of a bolus tail (T2 to T4). Functionally, this swallow is moderately impaired with reduced UES opening, a moderately increased pharyngeal postswallow residual of contrast (T4), and laryngeal penetration (T3) without aspiration. (From Williams RB, Wallace KL, Ali GN, et al. Biomechanics of failed deglutitive upper esophageal sphincter [UES] relaxation in patients with neurogenic dysphagia. *Am J Physiol* 2002;283:G16–G26, with permission.)

Most surgical procedures in the dysphagic patient aim to reduce or eliminate aspiration (275,276). The more conservative procedures (laryngeal suspension, vocal fold augmentation or medialization, and epiglottoplasty) preserve voice. The more destructive procedures, which achieve tracheoesophageal separation, render the patient unable to phonate. Such procedures include glottic closure, tracheoesophageal diversion, laryngotracheal separation, and total laryngectomy. There are virtually no reliable efficacy data upon which to base recommendations and indications for such therapies.

Botulinum Toxin Injection

Botox injection, either endoscopically or transcutaneously, has been reported in small case series to be of benefit (275,277–279). Whereas these studies attempted to target cricopharyngeal disorders, optimal identification of failed cricopharyngeal relaxation (using EMG or even manometry) was not adopted in those studies. Diffusion of the toxin to adjacent muscles may worsen dysphagia, and vocal cord dysfunction has also been observed following Botox injection. More systematic evaluation of safety and efficacy is needed before this therapy might be used to target particular dysphagic populations.

Dietary Modification and Swallow Therapy

Current swallow therapy strategies include dietary modification, manipulation of swallowing posture, or adjustment of swallowing technique. Modifications of swallowing technique are intended to strengthen weak oropharyngeal muscle groups, thereby improving their speed and range of movement, or to selectively modify the mechanics of the swallow to facilitate bolus flow and minimize aspiration. In applying swallow therapies, the speech-language pathologist uses videofluoroscopy to define the relevant mechanism of dysfunction and examines the acute effects of therapeutic strategies designed to eliminate or compensate for that dysfunction (31). Simple dietary modification has been shown in a single randomized, controlled trial to reduce the risk of aspiration pneumonia and should be instituted if an aspiration risk is apparent (161). Most of the studies in this field have focused on poststroke dysphagia. Reasonable data support the biological plausibility of the remaining swallow strategies, but the limited controlled efficacy data are inconclusive (11,280). There is only one published randomized, controlled trial of swallow therapy (281). Twelve months after acute stroke, 15% of that study population developed one or more of the study endpoints, thus failing to show benefit for intensive swallow rehabilitation. On the other hand, swallow therapy has not been proven to be ineffective. Based on the demonstration of biological plausibility for specific therapeutic techniques, the consistency of the low-grade evidence suggesting efficacy, the relatively low cost, and the absence of either risk or any better alternative in many instances, it is appropriate to institute swallow therapy under the supervision of a speech-language pathologist. Large-scale controlled trials are necessary to clarify the appropriateness of all current treatment strategies in neurogenic oropharyngeal dysphagia.

Percutaneous Endoscopic Gastrostomy Tube Placement

Percutaneous endoscopic gastrostomy (PEG) tube and nasogastric tubes are frequently used to feed stroke patients enterally to avoid aspiration. Four studies have compared the two techniques (282–284). Whereas PEG seems to be superior in terms of reliable delivery of prescribed calories, the PEG tube was not found to be superior to nasogastric tube in preventing aspiration in dysphagic patients following stroke. Indeed, feeding tubes have not yet been shown conclusively to reduce the risk of aspiration pneumonia, possibly because they provide no protection from bacteria within oral secretions and the feeding process itself can induce regurgitation (285). Although small numbers of subjects have been studied, PEG feeding may infer a lower case-fatality rate when compared with nasogastric feeding (280,284).

REFERENCES

1. Horner J, Massey EW, Riski JE, et al. Aspiration following stroke: clinical correlates and outcome. *Neurology* 1988;38: 1359–1362.
2. Young EC, Durant-Jones L. Developing a dysphagia program in an acute care hospital: a needs assessment. *Dysphagia* 1990; 5(3):159–165.
3. Barer DH. The natural history and functional consequence of dysphagia after hemisphere stroke. *J Neurol Neurosurg Psychiatry* 1989;52:236–241.
4. Gordon C, Hewer RL, Wade DT. Dysphagia in acute stroke. *BMJ* 1987;295:411–414.
5. Logemann JA, Blonsky ER, Boshes B. Dysphagia in Parkinsonism [Editorial]. *JAMA* 1975;231(1):69–70.
6. Horner J, Alberts MJ, Dawson DV, et al. Swallowing in Alzheimer's disease. *Alzheimer Dis Assoc Disord* 1994;8(3): 177–189.
7. Siebens H, Trupe E, Siebens A, et al. Correlates and consequences of eating dependency in institutionalized elderly. *J Am Geriatr Soc* 1986;34:192–198.
8. Groher ME. The prevalence of swallowing disorders in two teaching hospitals. *Dysphagia* 1986;1:3–6.
9. Smithard DG, O'Neill PA, Park C, et al. Complications and outcome after acute stroke: does dysphagia matter? [Erratum *Stroke* 1998;29(7):1480–1148]. *Stroke* 1996;27:1200–1204.
10. Smithard DG, O'Neill PA, England RE, et al. The natural history of dysphagia following a stroke. *Dysphagia* 1997;12(4): 188–193.
11. Cook IJ, Kahrilas PJ. American Gastroenterological Association technical review on management of oropharyngeal dysphagia. *Gastroenterology* 1999;116:455–478.
12. Logemann JA. *Evaluation and treatment of swallowing disorders.* San Diego: College Hill Press, 1983.
13. Polland WS, Bloomfield AL. Experimental referred pain from the gastrointestinal tract. Part I. The esophagus. *J Clin Invest* 1931;10(13):435–452.
14. Edwards D. Discriminatory value of symptoms in the differential diagnosis of dysphagia. *Clin Gastroenterol* 1976;5:49–57.
15. Wilcox CM, Alexander LN, Clark WS. Localization of an obstructing esophageal lesion. Is the patient accurate? *Dig Dis Sci* 1995;40(10):2192–2196.
16. Thompson W, Heaton K. Heartburn and globus on apparently healthy people. *CMA J* 1982;126:46–48.
17. Cook IJ. Globus—real or imagined? *Gullet* 1991;1:68–73.
18. Moser G, Vacariu-Granser G, Schneider C, et al. High incidence of esophageal motor disorder in consecutive patients with globus sensation. *Gastroenterology* 1991;101:1512–1521.
19. Schima W, Pokieser P, Schober E, et al. Globus sensation: value of static radiography combined with videofluoroscopy of the pharynx and oesophagus. *Clin Radiol* 1996;51(3):177–185.
20. Osterberg T, Landahl S, Hedegard M. Salivary flow, saliva, pH and buffering capacity in 70 year old men and women. *J Oral Rehabil* 1984;11:157.
21. Buchholz DW. Clinically probable brainstem stroke presenting primarily as dysphagia and nonvisualized by MRI. *Dysphagia* 1993;8(3):235–238.
22. Davies AE, Kidd D, Stone SP, MacMahon J. Pharyngeal sensation and gag reflex in healthy subjects. *Lancet* 1995;345: 487–488.
23. Leder SB. Gag reflex and dysphagia. *Head Neck* 1996;18(2): 138–141.
24. Leder SB. Videofluoroscopic evaluation of aspiration with visual examination of the gag reflex and velar movement. *Dysphagia* 1997;12(1):21–3.
25. Edwards LL, Pfeiffer RF, Quigley EMM, et al. Gastrointestinal symptoms in Parkinson's disease. *Mov Disord* 1991;6(2):151–156.
26. Leopold NA, Kagel MC. Pharyngo-esophageal dysphagia in Parkinson's disease. *Dysphagia* 1997;12:11–18.
27. Branski D, Levy J, Globus M, et al. Dysphagia as a primary manifestation of hyperthyroidism. *J Clin Gastroenterol* 1984;6 (5):437–440.
28. Splaingard ML, Hutchins B, Sulton LD, et al. Aspiration in rehabilitation patients: videofluoroscopy vs bedside clinical assessment. *Arch Phys Med Rehabil* 1988;69:637–640.
29. Logemann JA, Roa Pauloski B, Rademaker A, et al. Impact of the diagnostic procedure on outcome measures of swallowing rehabilitation in head and neck cancer patients. *Dysphagia* 1992;7:179–186.
30. Logemann JA. The role of the speech language pathologist in the management of dysphagia. *Otolaryngol Clin North Am* 1988;21(4):783–788.
31. Logemann JA. Role of the modified barium swallow in management of patients with dysphagia. *Otolaryngol Head Neck Surg* 1997;116(3):335–338.
32. Williams RB, Wallace KL, Ali GN, Cook IJ. Biomechanics of failed deglutitive upper esophageal sphincter (UES) relaxation in patients with neurogenic dysphagia. *Am J Physiol* 2002; 283:G16–G26.
33. Fenton JE, Hone S, Gormley P, et al. Hypopharyngeal tumours may be missed on flexible oesophagogastroscopy. *BMJ* 1995; 311:623–624.

34. Langmore SE, Schatz K, Olsen N. Endoscopic and videofluoroscopic evaluations of swallowing and aspiration. *Ann Otorhinolaryngol* 1991;100:678–681.

35. Murray J, Langmore SE, Ginsberg S, et al. The significance of accumulated oropharyngeal secretions and swallowing frequency in predicting aspiration. *Dysphagia* 1996;11:99–103.

36. Castell J, Dalton C, Castell D. Pharyngeal and upper esophageal sphincter manometry in humans. *Am J Physiol* 1990; 258:G173–G178.

37. Cook IJ. Cricopharyngeal function and dysfunction. *Dysphagia* 1993;8(3):244–251.

38. Olsson R, Castell JA, Castell DO, et al. Solid-state computerized manometry improves diagnostic yield in pharyngeal dysphagia: simultaneous videoradiography and manometry in dysphagia patients with normal barium swallows. *Abdom Imag* 1995;20(3):230–235.

39. Ali GN, Wallace KL, Schwartz R, et al. Mechanisms of oralpharyngeal dysphagia in patients with Parkinson's disease. *Gastroenterology* 1996;110:383–392.

40. Isberg A, Nilsson ME, Schiratzki H. Movement of the upper esophageal sphincter and a manometric device during deglutition, a cineradiographic investigation. *Acta Radiol Diagn* 1985; 26:381–388.

41. Kahrilas PJ, Clouse RE, Hogan WJ. American Gastroenterological Association technical review on the clinical use of esophageal manometry [Review]. *Gastroenterology* 1994;107(6): 1865–1884.

42. Sears VW, Castell JA, Castell DO. Radial and longitudinal asymmetry of human pharyngeal pressures during swallowing. *Gastroenterology* 1991;101:1559–1563.

43. Ergun GA, Kahrilas PJ, Logemann JA. Interpretation of pharyngeal manometric recordings: limitations and variability. *Dis Esoph* 1993;6:11–16.

44. Shaw DW, Cook IJ, Gabb M, et al. Influence of normal aging on oral-pharyngeal and upper esophageal sphincter function during swallowing. *Am J Physiol* 1995;268:G389–G396.

45. Shaker R, Lang I. Effect of aging on the deglutitive oral, pharyngeal, and esophageal motor function [Review]. *Dysphagia* 1994;9:221–228.

46. Meier-Ewart HK, van Herw MA, Gideon RM, et al. Effect of age on differences in upper esophageal sphincter and pharynx pressures between patients with dysphagia and control subjects. *Am J Gastroenterol* 2001;96(1):35–40.

47. McConnel FMS, Cerenko D, Hersh T, et al. Evaluation of pharyngeal dysphagia with manofluorography. *Dysphagia* 1988;2: 187–195.

48. Kahrilas PJ, Dodds WJ, Dent J, et al. Upper esophageal sphincter function during deglutition. *Gastroenterology* 1988;95:52–62.

49. Cook IJ, Dodds WJ, Dantas RO, et al. Opening mechanisms of the human upper esophageal sphincter. *Am J Physiol* 1989; 257:G748–G759.

50. Dantas RO, Cook IJ, Dodds WJ, et al. Biomechanics of cricopharyngeal bars. *Gastroenterology* 1990;99:1269–1274.

51. Cook IJ, Gabb M, Panagopoulos V, et al. Pharyngeal (Zenker's) diverticulum is a disorder of upper esophageal sphincter opening. *Gastroenterology* 1992;103:1229–1235.

52. Cook IJ, Wallace KL, Zagami AS, et al. Mechanisms of pharyngeal dysphagia in lateral medullary syndrome (LMS). *Gastroenterology* 1996;110(4):A650.

53. Taileffer R, Duranceau AC. Manometric and radionuclide assessment of pharyngeal emptying before and after cricopharyngeal myotomy in patients with oculopharyngeal dystrophy. *J Thorac Cardiovasc Surg* 1988;95:868–875.

54. Ali GN, Wallace KL, Laundl TM, et al. Predictors of outcome following cricopharyngeal disruption for pharyngeal dysphagia. *Dysphagia* 1997;12(3):133–139.

55. Mason RJ, Bremner CG, DeMeester TR, et al. Pharyngeal swallowing disorders: selection for and outcome after myotomy. *Ann Surg* 1998;228(4):598–608.

56. Hila A, Castell JA, Castell DO. Pharyngeal and upper esophageal sphincter manometry in the evaluation of dysphagia. *J Clin Gastroenterol* 2001;33(5):355–361.

57. Xue S, Katz PO, Castell JA, et al. Upper esophageal sphincter (UES) and pharyngeal manometry: which patients? *Gastroenterology* 2000;118(4):A410(abst).

58. Malhi-Chowla N, Achem SR, Stark ME, et al. Manometry of the upper esophageal sphincter and pharynx is not useful in unselected patients referred for esophageal testing. *Am J Gastroenterol* 2000;95(6):1417–1421.

59. Miller AJ. Neurophysiological basis of swallowing. *Dysphagia* 1986;1:91–100.

60. Shaker R, Ren J, Kern M, et al. Mechanisms of airway protection and upper esophageal sphincter opening during belching. *Am J Physiol* 1992;262:G621–G628.

61. Kahrilas P, Logemann J, Shezhang L, et al. Pharyngeal clearance during swallowing: a combined manometric and videofluoroscopic study. *Gastroenterology* 1992;103:128–136.

62. Kahrilas PJ, Lin S, Logemann JA, et al. Deglutitive tongue action: volume accommodation and bolus propulsion. *Gastroenterology* 1993;104(1):152–162.

63. Van Ruiswyk J, Cunningham C, Cerletty J. Obstructive manifestations of thyroid lymphoma. *Arch Intern Med* 1989;149(7): 1575–1577.

64. Close LG, Costin BS, Kim EE. Acute symptoms of the aerodigestive tract caused by rapidly enlarging thyroid neoplasms. *Otolaryngol Head Neck Surg* 1983;91(4):441–445.

65. Walther EK. Dysphagia after pharyngolaryngeal cancer surgery. Part 1: Pathophysiology of postsurgical deglutition. *Dysphagia* 1995;10:275–278.

66. Logemann JA, Pauloski BR, Rademaker AW, et al. Speech and swallow function after tonsil/base of tongue resection with primary closure. *J Speech Hear Res* 1993;36(5):918–926.

67. McConnel FM, Logemann JA, Rademaker AW, et al. Surgical variables affecting postoperative swallowing efficiency in oral cancer patients: a pilot study. *Laryngoscope* 1994;104(1):87–90.

68. Logemann JA, Gibbons P, Rademaker AW, et al. Mechanisms of recovery of swallow after supraglottic laryngectomy. *J Speech Hear Res* 1994;37(5):965–974.

69. Muller-Miny H, Eisele DW, Jones B. Dynamic radiographic imaging following total laryngectomy. *Head Neck* 1993;15(4): 342–347.

70. Welch RW, Luckmann K, Ricks PM, et al. Manometry of the normal upper esophageal sphincter and its alterations in laryngectomy. *J Clin Invest* 1979;63:1036–1040.

71. Stewart M, Johnston RA, Stewart I, et al. Swallowing performance following anterior cervical spine surgery. *Br J Neurosurg* 1995;9(5):605–609.

72. Buchholz DW. Oropharyngeal dysphagia due to iatrogenic neurological dysfunction [Review]. *Dysphagia* 1995;10(4): 248–254.

73. Ekberg O, Nylander G. Pharyngeal dysfunction after treatment for pharyngeal cancer with surgery and radiotherapy. *Gastrointest Radiol* 1983;8:97.

74. Gaze M, Wilson J, Gilmour H, et al. The effect of laryngeal irradiation on pharyngoesophageal motility. *Int J Rad Oncol Biol Phys* 1991;21:1315–1320.

75. Lazarus CL, Logemann JA, Pauloski BR, et al. Swallowing disorders in head and neck cancer patients treated with radiotherapy and adjuvant chemotherapy. *Laryngoscope* 1996;106: 1157–1166.

76. Shapiro BE, Rordorf G, Schwamm L, et al. Delayed radiation-induced bulbar palsy. *Neurology* 1996;46(6):1604–1606.

77. Ekberg O, Malmquist J, Lindgren S. Pharyngo-oesophageal webs in dysphageal patients. A radiologic and clinical investigation in 1134 patients. *ROFO: Fortschritte auf dem Gebiete der Rontgenstrahlen und der Nuklearmedizin* 1986;145(1):75–80.

78. Waldenstrom J, Kjellberg S. Roentgenologic diagnosis of sideropenic dysphagia (Plummer-Vinson syndrome). *Acta Radiol* 1939;20:618.

79. Chen TSN, Chen PSY. Rise and fall of the Plummer-Vinson syndrome [Review]. *J Gastroenterol Hepatol* 1994;9(6):654–658.

80. Chisolm M. The association between webs, iron, and post-cricoid carcinoma. *Postgrad Med J* 1974;50:215.

81. Seaman WB. Cineroentgenographic observations of the cricopharyngeus. *Am J Roentgenol* 1966;96:922–931.

82. Clements JL, Cox GW, Torres WE, et al. Cervical esophageal webs: a roentgen anatomic correlation. *Am J Roentgenol* 1974;121(2):221–231.

83. Ekberg O, Nylander B. Dysfunction of the cricopharyngeal muscle. *Radiology* 1982;143:481–486.

84. Curtis DJ, Cruess DF, Berg T. The cricopharyngeal muscle: a videorecording review. *Am J Roentgenol* 1984;142:497–500.

85. Jones B, Ravich WJ, Donner MW, et al. Pharyngoesophageal interrelationships: observations and working concepts. *Gastrointest Radiol* 1985;10:225–233.

86. Sokol EM, Heitmann P, Wolf BS, et al. Simultaneous cineradiographic and manometric study of the pharynx, hypopharynx, and cervical esophagus. *Gastroenterology* 1966;51:960–974.

87. Ekberg O. Dimension of the pharyngo-esophageal segment in dysfunction of the cricopharyngeal muscle. *Acta Radiolog Diagn* 1986;27(5):539–541.

88. Benedict EB, Sweet RH. Dysphagia due to hypertrophy of the cricopharyngeus muscle or hypopharyngeal bar. *N Engl J Med* 1955;253:1161–1162.

89. Watson WL, Bancroft FW. Hypertrophic cricopharyngeal stenosis. *Surg Gynecol Obstet* 1936;62:621–624.

90. Cruse JP, Edwards DAW, Smith JF, et al. The pathology of cricopharyngeal dysphagia. *Histopathology* 1979;3:223–232.

91. Cook IJ, Blumbergs P, Cash K, et al. Structural abnormalities of the cricopharyngeus muscle in patients with pharyngeal (Zenker's) diverticulum. *J Gastroenterol Hepatol* 1992;7:556–562.

92. Shapiro J, Martin S, DeGirolami U, et al. Inflammatory myopathy causing pharyngeal dysphagia: a new entity. *Ann Otol Rhinol Laryngol* 1996;105(5):331–335.

93. Horvath OP, Zombari J, Halmos L, et al. Pharyngeal dysphagia caused by isolated myogen dystrophy of musculus cricopharyngeus. *Acta Chir Hung* 1998;37(1-2):51–58.

94. Bachmann G, Streppel M, Krug B, et al. Cricopharyngeal muscle hypertrophy associated with florid myositis. *Dysphagia* 2001;16(4):244–248.

95. Georgalas C, Baer ST. Pharyngeal pouch and polymyositis: association and implications for aetiology of Zenker's diverticulum. *J Laryngol Otol* 2000;114(10):805–807.

96. Williams RB, Grehan MJ, Hersch M, et al. Biomechanics, diagnosis, and treatment outcome in inflammatory myopathy presenting as oropharyngeal dysphagia. *Gut* 2002 (*in press*).

97. Bonavina L, Khan NA, DeMeester TR. Pharyngoesophageal dysfunctions. The role of cricopharyngeal myotomy. *Arch Surg* 1985;120:541–549.

98. Shaw DW, Cook IJ, Jamieson GG, et al. Influence of surgery on deglutitive upper esophageal sphincter mechanics in Zenker's diverticulum. *Gut* 1996;38:806–811.

99. Lindgren S, Ekberg O. Cricopharyngeal myotomy in the treatment of dysphagia. *Clin Otolaryngol* 1990;15(3):221–227.

100. Jamieson GG, Duranceau AC, Payne WS. Pharyngo-oesophageal diverticulum. In: Jamieson GG, ed. *Surgery of the oesophagus.* Edinburgh: Churchill Livingstone Press, 1988:435–443.

101. Webb WA, McDaniel L, Jones L. Endoscopic evaluation of dysphagia in two hundred and ninety-three patients with benign disease. *Surg Gynecol Obstet* 1984;158(2):152–156.

102. Lindgren S. Endoscopic dilatation and surgical myectomy of symptomatic cervical esophageal webs. *Dysphagia* 1991;6:235–238.

103. Solt J, Bajor J, Moizs M, et al. Primary cricopharyngeal dysfunction: treatment with balloon catheter dilatation. *Gastrointest Endosc* 2001;54(6):767–771.

104. Bachman AL, Seaman WB, Macken KL. Lateral pharyngeal diverticula. *Radiology* 1968;91:774–782.

105. Liston SL. Lateral pharyngeal diverticula. *Otolaryngol Head Neck Surg* 1985;93:582–585.

106. Mantoni M, Ostri B. Acquired lateral pharyngeal diverticulum. *J Laryngol Otol* 1987;101:1092–1094.

107. Pace-Balzan A, Habashi SMZ, Nassar WY. View from within: radiology in focus. Lateral pharyngeal diverticulum. *J Laryngol Otol* 1991;105:793–795.

108. Zenker FA, von Ziemssen H. Dilatations of the esophagus. In: *Cyclopaedia of the practice of medicine.* London: Low, Marston, Searle and Rivington, 1878:46–68.

109. Ardran GM, Kemp FH, Lund WS. The aetiology of the posterior pharyngeal diverticulum: a cineradiographic study. *J Laryngol Otol* 1964;78:333–349.

110. Lichter I. Motor disorder in pharyngoesophageal pouch. *J Thorac Cardiovasc Surg* 1978;76:272–275.

111. Ellis FH, Schlegal JF, Lynch VP, et al. Cricopharyngeal myotomy for pharyngoesophageal diverticulum. *Ann Surg* 1969;170:340–349.

112. Hunt PS, Connell AM, Smiley TB. The cricopharyngeal sphincter in gastric reflux. *Gut* 1970;11:303–306.

113. Hurwitz AL, Nelson JA, Haddad JK. Oropharyngeal dysphagia: manometric and cine-esophagographic findings. *Am J Dig Dis* 1975;20:313–324.

114. Wilson CP. Pharyngeal diverticula, their cause and treatment. *J Laryngol Otol* 1962;76:151–180.

115. Knuff TE, Benjamin SB, Castell DO. Pharyngoesophageal (Zenker's) diverticulum: a reappraisal. *Gastroenterology* 1982;82:734–736.

116. Jackson C, Shallow TA. Diverticula of esophagus, pulsion, traction, malignant and congenital. *Ann Surg* 1926;83:1–19.

117. Siefert, A. Zur Behardlung beginnender hypopharynx-diverykel. *J Laryngol Rhinol Otol* 1932;23:256–262.

118. Lahey FH. Pharyngo-esophageal diverticulum: its management and complications. *Ann Surg* 1946;124:617–636.

119. Negus VE. The etiology of pharyngeal diverticula. *Johns Hopkins Hosp Bull* 1957;100:209–223.

120. Gullane PJ, Willett JM, Heenaman H, et al. Zenker's diverticulum. *Arch Otolaryngol* 1983;12:53–57.

121. Payne SW, King RM. Pharyngo-esophageal (Zenker's) diverticulum. *Surg Clin North Am* 1983;63:815–824.

122. Butcher RB, Larabee WF. Surgical treatment of hypopharyngeal (Zenker's) diverticulum. *Arch Otolaryngol* 1989;105:254–257.

123. Skinner DB, Altorki N, Ferguson M, et al. Zenker's diverticulum: clinical features and surgical management. *Dis Esoph* 1988;1(1):19–22.

124. Konowitz PM, Biller HF. Diverticulopexy and cricopharyngeal myotomy: treatment for the high risk patient with a pharyngoesophageal (Zenker's) diverticulum. *Otolaryngol Head Neck Surg* 1989;100:146–153.

125. Bingham DC. Cricopharyngeal achalasia. *Can Med Assoc J* 1963;89:1071–1073.

126. Harrison MS. The aetiology, diagnosis and surgical treatment of pharyngeal diverticula. *J Laryngol* 1958;72:523–534.

127. Ellis FH, Crozier RE. Cervical esophageal dysphagia. Indications for and results of cricopharyngeal myotomy. *Ann Surg* 1981;194(3):279–289.

128. Ekberg O, Lindgren S. Effect of cricopharyngeal myotomy on pharyngoesophageal function: pre and postoperative cineradiographic findings. *Gastrointest Radiol* 1987;12:1–6.

129. Duranceau A, Rheault MJ, Jamieson GG. Physiological response to cricopharyngeal myotomy and diverticulum suspension. *Surgery* 1983;94:655–662.

130. Lerut T, Van Raemdonck D, Guelinckx P. Pharyngo-oesophageal diverticulum (Zenker's). Clinical therapeutic and morphological aspects. *Acta Gastroenterol Belg* 1990;53: 330–337.

131. Barthlen W, Feussner H, Hannig C, et al. Surgical therapy of Zenker's diverticulum: low risk and high efficiency. *Dysphagia* 1990;5:13–19.

132. Witterick IJ, Gullane PJ, Yeung E. Outcome analysis of Zenker's diverticulectomy and cricopharyngeal myotomy. *Head Neck* 1995;17(5):382–388.

133. Dohlman G, Mattson O. The endoscopic operation for hyopharyngeal diverticula. *Arch Otolaryngol* 1960;71:744–752.

134. Mulder CJJ, den Hartog G, Robijn RJ, et al. Flexible endoscopic treatment of Zenker's diverticulum: a new approach. *Endoscopy* 1995;27:438–442.

135. Wouters B, van Overbeek JJ. Endoscopic treatment of the hypopharyngeal (Zenker's) diverticulum [see comments]. *Hepatogastroenterology* 1992;39(2):105–108.

136. Peracchia A, Bonavina L, Narne S, et al. Minimally invasive surgery for Zenker diverticulum: analysis of results in 95 consecutive patients. *Arch Surg* 1998;133(7):695–700.

137. Narne S, Cutrone C, Bonavina L, et al. Endoscopic diverticulotomy for the treatment of Zenker's diverticulum: results in 102 patients with staple-assisted endoscopy. *Ann Otol Rhinol Laryngol* 1999;108(8):810–815.

138. Baldwin DL, Toma AG. Endoscopic stapled diverticulotomy: a real advance in the treatment of hypopharyngeal diverticulum. *Clin Otolaryngol Allied Sci* 1998;23(3):244–247.

139. Cook RD, Huang PC, Richstmeier WJ, et al. Endoscopic staple-assisted esophagodiverticulostomy: an excellent treatment of choice for Zenker's diverticulum. *Laryngoscope* 2000;110 (12):2020–2025.

140. Jaramillo MJ, McLay KA, McAteer D. Long-term clinico-radiological assessment of endoscopic stapling of pharyngeal pouch: a series of cases. *J Laryngol Otol* 2001;115(6):462–466.

141. Bone RC, Nahum AM, Harris AS. Evaluation and correlation of dysphagia-producing cervical osteophytosis. *Laryngoscope* 1974;84:2045–2050.

142. Saffouri MH, Ward PH. Surgical correction of dysphagia die to cervical osteophytes. *Ann Otol* 1974;83:65–70.

143. Stuart D. Dysphagia due to cervical osteophytes. *Int Orthop* 1989;13(2):95–99.

144. Krause P, Castro WH. Cervical hyperostosis: a rare cause of dysphagia. Case description and bibliographical survey. *Eur Spine J* 1994;3(1):56–58.

145. Kodama M, Sawada H, Udaka F, et al. Dysphagia caused by an anterior cervical osteophyte: case report. *Neuroradiology* 1995;37(1):58–59.

146. Bridger AG, Stening WA, Bridger GP. Cervical osteophytes: an unusual cause of dysphagia. *Aust N Z J Surg* 1996;66(4): 261–264.

147. Sobol SM, Rigual NR. Anterolateral extrapharyngeal approach for cervical osteophyte induced dysphagia. *Ann Otol Rhinol Laryngol* 1984;93:498–503.

148. Papandoulos SM, Chen JC, Fledenzer JA, et al. Anterior cervical osteophytes as a cause of progressive dysphagia. *Acta Neurochirurgica* 1989;101:63–65.

149. Halama AR. Surgical treatment of oropharyngeal swallowing disorders. *Acta Otorhinolaryngol Belg* 1994;48(2):217–227.

150. Welsh LW, Welsh JJ, Chinnici JC. Dysphagia due to cervical spine injury. *Ann Otol Rhinol Laryngol* 1987;96:112–115.

151. Veis S, Logemann J. Swallowing disorders in persons with cerebrovascular accident. *Arch Phys Med Rehabil* 1985;66:372–375.

152. Horner J, Massey E. Silent aspiration following stroke. *Neurology* 1988;38:317–319.

153. Gresham SL. Clinical assessment and management of swallowing difficulties after stroke. *Med J Aust* 1990;153(7):397–399.

154. Zald DH, Pardo JV. The functional neuroanatomy of voluntary swallowing [see comments]. *Ann Neurol* 1999;46(3):281–286.

155. Hamdy S, Rothwell JC, Brooks DJ, et al. Identification of the cerebral loci processing human swallowing with H2 15 O PET activation. The American Physiology Society, 1999:1917–1926.

156. Hamdy S, Aziz Q, Rothwell JC, et al. The cortical topography of human swallowing musculature in health and disease [see comments]. *Nat Med* 1996;2(11):1217–1224.

157. Hamdy S, Aziz Q, Rothwell JC, et al. Recovery of swallowing after dysphagic stroke relates to functional reorganization in the intact motor cortex. *Gastroenterology* 1998;115(5):1104–1112.

158. Schmidt J, Holas M, Halvorson K, et al. Videofluoroscopic evidence of aspiration predicts pneumonia and death but not dehydration following stroke. *Dysphagia* 1994;9(1):7–11.

159. Anonymous. Diagnosis and treatment of swallowing disorders (dysphagia) in acute-care stroke patients. Rockville, MD: Agency for Health Care Policy and Research, March 1999. Report no. 99-E023.

160. Linden P, Siebens A. Dysphagia: predicting laryngeal penetration. *Arch Phys Med Rehabil* 1983;64:281–284.

161. Groher ME. Bolus management and aspiration pneumonia in patients with pseudobulbar dysphagia. *Dysphagia* 1987;1: 215–216.

162. Aviv JE, Sacco RL, Thomson J, et al. Silent laryngopharyngeal sensory deficits after stroke. *Ann Otol Rhinol Laryngol* 1997;106(2):87–93.

163. Mann G, Hankey GJ, Cameron D. Swallowing function after stroke. Prognosis and prognostic factors at six months. *Stroke* 2000;30:744–748.

164. Daniels SK, Foundas AL. Lesion localization in acute stroke patients with risk of aspiration. *J Neuroimaging* 1999;9(2): 91–98.

165. Daniels SK, Brailey K, Priestly DH, et al. Aspiration in patients with acute stroke. *Arch Phys Med Rehab* 1998;79(1):14–19.

166. Doggett DL, Tappe KA, Mitchell MD, et al. Prevention of pneumonia in elderly stroke patients by systematic diagnosis and treatment of dysphagia: an evidence-based comprehensive analysis of the literature. *Dysphagia* 2001;16(4):279–295.

167. Bushmann M, Dobmeyer SM, Leeker L, et al. Swallowing abnormalities and their response to treatment in Parkinson's disease. *Neurology* 1989;39:1309–1314.

168. Chen MYM, Peele VN, Donati D, et al. Clinical and videofluoroscopic evaluation of swallowing in 41 patients with neurologic disease. *Gastrointest Radiol* 1992;17:95–98.

169. Edwards LL, Eamonn BS, Quigley MM, et al. Gastrointestinal dysfunction in Parkinson's disease: frequency and pathophysiology. *Neurology* 1992;42:726–732.

170. Muller J, Wenning GK, Verny M, et al. Progression of dysarthria and dysphagia in postmortem-confirmed parkinsonian disorders. *Arch Neurol* 2001;58(2):259–264.

171. Hartelius L, Svensson P. Speech and swallowing symptoms associated with Parkinson's disease and multiple sclerosis: a survey. *Folia Phoniatr Logop* 1994;46(1):9–17.

172. Kuhlemeier KV. Epidemiology and dysphagia [Review]. *Dysphagia* 1994;9:209–217.

173. Johnston BT, Li Q, Castell JA, et al. Swallowing and esophageal

function in Parkinson's disease. *Am J Gastroenterol* 1995;90: 1741–1746.

174. Edwards LL, Quigley EM, Harned RK, et al. Characterization of swallowing and defecation in Parkinson's disease. *Am J Gastroenterol* 1994;89(1):15–25.

175. Li Q, Gideon MR, Castell JA, et al. Manometric evaluation of Sinemet effect on esophageal function in Parkinson's disease. *Gastroenterology* 1994;106:A530.

176. Robbins J, Logemann J, Kirshner H. Swallowing and speech production in Parkinson's disease. *Ann Neurol* 1986;19:283–287.

177. Leopold NA, Kagel MC. Prepharyngeal dysphagia in Parkinson's disease. *Dysphagia* 1996;11(1):14–22.

178. Bird MR, Woodward MC, Gibson EM, et al. Asymptomatic swallowing disorders in elderly patients with Parkinson's disease: a description of findings on clinical examination and videofluoroscopy in sixteen patients. *Age Ageing* 1994;23(3):251–254.

179. Weber J, Roman C, Hannequin D, et al. Esophageal manometry in patients with unilateral hemispheric cerebrovascular accidents or idiopathic Parkinsonism. *J Gastrointestinal Motility* 1991; 3(2):98–106.

180. Born LJ, Harned RH, Rikkers LF, et al. Cricopharyngeal dysfunction in Parkinson's disease: role in dysphagia and response to myotomy. *Mov Disord* 1996;11(1):53–58.

181. Calne DB, Shaw DG, Spiers AS, et al. Swallowing in Parkinsonism. *Br J Radiol* 1970;43(511):456–457.

182. Tison F, Wiart L, Guatterie M, et al. Effects of central dopaminergic stimulation by apomorphine on swallowing disorders in Parkinson's disease. *Mov Disord* 1996;11(6):729–732.

183. Hunter PC, Crameri J, Austin S, et al. Response of parkinsonian swallowing dysfunction to dopaminergic stimulation. *J Neurol Neurosurg Psychiatr* 1997;63:579–583.

184. Thomas M, Haigh RA. Dysphagia, a reversible cause not to be forgotten. *Postgrad Med J* 1995;71(832):94–95.

185. Fonda D, Schwarz J, Clinnick S. Parkinsonian medication one hour before meals improves symptomatic swallowing: a case study. *Dysphagia* 1995;10:165–166.

186. El-Sharkawi AL, Ramig L, Logemann JA, et al. Voice treatment (LSVT) and swallowing in Parkinson's disease. *Mov Disord* 1998;13[Suppl]:121.

187. Deane KH, Whurr R, Clarke CE, et al. *Non-pharmacological therapies for dysphagia in Parkinson's disease (Cochrane review).* Oxford: Update Software, 2002.

188. Mayberry JF, Atkinson M. Swallowing problems in patients with motor neuron disease. *J Clin Gastroenterol* 1986;8(3 Pt 1):233–234.

189. Tandan R, Bradley WG. Amyotrophic lateral sclerosis: part I. Clinical features, pathology, and ethical issues in management. *Ann Neurol* 1985;18:271–280.

190. Bowman K, Meurman T. Prognosis of amyotrophic lateral sclerosis. *Acta Neurol Scand* 1967;43:489–498.

191. Mulder De. *The diagnosis and treatment of amyotrophic lateral sclerosis.* Boston: Houghton Mifflin, 1980.

192. Bosma J, Brodie D. Disabilities of the pharynx in amyotrophic lateral sclerosis as demonstrated by cineradiography. *Radiology* 1969;92:97.

193. MacDougall G, Wilson JA, Pryde A, et al. Analysis of the pharyngoesophageal pressure profile in amyotrophic lateral sclerosis. *Otolaryngol Head Neck Surg* 1995;112(2):258–261.

194. Ertekin C, Aydogdu I, Yuceyar N, et al. Pathophysiological mechanisms of oropharyngeal dysphagia in amyotrophic lateral sclerosis. *Brain* 2000;123(Pt 1):125–140.

195. Borasio GD, Voltz R, Miller RG. Palliative care in amyotrophic lateral sclerosis. *Neurol Clin* 2001;19(4):829–847.

196. Strand EA, Miller RM, Yorkston KM, et al. Management of oral-pharyngeal dysphagia symptoms in amyotrophic lateral sclerosis. *Dysphagia* 1996;11(2):129–139.

197. Mazzini L, Corra T, Zaccala M, et al. Percutaneous endoscopic gastrostomy and enteral nutrition in amyotrophic lateral sclerosis. *J Neurol* 1995;242:695–698.

198. Chio A, Finocchiaro E, Meineri P, et al. Safety and factors related to survival after percutaneous endoscopic gastrostomy in ALS. ALS Percutaneous Endoscopic Gastrostomy Study Group. *Neurology* 1999;53(5):1123–1125.

199. Gelinas DF. Patient and caregiver communications and decisions. *Neurology* 1997;48[Suppl]:S9–S14.

200. Bhatia KP, Munchau A, Brown P. Botulinum toxin is a useful treatment in excessive drooling in saliva [letter]. *J Neurol Neurosurg Psychiatry* 1999;67(5):697.

201. Tan EK, Lo YL, Seah A, et al. Recurrent jaw dislocation after botulinum toxin treatment for sialorrhoea in amyotrophic lateral sclerosis. *J Neurol Sci* 2001;190(1-2):95–97.

202. Winterholler MG, Erbguth FJ, Wolf S, et al. Botulinum toxin for the treatment of sialorrhoea in ALS: serious side effects of a transductal approach. *J Neurol Neurosurg Psychiatry* 2001;70(3): 417–418.

203. Lueck W, Calligan J, Bosma JF. Persistent sequelae of bulbar poliomyelitis. *J Pediatr* 1952;41:549.

204. Baker AB, Matzke HA, Brown JR. Poliomyelitis III. Bulbar poliomyelitis; a study of medullary function. *Arch Neurol Psychiatry* 1950;62:257.

205. Bosma JF. Studies of the disabilities of the pharynx resultant from poliomyelitis. *Ann Otol Rhinol Laryngol* 1953;64:529.

206. Dalakas M, Elder G, Hallet M, et al. A long term follow-up study of patients with post-poliomyelitis neuromuscular symptoms. *N Engl J Med* 1986;314:954–963.

207. Buchholz D. Dysphagia in post-polio patients. *Birth Defects* 1987;23(4):55.

208. Silbergleit AK, Waring WP, Sullivan MJ, et al. Evaluation, treatment, and follow-up results of post polio patients with dysphagia. *Otolaryngol Head Neck Surg* 1991;104(3):333–338.

209. Coelho CA, Ferranti R. Incidence and nature of dysphagia in polio survivors. *Arch Phys Med Rehab* 1991;72(13):1071–1075.

210. Sonies BC, Dalakas MC. Dysphagia in patients with the post polio syndrome. *N Engl J Med* 1991;324:1162–1167.

211. Jones B, Buchholz DW, Ravich WJ, et al. Swallowing dysfunction in the postpolio syndrome: a cinefluorographic study. *Am J Roentgenol* 1992;158:283–286.

212. Ivanyi B, Phoa SS, de Visser M. Dysphagia in postpolio patients: a videofluorographic follow-up study. *Dysphagia* 1994;9(2):96–98.

213. Osserman KE, Genkins G. Studies in myasthenia gravis: review of a 20 year experience in over 1200 patients. *Mt Sinai J Med* 1971;38(6):497–537.

214. Dumitru D. *Electrodiagnostic medicine.* Philadelphia: Hanley and Belfus, 1995.

215. Viets HR. Diagnosis of myasthenia gravis in patients with dysphagia. *JAMA* 1947;134(12):987–992.

216. Grob D, Brunner NG, Namba T. The natural course of myasthenia gravis and effect of therapeutic measures. *Ann N Y Acad Sci* 1981;377:652–669.

217. Sanders DB, Howard JF. Disorders of neuromuscular transmission. In: Bradley WG, Daroff RB, Fenichel GM, et al, eds. *Neurology in clinical practice*, first ed. Massachusetts: Butterworth, Heinemann, 1991:1819–1842.

218. Kluin KJ, Bromberg MB, Feldman EL, et al. Dysphagia in elderly men with myasthenia gravis. *J Neurol Sci* 1996;138(1-2):49–52.

219. Simpson JA. Myasthenia gravis and myasthenic syndromes. In: Walton JN, ed. *Disorders of voluntary muscle*, fourth ed. London: Churchill Livingstone, 1981:585–624.

220. Newson-Davis J. Myasthenia gravis and related syndromes. In: Walton J, Karpati G, Hilton-Jones D, eds. *Disorders of voluntary*

muscle, sixth ed. Edinburgh: Churchill Livingstone, 1994:761–780.

221. Oh SJ, Kim DE, Kuruoglu R, et al. Diagnostic sensitivity of the laboratory tests in myasthenia gravis. *Muscle Nerve* 1992;15: 720–724.

222. Murray JP. Deglutition in myasthenia gravis. *Br J Radiol* 1962; 35:43–52.

223. Dalakas MC. Polymyositis, dermatomyositis and inclusion body myositis. *N Engl J Med* 1991;325:1487–1498.

224. Tymms KE, Webb J. Dermatopolymyositis and other connective tissue diseases: a review of 105 cases. *J Rheumatol* 1985;12: 1140–1148.

225. Hietaharju A, Jaaskelainen S, Kalimo H, et al. Peripheral neuromuscular manifestations in systemic sclerosis (scleroderma). *Muscle Nerve* 1993;16(11):1204–1212.

226. Johnson ER, McKenzie SW. Kinematic pharyngeal transit times in myopathy: evaluation for dysphagia. *Dysphagia* 1993;8:35–40.

227. Porubsky ES, Murray JP, Pratt LL. Cricopharyngeal achalasia in dermatomyositis. *Arch Otolaryngol* 1973;78:428–429.

228. Dietz F, Logeman JA, Sahgal V, et al. Cricopharyngeal muscle dysfunction in the differential diagnosis of dysphagia in polymyositis. *Arthritis Rheum* 1980;23(4):491–495.

229. Verma A, Bradley WG, Adesina AM, et al. Inclusion body myositis with cricopharyngeus muscle involvement and severe dysphagia. *Muscle Nerve* 1991;14:470–473.

230. Kilman WJ, Goyal RK. Disorders of pharyngeal and upper esophageal sphincter motor function. *Arch Intern Med* 1976; 136:592–601.

231. Scobey MW. Secondary motility disorders. In: Castell DO, Richter JE, Dalton CB, eds. *Esophageal motility testing*. Amsterdam: Elsevier, 1987:163.

232. Dalakas MC, Illa I, Dambrosia JM, et al. A controlled trial of high dose intravenous immune globulin infusions as treatment of dermatomyositis. *N Engl J Med* 1993;329:1993–2000.

233. Cherin P. Treatment of inclusion body myositis. *Curr Opin Rheumatol* 1999;11:456–461.

234. Dalakas MC, Sonies B, Dambrosia J, et al. Treatment of inclusion-body myositis with IVIG: a double-blind, placebo-controlled study [see comments]. *Neurology* 1997;48(3):712–716.

235. Darrow DH, Hoffman GT, Barnes GJ, et al. Management of dysphagia in inclusion body myositis. *Arch Otolaryngol Head Neck Surg* 1992;118:313–317.

236. Walton J, Karpati G, Hilton-Jones D. *Disorders of voluntary muscle*, sixth ed. Edinburgh: Churchill Livingstone, 1994.

237. Ming RH, Dreosti LM, Tim LO, et al. Thyrotoxicosis presenting as dysphagia. A case report. *South Afr Med J* 1982;61 (15):554.

238. Sweatman MC, Chambers L. Disordered oesophageal motility in thyrotoxic myopathy. Postgrad Med J 1985;61:619–620.

239. Ramsay ID. Thyrotoxic muscle disease. *Postgrad Med J* 1968; 44:385.

240. Taylor EW. Progressive vagus-glossopharyngeal paralysis with ptosis. *J Nerv Ment Dis* 1915;42:129.

241. Victor M, Hayes R, Adams RD. Oculopharyngeal muscular dystrophy: a familial disease of late life characterized by dysphagia and progressive ptosis of the eyelids. *N Engl J Med* 1962;267:1267–1272.

242. Dobrowski JM, Zajtchuk JT, LaPiana FG, et al. Oculopharyngeal muscular dystrophy: Clinical and histopathologic correlations. *Otolaryngol Head Neck Surg* 1986;9:131–142.

243. Blumbergs PC, Chin D, Burrows D, et al. Oculopharyngeal dystrophy: clinicopathologicical study of an Australian family. *Clin Exp Neurol* 1982;19:102–109.

244. Salvesen R, Brautaset NJ. Oculopharyngeal muscular dystrophy in Norway. Survey of a large Norwegian family. *Acta Neurol Scand* 1996;93(4):281–285.

245. Johnson CC, Kuwabara T. Oculopharyngeal muscular dystrophy. *Am J Ophthalmol* 1974;77:872–879.

246. Pauzner R, Blatt I, Mouallem M, et al. Mitochondrial abnormalities in oculopharyngeal muscular dystrophy [see comments]. *Muscle Nerve* 1991;14(10):947–952.

247. Pratt MF, Meyers PK. Oculopharyngeal muscular dystrophy: recent ultrastructural evidence for mitochondrial abnormalities. *Laryngoscope* 1986;96(4):368–373.

248. Duranceau A, Forand MD, Fateux JP. Surgery in oculopharyngeal muscular dystrophy. *Am J Surg* 1980;139:33–39.

249. Duranceau CA, Letendre J, Clermont RJ, et al. Oropharyngeal dysphagia in patients with oculopharyngeal muscular dystrophy. *Can J Surg* 1978;21(4):326–329.

250. Castell JA, Castell DO, Duranceau A. Pharyngeal and upper esophageal sphincter (UES) manometric characteristics of patients with oculopharyngeal muscular dystrophy (OPMD). *Gastroenterology* 1991;100(5):A39.

251. Castell JA, Castell DO, Duranceau CA, et al. Manometric characteristics of the pharynx, upper esophageal sphincter, esophagus, and lower esophageal sphincter in patients with oculopharyngeal muscular dystrophy. *Dysphagia* 1995;10:22–26.

252. Tiomny E, Khilkevic O, Korczyn AD, et al. Esophageal smooth muscle dysfunction in oculopharyngeal muscular dystrophy. *Dig Dis Sci* 1996;41(7):1350–1354.

253. Duranceau A, Lafontaine ER, Taillefer R, et al. Oropharyngeal dysphagia and operations on the upper esophageal sphincter. *Surg Annu* 1987;19:317–362.

254. Miller LG, Janovic J. Metoclopramide-induced movement disorders. *Arch Intern Med* 1989;149:2486.

255. Gregory RP, Smith PT, Rudge P. Tardive dyskinesia presenting as severe dysphagia. *J Neurol Neurosurg Psychiatry* 1992;55 (12):1203–1204.

256. Hayashi T, Nishikawa T, Koga I, et al. Life-threatening dysphagia following prolonged neuroleptic therapy. *Clin Neuropharmacol* 1997;20(1):77–81.

257. Bashford G, Bradd P. Drug-induced Parkinsonism associated with dysphagia and aspiration: a brief report. *J Geriatr Psychiatry Neurol* 1996;9(3):133–135.

258. Leopold NA. Dysphagia in drug-induced parkinsonism: a case report. *Dysphagia* 1996;11(2):151–153.

259. Wyllie E, Wyllie R, Cruse RP, et al. The mechanism of nitrazepam-induced drooling and aspiration. *N Engl J Med* 1986;314(1):35–38.

260. Lim HC, Nigro MA, Beierwaltes P, et al. Nitrazepam-induced cricopharyngeal dysphagia, abnormal esophageal peristalsis and associated bronchospasm: probable cause of nitrazepam-related sudden death. *Brain Dev* 1992;14(5):309–314.

261. Buchholz D, Jones B, Neumann W, et al. Two cases of benzodiazepine induced pharyngeal dysphagia. Proceedings of the Dysphagia Research Society Conference, McLean, VA, 1994 (abst).

262. Borodic GE, Joseph M, Fay L, et al. Botulinum A toxin for the treatment of spasmodic torticollis: dysphagia and regional toxin spread. *Head Neck* 1990;12:392–398.

263. Comella CL, Tanner CM, DeFoor HL, et al. Dysphagia after botulinum toxin injections for spasmodic torticollis: clinical and radiologic findings. *Neurology* 1992;42(7):1307–1310.

264. Buchholz DW, Neumann S. The swallowing side effects of botulinum toxin type A injection in spasmodic dysphonia. *Dysphagia* 1997;12(1):59–60.

265. Masters CL, Dawkins RL, Zilko PJ, et al. Penicillamine-associated myasthenia gravis, antiacetylcholine receptor and antistriational antibodies. *Am J Med* 1977;63:689–694.

266. Miller CD, Oleshansky MA, Gibson KF, et al. Procainamide-induced myasthenia-like weakness and dysphagia. *Ther Drug Monit* 1993;15(3):251–254.

267. May EF, Calvert PC. Aggravation of myasthenia gravis by erythromycin. *Ann Neurol* 1990;28(4):577–579.

268. Doyle DR, McCurley TL, Sergent JS. Fatal polymositis in D-penicillamine treated rheumatoid arthritis. *Ann Intern Med* 1983;98:327–330.

269. Dalakas MC, Illa I, Pezeshkpour GH, et al. Mitochondrial myopathy caused by long term zidovudine therapy. *N Engl J Med* 1990;322:1098–2105.

270. Dalakas MC. Inflammatory and toxic myopathies. *Curr Opin Neurol Neurosurg* 1992;5:645–654.

271. Berbegal J, Lluch V, Morera J, et al. Dysphagia as the presentation of amiodarone-induced hyperthyroidism [Letter]. *Med Clin* 1993;100(11):437–438.

272. London SF, Gross KF, Ringel SP. Cholesterol-lowering agent myopathy (CLAM). *Neurology* 1991;41:1159–1160.

273. Poirier NC, Bonavina L, Taillefer R, et al. Cricopharyngeal myotomy for neurogenic oropharyngeal dysphagia. *J Thorac Cardiovas Surg* 1997;113(2):233–241.

274. St Guily JL, Zhang K-X, Perie S, et al. Improvement of dysphagia following cricopharyngeal myotomy in a group of elderly patients. *Ann Otol Rhinol Laryngol* 1995;104:603–609.

275. Wisdom G, Blitzer A. Surgical therapy for swallowing disorders. *Otolaryngol Clin North Am* 1998;31(3):537–560.

276. Shin T, Tsuda K, Takagi S. Surgical treatment for dysphagia of neuromuscular origin. *Folia Phoniatr Logop* 1999;51(4-5):213–219.

277. Crary MA, Glowasky AL. Using botulinum toxin A to improve speech and swallowing function following total laryngectomy. *Arch Otolaryngol Head Neck Surg* 1996;122(7):760–763.

278. Atkinson SI, Rees J. Botulinum toxin for cricopharyngeal dysphagia: case reports of CT-guided injection. *J Otolaryngol* 1997;26(4):273–276.

279. Haapaniemi JJ, Laurikainen EA, Pulkkinen J, et al. Botulinum toxin in the treatment of cricopharyngeal dysphagia. *Dysphagia* 2001;16(3):171–175.

280. Bath PM, Bath FJ, Smithard DG. *Interventions for dysphagia in acute stroke (Cochrane review)*. Oxford: Update Software, 2002.

281. DePippo KL, Holas MA, Reding MJ, et al. Dysphagia therapy following stroke: a controlled trial. *Neurology* 1994;44:1655–1660.

282. Baeten C, Hoefnagels J. Feeding via nasogastric tube or percutaneous endoscopic gastrostomy. A comparison. *Scand J Gastroenterol Suppl* 1992;194:95–98.

283. Park RHR, Allison MC, Lang J, et al. Randomised comparison of percutaneous endoscopic gastrostomy and nasogastric tube feeding in patients with persisting neurological dysphagia. *BMJ* 1992;304:1406–1409.

284. Norton B, Homer WM, Donnelly MT, et al. A randomised prospective comparison of percutaneous endoscopic gastrostomy and nasogastric tube feeding after acute dysphagic stroke. BMJ 1996;312(7022):13–16.

285. Cole MJ, Smith JT, Molnar C, et al. Aspiration after percutaneous gastrostomy: assessment by Tc-99m labeling of the enteral feed. *J Clin Gastroenterol* 1987;9:90–95.

ACHALASIA

JOEL E. RICHTER

Achalasia is an esophageal disorder of unknown cause characterized by aperistalsis of the esophageal body and impaired relaxation of the lower esophageal sphincter (LES). Although uncommon, any individual specializing in esophageal diseases sees this disease with some frequency. The history is usually classic and the diagnosis easily made with a combination of barium esophagram and esophageal manometry. These patients generally have few comorbid illnesses, and their dysphagia and bland regurgitation respond well to a number of treatment modalities, including pneumatic dilatation, surgical myotomy, or drugs.

HISTORICAL PERSPECTIVES

The first case of achalasia was described in 1674 by Sir Thomas Willis, an English anatomist, who first described a network of arteries at the base of the brain (circle of Willis) and the eleventh cranial nerve (spinal accessory nerve, or nerve of Willis). In his description of a patient with achalasia, he noted, "the mouth of the stomach (i.e., cardia) being always closed either by tumour or palsie, nothing could be admitted into the ventricle (i.e., stomach) unless it was violently opened." The patient was treated with a primitive but effective dilator made from a whalebone with a small sponge at the tip. Over the next 15 years, the patient did well while performing postprandial dilations to force his food into the stomach (1).

Achalasia has been known by a variety of names, including *simple ectasia, cardiospasm, megaesophagus, diffuse dilatation of the esophagus without stenosis,* and *idiopathic dilatation of the esophagus.* In 1881, Von Mikulicz suggested that spasm of the esophagus (i.e., cardiospasm) was the etiologic cause of achalasia (2). Hurst and Rake in 1929, aware of the ease with which bougies could be passed into the stomach of patients with achalasia, questioned the spasm concept.

Instead, they coined the term *achalasia,* derived from a Greek word for "lack of relaxation" because they believed the LES was unable to open normally (3).

It is humbling to admit that the current treatments of achalasia, balloon dilation and surgical myotomy, are techniques that, although extensively modified, have nevertheless been used for more than a century. In 1898, Russel was the first to report success using a bag, or pneumatic, dilator made from a sausage-shaped silk bag containing a rubber bag. The rubber bag was connected to a hollow tube, which was inserted into the esophagus across the LES and inflated with air or water (4). Nearly all the surgical techniques for treating achalasia were developed in 20th century Germany. The most important operation, the long cardiomyotomy, was first described by Ernst Heller in 1914 when he was a senior surgical assistant at the University Surgical Clinic in Leipzig, Germany. His first patient was a 49-year-old man with a 30-year history of dysphagia, whose distal esophagus and cardia, at operation, reminded him of the multiple cases of pyloric stenosis that he had so often fixed with a simple pyloromyotomy. Heller's technique involved mobilizing the distal half of the esophagus completely and incising the muscular coat through to the mucosa. His incision was 8 cm in length, distally went just over the esophagogastric junction, and omentum was placed into the defect to maintain separation of the muscle layers. Seven years after the original procedure, his patient continued to do well (5).

EPIDEMIOLOGY

Achalasia is a disease that occurs with equal frequency among men and women. Case studies show an age distribution between birth and the ninth decade of life, occurring rarely during the first 2 decades of life. The mean ages for achalasia patients in case studies range between 30 and 60 years, with some studies suggesting an increased incidence with age, particularly after the seventh decade (6). Achalasia is an uncommon disease, but it is frequent enough to be encountered at least yearly by most gastroenterologists and

J.E. Richter: Department of Gastroenterology/Hepatology, Center for Swallowing and Esophageal Disorders, Cleveland Clinic Foundation, Cleveland, Ohio.

esophageal surgeons. The disease prevalence is approximately 10 cases per 100,000 population. Its incidence has been fairly stable over the last 50 years at about 0.5 cases per 100,000 population per year. There are, however, striking international differences with the disease. Achalasia is more common in North America, northwestern Europe, and New Zealand, with a reported incidence between 0.6 and 1.0, and it is rare in Singapore and Zimbabwe, where its incidence is less than 0.3 per 100,000 population per year (7). There is some evidence from human leukocyte antigen (HLA) studies that whites are at a greater risk than blacks (8,9). However, these data are relatively crude, with most published studies being retrospective, based on hospital records, and using less than optimal methods for diagnosing achalasia such as x-ray studies rather than esophageal manometry—all these techniques are likely to underestimate the true frequency of the disease (7). The only prospective review of the epidemiology of achalasia was performed in Edinburgh, Scotland (10). This study was conducted over a 5-year period and included only cases in which a manometric diagnosis of achalasia was made. Twenty men and 18 women presented throughout adult life with a mean age at the time of diagnosis of 44 years (range 17 to 76 years). The annual incidence was 0.8 cases per 100,000 population, comparable to other retrospective studies from the British Isles.

PATHOPHYSIOLOGY

Neuropathology

A wide variety of pathologic abnormalities have been described in patients with achalasia (11). Some of these changes may be primary (i.e., loss of ganglion cells and myenteric inflammation), whereas others (i.e., degenerative changes in the vagus nerve and dorsal motor nucleus of the vagus as well as mucosa and muscle changes) are likely secondary phenomena caused by longstanding esophageal obstruction and stasis. Probably as a result of vagal damage, other organs outside the esophagus may be involved in achalasia.

Abnormalities of Extrinsic Innervation

The vagal efferent nerves, with their cell bodies in the dorsal motor nucleus (DMN) of the vagus, initiate and modulate LES relaxation and esophageal peristalsis in response to swallows (12). By light microscopy, vagal fibers from the esophagus appear normal in achalasia patients. However, Cassella and colleagues (13) performed electron microscopic studies finding evidence of wallerian degeneration of the vagus nerve with disintegration of the axoplasm changes in Schwann cells and degeneration of the myelin sheath, changes that are characteristic of experimental nerve transection. In meticulous dissection studies

of the brain, both Kimura and co-workers (14) and Cassella (15) described degeneration and absolute reduction of the number of DMN neurons in four patients with advanced achalasia. It is plausible that these lesions in the DMN or vagus nerve are pathologic, because bilateral lesions in the cat DMN can produce dysfunction resembling achalasia (16). However, these changes were not invariably present (absent in one patient), and, unlike the pathologic changes in the myenteric plexus, were not associated with an inflammatory cell infiltration. It is likely that these changes in the vagus nerve and DMN are secondary phenomena, and as such they are not required for expression of the disease.

Abnormalities of Intrinsic Innervation

Nitrergic neurons within the myenteric plexus mediate inhibition along the esophageal body and LES that occurs at the onset of swallowing. This inhibition is crucial in producing an aborally increasing latency of contractions along the esophagus, resulting in peristalsis and relaxation of the LES. In classic achalasia, the intrinsic inhibitory esophageal nervous system is damaged with inflammation and loss of ganglion cells within the myenteric (Auerbach's) plexus. This was first reported by Lendrum (17) in a detailed autopsy study of 13 patients with cardiospasm and marked esophageal dilatation, in which he reported a 20-fold decrease in the number of ganglion cells per plexus. In the most comprehensive study to date, Goldblum and co-workers (18) examined 42 resected esophagi from patients with advanced disease. In all cases, myenteric ganglion cells were markedly diminished in number, with 20 specimens having none. Inflammation of varying intensity was present in the myenteric nerves of all specimens consisting primarily of lymphocytes and eosinophils, with a small number of plasma and mast cells. In addition, all cases had collagen deposition within the myenteric plexus. Subsequently, Goldblum and colleagues (19) reported on the histopathologic features in esophagomyotomy specimens from 11 patients with less advanced disease. As in the end-stage cases, myenteric plexus inflammation was present in all cases, with most cells staining positive with Leu-22, a pan T-cell lymphocyte marker. Ganglion cells were absent or markedly decreased in 8 of the 11 patients (all with classic achalasia by manometry), and the extent of ganglion cell loss correlated inversely with the degree of myenteric fibrosis (Fig. 11.1A–B). Interestingly, the three patients with normal ganglion cell numbers all had manometric criteria of vigorous achalasia with minimal esophageal dilatation (Fig. 11.1C). Two earlier studies (15,20) had also noted a small number of patients with early stage disease, characterized by nondilated esophagus or short symptom duration, and a normal number of ganglion cells within the myenteric

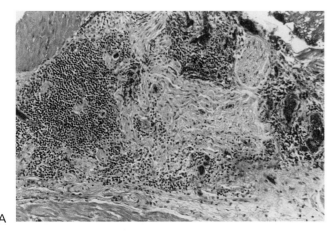

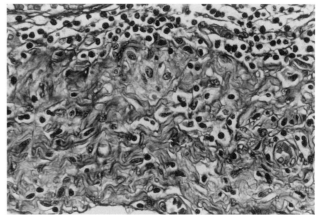

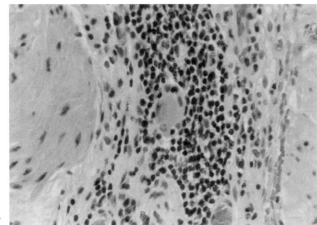

FIGURE 11.1. A: Myenteric plexus from patient with classic achalasia showing rare ganglion cells and increased lymphocytic inflammation. **B:** High-magnification view of a trichome-stained section from a patient with classic achalasia. This nerve is markedly scarred and a small amount of residual lymphocytic inflammation is seen both within and surrounding the residual nerve. (Courtesy of John Goldblum, M.D.). **C:** High magnification view of myenteric plexus from a patient with vigorous achalasia showing moderate degree of inflammation, predominantly lymphocytic, surrounding both myenteric nerves (*left*) and ganglion cells (*center*). In this case, a normal number of ganglion cells was seen and there was minimal fibrous scarring. (Courtesy of John Goldblum, M.D.)

plexus. Taken together, these studies suggest that an inflammatory process involving the myenteric plexus is present in the early stages of achalasia, and only later over years is there a loss of ganglion cells and myenteric fibrosis. Along with the destruction of ganglion cells, there is also reduction in the nerve fibers within the walls of the achalasia esophagus (21).

Immunohistochemical studies have provided insight into the neurotransmitter content of affected myenteric plexus nerves in achalasia. There is a marked reduction of vasoactive intestinal peptide (VIP) staining neurons (22,23) as well as the concentration of VIP (22) in the esophagus of achalasia patients compared with control subjects, usually obtained from the tumor-free portion of the lower esophagus of patients with esophageal or gastric carcinoma. These initial observations were described at a time when VIP was believed to be the nonadrenergic, noncholinergic inhibitory neurotransmitter in the esophagus. Later, nitric oxide (NO), which co-localizes to the same neurons as VIP, was established as the primary esophageal inhibitory neurotransmitter with subsequent studies confirming that intrinsic nitrergic neurons are either lost or markedly diminished in achalasia (24,25) (Fig. 11.2). Loss of intrinsic neuropep-

tide Y–immunoreactive nerves has also been reported in achalasia (23), but the functional significance of this is unknown. To date, no morphologic studies on intrinsic cholinergic neurons in achalasia patients have been reported.

Abnormalities of Esophageal Smooth Muscle

The muscularis propria, especially the circular smooth muscle, is usually thickened in patients with achalasia. Goldblum and colleagues (17) described in detail the various muscular abnormalities in patients with advanced achalasia undergoing esophagectomy. Muscular hypertrophy was present in all cases, and 79% of specimens had evidence of muscle degeneration usually involving fibrosis but also including liquefactive necrosis, vacuolar changes, and dystrophic calcification. Nearly half of the specimens also had eosinophilia of the muscularis propria. The authors speculated that the degenerative changes were caused by the muscles outgrowing their blood supply due to longstanding obstruction and esophageal dilatation. Another possibility was that muscle hypertrophy is a reaction to loss of innervation (26).

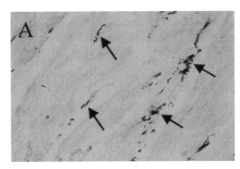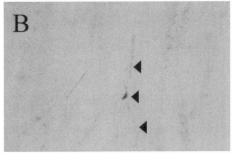

FIGURE 11.2. Immunostaining for NADPH diaphorase (which stains NO synthase) from the lower esophageal sphincter in a control subject (**A**) and in patients with achalasia (**B**). There is abundant labeling of NADPH diaphorase nerve profiles in the control section (*arrows*), but near absence of labeling in achalasia patients (*arrowheads*). (From DeGiorgio R, Di Simone MP, Stanghellini V, et al. Esophageal and gastric nitric acids synthesizing innervation in primary achalasia. *Am J Gastroenterol* 1999;94:2357–2362, with permission.)

Abnormalities of Esophageal Mucosa

Mucosal abnormalities, presumably secondary to chronic luminal stasis, have been described in achalasia. In another series from Goldblum's group (27), squamous alterations in 35 esophagectomy specimens from patients with end-stage achalasia were compared with the squamous mucosa near the esophagogastric junction from pediatric autopsies (less than 18 years of age) from patients with no esophageal disease. In all cases, the squamous mucosa from the achalasia patients was markedly hyperplastic with papillomatosis and basal cell hyperplasia. In addition, *p53* staining in the squamous mucosa was seen in nearly all specimens and CD3+ cells (pan T-cell marker) always far outnumbered CD20+ cells (pan B-cell markers). These latter changes have clinical significance in that chronic inflammation may be related to the increased risk of squamous cell carcinoma in these patients.

Abnormalities Outside the Smooth Muscle Esophagus

Striated muscle function in the proximal esophagus and upper esophageal sphincter (UES) may be impaired in achalasia patients. Although peristalsis is intact in the striated muscle, the amplitude of contractions may be diminished (28). Massey and co-workers (29) reported that the belch reflex was impaired in achalasia patients with an increase, rather than decrease, in UES pressure with rapid infusion of air into the esophagus. This impairment may contribute to the massive esophageal dilatation and acute airway obstruction occasionally reported in patients with achalasia (30).

Motility abnormalities in the gallbladder (31), small intestine (32), and sphincter of Oddi (33) have rarely been reported in achalasia patients, but their clinical significance is unknown. On the other hand, abnormalities of stomach function have been reported in up to 50% of achalasia patients. Reported pathologic abnormalities include decreased myenteric ganglion cells (18), a loss of NADPH

diaphorase (a marker for NO synthase) neural staining (24) in the proximal stomach, and loss of ganglion cells and myenteric plexus inflammation in the mid-stomach (20). These findings are consistent with the loss of inhibitory innervation to the proximal stomach, which, in some achalasia patients, has been associated with rapid gastric emptying of liquid (34) and abnormal fundic relaxation (35). Lastly, sensory and extrinsic autonomic nervous system dysfunction has been described in some patients with achalasia (36).

Neurophysiologic Abnormalities

In the healthy esophagus, the excitatory cholinergic neurons releasing acetylcholine promote muscle contractions and resting LES tone, whereas the inhibitory NO/VIP neurons mediate inhibition along the esophageal body in response to swallowing, which creates a latency gradient necessary for esophageal peristalsis and LES relaxation. The key abnormality in achalasia is impairment of the postganglionic inhibitory neurons to the circular LES muscles.

Studies from isolated LES muscle strips from achalasia patients suggest that the absence of ganglionic inhibitory stimulation results in unopposed LES contractions (37). Similarly, during electrical field stimulation, Tottrup and colleagues (38) observed contractions rather than relaxation of circular muscle strips from achalasia patients, whereas stimulation of the longitudinal muscle in these patients and in control subjects resulted in relaxation. Further evidence of denervation is supported by the abnormal response to various drugs in achalasia patients when compared with healthy volunteers. For example, cholecystokinin, which normally causes LES relaxation, produces a paradoxical increase in sphincter pressure in achalasia patients (39). This can be explained by the observation that cholecystokinin receptors are present on both intrinsic inhibitory nerves (to cause relaxation) and circular smooth muscle of the LES (to cause contractions). Normally, activation of inhibitory neurons predominate, promoting LES relaxation, but if they are destroyed or dysfunctional, the direct excitatory effect on the muscle predominates. Also, in keeping with the loss of intrinsic inhibitory innervation, the LES in achalasia patients have been reported to be supersensitive (i.e., denervation hypersensitivity) to intravenous gastrin (40), intravenous VIP (41), or an NO donor (42), and intravenous acetylcholine (37,43). The latter drug, in the form of the Mecholyl test, was used in the past to help diagnose achalasia as an injection, which resulted in a marked increase in esophageal and LES baseline pressure with spontaneous contractions and retrosternal pain (43). On the other hand, morphine and secretin decrease LES pressure in achalasia patients, although the degree may be greater than that noted in healthy control subjects (44). Finally, consistent with the muscle strip studies, Holloway and co-workers (45) found evidence *in vivo* that postganglionic cholinergic innervation was either normal or only minimally impaired in achalasia patients. These conclusions were based on the observations that atropine significantly decreased resting LES pressure in achalasia patients similar to that in control subjects, and edrophonium, by promoting the availability of acetylcholine, increased LES pressure.

Several novel human studies give a better understanding of the abnormalities in peristalsis seen in achalasia patients and the important role of NO. Using a partially inflated esophageal balloon to measure esophageal inhibition during primary peristalsis, Sifrim and colleagues (46) noted absent or impaired initial inhibition in patients with achalasia. It is known from animal studies that this initial inhibition is mediated by intrinsic nitrergic innervation. The generation of secondary peristalsis in response to balloon distention is also impaired in patients with achalasia. In healthy subjects, balloon distention in the midesophagus produces contractions above the balloon and inhibition in both the esophageal body below and the LES. In achalasia patients, balloon distention-induced relaxation is markedly impaired and paradoxical contractions are often recorded below the balloon in the esophageal body, but contractions in the smooth muscle esophagus above the balloon are maintained (47). From animal studies, the distal esophageal response is consistent with a loss of intrinsic inhibitory neurons, whereas the proximal contractions are maintained because they involve vagal cholinergic mechanisms (48). Finally, Murray and colleagues (49), in a serendipitous experiment, noted that the infusion of synthetic recombinant human hemoglobin, which is known to bind and inactivate NO, caused impairment in LES relaxation, simultaneous swallow-induced contractions, and sometimes chest pain when infused in human volunteers. This pattern was identical to the manometric findings in achalasia, confirming the critical role of NO in promoting normal LES relaxation and peristalsis.

Lastly, Singaram and co-workers (50) have created an opossum model of achalasia by destroying the esophageal myenteric plexus using benzalkonium compounds. The LESs of these esophagi were unresponsive to infused argi-

nine and showed a decrease in NADPH diaphorase activity but an increase in cholinergic nerve bundles, suggesting greater cholinergic input in the face of a markedly damaged NO system, which resulted in a hypertensive LES (50,51).

ETIOLOGY

Pathologic and pathophysiologic studies strongly point to an inflammatory injury to the myenteric plexus as the crucial insult in achalasia. The underlying cause is unknown and remains an area of intense interest and speculation. One of the major obstacles faced in elucidating its etiology is that achalasia is an insidious, gradually progressive disease. The initial insult likely occurs years before the patients come to clinical attention. Available data have suggested hereditary, infectious, autoimmune, and degenerative factors as possible causes of achalasia.

Genetic Theory

Reports of achalasia occurring in family members has led to the suggestion that achalasia might be inherited. Familial achalasia probably accounts for only 1% to 2% of the achalasia population (52,53). About 86 familial achalasia cases have been reported, with many being linked to consanguinity. Most reported familial cases are horizontally transmitted, occurring in the pediatric age group, and between siblings and even monozygotic twins (52–55). With an early childhood presentation, usually before age 5 years, associated anomalies can occur, including adrenocorticotropic hormone insensitivity, alacrima (lack of tears), microcephaly, Sjögren's syndrome, short stature, nerve deafness, vitiligo, hyperlipoproteinemia, and autonomic and motor neuropathy (54). The mode of inheritance is most likely autosomal recessive, with full penetrance in the homozygote form. In a recent linkage study, the gene for the triple A syndrome was localized to chromosome 12q13 near the type II keratin gene cluster (56). Five vertically transmitted cases of achalasia have been reported, with these being in children of both sexes and their father or mother (2,57–59). Unlike the horizontally transmitted cases, these cases present at an older age (range 37 to 72 years, mean age 56 years). On the other hand, the rarity of a hereditary form of achalasia was noted in a survey of 1,012 first degree relatives of 159 patients with achalasia, including 447 siblings and 247 children, in which not a case was found (60). According to mendelian principles, if achalasia was an autosomal recessive disorder, 112 of the 447 siblings should be affected.

Infectious Theory

Epidemiologic studies demonstrate geographic variations in the prevalence of achalasia that might be caused by infectious or environmental factors. Implicated factors include bacteria (diphtheria pertussis, clostridia, tuberculosis, and syphilis), viruses (herpes, varicella zoster, polio, and measles), toxic agents (combat gas), esophageal trauma, and ischemic esophageal damage *in utero* during gut rotation (61). The strongest evidence to date suggests that a neurotropic infectious agent could be the involved etiologic factor: First, the specific localization of the disease to the esophagus and the fact that the esophagus is the only part of the gut where a smooth muscle is covered by squamous epithelium make it plausible that certain infectious agents with an affinity for squamous mucosa could be involved (62). The herpes viruses, for example, have a predilection for squamous mucosa but rarely involve the columnar mucosa of the gastrointestinal tract (62,63). Furthermore, an infectious agent, *Trypanosoma cruzi* can cause a form of achalasia that has many of the features seen in idiopathic achalasia (64). Second, many of the pathologic changes seen in achalasia could be explained by an infectious, process particularly those caused by neurotropic viruses (18). Third, serologic studies in achalasia patients, compared with age- and gender-matched control subjects, show an association with measles and varicella zoster viruses (63,65). Additionally, a recent case report identified a patient with varicella infection who soon afterward developed achalasia (66). However, the major argument against an infectious etiology has been the general failure to demonstrate an infectious agent in tissue samples from achalasia patients. Robertson and colleagues (63), using *in situ* DNA hybridization, demonstrated varicella zoster virus—DNA in esophageal tissue obtained at cardiomyotomy, in three of nine achalasia patients but in none of the 20 controls. However, using more advanced methodology, including polymerase chain reaction techniques, my group and others (67,68) failed to find evidence of DNA or RNA from a variety of human viruses including herpes simplex, measles, cytomegalovirus, Epstein-Barr, varicella zoster, and human papilloma virus.

Autoimmune Theory

Evidence of an autoimmune etiology for achalasia comes from several sources. First, the inflammatory response in the esophageal myenteric plexus is usually dominated by T lymphocytes, which are known to be involved in autoimmune diseases (18). Second, a higher prevalence of certain class II histocompatibility antigens, which are known to be associated with other autoimmune disorders, have been reported in achalasia. Wong and colleagues (8) first reported a higher than expected prevalence of the DQw1 antigen, whereas subsequent investigators, using molecular techniques to subtype alleles, reported an association with HLA-DQA1*0101 (69) and DQB1*0602 (9). These associations were present in white but not black patients. Finally, several recent reports have found autoantibodies to myenteric plexus neurons in some achalasia patients. Storch and colleagues (70), found IgG-antibodies directed against the cytoplasm of the myen-

teric plexus in 37 of 58 patients with achalasia with variable stages of disease but in only 4 of 54 healthy subjects and 2 of 48 disease control subjects. Using a double-label, indirect immunofluorescence technique, Verne and co-workers (71) found that the sera from 7 of 18 achalasia patients stained neurons within the myenteric plexus from rat esophagus and intestine; this was not observed in 22 disease-free control subjects. These autoantibodies and HLA markers are only reported in about half of achalasia patients. Furthermore, they may be a nonspecific reaction to neurons that have been altered by some other causative agent.

Degenerative Theory

An epidemiologic study from the United States suggested that achalasia was associated with older subjects having various neurologic or psychiatric diseases, such as Parkinson's disease and depression (72). Case reports have associated achalasia with neurologic disorders such as hereditary cerebellar ataxia and neurofibromatosis (73,74). Additionally, some studies demonstrate Lewy bodies in the myenteric plexus and dorsal motor nucleus of the vagus in achalasia patients as well as in patients with Parkinson's disease having dysphagia (75). These studies suggest that a small population of elderly patients may have achalasia secondary to degenerative neurologic disorders.

Figure 11.3 summarizes the pathogenesis of idiopathic achalasia recently suggested by Paterson (11). He conceptualizes that achalasia is a disease that initially and primarily affects the nitrergic myenteric plexus neurons of the LES and esophageal body of the smooth muscle esophagus. An initiating insult, be it viral infection, a toxin, or some other unknown factor, likely occurs long before the patient comes to clinical attention. This injury triggers a chronic inflammatory response within the myenteric plexus, damaging but not destroying primarily NO-containing neurons. At this stage, a functional motility disorder of variable severity may be produced, including diffuse esophageal spasm, nutcracker esophagus, and vigorous achalasia, all of which have been rarely reported to progress to achalasia (76,77). Over time, probably measured in years, the inflammation results in death and destruction of the myenteric ganglion cells with fibrous tissue replacement, producing the classic manometric features of achalasia associated with progressive esophageal dilatation. Secondary muscle hypertrophy may occur as a result of chronic obstruction and dilatation, and eventually muscle degeneration evolves. Secondary inflammatory changes within the esophageal mucosa occur because of chronic stasis. Finally, in some patients, degeneration of vagal efferent neurons and their cell bodies in the DMN of the vagus may occur. This may be a consequence of loss of functional contact of these extrinsic nerves with their myenteric plexus effector neurons, but a primary insult to these neurons cannot be excluded. In fact, it is possible in this model that idiopathic achalasia may be the end result of more than one etiologic and pathophysiologic mechanism.

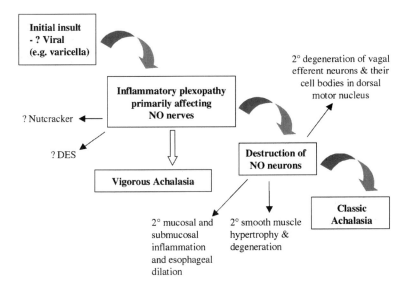

FIGURE 11.3. Overview of possible etiopathogenesis of idiopathic achalasia. (From Paterson WG. Etiology and pathogenesis of achalasia. *Gastrointest Endosc Clin North Am* 2001;11:249–265, with permission.)

CLINICAL PRESENTATION

The most common symptoms for achalasia are summarized in Table 11.1 (61). Most patients are symptomatic for years before seeking medical attention, probably because they learn to adapt to their slowly worsening symptoms, but some patients present early with severe symptoms. The mean duration of symptoms in 12 studies involving more than 1,200 patients was 4.6 years (10,78–86). The duration of symptoms ranged from as short as 1 month to as long as 67 years. Many patients see several physicians before the correct diagnosis is made, sometimes because their complaints are vague but more likely because many physicians lack an appreciation of functional esophageal disorders (87). Common antecedent misdiagnoses include gastroesophageal reflux, peptic stricture, esophageal spasm, presbyesophagus, allergies, and eating disorder (87). Others are misdiagnosed because improper tests are done, especially the initial use of endoscopy as a diagnostic tool in all patients with dysphagia. On the other hand, a recent study from Scotland found that the current widespread use of esophageal manometry resulted in more cases of early achalasia and milder symptoms being diagnosed and treated (10).

TABLE 11.1. SYMPTOMS IN ACHALASIA PATIENTS

Symptoms	Patients Studied	Mean %	Mean Range %
Dysphagia	1,930	97	82–100
Regurgitation	1,892	75	56–97
Weight loss	1,675	58	30–91
Chest pain	1,894	43	17–95
Heartburn	127	36	27–42
Cough	732	30	11–46

From Birgisson S, Richter JE. Achalasia: what's new in diagnosis and treatment. *Dig Dis* 1997;15[Suppl]:1–27.

Dysphagia

Dysphagia is reported by most patients with achalasia. In many patients, the dysphagia is initially more for solids than liquids, but by the time of presentation as many as 70% to 97% of patients have troubling dysphagia for liquids (10,78–86). In contrast to patients with organic and obstructing esophageal lesions, patients with achalasia report their symptoms not only during the intake of solid food, but perhaps more frequently when drinking liquids between meals. The onset of dysphagia is usually gradual, being described initially as an infrequent "fullness in the chest" or "sticking sensation" but usually occurs daily or with every meal by the time of presentation to a physician. Some patients correctly locate their dysphagia to the xiphoid area, but in my personal experience many complain of dysphagia referred to the region of the cervical esophagus. In many patients, the dysphagia seems to increase in severity, reaching a plateau over time, whereas other patients note increasing symptoms that lead to significant weight loss. Occasionally, the patient does not complain of dysphagia, although family members note the prolonged time required to complete a meal. Patients over the years learn to accommodate to their dysphagia using various maneuvers, including throwing the shoulders back, lifting the neck or using the headback position and simultaneously performing the Valsalva maneuver in an upright position to help empty the esophagus (85). Other patients may try to increase intraesophageal pressure by using slow deliberate swallowing during a meal or by drinking large volumes of liquids, especially carbonated beverages (88). All of these maneuvers attempt to increase intraesophageal pressure by 10 to 20 mm Hg, thereby encouraging esophageal emptying (86). Other remedies reported to improve dysphagia including drinking alcohol, warm liquids, or smoking marijuana, all of which relax the patient or the LES (85).

Regurgitation

Regurgitation of undigested, retained food or accumulated saliva occurs in about 75% of patients with achalasia (10,78–86,89). The material brought up is often recognized as food that has been eaten many hours previously. It tends to be nonbilious and not have an acid taste. However, fermented intraesophageal contents may taste and become acidic over time (90). Unprovoked regurgitation often occurs during or shortly after a meal. It is not unusual for some patients to induce vomiting manually to relieve chest discomfort. Other patients complain of thick white phlegm in their mouth, the result of regurgitated swallowed saliva. This sometimes leads to the initial misdiagnosis of allergies or sinus problems. Typically, patients note food or saliva backing up in the mouth while asleep. Nocturnal regurgitation can be annoying or severe. Regurgitated food or saliva may end up on the pillow case, cause audible gurgling sounds, or sometimes be aspirated into the trachea, producing severe bouts of coughing and choking. Respiratory complications, such as aspiration pneumonia or lung abscess may occur, particularly in older patients (72,91). Many achalasia patients learn to adapt to these problems by elevating the head of the bed at night and not eating large meals for several hours before bedtime. Occasionally in young women, these symptoms of regurgitation may be confused with those of an eating disorder, such as anorexia nervosa or bulimia (92).

Chest Pain

Chest pain or retrosternal discomfort is reported by nearly 40% of patients with achalasia; however, it is rarely the major complaint (10,78–86,89). Pain episodes mainly affect younger patients (93) and are usually described as being cramping in nature and as radiating to the back and lower jaw, sometimes mimicking angina pectoris. Symptoms can last for minutes to all day. Chest pain is often precipitated by eating, can awake the patient at night, and may be so severe as to cause decreased food intake and weight loss. Prominent pain occurs more frequently early in the course of achalasia, usually when the esophagus is only minimally dilated. As the esophagus dilates, the pain usually lessens and sometimes resolves (93). The mechanism of chest pain is unknown, but it is not simply repetitive episodes of simultaneous contractions causing the esophageal lumen to be occluded (93). Some patients practice self-induced vomiting to relieve their pain, whereas others believe cold beverages help their symptoms. Calcium channel blockers, nitrates, and acid suppressive medications do not predictably relieve the chest pain (85). Whereas pneumatic dilatation or surgery usually relieves dysphagia and regurgitation, the chest pain in achalasia patients responds much more unpredictably. In the first few weeks following dilatation, some patients even describe an increase in chest pain frequency and less than 20% notice a major improvement in this symptom (93). Other causes of chest pain in achalasia are pill-induced esophagitis, candidal esophagitis, and impairment of the belch reflex, causing increased intraesophageal pressure from trapped air (29).

Heartburn

Heartburn is not an uncommon complaint in achalasia patients (Table 11.1), although one would expect the contrary based on the high LES pressure and impaired relaxation (10,85,86,89). Characteristically, the heartburn is not immediately postprandial and responds poorly to acid-suppressing medications including proton pump inhibitors (10). The etiology of heartburn in achalasia is controversial and unresolved. Some have reported patients with well-defined gastroesophageal reflux disease (GERD) progressing to diffuse esophageal spasm and achalasia (94). Smart and co-workers (95), noted that four of their five patients had hiatal hernias and postulated that the progression from gastroesophageal reflux to achalasia may be secondary to acid damage to the autonomic nervous system. Spechler and colleagues (96) noted that achalasia patients complaining of heartburn had lower LES pressures than those without heartburn and that in some patients heartburn disappeared with the onset of dysphagia, suggesting that GERD was present before the development of achalasia. On the other hand, these isolated cases do not explain the patients with current symptoms of heartburn. Several studies using prolonged pH monitoring found evidence of excessive acid exposure, but the pattern was characterized by a slow steady drift to less than pH 4, rather than the abrupt pH decreases with slow clearance seen in classic GERD (90,97). This abnormal acid response is likely secondary to the slow clearance of exogenous ingested acidic materials, such as carbonated drinks, or *in situ* production of lactic acid from retained food in a dilated esophagus (98).

Weight Loss

More than half of patients with achalasia report weight loss (Table 11.1). The weight loss is usually mild and occurs over several months to years, but some patients have marked weight loss up to 100 to 150 pounds. In the latter group, significant weight loss over a short period of time associated with progressive dysphagia should raise the suspicion of secondary achalasia (99,100). On the other hand, many patients do not lose weight and some are obese.

Miscellaneous Symptoms

Although most presentations of achalasia are typical, important complications of achalasia can occur in patients with megaesophagus and longstanding disease. These complications are associated with three major physiologic processes: (a) displacement of mediastinal structures by the esophagus, (b) esophageal ulcerations and perforation through the esophageal wall, and (c) aspiration of esophageal contents

TABLE 11.2. COMPLICATIONS OF ACHALASIA

Aspiration pneumonia
Bezoar of the esophagus
Bronchitis
Distal esophageal diverticulum
Esophagocardiac fistula
Esophageal bleed
Esophagobronchial fistula
Esophageal foreign body
Esophageal perforation
Esophageal squamous cell cancer
Esophageal varices
Gastroesophageal intussusception
Hiccups
Lung abscess
Neck mass (bull frog neck)
Pneumopericardium
Postmyotomy Barrett's esophagus
Pulmonary *Mycobacterium fortuitum*
Small cell carcinoma
Stridor with upper airway obstruction
Sudden death
Supprative pericarditis

Modified from Wong RKH, Maydonovitch CL. Achalasia. In Castell DO, Richter JE. *The esophagus,* third ed. Philadelphia: Lippincott Williams and Wilkins, 1999:185–404.

(85) (Table 11.2). Approximately 10% of achalasia patients have significant bronchopulmonary complications as a result of regurgitation of material from the esophagus (78). Patients with esophageal symptoms of long duration may actually come to medical attention because of pulmonary complications. Organisms involved most commonly are aerobic and anaerobic oropharyngeal flora, which are aspirated, leading to bronchitis, pneumonia, or lung abscess. There is also an apparent increased incidence of pulmonary infection with mycobacteria in achalasia (91). Rarely, the dilated, fluid-filled esophagus can lead to hypopharyngeal displacement (bull frog neck) and acute obstruction of the airway, usually the trachea (101–103). Such patients may be difficult to intubate endotracheally, requiring decompression of the esophagus by a nasogastric tube (101) or rarely by pharyngotomy (102). Some achalasia patients have hiccups, which usually occur during meals and disappear after ingestion of liquids or following forced regurgitation. It has been speculated that hiccups are the consequence of esophageal distention and stimulation of afferent vagal fibers (104). Bleeding is rare in achalasia, although there has been one report of massive bleeding from an esophagopericardial fistula (105).

DIAGNOSTIC EVALUATION

Achalasia is suspected from a compatible history and the diagnosis usually is not difficult. Early cases may be misdiagnosed because screening barium x-ray studies fail to reveal esophageal dilatation and peristalsis is not evaluated, or

endoscopy is used as the sole test for the patient presenting with dysphagia. However, the diagnosis is made correctly in virtually all cases if a systematic approach, including esophageal manometry, is taken for patients with symptoms suggestive of this motility disorder.

Radiographic Studies

The plain chest x-ray film may suggest achalasia. The classic sign of an absent gastric air bubble in the upright position, present in almost all healthy individuals, may be found in 50% of achalasia patients (78,106,107). The plain chest film may also show an air-fluid level in the posterior mediastinum from retained secretions, widened mediastinum from esophageal dilation and chronic parenchymal lung changes, and lung abscesses from chronic aspiration (108) (Fig. 11.4).

A *barium esophagram with fluoroscopy* may be the *single best* diagnostic test for achalasia (Fig. 11.5A). The classic features are esophageal dilation, aperistalsis, impaired esophageal emptying in the upright position, and symmetric tapering at the esophagogastric junction (bird's beak appearance). Aperistalsis results in failure to clear the barium bolus from the esophagus in the supine position, and subsequent barium boluses cause to-and-fro movement with esophageal dilation (109). In the upright position, retained food and saliva causes a heterogeneous air-fluid level at the top of the barium column. This upright position also can be used to assess barium emptying (110). Healthy subjects should empty a barium bolus challenge of 150 to 250 mL within 1 minute. Most patients with achalasia have residual barium in the esophagus at the end of 5 minutes. Early in the disease,

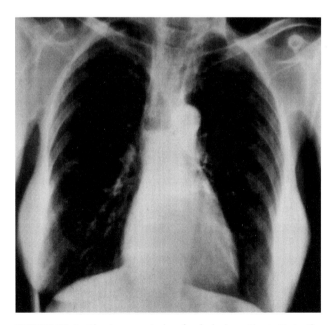

FIGURE 11.4. Chest x-ray study of achalasia patient. Note the air-fluid level from retained secretions across from the aortic arch and the widened mediastinum from esophageal dilation.

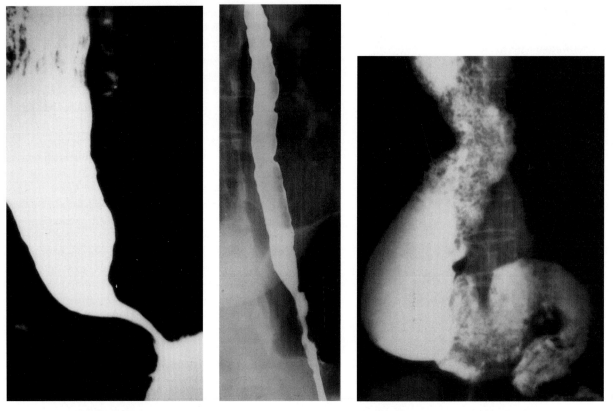

A,B   C

FIGURE 11.5. Barium esophagrams in patients with achalasia. **A:** Classic features of esophageal dilation, retention of liquids and secretions, and symmetric smooth tapering at the esophagogastric junction known as a bird's beak. **B:** In early disease, the esophagus may not be dilated and the distal tapering at the esophagogastric junction may be confused for a peptic stricture. However, on fluoroscopy, aperistalsis is usually present. This patient was originally referred for antireflux surgery. **C:** Chronic end-stage achalasia with marked dilation and sigmoid-like left angle distortion.

the esophagus may be minimally dilated and, with the distal tapering at the esophagogastric junction, confused for a peptic stricture (Fig. 11.5B). However, a careful fluoroscopic evaluation of esophageal peristalsis always finds evidence of simultaneous contractions and failure of the primary esophageal wave to clear the esophagus of barium (108,109). As the disease progresses, the esophagus becomes more dilated generally in the range of 3 to 8 cm, sometimes with a sigmoid-like left angle deviation of the distal esophagus. In chronic end-stage cases, the esophagus becomes massively dilated, (greater than 9 cm) and may resemble a sigmoid colon with stool (the inhomogeneous barium from the residual food) (Fig. 11.5C). In classic achalasia, the distal esophagus has a smooth tapering resembling a bird's beak. On spot films, this may appear to be a fixed obstruction, but fluoroscopy reveals intermittent partial opening of the esophagogastric junction allowing the barium to trickle or sometimes spurt into the stomach.

We and others have found that these classic radiologic features of achalasia show some correlation with symptoms (111,112). The height of the barium column in the upright position is related to the degree of regurgitation, whereas chest pain is inversely correlated with esophageal dilation (111). The severity of dysphagia may parallel the decline of

esophageal emptying over 5 minutes in the upright position (111). The overall degree of esophageal dilation and the development of a sigmoid esophagus shows little relationship to the severity of symptoms or the presence of weight loss. In fact, rare patients with massive esophageal dilation present serendipitously with no esophageal symptoms and only because of their cough or pneumonia from silent aspiration.

Other less common radiologic abnormalities in achalasia include an epiphrenic diverticulum and hiatal hernia. The unexpected presence of an epiphrenic diverticulum in the distal esophagus strongly suggests the associated diagnosis of achalasia (113). Hiatal hernias are infrequently found in achalasia patients (1.2% to 14%) compared with a higher prevalence (20% to 50%) in the general population (114–116). These hernias are generally small (<2 cm), although in elderly patients they can be large. Some believe the presence of a hiatal hernia increases the chance of perforation during dilatation (114). Spot films of the gastric cardia should always be done looking for a tumor of the cardia or gastroesophageal junction. However, compiled data from five studies found that the barium x-ray studies detected tumors of the gastroesophageal junction in only 28% (10/36) of patients with pseudoachalasia (100,101, 117–119).

TABLE 11.3. MANOMETRIC FINDINGS IN ACHALASIA

Lower esophageal sphincter
  Elevated resting pressure
  Abnormal relaxation
    Absent
    Incomplete
    Short but complete
Esophageal body
  Aperistalsis
    Isobaric simultaneous waves
    Simultaneous contractions
  Repetitive waves
  Increased intraesophageal pressure
Upper esophageal sphincter
  Elevated resting pressure
  Shortened duration of relaxation
  Spontaneous repetitive contractions
  Abnormal belch reflex

Esophageal Manometry

Esophageal manometry is the gold standard for diagnosing achalasia. Table 11.3 reviews the manometric findings in achalasia. Although the diagnosis of achalasia is often sug-gested by the barium esophagram or sometimes endoscopy, the diagnosis is confirmed by esophageal manometry. It is an *essential test* before pneumatic dilatation or surgical myotomy, in which there are potential treatment risks for the patient. Manometry may not be necessary when the symptoms and x-ray findings are classic and less invasive treatments such as botulinum toxin (BTX) or drug therapies are planned. Place-ment of the manometry catheter may be difficult in the very dilated or tortuous esophagus. The author has found that these patients can have manometry completed by passing a water-perfused motility catheter over a guidewire endoscopi-cally placed in the stomach. The decision to perform endos-copy for manometric catheter placement is based on the appearance of the barium esophagram.

Although occasional peristaltic and retrograde contrac-tions may be seen on prolonged ambulatory manometry studies (120), standard manometric studies in achalasia always show aperistalsis in the distal smooth muscle portion of the esophagus. This means that all swallows in response to a water bolus are followed by simultaneous contractions. The contractions (or more correctly waves) are classically identical to each other (isobaric or mirror images) as a result of a com-mon cavity or closed chamber phenomena (Fig. 11.6A). The contractile pressures are typically low (10 to 40 mm Hg), and

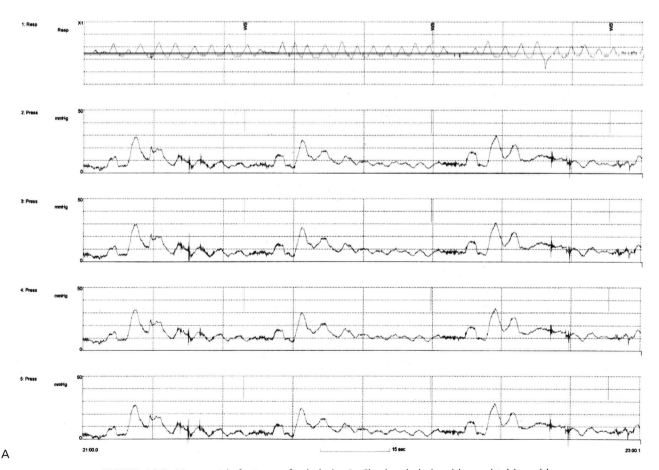

FIGURE 11.6. Manometric features of achalasia. **A:** Classic achalasia with aperistalsis and low-amplitude isobaric waves after all wet swallows.

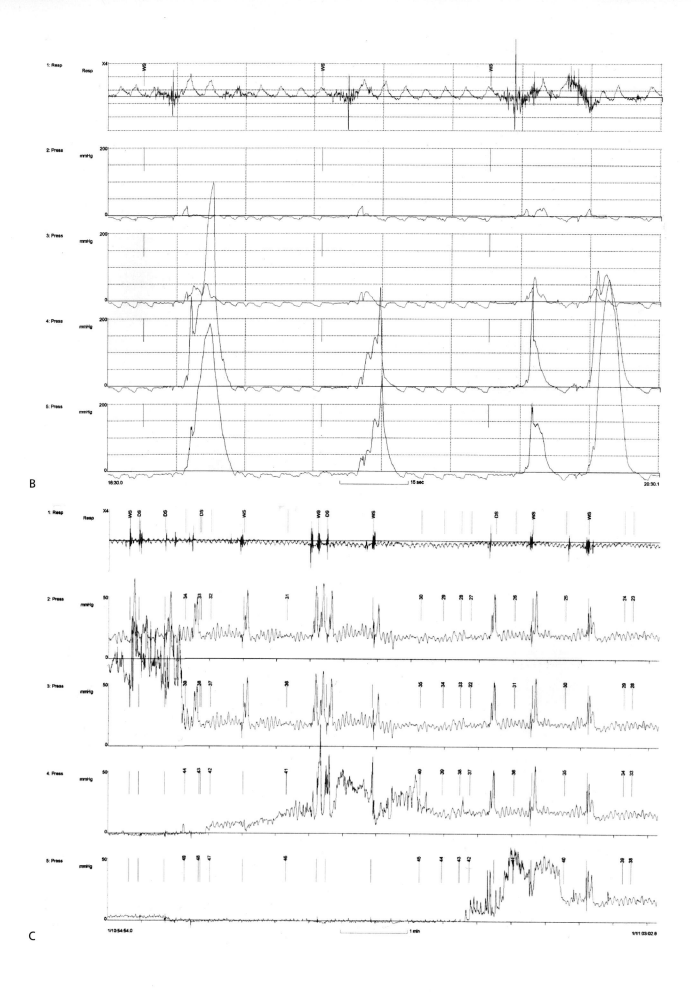

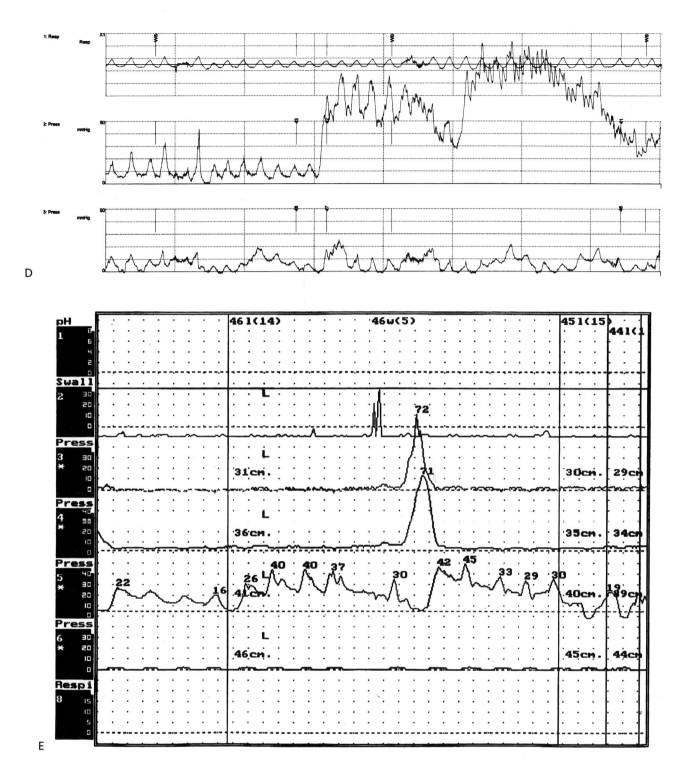

FIGURE 11.6 (continued). Manometric features of achalasia. **B:** Vigorous achalasia with aperistalsis and simultaneous high-amplitude (some greater than 200 mm Hg) contractions. Note that these contractions do not have the mirror-image quality seen in classic achalasia. **C:** Achalasia with intraesophageal pressure exceeding intragastric pressure best seen in the fourth tracing from the top. There is also evidence of incomplete lower esophageal sphincter (LES) relaxation. **D:** Achalasia with incomplete LES relaxation and increased residual pressure of 30 mm Hg. In this lead, LES pressure is also elevated measuring 60 to 80 mm Hg. **E:** Complete but short duration LES relaxation in achalasia. Relaxation to baseline for only 3 to 4 seconds duration is not adequate for normal esophageal emptying.

repetitive, prolonged waves are frequently observed (121). Physiologically, the low-amplitude waves represent simultaneous fluid movement in a fluid-filled dilated esophagus, rather than true lumen occluding contractions. In contrast, the term *vigorous achalasia* is sometimes used when there is aperistalsis with higher than normal contraction amplitudes (usually defined as greater than 37 to 40 mm Hg) (122–124). These simultaneous contractions can be high, sometimes reaching 100 to 200 mm Hg (121,124). These contractions are usually not mirror images of each other (Fig. 11.6B), because the esophagus is actually contracting and occluding the lumen of the minimally dilated esophagus. Patients with vigorous achalasia have less esophageal dilatation on barium esophagram but otherwise do not differ from patients with classic achalasia (122,123). In several series, including our own experience, the diagnosis of vigorous achalasia is made in up to one third of patients with achalasia (122–124). Several other variations of aperistalsis may be seen. In the usual patient, aperistalsis is confined to the distal 2 to 3 manometric sites recording from the smooth muscle esophagus. In patients with a markedly dilated esophagus to the level of the UES, recording sites throughout the esophagus show aperistalsis as lumen occluding waves cannot be generated. Recently, a patient with classic symptoms of achalasia and a poorly relaxing hypertensive LES was reported with aperistalsis confined to the distal 3 cm of the esophagus (121). The patient did well with a surgical myotomy. It has been reported that peristaltic contractions may be restored in some (up to 15%) patients with achalasia after treatment by myotomy or pneumatic dilatation (125). In the future, impedance studies may help to define whether this represents the actual return of peristalsis with intermittent normal bolus clearance. If true, then it suggests that functional obstruction of the LES may play a role in the esophageal aperistalsis seen in some achalasia patients. This would be similar to the model of an achalasia-like syndrome generated in animals by tying off the esophagogastric junction (126) or in patients with a pseudoachalasia-like syndrome after a tight antireflux fundoplication (127). Lastly, intraesophageal pressure exceeds intragastric pressure in some achalasia patients, probably because of retained food and saliva (Fig. 11.6C), because the pressure gradient returns to normal with evacuation of the esophagus.

Manometric abnormalities of the LES are always present in achalasia. The LES resting pressure is normal (10 to 45 mm Hg) in up to 40% of achalasia patients; therefore, an elevated resting pressure is not required for the diagnosis (46,122). It has been speculated that the subset of achalasia patients with GERD preceding the onset of dysphagia may have normal resting LES pressure, especially in patients who experience cessation of heartburn as their dysphagia progresses (96). A low LES pressure is never seen in untreated achalasia patients. The constellation of a low LES pressure and aperistalsis should raise the question of scleroderma or severe GERD.

Abnormal LES relaxation is seen in all achalasia patients (128–130). About 70% to 80% of patients have absent or incomplete LES relaxation with wet swallows (129) (Fig. 11.6D). Normally, LES relaxation exceeds 90% but averages only 40% in achalasia patients (129). Incomplete relaxation can be seen in normal individuals after dry swallows, so wet swallows should be used to evaluate LES relaxation (131). Studies, using the Dent sleeve (121) or computerized assessment of LES relaxation (131), suggest that residual or nadir LES pressure may be the best manometric indicator of impaired relaxation with values exceeding 8 to 10 mm Hg being abnormal. In the elderly achalasia patient (older than 75 years), resting LES pressure and esophageal body contraction amplitudes do not differ from those in younger patients, but residual LES pressure may be significantly lower, possibly confusing the diagnosis (132). On the other hand, complete LES relaxation does not exclude achalasia and can be seen in 20% to 30% of these patients (130). These relaxations are complete to the gastric baseline but of short duration (usually less than 6 seconds) and functionally inadequate as assessed by nuclear emptying studies (Fig. 11.6E). They are probably artifacts related to the small diameter of the manometry catheter or movement allowing the manometry orifice to drop into the stomach. Patients with apparent complete LES relaxation usually have early stage achalasia in that their duration of symptoms and esophageal dilatation are less than in patients with classic achalasia (130). Other reports have found evidence of intermittent transient LES relaxation but absence of swallow-induced LES relaxation (120,121,133). This finding suggests the possibility that transient LES relaxations and deglutitive LES relaxation may involve distinct neuropathways. Finally, a rare patient has been reported with aperistalsis and complete LES relaxation as the earliest stage of achalasia. At myotomy, preservation of the myenteric ganglions was seen but there was myenteric inflammation involving some of the ganglion cells and the patient's symptoms improved after myotomy (121).

UES and striated muscle function can be abnormal in achalasia. Although peristalsis is intact in the striated muscle, the amplitude of contractions may be diminished (28). Using solid-state or sleeve techniques, increased UES residual pressure, shortened duration of relaxation, repetitive spontaneous UES contractions, and impaired belch reflex have been recorded in some achalasia patients (29,134). UES changes may represent a reflex measure to prevent aspiration.

Endoscopy

Endoscopic examination of the esophagus is required to exclude neoplastic processes at the level of the gastroesophageal junction and evaluate the esophageal mucosa before therapeutic manipulations (85,100,117). Practically, it is usually done immediately before pneumatic dilatation unless there is a high suspicion of associated tumor. Patients with a markedly dilated esophagus may need to be lavaged or kept on a clear liquid diet for several days before endoscopy to avoid aspiration and allow complete visualization of the esophagus. The esophageal body usually appears dilated, atonic, and often tortuous with normal-appearing mucosa. Sometimes the mucosa is reddened, friable, thickened, or even superficially ulcerated as a result of chronic stasis, pills, or candidal esophagitis (Color Plate 11.7A and B). White plaques may suggest the presence of a fungal infection and, if confirmed by mucosal biopsies, topical antifungal therapy before pneumatic dilatation is recommended as prophylaxis against mediastinal contamination in case perforation occurs. The LES appears puckered and remains closed with air insufflation; however, the endoscope usually passes into the stomach with gentle pressure (Color Plate 11.7C). In some patients a "pop" is noted but this is uncommon. If excessive pressure is required, the presence of pseudoachalasia should be highly suspected (117), although benign strictures, usually from pills, are another possible etiology. In four studies involving 20 patients with pseudoachalasia resulting from tumors of the gastroesophageal junction, difficulty in passing the endoscope through to the LES was noted in 55% of patients (99,100,117,119). Retroflex view of the cardia and gastroesophageal junction should always be done and biopsy samples obtained from suspicious areas to exclude a malignancy before treatment (Color Plate 11.7D). Endoscopy is not infallible in that tumors of the gastroesophageal junction can be missed in about 35% of patients with pseudoachalasia (99,100,117,119).

Endoscopic Ultrasound and Computed Tomography Scan

Both endoscopic ultrasound and computed tomography (CT) scan may be helpful in evaluating the patient with suspected pseudoachalasia. Using a 20-mHz probe, endoscopic ultrasound (EUS) reveals a thickened LES muscle in achalasia patients, measuring 31 mm rather than 22 mm for normal subjects (135). In patients with cancer of the distal esophagus or cardia causing secondary achalasia, EUS may show thickening of the second and third hypoechoic layers (mucosa and submucosa) as well as enlargement of adjacent lymph nodes (136). Thoracic CT may detect asymmetric esophageal wall thickening or nodularity, extrinsic masses, or lymphadenopathy in addition to esophageal dilation in pseudoachalasia (137). However, EUS is better for evaluating a submucosal etiology of achalasia and CT scan may have difficulty in differentiating a mass from a hiatal hernia or tortuous redundant sigmoid esophagus. Neither can be recommended as a routine test in achalasia (138), and EUS is preferred to CT scanning for the initial evaluation of a patient with suspected pseudoachalasia (139).

Esophageal Transit Scintigraphy

Esophageal scintigraphy measures the rate at which a radiopaque liquid or solid test meal empties from the esophagus. In the supine position with minimal radiation, scintigraphy shows an adynamic pattern because the material lays in the atonic esophagus (140). However, esophageal emptying also is abnormally slow in other disorders of esophageal peristalsis and anatomic obstruction of the esophagus. Therefore, the test lacks specificity and has not been widely used. On the other hand, esophageal emptying of a semisolid meal (usually egg salad sandwich, oatmeal, or beef stew) in the upright position may be a useful diagnostic and therapeutic test (141–143). In achalasia patients, retention of the meal is prolonged when compared with normal subjects and retention is also abnormal in patients with early achalasia and apparent complete LES relaxation (130). Furthermore, it can be repeated after treatment to assess the degree of improvement, which generally correlates with the changes in LES pressures (141,142). False-positive results have occasionally been seen in patients with isolated hypertensive LES sphincter or a stricture, and, rarely, untreated achalasia patients may have a normal test.

DIFFERENTIAL DIAGNOSIS

As shown in Table 11.4, a number of disorders are associated with achalasia-like syndromes with esophageal manometry and barium esophagram being indistinguishable from primary achalasia (87,99,100,117). The most

TABLE 11.4. SECONDARY CAUSES OF ACHALASIA

Malignancies (pseudoachalasia)
Involving the gastroesophageal junction
  Adenocarcinomas (breast, gastric, prostate, lung)
  Esophageal squamous cell carcinoma
  Lymphoma (gastric, esophageal)
  Esophageal lymphangioma
Remote from the gastroesophageal junction
  Brainstem metastasis
  Hodgkin's disease
  Hepatocellular carcinoma
  Gastric adenocarcinoma
  Poorly differentiated lung cancer
  Reticular cell sarcoma
  Peritoneal mesothelioma
Nonmalignant esophageal infiltrative disorders
  Amyloidosis
  Leiomyomatosis
  Eosinophilic esophagitis
  Sarcoidosis
  Sphingolipidiosis (Anderson-Fabry's disease)
Miscellaneous
  Chagas' disease
  Congenital lower esophageal diaphragmatic web
  Diabetes mellitus
  Familial adrenal insufficiency with alacrima
  Multiple endocrine neoplasia, type IIB
  Pancreatic pseudocysts
  Postvagotomy

Modified from Birgisson S, Richter JE. Achalasia: what's new in diagnosis and treatment. *Dig Dis* 1997;15[Suppl]:1–27.

common disorders mimicking primary achalasia are malignancies (100,119,144–154) and Chagas' disease (64), with the others being rare case reports (155–160).

Secondary achalasia related to malignancies, "pseudoachalasia," represents about 3% of all achalasia cases and about 9% of achalasia patients older than 60 years of age (87,99,100,117). Most commonly, these tumors are adenocarcinomas of the gastroesophageal junction, but reports exist of pancreatic, oat cell, squamous cell of the esophagus, prostate, and lymphoma invading the region of the LES (144,147–151). These tumors usually produce achalasia as a result of one or two mechanisms: (a) the tumor mass encircles or compresses the distal esophagus producing a constricting segment or (b) malignant cells infiltrate the esophageal myenteric plexus (161). However, there are other reports of apparently nonneurogenic involvement by tumors such as Hodgkin's disease, poorly differentiated bronchogenic carcinoma, small cell carcinoma, and hepatoma that cause achalasia from a distance, probably as a result of a paraneoplastic syndrome (145,146,150–155). In 1978, Tucker and colleagues (99) identified three clinical criteria that could distinguish pseudoachalasia from primary achalasia, that is, age older than 50 years, duration of symptoms less than 1 year, and weight loss greater than 6.8 kg. However, others found that the positive predictive value of these symptoms was only 18%, with the sensitivity and specificity being 100% and 55% to 85% respectively (107). Clinically, this symptom triad is not very helpful because four out of five cases of older patients with achalasia would be mistaken for pseudoachalasia (107). Barium studies reveal classic findings of secondary achalasia with an eccentric, nodular, or shoulder segment of distal esophageal narrowing in about 40% of patients with this condition. In the remaining patients, the narrowed segment is smooth and symmetric with tapered proximal borders. A recent report identified two additional radiologic findings seen in more than 80% of patients with pseudoachalasia and not in patients with idiopathic achalasia. These findings included a narrowed distal esophageal segment that was longer than 3.5 cm and a minimal degree of esophageal dilatation of 4 cm or less (162). Additionally, amyl nitrate inhaled during barium examination may aid in distinguishing pseudoachalasia from primary achalasia (163). Amyl nitrate does not affect LES diameter in pseudoachalasia, but usually causes 2 mm or more increase in diameter in patients with primary achalasia. Endoscopy with biopsies results in the diagnosis of pseudoachalasia in most patients. Ominous endoscopic findings include mucosal ulcerations or nodularity, reduced compliance of the esophagogastric junction, or the inability to pass the endoscope into the stomach. However, as many as 25% of patients with pseudoachalasia have a normal endoscopic examination because of submucosal involvement by the malignancy (87,99,100,117). EUS is helpful in selected cases (139), but CT scans usually find only nondiagnostic features unless massive tumor involvement is present. Successful treatment of the underlying tumor sometimes cures the pseudoachalasia (147,148,150).

Chagas' disease (American trypanosomiasis) is a multisystem infectious disease caused by the protozoan *Trypanosomas cruzi* and transmitted by bites from reduviid (kissing) bugs. The disease is endemic in Central and South America, affecting millions of people (164,165). Latin American immigrants and travelers to endemic areas are increasingly seen with this disease (166). Ganglion cells are destroyed throughout the body, resulting in megaesophagus, megaduodenum, megacolon and rectum, in addition to cardiac involvement, the leading cause of death in Chagas' patients (164). The clinical presentation, radiographic and manometric features, and treatment for Chagas' disease are no different from those for primary achalasia (64). The clinical suspicion of Chagas' disease is confirmed with a positive serologic complement fixation or hemagglutination reaction (64). (See Chapter 37 for more details.)

TREATMENT OF ACHALASIA

The degenerative neural lesion of achalasia cannot be corrected. Therefore, treatment is directed at palliation of symptoms and prevention of complications. This is mainly accomplished by reducing LES pressure because peristalsis rarely, if ever, returns with therapy (125). LES pressure can be reduced by three modalities: drug therapy, forceful pneumatic dilation, and surgical myotomy. These therapies intend to overcome the obstructing LES pressure by improving gravitational esophageal emptying through reduction of sphincter tone while maintaining an adequate barrier against gastroesophageal reflux. Abnormal LES relaxation is not improved by any form of therapy. In most patients, swallowing can return to near normal quality and regurgitation is eliminated. Improvement and normalization of esophageal emptying in the upright position usually parallels symptom relief and may predict long-term success. Adequate decompression of the esophagus is key to preventing the development of complication, especially megaesophagus.

Assessment of Treatment Success

Traditionally, the success of medical and surgical treatments for achalasia is based on the patient's report of improved symptoms after therapy (61). This type of follow-up relies on subjective symptoms and not objective evaluation of esophageal function. Proponents of symptom follow-up argue that objective evaluation is not important if treatment relieves the complaints of dysphagia and regurgitation, the driving force in the initial presentation to the physician. Furthermore, it can be argued that the complications associated with treatment may preclude pushing for improvement other than symptom relief. However, these arguments are only valid if symptom relief parallels improvement in esophageal emptying. Recent data show that 30% of patients treated with a pneumatic dilation who experience complete or near complete resolution of symptoms still have poor esophageal emptying as suggested by barium x-ray studies (167). This group of patients is likely to have symptom recurrence earlier than those who have both subjective and objective improvement after therapy (168). More importantly, ignoring poor esophageal emptying in the setting of improved symptoms can result in worsening of esophageal function with the development of megaesophagus (Fig. 11.8).

Potential esophageal tests for assessing treatment success include esophageal manometry, radionuclide esophageal emptying test, and the barium esophagram. Manometric studies have reported a correlation between symptom improvement, especially in those patients experiencing at least a 40% to 50% reduction in baseline LES pressure (169,170) or in those with a posttreatment LES pressure less than 10 mm Hg (171,172). The latter criteria was shown to be the single most valuable predictor ($p < .005$) of long-term clinical success over 5 years in a large study of 54 achalasia patients treated with pneumatic dilation by Eckardt and colleagues (171). Similarly, several surgical series found that postmyotomy LES pressures less than 10

mm Hg favored long-term success (173,174). However, several recent pneumatic dilation studies using the new Rigiflex balloons failed to identify any manometric predictors of symptom response (175,176). Additionally, patients do not like serial manometric studies, and manometry may be difficult and requires repeat endoscopy in patients with megaesophagus.

Radionuclide esophageal emptying tests have the capability of assessing either liquid or solid food emptying in the upright position. Radiation exposure is limited, the test is acceptable to patients for serial testing, and the procedure is available in most nuclear medicine laboratories. However, the test is expensive and there is a high degree of technical variability, which is institutional dependent. The results of pretherapy and posttherapy scintigraphy for the evaluation of treatment response in achalasia patients are mixed. Holloway and co-workers (141) found that symptom improvement after pneumatic dilation or surgical myotomy significantly ($p < .05$) correlated with scintigraphic improvement in esophageal emptying (r = .70). Similarly, Gelfand and Kozarek (169) reported that an improvement of scintigraphic esophageal emptying of greater than 25% corresponded well with symptom improvement. On the other hand, Eckardt and colleagues (171) and others (175,176), found that, despite good correlation between symptom

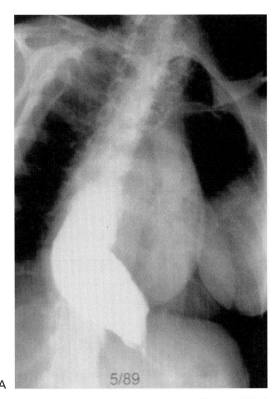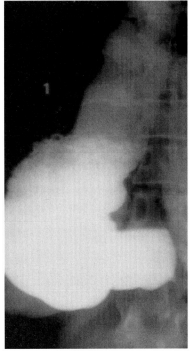

A

B

FIGURE 11.8. Progressive esophageal dilation with development of megaesophagus over nearly 10 years. **A:** Initial barium esophagram in May 1989 with early sigmoid deviation. The patient was treated with single pneumatic dilation and was lost to follow-up. **B:** Nearly 10 years later, the patient presented with primarily symptoms of regurgitation and recurrent pneumonias. Laparoscopic Heller myotomy gave only minimal relief and esophagectomy was finally required.

relief and scintigraphic emptying short-term, this technique did not predict long-term clinical response. The reason for the dichotomy between short- and long-term studies is unknown.

Assessment of barium emptying in the upright position is simple, widely available, inexpensive, acceptable to the patient for serial testing, and associated with very little radiation exposure. Although emptying of liquids is usually assessed, foods and pills can also be evaluated. Early studies reported that posttreatment predictors of success included an esophageal diameter less than 3 cm, barium height less than 1 cm at 5 minutes, or an esophagogastric diameter of 8 to 10 mm (177–179). However, other studies have not shown a good correlation between symptom improvement and barium findings (175,176,180,181). The conflicting data may be because of varying time intervals after pneumatic dilation when barium esophageal emptying was measured, the use of different dilators for pneumatic dilation, or differences in radiographic techniques. For example, barium emptying results may be affected if patients are tested only 1 day after therapy, as performed by Cohen (178) and Lee and colleagues (180), because considerable edema and spasm may still be present. A standardized approach may clarify the role of barium esophagram in the objective assessment of achalasia after therapy.

Recently, we developed a timed-barium esophagram, which is a simple and reproducible means of assessing esophageal function before and after treatment of achalasia (182). The technique is as follows:

1. The patient stands.
2. The patient ingests 100 to 200 ml of low-density barium (45% weight and volume) over 30 to 45 seconds. The volume ingested is based on patient tolerance.

3. Three-on-one spot films (35 × 35 cm) are obtained at 1, 2, and 5 minutes after ingestion, with the patient in a left posterior oblique position. The distance of the fluoroscope carriage from the patient is kept constant for all spot films. The 2-minute film is optional, but fluoroscopy at 2 minutes is performed to determine the state of emptying.
4. The degree of emptying is estimated qualitatively by comparing the 1- and 5-minute films. The degree of emptying may also be estimated by measuring the height and width for films, calculating the rough area for both, and determining the percentage of change in the area.
5. On subsequent follow-up studies, the same volume of barium is used for accurate serial assessment.

We routinely follow up patients 1 month after pneumatic dilation and surgery with an assessment of symptoms and objective measurements of esophageal diameter and emptying by barium esophagram (Fig. 11.9). This test is better tolerated than repeat esophageal manometry. It is more physiologic because it allows assessment of both changes in diameter and improvement of esophageal emptying (both measures of decreased LES resistance) and can be performed easily in small clinics and hospitals where esophageal manometry may not be available.

Using this method, we have shown that both short-term and long-term clinical response after pneumatic dilations have good correlation with esophageal barium emptying. This was accomplished by evaluating the symptom response and barium esophagram results of 61 pneumatic dilations in 37 achalasia patients who were treated using the Rigiflex pneumatic balloons (167). There was a significant association (r = .61; *p* < .001) between improvement in patient's symptoms and barium emptying. Short-term symptom improvement at 1 month and esophageal barium emptying

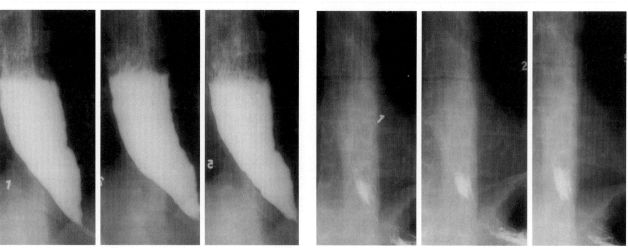

FIGURE 11.9. A timed barium esophagram in a 33-year-old man before (**A**) and 1 month after (**B**) pneumatic dilation with the 3.0-cm Rigiflex balloon. He had complete symptom relief and excellent esophageal emptying at 5 minutes.

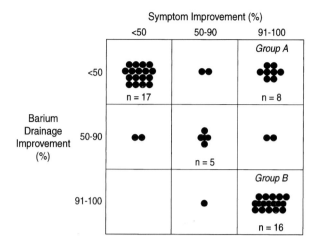

FIGURE 11.10. The association between degree of symptom improvement and barium drainage after 61 pneumatic dilations in 37 achalasia patients. Note that 10 of 34 patients (30%; group A) reporting complete symptoms relief had barium esophagram emptying that was less than 50% improved as assessed by barium height. In subsequent follow-up, group A patients were much more likely to relapse than group B patients, who had concordance between symptoms and esophageal emptying. (From Vaezi MF, Baker ME, Richter JE. Assessment of esophageal emptying post-pneumatic dilation: use of timed barium esophagram. *Am J Gastroenterol* 1999;94:1802–1807, with permission.)

were similar in 44 of 61 patients (72%). Ten of 34 patients (30%), however, who reported almost complete symptom resolution, had barium esophagram emptying that was less than 50% improved as assessed by barium height (Fig. 11.10). The latter group was older than their successfully treated colleagues, suggesting a possible disturbance in esophageal sensation. Importantly, we followed these two groups of patients for several years, finding that patients with both symptomatic and objective improvement at 1 month were significantly (*p* < .001) more likely to be in remission long term than those who had poor objective emptying 1 month after pneumatic dilatation (168). Eighteen of 22 (82%) of the former group and only 1 of 10 (10%) of the latter group were in remission on follow-up. The patients doing well at follow-up usually continued to have good esophageal emptying. We believe the results of these studies emphasize the need for objective assessment of achalasia patients after pneumatic dilation rather than reliance solely on the patient's reported improvement in symptoms.

Pharmacologic and Other Medical Treatment

Smooth Muscle Relaxants

The two most common drug classes used in treating achalasia are nitrates and calcium channel blockers. Nitrates increase the nitric oxide concentration in smooth muscle cells, which subsequently increases cyclic guanosine

monophosphate (GMP) levels and result in muscle relaxation. Calcium is necessary for esophageal smooth muscle contractions and its action is blocked by calcium antagonists (183). Both drug classes are effective in reducing LES pressure and temporarily relieving dysphagia, but do not improve LES relaxation or improve peristalsis. These drugs are best used sublingually 15 to 45 minutes before meals with doses ranging from 10 to 30 mg for nifedipine, the most effective calcium channel blocker, and 5 to 20 mg for isosorbide dinitrate (Isordil) (183). Nitrates and calcium channel blockers decrease LES pressure in a dose-dependent manner with a maximum effect of approximately 50%, with the long-acting nitrates having a shorter time to maximum effect (3 to 27 minutes) compared with sublingual nifedipine (30 to 120 minutes) (184–188). Overall, sublingual nitrates result in symptom improvement in 53% to 87% of patients with achalasia (184,187,189), whereas calcium channel blockers improve symptoms in 53% to 77% of similar patients (185,187,188,190). Comparative studies suggest that sublingual isosorbide dinitrate (5 mg) is more effective than 20 mg of sublingual nifedipine (85% vs. 50%) (187). On the other hand, nifedipine has been shown to be more effective than both diltiazem and verapamil (191,192). The clinical response to these drugs are short-lived, they usually do not provide complete relief, and efficacy decreases with time. For example, Bortolotti (193) recently published his 20-year experience with nifedipine 10 to 20 mg. Thirty-nine of 56 patients with achalasia were selected for long term treatment based on a good mano metric response to nifedipine administration (defined by a decrease in LES pressure greater than 30% for at least one episode of 10 minutes). Even in this select group of patients, only one third of the patients were still on therapy after an average follow-up of about 4 years. Both nitrates and calcium channel blockers are associated with frequent side effects, including headaches, dizziness, and pedal edema. This is a major factor limiting the use of these drugs as is the frequent development of tolerance to their beneficial effects.

Other medications that have been used to decrease LES pressure in achalasia patients include anticholinergics (cimetropium), β-adrenergic agonists (terbutaline and carbuterol), and peripheral opioid agonists (loperamide) (194–197). Most of these reports are small short-term studies without placebo controls in which route of administration and side effects often limited their widespread application in patients. Cimetropium bromide was evaluated in a double-blind, placebo-controlled trial and was found to reduce LES pressure by 70% for a duration of about 40 minutes (194). This was accompanied by improvement in esophageal transit time and few cardiovascular side effects. Improvement in achalasia symptoms was not evaluated. Most recently, sildenafil (Viagra), best known for its use in impotence, was evaluated in achalasia patients. Sildenafil blocks phosphodiesterase-type 5 (the enzyme responsible for degradation of cyclic GMP), which results in increased cyclic GMP levels within the muscles resulting in relaxation. In a placebo-controlled study involving 14 achalasia patients, sildenafil 50 mg by mouth significantly decreased LES pressure, residual pressure, and wave amplitude with its maximum inhibitory effect (about 50%) reached in 15 to 20 minutes after ingestion and lasting for up to 1 hour (198).

Other intriguing methods to relax LES pressure have included transcutaneous electrical nerve stimulation (TENS) and behavioral pain management. It has been suggested that the response to low-frequency TENS stimulation may be mediated by a nonadrenergic, noncholinergic pathway in which the release of VIP is responsible for smooth muscle relaxation. In a study of six achalasia patients, Guelrud and colleagues (199) observed that after 1 week of TENS therapy there was a significant decrease in LES pressure by 28%, improved LES relaxation, and increased VIP plasma levels, but symptom relief was not assessed (199). Shabsin and co-workers (200) reported complete relief of chest pain in a patient with vigorous achalasia following behavioral pain management, suggesting that psychophysiologic mechanisms can be recruited to improve esophageal symptoms and emptying.

Botulinum Toxin

BTX is a potent inhibitor of acetylcholine release from nerve endings. The inactive form of BTX is synthesized by the *Clostridium botulinum* species as a single-chain polypeptide. The active form is a protein that consists of a light chain and a heavy chain, linked by a disulfide bond. It cleaves SNAP-25, a cytoplasmic protein involved in the fusion of acetylcholine-containing presynaptic vesicles with the neuronal plasma membrane. Once BTX cleaves SNAP-

25, exocytosis of acetylcholine is inhibited and paralysis of the innervated muscle occurs (201). Because the pathophysiologic derangement underlying achalasia results in relatively unopposed stimulation of the LES by cholinergic neurons, BTX helps restore the LES to a lower resting pressure by blocking the release of acetylcholine.

Recognizing the pharmacologic attributes of BTX, Pasricha and colleagues (202) were the first to describe the successful use of BTX in reducing the LES pressure by 60% in piglets. Subsequently, the same investigators performed a pilot study on ten achalasia patients using 80 units of BTX endoscopically injected into the LES (203). One week after injection, there was a significant reduction in symptom scores (87%), LES pressure (43%), esophageal diameter (17%), and esophageal retention (25%). Later, Pasricha and colleagues (204) published a double-blind, placebo-controlled trial in 21 achalasia patients. BTX was significantly more effective than placebo at 1 week in 82% (9/14) of the drug-treated patients compared to 10% (1/10) of the placebo group. Long-term follow-up by this group found that 70% of their 31 patients had symptomatic and objective improvement with a median follow-up of 18 months (205). However, 40% needed more than one injection.

Similar results had been reported in a number of other studies in which the overall efficacy of one BTX injection was evaluated from 1 month to more than 24 months (206–217) (Table 11.5). Overall, 76% of achalasia patients initially responded to BTX, but symptoms recurred in more than 50% of patients within 6 months, possibly because of regeneration of the affected receptors (201). In those responding to the first injection, 75% respond to a second BTX injection, but some report a decreased response to further injections, probably from antibody production to the foreign protein (201). Less than 20% of patients failing to respond to the initial injection respond to a second BTX

TABLE 11.5. BOTULINUM TOXIN TREATMENT FOR ACHALASIA

Author	# Patients	% Symptomatic Improvement after 1 Injection				% Responding to Repeat Injections
		1 Mo or less	6 Mo	12 Mo	24 Mo	
Pasricha (204,205)	31	90	55			27
Cuillere (206)	55	75	50			33
Rollan (207)	3	100	66			
Fishman (208)	60	70		36		86
Annese (209)	8	100	13			100
Gordon (210)	16	75	44			
Muenhldorfer (211)	12	75	50	25	10	
Vaezi (212)	22	63	36	32		
Annese (213)	118	82		64		100
Kolbasnik (214)	30	77	57	39	25	100
Mikaeli (215)	20	65	25	15		60
Allescher (216)	23	74		45	30	
Neubrand (217)	25	65			36	0

Modified from Hoogerwerf WA, Pasricha PJ. Pharmacologic therapy in treating achalasia. *Gastrointest Endosc Clin North Am* 2001;11:311–323, with permission.

injection (208). Many patients in the aforementioned studies were treated with BTX after failing pneumatic dilation or Heller myotomy. In some reports, patients older than 60 years (205,208,217) and those with vigorous achalasia (205,206,212) were found more likely to have a sustained response (up to 1.5 years) to BTX injections. Most studies (204,206,209,210,212,214) assessing both subjective symptoms and esophageal function tests (i.e., LES pressure, esophageal emptying by barium or nuclear scintigraphy) found that symptom relief of dysphagia and regurgitation was much more striking than the improvement in esophageal function. This raises the possibility that BTX is also affecting sensory neurons and raises concerns that its chronic use for symptom relief may obscure a marginal improvement in esophageal function (212). BTX has also been reported to help some patients with pseudoachalasia (208,218) and may be used as a diagnostic test in patients with achalasia-like symptoms but atypical manometric features (219).

BTX (Allergen, Inc., Irvine, CA) is injected during a routine outpatient endoscopy. It is kept at −5° C prior to reconstitution and is gently diluted with 5 mL of preservative-free, sterile saline, being careful not to agitate the solution by forming bubbles during the mixing process, which could decrease the potency of the toxin (85). Once reconstituted, the toxin should be kept at 2° C to 8° C and used within 4 hours. Injections are contraindicated in patients allergic to egg proteins and should be administered cautiously to patients receiving aminoglycosides because these medications may potentiate the effect of the toxin (85). The average total dose used per session ranges between 80 and 100 units, with a concentration of 20 to 25 units per milliliter injected into each quadrant of the LES. Endoscopically, BTX is injected using a sclerotherapy needle inserted at a 45-degree angle into the esophageal wall, entering the mucosa approximately 1 to 2 cm above the squamocolumnar junction. This location places the needle just above the proximal margin of the LES with the toxin injected caudad into the sphincter. EUS may help identify the LES and allow for more precise injection of the BTX, but there is no evidence that this approach improves efficacy (220). BTX dose and dosing schedule may be important in prolonging the duration of response. In a study of nearly 200 patients receiving one of three doses of BTX (50, 100, or 200 units), those receiving 100 units followed by a second injection of 100 units 30 days later did the best. After 12 months, patients who received this two-dose regimen were more likely to be in remission (80% vs. 55% for the other two groups) (213).

Complications after BTX injections are mild and infrequent, usually consisting of chest pain in 16% to 25% of patients (85). There is some concern regarding the effects of prior BTX treatments on the success of subsequent Heller myotomy. Three surgical series (221,222,307) report difficulty in the dissection of the submucosal plane with increased intraoperative mucosal perforation rate in patients receiving prior BTX treatment. However, there was no difference in time of hospitalization or postoperative symptom improvement, although two patients in one series had persistent dysphagia (307).

Pneumatic Dilation

Balloon dilation is considered the most effective nonsurgical therapy for achalasia. The aim is to produce a controlled tear of the LES, resulting in relief of the distal esophageal obstruction and clinical improvement without perforating the esophagus. The first reported case of achalasia was treated with self-bougienage using a whalebone attached to a sponge (1). Although bougie dilation with a large Hurst or Maloney dilator can transiently relieve symptoms (223,224), pneumatic dilation has become the dilation procedure of choice for treating patients with achalasia.

Older Dilators

Early metal dilators (Starck) were modified in the early 1900s such that expanding bags and balloons were incorporated onto flexible shafts so that they could be placed across the LES to dilate it forcefully. The first balloon was the Plummer hydrostatic dilator, which used water to expand the balloon (225). Subsequent dilators replaced the water with air and were called *pneumatic* dilators (226,227). The Browne-McHardy and Hurst-Tucker pneumatic dilators consisted of a mercury filled tube with a rubber covered silk bag at the distal end. The Mosher bag contained barium strips impregnated into the wall of the bag for easy visualization at fluoroscopy. The Rider-Mueller dilator contained a dumbbell-shaped bag that could be positioned across the gastroesophageal junction by a guidewire and was the first dilator available in variable sizes. The Sippy pneumatic dilator had two latex balloons covered by a nylon bag to limit expansion of the balloon. Progressively larger balloons were used until symptom relief was obtained. All these dilators require fluoroscopy for proper positioning before dilation, and balloon size, when expanded, ranged from 2.5 to 4.5 cm (227).

There is a significant experience reported in the literature using the older dilators. Results of five prospective studies (171,228–231) in 235 achalasia patients using the older type dilators reported a good to excellent symptomatic response (defined as greater than 50% improvement in dysphagia) varying between 61% and 100%, with a cumulative mean of 85%. The follow-up of these studies ranged from a few months to more than 9 years with a mean of nearly 3 years. The overall perforation rate when reported was 2%. Results of 15 retrospective studies (227) in nearly 2,200 patients found a similar overall good to excellent symptomatic response averaging 71% (range 34% to 96%). The mean follow-up in these studies was 5 years with an esophageal perforation rate of 3%. However, this information is only of historical interest because most of these older dilators are no longer in use. The Browne-McHardy dilator, once the most commonly used dilator in the United States, is no longer manufactured.

Newer Dilators

Two newer type pneumatic dilators are available worldwide. The most commonly used balloon is the Rigiflex dilator (Boston Scientific Corp., Boston, MA), which is made of a modified polyethylene polymer mounted on a flexible catheter similar in design to the Gruentzig angioplasty catheter. The Rigiflex balloon is 10 cm long and comes in three diameters, 3.0, 3.5, and 4.0 cm (Fig. 11.11). It is not visible under fluoroscopy but has several radiopaque markers on the shaft that define the upper, middle, and distal borders of the balloon. The Rigiflex balloon is noncompliant, meaning that it inflates maximally to its designated diameter only. Further inflation pressure increases the pounds per square inch (psi) within the lumen but not the balloon diameter. Once the maximum psi for any balloon is exceeded, it simply ruptures without ever increasing the diameter. The other pneumatic dilator is the Witzel dilator (U.S. Endoscopy, Mentor, OH), which is made of a 20-cm long polyvinyl tube surrounded by a 15-cm long polyurethane balloon, which is passed in a retrograde fashion over an endoscope (Fig. 11.12). The Witzel dilator has the advantage of direct endoscopic visualization of the balloon position during dilation; however, its utility is limited because it comes in only one size, a 4.0-cm balloon diameter. In the United States, the vast majority of dilations are done with the Rigiflex balloons.

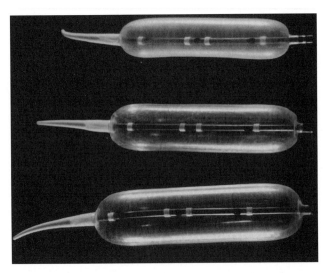

FIGURE 11.11. Rigiflex pneumatic balloons with three diameter sizes: 3.0, 3.5, and 4.0 cm.

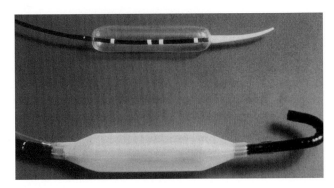

FIGURE 11.12. Rigiflex pneumatic balloon (3.0 cm diameter) compared to the Witzel over-the-scope pneumatic balloon, which comes in only the 4.5-cm diameter size.

Technique of Pneumatic Dilation

The technique used for pneumatic dilation varies at different institutions depending on the experience of the individuals performing the procedure. For the last 15 years, I have used the Rigiflex balloon dilators exclusively, using the technique outlined in Table 11.6. Several additional points regarding the procedure follow:

1. Screening endoscopy to exclude cancer is usually performed at the same time as pneumatic dilation unless there is a high suspicion of malignancy.

2. The smallest balloon size (3.0 cm) is usually used first. If there is no response, a 3.5-cm balloon is used after 4 weeks or longer, and then the 4.0-cm balloon is used, if necessary. In patients with prior pneumatic dilation or Heller myotomy who are still symptomatic, I begin with the 3.5-cm balloon.

3. The positioning of the Rigiflex balloon may be difficult, especially if a good waist caused by the hypercontracting LES is not easily seen. Partial inflation and repositioning may be required to get the balloon in proper position, that is, with half of the partially inflated balloon above the waist and half below the waist. This is the "key" step in the dilation procedure.

4. As the balloon is inflated, there is a tendency for the dilator to be pulled down into the stomach. Therefore, the individual holding the balloon must apply appropriate upward traction at the mouthpiece to keep the balloon in proper position.

5. The duration of balloon inflation does not appear to be as important as making sure the waist is obliterated. This was recently confirmed in a study comparing the efficacy of 6- or 60-second balloon distention times (232). Some authors suggest repeat inflation for up to 3 minutes, but none of these variables have been prospectively studied.

6. Blood on the balloon indicates a mucosal tear but does not always indicate a successful dilatation.

7. The Gastrografin swallow is followed by the heavier barium swallow if no perforation is noted. This study may

TABLE 11.6. THE AUTHOR'S TECHNIQUE FOR PNEUMATIC DILATION USING RIGILEX BALLOONS

1. Fasting for at least 12 hours before endoscopy.
2. Esophageal lavage with Ewald tube (if needed).
3. Standard conscious sedation and upper endoscopy in left lateral position.
4. Savary guidewire placed in stomach and Rigiflex balloon passed over it.
5. Accurate placement of the balloon with it centered across the gastroesophageal junction by fluoroscopy with the patient in the supine position. (This is key to a successful dilation).
6. Balloon distended, usually to 7 to 12 psi, enough to obliterate the waist and maintained for 60 seconds.
7. Patient repositioned in the left lateral position and the balloon carefully removed after deflating.
8. The patient sent for Gastrografin followed by barium swallow after recovery from conscious sedation to exclude esophageal perforation.
9. Observation for 4 hours for chest pain or fever. Patient discharge home after drinking fluids without difficulty.
10. Clinic follow-up in 1 month to assess symptoms and esophageal emptying with timed barium esophagram.
11. If symptoms and/or barium emptying not improved, then repeat dilation with the next larger size balloon.

not show good esophageal emptying secondary to edema and LES spasm; it is done solely to identify early esophageal perforation (180,181). Some, however, do not recommend obtaining barium x-ray films unless clinically indicated (233).

8. Before 1994, I used to observe all our achalasia patients overnight in the hospital after dilation, but since the report of Barkin and colleagues (234), most patients are discharged after 4 hours of outpatient observation.

Efficacy of Treatment—Short and Long Term

The efficacy and complication rates with the two pneumatic dilators are not comparable. The results of the six studies (172,179,235–238) using the Witzel dilator for the treatment of achalasia in 266 patients only reported good to excellent symptomatic response in 66% of the subjects with an average follow-up of 11 months. In the largest series, Ponce and colleagues (172) reported symptom improvement in 59% of 157 patients, which is the lowest response among all six studies (others ranged from 78% to 94% improvement). Furthermore, the perforation rate was high in five of the six series (mean 6% with a range from 0% to 13%). This perforation rate is two to three times higher than reported for the older dilators and the Rigiflex balloons.

Using the Rigiflex dilators, good to excellent symptomatic relief was reported in 74% to 93% (mean 82%) of nearly 600 patients with an average follow-up of 17 months evaluated in 17 studies (169,175,176,180,227,230,234, 239–248). See Table 11.7. These studies found that the clinical response improves in a graded fashion with increasing size of the balloon diameter. Cumulatively, dilation with

3.0, 3.5, and 4.0 cm balloon diameters resulted in good to excellent symptom response in 74%, 86% and 90% of treated patients, respectively. The overall perforation rate with the Rigiflex balloon was 2.3% (13 of 559 patients). We recently reviewed my experience using the Rigiflex pneumatic dilator at the Cleveland Clinic Foundation from 1994 to 2002 (249). Of the 100 patients initially treated with pneumatic dilatation, the success rate was 82% with a maximum balloon size needed of 3.0 cm (59% of patients), 3.5 cm (31%), and 4.0 cm (10%). Esophageal perforations occurred in 2 of 100 (2%) patients or in 2 of 146 (1.4%) pneumatic dilations (one with a 3.0-cm and another with a 3.5-cm balloon).

Although the results of pneumatic dilation are good in the aforementioned series with the Rigiflex dilators, only three series have follow-up data longer than 2 years and none longer than 5 years. Several authors have reported the results of long-term success with a variety of old and new pneumatic dilators, but the assessments were limited to symptom relief or the need for repeat treatment, and efficacy may deteriorate over time. Csendes and co-workers (229) followed up 39 patients who were part of a randomized trial of dilation versus surgery for a median of 58 months, reporting an overall success rate of 65% for pneumatic dilation. Thirty percent of the patients initially dilated subsequently required myotomy. Eckhardt and colleagues (171) followed up 54 patients for a median of 46 months, reporting an 89% success rate for improvement in dysphagia with up to three dilations. Parkman and colleagues (251) followed up 123 patients for a median of 46 months, reporting an 88% success rate, defined as needing no additional treatment other than pneumatic dilation. Katz and co-workers (252) reported their follow-up of 72 of a possible 113 achalasia patients responding to a mailed

TABLE 11.7. RIGIFLEX PNEUMATIC BALLOON DILATION FOR ACHALASIA

Author	No. of Patients	Study Design	Dilator Size (cm)	% with Exc/Good Response	F/U in Months (Mean)	Perforation Rate (%)
Cox (239)	7	P	3	86	9	0
Gelfand (169)	24	P	3, 3.5	93	NR	0
Barkin (234)	50	P	3, 3.5, 4	90	20	2
Stark (230)	10	P	3.5	74	6	0
Markela (240)	17	R	3, 3.5, 4	75	6	5.9
Levine (241)	62	R	3, 3.5, 4	85	NR	0
Kim (176)	14	P	3, 3.5	75	4	0
Lee (180)	28	P	3, 3.5, 4	87	NR	0
Abid (242)	36	P	3, 3.5, 4	88	27	6.6
Wehrmann (243)	40	R	3, 3.5	87	NR	2.5
Lambroza (244)	27	P	3, 3.5, 4	89	21	0
Muehldorfer (245)	12	R	3.5	83	18	8.3
Bhatnager (246)	15	R	3, 3.5	84	14	0
Gideon (247)	24	R	3, 3.5	NR	6	4
Khan (248)	9	P	3.5	85	NR	0
Kadakia (175, 227)	56	P	3, 3.5, 4	88	59	0
Vela (249)	100	P	3, 3.5, 4	82	24	2
Total	597			82%	17	2.3%

Exc, excellent; F/U, follow-up; P, prospective; R, retrospective; NR, not recorded.
Data modified and updated from references 231 and 250.

questionnaire assessing swallowing status and patient satisfaction. With a mean follow-up of 6.5 years, 85% reported their initial pneumatic dilatation was successful, whereas 11 (15%) patients required further treatment with either BTX or surgical myotomy. Only four of the satisfied patients required a second pneumatic dilatation over this time interval.

On the other hand, not all reports are so optimistic about the long-term success of pneumatic dilation. The group at the Academic Medical Center in Amsterdam recently reported their long-term follow-up of 125 achalasia patients from a series of 249 patients treated at their center over the last 30 years (253). Treatment success was defined as only occasional dysphagia (less than once a week) or pain of short duration defined as retrosternal hesitation of food lasting for 2 to 3 seconds to 2 to 3 minutes and disappearing after drinking fluids. In the responding group, the mean follow-up was 12 years with a therapeutic success of 50% obtained after a median of four dilations. For the group treated 5 to 9 years ago, the success rate was 60%; in the group treated between 10 and 14 years ago, the success rate was 50%; in the group treated more than 15 years ago (25 patients), it was only 40%. Only one series of pneumatic dilations was required in 13% of the patients. On average, the patients were re-treated after 2.3 years with some patients having undergone up to 14 dilations. Similar results were found when we reviewed our experience with both pneumatic dilation using the Browne-McHardy dilator and Heller myotomy through the chest between 1986 and 1990 (254). Overall, more than 60% of our patients had recurrent symptoms, but only half of this group had

sought further treatment, claiming their symptoms were not bothersome, they did not like the treatment alternatives, or they did not know any other therapies were available. These experiences from reputable high-volume esophageal centers suggests that achalasia patients need closer follow-up and may benefit from early intervention with a variety of treatments based on objective tests rather than symptoms alone (253,254).

Predictors of Success

Pneumatic dilation does not improve LES relaxation but decreases basal LES pressure by 39% to 68% (128,169,175,176,243). Partial return of peristalsis is reported in 20% of patients (255–257), but peristalsis does not correlate with symptom improvement or esophageal emptying. Over time, LES pressure seems to increase to a varying degree (169). Predictors of success for pneumatic dilation have been evaluated in some studies but the results generally are inconsistent. Many investigators (83,171,172, 251,258,259) agree that older patients (usually older than 40 years of age) respond better to pneumatic dilation when compared with younger patients, with one study reporting contrary results (260). In a further refinement on this theme, we recently found that young men do not do as well with pneumatic dilation as young women (259). Vantrappen and colleagues (258) reported better results among patients with a long history of dysphagia (mean duration 8.2 years) than in patients with a mean dysphagia history of only 2.5 years. Also, this group found the best long-term results in patients with a moderately dilated esophagus with a diameter of 5 to 8 cm (258). Surprisingly, the technique of balloon dilation with the exception of the diameter of the balloon (diameter greater than 3.6 cm with a Browne-McHardy dilator) does not seem to predict long-term success (171). Finally, a few postprocedure physiologic studies may predict long-term success. Eckardt and colleagues reported that all patients in whom an LES pressure of ≤ 10 mm Hg was attained remained in remission for at least 2 years after pneumatic dilation with the Browne-McHardy dilators (171). Using the timed barium esophagram, we found that patients with complete symptom relief correlating with marked improvement in esophageal emptying were more likely to be doing well at 3 years than those with symptom relief but poor esophageal emptying (82% vs. 10%, respectively) (168).

Complications

Complications after pneumatic dilation are reported in up to 33% of patients with most complications being minor (261). In a prospective study with long-term follow-up by Eckardt and colleagues (261), prolonged postdilation chest pain was reported in 15% of patients. The intensity and long duration of chest pain in this study, however, may be caused by lack of routine use of conscious sedation. This has not been my experience or that of others (227) when conscious sedation is administered for pneumatic dilation. Other usually minor complications after pneumatic dilation include aspiration pneumonia, hematemesis without a decrease in hemoglobin, fever that resolves spontaneously, esophageal mucosal tear without perforation, esophageal hematoma, and angina (261,262).

The most significant and serious complication after pneumatic dilation is esophageal perforation. Although the perforation rate varies from 0% to 16%, the overall perforation rate of 2.3% with the new Rigiflex balloon dilators is acceptable (Table 11.7). In my experience with these dilators, we began by using the 3.5-cm balloon because it was comparable in diameter to the Browne-McHardy dilator, but our perforation rate was unacceptably high at 10.6% (230). Currently, beginning with the 3.0-cm balloon, our perforation rate has been 2% in our last 200 patients. This observation confirms the safety of a graded approach to pneumatic dilation (175). Some researchers have suggested that patients with vigorous achalasia, associated epiphrenic diverticulum or hiatal hernia, malnutrition, or more than one previous dilation may have an increased risk of perforation (76,263). However, a retrospective study of 237 patients by Metman and co-workers (264) found no difference in clinical, endoscopic, manometric, or radiographic characteristics among seven patients who had perforations and 230 patients who did not. Furthermore, I have performed pneumatic dilation on all these subsets of achalasia patients without perforation and find the only contraindication to pneumatic dilation to be in the patient who can-

not undergo safely the anesthesia required to perform the procedure comfortably or who cannot tolerate surgery if a perforation occurs. After pneumatic dilation, all my patients undergo a Gastrografin x-ray study followed by a more careful barium study to exclude obvious and subtle perforations. Others suggest a more selected approach (233), obtaining x-ray films only if patients have prolonged chest pain, tachycardia, dyspnea, or fever (262). Patients with free perforation into the mediastinum, pleural ,or peritoneal space should undergo surgery to close the perforation, preferably through an open posterior thoracotomy. If performed within the first 8 to 12 hours, a myotomy on the contralateral esophageal wall also can be done. Perforations that seem contained within the muscle wall can be treated medically with nasogastric suction, parenteral alimentation, and intravenous antibiotics for 10 to 14 days (76,265,266). When the perforation was recognized early, Schwartz and colleagues (267) found no difference in the duration of the operation, intensive care stay, hospitalization days, or the long-term outcome in seven patients who had surgical repair for pneumatic perforation compared with those outcomes in five patients undergoing elective myotomy during the same period. However, surgical myotomy in these patients was an open rather than laparoscopic myotomy, which has become more common in recent years.

The incidence of gastroesophageal reflux after pneumatic dilation has been poorly studied. Older reports suggest this is a minor problem, with less than 20% of patients experiencing symptomatic heartburn with rare cases of esophagitis or peptic stricture (226,229,258). Two recent studies (268,269) evaluated patients before and after pneumatic dilation, finding that 25% to 33% had abnormal pH values not noted before treatment, but most were asymptomatic. The importance of this asymptomatic reflux is unknown. In our recent follow-up of 100 patients undergoing pneumatic dilation (249), 15% had heartburn symptoms requiring proton pump inhibitors with an average follow-up of nearly 4 years.

Surgical Cardiomyotomy

The first successful surgery for achalasia was performed in 1913 by the German surgeon Ernest Heller (5). The surgery consisted of an anterior and posterior (double) lower esophageal myotomy through a laparotomy. Heller's myotomy was successfully modified by the Dutch surgeon, Zaaijer (270) in 1923, using a single anterior lateral myotomy incision. Until the mid-1990s, the modified Heller myotomy, usually performed via a left posterior thoracotomy, was the primary surgical operation for achalasia. Good to excellent results were obtained in about 83% (range 60% to 94%) of achalasia patients followed up for 1 to 36 years (250). In 1992, Pellegrini and co-workers (271) reported the first series of achalasia patients who underwent minimally invasive Heller myotomy via the thorascopic approach. The benefits of a shorter hospital stay with decreased morbidity and earlier resumption of normal activity compared with the open operation has led to the widespread popularity of minimally invasive Heller myotomy, especially performed laparoscopically, over the last decade. Oelschlager, Eubanks, and Pellegrini in Chapter 18 review the surgical treatments of esophageal motor disorders in detail. In this section, I highlight some of these areas and help position laparoscopic Heller myotomy in our armamentarium of treatments for achalasia.

Esophageal myotomy lowers LES pressure more consistently than pneumatic dilation (229,272,273). Depending on the distal extent of the myotomy onto the cardia, LES pressure is lowered by 55% to 75% with the remaining residual pressure usually being less than 10 mm Hg (229,272,273). Myotomy also lowers intraesophageal pressure but does not improve LES relaxation (229). Partial return of peristalsis is reported in up to 20% of patients after myotomy, but these are usually manometric reports without correlation with barium clearance or impedance studies (274–276). One study (276) suggested the patients with return of peristalsis were more likely to have a shorter duration of dysphagia, less preoperative esophageal dilation, and greater contractile activity. Solid esophageal emptying studies are markedly improved, LES maximal diameter increases significantly, and esophageal diameter measured by the barium esophagram decreases after a successful myotomy (111,229,277).

Thorascopic versus Laparoscopic Heller Myotomy

The minimally invasive experience with the thorascopic myotomy is limited (278–282) with good to excellent symptom relief reported cumulatively in 82% of 103 treated patients (Table 11.8). However, the high rate of persistent dysphagia (up to 18% of patients) and secondary GERD (42%) resulted in this procedure being abandoned by most in favor of the laparoscopic approach. Additional problems with the thorascopic operation included the need for double lumen endotracheal intubation, the more demanding performance of the myotomy in the perpendicular plane of the esophagus, the difficulty in judging the appropriate extent of the myotomy onto the stomach, and the greater postoperative pain and longer hospital stay after a thorascopic compared with the laparoscopic operation (278–282).

The first laparoscopic Heller myotomy was performed in 1989 by Cuschieri and colleagues (283). Over the next 10 years, this operation became the preferred surgical approach for achalasia because it is less invasive, the hospital stay is shorter (usually 2 to 5 days), there is less incisional pain, and most patients can return to nearly normal activity in about 2 weeks (250,284). Furthermore, it is a less demanding and better operation because there is excellent mobilization of the cardioesophageal junction, allowing instruments to work parallel to the axis of the esophagus, the longer intraabdominal LES is more accessible through the abdomen, complex anesthesia is not required, there is no need for an uncomfortable chest tube postoperatively, and the abdominal approach is easier for adding an effective antireflux procedure (284).

As summarized in Table 11.9, 21 studies containing at least ten patients each (280,282,285–303) found that laparoscopic Heller myotomy has a cumulative good to excellent symptom improvement rate of 87.5% in 924 patients (range 52% to 100%). Three of the more recent studies (300,302,303) found that improvement in esophageal symptoms was associated with improvement in patient quality of life comparable to that of control populations in the United States and Europe. All but five of these studies combined the myotomy with an antireflux operation, usually a Dor (anterior) fundoplication. Troublesome GERD was reported in 13% of patients and there were two operative deaths. In the three studies without a fundoplication (290,294,299), the symptomatic improvement rate (52% to 88%) tended to be lower than the operations adding an antireflux procedure and the GERD rate was higher (13% to 38%). The average follow-up of these patients in the 21 series was 19 months, nearly identical to the follow-up of patients undergoing pneumatic dilation with the Rigiflex balloons in which

TABLE 11.8. SURGICAL MYOTOMY FOR ACHALASIA—THE THORASCOPIC APPROACH

Author	No. of Patients	Antireflux Procedure	% Symptoms Improve Good/Excellent	F/U in Months (Mean)	% Complication GERD
Patti (278)	30	No	87	—	—
Cade (279)	12	No	92	3	18
Raiser (280)	10	Yes	62	15	57
Pellegrini (281)	35	No	87	12	60
Ramacciato (282)	16	No	63	35	31
Total	103		82%	16	42%

F/U, follow-up; GERD, gastroesophageal reflux disease.
Data modified and updated from Vaezi MF, Richter JE. Current therapies for achalasia. Comparison and efficacy. *J Clin Gastroenterol* 1998;27:21–35.

TABLE 11.9. SURGICAL MYOTOMY FOR ACHALASIA—THE LAPAROSCOPIC APPROACH IN SERIES WITH MORE THAN 10 PATIENTS

Author	No. of Patients	Antireflux Procedure	% symptoms Improve Good/Excellent	F/U in Months (Mean)	% Complication GERD
Rosati (285)	25	Yes	96	12	—
Ancona (286)	17	Yes (Dor)	100	8	6
Mitchell (287)	14	Yes (Dor)	86	—	7
Swanstrom (288)	12	Yes (Toupet)	100	16	16
Raiser (280)	39	Yes (Dor/Toupet)	63	26	27
Morino (289)	18	Yes (Dor)	100	8	6
Robertson (290)	10	No	88	14	13
Bonovina (291)	33	Yes (Dor)	97	12	—
Delgado (292)	12	Yes (Dor)	83	4	—
Hunter (293)	40	Yes (Dor/Toupet)	90	13	18
Kjellin (294)	21	No	52	22	38
Ackroy (295)	82	Yes (Dor)	87	24	5
Yamamura (296)	24	Yes (Dor)	88	17	0
Patti (297)	102	Yes (Dor)	89	25	—
Pechlivanides (298)	29	Yes (Dor)	90	12	10
Sharp (299)	100	No	87	10	14
Donahue (300)	81	Yes (Dor)	84	45	26
Zaninotto (301)	113	Yes (Dor)	92	12	5
Ramacciato (282)	17	Yes (Dor)	94	18	6
Luketich (302)	62	Yes (Toupet/Dor)	92	19	9
Decker (303)	73	Yes (Toupet/Dor)	83	31	11
Total	924		87.5%	19	13%

F/U, follow-up; GERD, gastroesophageal reflux disease.
Data modified and updated from Vaezi MF, Richter JE. Current therapies for achalasia. Comparison and efficacy. *J Clin Gastroenterol* 1998;27:21–35.

the success rate was 82%, and troublesome GERD developed in 5.0% of patients. Although the anterior (Dor) fundoplication was the most popular antireflux operation, some authors preferred the Toupet (280,293,302,303) as a more effective antireflux barrier. Hunter and colleagues (293) used the Toupet routinely but switched to the Dor fundoplication in patients with markedly dilated esophagi, because they found the posterior fundoplication can cause a relative outlet obstruction by excessively angling the gastroesophageal junction anteriorly. Only one of the studies addressed the learning curve for this procedure. Sharp and colleagues (299) observed that most of the complications occurred in the first 50 operations and the operative time decreased significantly in the last 20 procedures in a series of 100 operations compared with the first 20, from 144 ± 7 minutes to 110 ± 5 minutes. No study or society identifies the number of procedures to be performed yearly to maintain competency with laparoscopic Heller myotomy.

Failure of Primary Myotomy and Need for Esophagectomy

Recurrence of dysphagia after laparoscopic myotomy is reported to range from 8% to 31% (297,301,304,311), with more than half of these patients requiring more

surgery. Early postoperative dysphagia is usually the result of incomplete myotomy, periesophageal scarring, obstructing fundoplication, or megaesophagus and usually manifests within 3 years after surgery (304). Incomplete myotomy may be prevented by extending the incision at least 1.5 cm to 3 cm onto the stomach to ensure transection of the gastric sling fibers and separating the cut edges of the myotomy by at least 30% of the esophageal circumference. Perihiatal scarring may be prevented by minimizing the amount of electrocautery injury to the crura. An obstructing fundoplication may be almost impossible to distinguish from an incomplete myotomy by either manometry, barium esophagram, or endoscopy. For this reason, some experts (305,306) suggest using intraoperative manometry to help guide the completeness of the myotomy and the snugness of the fundoplication. BTX injection or pneumatic dilation can be performed postoperatively with prolonged improvement of symptoms favoring the diagnosis of an incomplete myotomy. Although BTX injection affects the surgical treatment of achalasia in some cases (221, 222,309), most reports (307–310), but not all (306), find that previous pneumatic dilations do not affect the results of myotomy. Postoperatively, pneumatic dilation can be safely performed for persistent or recurrent achalasia. Theoretically, pneumatic dilatation seems dangerous after surgical myotomy because only the mucosa stands between the balloon and the mediastinum or the peritoneal cavity. However, my experience in 15 patients after Heller myotomy and the experience of others (301) suggests that this is not the case as long as the dilation is performed no sooner than 3 to 4 months after the initial surgery. The 3.0-cm Rigiflex balloon is rarely successful in these cases (301), and I routinely begin with the 3.5-cm balloon in these individuals. On the other hand, pneumatic dilation is not as successful in this subset of achalasia patients with improvement in the range of 50% to 70% (249,301). If dilation is not available or if it fails to resolve the dysphagia, 70% to 80% of patients respond to a repeat myotomy, which, in many cases, can be done laparoscopically (229,311).

Late recurrences of dysphagia are usually secondary to GERD or the recurrence of achalasia, with the latter reported to occur from 8% to 13% of the time (301,312). As Table 11.9 shows, 5% to 38% (mean 13%) of patients after surgical myotomy may suffer from troubling heartburn requiring H_2 receptor antagonists or proton pump inhibitors. These values may be a gross underestimation as the group from the University of Washington recently reported (see Chapter 18). After a laparoscopic Heller-Dor or Heller-Toupet procedure, 19% of patients had heartburn more than once a week, but of the subset of patients undergoing postoperative 24 hour pH studies, more than twice that number (35%) had abnormal acid reflux values. This chronic gastroesophageal reflux over time can potentially cause esophagitis, peptic stricture, and even Barrett's esophagus with adenocarcinoma. Jaakkola and co-workers (314) found that Barrett's esophagus developed in 4 of 46 patients following Heller's myotomy after an average follow-up of 13 years. In a recent review of the literature, Guo and colleagues (315) reported 30 cases of Barrett's esophagus in patients with achalasia; 73% (22 cases) were after Heller myotomy. In 20% of the cases (six subjects), dysplasia and adenocarcinoma developed in the Barrett's esophagus. For these reasons, some authorities are suggesting routine 24-hour pH testing after surgical myotomy with chronic medical antireflux therapy if abnormal gastroesophageal reflux is identified (see Chapter 18).

Some patients with achalasia and a megaesophagus may require esophagectomy to relieve their symptoms of dysphagia and regurgitation. The definition of a megaesophagus varies, but it is suggested by a sigmoid configuration, especially when the maximum esophageal diameter exceeds 6 to 9 cm (293,316). Several series (298,301) have suggested that many of these patients will not do well after a surgical myotomy. However, Patti and colleagues (316) recently reported that 19 patients with megaesophagus (greater than 6 cm), some with sigmoid deviation, did as well after Heller myotomy as those with mild esophageal dilation. Therefore, we recommend initial treatment with a laparoscopic myotomy with either no or minimal (Dor) fundoplication in all our patients with untreated achalasia and a megaesophagus. In these patients, failure of the initial

myotomy or failure of repeat myotomy in other achalasia patients with persistent symptoms may require esophageal resection as the only surgical alternative, especially if these patients are otherwise healthy. On the other hand, more debilitated patients may do better with alternative therapies, including repeat pneumatic dilatation, BTX injection, calcium channel blockers, and even the placement of a percutaneous endoscopic gastrostomy tube for nutrition. If an esophagectomy is considered, then the surgical team must be skilled because the mortality rate ranges between 2% and 8%, but good to excellent results can be expected in 78% to 90% of patients (317–319). The operation of choice is a transhiatal esophagectomy and the conduit for this operation is discussed elsewhere, but we prefer using the stomach whenever possible.

Comparison of Medical and Surgical Treatment of Achalasia

Pneumatic Dilation versus Heller Myotomy

There are no data in the literature comparing pneumatic dilation with the Rigiflex balloon and laparoscopic myotomy, the two current most definitive treatments for achalasia. However, there are 12 studies, mostly retrospective, comparing open Heller myotomy and pneumatic dilation using older balloon dilators (Browne-McHardy, Mosher, or Rider-Mueller) (320). Overall, 1,199 patients received pneumatic dilation, but only one study used the newer Rigiflex balloons (242). In the surgical series, 2,549 patients were studied; however, 72% came from the multicenter European study by Gonzales and colleagues (321). All the surgical studies were classic Heller myotomy by either a thoracotomy or laparotomy, except for one small thorascopic study (278). The cumulative symptomatic success rate, defined as a good to excellent response, was 65% (range 38% to 89%) for pneumatic dilation compared with 86% (range 63% to 95%) for surgical myotomy with an average follow-up for both groups of about 4 years. In these comparison studies, the perforation rate for pneumatic dilation was 5%, whereas GERD developed in approximately 25% of surgical patients.

The only prospective randomized study comparing pneumatic dilation and Heller myotomy was reported by Csendes and colleagues (229) in 1989. This was a single center study in which the same surgeon performed both the open Heller myotomies through the abdomen and the pneumatic dilations with an older Mosher bag. He found that 95% of 41 patients treated with Heller myotomy were improved with a mean follow-up of 62 months, which was significantly better ($p < 0.01$) than the 65% improvement rate observed in the 39 patients undergoing pneumatic dilation with a mean follow-up of 58 months. Two patients (5.6%) had an esophageal perforation. Gastroesophageal reflux was reported in 8% of the dilation group and in 28%

after surgery. This study clearly found a better outcome after surgery compared with that after pneumatic dilation, but the technique of balloon dilation and patient selection has been criticized. The Mosher balloon was only distended to 5.4 psi for a short duration (10 to 20 seconds), no comments were made about obliteration of the waist, atropine used for premedication may have reduced LES pressure at the time of dilation, and 14% of the patients had Chagas' disease.

Two of the older retrospective studies by Okike and colleagues (322) and by Parkman (257) involved a large number of patients (431 and 223, respectively) undergoing pneumatic dilation who were compared with patients undergoing surgical myotomy in the same institution. In these series, pneumatic dilation was generally comparable to surgery (i.e., 65% and 85%, respectively, in Okike's experience and 89% and 80%, respectively, in Parkman's series). Similarly, we found pneumatic dilation with the newer Rigiflex balloons was 88% successful in 36 patients, which was identical to the 89% success rate among nine patients undergoing a thoracic Heller myotomy by a single experienced thoracic surgeon (242). These results may be more representative of the true success rate with pneumatic dilation when performed by gastroenterologists experienced with this procedure and who do it with some frequency.

Heller Myotomy versus Botulinum Toxin

Only one study has compared surgical myotomy with endoscopic injections of BTX. In the study by Andrews and co-workers (323), 22 achalasia patients were given a choice of treatment: laparoscopic Heller myotomy or 100 units of BTX. Eighteen patients chose BTX as the initial treatment; 78% required a second or further injections. Over time, the interval between each BTX injection decreased (i.e., 324-day mean intervals between first and second injection versus 130 days between the third and fourth injections). Both treatments significantly improved symptoms to the same degree; however, only laparoscopic Heller myotomy significantly decreased basal LES pressure and improved esophageal emptying by barium esophagram. Overall, 5 of 18 (28%) patients in the BTX group switched to Heller myotomy after an average of 1.5 years because of treatment failure. There were no treatment failures in the laparoscopic Heller myotomy group or in the patients who had surgery after failing BTX injection, with an average follow-up of 1.5 years for both groups.

Botulinum Toxin versus Pneumatic Dilation

Table 11.10 summarizes the five prospective published studies comparing endoscopic injection of BTX with pneumatic dilation in the treatment of achalasia (209,211,212,215,216). All five reports were randomized studies involving about 75 patients in each treatment arm. In two studies, one or two BTX injections were given and the responders were followed up until symptoms relapsed (211,212). Repeat injections were administered in the three other studies (209,215,216), but subset analysis allowed determination of response rates for single injections versus serial injections. All but one study used the Rigiflex balloons (211) with pneumatic dilation performed once or twice, and then the patients were followed up until symptoms relapsed. As Table 11.10 shows, the initial response for BTX and pneumatic dilation are similar, but a single successful injection of BTX does not have the durability of pneumatic dilation, with the average injection lasting about 6 to 7 months. Whereas the success after pneumatic dilation gradually deteriorates over the 30-month follow-up from 85% to 50%, BTX showed a dramatic deterioration in success by 6 months (32%) with only 8% of the remaining patients having symptom relief after 30 months. Two of these studies permitted a critical assessment of pneumatic dilation versus BTX when re-treatment of relapses was allowed, but here again pneumatic dilation seems superior. Mikaeli and colleagues (215) observed that all 12 patients in the pneumatic dilation group requiring re-treatment were in symptomatic remission at 12 months versus 12 of 20 BTX patients (60%). In the study by Allescher (216), there was no significant difference at 1 year among those treated once or requiring re-treatment in either the pneumatic dilation or BTX groups. However, after 24, 36, and 48 months, a single pneumatic dilation was significantly

TABLE 11.10. BOTULINUM TOXIN VERSUS PNEUMATIC DILATION FOR ACHALASIA: PROSPECTIVE STUDIES

Author	Pneumatic Dilation Symptom Improvement (%)					Botulinum Toxin Symptom Improvement (%)					
	# Patients	Initial	6 Mo	12 Mo	>30 Mo	# Patients	Dose (Units)	Initial	6 Mo	12 Mo	>30 Mo
Annese (209)	8	100	—	—	—	8	100	100	13	—	—
Vaezi (212)	20	75	75	70	—	22	100	64	36	32	—
Muehldorfer (211)	12	83	75	66	50	12	80	75	50	25	0
Mikali (215)	20	90	75	53		20	200	65	25	15	—
Allescher (216)	14	78	—	65	50	23	100	74		45	15
Total	74	85%	75%	64%	50%	85	75%	31%	29%	8%	

superior to a single BTX injection, and after 36 and 48 months, a single pneumatic dilation was even superior to repeat BTX injections.

Cost Analysis and Quality of Life Comparisons between Treatments

Three studies addressing some form of cost analysis in the treatment of achalasia are summarized in Table 11.11. Only the study by Parkman and co-workers (251) is a true cost analysis in an actual series of patients, whereas the other studies are decision models.

Parkman and co-workers (251) attempted to address the direct and indirect costs of pneumatic dilation versus open Heller myotomy in a large series of patients treated at the University of Pennsylvania from 1976 to 1986. Direct medical costs of the procedures, hospitalization, and post-treatment care were estimated from the actual costs paid as determined from hospital financial records. Indirect non-medical costs for transportation, family care, and lost time from work were estimated from a questionnaire given to all patients. The initial cost of Heller myotomy was five times greater than the cost of pneumatic dilation. When costs were analyzed over 7 years to include subsequent treatment of symptomatic patients, the total expectant cost of treatment initially with a surgical myotomy remained 2.4 times greater than treating initially with pneumatic dilation ($20,064 vs. $8,474).

The decision model by Panaccione and colleagues (324) is a cost minimization analysis based on this Canadian group's 10-year experience with pneumatic dilation and the early, more optimistic literature on BTX injections. Direct costs were considered from a third party payor perspective and derived by summing inpatient and outpatient hospital costs, including supplies, nursing costs, and physician fees. Cost of the pneumatic dilation included an overnight hospital stay, whereas BTX injections were done as an outpatient procedure. BTX was significantly more costly at $3,271 compared with $2,345 for the pneumatic dilation strategy. Sensitivity analysis showed that the probability of requiring repeat BTX injections would have to decrease from 95% to 51%, the interval between injections would have to increase from 1.3 years to 5 years, or the success rate for

pneumatic dilation would have to diminish from 92% to 34% for the cost of the two strategies to equalize—all unlikely probabilities. BTX injection strategy was only less costly if the life expectancy of the patient was less than 2 years.

The second decision model by Imperiale and colleagues (325) compared BTX injections, pneumatic dilation using a Rigiflex balloon, and laparoscopic Heller myotomy over a 5-year horizon. Only direct costs were considered and these values were derived from hospital accounting department and Medicare allowable payments. Under these conditions, the respective cost per cure for pneumatic dilation, BTX injection, and laparoscopic Heller myotomy were $3,111, $3,723, and $10,792, respectively. Despite efficacy rates of 95%, laparoscopic Heller myotomy remained the most costly strategy. In one-way sensitivity analysis, laparoscopic Heller myotomy was less costly than BTX injections only when the myotomy cost was less than $3,244, a highly unlikely scenario. Pneumatic dilation remained less costly than BTX, as long as the rate of pneumatic dilation efficacy and perforation rates were greater than 70% or less than 9.5%, respectively, and the cost of BTX injections including endoscopy was greater than $450.

Other authors have recently used decision analysis modeling to address the gain in quality-adjusted life expectancy, the product of the duration of survival in a particular health state and the quality of life (0—dead to 1—perfect health) associated with state of health, to compare treatments for achalasia. Urbach and co-workers (326) calculated that laparoscopic Heller myotomy with a partial fundoplication was associated with the longest quality-adjusted life-years, but this only occurred after 10 years. However, the differences between this strategy and pneumatic dilation were small, with pneumatic dilation becoming the preferred strategy when the effectiveness of laparoscopic surgery was less than 90%, the operative mortality greater than 0.7%, or the probability of reflux after pneumatic dilation was less than 19%.

Limitations of these studies are similar and include relatively short follow-up periods in the life of a patient with achalasia, modeled data rather than actual cost analysis for BTX injections and laparoscopic Heller myotomy, and no consideration for patient preference.

TABLE 11.11. COST ANALYSIS FOR ACHALASIA TREATMENT

	Pneumatic Dilation	Myotomy	Botulinum Toxin	Time Horizon
Parkman (251)	$8,474	$20,064[a]	—	7 yr
Panaccione (324)	$2,345	—	$3,271	10 yr
Imperiale (325)	$3,111	$10,792	$3,723	5 yr

[a]Open myotomy; other studies laparoscopic Heller myotomy.
Amounts converted to U.S. dollars.

GENERAL RECOMMENDATIONS AND THE CLEVELAND CLINIC EXPERIENCE

For the newly diagnosed patient with achalasia, a suggested treatment algorithm is shown in Figure 11.13 (327). Symptomatic healthy patients with achalasia should be given the option of graded pneumatic dilation or laparoscopic Heller myotomy in that my review (Tables 11.7 and 11.9) and experience suggests relatively similar efficacies in the hands of experienced gastroenterologists and surgeons. Pneumatic dilation has the advantage of being an outpatient procedure, the pain is minimal, GERD is an infrequent problem, pneumatic dilation can be performed in any age group (children to 90 years of age) and during pregnancy (328,329), pneumatic dilation does not hinder the performance of a future myotomy, and all cost analyses find it less expensive than Heller myotomy over 5 to 7 years. On the other hand, laparoscopic Heller myotomy has the advantage of being a single procedure, the dysphagia relief may be greater at the cost of more troubling heartburn, and a myotomy may be more effective treatment than pneumatic dilation in adolescents and young adults, especially men. Myotomy is definitely the treatment of choice in uncooperative patients and patients in whom pseudoachalasia cannot be excluded. In healthy subjects who are good surgical candidates, I do not offer BTX as an option, because the treatment is not definitive and the duration of relief short term. On the other hand, BTX injections are my treatment of choice in patients who are poor surgical candidates or older than 80 years, because it is safe, improves symptoms, and

generally elderly patients require re-treatment no more frequently than once a year. Nifedipine or isosorbide dinitrate are at best second-line treatments, being rarely used because of drug side effects. If medical therapy fails, a "gentle" pneumatic dilatation can be performed with a 3.0-cm Rigiflex balloon.

Figure 11.14 summarizes my personal experience treating 223 achalasia patients at the Cleveland Clinic from 1994 to 2002 (249). Nearly 80% of these patients had newly diagnosed achalasia or were diagnosed and treated unsuccessfully elsewhere with drugs, BTX, or pneumatic dilation. Very old patients or those with severe comorbid illnesses (21 patients—12%) received BTX injections as initial treatment. Healthy patients were offered either graded pneumatic dilation or laparoscopic Heller myotomy by my best esophageal surgeon, Thomas Rice. Seventy-six patients (44%) were successfully treated with pneumatic dilatation and 43 patients (25%) underwent successful Heller myotomy. Overall, good to excellent symptom relief at last follow-up for pneumatic dilation and surgical myotomy were remarkably similar (82% vs. 80%, respectively). My esophageal perforation rate was 2%; 15% of my patients undergoing pneumatic dilation had troubling heartburn requiring proton pump inhibitors, and 15 patients eventually required myotomy to relieve their dysphagia. In the patients treated with laparoscopic myotomy, two patients (3%) required repeat myotomy, four patients (6%) required subsequent pneumatic dilations, and 51% of patients had troubling heartburn requiring proton pump inhibitors. Our high rate of GERD is bothersome but is representative of

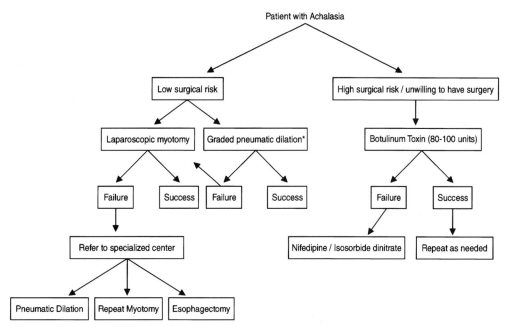

FIGURE 11.13. Suggested algorithm for the treatment of achalasia. (From Vaezi MF, Richter JE. American College of Gastroenterology Practice Guidelines: Diagnosis and management of achalasia. *Am J Gastroenterol* 1999;94:3406–3412, with permission.

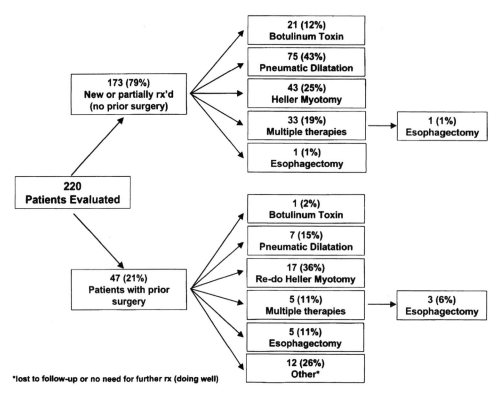

FIGURE 11.14. The author's personal experience treating 220 patients with achalasia at the Cleveland Clinic Foundation from 1994 to 2002. Note the multiple therapies required in the treatment of many of these achalasia patients.

our personal evolution with the technique of laparoscopic Heller myotomy. Initially, our operation was done with a Toupet fundoplication, but several patients required wrap modification or takedown because of dysphagia. Next, the myotomy was performed without a fundoplication with minimal dissection of the hiatus and a gastropexy. As a result of the high rate of heartburn, we have added a Dor fundoplication, which has resulted in fewer gastroesophageal reflux problems. Forty-seven patients (21%) with achalasia were referred to me after failing surgery; 93% had prior Heller myotomy (more than 60% via the thoracic approach) and 7% were initially misdiagnosed with GERD and underwent antireflux surgery. The success rate for either pneumatic dilation (67%) or repeat Heller myotomy (65%) was significantly less in this group of patients than for untreated achalasia patients. In the patients with prior surgery, eight patients (17%) eventually needed an esophagectomy with gastric pullup and in my entire 223 patient experience, ten patients (4.5%) ultimately required esophagectomy.

This experience with complicated achalasia patients confirms our recommendation in the algorithm (327) that patients failing initial laparoscopic myotomy need referral to specialized esophageal centers with expertise in pneumatic dilation, repeat myotomy, and esophagectomy. Fur-

thermore, my ongoing long-term follow-up of these patients, both symptomatically and objectively with the timed barium esophagram, suggests that the vast majority of individuals can be helped with general relief of their dysphagia and good quality of life. However, as we and others have reported (253,254), few patients are "cured" with a single procedure, and intermittent "tune-up" procedures (especially pneumatic dilation and occasionally repeat myotomy) may be required.

ESOPHAGEAL CANCER

In 1872, Fagge (330) first described the relationship between achalasia and esophageal cancer in an 84-year-old patient suffering from dysphagia for more than 40 years. Over the past 30 years, 15 studies have addressed this issue, showing an overall prevalence rate of 0% to 6.7% with a mean of 3%. Among these studies, five found no correlation but the remainder had incidences that ranged from 1% to 20% (mean 7.5%) with the average risk being 197 cases per 100,000 achalasia patients (331). In the most careful endoscopic follow-up of achalasia, Meijssen and colleagues (332) prospectively studied 195 patients with surveillance endoscopy at 3 months and at 1, 2, 7, and 10 years after dilation. Squamous cell carcinoma was discovered in the middle of the esophagus in three patients at 5, 19, and 28 years following the onset of dysphagia, with the age of the patients being 89, 37, and 77 years, respectively.

Achalasia patients with esophageal cancer average 60 years of age. They are four times more likely to be men, despite the prevalence of achalasia being equal between genders (331). Compared with the general population presenting with esophageal cancer, achalasia patients have a poorer prognosis and have more unresectable disease (50% vs. 80%) (332). This difference is most likely related to the more dilated esophagi and large tumor mass necessary to produce symptoms as well as a lack of patient and physician alarm when new dysphagia complaints present. Cancer presents in the midesophagus in 50% of cases, lower third in 38%, and upper esophagus in 12% of patients with more than 90% having a predominant histologic type of squamous cell carcinoma. Adenocarcinoma more commonly occurs following myotomy and comprises less than 10% of cases (331). Most cancers occur in patients with a megaesophagus (333). The malignancy rarely occurs at the stenotic area and is more common in the dilated esophagus. It is theorized that stasis of esophageal contents causes chronic esophagitis, which progresses to chronic ulcerations. Over time, the ulcerations can heal to form epithelial hyperplasia and benign papillomas. As the irritation continues in the poorly emptying esophagus, the opportunity for malignant degeneration occurs (334). This theory has been confirmed in two large esophageal resection studies (18,335).

The diagnosis of esophageal cancer in an achalasia patient is best made by careful endoscopy after the subject has been on a clear liquid diet for several days. The right wall of the lower third of the esophagus should be inspected carefully, because this area is most susceptible to malignant changes (336). Lugol staining to help direct biopsies (337) and brush cytology may help in patients without obvious masses. Overall survival in achalasia patients after the diagnosis of esophageal cancer generally is not good because of the large tumor burden with extensive regional and distant spread. Only 20% of these patients are suitable for surgery (332). In a study of 167 cases of achalasia and cancer, only 5 of the 38 subjects undergoing surgery could be resected and no patient was alive beyond 5 years (336). Over the past 30 years, 5-year survival rates for esophageal cancer in the general population have significantly improved, varying from 25% to 40% (338), whereas the mean survival for achalasia patients with cancer is approximately 10 months, with most patients living less than 6 months (331).

Because the data are overwhelming confirming the risk of squamous cell carcinoma in achalasia, the key is prevention and early detection. Although Ronald Belsey in 1958 (339) suggested that "procrastination and the extended trial of less than satisfactory procedures, such as repeated attempts at dilation, can only increase the risk of malignant generation," there are many examples in the literature of squamous cell cancer after myotomy (331). Because most patients have megaesophagus, this suggests the need for careful follow-up of patients monitoring esophageal diameter and emptying time, perhaps with a timed barium swallow (182), independent of the patient's complaints about dysphagia or regurgitation. Despite this cancer risk, the most recent guidelines from the American Society of Gastrointestinal Endoscopy do not recommend routine endoscopic surveillance for squamous cell cancer in achalasia patients (340). Without guidelines, this is an area of debate and further intervention studies are unlikely because the disease (cancer in achalasia) is rare and would require long-term and probably multicenter studies. I agree with others that older patients with longstanding disease and megaesophagus are the best candidates for a surveillance program (253,331,332). The endoscopy interval is unknown but probably should be every 2 to 3 years.

FUTURE INVESTIGATIONS

Despite our expanding knowledge about achalasia over the last 30 years, much still is to be learned. Is this a genetically modulated autoimmune disease or the result of a viral insult? Should success of therapy be based on symptoms alone or should objective improvement in esophageal emptying be routinely evaluated? Does aggressive therapy with the goal of dramatically improving esophageal emptying result in better long-term results? What is the best treatment for achalasia or will treatment vary based on subsets of patients? Should young patients preferentially be treated with laparoscopic Heller myotomy, patients older 40 years with pneumatic dilation, and the elderly with BTX injections? If a fundoplication is added to the Heller myotomy, which procedure results in the best long-term gastroesophageal reflux relief without the risk of dysphagia? Will routine intraoperative manometry improve the success of surgical myotomy? Can modifications of BTX or its regimen of injections result in longer symptom relief and better esophageal emptying in young achalasia patients? Are any of these treatments really "curative" for achalasia or does the disease gradually deteriorate over time, requiring frequent "tune-up" treatments? What is the role of endoscopy in the surveillance for squamous cell cancer in these patients? These and other basic and clinical questions will keep investigators busy for many years to come. Hopefully, multidiscipline teams of basic scientists, gastroenterologists, and surgeons working in esophageal centers of excellence or in multicenter research studies will answer most of these questions in the next 30 years.

ACKNOWLEDGMENT

This work was supported by the Pier Borra Family Endowment for Esophageal and Swallowing Disorders.

REFERENCES

1. Willis T. *Pharmaceutic Rationalis: Sive Diatriba de Medicamentorum; Operatimibus in Humano Corpore*. London, Hagae-Comitis, 1674.
2. Von Mikulicz J, Ueber Gastroskopic und Oesophagoskopic. *Miu Ver Aeszte Niedes Orst Wein*. 1882;8:41-4.
3. Hurst AF. Achalasia of the cardia. *Q J Med* 1915;8:200–202.
4. Russel JC. Diagnosis and treatment of spasmodic strictures of the esophagus. *BMJ* 1898;1:1450–1454.
5. Heller E. Extramukoese cardinplastik bein chronischen cardiopsasmus mit dilation des oesophagus. *Mitt Grenzgeb Med Chir* 1914;27:141–145.
6. Mayberry JF, Atkinson M. Variations in the prevalence of achalasia in Great Britain and Ireland: an epidemiological study based on hospital admissions. *Q J Med* 1987;62:67–71.
7. Mayberry JF. Epidemiology and demographics of achalasia. *Gastrointest Endosc Clin North Am* 2001;11:235–247.
8. Wong RK, Maydonovitch CL, Metz SJ, et al. Significant DQwl association in achalasia. *Dig Dis Sci* 1989;34:349–354.
9. Verne GN, Hahn AB, Pineau BC, et al. Association of HLA-DR and –DQ alleles with idiopathic achalasia. *Gastroenterology* 1999;117:26–31.
10. Howard PJ, Maker L, Pryde A, et al. Five year prospective study of the incidence, clinical features, and diagnosis of achalasia in Edinburgh. *Gut* 1992;33:1011–1015.
11. Paterson WG. Etiology and pathogenesis of achalasia. *Gastrointest Endosc Clin North Am* 2001;11:249–265.
12. Goyal RK, Paterson WG. Esophageal motility. In Woods JD, ed. *Handbook of physiology*. New York: Oxford Press, 1989:865–882.
13. Cassella RR, Ellis FH, Brown AL. Fine structure changes in achalasia of the esophagus. I. Vagus nerves. *Am J Pathol* 1965;279:46–54.
14. Kimura K. The nature of idiopathic esophagus dilatation. *Jpn J Gastroenterol* 1929;1:199–201.
15. Casella RR, Brown AL, Sayre GP, et al. Achalasia of the esophagus: pathologic and etiologic observations. *Ann Surg* 1964;160:474–480.
16. Higgs B, Kerr FWL, Ellis FH. The experimental production of esophageal achalasia by electrolytic lesions in the medulla. *J Thorac Cardiovasc Surg* 1965;50:613–617.
17. Lendrum FC. Anatomic features of the cardiac orifice of the stomach with special reference to cardiospasm. *Arch Intern Med* 1937;59:474–478.
18. Goldblum JR, Whyte RI, Orringer MB, et al. Achalasia: a morphologic study of 42 resected specimens. *Am J Surg Pathol* 1994;18:327–337.
19. Goldblum JR, Rice TW, Richter JE. Histopathologic features in esophagomyotomy specimens from patients with achalasia. *Gastroenterology* 1996;111:648–654.
20. Csendes A, Smok G, Braghetto I, et al. Histological studies of Auerbach's plexuses of the oesophagus, stomach, jejunum, and colon in patients with achalasia of the esophagus: correlation with gastric acid secretion, presence of parietal cells and gastric emptying of solids. *Gut* 1992;33:150–155.
21. Friesen DL, Henderson RD, Hanna W. Ultrastructure of the esophageal muscle in achalasia and diffuse esophageal spasm. *Am J Clin Pathol* 1983;79:319–322.
22. Aggestrup S, Uddman R, Sandler F, et al. Lack of vasoactive intestinal polypeptide nerves in esophageal achalasia. *Gastroenterology* 1983;84:924–927.
23. Wattchow DA, costa M. Distribution of peptide-containing nerve fibers in achalasia of the esophagus. *J Gastroenterol Hepatol* 1996;11:478–482.
24. DeGiorgio R, Di Simone MP, Stanghellini V, et al. Esophageal and gastric nitric acids synthesizing innervation in primary achalasia. *Am J Gastroenterol* 1999;94:2357–2362.
25. Mearin F, Mourelle M, Guarner F, et al. Patients with achalasia lack nitric oxide synthase in the gastro-oesophageal function. *Eur J Clin Invest* 1993;23:724–728.
26. Blennerhassett MG, Lourenssen S. Neural regulation of intestinal smooth muscle growth. *Am J Physiol* 2000;279:6511–6517.
27. Lehman MB, Clark SB, Ormsby AH, et al. Squamous mucosal alterations in esophagectomy specimens from patients with end-stage achalasia. *Am J Surg Pathol* 2001;25:1413–1418.
28. Dunaway PM, Maydonovitch CL, Wong RKH. Characterization of esophageal muscle in patients with achalasia. *Dig Dis Sci* 2000;45:285–290.
29. Massey BT, Hogan WJ, Dodds WJ, et al. Alteration of upper esophageal sphincter belch reflex in patients with achalasia. *Gastroenterology* 1992;103:1574–1579.
30. Ali GN, Hunt DR, Jorgensen JO, et al. Esophageal achalasia and coexistent upper esophageal sphincter relaxation disorder presenting with airway obstruction. *Gastroenterology* 1995;109:1328–1332.
31. Annese V, Caruso N, Accadia L, et al. Gallbladder function and gastric liquid emptying in achalasia. *Dig Dis Sci* 1991;36:1116–1120.
32. Schmidt T, Pfeiffer A, Hachelsberger N, et al. Dysmotility of the small intestine in achalasia. *Neurogastroenterol Motil* 1999;11:11–15.
33. Hagenmuller F, Classen M. Motility of Oddi's sphincter in Parkinson's disease, progressive systemic sclerosis and achalasia. *Endoscopy* 1988;20[Suppl 1]:189–192.
34. Eckardt WF, Krause I, Belle D. Gastrointestinal transit and gastric acid secretion in patients with achalasia. *Dig Dis Sci* 1989;34:665–670.
35. Mearin F, Papo M, Malagelda JR. Impaired gastric relaxation in patients with achalasia. *Gut* 1995;36:363–368.
36. Olk W, Kiesewalter B, Aver P, et al. Extraesophageal autonomic dysfunction in patients with achalasia. *Dig Dis Sci* 1999;44:2088–2092.
37. Misiewicz J, Waller SC, Anthony PP, et al. Pharmacology and histopathology of isolated cardiac sphincter muscle from patients with and without achalasia. *Q J Med* 1969;38:17–20.
38. Tottrup A, Forman A, Funch-Jensen P, et al. Effects of postganglionic nerve stimulation in oesophageal achalasia: an *in vitro* study. *Gut* 1990;31:17–20.
39. Dodds WJ, Dent J, Hogan WJ, et al. Paradoxical lower esophageal sphincter contraction induced by cholecystokinin-octapeptide in achalasia. *Gastroenterology* 1981;80:27–33.
40. Cohen S, Fisher R, Tuch A. The site of denervation in achalasia. *Gut* 1972;13:556–559.
41. Guelrud M, Rossiter A, Souney E, et al. The effect of vasoactive intestinal polypeptide on the lower esophageal sphincter in achalasia. *Gastroenterology* 1992;103:377–382.
42. Gonzales M, Mearin F, Vasconez JR, et al. Oesophageal tone in patients with achalasia. *Gut* 1997;41:291–296.
43. Kramer P, Ingelfinger FJ. Esophageal sensitivity to Mecholyl in achalasia. *Gastroenterology* 1951;19:242–244.
44. Penagini R, Bartesaghi B, Zannini P, et al. Lower esophageal

sphincter hypersensitivity to opioid receptor stimulation in patients with idiopathic achalasia. *Gut* 1993;34:16–20.

45. Holloway RH, Dodds WJ, Helm JF, et al. Integrity of cholinergic innervation to the lower esophageal sphincter in achalasia. *Gastroenterology* 1986;90:924–929.

46. Sifrim D, Janssen J, Vantrappen G. Failing deglutitive inhibition in primary esophageal motility disorders. *Gastroenterology* 1994;106:875–882.

47. Paterson WG. Esophageal and lower esophageal sphincter response to balloon distention in patients with achalasia. *Dig Dis Sci* 1997;42:106–110.

48. Paterson WG. Neuromuscular mechanisms of esophageal response at and proximal to a distending balloon. *Am J Physiol* 1991;42:106–110.

49. Murray JA, Ledlow A, Launspach J, et al. The effects of recombinant human hemoglobin on esophageal motor function in humans. *Gastroenterology* 1995;109:1241–1248.

50. Singarum C, Snipes RL, Bass P, et al. Evaluation of early events in the creation of amyenteric opossum model of achalasia. *Neurogastroenterol Motil* 1996;8:351–357.

51. Gaumnitz EA, Bass P, Osinski M, et al. Electrophysiological and pharmacological responses of chronically denervated LES of the opossum. *Gastroenterology* 1995;109:789–799.

52. Zimmerman FH, Rosensweig NS. Achalasia in a father and son. *Am J Gastroenterol* 1984;79:506–508.

53. Bosher LP, Shaw A. Achalasia in siblings. Clinical and genetic aspects. *Am J Dis Child* 1981;135:709–710.

54. Ehrich E, Aranoff G, Johnson WG. Familial achalasia associated with adrenocortical insufficiency, alacrima, and neurological abnormalities. *Am J Med Genet* 1987;26:637–644.

55. Stein DT, Knauer M. Achalasia in monozygote twins. *Dig Dis Sci* 1982;27:636–640.

56. Weber A. Linkage of the gene for the triple A syndrome to chromosome 12q13 near the type 11 keratin gene cluster. *Hum Mol Genet* 1996;5:2061–2067.

57. Chawla K, Chawla SK, Alexander LL. Familial achalasia of the esophagus in mother and son: a possible pathogenic relationship. *J Am Geriatr Soc* 1979;27:519.

58. Kilpatrick ZM, Milles S. Achalasia in mother and daughter. *Gastroenterology* 1972;62:1042–1046.

59. Machler D, Schneider R. Achalasia in a father and son. *Dig Dis Sci* 1978;23:1042–1045.

60. Mayberry JF, Atkinson M. A study of swallowing difficulties in first-degree relatives of patients with achalasia. *Thorax* 1985;40: 391–393.

61. Birgisson S, Richter JE. Achalasia: what's new in diagnosis and treatment. *Dig Dis* 1997;15[Suppl]:1–27.

62. Atkinson M. Antecedents of achalasia. *Gut* 1994;35:861–862.

63. Robertson CS, Martin BA, Atkinson M. Varicella-zoster virus DNA in the oesophageal myenteric plexus in achalasia. *Gut* 1993;34:299–302.

64. Oliveira RB, Filho RJ, Dantas RO, et al. The spectrum of esophageal motor disorders in Chagas' disease. *Am J Gastroenterol* 1995;90:119–124.

65. Jones DB, Mayberry JF, Rhodes J, et al. Preliminary report of an association between measles virus and achalasia. *J Clin Pathol* 1983;36:655–657.

66. Castex F, Guillemot F, Talbode N, et al. Association of an attack of varicella and achalasia. *Am J Gastroenterol* 1995;90: 1188–1189.

67. Niwamoto H, Okamoto E, Fujmoto J, et al. Are human herpes viruses or measles virus associated with esophageal achalasia? *Dig Dis Sci* 1995;40:859–864.

68. Birgisson S, Galinski MS, Goldblum JR, et al. Achalasia is not associated with measles as known herpes or human papilloma viruses. *Dig Dis Sci* 1997;42:300–306.

69. De la Concha EG, Fernandez-Arquero M, Mendoza JL, et al. Contribution of HLA class II genes to susceptibility in achalasia. *Tissue Antigens* 1998;52:3812–3815.

70. Storch WB, Eckardt VF, Wienbeck M, et al. Autoantibodies to Auerbach's plexus in achalasia. *Cell Mol Biol* 1995;41: 1033–1038.

71. Verne GN, Sallustio JE, Eaker EY. Anti-myenteric neuronal antibodies in patients with achalasia. *Dig Dis Sci* 1997;42: 302–313.

72. Sonnenberg A, Massey BT, McCarty DJ, et al. Epidemiology of hospitalization for achalasia in the United States. *Dig Dis Sci* 1993;38:233–244.

73. Murphy MS, Gardner-Medwin D, Eastham EJ. Achalasia of the cardia associated with hereditary cerebellar ataxia. *Am J Gastroenterol* 1989;84:1329–1330.

74. Foster PN, Stewart M, Lowe JS, et al. Achalasia-like disorder of the oesophagus in von Recklinghausen's neurofibromatosis. *Gut* 1987;28:1522–1526.

75. Qualman SJ, Hupt HM, Yang P, et al. Esophageal Lewy bodies associated with ganglion cell loss in achalasia. Similarity to Parkinson's disease. *Gastroenterology* 1984;87:848–856.

76. Vantrappen G, Janssen J, Hellemans J, et al. Achalasia, diffuse spasm and related motility disorders. *Gastroenterology* 1979;76: 450–459.

77. Paterson WG, Beck IT, DaCosta TR. Transition from nutcracker esophagus to achalasia. A case report. *J Clin Gastroenterol* 1991;13:554–555.

78. Vantrappen G, Hellemans J, Deloof W, et al. Treatment of achalasia with pneumatic dilatation. *Gut* 1971;12:268–275.

79. Grimes R, Stephens HB, Margulis AR. Achalasia of the esophagus. *Am J Surg* 1970;120:198–202.

80. Black J, Vorbach AW, Collis J. Results of Heller operation for achalasia of the esophagus: the importance of hiatal hernia. *Br J Surg* 1976;63:649–653.

81. Menzies-Gow N, Gummes WP, Edward DAW. Results of Heller's operation for achalasia of the cardia. *Br J Surg* 1978; 65:483–485.

82. Sawyer JG, Foster JH. Surgical consideration in the management of achalasia of the esophagus. *Ann Surg* 1967;165:780–783.

83. Fellows IW, Ogilivie AL, Atkinson M. Pneumatic dilation in achalasia. *Gut* 1983;1020–1023.

84. Clouse RE, Abramson BK, Todorszuk JR. Achalasia in the elderly. Effect of aging on clinical presentation and outcome. *Dig Dis Sci* 1991;36:225–228.

85. Wong RKH, Maydonovitch CL. Achalasia. In Castell DO, Richter JE, eds. *The esophagus*, third ed. Philadelphia: Lippincott Williams and Wilkins, 1999:185–404.

86. Eckardt VF. Clinical presentation and complications of achalasia. *Gastroint Endosc Clin North Am* 2001;11:281–292.

87. Rosenzweig S, Traube M. The diagnosis and misdiagnosis of achalasia. *J Clin Gastroenterol* 1989;11:147–153.

88. Yang P, Ravich WJ, Espinola D, et al. The effect of carbonated beverages on esophageal clearance in achalasia. *Gastroenterology* 1982;82:1215A.

89. Reynolds JC, Parkman HP. Achalasia. *Gastroenterol Clin North Am* 1989;18:223–255.

90. Crookes PF, DeMeester TF, Corkill S. Gastroesophageal reflux in achalasia. When is reflux really reflux? *Dig Dis Sci* 1997; 42:1354–1359.

91. Aronchick JM, Miller WT, Epstein DM, et al. Association of achalasia and pulmonary *Mycobacterium fortuitum* infection. *Radiology* 1986;160:85–86.

92. Stacher G, Kiss A, Wiesnagrotzki S, et al. Oesophageal and gastric motility disorders in patients categorized as having primary anorexia nervosa. *Gut* 1986;27:1120–1126.

93. Eckardt VF, Stauf B, Bernhard G. Chest pain in achalasia:

patient characteristics and clinical course. *Gastroenterology* 1999;116:1300–1304.

94. Robson K, Rosenberg S, Lembo T. GERD progressing to diffuse esophageal spasm and then achalasia. *Dig Dis Sci* 200;45: 110–113.

95. Smart HC, Mayberry JF, Atkinson M. Achalasia following gastro-oesophageal reflux. *J R Soc Med* 1986;79:71–73.

96. Spechler SJ, Souza RF, Rosenberg SJ, et al. Heartburn in patients with achalasia. *Gut* 1995;37:305–308.

97. Shoenut JP, Micflikier AB, Yaffe CS, et al. Reflux in untreated achalasia patients. *J Clin Gastroenterol* 1995;20:6–11.

98. Smart HL, Foster PN, Evans DF, et al. Twenty-four hour oesophageal acidity in achalasia before and after pneumatic dilation. *Gut* 1987;28:883–887.

99. Tucker HJ, Snape WJ, Cohen S. Achalasia secondary to carcinoma: manometric and clinical features. *Ann Intern Med* 1978;89:315–318.

100. Rozman RW, Achkar E. Features distinguishing secondary achalasia from primary achalasia. *Am J Gastroenterol* 1990;85: 1327–1330.

101. Dominguez F, Hernandes-Ranz F, Boixeda D, et al. Acute upper airway obstruction in achalasia of the esophagus. *Am J Gastroenterol* 1987;82:362–364.

102. Collins MP, Rabie S. Sudden airway obstruction in achalasia. *J Laryngol Otol* 1984;98:701–711.

103. Becker DJ, Castell DO. Acute airway obstruction in achalasia: possible role of defective belch reflex. *Gastroenterology* 1989; 97:1323–1326.

104. Seeman H, Traube M. Hiccups and achalasia. *Ann Intern Med* 1991;115:711–712.

105. Breatnach E, Han SY. Pneumopericardium occurring as a complication of achalasia. *Chest* 1986;90:292–294.

106. Siriser F, Bardaxaglow E, Lebeau S, et al. A long-term clinical study of the effectiveness of myotomy for achalasia. *Gullet* 1992;2:124–128.

107. Orlando RC, Call DL, Beam CA. Achalasia and absent gastric air bubble. *Ann Intern Med* 1978;88:60–61.

108. Stewart ET. Radiographic evaluation of the esophagus and its motor disorders. *Med Clin North Am* 1981;65:1173–1190.

109. Schima W, Ryan JM, Harisinghani M, et al. Radiographic detection of achalasia: diagnostic role of video fluoroscopy. *Clin Radiol* 1998;53:372–375.

110. DeOliveira JMA, Birgisson S, Doinoff C, et al. Timed-barium swallow: a simple technique for evaluating esophageal emptying in patients with achalasia. *Am J Roentgenol* 1997;169:473–479.

111. Kostic SV, Rice TW, Baker ME, et al. Timed barium esophagram: a simple physiologic assessment for achalasia. *J Thorac Cardiovasc Surg* 2000;120:935–946.

112. Meshkinpour H, Kaye L, Elias A, et al. Manometric and radiologic correlations in achalasia. *Am J Gastroenterol* 1992;87: 1567–1570.

113. Debas HT, Payne WS, Cameron AJ, et al. Physiopathology of the lower esophageal diverticulum and its implications for treatment. *Surg Gynecol Obstet* 1980;151(5):593–600.

114. Taub W, Achkar E. Hiatal hernia in patients with achalasia. *Am J Gastroenterol* 1987;82:1256–1258.

115. Goldenberg SP, Vos C, Burrell M, et al. Achalasia and hiatal hernia. *Dig Dis Sci* 1992;37:528–531.

116. Ott DJ, Hodge RG, Chen MYM, et al. Achalasia associated with hiatal hernia: prevalence and potential implications. *Abdom Imaging* 1993;18:7–9.

117. Kahrilas PJ, Kishk SM, Helm JF, et al. Comparison of pseudoachalasia and achalasia. *Am J Med* 1987;82:439–446.

118. Tracey JP, Traube M. Difficulties in the diagnosis of pseudoachalasia. *Am J Gastroenterol* 1994;89:2014–2018.

119. Sandler RS, Bozymski EM, Orlando RC. Failure of clinical cri-

teria to distinguish between primary achalasia and achalasia secondary to tumor. *Dig Dis Sci* 1982;27:209–213.

120. Herwaarden MAV, Samson M, Smout AJPM. Prolonged manometric recordings of oesophagus and lower oesophageal sphincter in achalasia patients. *Gut* 2001;49:813–821.

121. Hirano I, Tatum RP, Shi G, et al. Manometric heterogeneity in patients with idiopathic achalasia. *Gastroenterology* 2001;120: 789–798.

122. Goldenberg SP, Burell M, Fette GG, et al. Classic and vigorous achalasia: a comparison of manometric, radiographic, and clinical findings. *Gastroenterology* 1991;101:743–748.

123. Todorczuk JR, Aliperti G, Staiano A, et al. Reevaluation of manometric criteria for vigorous achalsia. Is this a distinct clinical disorder? *Dig Dis Sci* 1991;36:274–278.

124. Camacho-Lobato L, Katz PO, Eveland J, et al. Vigorous achalasia. Original description requires minor change. *J Clin Gastroenterol* 2001;33:375–377.

125. Vantrappen G, Hellemans J. Treatment of achalasia and related motor disorders. *Gastroenterology* 1980;79:144–154.

126. Schneider JH, Peters JH, Kirkman E, et al. Are the motility abnormalities of achalasia reversible? An experimental outflow obstruction in the feline model. *Surgery* 1999;125:498–503.

127. Parilla P, Aguayo JR, Martinex DHL, et al. Reversible achalasia-like motor pattern of esophageal body secondary to postoperative stricture of gastroesophageal junction. *Dig Dis Sci* 1992; 37:1781–1784.

128. Vantrappen G, Van Goidsenhoven GE, Verbekke S, et al. Manometric studies in achalasia of the cardia, before and after pneumatic dilation. *Gastroenterology* 1963;45:317–325.

129. Cohen S, Lipschutz W. Lower esophageal sphincter dysfunction in achalasia. *Gastroenterology* 1971;61:814–820.

130. Katz PO, Richter JE, Cowan R, et al. Apparent complete lower esophageal sphincter relaxation in achalasia. *Gastroenterology* 1986;90:978–983.

131. Castell JA, Dalton CB, Castell DO. On-line computer analysis of human lower esophageal sphincter relaxation. *Am J Physiol* 1988;255:G794–G799.

132. Clouse RE, Abramson BK, Todorczuk JR. Achalasia in the elderly. Effects of age on clinical presentation and outcome. *Dig Dis Sci* 1991;36:225–228.

133. Holloway RH, Wyman JB, Dent J. Failure of transient lower oesophageal sphincter relaxation in response to gastric distension in patients with achalasia: evidence for neural mediation of transient lower oesophageal sphincter relaxation. *Gut* 1989;30: 762–767.

134. Dudnick RS, Castell JA, Castell DO. Abnormal upper esophageal sphincter function in achalasia. *Am J Gastroenterol* 1992;87:1712-1715.

135. Liu JB, Miller LS, Goldberg BB, et al. Transnasal ultrasound of the esophagus: preliminary morphologic and function studies. *Radiology* 1992;184:721–727.

136. Miller LS, Liu JB, Klenn PJ, et al. High-resolution endoluminal sonography in achalasia. *Gastrointest Endosc* 1995;42:545–549.

137. Carter M, Deckmann RC, Smith RC, et al. Differentiation of achalasia from pseudoachalasia by computed tomography. *Am J Gastroenterol* 1997;92:624–628.

138. Van Dam J, Falk GW, Sivak MV, et al. Endosonographic evaluation of the patient with achalasia: appearance of the esophagus using the echoendoscope. *Endoscopy* 1995;27: 185–190.

139. Deviere J, Dunham F, Rickaert F, et al. Endoscopic ultrasonography in achalasia. *Gastroenterology* 1989;96:1210–1213.

140. Russell COH, Hill LD, Holmes ER. Radionuclide transit: a sensitive screening test for esophageal dysfunction. *Gastroenterology* 1981;80:887–891.

141. Holloway RH, Krosin G, Lange RC, et al. Radionuclide

esophageal emptying of a solid meal to quantitate results of therapy in achalasia. *Gastroenterology* 1983;84:771–776.

142. Rosen P, Gelfond M, Zalzman S, et al. Dynamic, diagnostic, and pharmacological radionuclide studies of the esophagus in achalasia. *Radiology* 1982;144:587–590.

143. Gross R, Johnson LF, Kaminski RJ. Esophageal emptying in achalasia quantitated by a radioisotope technique. *Dig Dis Sci* 1979;24:945–949.

144. Fredens K, Tottrup A, Kristensen IB, et al. Severe destruction of esophageal nerves in a patient with achalasia secondary to a gastric cancer. A possible role of eosinophil neurotropic protein. *Dig Dis Sci* 1989;34:297–303.

145. Benjamin SB, Castell DO. Achalasia and Hodgkin's disease. A chance association. *J Clin Gastroenterol* 1981;3:175–178.

146. Roark G, Shabot M, Patterson M. Achalasia secondary to hepatocellular carcinoma. *J Clin Gastroenterol* 1983;5:255–258.

147. Kline MM. Successful treatment of vigorous achalasia associated with gastric lymphoma. *Dig Dis Sci* 1980;25:311–213.

148. Goldin NR, Butud TW, Ferrante WA. Secondary achalasia: association with adenocarcinoma of the lung and reversal with radiation therapy. *Am J Gastroenterol* 1983;78:203–205.

149. Eaves R, Lambert J, Rees J, et al. Achalasia secondary to carcinoma of the prostate. *Dig Dis Sci* 1983;28:278–284.

150. Davis JA, Kantrowitz PA, Chandler HL, et al. Reversible achalasia due to reticulum-cell sarcoma. *N Engl J Med* 1975;293:130–132.

151. Rock LA, Latham PS, Hankins JR, et al. Achalasia associated with squamous cell carcinoma of the esophagus. *Am J Gastroenterol* 1985;80:526–528.

152. Goldschmiedt M, Peterson WL, Spielberger R, et al. Esophageal achalasia secondary to mesothelioma. *Dig Dis Sci* 1989;34:1285–1288.

153. Herrera JL. Esophageal metastasis from breast carcinoma presenting as achalasia. *Am J Med Sci* 1992;303:321–323.

154. Manela FD, Quiqley EMM, Paustian FF, et al. Achalasia of the esophagus in association with renal cell carcinoma. *Am J Gastroenterol* 1991;86:1812–1816.

155. Lefkowitz JR, Brand DL, Schuffler MD, et al. Amyloidosis mimics achalasia's effect on lower esophageal sphincter. *Dig Dis Sci* 1989;34:630–635.

156. Dufresne CR, Jeyasingham K, Baker RR. Achalasia of the cardia associated with pulmonary sarcoidosis. *Surgery* 1983;94:32–35.

157. Roberts DH, Gilmore IT. Achalasia in Anderson-Fabry's disease. *J R Soc Med* 1984;77:430–431.

158. Hollis JR, Castell DO, Braddom RL. Esophageal function in diabetes mellitus and its relation to peripheral neuropathy. *Gastroenteroogy* 1977;73:1098–1102.

159. Woods CA, Foutch PG, Waring JP, et al. Pancreatic pseudocyst as a cause for secondary achalasia. *Gastroenterology* 1989;96:235–239.

160. Duntemann TJ, Dresner DM. Achalasia-like syndrome presenting after highly selective vagotomy. *Dig Dis Sci* 1995;40:2081–2083.

161. Liu W, Fackler W, Rice TW, et al. The pathogenesis of pseudoachalasia: a clinicopathologic study of 13 cases of a rare entity. *Am J Surg Pathol* 2002;26:784–788.

162. Woodfield CA, Levine MS, Rubesin SE, et al. Diagnosis of primary versus secondary achalasia: reassessment of clinical and radiographic criteria. *Am J Roentgenol* 2000;175:727–731.

163. Dodds WJ, Stewart ET, Kishk SM, et al. Radiologic amyl nitrite test for distinguishing pseudoachalasia from idiopathic achalasia. *Am J Roentgenol* 1986;146:21–23.

164. Koberle F, Chagas' disease and Chagas' syndrome: the pathology of American trypanosomiasis. *Adv Parasitol* 1968;6:63–73.

165. World Health Organization. Chagas' disease: frequency and geographic distribution. *Weekly Epidemiol Res* 1990;65:257–264.

166. Kirchoff LV. American trypanosomiasis (Chagas' disease): a tropical disease now in the United States. *N Engl J Med* 1993;329:639–644.

167. Vaezi MF, Baker ME, Richter JE. Assessment of esophageal emptying post-pneumatic dilation: use of timed barium esophagram. *Am J Gastroenterol* 1999;94:1802–1807.

168. Vaezi MF, Baker MF, Achkar E, et al. Timed barium esophagram: better predictor of long-term success after pneumatic dilation than symptoms assessment. *Gut* 2002;50:765–770.

169. Gelfand MD, Kozarek RA. An experience with polyethylene balloon for pneumatic dilation for achalasia. *Am J Gastroenterol* 1989;84:924–927.

170. Alonso P, Gonzalez-Conde B, Macenille R, et al. Achalasia: the usefulness of manometry for evaluation of treatment. *Dig Dis Sci* 1999;44:536–541.

171. Eckardt VF, Aignherr C, Bernhard G. Predictors of outcome in patients with achalasia treated by pneumatic dilation. *Gastroenterology* 1992;103:1732–1738.

172. Ponce J, Garrigues V, Pertejo V, et al. Individual prediction of response to pneumatic dilation in patients with achalasia. *Dig Dis Sci* 1996;41:2135–2141.

173. Rosati R, Fumagolli U, Bona S, et al. Evaluating results of laparoscopic surgery for esophageal achalasia. *Surg Endosc* 1998;12:270–273.

174. Anselmino M, Zaniotto G, Costantini M. One year follow-up after laparoscopic Heller-Dor operation for esophageal achalasia. *Surg Endosc* 1997;11:3–7.

175. Kadakia SC, Wong RKH. Graded pneumatic dilation using Rigiflex achalasia dilators in patients with primary esophageal achalasia. *Am J Gastroenterol* 1993;88:34–38.

176. Kim CH, Cameron AJ, Hsu JJ, et al. Achalasia: prospective evaluation of relationship between lower esophageal sphincter pressure, esophageal transit, and esophageal diameter and symptoms in response to pneumatic dilation. *Mayo Clin Proc* 1993;68:1067–1073.

177. Sultan M, Norton RA. Esophageal diameter and the treatment of achalasia. *Am J Dig Dis* 1969;14:611–618.

178. Cohen NN. An endpoint for pneumatic dilation of achalasia. *Gastrointest Endosc* 1975;22:29.

179. Agha FP, Lee HH. The esophagus after endoscopic pneumatic balloon dilation for achalasia. *Am J Roentgenol* 1986;146:25–29.

180. Lee JD, Cecil BD, Brown PE, et al. The Cohen test does not predict outcome in achalasia after pneumatic dilation. *Gastrointest Endosc* 1992;39:157–160.

181. Ott DJ, Donati D, Wu WC, et al. Radiographic evaluation of achalasia immediately after pneumatic dilation with the Rigiflex dilator. *Gastrointest Radiol* 1991;16:279–282.

182. DeOliveira JMA, Birgisson S, Doinoff C, et al. Timed-barium swallow: a simple technique for evaluating esophageal emptying in patients with achalasia. *Am J Roentgenol* 1997;169:473–479.

183. Hoogerwerf WA, Pasricha PJ. Pharmacologic therapy in treating achalasia. *Gastrointest Endosc Clin North Am* 2001;11:311–323.

184. Gelfand M, Rozen P, Keren S, et al. Effect of nitrates on LOS pressure in achalasia: a potential therapeutic aid. *Gut* 1981;22:312–318.

185. Bortolotti M, Labo G. Clinical and manometric effects of nifedipine in patients with esophageal achalasia. *Gastroenterology* 1981;80:39–44.

186. Berger K, McCallum RW. Nifedipine in the treatment of achalasia. *Ann Intern Med* 1982;96:61–62.

187. Gelfand M, Rozen P, Gilat T. Isosorbide dinitrate and nifedipine treatment of achalasia: a clinical, manometric and radionuclide evaluation. *Gastroenterology* 1982;83:963–969.

188. Traube M, Dubovik S, Lange RC, et al. The role of nifedipine

therapy in achalasia: results of a randomized, double-blind, placebo-controlled study. *Am J Gastroenterol* 1989;84:1259–1262.

189. Rozen P, Gelfand M, Salzman S, et al. Radionuclide confirmation of the therapeutic value of isosorbide dinitrate in relieving dysphagia in achalasia. *J Clin Gastroenterol* 1982;4:17–22.

190. Coccia G, Bortolotti M, Michetti P, et al. Prospective clinical and manometric study comparing pneumatic dilation and sublingual nifedipine in the treatment of oesophageal achalasia. *Gut* 1991;32:604–606.

191. Becker BS, Burakoff R. The effect of verapamil on the lower esophageal sphincter pressure in normal subjects and in achalasia. *Am J Gastroenterol* 1983;78:773–776.

192. Triadafilopoulos G, Aaronson M, Sackel S, et al. Medical treatment of esophageal achalasia. Double-blind crossover study with oral nifedipine, verapamil and placebo. *Dig Dis Sci* 1991; 36:260–267.

193. Bortolotti M. Medical therapy of achalasia. A benefit reserved for few. *Digestion* 1999;60:11–16.

194. Marzio L, Grossi L, DeLaurentilis MF, et al. Effect of cimetropium bromide on esophageal motility and transit in patients affected by primary achalasia. *Dig Dis Sci* 1994; 39:1389–1394.

195. DiMarino AJ, Cohen S. Effect of an oral beta 2-adrenergic agonist on lower esophageal sphincter pressure in normals and in a patient with achalasia. *Dig Dis Sci* 1982;27: 1063–1066.

196. Wong RKH, Maydonovitch C, Garcia JE, et al. The effect of terbutaline sulfate, nitroglycerin, and aminophylline on lower esophageal sphincter pressure and radionuclide esophageal emptying in patients with achalasia. *J Clin Gastroenterol* 1987; 9:386–340.

197. Penagini R, Bartesaghi B, Negri G, et al. Effect of loperamide on lower esophageal sphincter pressure in idiopathic achalasia. *Scand J Gastroenterol* 1994;29:1057–1060.

198. Bortolotti M, Mari C, Lopilato C, et al. Effects of sildenafil on esophageal motility of patients with idiopathic achalasia. *Gastroenterology* 2000;118:253–257.

199. Guelrud M, Rossiter A, Souney PF, et al. Transcutaneous electrical nerve stimulation decreases lower esophageal sphincter pressure in patients with achalasia. *Dig Dis Sci* 1991;36: 1029–1033.

200. Shabsin HS, Katz PO, Schuster MM. Behavioral treatment of intractable chest pain in a patient with vigorous achalasia. *Am J Gastroenterol* 1988;83:970–973.

201. Tsai JKC. Botulinum toxin as a therapeutic agent. *Pharmacol Ther* 1996;72:13–24.

202. Pasricha PJ, Ravich WJ, Kalloo AN. Effects of intrasphincteric botulinum toxin on the lower esophageal sphincter in piglets. *Gastroenterology* 1993;105:1045–1049.

203. Pasricha PJ, Ravich WJ, Hendrix TR, et al. Treatment of achalasia with intrasphincteric injection of botulinum toxin. A pilot trial. *Ann Intern Med* 1994;121:590–591.

204. Pasricha PJ, Ravich WJ, Hendrix TR, et al. Intrasphincteric botulinum toxin for the treatment of achalasia. *N Engl J Med* 1995;322:774–778.

205. Pasricha PJ, Rai R, Ravich WJ, et al. Botulinum toxin for achalasia: Long-term outcome and predictor of response. *Gastroenterology* 1996;110:1410–1415.

206. Cuilliere C, Ducrotte P, Zerbib F, et al. Achalasia: outcome of patients treated with intrasphincteric injection of botulinum toxin. *Gut* 1997;41:87–92.

207. Rollan A, Gonzales R, Carvajal S, et al. Endoscopic intrasphincteric injection of botulinum toxin for the treatment of achalasia. *J Clin Gastroenterol* 1995;20:189–191.

208. Fishman VM, Parkman HP, Schiano TD, et al. Symptomatic improvement in achalasia after botulinum toxin injection of the lower esophageal sphincter. *Am J Gastroenterol* 1996;91: 1724–17230.

209. Annese V, Basciani M, Perri F, et al. Controlled trial of botulinum toxin injection versus placebo and pneumatic dilation in achalasia. *Gastroenterology* 1996;111:1418–1424.

210. Gordon JM, Eaker EY. Prospective study of esophageal botulinum toxin injection in high-risk achalasia patients. *Am J Gastroenterol* 1997;92:1812–1816.

211. Muchldorfer SM, Schneider TH, Hochberger J, et al. Esophageal achalasia: intrasphincter injection of botulinum toxin versus balloon dilation. *Endoscopy* 1999;31:517–521.

212. Vaezi MJ, Richter JE, Wilcox CM, et al. Botulinum toxin versus pneumatic dilation in the treatment of achalasia: a randomized trial. *Gut* 1999;44:231–239.

213. Annese V, Bassotti G, Coccia G, et al. A multicenter randomized study of intrasphincteric botulinum toxin in patients with oesophageal achalasia. *Gut* 2000;46:597–600.

214. Kolbasnik J, Waterfall WE, Fachnie B, et al. Long-term efficacy of botulinum toxin in classical achalasia; a prospective study. *Am J Gastroenterol* 1999;94:3434–3439.

215. Mikaeli J, Fazel A, Montazeri G, et al. Randomized controlled trial comparing botulinum toxin injection to pneumatic dilation for the treatment of achalasia. *Aliment Pharmacol Ther* 2001;15:1389–1396.

216. Allescher HD, Storr M, Seige M, et al. Treatment of achalasia: botulinum toxin injection vs pneumatic balloon dilation. A prospective study with long-term follow-up. *Endoscopy* 2001; 33:1007-1017.

217. Neubrand M, Scheurlen C, Schepke M, et al. Long-term results and prognostic factors in the treatment of achalasia with botulinum toxin. *Endoscopy* 2002;34:519–523.

218. Vallera RZ, Brazer SR. Botulinum toxin for suspected pseudoachalasia. *Am J Gastroenterol* 1995;90:1319–1321.

219. Katzka DA, Castell DO. Use of botulinum toxin as a diagnostic/therapeutic trial to help clarify and indication for definitive therapy in patients with achalasia. *Am J Gastroenterol* 1999; 94:637–642.

220. Hoffman BJ, Knapple WL, Bhutani MS, et al. Treatment of achalasia by injection of botulinum toxin under endoscopic ultrasound guidance. *Gastrointestinal Endosc* 1997;45:77–79.

221. Bonavina L, Incarbone R, Antoniazzi L, et al. Previous endoscopic treatment does not affect complication rate and outcome of laparoscopic Heller myotomy and anterior fundoplication for achalasia. *Ital J Gastroenterol Hepatol* 1999;31:827–830.

222. Horgan S, Hudda K, Eubanks T, et al. Does botulinum toxin injection make esophagomyotomy a more difficult operation? *Surg Endosc* 1999;13:576–579.

223. Mandelstam P, Block C, Newell L, et al. The role of bougienage in the management of achalasia—the need for reappraisal. *Gastrointest Endosc* 1982;28:169–172.

224. McJunkin B, McMillian WO, Duncan HE, et al. Assessment of dilation methods in achalasia: large diameter mercury bougienage followed by pneumatic dilation as needed. *Gastrointest Endosc* 1991;37:18–21.

225. Olsen AM, Harrington SW, Moersch HJ, et al. Treatment of cardiospasm: analysis of a twelve-year experience. *J Thorac Surg* 1951;22:164–169.

226. Bennett JR, Hendrix TR. Treatment of achalasia with pneumatic dilatation. *Mod Treat* 1970;7:1217–1228.

227. Kadakia SC, Wong RKH. Pneumatic balloon dilation for esophageal achalasia. *Gastrointest Endosc Clin North Am* 2001; 11:325–345.

228. Heimlich HU, O'Connor TW, Fiores DC. Case for pneumatic dilation for achalasia. *Ann Otol* 1978;87:519–522.

229. Csendes A, Braghetto I, Henriques A, et al. Late results of a prospective randomized study comparing forceful dilatation

and esophagomyotomy in patients with achalasia. *Gut* 1989; 30:299–305.

230. Stark GA, Castell DO, Richter JE, et al. Prospective randomized comparison of Browne-McHardy and microvasive balloon dilator in the treatment of achalasia. *Am J Gastroenterol* 1990; 85:1322–1326.

231. Wong RKH, Maydonovitch C. Utility of parameters measured during pneumatic dilation as predictors of successful dilation. *Am J Gastroenterol* 1996;91:1126–1129.

232. Khan AA, Shah SWH, Alam A, et al. Pneumatic balloon dilation in achalasia: a prospective comparison of balloon distention time. *Am J Gastroenterol* 1998;93:1064–1067.

233. Ciarolla DA, Traube M. Achalasia. Short-term clinical monitoring after pneumatic dilation. *Dig Dis Sci* 1993;38:1905–1908.

234. Barkin JS, Guelrud M, Reiner DK, et al. Foreceful balloon dilation: an outpatient procedure for achalasia. *Gastrointest Endosc* 1990;36:123–125.

235. Elta GH, Nostrant TT, Wilson JAP. Treatment of achalasia with the Witzel pneumatic dilator. *Gastrointest Endosc* 1987;33:101–103.

236. Barnett JL, Eisenman R, Nostrant TT, et al. Witzel pneumatic dilation for achalasia: safety and long-term efficacy. *Gastrointest Endosc* 1990;36:482–485.

237. Johnston BT, Collins BJ, Collins JSA, et al. Perendoscopic pneumatic dilatation in achalasia: assessment of outcome using esophageal scintigraphy. *Dysphagia* 1992;7:201–204.

238. Mearin F, Armengol JR, Chicharro L, et al. Forceful dilatation under endoscopic control in the treatment of achalasia: a randomized trial of pneumatic vs metallic dilator. *Gut* 1994;35: 1360–1362.

239. Cox J, Buckton GK, Bennett JR. Balloon dilatation in achalasia: a new dilator. *Gut* 1986;27:986-9.

240. Makela J, Kiviniemi H, Laitinen S. Heller's cardiomyotomy compared with pneumatic dilation for the treatment of oesophageal achalasia. *Eur J Surg* 1991;157:411–414.

241. Levine ML, Moskowitz GW, Dorf BS, et al. Pneumatic dilation in patients with achalasia with a modified Gruntzig dilator (Levine) under direct endoscopic control. Results after 5 years. *Am J Gastroenterol* 1991;86:1581–1584.

242. Abid S, Champion G, Richter JE, et al. Treatment of achalasia: the best of both worlds. *Am J Gastroenterol* 1993;89:979–985.

243. Wehrmann T, Jacobi V, Jung M, et al. Pneumatic dilation in achalasia with a low-compliance balloon. Results of a 5 year prospective evaluation. *Gastrointest Endosc* 1995;42:31–36.

244. Lambroza A, Schuman RW. Pneumatic dilation for achalasia without fluoroscopic guidance: safety and efficacy. *Am J Gastroenterol* 1995;90:1226–1229.

245. Muehldorfer SM, Hahn EG, Eli C. High- and low-compliance balloon dilators in patients with achalasia: a randomized prospective comparion trial. *Gastrointest Endosc* 1996;44: 398–403.

246. Bhatnager MS, Nanivadekar SA, Sawant P, et al. Achalasia cardia dilation using polyethylene balloon (Rigiflex) dilator. *Ind J Gastroenterol* 1996;15:49–51.

247. Gideon RM, Castell DO, Yarze J. Prospective randomized comparison of pneumatic dilation techniques in patients with idiopathic achalasia. *Dig Dis Sci* 1999;44:1853–1857.

248. Khan AA, Shah WH, Alam A, et al. Massively dilated esophagus in achalasia: response to pneumatic balloon dilation. *Am J Gastroenterol* 1999;94:2363–2366.

249. Vela MF, Richter JE. Management of achalasia at a tertiary center—a complicated disease. *Gastroenterology* 2003;124:S1635.

250. Vaezi MF, Richter JE. Current therapies for achalasia. Comparison and efficacy. *J Clin Gastroenterol* 1998;27:21–35.

251. Parkman HP, Reynolds JC, Ouyang A, et al. Pneumatic dilatation or esophagomyotomy treatment for idiopathic achalasia: clinical outcome and cost analysis. *Dig Dis Sci* 1993;38:75–85.

252. Katz PO, Gilbert J, Castell DO. Pneumatic dilatation is effective long-term treatment for achalasia. *Dig Dis Sci* 1998;43: 1973–1977.

253. West RC, Hirsch DP, Bartelsman JFWM, et al. Long term results of pneumatic dilation in achalasia followed for more than 5 years. *Am J Gastroenterol* 2002;97:1346–1351.

254. Torbey CF, Achkar E, Rice TW, et al. Long-term outcome of achalasia treatment: the need for closer follow-up. *J Clin Gastroenterol* 1994:28:125–130.

255. Lamet H, Fleshler B, Achkar E. Return of peristalsis in achalasia after pneumatic dilation. *Am J Gastroenterol* 1985;80:602–604.

256. Mellow MH. Return of esophageal peristalsis in idiopathic achalasia. *Gastroenterology* 1976;70:1148–1151.

257. Bielefeldt K, Enck P, Erckenbrecht F. Motility changes in primary achalasia following pneumatic dilation. *Dysphagia* 1990; 5:152–158.

258. Vantrappen G, Hellemans J, Deloof W, et al. Treatment of achalasia with pneumatic dilation. *Gut* 1971;12:268–275.

259. Farhoomand KS, Richter JE, Achkar E, et al. A new predictor of outcome of pneumatic dilation in achalasia. *Gastroenterology* 2003;124:S1626.

260. Ghosh S, Palmer KR, Heading RC. Achalasia of the esophagus in elderly patients responds poorly to conservative therapy. *Age Ageing* 1994;4:280–282.

261. Eckardt VF, Kanzler G, Westermeier T. Complications and their impact after pneumatic dilation for achalasia: prospective long-term follow-up study. *Gastrointest Endosc* 1997;45:349–353.

262. Nair LA, Reynolds JC, Parkman HP, et al. Complications during pneumatic dilation for achalasia and diffuse esophageal spasm: analysis of risk factors, early clinical characteristics and outcome. *Dig Dis Sci* 1993;38:1893–1904.

263. Borotto E, Gaudric M, Daniel B, et al. Risk factors of oesophageal perforation during pneumatic dilation for achalasia. *Gut* 1996;39:9–12.

264. Metman EH, Lagasse JP, Alteroche L, et al. Risk factors for immediate complications after progressive pneumatic dilation for achalasia.. *Am J Gastroenterol* 1999;94:1179–1185.

265. Michel L, Grillo HC, Malt RA. Operative and non-operative management of esophageal perforation. *Ann Surg* 1981;194: 57–63.

266. Swedlund A, Traube M, Siskind BN, et al. Nonsurgical management of esophageal perforation from pneumatic dilation in achalasia. *Dig Dis Sci* 1989;34:379–384.

267. Swartz AM, Cahow CE, Traube M. Outcome after perforation sustained during pneumatic dilation for achalasia. *Dig Dis Sci* 1993;38:1409–1413.

268. Shoenut JP, Duerksen D, Yaffe CS. A prospective assessment of gastroesophageal reflux before and after treatment of achalasia patients: Pneumatic dilation vs transthoracic limited myotomy. *Am J Gastroenterol* 1997;92:1109–1112.

269. Burke CA, Achkar EA, Falk GW. Effect of pneumatic dilation on gastroesophageal reflux in achalasia. *Dig Dis Sci* 1997;42: 998–1002.

270. Zaaijer JH, Cardiospasm in the aged. *Ann Surg* 1923;77:615–617.

271. Pelligrini C, Wetter LA, Patti M, et al. Thoracoscopic esophagomyotomy. Initial experience with a new approach for achalasia. *Ann Surg* 1992;216:291–296.

272. Ellis FH, Crozier RE, Watkins E. Operation for esophageal achalasia. Result of esophagomyotomy without an antireflux operation. *J Thorac Cardiovas Surg* 1984;88:344–351.

273. Little AG, Soriano A, Fergusson MK, et al. Surgical treatment of achalasia: results with esophagomyotomy and Belsey repair. *Ann Thorac Surg* 1988;45:489–494.

274. Ponce J, Miralbes M, Garriques V, et al. Return of esophageal peristalsis after Heller's myotomy for idiopathic achalasia. *Dig Dis Sci* 1986;31:545–547.

275. Bianco A, Cagossi M, Scrimieri D, et al. Appearance of esophageal peristalsis in treated idiopathic achalasia. *Dig Dis Sci* 1986;31:40–48.

276. Parilla P, Martinez de Haro LF, Ortiz A, et al. Factors involved in the return of peristalsis in patients with achalasia of the cardia after Heller's myotomy. *Am J Gastroenterol* 1995;90: 713–717.

277. Csendes A, Larrain A, Strauszer R, et al. Long-term clinical, radiological and manometrical follow-up of patients with achalasia fo the esophagus treated with esophagomyotomy. *Digestion* 1975;13:27–32.

278. Patti MG, Pelligrini CA, Arcerito M, et al. Comparison of medical and minimally invasive surgical therapy for achalasia. *Arch Surg* 1997;132:233–240.

279. Cade RJ, Martin CJ. Thoracoscopic cardiomyotomy for achalasia. *Aust N Z J Surg* 1996;66:107–109.

280. Raiser F, Perdikis G, Hinder RA, et al. Heller myotomy via minimal access surgery: an evaluation of anti-reflux procedure. *Am J Surg* 1995;169:424–427.

281. Pellegrini CA, Leichter R, Patti M, et al. Thoracoscopic esophageal myotomy in the treatment of achalasia. *Ann Thorac Surg* 1993;56:680–682.

282. Ramacciato G, Mercantini P, Amodio PM, et al. The laparoscopic approach with antireflux surgery is superior to the thoracoscopic approach for the treatment of esophageal achalasia. *Surg Endosc* 2002;16:1431–1437.

283. Shimi S, Nathanson LK, Cuschieri A. Laparoscopic cardiomyotomy for achalasia. *J R Coll Surg Edinburgh* 1991;36:152–154.

284. Ali A, Pellegrini CA. Laparoscopic myotomy. Technique and efficacy in treating achalasia. *Gastrointest Endosc Clin North Am* 2001;11:347–357.

285. Rosati R, Fumagalli U, Bonavina L, et al. Laparoscopic approach to esophageal achalasia. *Am J Surg* 1995;169:424–427.

286. Ancona E, Anselmino M, Zaninotto G, et al. Esophageal achalasia: laparoscopic vs conventional open Heller-Dor operation. *Am J Surg* 1995;170:265–270.

287. Mitchell PC, Watson DI, Devitt PG, et al. Laparoscopic cardiomyotomy with a Dor patch for achalasia. *Can J Surg* 1995; 38:445–449.

288. Swanstrom LL, Pennings J. Laparoscopic esophagomyotomy for achalasia. *Surg Endosc* 1995;9:286–272.

289. Morino M, Rebecchi F, Festa V, et al. Laparoscopic Heller cardiomyotomy with intraoperative manometry in the management of oesophageal achalasia. *Int Surg* 1995;80:332–335.

290. Robertson GSM, Lloyd DM, Wicks ACB, et al. Laparoscopic Heller's cardiomyotomy without an antireflux procedure. *Br J Surg* 1995;82:957–959.

291. Bonovina L, Rosati P, Segalin A, Peracchia A. Laparoscopic Heller-Dor operation for the treatment of oesophageal achalasia: technique and early results. *Ann Chir Gynaecol* 1995;84: 165—168.

292. Delgado F, Bolufer JM, Martinex-Abad M, et al. Laparoscopic treatment of esophageal achalasia. *Surg Laparasc Endosc* 1996; 2:83–90.

293. Hunter JG, Trus TL, Branum GD, et al. Laparoscopic Heller myotomy and fundoplication for achalasia. *Ann Surg* 1997; 225:655-665.

294. Kjellin AP, Granquist S, Ramel S, et al. Laparoscopic myotomy without fundoplication in patients with achalasia. *Eur J Surg* 1999;165:1162–1166.

295. Ackroyd R, Watson DI, Devitt PG, et al. Laparoscopic cardiomyotomy and anterior partial fundoplication for achalasia. *Surg Endosc* 2001;15:683–686.

296. Yamamura MS, Gilster JC, Myers BS, et al. Laparoscopic Heller myotomy and anterior fundoplication for achalasia results in a high degree of patient satisfaction. *Arch Surg* 2000;135:902–906.

297. Patti MG, Molena D, Fisichella PM, et al. Laparoscopic Heller myotomy and Dor fundoplication for achalasia. Analysis of successes and failures. *Arch Surg* 2001;136:870–877.

298. Pechlivanides G, Chryos E, Athanasakis E, et al. Laparoscopic Heller cardiomyotomy and Dor fundoplication for esophageal achalasia. *Arch Surg* 2001;136:1240–1243.

299. Sharp KW, Khaitan L, Scholz S, et al. 100 consecutive minimally invasive Heller myotomies: lessons learned. *Ann Surg* 2002;235:631–639.

300. Donahue PE, Horgan S, Liu KJM, et al. Floppy Dor fundoplication after esophagocardiomyotomy for achalasia. *Surgery* 2002;132:716–722.

301. Zaninotto G, Costantini M, Portale G, et al. Etiology, diagnosis and treatment of failures after laparoscopic Heller myotomy for achalasia. *Ann Surg* 2002;235:186–192.

302. Luketich JD, Fernando HC, Christie, et al. Outcome after minimally invasive esophagomyotomy. *Ann Thorac Surg* 2001;72: 1909–1913.

303. Decker G, Borie F, Bouamirrene D, et al. Gastrointestinal quality of life before and after laparoscopic Heller myotomy with partial posterior fundoplication. *Surgery* 2002;236: 750–758.

304. Di Simone MP, Felice V, D'Errico A, et al. Onset timing of delayed complications and criteria of follow-up after operation for esophageal achalasia. *Ann Thorac Surg* 1996;61: 1106–1111.

305. Nussbaum MS, Jones MP, Pritts TA, et al. Intraoperative manometry to assess the esophagogastric junction during laparoscopic fundoplication and myotomy. *Surg Laparosc Endosc Percutan Tech* 2001;11:294–300.

306. Tatum RP, Kahrilas PJ, Manka M, et al. Operative manometry and endoscopy during laparoscopic Heller myotomy. An initial experience. *Surg Endosc* 1999;13:1015–1020.

307. Fergunson MK, Reeder GB, Olak J. Results of myotomy and partial fundoplication after pneumatic dilation for achalasia. *Ann Thorac Surg* 1996;62:327–330.

308. Ponce J, Juan M, Garriques V, et al. Efficacy and safety of cardiomyotomy in patients with achalasia after failure of pneumatic dilatation. *Dig Dis Sci* 1999;44:2277–2282.

309. Patti MG, Feo CV, Arcerito M, et al. Effects of previous treatment on results of laparoscopic Heller myotomy for achalasia. *Dig Dis Sci* 1999;44:2270–2276.

310. Morino M, Rebecchi F, Festa V, et al. Preoperative pneumatic dilatation represents a risk factor for laparoscopic Heller myotomy. *Surg Endosc* 1997;11:359–361.

311. Gorecki PJ, Hinder RA, Libbey JS, et al. Redo laparoscopic surgery for achalasia. Is it feasible? *Surg Endosc* 2002;16: 772–776.

312. Johnson O. Achalasia of the cardia: experience of extramucosal cardiomyotomy during a ten-year period. *Ethiopian Med J* 1994;32:89–91.

313. Deleted in press.

314. Jaakkola A, Reinikainen P, Ovaska J, et al. Barrett's esophagus after cardiomyotomy for esophageal achalasia. *Am J Gastroenterol* 1994;89:165–169.

315. Guo JP, Gilman PB, Thomas RM, et al. Barrett's esophagus and achalasia. *J Clin Gastroenterol* 2002;34:439–443.

316. Patti MG, Feo CV, Diener U, et al. Laparoscopic Heller myotomy relieves dysphagia in achalasia when the esophagus is dilated. *Surg Endosc* 1999;13:843–846.

317. Miller DL, Allen MS, Trastek VF, et al. Esophageal resection for recurrent achalasia. *Ann Thorac Surg* 1995;60:922–928.

318. Banbury MK, Rice TW, Goldblum JR, et al. Esophagectomy with gastric reconstruction for achalasia. *J Thorac Cardiovasc Surg* 1997;117:1077–1085.

319. Devaney EJ, Iannettoni M, Orringer MB, et al. Esophagectomy

for achalasia: patient selection and clinical experience. *Ann Thorac Surg* 2001;72:854–858.

320. Richter JE. Comparison and cost analysis of different treatments. *Gastrointest Endosc Clin North Am* 2001;11:359–369.

321. Gonzales EM, Alvarez AG, Garcia IL, et al. Results of surgical treatment of esophageal achalasia: multicenter retrospective study of 1856 cases. *Int Surg* 1998;73:69–73.

322. Okike N, Payne WS, Newfeld DM, et al. Esophagomyotomy versus forceful dilation for achalasia of the esophagus. Results in 899 patients. *Ann Thorac Surg* 1979;31:517–525.

323. Andrews CN, Anvari M, Dobranowski J. Laparoscopic Heller's myotomy or botulinum injection for management of achalasia. *Surg Endosc* 1999;13:742–746.

324. Panaccione R, Gregor JC, Reynolds RPE, et al. Intrasphincteric botulinum toxin versus pneumatic dilatation for achalasia: a cost minimization analysis. *Gastrointest Endosc* 1999;50:492–498.

325. Imperiale TF, O'Connor B, Vaezi MF, et al. A cost-minimization analysis of alternative treatment strategies for achalasia. *Am J Gastroenterol* 2000;95:2737–2745.

326. Urbach DR, Hansen PD, Khajanchee YS, et al. A decision analysis of the optimal initial approach to achalasia: laparoscopic Heller myotomy with partial fundoplication, thoracoscopic Heller myotomy, pneumatic dilatation, or botulinum toxin injection. *J Gastrointest Surg* 2001;5:191–205.

327. Vaezi MF, Richter. American College of Gastroenterology practice guidelines: diagnosis and management of achalasia. *Am J Gastroenterol* 1999;94:3406–3412.

328. Mayberry JF, Atkinson M. Achalasia and pregnancy. *Br J Obstet Gynaecol* 1987;94:855–859.

329. Fiest TC, Foong A, Chokhavatia S. Successful balloon dilation of achalasia during pregnancy. *Gastrointest Endosc* 1993;39:810–812.

330. Fagge CH. A case of simple stenosis of the oesophagus, followed by epithelioma. *Guys Hosp Report* 1872;108:75–77.

331. Dunaway PM, Wong RKH. Risk and surveillance intervals for squamous cell carcinoma in achalasia. *Gastrointest Clin North Am* 2001;11:425–433.

332. Meijssen MAC, Tilanus HW, Blakenstein MV, et al. Achalasia complicated by oesophageal squamous cell carcinoma: a prospective study in 195 patients. *Gut* 1992;33:155–158.

333. Barrett NR. Achalasia of the cardia: Reflections upon a clinical study of over 100 cases. *BMJ* 1964;1:1135–1138.

334. Rake G. Epithelioma of the oesophagus in association with achalasia of the cardia. *Lancet* 1931;2:262–267.

335. Camara-Lopes LK. Carcinoma of the esophagus as a complication of megaesophagus: an analysis of seven cases. *Am J Dig Dis* 1961;6:741–746.

336. Just-Viera JO, Haight C. Achalasia and carcinoma of the esophagus. *Surg Gynecol Obstet* 1969;128:1081–1084.

337. Loviscek LF, Cenoz MC, Badaloni AE, et al. Early cancer in achalasia. *Dis Esophagus* 1998;11:239–243.

338. Lerut T, Coosemans W, DeLeyn P, et al. Treatment of esophageal carcinoma. *Chest* 1999;116:463–465.

339. Belsey RHR. Discussion. In Tuttle WM, Crowley RT, Barrett RJ, eds. Achalasia of the esophagus. Further thoughts on surgical management. *J Thorac Surg* 1958;36:453–455.

340. American Society of Gastrointestinal Endoscopy Guidelines. The role of endoscopy in surveillance of premalignant conditions of the upper gastrointestinal tract. *Gastrointest Endosc* 1998;48:663–668.

NONACHALASIA ESOPHAGEAL MOTILITY ABNORMALITIES

STUART JON SPECHLER
DONALD O. CASTELL

Esophageal motility studies are used to evaluate patients who have dysphagia that is not explained by esophageal strictures and inflammation, or who have chest pain that is not explained by heart disease and other disorders (1). Manometry frequently reveals aberrant esophageal motility patterns in these patients (2), but the importance of these manometric abnormalities has been disputed for decades (3,4). Although a number of classification systems have been proposed for the putative esophageal motility disorders, there is no clear consensus regarding which system is the most appropriate (5–7).

The following factors have contributed to confusion about the esophageal motility disorders and have confounded attempts to devise a meaningful classification system:

1. The cause of most esophageal motility abnormalities is not known (8); thus, there can be no ideal classification system based on an understanding of the underlying pathophysiology.
2. Some manometric abnormalities have no apparent physiologic or clinical consequences (9). For example, the high-amplitude, peristaltic waves that characterize the so-called nutcracker esophagus cause no demonstrable radiographic or endoscopic abnormalities, do not affect esophageal emptying, and often do not correlate with episodes of dysphagia and chest pain (10).
3. Symptoms may not respond to therapies that correct the manometric abnormalities. For example, patients who have nutcracker esophagus and chest pain often get no pain relief from treatment with agents like calcium channel blockers that cause significant reductions in peristaltic wave amplitudes (11). Consequently, it is not clear that certain "esophageal motility disorders" are

clinical disorders at all. The observed esophageal motor disturbances may be merely epiphenomena (i.e., inconsequential associated abnormalities or effects) rather than causes of the symptoms.
4. Some putative disorders, like nutcracker esophagus, have been defined solely on the basis of manometric features. For such conditions, there is no extramanometric means to validate the diagnosis.

Considering the aforementioned factors, we prefer to use the term *esophageal motility abnormalities* rather than *esophageal motility disorders* when referring to these aberrant motility patterns.

Despite the controversy regarding the clinical importance and classification of esophageal manometric abnormalities, a large body of literature dealing with the putative esophageal motility disorders has accumulated over the past few decades (12). Whereas different investigators have used different manometric criteria to identify the same putative disorder, comparisons among studies are problematic (13). Recently, we suggested a general operational scheme for the classification of esophageal motility abnormalities and proposed standardized manometric criteria for the abnormal esophageal motility patterns (6). Those criteria are summarized in this chapter.

Fulfillment of the manometric criteria for a putative motility disorder does not establish that the motility abnormality has clinical importance or that the manometric phenomena are manifestations of a disease process. The ultimate diagnosis of a motility *disorder* requires consideration of clinical as well as manometric data. By applying the guidelines summarized in this chapter, the clinician can determine only whether a patient fulfills the manometric, not the clinical, criteria for a given motility abnormality.

The chest pain associated with some of the esophageal motility disorders can mimic the pain of angina pectoris related to ischemic heart disease, including its relief by nitroglycerin. Coronary artery disease is common and potentially lethal, whereas the esophageal motility disorders

S. J. Spechler: Department of Medicine, Dallas VA Medical Center and University of Texas Southwestern Medical Center, Dallas, Texas.

D. O. Castell: Department of Medicine, Medical University of South Carolina, Charleston, South Carolina.

generally are not life threatening. Consequently, the clinician must exclude heart disease before pursuing a workup for esophageal motility disorders in patients who complain of chest pain.

GENERAL CLASSIFICATION OF ESOPHAGEAL MANOMETRIC ABNORMALITIES

The four major patterns of esophageal manometric abnormalities are summarized in Table 12.1. Inadequate lower esophageal sphincter (LES) relaxation (i.e., relaxation that is incomplete in amplitude or too short in duration) results from processes that disrupt the inhibitory innervation of the LES or that restrict LES opening (e.g., postfundoplication) (12,14). Abnormal motility in the body of the esophagus is manifested by contractions that are uncoordinated or by contractions that are abnormally strong (hypercontraction) or weak (hypocontraction) (7). For patients with motility problems that cause both inadequate LES relaxation and abnormal motility in the esophageal body (e.g., classic achalasia), symptoms often are caused primarily by the abnormality in LES relaxation. Inadequate LES relaxation delays esophageal clearance, and patients with this abnormality often respond to treatments that reduce LES pressure through pharmacologic or mechanical means. Therefore, the finding of inadequate LES relaxation has clear-cut physiologic importance and therapeutic implications. For clinical purposes, patients who exhibit this abnormality can be categorized as having a disorder of inadequate LES relaxation, regardless of the motility pattern observed in the body of the esophagus. Classic achalasia is included in this category of inadequate LES relaxation, as are a number of other disorders that do not exhibit the abnormalities in esophageal body function that are characteristic of classic achalasia.

Contractions in the body of the esophagus that are not peristaltic and aborally directed (e.g., simultaneous, retrograde, segmental contractions) can be considered uncoordinated (or spastic). Such contractions can interfere with esophageal emptying (15). Uncoordinated (simultaneous) esophageal contraction is the key manometric feature of diffuse esophageal spasm.

Hypercontraction abnormalities are those characterized by esophageal muscle contractions that are of abnormally high amplitude, long duration, or both. It is not clear that such contractions have any physiologic or clinical consequences, however, and the putative disorders of hypercontraction (e.g., nutcracker esophagus, isolated hypertensive LES) are perhaps the most controversial of the abnormal esophageal motility patterns. In contrast, hypocontraction abnormalities that result from weak (abnormally low-amplitude) muscle contractions clearly can have important physiologic and clinical consequences. Hypocontraction can cause ineffective esophageal motility that delays esophageal emptying and LES hypotension that can result in gastroesophageal reflux disease (GERD).

Most esophageal motility abnormalities fall predominantly into one of the four major categories listed in Table 12.1, although there can be considerable overlap, with some conditions exhibiting features of more than one category. Nevertheless, this classification has clinical implications that may be helpful in patient management. For example, patients with inadequate LES relaxation often benefit from pharmacologic or mechanical therapies aimed at reducing LES pressure. Conversely, patients with hypocontraction abnormalities may need treatment for GERD and may benefit from prokinetic agents that enhance muscle contraction in the LES and esophageal body.

ESOPHAGEAL MANOMETRIC PROCEDURE

A well-performed esophageal manometric study is crucial for identifying and categorizing the esophageal motility disorders. To use the general classification system proposed earlier, the manometry must provide at least an assessment of the completeness of LES relaxation and an evaluation of the adequacy of peristalsis in the esophageal body. This can be accomplished as follows (16): The motility catheter is passed through the nose or mouth until the pressure sensors are positioned in the stomach, and gastric baseline pressure is recorded. While the patient breathes quietly, a slow, station pull-through is performed for evaluation of LES pressure. LES pressure is measured as the midrespiratory level in the area of maximal pressure (compared to gastric baseline pressure). With the pressure sensor positioned in the LES, the patient is asked to perform at least five separate, wet swallows (5 mL water) to assess the completeness of swallow-induced LES relaxation. Completeness of relaxation is determined by measuring the residual LES pressure, that is, the difference between the pressure recorded at the nadir of LES relaxation and gastric baseline pressure. Next, peristalsis is eval-

TABLE 12.1. CLASSIFICATION OF ESOPHAGEAL MOTILITY ABNORMALITIES

Inadequate LES relaxation
Classic achalasia
Atypical disorders of lower esophageal sphincter (LES)
relaxation
Uncoordinated contraction
Diffuse esophageal spasm
Hypercontraction
Nutcracker esophagus
Isolated hypertensive LES
Hypocontraction
Ineffective esophageal motility

Adapted from Spechler SJ, Castell DO. Classification of oesophageal motility abnormalities. *Gut* 2001;49:145–151, with permission.

TABLE 12.2. NORMAL ESOPHAGEAL MANOMETRIC FEATURES

Basal lower esophageal sphincter (LES) pressure	10–45 mm Hg (midrespiratory pressure measured by station pull-through technique)
LES relaxation with swallow	Complete (to a level <8 mm Hg above gastric pressure)
Wave progression	Peristalsis progressing from upper esophageal sphincter through LES at a rate of 2 to 8 cm per second
Distal wave amplitude	30–180 mm Hg (average of 10 swallows at two recording sites positioned 3 and 8 cm above the LES)

Values from Richter JE, Wu WC, Hohns DN, et al. Esophageal manometry in 95 healthy adult volunteers. Variability of pressures with age and frequency of "abnormal" contractions. *Dig Dis Sci* 1987;32:583–592.

uated by positioning at least three pressure sensors separated by intervals of 5 cm in the body of the esophagus. The distal sensor is positioned at a level 3 cm above the LES, and a series of ten wet swallows is performed. The swallows are separated by an interval of at least 30 seconds, and pressure wave amplitude, duration, and velocity are measured.

Normal values for esophageal manometry in 95 healthy adult volunteers derived from a study (17) that used the manometry protocol described are provided in Table 12.2. The range of normal values shown comprise two standard deviations (SD) above and below the mean.

ATYPICAL DISORDERS OF LES RELAXATION

Achalasia is a Greek term that means "does not relax," and, although there are severe abnormalities in esophageal body function in classic achalasia, dysphagia is primarily due to inadequate LES relaxation (18). Refer to Chapter __ for a detailed discussion of classic achalasia. The key manometric features required for a diagnosis of classic achalasia are (a) incomplete relaxation of the LES (defined as a mean swallow-induced decrease in resting LES pressure to a nadir value greater than 8 mm above gastric pressure) (Fig. 12.1A) and (b) aperistalsis in the body of the esophagus characterized either by simultaneous esophageal contractions with amplitudes less than 40 mm Hg or by no apparent esophageal contractions (Fig. 12.1).

Patients with atypical disorders of LES relaxation have symptoms suggestive of classic achalasia (e.g., dysphagia for liquids as well as solids), but have one or more manometric features that preclude a diagnosis of classic achalasia such as (a) preserved peristalsis, (b) esophageal contractions with amplitudes greater than 40 mm Hg, and (c) LES relaxation that is complete but of inadequate duration (19,20–22). The barium swallow may appear normal, or it may show features suggestive of classic achalasia with a dilated esophagus that terminates in a beaklike narrowing caused by persistent LES contraction. The clinical feature common to all

of the atypical disorders of LES relaxation is that affected patients have dysphagia that responds to treatments that decrease resting LES pressure. Clinical and experimental data suggest that some of these atypical disorders may be early manifestations of the same enteric neuropathy that causes classic achalasia, and some patients may develop classic achalasia over time (20,21).

By definition, evidence of inadequate LES relaxation must be found in all patients with atypical disorders of LES relaxation. However, the LES dysfunction may be subtle and may not be apparent by standard manometric analyses. For example, some patients exhibit LES relaxation that is complete in amplitude but inadequate in duration (i.e., the LES contracts before the peristaltic wave has passed) (22). Duration of LES relaxation is not reported routinely by most motility laboratories. Although the atypical disorders of LES relaxation can be suspected on the basis of symptoms and manometric features, confirmation of the diagnosis ultimately requires relief of dysphagia by a treatment that decreases resting LES pressure such as pneumatic dilation, Heller myotomy, or botulinum toxin injection.

Some patients with atypical disorders of LES relaxation have abnormalities in esophageal body function that are not characteristic of classic achalasia. It is not clear that these abnormalities have any specific clinical or therapeutic implications, however. Some investigators have proposed that chest pain might be more prominent in patients with a variant of achalasia in which esophageal contractions have amplitudes greater than 40 mm Hg (so-called vigorous achalasia), whereas others have found that such patients cannot be distinguished clinically from those with classic achalasia (19). Some have reported that botulinum toxin injection is more effective for treating vigorous than classic achalasia (23), whereas others have found no such difference in the response to toxin injection (24). Rather than assigning names of dubious significance (e.g., vigorous achalasia) to the atypical disorders of LES relaxation, we prefer to use descriptive terms (e.g., inadequate LES relaxation with preserved peristalsis, inadequate LES relaxation

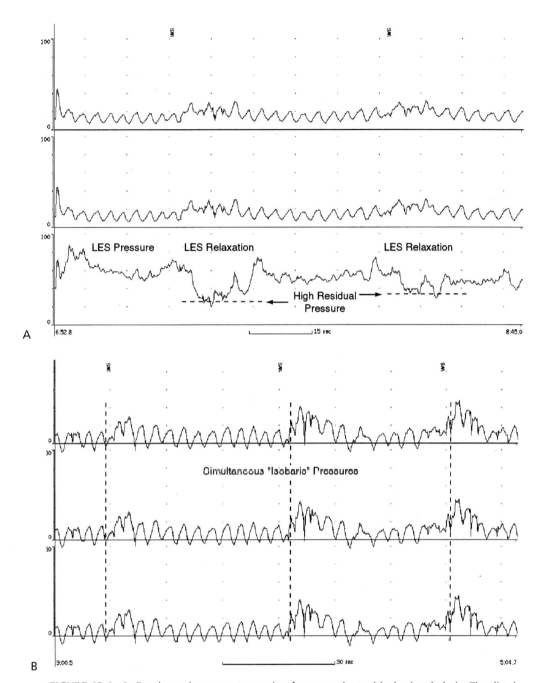

FIGURE 12.1. A: Esophageal manometry tracing from a patient with classic achalasia. The distal recording site, positioned in the lower esophageal sphincter (LES), shows high basal LES pressure (approximately 60 mm Hg). Note that the two wet swallows (WS) are followed by incomplete relaxation of the LES, with residual pressure values of 24 and 36 mm Hg. The two proximal recording sites, located 3 and 8 cm above the LES, show that wet swallows are not attended by peristalsis. **B:** Esophageal manometry tracing from a patient with classic achalasia. The three recording sites are positioned 3, 8, and 13 cm above the LES. Note that wet swallows (WS) are not followed by peristaltic contractions and that the pressure changes recorded in the esophageal body are simultaneous, low-amplitude, and identical in appearance (isobaric).

with preserved peristalsis, and esophageal contractions with amplitudes greater than 40 mm Hg).

UNCOORDINATED ESOPHAGEAL CONTRACTION

Diffuse Esophageal Spasm

Diffuse esophageal spasm is an uncommon condition of unknown etiology that is manifested clinically by episodes of dysphagia and chest pain, radiographically by tertiary (purposeless) contractions of the esophagus, and manometrically by uncoordinated ("spastic") activity in the smooth muscle portion of the esophagus (25). One could argue that a more appropriate term for the abnormality is *distal esophageal spasm*, because the motor abnormalities involve the lower half of the esophagus (the smooth muscle portion) almost exclusively. Patients typically are older than 50 years of age at the time of diagnosis, and the chest pain can mimic the angina of coronary artery disease (including relief by nitroglycerin, which relaxes the spastic esophageal smooth muscle). The pathophysiology and natural history of the disorder are poorly understood. Some patients show evidence of hypersensitivity to cholinergic stimuli (26), similar to patients with classic achalasia, and, in some patients initially found to have diffuse esophageal spasm, classic achalasia develops over time (20).

Two recent publications have suggested that the abnormal motility of diffuse esophageal spasm may be caused by defects in the nitric oxide–mediated neuromuscular signaling system that affects normal peristalsis in the esophagus (27,28). After the intravenous infusion of recombinant human hemoglobin (rHb1.1; a scavenger of nitric oxide) in healthy volunteers, Murray and colleagues (27) found that swallowing induced simultaneous esophageal contractions of high amplitude and long duration. In eight of nine volunteers, the simultaneous contractions also occurred spontaneously, a phenomenon that is often observed in diffuse esophageal spasm. In five patients with diffuse esophageal spasm, Konturek and colleagues (28) performed esophageal motility studies after the infusion of graded doses of glyceryl trinitrate (a nitric oxide donor). Compared with saline infusion, the glyceryl trinitrate caused a significant dose-dependent elongation of the latency period for distal esophageal contractions and a decrease in the mean duration of contraction. These observations suggest that defects in nitric oxide–mediated neuromuscular signaling may underlie diffuse esophageal spasm and support a role for nitrate therapy in patients with this condition.

Authorities have disagreed on the manometric criteria for spastic activity in the esophagus, and comparisons among studies on diffuse esophageal spasm have been compromised by the lack of universally accepted diagnostic criteria. Published manometric criteria have differed regarding the requirement for spontaneous and repetitive contrac-

tions and the need for high-amplitude esophageal contractions. However, simultaneous esophageal contractions have been found in most patients in published reports. In 1984, Richter and Castell called for a reappraisal of the diagnostic criteria for diffuse esophageal spasm based on their experience and review of published series (25). They proposed that simultaneous esophageal contractions induced by wet swallows should be the key diagnostic criterion for diffuse esophageal spasm (25,29).

Simultaneous contractions similar to those seen in idiopathic diffuse esophageal spasm can be found in a variety of disorders, including diabetes mellitus, alcoholism, amyloidosis, and scleroderma, as well as in patients who have GERD without other diseases (30). The physiologic and clinical consequences of the low-amplitude simultaneous contractions of scleroderma may differ substantially from those of the normal or high-amplitude simultaneous contractions seen in patients with idiopathic diffuse esophageal spasm. Consequently, it may be inappropriate to include patients with low-amplitude simultaneous contractions under the rubric of "diffuse esophageal spasm" (31).

A primary focus on the finding of simultaneous esophageal contractions also can cause confusion in distinguishing diffuse esophageal spasm from achalasia. Simultaneous contractions are a hallmark of achalasia, whereas inadequate LES relaxation has been described in diffuse esophageal spasm. Normal peristalsis is not found in classic achalasia, and the finding of an occasional normal peristaltic sequence has been used to distinguish achalasia from diffuse esophageal spasm (31). However, this distinction can be arbitrary and somewhat artificial. For a patient who has the clinical and radiographic features of classic achalasia, whose manometric examination shows inadequate LES relaxation and simultaneous esophageal contractions, and whose dysphagia resolves with pneumatic dilation, it seems inappropriate to call the disorder diffuse esophageal spasm simply because there are occasional normal peristaltic sequences. This constellation of findings is better characterized as an atypical disorder of LES relaxation (see earlier discussion).

The manometric features required for a diagnosis of diffuse esophageal spasm are (a) simultaneous contractions associated with more than 10% of wet swallows and (b) mean simultaneous contraction amplitude greater than 30 mm Hg (Fig. 12.2). Features that can be found commonly but are not required for the manometric diagnosis include

- Spontaneous contractions
- Repetitive contractions
- Multiple peaked (>2) contractions
- Intermittent normal peristalsis

If there is incomplete relaxation of the LES (defined as a mean swallow-induced decrease in resting LES pressure to a nadir value greater than 8 mm above gastric pressure), the condition is better classified as an atypical disorder of LES relaxation.

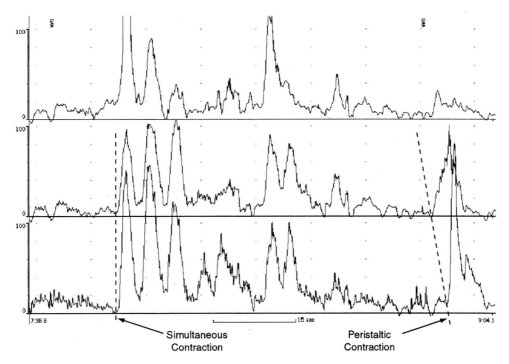

FIGURE 12.2. Esophageal manometry tracing from a patient with diffuse esophageal spasm. The recording sites are positioned 3, 8, and 13 cm above the lower esophageal sphincter (LES). Note that the first wet swallow (WS) is followed by esophageal contractions that are simultaneous and repetitive. However, some peristaltic activity is preserved as evidenced by the peristaltic contraction of the esophageal body shown in the sequence on the right.

Treatments available for diffuse esophageal spasm are listed in Table 12.3. Patients with chest pain resulting from diffuse esophageal spasm often are concerned that they have heart disease, and reassurance that their pain is esophageal and not cardiac in origin can be helpful in managing the syndrome (32). Few studies have dealt specifically with the contribution of GERD to chest pain in diffuse esophageal spasm, but data suggest that some patients improve with antireflux therapy such as proton pump inhibitors (33). An empirical trial of such therapy is warranted in most cases. Treatments aimed at relaxing esophageal smooth muscle (e.g., nitrates, calcium channel blockers, and antimuscarinic agents) decrease the amplitude of esophageal contractions, but do not reliably improve chest pain (28,34–36). Antidepressant medications have been helpful in some patients, perhaps through effects on the perception of visceral pain (37,38). Injection of botulinum toxin into the LES has resulted in pain relief in a substantial number of patients, even those with apparently normal LES function (39). The mechanism underlying this benefit is not clear. Pneumatic dilation and Heller myotomy have been used to treat diffuse esophageal spasm associated with LES dysfunction, but there seems to be little reason to use these invasive treatments if LES relaxation is normal (40). (As discussed earlier, by our proposed criteria, a patient with inadequate LES relaxation would be categorized as having an atypical disorder of LES relaxation rather than diffuse esophageal spasm.) Finally, although good results have been reported for some patients with diffuse esophageal spasm who were treated with long surgical myotomy (41), this invasive and potentially hazardous procedure should be used with great caution, and its role remains controversial (42).

TABLE 12.3. TREATMENTS FOR PATIENTS WITH UNCOORDINATED CONTRACTION AND HYPERCONTRACTION ABNORMALITIES

Reassurance that the condition is not life threatening

Antireflux therapy for gastroesophageal reflux disease

Agents that relax esophageal smooth muscle
  Nitrates
    Nitroglycerin 0.4 mg SL prn pain
    Isosorbide dinitrate 10–30 mg bid
  Calcium channel blockers
    Nifedipine 10–30 mg qid
    Diltiazem 90 mg qid
  Antimuscarinics
    Dicyclomine 10–20 mg qid

Psychotropic medications
  Trazodone 100–150 mg qd
  Imipramine 50 mg qd

Botulinum toxin injection

Long myotomy

ESOPHAGEAL HYPERCONTRACTION

Nutcracker Esophagus

Castell coined the term "nutcracker esophagus" to describe the condition in which patients with noncardiac chest pain had distal esophageal peristaltic waves whose mean amplitudes exceeded normal levels by more than 2 SD (43). Although high-amplitude peristaltic sequences have been the most common motility abnormalities observed in patients with noncardiac chest pain (2), the clinical and physiologic importance of these sequences remains disputed (3–8). Dysphagia has been reported in patients with nutcracker esophagus, but far less frequently than has chest pain. The contribution of the hypercontracting esophagus to the symptoms associated with this putative motility disorder has yet to be established.

The nutcracker esophagus has been defined by the presence of peristaltic waves in the distal esophagus with mean amplitudes of more than 2 SD above normal. Consequently, the amplitudes required for the diagnosis vary with the data used to establish normal values. In the initial report of the condition by Benjamin and co-workers in 1979 (44), the mean distal esophageal peristaltic wave amplitude in 40 healthy subjects was 81 ± 15 mm Hg (1 SD) (44). These authors suggested a cutoff value of 120 mm Hg (slightly more than 2 SD above the mean value) as the diagnostic criterion for high-amplitude peristalsis. A subsequent study of 95 healthy adults found that the mean amplitude of peristaltic waves at two recording sites in the distal esophagus (i.e., distal esophageal amplitude) was 99 ± 40 mm Hg (1 SD) (45) and, based on this report, a number of subsequent reports on nutcracker esophagus have used 180 mm Hg as the diagnostic criterion (30).

Peristaltic wave amplitude varies considerably from region to region within the esophagus (17,45). Therefore, the location of the recording sensors is an important factor in establishing a diagnosis of nutcracker esophagus. A number of studies have used the average value of the peristaltic wave amplitudes measured at two distal recording sites to determine the mean distal esophageal peristaltic wave amplitude. Some investigators have used recording sites positioned at 3 and 8 cm above the LES (43,46), whereas others have used sites positioned at 2 and 7 cm above the LES for the estimation of mean distal esophageal peristaltic wave pressure (47). Some studies have shown that high-amplitude contractions may involve the esophagus in a segmental fashion, with high-amplitude peristaltic waves found in only one of the two recording sites in the distal esophagus (46,47). The importance of these segmental high-amplitude contractions is not clear.

In the aforementioned manometric study of 95 healthy adults, the mean duration of peristaltic waves in the distal esophagus was 3.9 ± 0.9 seconds (1 SD) (17). Accordingly, a contraction duration of more than 6 seconds (slightly more than 2 SD above the mean value) can be regarded as abnormal. Patients with nutcracker esophagus often exhibit peristaltic contractions with average durations that exceed 6 seconds (30). Conceivably, such prolonged contractions could interfere with esophageal blood flow, causing transient ischemia that triggers pain. Indeed, patients have been described who have chest pain associated with peristaltic contractions of long duration but normal amplitude (48). Investigators generally have not used prolonged peristaltic contraction durations as a requisite diagnostic criterion for nutcracker esophagus, and the physiologic and clinical consequences of such contractions are not clear. Finally, high resting pressures in the LES have been found in some patients with nutcracker esophagus (30).

We have proposed that the sole manometric feature required for a diagnosis of nutcracker esophagus is a mean distal esophageal peristaltic wave amplitude greater than 180 mm Hg (measured as the average amplitude of ten swallows at two recording sites positioned 3 and 8 cm above the LES) (Fig. 12.3). Although peristaltic contractions of long duration are found commonly, they are not required for the manometric diagnosis of nutcracker esophagus. Resting pressure in the LES is usually normal, but it may be elevated, in which case patients are categorized as having nutcracker esophagus with a hypertensive LES. If there is inadequate LES relaxation associated with high-amplitude peristalsis, we believe that the patient should be categorized as having an atypical disorder of LES relaxation, with initial treatment directed at the LES dysfunction.

Treatment of nutcracker esophagus is similar to that described earlier for the treatment of diffuse esophageal spasm (Table 12.3). Reassurance and empirical treatment for GERD appear to be particularly important. For patients who do not respond to these measures, antidepressant medications can be useful. Sildenafil, which relaxes esophageal smooth muscle by blocking the phosphodiesterase enzyme that degrades cyclic guanine monophosphate, recently was found to improve symptoms in some patients with esophageal hypercontraction in a small, uncontrolled study (49). Frequent side effects limit the utility of sildenafil therapy, however.

Isolated Hypertensive LES

The hypertensive LES was described by Code more than 40 years ago (50), but it remains unclear whether this condition has any clinical or physiologic consequences. Published studies on the hypertensive LES have included patients with normal peristalsis who have any or all combinations of three LES abnormalities: (a) abnormally elevated resting LES pressure (>2 SD above the normal mean value) (51), (b) exaggerated contraction of the LES after relaxation (aftercontraction) (52), and (c) incomplete LES relaxation (53). It is not clear how the former two LES abnormalities cause symptoms, or even whether they do. Incomplete LES relaxation, however, clearly can cause symptoms by inter-

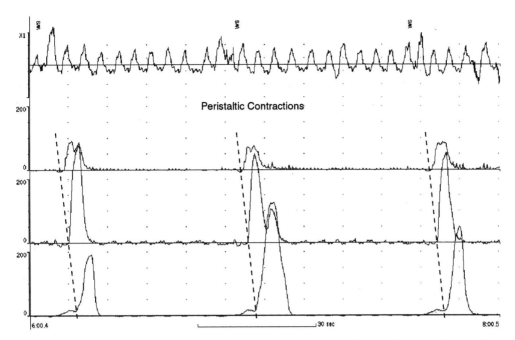

FIGURE 12.3. Esophageal manometry tracing from a patient with nutcracker esophagus. The recording sites are positioned 3, 8, and 13 cm above the lower esophageal sphincter (LES). Note the high amplitude peristaltic contractions initiated by wet swallows (WS).

fering with esophageal clearance. We think that it is inappropriate to include patients with incomplete LES relaxation in the category of "hypertensive LES." Such patients are better categorized as having an atypical disorder of LES relaxation.

A hypertensive LES is one with a resting pressure value greater than 2 SD above the normal mean value. By this definition, therefore, the pressure value used to define a hypertensive LES varies among series and among the techniques used to measure resting LES pressure (rapid pull-through versus station pull-through; end-expiratory, midrespiratory, end-inspiratory). Published values used for the lower limit of resting LES pressure in this condition have ranged from 26.5 to 45 mm Hg (54,55). If midrespiratory LES pressure is measured using the station pull-through technique, then a hypertensive LES can be defined as one with a resting pressure of more than 45 mm Hg (30,55,56).

We believe that the sole manometric feature required for a diagnosis of isolated hypertensive LES is a mean resting LES pressure of more than 45 mm Hg measured in midrespiration using the station pull-through technique. Patients who also have a mean distal esophageal peristaltic wave amplitude greater than 180 mm Hg are categorized as having nutcracker esophagus with a hypertensive LES. Patients with incomplete LES relaxation are categorized as having an atypical disorder of LES relaxation. Treatment for patients with an isolated hypertensive LES is similar to that described for diffuse esophageal spasm and nutcracker esophagus (Table 12.3).

ESOPHAGEAL HYPOCONTRACTION

Scleroderma (progressive systemic sclerosis) is the paradigm disorder for esophageal hypocontraction. In scleroderma, there is fibrosis and vascular obliteration of esophageal muscle and its innervation (57). This process weakens the LES, thereby predisposing to GERD, and causes muscle atrophy in the body of the esophagus that results in feeble contractions. Esophageal clearance is compromised significantly when the amplitude of peristaltic contractions decreases to values less than 30 mm Hg (58,59). With advanced disease, the combination of neural and muscular damage in the esophagus may result in a complete loss of peristalsis. Scleroderma affects the smooth muscle of the distal esophagus predominantly, but the striated muscle of the proximal esophagus may be involved in some cases (60). Manometric evidence of esophageal dysfunction can be found in approximately 80% of patients with scleroderma (61).

Although scleroderma clearly can obliterate LES muscle and cause severe LES hypotension (60,62), mean LES pressures are only moderately reduced in most patients with this disorder. In a recent study of 36 patients with progressive systemic sclerosis, for example, the mean resting LES pressure (measured in midrespiration) was 15.8 ± 1.2 mm Hg in the patients compared with 26.0 ± 2.1 mm Hg in normal control subjects (63). If peristalsis is preserved, the peristaltic waves often are of low amplitude (<30 mm Hg) (62,63). The low-amplitude waves may involve the esophagus in a patchy fashion. Abnormalities in the progression of peristalsis are observed frequently and include (a) failed peristalsis in which the peristaltic wave progresses through the pharynx and proximal esophagus but fails to traverse the entire length of the distal esophagus, (b) simultaneous esophageal contractions of low amplitude, and (c) absent esophageal contractions (i.e., swallowing results in no discernible contractions) (58–64).

It is important for the clinician to appreciate that the manometric features of scleroderma are by no means specific for this disorder. Identical manometric abnormalities can be found in patients with other collagen vascular disorders such as mixed connective tissue disease, rheumatoid arthritis, and systemic lupus erythematosus (65). Patients with certain nonrheumatic diseases such as diabetes mellitus, amyloidosis, alcoholism, myxedema, and multiple sclerosis also can exhibit hypocontraction in the distal esophagus indistinguishable from that of scleroderma. Perhaps most importantly, many otherwise healthy patients who have GERD can exhibit all of the manometric features of scleroderma esophagus (65). In one study on the natural history of patients who had "scleroderma-like" esophageal motility abnormalities with no apparent rheumatic disease at baseline, rheumatic disease did not develop over a follow-up period of more than 5 years (65). For these reasons, we discourage use of the term *scleroderma esophagus*. Patients who are told that they have a scleroderma esophagus often are horrified to see pictures of patients with advanced scleroderma when they investigate the condition on the Internet. If used at all, the term *scleroderma esophagus* should be restricted only to patients who actually have scleroderma that involves the esophagus. The term *ineffective esophageal motility*' is preferable to describe patients who have no rheumatic disease but have the constellation of findings typical of scleroderma. Although uncoordinated contractions of normal or high amplitude also can impair esophageal motility and thus might be considered "ineffective," the term *ineffective esophageal motility* is used to describe abnormalities characterized by hypocontraction.

Leite and colleagues (66) recently identified a group of 61 patients who had been diagnosed as having nonspecific esophageal motility disorders because their pattern of manometric abnormalities did not fall into any well-defined category (66). A detailed review of this group showed that, in 60 of the 61 patients, the motility pattern was one of esophageal hypocontraction that resulted in ineffective esophageal motility. This phenomenon is observed commonly in patients with GERD in whom it may contribute to poor esophageal clearance of acid.

The manometric features of ineffective esophageal motility are evidence of hypocontraction in the distal esophagus with at least 30% of wet swallows exhibiting any combination of the following abnormalities:

1. Distal esophageal peristaltic wave amplitude less than 30 mm Hg (Fig. 12.4)
2. Simultaneous contractions with amplitudes less than 30 mm Hg
3. Failed peristalsis in which the peristaltic wave does not traverse the entire length of the distal esophagus (Fig. 12.4)
4. Absent peristalsis

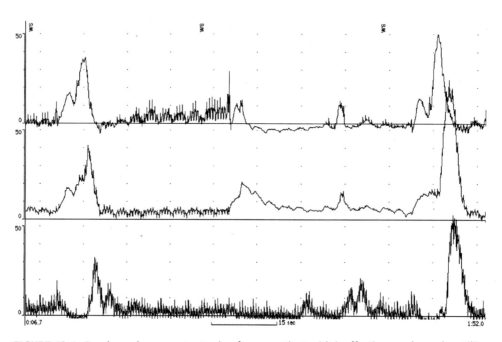

FIGURE 12.4. Esophageal manometry tracing from a patient with ineffective esophageal motility. The recording sites are positioned 3, 8, and 13 cm above the LES. Note that the first and third wet swallows (WS) result in normal peristaltic sequences. However, the second wet swallow stimulates only low-amplitude contractions in the proximal two leads, and no contraction in the distal lead (nontransmitted contraction or "failed peristalsis").

TABLE 12.4. MANOMETRIC FEATURES OF NAMED ESOPHAGEAL MOTILITY ABNORMALITIES

	Basal LESP	LES Relaxation	Wave Progression	Distal Wave Amplitude
Achalasia	Usually high, may be normal, rarely low	Incomplete	Simultaneous or absent, no peristalsis	Low or normal
Atypical disorders of lower esophageal sphincter (LES) relaxation	Low, normal, or high	Inadequate (incomplete or short duration)	Some normal peristalsis, may have simultaneous or absent sequences	Low, normal, or high
Isolated hypertensive LES	High	Complete	Normal	Normal
Diffuse esophageal spasm	Low, normal, or high	Complete	Simultaneous in >10% of swallows	Normal or high
Nutcracker esophagus	Low, normal, or high	Complete	Normal	High
Ineffective esophageal motility	Low or normal	Complete	Normal, simultaneous, or absent	Low in ≥30% of wet swallows

Adapted from Spechler SJ, Castell DO. Classification of oesophageal motility abnormalities. *Gut* 2001;49:145–151, with permission.

Patients with ineffective esophageal motility often have LES hypotension. The LES hypotension may not be severe, however, and studies suggest that abnormal esophageal acid exposure in patients with ineffective esophageal motility may correlate better with the abnormalities in peristaltic function than with the resting LES pressure. For these reasons, LES hypotension is not required as a diagnostic criterion for ineffective esophageal motility.

There is no treatment, medical or surgical, that reliably restores smooth muscle contractility for patients with ineffective esophageal motility. Prokinetic agents (e.g., metoclopramide) have limited efficacy and frequent side effects. Most patients with ineffective esophageal motility have little or no dysphagia. The presence of troublesome dysphagia in this condition suggests that there is a complicating disorder such as a peptic esophageal stricture or reflux esophagitis. Medical antireflux therapy usually is highly effective for controlling GERD in patients with ineffective esophageal motility. When fundoplication surgery is used to treat GERD in these patients, it has been traditional in many centers to "tailor" the operation according to the severity of the motility disorder. For example, a patient with substantial ineffective esophageal motility might be treated with a "loose" fundoplication, such as a Toupet procedure (a 270-degree wrap), rather than a "tight" fundoplication, such as a Nissen procedure (a 360-degree wrap) for fear that the tight procedure would cause severe postoperative dysphagia. Although this rationale sounds reasonable, studies have not shown that ineffective esophageal motility affects the surgical outcome (67). In one study of 200 patients with GERD who were randomly assigned to receive either Nissen or Toupet fundoplication, for example, the two groups had similar clinical outcomes regardless of the results of preoperative esophageal manometry (68).

NONSPECIFIC ESOPHAGEAL MOTILITY ABNORMALITIES

The conditions discussed earlier are those that have been recognized and named by investigators and for which there are published series. The minimal requisite features for establishing a manometric diagnosis of the named esophageal motility abnormalities are summarized in Table 12.4. As discussed, most patients previously categorized as having "nonspecific esophageal motility disorders" would now be included in the category of "ineffective esophageal motility" (66). Nevertheless, one occasionally encounters patients who have esophageal motility abnormalities with manometric features that do not meet the requisite criteria for any of the recognized conditions. Pending further advances in our understanding of the

pathophysiology of motility abnormalities, we recommend that nonspecific esophageal motility abnormalities be reported descriptively.

REFERENCES

1. Alrakawi A, Clouse RE. The changing use of esophageal manometry in clinical practice. *Am J Gastroenterol* 1998;93: 2319–2320.
2. Katz PO, Dalton CB, Richter JE, et al. Esophageal testing in patients with noncardiac chest pain or dysphagia: results of three years' experience with 1161 patients. *Ann Intern Med* 1987;106: 593–597.
3. Cohen S. Esophageal motility disorders and their response to calcium channel antagonists. The sphinx revisited. *Gastroenterology* 1987;93:201–203.
4. Kahrilas PJ. Esophageal motility disorders: current concepts of pathogenesis and treatment. *Can J Gastroenterol* 2000;14: 221–231.
5. Richter JE. Oesophageal motility disorders. *Lancet* 2001;358: 823–828.
6. Spechler SJ, Castell DO. Classification of oesophageal motility abnormalities. *Gut* 2001;49:145–151.
7. Clouse RE, Staiano A. Manometric patterns using esophageal body and lower sphincter characteristics. Findings in 103 patients. *Dig Dis Sci* 1992;37:289–296.
8. Richter JE, Bradley LA, Castell DO. Esophageal chest pain: current controversies in pathogenesis, diagnosis, and therapy. *Ann Intern Med* 1989;110:66–78.
9. Song CW, Lee SJ, Jeen YT, et al. Inconsistent association of esophageal symptoms, psychometric abnormalities and dysmotility. *Am J Gastroenterol* 2001;96:2312–2316.
10. Kahrilas PJ. Nutcracker esophagus: an idea whose time has gone? *Am J Gastroenterol* 1993;88:167–169.
11. Richter J, Dalton C, Bradley L, et al. Oral nifedipine in the treatment of noncardiac chest pain in patients with the nutcracker esophagus. *Gastroenterology* 1987;93:21–28.
12. Diamant NE. Regulation and dysregulation of esophageal motor function. In: Janssens J, ed. *Progress in understanding and management of gastrointestinal motility disorders.* Belgium: University of Leuven, 1993:85–103.
13. Pilhall M, Borjesson M, Rolny P, et al. Diagnosis of nutcracker esophagus, segmental or diffuse hypertensive patterns, and clinical characteristics. *Dig Dis Sci* 2002;47:1381–1388.
14. Spechler SJ, Souza RF, Rosenberg SJ, et al. Heartburn in patients with achalasia. *Gut* 1995;37:305–308.
15. Kahrilas PJ, Dodds WJ, Hogan WJ. Effect of peristaltic dysfunction on esophageal volume clearance. *Gastroenterology* 1988;94: 73—80.
16. Castell DO, Diederich LL, Castell JA, eds. *Esophageal motility and pH testing. Technique and interpretation,* third ed. Colorado: Sandhill Scientific, 2000.
17. Richter JE, Wu WC, Hohns DN, et al. Esophageal manometry in 95 healthy adult volunteers. Variability of pressures with age and frequency of "abnormal" contractions. *Dig Dis Sci* 1987; 32:583–592.
18. Spechler SJ. AGA technical review on treatment of patients with dysphagia caused by benign disorders of the distal esophagus. *Gastroenterology* 1999;117:233–254.
19. Goldenberg SP, Burrell M, Fette GC, et al. Classic and vigorous achalasia: a comparison of manometric, radiographic, and clinical findings. *Gastroenterology* 1991;101:743–748.
20. Vantrappen G, Janssens J, Hellemans J, et al. Achalasia, diffuse

esophageal spasm, and related motility disorders. *Gastroenterology* 1979;76:450–457.

21. Goldblum JR, Rice TW, Richter JE. Histopathologic features in esophagomyotomy specimens from patients with achalasia. *Gastroenterology* 1996;111:648–654.

22. Katz PO, Richter JE, Cowan R, et al. Apparent complete lower esophageal sphincter relaxation in achalasia. *Gastroenterology* 1986;90:978–983.

23. Pasricha PJ, Rai R, Ravich WJ, et al. Botulinum toxin for achalasia: long-term outcome and predictors of response. *Gastroenterology* 1996;110:1410–1415.

24. Cuilliere C, Ducrotte P, Zerbib F, et al. Achalasia: outcome of patients treated with intrasphincteric injection of botulinum toxin. *Gut* 1997;41:87–92.

25. Richter JE, Castell DO. Diffuse esophageal spasm: a reappraisal. *Ann Intern Med* 1984;100:242–245.

26. Richter JE, Hackshaw BT, Wu WC, et al. Edrophonium: a useful provocative test for esophageal chest pain. *Ann Intern Med* 1985;103:14–21.

27. Murray JA, Ledlow A, Launspach J, et al. The effects of recombinant human hemoglobin on esophageal motor function in humans. *Gastroenterology* 1995;109:1241–1248.

28. Konturek JW, Gillessen A, Domschke W. Diffuse esophageal spasm: a malfunction that involves nitric oxide? *Scand J Gastroenterol* 1995; 30:1041–1045.

29. Dalton CB, Castell DO, Hewson EG, et al. Diffuse esophageal spasm. A rare motility disorder not characterized by high-amplitude contractions. *Dig Dis Sci* 1991;36:1025–1028.

30. Achem SR, Benjamin SB. Esophageal dysmotility (spastic dysmotility). In: Castell DO, ed. *The esophagus*, second ed. Boston: Little, Brown, 1995:247–268.

31. Allen ML, DiMarino AJ. Manometric diagnosis of diffuse esophageal spasm. *Dig Dis Sci* 1996;41:1346–1349.

32. Ward BW, Wu WC, Richter JE, et al. Long-term follow-up of symptomatic status of patients with noncardiac chest pain: is diagnosis of esophageal etiology helpful? *Am J Gastroenterol* 1987;82:215–218.

33. Achem SR, Kolts BE, MacMath T, et al. Effects of omeprazole versus placebo in treatment of noncardiac chest pain and gastroesophageal reflux. *Dig Dis Sci* 1997;42:2138–2145.

34. Orlando RC, Bozymski EM. Clinical and manometric effects of nitroglycerin in diffuse esophageal spasm. *N Engl J Med* 1973;289:23–25.

35. Davies HA, Lewis MJ, Rhodes J, et al. Trial of nifedipine for prevention of oesophageal spasm. *Digestion* 1987;36:81–83.

36. Hongo M, Traube M, McCallum RW. Comparison of effects of nifedipine, propantheline bromide, and the combination on esophageal motor function in normal volunteers. *Dig Dis Sci* 1984;29:300–304.

37. Clouse RE, Lustman PJ, Eckert TC, et al. Low-dose trazodone for symptomatic patients with esophageal contraction abnormalities. A double-blind, placebo-controlled trial. *Gastroenterology* 1987;92:1027–1036.

38. Cannon RO 3rd, Quyyumi AA, Mincemoyer R, et al. Imipramine in patients with chest pain despite normal coronary angiograms. *N Engl J Med* 1994;330:1411–1417.

39. Miller LS, Pullela SV, Parkman HP, et al. Treatment of chest pain in patients with noncardiac, nonreflux, nonachalasia spastic esophageal motor disorders using botulinum toxin injection into the gastroesophageal junction. *Am J Gastroenterol* 2002;97:1640–1646.

40. Ebert EC, Ouyang A, Wright SH, et al. Pneumatic dilatation in patients with symptomatic diffuse esophageal spasm and lower esophageal sphincter dysfunction. *Dig Dis Sci* 1983;28:481–485.

41. Henderson RD, Ryder D, Marryatt G. Extended esophageal myotomy and short total fundoplication hernia repair in diffuse esophageal spasm: five-year review in 34 patients. *Ann Thorac Surg* 1987;43:25–31.

42. Ellis FH Jr. Long esophagomyotomy for diffuse esophageal spasm and related disorders: an historical overview. *Dis Esophagus* 1998;11:210–214.

43. Dalton CB, Castell DO, Richter JE. The changing faces of the nutcracker esophagus. *Am J Gastroenterol* 1988;83:623–628.

44. Benjamin SB, Gerhardt DC, Castell DO. High amplitude, peristaltic esophageal contractions associated with chest pain and/or dysphagia. *Gastroenterology* 1979;77:478–483.

45. Clouse RE, Staiano A. Topography of normal and high-amplitude esophageal peristalsis. *Am J Physiol* 1993;265:G1098-107.

46. Achem SR, Kolts BE, Burton L. Segmental versus diffuse nutcracker esophagus: an intermittent motility pattern. *Am J Gastroenterol* 1993;88:847–851.

47. Freidin N, Mittal RK, Traube M, et al. Segmental high amplitude peristaltic contractions in the distal esophagus. *Am J Gastroenterol* 1989;84:619–623.

48. Herrington JP, Burns TW, Balart LA. Chest pain and dysphagia in patients with prolonged peristaltic contractile duration of the esophagus. *Dig Dis Sci* 1984;29:134–140.

49. Eherer AJ, Schwetz I, Hammer HF, et al. Effect of sildenafil on oesophageal motor function in healthy subjects and patients with oesophageal motor disorders. *Gut* 2002;50:758–764.

50. Code CF, Schlegel JF, Kelley ML, et al. Hypertensive gastroesophageal sphincter. *Proc Mayo Clin* 1960;35:391–399.

51. Bassotti G, Alunni G, Cocchieri M, et al. Isolated hypertensive lower esophageal sphincter. Clinical and manometric aspects of an uncommon esophageal motor abnormality. *J Clin Gastroenterol* 1992;14:285–287.

52. Garrett JM, Godwin DH. Gastroesophageal hypercontracting sphincter. Manometric and clinical characteristics. *JAMA* 1969; 208:992–998.

53. Freidin N, Traube M, Mittal RK, et al. The hypertensive lower esophageal sphincter. Manometric and clinical aspects. *Dig Dis Sci* 1989;34:1063–1067.

54. Katada N, Hinder RA, Hinder PR, et al. The hypertensive lower esophageal sphincter. *Am J Surg* 1996;172:439–443.

55. Katzka DA, Sidhu M, Castell DO. Hypertensive lower esophageal sphincter pressures and gastroesophageal reflux: an apparent paradox that is not unusual. *Am J Gastroenterol* 1995; 90:280–284.

56. Waterman DC, Dalton CB, Ott DJ, et al. Hypertensive lower esophageal sphincter: what does it mean? *J Clin Gastroenterol* 1989;11:139–146.

57. Lock G, Holstege A, Lang B, Schölmerich J. Gastrointestinal manifestations of progressive systemic sclerosis. *Am J Gastroenterol* 1997; 92:763–771.

58. Richter JE, Blackwell JN, Wu WC, et al. Relationship of radionuclide liquid bolus transport and esophageal manometry. *J Lab Clin Med* 1987;109:217–224.

59. Turner R, Lipshutz W, Miller W, et al. Esophageal dysfunction in collagen disease. *Am J Med Sci* 1973;265:191–199.

60. Cohen S, Laufer I, Snape WJ Jr, et al. The gastrointestinal manifestations of scleroderma: pathogenesis and management. *Gastroenterology* 1980;79:155–166.

61. Bassotti G, Battaglia E, Debernardi V, et al. Esophageal dysfunction in scleroderma. Relationship with disease subsets. *Arthrit Rheum* 1997;40:2252–2259.

62. Cohen S. Motor disorders of the esophagus. *N Engl J Med* 1979; 301:184–192.

63. Yarze JC, Varga J, Stampfl D, et al. Esophageal function in sys-

temic sclerosis: a prospective evaluation of motility and acid reflux in 36 patients. *Am J Gastroenterol* 1993;88:870–876.

64. Zamost BJ, Hirschberg J, Ippoliti AF, et al. Esophagitis in scleroderma. Prevalence and risk factors. *Gastroenterology* 1987;92: 421–428.

65. Schneider HA, Yonker RA, Longley S, et al. Scleroderma esophagus: a nonspecific entity. *Ann Intern Med* 1984;100:848–850.

66. Leite LP, Johnston BT, Barrett J, et al. Ineffective esophageal motility (IEM). The primary finding in patients with non-specific esophageal motility disorder. *Dig Dis Sci* 1997;42: 1859–1865.

67. Castell DO. Esophageal manometry prior to antireflux surgery: required, preferred, or even needed? *Gastroenterology* 2001;121: 214–216.

68. Fibbe C, Layer P, Keller J, et al. Esophageal motility in reflux disease before and after fundoplication: a prospective, randomized, clinical, and manometric study. *Gastroenterology* 2001; 121:5–14.

TUMORS OF THE ESOPHAGUS

GREGORY ZUCCARO, JR.

BENIGN TUMORS

Benign neoplasms of the esophagus are rare. When encountered, they are most commonly asymptomatic, discovered incidentally during evaluation for some other problem in the upper gastrointestinal tract. Benign neoplasms may arise from the mucosa, submucosa, or muscularis propria of the esophagus. Their premalignant potential is small. Benign neoplasms are most commonly diagnosed by endoscopy, but may also be seen on videoesophagram. For those arising in the submucosal or muscularis propria layer of the esophageal wall, endosonography often provides key diagnostic information. This section focuses on the clinical presentation, histopathology, diagnosis, and management of the more common benign neoplasms of the esophagus encountered in practice. Afterward, a brief summary of the most rare lesions is presented.

Neoplasms Arising from the Mucosal Layer

Fibrovascular Polyps

Clinical Presentation
These lesions are found primarily in the proximal esophagus, and therefore may become symptomatic as they enlarge. Eventually, dysphagia develops in most patients, although respiratory symptoms and even regurgitation of the polyp with aspiration has been reported (1).

Histopathology. The fibrovascular polyp is a collection of adipose and fibrovascular connective tissue that is covered with normal squamous epithelium. If the overlying mucosa becomes abnormal, it is usually due to trauma from prolapse as the lesion enlarges. These lesions may be highly vascular. As they enlarge just distal to the cricopharyngeus,

they undergo traction and elongation as a result of peristalsis, and they may become pedunculated.

Diagnosis. These lesions may be identified by videoesophagram as mass lesions with smooth overlying mucosa. It is possible to overlook the fibrovascular polyp at endoscopy because of its proximal nature and normal overlying mucosa. With the larger pedunculated polyp, care must be taken to not retract the polyp into the hypopharynx at the completion of the endoscopy. When possible, the exact extent and site of attachment of the symptomatic fibrovascular polyp should be noted, because this information guides the optimal surgical approach. There is a limited role for esophageal endosonography, which may both identify the layer of origin of the lesion (thus helping to confirm the diagnosis) and characterize the vascularity of its stalk.

Management. The symptomatic lesion should be resected. Endoscopic resection of smaller fibrovascular polyps has been reported (2). The literature is not extensive enough to determine whether endosonography is a helpful adjunct in determining the degree of vascularity within the stalk when an endoscopic resection is contemplated. Larger lesions are best handled with surgery. Even for the asymptomatic proximal lesion, a case can be made for resection, because there is a possibility of regurgitation and resultant aspiration if the fibrovascular polyp increases in size over time.

Squamous Papilloma

Clinical Presentation
These are typically less than 1 cm in size, sessile, wartlike projections seen more commonly in the distal esophagus. They are most commonly an incidental finding, although the very rare large lesion may cause dysphagia (3) (Color Plate 13.1). According to autopsy studies, the prevalence of the squamous papilloma is approximately 0.02% (4). The etiology of these lesions is unknown, although the human papilloma virus has been implicated (5).

G. Zuccaro: Dept. of Gastroenterology and Hepatology, Cleveland Clinic Foundation, Cleveland, Ohio.

Histopathology. Squamous papillomas are projections of connective tissue emanating from the lamina propria. They are often covered with hyperplastic squamous epithelium.

Diagnosis. Squamous papillomas are typically diagnosed on forceps biopsy. At times, these can be mistaken for early squamous cell carcinoma when there is a question of invasion into the submucosal layer.

Management. The asymptomatic lesion may be observed. In the rare circumstance when the lesion is large and obstructing, it may be removed surgically or endoscopically (3). Resection is also indicated when there is any question about the diagnosis or when the lesion may be an early squamous cell cancer.

Esophageal Cysts

Clinical Presentation

The esophageal cyst is typically asymptomatic and discovered incidentally. Even large cysts are often compliant and therefore asymptomatic. However, the enlarging cyst may sometimes cause dysphagia, chest pain, or pulmonary symptoms.

Histopathology. Some cysts are epithilium-lined cysts that arise from the lamina propria and have normal overlying squamous epithelium (6). Inflammation within the glands is the suspected cause. Duplication cysts may also be found within or outside the esophageal wall. They may be lined with several types of epithelium, including squamous, columnar, or even respiratory epithelium.

Diagnosis. Cysts are identified on endoscopy as masslike bulges in the esophageal wall that are covered with normal-appearing epithelium (Color Plate 13.2). Biopsy of the mucosal cyst may allow for its diagnosis, but this is rarely done because the endoscopist often cannot rule out a vascular nature to the lesion and is typically reluctant to perform a biopsy. Forceps biopsy is not useful in diagnosing the duplication cyst. Computed tomography (CT) or magnetic resonance imaging (MRI) of the chest may often identify the duplication cyst. Endosonography is especially helpful, in that the lesion may be identified as a cyst, the layer of the esophageal wall with which it is associated may be identified, or it may be seen as an extrinsic compression of a normal esophageal wall (Fig. 13.3). Fine needle aspiration (FNA) may be performed if there is any question about the diagnosis, but this is infrequently necessary.

Management. In the asymptomatic patient, the lesion may be observed. However, in the presence of symptoms or if there is any doubt about the diagnosis, surgery

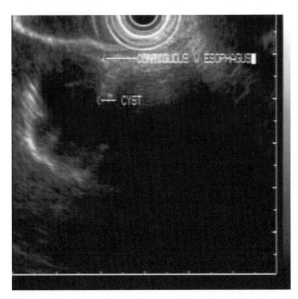

FIGURE 13.3. Endoscopic ultrasound image of a large foregut cyst contiguous with the esophageal wall.

should be undertaken. There are rare reports of transesophageal drainage of a foregut cyst, but because the epithelial lining of the cyst remains, the lesion may theoretically recur (7).

Neoplasms Arising from the Submucosal Layer

Granular Cell Tumor

Clinical Presentation

These lesions are generally found incidentally and are asymptomatic. In longitudinal studies, these lesions generally are stable over time (8). There is a suggestion in the literature that they may occur more frequently in the distal esophagus, although they can be found anywhere in the esophagus (9). They are typically less than 1 cm in diameter.

Histopathology. These lesions are thought to arise from the Schwann cell; that is, they are neural in origin. In a series published from our institution, the tumors were typically comprised of nests of cells with pyknotic nuclei, abundant granular cytoplasm, and an absence of mitotic figures with strong S-100 protein positivity (10) .

Diagnosis. Granular cell tumors appear pale (almost yellow) on endoscopy and have a smooth overlying mucosa (Color Plate 13.4). They are firm to touch with the forceps, and a diagnosis can be made typically with precise forceps biopsy. On endosonography, these lesions are hyperechoic and arise from the third ultrasound layer (submucosa).

Management. These lesions are rarely symptomatic, and the likelihood of malignancy is low. In our series, only 1 of 11 tumors showed any characteristics of malignant change; this was a tumor several centimeters in size. Therefore, the smaller lesions may be followed up periodically, with surgery reserved only for the rare enlarging or symptomatic granular cell tumor.

Neoplasms Arising from the Muscle Layer

Smooth Muscle Tumors

Clinical Presentation

These are the most common of the benign neoplasms of the esophagus, accounting for approximately 70% of such lesions. They most commonly arise from the circular layer of the muscularis propria, but they may also arise from the muscularis mucosae. These lesions are most commonly discovered incidentally. However, when they are sufficient in size, they may cause dysphagia, pain, or gastrointestinal bleeding. Lesions causing esophageal obstruction are typically large, approximately 5 cm or more in diameter (11). Smooth muscle tumors in the distal esophagus may be associated with symptoms of gastroesophageal reflux disease. Rarely, these tumors may grow in a spiral and elongated fashion, mimicking a peptic or malignant stricture (12).

Histopathology. These lesions consist of muscle cells in a cascade or whirl type pattern surrounded by a fibrous tissue capsule. Nerve fragments and ganglion cells may also be detected. The muscle cells are elongated with eosinophilic cytoplasm. Larger tumors contain more collagen. The distinction between benign and malignant smooth muscle tumors may be problematic; increased cellularity, nuclear atypia, necrosis, and an abundance of mitotic figures may all be associated with malignancy.

Diagnosis. On videoesophagram, these lesions are seen as smooth, often rounded filling defects. Similarly, on esophagoscopy, these lesions are seen as firm, discrete nodules with normal overlying mucosa (Color Plate 13.5). It may be difficult to distinguish these lesions from extrinsic esophageal compression. Forceps biopsy is rarely helpful; an exception is when the tumor arises from the muscularis mucosae where a "bite on bite" technique may provide a histologic diagnosis. Endosonography is the technique most helpful in the evaluation and management of smooth muscle tumors of the esophagus. Endosonography is unique in its ability to provide a detailed view of the layers of the esophageal wall. The smooth muscle tumor appears hypoechoic and may be seen to arise from the muscle layer of the esophageal wall, confirming the diagnosis (Fig. 13.6).

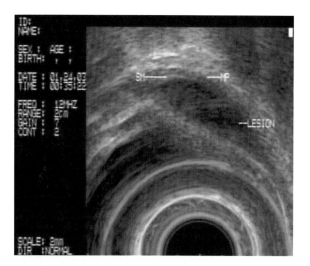

FIGURE 13.6. Endoscopic ultrasound of an esophageal leiomyoma. It is contiguous with the muscularis mucosae layer of the esophageal wall. Note the homogeneous internal echo pattern and smooth borders, both consistent with a benign lesion. An intact submucosal layer and muscularis propria layer are seen beneath the lesion. MP, muscularis propria; SM, submucosa.

Management. These lesions grow slowly and may be stable in size during observation over many years (13). Malignant smooth muscle tumors of the esophagus are exceedingly rare (14). However, it may be difficult to distinguish the benign from the malignant esophageal smooth muscle tumor. Size greater than 4 cm in the intestine and size greater than 6 cm in the stomach are associated with increased risk of malignancy, but it is unclear whether these parameters hold true for esophageal smooth muscle tumors. Benign esophageal smooth muscle tumors up to 10 cm in size have been reported (15). Certain endosonographic features, including mixed internal echo patterns, irregular borders, and associated lymphadenopathy, are suggestive of but not pathognomonic for malignant degeneration. Endosonographically guided FNA of the primary lesion is not typically helpful, because cytology does not provide the architecture necessary to make this distinction. Cytologic aspiration of enlarged lymph nodes can establish a diagnosis of malignant smooth muscle tumor (Fig. 13.7 and Color Plate 13.8).

The symptomatic lesion should be surgically resected. Benign lesions may be removed with simple enucleation, with more extensive operations being reserved for malignant lesions. The asymptomatic lesion (if less than 4 cm in size) with benign-appearing features on endosonography may be followed up with surveillance examinations every 1 to 2 years. Surgery should be undertaken for the asymptomatic smooth muscle tumor clearly growing in size over time or if worrisome endosonographic features are detected. Whereas lesions 4 cm or greater in size are still most likely benign, surgery should be considered.

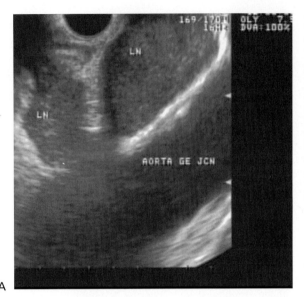 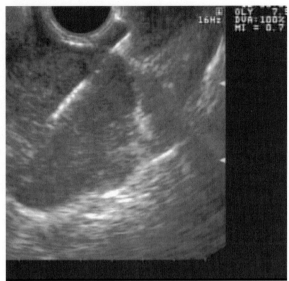

FIGURE 13.7. Endoscopic ultrasound of enlarged periesophageal lymph nodes in a patient with a malignant smooth muscle tumor of the esophagogastric junction. A needle is passed into a node under ultrasound guidance.

Other Benign Esophageal Tumors

Esophageal lipomas have a pale or yellow appearance, have normal overlying mucosa, and are soft or "pillow-like" when probed with a biopsy forceps. Endosonography is generally unnecessary to establish the diagnosis, but if it is performed, it reveals a homogenous, hyperechoic lesion arising in the third ultrasound layer. *Fibromas* are more firm to touch and are less hyperechoic on endoscopic ultrasound (EUS). *Hemangiomas* are cavernous, sometimes large endothelium-lined entities that appear cystic and may have a blue-purple hue.

Summary

Benign lesions of the esophagus are rare and frequently are of little clinical significance. The differential diagnosis

TABLE 13.1. COMMON NEOPLASMS OF THE ESOPHAGUS

Associated with the mucosal layer
Fibrovascular polyps
Squamous papilloma
Esophageal cysts
Smooth muscle tumor (arising from the muscularis mucosa)
High grade dysplasia/intramucosal cancer

Associated with the submucosal layer
Granular cell tumor
Fibroma
Lipoma
T1 cancer

Associated with the muscularis propria layer
Smooth muscle tumor
T2 cancer

includes neoplastic and nonneoplastic lesions. A summary of common lesions is listed in Table 13.1. Often, forceps biopsy is insufficient to establish the correct diagnosis. EUS allows visualization of the layers of the gastrointestinal wall and surrounding tissues. EUS is therefore well suited to assist in establishing the nature of these lesions, because the layer of origin and echo characteristics of a lesion often confirms the diagnosis.

ESOPHAGEAL CANCER

Overview of Esophageal Cancer

The two main histologic types of esophageal cancer are squamous cell cancer and adenocarcinoma. Because the esophagus is lined with squamous mucosa, it is reasonable to expect that squamous cell cancer should be the most common type of malignancy within the esophagus. Indeed, worldwide, this is the case; cancer of the esophagus is one of the ten most common malignancies worldwide. However, in the United States, adenocarcinoma has overtaken squamous cell carcinoma as the most common malignancy of the esophagus and gastroesophageal junction in white men (16,17). There are regions in the world where the incidence of esophageal cancer is strikingly high, including certain parts of China, Iran, and Southern Africa (18–21). This likely reflects an interaction between genetics and environment, but the true causes of esophageal cancer are unknown.

Several factors are associated with the development of esophageal cancer (Table 13.2). Esophageal cancer risk increases with age (22). Gender also plays a role: women are at decreased risk for adenocarcinoma of the esophagus com-

TABLE 13.2. POSSIBLE ETIOLOGIC FACTORS ASSOCIATED WITH ESOPHAGEAL CANCER

Factor	Comment
Age	Risk increases with advancing age
Race	Associated for both adenocarcinoma and squamous cell cancer
Gender	Males > females
Alcohol/tobacco	Likely for squamous cancer
Diet	All putative factors: High carbohydrate, low fruit/vegetables High fat/cholesterol intake Deficiency in vitamin A Intake of nitrosamines
Genetics	Associated with tylosis, Plummer-Vinson syndrome, among others
Acquired disease	Untreated achalasia, lye stricture
Gastroesophageal reflux disease	Associated with adenocarcinoma, not squamous cell cancer
Helicobacter pylori	May be protective for adenocarcinoma

pared with men (23). However, women who have undergone radiation treatment for breast cancer are at increased risk for development of esophageal cancer (24). Race and ethnic differences exist as well. For example, in the United States, the incidence of adenocarcinoma is increasing among white men, whereas African-American men are at greater risk for squamous cell carcinoma(17,25,26). Dietary factors implicated in the development of esophageal cancer include a diet high in carbohydrates or animal fat, diets low in protein, fruit, or vegetables, diet deficient in vitamin A, and diets high in nitrosamines (27–36). Alcohol and tobacco use have been implicated in the development of esophageal cancer, more so for squamous cell carcinoma (37–46). With respect to adenocarcinoma, there is a strong causal relationship with chronic gastroesophageal reflux disease. Lagergren and colleagues (47) interviewed 189 patients with esophageal adenocarcinoma, 262 with adenocarcinoma of the cardia, 167 with esophageal adenocarcinoma, and 820 control subjects from the general population. Patients with esophageal adenocarcinoma were more than seven times more likely to have symptoms of gastroesophageal reflux disease than patients who did not have esophageal adenocarcinoma. Patients with long duration of severe gastroesophageal reflux were more than 43 times more likely to have adenocarcinoma of the esophagus. The association between gastroesophageal reflux and adenocarcinoma of the gastric cardia was less strong. There was no association between gastroesophageal reflux and squamous cell carcinoma (47). Prolonged gastroesophageal reflux disease does predispose an individual to the development of Barrett's esophagus. The pathogenesis of Barrett's esophagus and association with the development of adenocarcinoma is discussed elsewhere in this textbook. Many genetic and acquired conditions are associated with an increased risk of esophageal cancer, including tylosis, Plummer-Vinson syndrome, and untreated achalasia (48–50). The role of *Helicobacter pylori* is controversial, with some suggestion that it may be protective for adenocarcinoma of the esophagus, but perhaps causative for cancer of the gastroesophageal junction and gastric cardia (51,52).

Clinical Presentation and Diagnosis

Most cases of newly diagnosed esophageal cancer present relatively late in the course of the disease, when solid-food dysphagia and weight loss manifest. Patients may present with other symptoms or signs, such as overt gastrointestinal bleeding, anemia, or pain. An increasing number of early cancers are diagnosed according to multiple factors, including screening of patients in high endemic areas with balloon cytology or endoscopy, screening of patients with chronic gastroesophageal reflux disease for the presence of Barrett's esophagus, and surveillance programs of patients with known Barrett's esophagus. Nevertheless, in most cases, the clinician is faced with the challenge of managing the patient presenting with a relatively late stage of esophageal cancer.

Endoscopy is the mainstay in establishing the diagnosis of esophageal cancer. It allows visualization of the tumor mass as well as an opportunity to confirm the diagnosis with cytology or biopsy. On rare occasions, establishing the diagnosis may be difficult because of a tight stricture with no obvious tumor at the proximal aspect of the stricture. It may be difficult to procure tissue from such lesions, particularly if they occur in the very proximal esophagus. There are various techniques to overcome this technical difficulty. One is the simple passage of a cytology brush into the lumen of the malignant stricture. A second technique involves careful dilation of the malignant stricture with a balloon or solid dilator passed over a wire to allow passage of the endoscope into or through the stricture. An unguided bougie dilator should not be passed in such circumstances, even with fluoroscopic guidance, because the tip of the dilator may become lodged and result in excessive force on the esophageal wall, proximal to the stricture, leading to perforation. When the clinician suspects a tight stricture in the proximal esophagus, a careful barium esophagram obtained before endoscopy may allow for additional planning, including availability of fluoroscopy for placement of a guidewire through the tight stricture.

Staging of Esophageal Cancer

There are three reasons to perform staging of newly diagnosed esophageal cancer (Table 13.3):

1. Prognosis for the individual patient depends on the stage at the time of presentation. Certainly, patients with cancers associated with distant metastases or lymph node metastases have far lower rates of survival compared with patients without distant metastases or lymph node or regional lymph node metastases.
2. Interpretation of clinical trials in which two modes of treatment are compared can only be interpreted if the patients are matched with accurate pretreatment clinical staging. For example, Urba and co-workers (53) randomized 100 patients to either surgery alone or chemoradiotherapy followed by surgery in the treatment of patients with newly diagnosed esophageal cancer. They concluded that there was no statistically significant difference in survival (53). Walsh and colleagues (54) performed a similar study on 113 patients with esophageal cancer, but concluded that there was a survival advantage if pretreatment chemoradiotherapy was offered. Bosset and colleagues (55) found no overall survival advantage to presurgical chemoradiotherapy, but did find increased disease-free survival and survival free of local disease when chemoradiotherapy was offered before surgery. There

are several possible reasons why clinical trials such as these draw such different conclusions. One reason is that the patients may not have been well matched as to their true clinical stage before enrollment in the two arms of each study. In these three studies, clinical staging was performed by physical examination, standard barium x-ray study, laboratory workup, endoscopy, and either abdominal ultrasound or chest and abdominal CT scan. In none of these trials was EUS used. Therefore, it is likely that patients in these trials were not well matched as to their true pretreatment clinical stage. Accurate clinical staging is necessary to properly interpret the conclusions drawn from studies such as these.
3. Accurate staging of patients with newly diagnosed esophageal cancer guides therapy for the individual patient. Clearly, the patient with diffuse metastases should not undergo aggressive surgery or chemoradiotherapy in an attempt to cure. Conversely, patients with superficial cancer need not undergo potentially toxic chemoradiotherapy if surgery alone will provide the highest chance of long-term survival.

Methods of Clinical Staging

The clinical staging system for newly diagnosed esophageal cancer follows the TNM classification system, where *T* refers to depth of tumor invasion, *N* to the presence or absence of regional lymph node metastases, and *M* to the presence or absence of distant metastases (Table 13.4). Various TNM stages may be put together into stage groupings (I through IV) in which each group represents similar prognosis.

For the patient with esophageal cancer, many tests are performed for the purpose of clinical staging. Physical examination is typically not helpful except in rare instances when distant spread can be detected (e.g., a palpable supraclavicular lymph node). For the gastroenterologist, the main tests ordered are endoscopy, CT scan, and endosonog-

TABLE 13.3. RATIONALE FOR STAGING ESOPHAGEAL CANCER

Reason for Staging	Comment
Determine prognosis	Distant metastases, regional lymph node metastases associated with very poor prognosis
Evaluate clinical trials	In major trials comparing chemoradiotherapy plus surgery with surgery alone, endosonography is not used for preoperative staging; raises possibility that patients are not evenly matched before randomization
Determine therapy	For cancer confined to the esophageal wall, surgery as first intervention is appropriate; for cancer extending through the esophageal wall, chemoradiotherapy followed by surgery is appropriate

TABLE 13.4. TNM CLASSIFICATION FOR CLINICAL STAGING OF ESOPHAGEAL CANCER

T Stage	
T0	No detectable cancer
Tis	Carcinoma *in situ*
T1	Tumor extends to, not through, lamina propria (T1m) or submucosa (T1sm)
T2	Tumor extends to, not through, muscularis propria
T3	Tumor extends into adventitia
T4	Tumor invades adjacent organs (pericardium, aorta)

N Stage	
N0	No evidence of regional lymph node metastases
N1	Evidence of regional lymph node metastases

M Stage	
M0	No evidence of distant metastases
M1	Evidence of distant metastases

raphy; newer tests are still in the investigational stage. A summary of the common imaging tests and their attributes is presented in Table 13.5.

Endoscopy is the most helpful test in the evaluation of the patient with esophageal cancer, because the tumor can be visualized and characterized, and biopsy or brush cytology may be obtained for confirmation of the diagnosis (Color Plate 13.9). Can more be learned about the T, N, or M stage of esophageal cancer by endoscopy alone? Little direct information can be ascertained regarding N stage from standard endoscopy. Similarly, it is rare for M stage to be confirmed by endoscopy. However, indirect information about T stage can be gathered from endoscopy alone (Color Plate 13.10). At the Cleveland Clinic, Van Dam and colleagues (56) studied patients with esophageal cancer and malignant stenosis, and found that 91% of malignant stenoses represented T3 or T4 cancers. Bhutani and coworkers (57) reported on a group of 35 patients with esophageal cancer. They found that, for tumors greater than 5 cm in length or those with luminal stenosis, it was extremely likely for them to be pathologic T3 or T4 (57). Vickers and Elderson (58) also noted that most patients with malignant stenoses had T3 tumors. If information on

T stage can be gathered from endoscopy alone, then N stage can also be predicted from endoscopy alone with some accuracy, because advancing T stage correlates strongly with the presence of regional lymph node metastases. Our esophageal research group reported on 359 patients with esophageal cancer and indeed found that the likelihood of regional lymph node metastases increased with increasing depth of tumor invasion. For example, 77% of T3 tumors were associated with regional lymph node metastases (59). In summary, in some tumors, endoscopy alone can predict a strong likelihood of loco regionally advanced cancer. However, such endoscopic scoring systems are not sufficiently developed to discriminate a T3 from a T4 cancer, nor can they determine the likelihood of distant metastases, such as metastases to the celiac axis from an intrathoracic cancer.

Once a diagnosis of esophageal cancer is established by endoscopy and biopsy, what test should be performed next? CT scan is typically the test ordered, because it determines the presence of distant metastatic disease (e.g., liver metastases). In fact, this is the standard of care at the present time. However, this viewpoint may change as other modalities are investigated and improved. For example, EUS can

TABLE 13.5. ATTRIBUTES OF COMMONLY UTILIZED IMAGING STUDIES FOR ESOPHAGEAL CANCER STAGING

Imaging Study	Comment
Endoscopy	Able to visualize tumor, establish tissue diagnosis. Longer tumors with tight stenosis more likely to be advanced through esophageal wall.
Computed tomography scan	Visualize distant metastases. Somewhat insensitive for T and N stage.
Endoscopic	Visualize layers of esophageal wall and adjacent tissues; ideal for T staging.
Ultrasound	Fine needle aspiration can establish N stage with greater confidence.
Positron emission tomography scanning	Data limited; may be more accurate than computed tomography scan for detection of distant metastases.

TABLE 13.6. ATTRIBUTES OF ECHOENDOSCOPES

Echoendoscope	Comments
Radial scanning	Commonly used to determine T and N stage; provides 360-degree view of wall and surrounding tissues; cannot be used for fine needle aspiration (FNA).
Linear scanning	Used for FNA of lymph nodes; can be used for T staging but is technically demanding because 360-degree view of tumor is not provided at one time.
High-frequency probes	Through the endoscope channel, probe frequency may be as high as 30 mHz. Used primarily for staging of small/superficial cancers.

visualize many structures such as the liver and can even obtain FNA of suspected distant metastases in the liver and elsewhere (60). Besides distant metastases, many centers also consider T4 disease or the presence of celiac axis lymph nodes from intrathoracic cancers a reason to offer palliation rather than aggressive therapy intended toward cure. Advocates of both CT scan and EUS believe their test is helpful in the detection of T4 disease (61,62). With respect to celiac axis lymphadenopathy, it is acknowledged that CT scan is relatively insensitive for its detection. F-fluorodeoxyglucose positron emission tomography (FDG PET) scanning has been advocated as helpful in detection of metastatic disease. Lerut and co-workers (63) studied 42 patients with esophageal cancer detected by CT scan, EUS, and FDG PET scanning followed by surgery. They found that, for regional lymph nodes, CT and EUS were superior to PET scan, but for detection of distant nodal metastases, the PET scan was superior (63). In a similar study by Choi and colleagues (64) in patients with squamous cell cancer of the esophagus, FDG PET scan was also superior for the detection of distant lymph node metastases. Laparoscopy may be helpful in the staging of adenocarcinoma of esophageal cancer because of its ability to detect occult peritoneal metastases. Using laparoscopic ultrasound, Finch and colleagues (65) reported TNM assessment equivalent to published results for EUS. Thoracoscopy has been reported to correctly stage 88% of patients undergoing resection of esophageal cancers. Accurate in defining N, it is less accurate in the assessment of T (66). A cost minimization analysis has raised the questions as to whether EUS might be superior to CT scan as the next staging step in patients with newly diagnosed esophageal cancer (67). However, it is generally accepted that CT scan is the next appropriate test once the diagnosis is made by endoscopy and biopsy.

Endoscopic Ultrasound in the Staging of Esophageal Cancer

EUS represents a major technologic breakthrough in the staging of esophageal cancer. The ability to visualize layers of the esophageal wall in vivid detail, as well as the tissues and structures immediately adjacent to the esophagus and proximal stomach, have had a significant impact on T and N staging of esophageal cancer. A summary of the types of echoendoscopes used for imaging the esophagus is presented in Table 13.6.

EUS is highly accurate in determination of T stage (Fig. 13.12 and Color Plate 13.11). Most clinical series report T stage accuracy of 75% to 92% (68–79) (Table 13.7). It has been shown that EUS is superior to CT scan in determination of T and N stage (80). There are some potential limitations to accurate determination of T stage, however. In most series on esophageal cancer staging, there is a subset of patients with malignant stenosis that is not passable by the echoendoscope. Although, as stated earlier, most of these patients had advanced disease, often more information can be determined if the entire length of the tumor and distal structures can be examined. For example, a tumor may be T3 at its proximal end but a T4

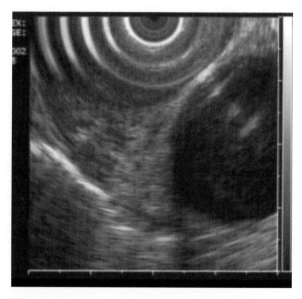

FIGURE 13.12. Endoscopic ultrasound image of a T4 cancer, with invasion of the thoracic aorta.

TABLE 13.7. ACCURACY OF ENDOSCOPIC ULTRASOUND IN T STAGING OF ESOPHAGEAL CANCER: REPRESENTATIVE CLINICAL SERIES

Author	Number of Patients	Reported Accuracy (%)
Takemoto (1986)	16	75
Tio (1989)	74	89
Ziegler (1991)	37	89
Botet (1991)	50	92
Grimm (1993)	63	86
Dittler (1993)	167	86
Murata (1994)	328	83
Binmoeller (1995)	87	89

when viewed from the mid or distal end. Likewise, presence of celiac axis nodes can only be ascertained if EUS is performed at that level. An early report on staging of patients with malignant stenoses suggested that esophageal dilation is associated with an unacceptably high risk of perforation (56). Subsequent series have indicated that dilation can safely be performed (81). Use of a 7.9-mm probe, which can provide a radial EUS image but no video information, has been reported with passage over a guidewire and reasonably accurate staging information provided. However, FNA cannot be performed using a radial system (68).

Another potential limitation of conventional EUS is in the evaluation of superficial adenocarcinoma. Most patients with newly diagnosed esophageal cancer present with malignant dysphagia and weight loss, and have advanced disease at the time of initial presentation. EUS is accurate in this setting. There are fewer data on the accuracy of EUS staging in early or less invasive esophageal cancer, and these data are somewhat contradictory. Tio and colleagues (82) reported on 66 cases undergoing EUS followed by surgery in which pathologic stage was determined; 17 of 66 (26%) of these patients had tumor confined to the esophageal wall (T1 or T2), and EUS accurately determined T stage in 14 of 17 (82%). Grimm and colleagues (70) reported on 68 cases undergoing EUS and then surgery in which pathologic stage was determined; 25 of 68 (37%) of these patients had tumor confined to the esophageal wall (T1 or T2), and EUS accurately determined T stage in 21 of 25 (84%). However, Hiele and co-workers (83) reported on 78 cases undergoing EUS and then surgery in which pathologic stage was determined; 19 of 78 (24%) of these patients had tumor confined to the esophageal wall (T1 or T2), and EUS accurately determined T stage in only 2 of 19 (11%). An increased accuracy of T staging in superficial esophageal cancer has been reported with the use of higher frequency ultrasound probes, rather than conventional echoendoscopes, to stage patients with esophageal cancer (84).

The reported N stage accuracy of EUS for esophageal cancer is 69% to 90% (68–79) (Table 13.8). Early reports using radial scanners relied on the descriptive features of lymph nodes, including size, shape, border characteristics, and internal echo pattern (Table 13.9). Using these criteria, Catalano and co-workers (85) reported overall N stage accuracy of 94%. However, with the advent of curvilinear echoendoscopy and the ability to perform FNA, there has been a shift toward FNA to document the presence or absence of regional or distant lymph node metastases (Fig. 13.13 and Color Plate 13.14). Wiersema and colleagues (86) compared EUS descriptive criteria for lymph nodes to EUS with FNA in the evaluation of malignant lymphadenopathy. Histologic confirmation was available for

TABLE 13.8. ACCURACY OF ENDOSCOPIC ULTRASOUND IN N STAGING OF ESOPHAGEAL CANCER: REPRESENTATIVE CLINICAL SERIES

Author	Number of Patients	Reported Accuracy (%)
Takemoto (1986)	16	NR
Tio (1989)	74	80
Ziegler (1991)	37	69
Botet (1991)	50	88
Grimm (1993)	63	90
Dittler (1993)	167	73
Murata (1994)	328	88
Binmoeller (1995)	87	79

TABLE 13.9. ENDOSONOGRAPHIC FEATURES OF LYMPH NODES SUGGESTIVE OF METASTATIC INVOLVEMENT

Criteria	Comment
Internal echo pattern	A hypoechoic node is more likely to be associated with malignant involvement.
Border	A sharp border is more likely to be associated with malignant involvement.
Shape	A round node is more likely to be associated with malignant involvement.
Size	Likelihood of malignant involvement is proportional to lymph node size.

192 lymph nodes. Sensitivity for regional lymph node metastases for EUS size criteria and EUS-FNA were similar (86% and 92%, respectively). However, specificity was superior for EUS-FNA (93% vs. 24%), as was accuracy (92% vs. 69%). Vazquez-Sequeiros and colleagues (87) found that the sensitivity for regional lymph node metastases improved from 63% to 93% with FNA compared to descriptive EUS alone, with accuracy increasing from 70% to 93% (87). Reed and colleagues (88) described 54 patients with esophageal cancer, 23 of whom had celiac lymphadenopathy. EUS with FNA was able to document the presence of lymph node metastases in 15 of 23 patients. In seven of the false-negative cases by EUS, micrometastases were found. From the same institution, Eloubeidi and colleagues (89) reported a sensitivity of EUS for celiac axis lymph node metastases of 77%, with 98% accuracy of FNA in documentation of malignant spread when lymph nodes were visualized by EUS. Nevertheless, there are limitations of EUS with FNA, including the aforementioned presence of micrometastases and the inability to sample some lymph nodes if the only potential path for the needle travels through the primary tumor. There are no commercially available reliable shielded needles that can pass through the primary tumor and sample only the lymph node beyond it. Such practice should not be performed because it is possible that contamination from the primary tumor may lead to a false-positive staging of the regional lymph node.

Staging after Chemoradiotherapy

The clinician should determine the patient's response to chemoradiotherapy, because this might influence the decision on surgery, and it certainly has implications for the

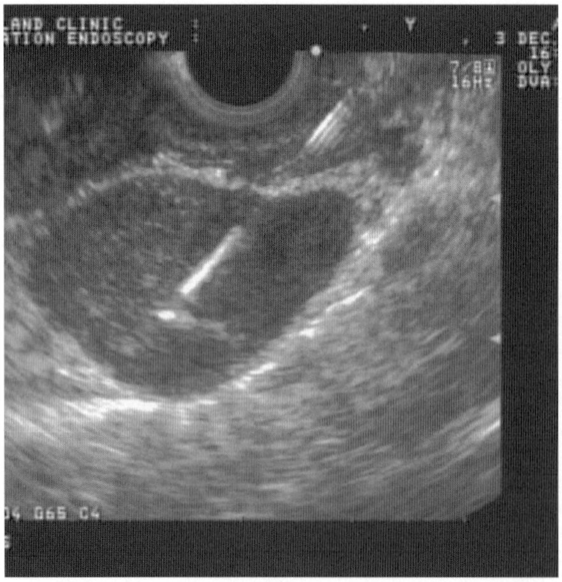

FIGURE 13.13. Endoscopic ultrasound–guided fine needle aspiration of an enlarged lymph node adjacent to an esophageal adenocarcinoma.

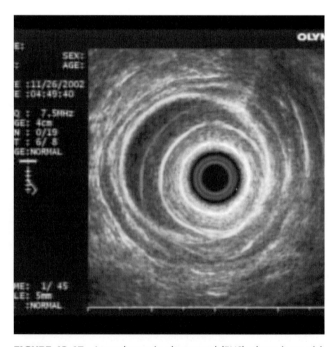

FIGURE 13.17. At endoscopic ultrasound (EUS), there is no visible tumor, and the wall layers are intact. EUS predicted pathologic T0, and, indeed, at surgery this patient was pathologic T0, due to the effect of induction chemoradiotherapy.

patient's prognosis. Multiple series on EUS staging of patients with esophageal cancer after chemoradiotherapy have shown that EUS was only accurate in the staging of patients with advanced cancer and no response. For patients who did respond to chemoradiotherapy, EUS typically overstaged those patients, because EUS was unable to distinguish fibrosis or necrotic tumor from viable tumor (90) (Color Plates 13.15 and 13.16, Fig. 13.17). Recent clinical series have suggested that a pre- and post-chemoradiotherapy measurement of cross-sectional tumor area may predict which patients will have improved survival outlook after surgery (91,92). The role of EUS in this setting has not yet been completely defined.

Palliation of Malignant Dysphagia

When patients with esophageal cancer present with distant metastases, or when attempts at curative chemoradiotherapy or surgery fail, palliation is often appropriate. Part of the palliative process involves restoring as best as possible the patient's ability to swallow. The attributes and limitations of endoscopic palliation are listed in Table 13.10.

Dilation

Dilation with balloons or bougie-type dilators is helpful, but unlike the longer effects in patients with peptic disease, the effects last only a few days. The reported perforation rate is only slightly higher than that of benign strictures, as long as a prudent, stepwise approach is taken (93). Wire-guided bougies are most frequently used, because an unguided bougie may catch on an exophytic portion of the tumor and make perforation more likely. The endoscopist is wise to begin with a dilator slightly above the estimated luminal circumference and to increase in 1- to 2-mm increments, concluding the session when a moderate amount of resistance is encountered. In most circumstances, dilation is performed in conjunction with other methods to treat malignant dysphagia. Dilation can be performed during or after external beam radiation therapy, but even more caution must be exercised, because surgical repair is often not possible in a radiated field.

Tumor Ablation

There are both thermal-based and non–thermal-based methods of tumor ablation. They are all effective, and the choice often depends on local expertise and availability. Multiple agents, such as absolute alcohol, polidocanol, and a combination of sodium morrhuate and 5 flurouracil (5 F-U), may be used to induce tumor necrosis. Using absolute alcohol, improvement in dysphagia score can be anticipated in virtually all cases. The typical technique is to inject in 0.5-mL aliquots, for a total injection of 7.5 to 10 mL, depending on the overall tumor length. Complications include perforation and mediastinitis. This technique should be reserved for exophytic tumors (94,95).

Direct application of thermal energy, using devices such as the Nd-YAG laser, BICAP tumor probe, or argon plasma coagulator, can improve swallowing in up to 90% of patients (96–99). Typically, multiple sessions are necessary, because the palliative effect lasts only a few weeks. These techniques are often performed after endoscopic dilation, particularly with the laser or argon plasma coagulator (Color Plate 13.18). A retrograde approach to tumor ablation is generally safer than an antegrade approach. Complications include perforation, formation of a tracheoesophageal fistula, bleeding, and sepsis. When compared with placement of a plastic prosthesis, laser therapy is associated with an increased number of hospital days and increased need for additional procedures (100).

Another method of thermal-based tissue destruction is photodynamic therapy. With this technique, patients are first injected with a photosensitizing agent, which is preferentially absorbed by the tumor. The most commonly used agent at the time of this writing is porfimer sodium. The

TABLE 13.10. METHODS OF PALLIATION OF MALIGNANT DYSPHAGIA

Method	Advantages	Disadvantages
Dilation	Easy, fast	Risk of perforation Effect not long-lasting
Alcohol	Easy, inexpensive	Mediastinitis/perforation No control of injury depth
Laser/APC	Effective, fast	Risk of perforation Not universally available May require dilation
Photodynamic therapy	Effective, no dilation for tight strictures	Photosensitivity Multiple endoscopic procedures necessary
Metal stents	Requires one procedure Very effective Can cover tracheoesophageal fistulae	May increase pain/GERD Expensive Complications may be more likely if radiation therapy also provided

APC, argon plasma coagulator; GERD, gastroesophageal reflux disease.

tumor is exposed to laser light of a specific wavelength 48 and 96 hours after injection of the photosensitizing agent. This combination of photosensitizer and laser light exposure induces a biochemical reaction that leads to tumor necrosis; specifically, photoactivation leads to production of singlet oxygen radicals, causing tumor necrosis via vascular occlusion mediated by thromboxane A2 release. The specific laser light generally chosen is 630 nm. New diode technology in currently available lasers allow for a portable laser system. The cylindrical probes used to treat the tumor may be obtained in 1-, 2.5-, or 5-cm lengths. Improvement in malignant dysphagia is generally observed. Compared to Nd-YAG laser treatment, there is less risk of esophageal perforation with photodynamic therapy, but there are more proble (101,102). A major ms with photosensitivity, which can occur even up to 30 to 40 days after injection advantage for photodynamic therapy is in the treatment of proximal tumors or extremely tight strictures. Using other thermal ablative methods, dilation must be performed to visualize the tumor length and pass the endoscope through before treatment. However, with photodynamic therapy, the very thin probe can be passed through the endoscope channel and into the tight stricture and treatment applied. A repeat endoscopy in 48 hours usually reveals an increase in luminal size, allowing for passage of the endoscope and a second treatment to take place, without the risk of endoscopic dilation.

Stent Placement

Plastic stents are no longer used in most settings. To place a plastic, nonexpanding stent, endoscopic dilation to 18 to 20 mm in diameter was frequently necessary. This dilation and placement of a stent of this diameter was associated with perforation rates of approximately 10%, significant bleeding in 1% to 5% of patients, and death in 4% to 16% of patients (103–107). Self-expanding metal stents do not require this degree of aggressive dilation before placement, which can be achieved in a single setting. Self-expanding metal stents are superior to plastic stents in terms of complication rates and need for hospital stay (108–110).

There are many advantages to stents over other methods for palliation of malignant dysphagia. The procedure may be done on an outpatient basis and requires only one endoscopic intervention. The covered stents may be used to seal over a tracheoesophageal fistula (Color Plate 13.19). Even if dilation is performed before stent placement and a perforation occurs, placement of the covered stent usually seals the perforation, and along with intravenous antibiotics, can avoid the need for surgery (Color Plates 13.20 through 13.22). In fact, an appropriate treatment for an unexpected perforation during laser or argon plasma coagulation therapy, or during endoscopic dilation of a tumor, is placement of a stent. Disadvantages of stent placement include pain after placement, gastroesophageal reflux if the stent is placed across the esophagogastric junction, and inability to use stents for very proximal tumors.

There are other potential disadvantages of stent placement. Airway compromise (i.e., compression of the trachea or left mainstem bronchus) may occur if a stent is placed into the esophagus to palliate a tumor that also involves the airway. Dual stenting involving the placement of stents into the airway and the esophagus at the same setting can often prevent this problem, which was more evident when the larger, nonexpanding plastic stents were used (111–112). Another potential disadvantage relates to a possible incompatibility of stents with radiation therapy; there may be an increased complication rate of self-expanding metal stent placement if prior radiation therapy was provided for the patient (113–115).

Other Malignancies of the Esophagus

Involvement of the esophagus with other malignancies is rare. Malignant melanoma or breast cancer metastases may involve the esophagus. Both Hodgkin's and non-Hodgkin's lymphoma may involve the esophagus. Other rare tumors, including adenoid cystic carcinoma, solitary plasmacytoma, sarcoma, and small cell carcinoma have been reported.

SUMMARY

There are many benign lesions of the esophagus that may be encountered. In most cases, these are incidental findings of no consequence to the patient. Forceps biopsy is important for the mucosally based lesions to rule out early malignancy. Endosonography may provide invaluable information as to the nature of the lesion. Both squamous cell cancer and adenocarcinoma of the esophagus may be encountered in clinical practice. Endoscopy is essential to establish the tissue diagnosis. Endosonography and CT scan provide complementary staging information. The results of staging with EUS often guide therapy, with surgery being provided for tumors limited to the esophageal wall and chemoradiotherapy followed by surgery for tumors extending beyond the esophageal wall. Various endoscopically based methods of palliation of malignant dysphagia are available for patients with distant metastases or those unable to undergo surgery or chemoradiotherapy.

REFERENCES

1. Levine MS, Buck JL, Pantongrag-Brown L, et al. Fibrovascular polyps of the esophagus: clinical, radiographic, and pathologic findings in 16 patients. *Am J Roentgenol* 1996;166:781–787
2. Tasaka Y. Makimoto K, Yamauchi M, et al. Benign pedunculated intraluminal tumor of the esophagus. *J Otolaryngol* 1982; 1:111.

3. Dumot JA, Vargo J, Zuccaro G. Esophageal squamous papilloma causing dysphagia. *Gastrointest Endosc* 2000;52:660.

4. Weitzner S, Hentel W. Squamous papilloma of the esophagus: case report and review of the literature. *Am J Gastroenterol* 1968;50:391.

5. Winkler B, Capo V. Reumann W, et al. Human papillomavirus infection of the esophagus: a clinicopathologic study with demonstration of papilloma virus antigen by the immunoperoxidase technique. *Cancer* 1985;55:149.

6. Hover AR, Brady CE III, Williams JR, et al. Multiple retention cysts of the lower esophagus. *J Clin Gastroenterol* 1982;4:209–212.

7. Kuhlman JE, Fishman EK, Wang KP, et al. Esophageal duplication cyst: CT and transesophageal needle aspiration. *Am J Roentgenol* 1985;145:531–532.

8. Brady PG, Nord H, Connar RG. Granular cell tumor of the esophagus: natural history, diagnosis, and therapy. *Dig Dis Sci* 1988;33:1329.

9. Andrade J, Bambirra EA, De Oliverira CA. Granular cell tumor of the esophagus: a study of seven cases diagnosed by histologic examination of endoscopic biopsies. *South Med J* 1987;80:852.

10. Goldblum JR, Rice TW, Zuccaro G, et al. Granular cell tumors of the esophagus: a clinical and pathologic study of 13 cases. *Ann Thorac Sug* 1996;62:860–865.

11. Schmidt HW, Clagett OT, Harrison EG Jr. Benign tumors and cysts of the esophagus. *J Thorac Cardiovasc Surg* 1961;41:717.

12. Seremetis MG, Lyons WS, Defuzman VC, et al. Leiomyomata of the esophagus: an analysis of 838 cases. *Cancer* 1961;41:717.

13. Glanz I, Grunebaum M. The radiological approach to leiomyoma of the oesophagus with a long-term follow-up. *Clin Radiol* 1977;28:197.

14. Ueyama T, Guo K, Hashmoto H, et al. A clinicopathologic and immunohistochemical study of gastrointestinal stromal tumors. *Cancer* 1992;69:947.

15. Bardini R, Segalin A, Ruol A, et al. Videothoracoscopic enucleation of esophageal leiomyoma. *Ann Thorac Surg* 1992;54:576–577.

16. Blot WJ, Fraumeni JF. Trends in esophageal cancer mortality among U.S. blacks and whites. *Am J Public Health* 1987;77:296.

17. Devesa SS, Blot WJ, Fraumeni JF Jr. Changing patterns in the incidence of esophageal and gastric cancer in the United States. *Cancer* 1998;83:2049–2053.

18. FeJong UW, Breslow N, Hong JG, et al. Aetiological factors in oesophageal cancer in Singapore Chinese. *Int J Cancer* 1974;13:291.

19. Mahboudi EO, Aramesh B. Epidemiology of esophageal cancer in Iran, with special reference to nutritional and cultural aspects. *Prev Med* 1980;9:613.

20. Rose EF. Cancer of the oesophagus. *S Afr J Hosp Med* 1978;4:110.

21. Yang CS. Research on esophageal cancer in China: a review. *Cancer Res* 1980;40:2633.

22. Yang PC, Davis S. Incidence of cancer of the esophagus in the U.S. by histologic type. *Cancer* 198861:612.

23. Cheng KK, Sherp L, McKinney PA, et al. A case-control study of oesophageal adenocarcinoma in women: a preventable disease. *Br J Surg* 2000;83:127–132.

24. Ahsan H, Neugut AI. Radiation therapy for breast cancer and increased risk for esophageal carcinoma. *Ann Intern Med* 1998;128:114–117.

25. Schottenfeld D. Epidemiology of cancer of the oesophagus. *Semin Oncol* 1984;11:92.

26. Silber W. Carcinoma of the oesophagus: aspects of epidemiology and aetiology. *Proc Nutr Soc* 1985;44:101.

27. Ziegler RG, Morris LE, Blot WJ, et al. Esophageal cancer among black men in Washington DC: I. Role of nutrition. *J Natl Cancer Inst* 1981;67:1199.

28. Decarli A, Liati P, Negri E, et al. Vitamin A and other dietary factors in the etiology of esophageal cancer. *Nutr Cancer* 1987;10:29.

29. Gabrial GN, Schriazder TF, Newberne PM. Zinc deficiency, alcohol, and da retinoid: association with esophageal cancer in rats. *J Natl Cancer Inst* 1982;68:785.

30. Launoy G, Milan C, Day NE, et al. Diet and squamous cell cancer of the oesophagus: a French multicentre case-control study. *Int J Cancer* 1989;43:755.

31. Sporn MB, Newton DL. Chemoprevention of cancer with retinoids. *FASEB J* 1979;38:2528.

32. Lu SH, Ruggero M, Zhang MS, et al. Relevance of N-nitrosamines to esophageal cancer in China. *J Cell Physiol* 1986;4:51.

33. Siddiqui M, Preussmann R. Esophageal cancer in Kashmir—an assessment. *J Cancer Res Clin Oncol* 1989;115:111.

34. Chanvitan A. *Oesophageal cancer studies in Southern Thailand.* Bangkok: Medial Media Publisher, 1990.

35. Terzaghi M, Nettesheim P, Yarita T, et al. Epithelial focus assay for early detection of carcinogen-altered cells in various organs of rats exposed in situ to N-nitrosoheptamethyleneimine. *J Natl Cancer Inst* 1981;67:1057.

36. Yang CS. Research on esophageal cancer in China: a review. *Cancer Res* 1980;40:2633.

37. Bradshaw E, Schonland M. Smoking, drinking, and oesophageal cancer in African males in Johannesburg, South Africa. *Br J Cancer* 1974;30:157.

38. Franceschi S, Talamini R, Barra S, et al. Smoking and drinking in relation to cancer of the oral cavity, pharynx, larynx, and esophagus in northern Italy. *Cancer Res* 1990;50:6502.

39. Dean G, Maclennan R, McLoughlin H, et al. Causes of death of blue collar workers at a Dublin brewery. *Br J Cancer* 1979;40:581.

40. Schmidt W, Popham RE. The role of drinking and smoking in mortality from cancer and other causes in male alcoholics. *Cancer* 1981;47:1031.

41. Hakulinen T, Lehtimaki L, Lehtonen M, et al. Cancer morbidity among two male cohorts with increased alcohol consumption. *J Natl Cancer Inst* 1974;52:1711.

42. Jensen OM. Cancer morbidity and causes of death among Danish brewery workers. *Int J Cancer* 1979;23:454.

43. Doll R, Peto R. Mortality in relation to smoking: 20 years observation on male British doctors. *BMJ* 1976;2:1525.

44. Rogot E., Murray JL. Smoking and causes of death among U.S. veterans: 16 years of observation. *Public Health Rep* 1980;95:127.

45. Tuyns AJ. Oesophageal cancer in non-smoking drinkers and non-drinking smokers. *Int J Cancer* 1983;32:443.

46. Hammond EC. Smoking in relation to death rates of one million men and women. *Natl Cancer Inst Monogr* 1966;19:127.

47. Lagergren J, Bergstrom R, Lindgren A, et al. Symptomatic gastroesophageal reflux as a risk factor for esophageal adenocarcinoma. *N Engl J Med* 1999;340:825.

48. Wychulis AR, Cunnulangsson GH, Lagett OT. Carcinoma occurring in pharyngeal-oesophageal diverticulum. *Surgery* 1969;66:976.

49. Larson LG, Sandstrom A, Westling P. Relationship of Plummer-Vinson disease to cancer of the upper alimentary tract in Sweden. *Cancer Res* 1975;35:3308.

50. Harper PAS, Harper RMJ, Howel-Evans AW. Carcinoma of the esophagus with tylosis. *Q J Med* 1970;34:317.

51. Vieth M, Masoud B, Meining A, et al. *Helicobacter pylori* infection: protection against Barrett's mucosal and neoplasia. *Digestion* 2000;62:225–231.

52. Goldblum JR, Richter JE, Vaezi M, et al. *Helicobacter pylori* infection, not gastroesophageal reflux, is major cause of inflammation and intestinal metaplasia of gastric cardia mucosal. *Am J Gastroenterol* 2002;97:302–311.

53. Urba SG, Orringer MB, Turrisi A, et al. Randomized trial of preoperative chemoradiation versus surgery alone in patients with locoregional esophageal carcinoma. *J Clin Oncol* 2001;19(2):305–313.

54. Walsh TN, Noonan N, Hollywood D, et al. A comparison of multimodal therapy and surgery for esophageal adenocarcinoma. *N Engl J Med* 1996;335:462–467.

55. Bossett J-F, Gignoux M, Triboulet J-P, et al. Chemoradiotherapy followed by surgery compared with surgery alone in squamous cell cancer of the esophagus. *N Engl J Med* 1997;337:161–167.

56. Van Dam J, Rice TW, Sivak MV, et al. Malignant esophageal stricture is predictive of tumor stage and a contraindication of endosonography using dedicated echoendoscopes. *Cancer* 1993;71:2190–2197.

57. Bhutani MS, Barde CJ, Markert RJ, et al. Length of esophageal cancer and degree of luminal stenosis during upper endoscopy predict T stage by endoscopic ultrasound. *Endoscopy* 2002;34(6):461–3.

58. Vickers J, Alderson D. Influence of luminal obstruction on oesophageal cancer staging using endoscopic ultrasonography. *Br J Surg* 1998;85:999–1001.

59. Rice TW, Zuccaro G Jr, Adelstein DJ, et al. Esophageal carcinoma: depth of tumor invasion is predictive of regional lymph node status. *Ann Thorac Surg* 1998;65:787–792.

60. Nguyen P, Feng JC, Chang KJ. Endoscopic ultrasound (EUS) and EUS-guided fine-needle aspiration (FNA) of liver lesions. *Gastrointest Endosc* 1999;50:357–361.

61. Chak A, Canto M, Gerdes H, et al. Prognosis of esophageal cancers preoperatively staged to be locally invasive (T4) by endoscopic ultrasound (EUS): a multicenter retrospective cohort study. *Gastrointest Endosc* 1995;42:501–506.

62. Fockens P, Kisman K, Merkus MP, et al. The prognosis of esophageal carcinoma staged irresectable (T4) by endosonography. *J Am Coll Surg* 1998;186:17–23.

63. Lerut T, Flamen P, Ectors N, et al. Histopathological validation of lymph node staging with FDG-PET in cancer of the esophagus and gastroesophageal junction. *Ann Surg* 2000;232:743–752.

64. Choi JY, Lee KH, Shim YM, et al. Improved detection of individual nodal involvement in squamous cell carcinoma of the esophagus by FDG PET. *J Nucl Med* 2000;41:808–815.

65. Finch MD, John TG, Garden OJ, et al. Laparoscopic ultrasonography for staging gastroesophageal cancer. *Surgery* 1997;121:10–17.

66. Krasna MJ, Reed CE, Jaklitsch MT, et al. Thoracoscopic staging of esophageal cancer: a prospective, multiinstitutional trial. Cancer and Leukemia Group B Thoracic Surgeons. *Ann Thorac Surg* 1995;60:1337–1340.

67. Hadzijahic N, Wallace MB, Hawes RH, et al. CT or EUS for the initial staging of esophageal cancer? A cost minimization analysis. *Gastrointest Endosc* 2000;52:715–720.

68. Binmoeller KF, Seifert H, Seitz U, et al. Ultrasonic esophagoprobe for TNM staging of highly stenosing esophageal carinoma. *Gastrointest Endosc* 1995;41:547–552.

69. Dittler HJ, Siewart JR. Role of endoscopic ultrasonography in esophageal carcinoma endoscopy. *Endoscopy* 1993;25:156–161.

70. Grimm H, Binmoeller KF, Hamper K, et al. Endosonography for preoperative locoregional staging of esophageal and gastric cancer. *Endoscopy* 1993;25:224–230.

71. Heintz A, Hohne U, Schweden F, et al. Preoperative detection of intrathoracic tumor spread of esophageal cancer: endosonography versus computer tomography. *Surg Endosc* 1991;5:75–78.

72. Hunerbein M, Dohmoto M, Rau B, et al. Endosonography and endosonography guided biopsy of upper GI tract tumors using a curved array echoendoscope. *Surg Endosc* 1996:10:1205–1209.

73. Manzoni G. Endosonography and CT in the evaluation of tumor invasion. In *Recent advances in diseases of the esophagus*. Nabeya C, Hanaoka T, Nogami H, eds. New York: Springer-Verlag;1993:532–539.

74. Murata Y, Suzuki S, Hashimoto H. Endoscopic ultrasonography of the upper gastrointestinal tract. *Surg Endosc* 1988;2:180–183.

75. Murata Y, Hayashi K, Kobayashi A, et al. Pre-operative staging of oesophageal carcinoma by ultrasound. *Asian Surg* 1993;17:200–207.

76. Peters JH, Hoeft SF, Heimbucher J, et al. Selection of patients for curative or palliative resection of esophageal cancer based on preoperative endoscopic ultrasonography. *Arch Surg* 1994;129:534–539.

77. Takemoto T, Ito T, Aibe T, et al. Endoscopic ultrasonography in the diagnosis of esophageal carcinoma, with particular regard to staging for operability. *Endoscopy* 1986;18[Suppl 3]:22–25.

78. Ziegler K, Sanft C, Friedrich M, et al. Evaluation of endosonography in TN staging of oesophageal cancer. *Gut* 1991;32:16–20.

79. Kelly S, Harris KM, Berry E, et al. A systematic review of the staging performance of endoscopic ultrasound in gastro-oesophageal carcinoma. *Gut* 2001;49(4):534–539.

80. Botet JF, Lightdale CJ, Zauber AG, et al. Preoperative staging of esophageal cancer: comparison of endoscopic US and dynamic CT. *Radiology* 1991;181:419–425.

81. Wallace MB, Hawes RH, Sahai AV, et al. Dilation of malignant esophageal stenosis to allow EUS-guided fine-needle aspiration: safety and effect on patient management. *Gastrointest Endosc* 2000;51:309–313.

82. Tio TL, Cohen P, Coene PP, et al. Endosonography and computer tomography of esophageal carcinoma: preoperative classification compared to the new (1987) TNM system. *Gastroenterology* 1989;96:1478–1486.

83. Hiele M, DeLeyn P, Schurmans P, et al. Relation between endoscopic ultrasound findings and outcome of patients with tumors of the esophagus or esophagogastric junction. *Gastrointest Endosc* 1997;45:381–386.

84. Hasegawa N, Niwa Y, Arisawa T, et al. Preoperative staging of superficial carcinoma: comparison of a standard probe and standard endoscopic ultrasonography. *Gastrointest Endosc* 1996;44:388–393.

85. Catalano MF, Sivak MV, Rice T, et al. Endosonographic features predictive of lymph node metastasis. *Gastrointest Endosc* 1994;40:442–446.

86. Wiersema MJ, Vilmann P, Giovanini M, et al. Endosonogrpahy-guided fine-needle aspiration biopsy: diagnostic accuracy and complication assessment. *Gastroenterology* 1997;112:1087–1095.

87. Vazquez-Sequerios E, Norton ID, Clain JE, et al. Impact of EUS-guided fine needle aspiration on lymph node staging in patients with esophageal carcinoma. *Gastrointest Endosc* 2001;53:751–757.

88. Reed CE, Mishra G, Sahai AV, et al. Esophageal cancer staging: improved accuracy by endoscopic ultrasound of celiac lymph nodes. *Ann Thorac Surg* 1999;67:319–321.

89. Eloubeidi MA, Wallace MB, Reed CE, et al. The utility of EUS and EUS-guided fine needle aspiration in detecting celiac lymph node metastasis in patients with esophageal cancer: a single center experience. *Gastrointest Endosc* 2001;54:714–719.

90. Zuccaro G Jr, Rice TW, Goldblum J, et al. Endoscopic ultrasound cannot determine suitability for esophagectomy after aggressive chemoradiotherapy for esophageal cancer. *Am J Gastroenterol* 1999;94(4):906–912.

91. Chak A, Canto MI, Cooper GS, et al. Endosonographic assessment of multimodality therapy predicts survival of esophageal carcinoma patients. *Cancer* 2000;88:1788–1795.

92. Willis J, Cooper GS, Isenberg G, et al. Correlation of EUS measurement with pathologic assessment of neoadjuvant therapy response in esophageal carcinoma. *Gastrointest Endosc* 2002;55:655–661.

93. Heit HA, Johnson LF, Sigel SR, et al. Palliative dilation for esophageal carcinoma. *Ann Intern Med* 1978;89:629–631.

94. Chung SCS, Leong HT, Choi CYC, et al. Palliation of malignant oesophageal obstruction by endoscopic alcohol injection. *Endoscopy* 1994;26:275–277.

95. Nwokolo CU, Payne-James JJ, Silk DBA, et al. Palliation of malignant dysphagia by ethanol induced tumor necrosis. *Gut* 1994;35:299–303.

96. Mellow MH, Pinkas H. Endoscopic laser therapy for malignancies affecting the esophagus and gastroesophageal junction. *Arch Intern Med* 1985;145:1443–1446.

97. Jensen DM, Machicado G, Randal G, et al. Comparison of low-power YAG laser and BICAP tumor probe for palliation of esophageal cancer strictures. *Gastroenterology* 1988;94:1263–1270.

98. Robertson GSM, Jamieson MJT, Veitch PS, et al. Palliation of oesophageal carcinoma using the argon beam coagulator. *Br J Surg* 1996;83:1769–1777.

99. Heindorff H, Wojdemann M, Bisgaard L, et al. Endoscopic palliation of inoperable cancer of the oesophagus or cardia by argon electrocoagulation. *Scand J Gastroenterol* 1998;63:21–23.

100. Loizou LA, Grigg D, Atkinson M, et al. A prospective comparison of laser therapy of intubation in endoscopic palliation for malignant dysphagia. *Gastroenterology* 1991;100:1303–1310.

101. McCaughan JS, Nims TS, Guy JT, et al. Photodynamic therapy for esophageal tumors. *Arch Surg* 1989;124:74–80.

102. Lightdale CJ, Heier SK, Marcon NE, et al. Photodynamic therapy with porfimer sodium versus thermal ablation with Nd:YAG laser for palliation of esophageal cancer: a multicenter randomized trial. *Gastrointest Endosc* 1995:42:507–512.

103. Scheider DM, Siements M, Cirocco M, et al. Esophageal prosthesis for neoplastic stenosis. *Cancer* 1986;57:1426–1431.

104. Cavy AL, Rougier PM, Pieddeloup SA, et al. Esophageal prosthesis for neoplastic stenosis. *Cancer* 1986;57:1426–1431.

105. Hegarty MM, Angorn IB, Bryer JV, et al. Pulsion intubation for palliation of carcinoma of the esophagus. *Br J Surg* 1977;64:160–165.

106. Oglivie AL, Dronfield MW, Ferguson R, et al. Palliative intubation of oesophagogastric neoplasms at fiberoptic endoscopy. *Gut* 1982;23:1060–1067.

107. Tytgat GN. Endoscopic methods of treatment of gastrointestinal and biliary stenoses. *Endoscopy* 1980;[Suppl]:57–68.

108. Knyrim K, Wagner HJ, Bethge N, et al. A controlled trial of an expansible metal stent for palliation of esophageal obstruction due to inoperable cancer. *N Engl J Med* 1993;329:1302–1307.

109. De Palma GD, di Matteo E, Romano G, et al. Plastic prosthesis versus expandable metal stents for palliation of inoperable esophageal carcinoma: a controlled prospective study. *Gastrointest Endosc* 1996;43:478–482.

110. Siersema, PD, Wim CJ, Dees J, et al. Coated self-expanding metal stents versus latex prosthesis for esophagogastric cancer with special reference for prior radiation and chemotherapy: a controlled, prospective study. *Gastrointest Endosc* 1998;47:113–120.

111. Ciolt HG, Meric B, Dumon JF. Double stents for cancer of the esophagus invading the tracheo-bronchial tree. *Gastrointest Endosc* 1992;38:485–489.

112. Freitag L, Tekolf E, Steveling H, et al. Management of malignant esophagotracheal fistulas with airway stenting and double stenting. *Chest* 1996;110:1155–1160.

113. Kinsman KJ, DeGregorio BT, Kanton RM, et al. Prior radiation and chemotherapy increase the risk of life-threatening complications after insertion of metallic stents for esophagogastric malignancy. *Gastrointest Endosc* 1996;43:196–203.

114. Kozarek RA, Ball TJ, Brandabur JJ, et al. Expandable versus conventional esophageal prostheses: easier insertion may not preclude subsequent stent-related problems. *Gastrointest Endosc* 1996;43:204–208.

115. Raijman I, Siddique I, Lynch P. Does chemoradiation therapy increase the incidence of complications with self-expanding metal stents in the management of malignant esophageal strictures? *Am J Gastroenterol* 1997;92:2192–2195.

SURGERY FOR CANCER OF THE ESOPHAGUS AND ESOPHAGOGASTRIC JUNCTION

THOMAS W. RICE

Surgery for carcinoma of the esophagus and esophagogastric junction evolved from cervical esophageal bypass for palliation of dysphagia to curative resection and reconstruction in a little over 125 years. Early surgery carried significant morbidity and mortality with minimal hope for cure. This led to use of radiation as definitive, yet palliative, therapy. With advances in staging, better preoperative evaluation and preparation, alternative surgical technique, and improved postoperative care, surgery is now the principal curative therapy for esophageal cancer.

Although these evolutionary changes seem only natural, they were not direct or easy. Innovative therapy or technique always gives rise to controversy. Manuscripts and dissertations address topics such as best therapy for a specific cancer, criteria for a good surgical candidate, optimal surgical technique, qualifications needed to perform surgery, and role of adjuvant therapy. Despite uncertainties, surgical management of cancer of the esophagus and esophagogastric junction must begin with accurate assessment of both the tumor and the patient.

THE TUMOR

Diagnosis

Clinical diagnosis of esophageal carcinoma includes history, physical examination, and barium esophagram. Solid dysphagia in a middle-aged to older white man with a longstanding history of reflux and a known hiatal hernia is the classic presentation in the western hemisphere. It is best treated as an esophageal adenocarcinoma of the distal esophagus or esophagogastric junction unless proven otherwise. Typically, physical examination reveals a robust middle-aged to older white man with potential comorbidities, without weight loss, and without clinically detectable metastases to nonregional lymph nodes (supraclavicular) or distant sites (e.g., liver, pleura). In contradistinction, squamous cell carcinoma is found in the midthoracic esophagus in slightly younger nonwhite men, usually from an endemic area and a lower socioeconomic class. History is typically of dysphagia, weight loss, and heavy smoking and drinking, and examination usually reveals an advanced stage carcinoma.

In many centers, flexible fiberoptic videoesophagoscopy (Color Plate 14.1) has replaced barium esophagram (Fig. 14.2) as the first investigation in the evaluation of dysphagia and the clinical diagnosis of esophageal carcinoma. However, in patients with esophageal carcinoma, reports show that modern barium esophagram detects a lesion in 98% of barium studies, is suggestive or diagnostic of esophageal carcinoma in 96%, and has an estimated positive predictive value of 42% (1). For many physicians, barium esophagram remains the principal test for the clinical diagnosis of esophageal carcinoma.

Clinical diagnosis of esophageal carcinoma requires tissue confirmation. For the pathologic diagnosis of esophageal carcinoma, flexible esophagoscopy is the procedure of choice. Cytology brushings followed by multiple biopsies are diagnostic in most patients (Color Plates 14.3 and 14.4). Useful in the diagnosis of malignant strictures that are not endoscopically accessible are endoscopic esophageal ultrasound (EUS) and fine needle aspiration (EUS FNA) of the abnormal esophageal wall (2). FNA or open biopsy of distant metastases can provide both a pathologic diagnosis and crucial staging.

In North America, patients with a columnar-lined esophagus should have esophagoscopy and biopsy (four quadrant biopsies every 2 cm) every 3 years. Surveillance of these high-risk groups allows diagnosis of early stage disease

T. W. Rice: Section of General Thoracic Surgery, Department of Thoracic and Cardiovascular Surgery, The Cleveland Clinic Foundation, Cleveland, Ohio.

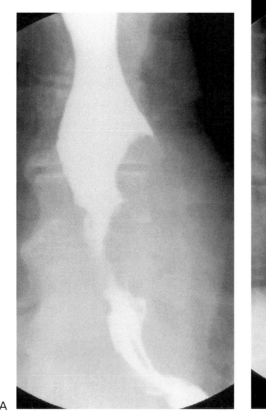
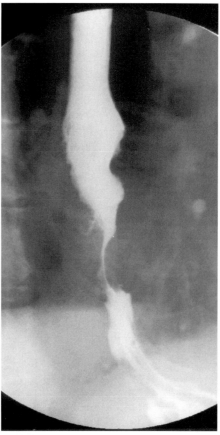

A

B

FIGURE 14.2. Barium esophagram of a malignant esophageal stricture. This long, irregular stricture has mucosal destruction and irregular filling defects obstructing the esophageal lumen. It occurs above a hiatal hernia.

in asymptomatic patients and is cost-effective compared to other cancer surveillance programs (3,4).

Staging

TNM staging of esophageal carcinoma is obtained by evaluation of primary tumor invasion (T), the status of regional lymph nodes (N), and distant sites (M) (5) (Table 14.1). Depth of tumor invasion defines the primary tumor (T) (Fig. 14.5). Tis tumors are intraepithelial malignancies confined to the epithelium without invasion of the basement membrane (high-grade dysplasia). T1 tumors breach the basement membrane to invade the lamina propria, muscularis mucosa, or the submucosa but do not invade beyond the submucosa. T2 tumors invade into but not beyond the muscularis propria. T3 tumors invade beyond the esophageal wall into the periesophageal tissue but do not invade adjacent structures. T4 tumors directly invade structures in the vicinity of the esophagus. The broad definition of T1 carcinomas prompted the practical subdivision of this subset into T1 intramucosal carcinomas (T1a), which invade the lamina

propria or muscularis mucosa, and T1 submucosal carcinomas (T1b) (6) (Fig. 14.5).

Regional lymph nodes (N) are either free of (N0) or involved by (N1) metastatic cancer (Table 14.1 and Fig. 14.5). Distinction of a regional lymph node from a nonregional lymph node may be problematic despite the broad and overlapping definitions in the staging manual (5) (Table 14.2). The regional lymph node map is crucial for clinical and pathologic staging (Fig. 14.6). Lack of subclassification of N1 is a shortcoming of the present staging system. N1 lymph node burden is a prognosticator and many physicians substage N1 depending upon the total number of N1 nodes and percent of resected lymph nodes that are N1 (6–9).

Similarly, distant sites (M) are either free of (M0) or involved by (M1) metastatic cancer (Table 14.1). Recent revision of the staging system for esophageal carcinoma subdivides distant metastatic carcinomas (M1) into M1a (distant, nonregional lymph node metastases) and M1b (other distant metastases) (5). M1a disease is classified further by tumor location: M1a tumors of the upper thoracic esophagus metastasized to supraclavicular nodes and M1a tumors

TABLE 14.1. TNM STAGING OF ESOPHAGEAL CARCINOMAS

T: Primary Tumor

TX   Tumor cannot be assessed.
T0   No evidence of tumor.
Tis   High-grade dysplasia.
T1   Tumor invades the lamina propria, muscularis mucosa, or submucosa. It does not breach the submucosa.
T2   Tumor invades into but not beyond the muscularis propria.
T3   Tumor invades the paraesophageal tissue but does not invade adjacent structures.
T4   Tumor invades adjacent structures.

N: Regional Lymph Nodes

NX   Regional lymph nodes cannot be assessed.
N0   No regional lymph node metastases.
N1   Regional lymph node metastases.

M: Distant Metastasis

MX   Distant metastases cannot be assessed.
M1a   Upper thoracic esophagus metastatic to supraclavicular lymph nodes.
      Lower thoracic esophagus metastatic to celiac lymph nodes.
M1b   Upper thoracic esophagus metastatic to other nonregional lymph nodes or other distant sites.
      Midthoracic esophagus metastatic to either nonregional lymph nodes or other distant sites.
      Lower thoracic esophagus metastatic to other nonregional lymph nodes or other distant sites.

Stage Groupings	T	N	M
Stage 0	Tis	N0	M0
Stage I	T1	N0	M0
Stage IIA	T2	N0	M0
	T3	N0	M0
Stage IIB	T1	N1	M0
	T2	N1	M0
Stage III	T3	N1	M0
	T4	Any N	M0
Stage IVA	Any T	Any N	M1a
Stage IVB	Any T	Any N	M1b

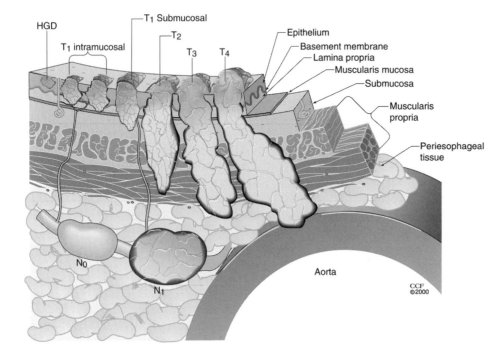

FIGURE 14.5. Primary tumor status is defined by depth of tumor invasion (T). Regional lymph node status (N) is defined by the absence (N0) or presence (N1) of regional nodal metastases. HGD is high-grade dysplasia (Tis).

TABLE 14.2. REGIONAL LYMPH NODES

Cervical Esophagus
    Scalene
    Internal jugular
    Upper and lower cervical
    Periesophageal
    Supraclavicular
Intrathoracic Esophagus (Upper, middle and lower)
    Upper periesophageal (above the azygous vein)
    Subcarinal
    Lower periesophageal (below the azygous vein)
Gastroesophageal Junction
    Lower periesophageal (below the azygous vein)
    Diaphragmatic
    Pericardial
    Left gastric
    Celiac

of the lower thoracic esophagus metastasized to celiac lymph nodes. No M1a subdivision for midthoracic esophageal carcinomas exists because these tumors metastatic to nonregional lymph nodes have an equivalent prognosis to those metastatic to other distant sites. Although this subclassification has anatomic and statistical significances, the clinical relevance is questionable in North America (10).

TNM descriptors are grouped into stages to assemble subgroups with similar behavior and prognosis (Table 14.1). Despite shortcomings, the present staging system is an essential tool in the evaluation and treatment of esophageal carcinoma (6,9).

Clinical Staging

Physical examination, imaging, esophagoscopy, laparoscopy, thoracoscopy, biopsy, and needle aspiration are necessary to establish clinical stage (cTNM). Clinical stage provides the baseline for treatment evaluation and rational treatment decisions.

Determination of cT

EUS is the only clinical tool that provides detailed examination of the esophageal wall. It is the procedure of choice for determining cT. The muscularis propria (fourth ultrasound layer) is vital in differentiating T1, T2, and T3 tumors (Fig. 14.7). Tumors are defined as cT1 if there is no invasion of the muscularis propria (fourth ultrasound layer); cT2, if invasion is into the muscularis propria; or cT3, if invasion is beyond the muscularis propria. EUS evaluates the interface between the primary tumor and adjacent structures. If invasion is detected, the tumor is cT4. In a review of 21 series, the accuracy of EUS for T determination was 84% (11). Accuracy is not constant and varies with T. In this metaanalysis, accuracy for T1 carcinomas was 83.5% with 16.5% of tumors over-

staged; accuracy for T2 was 73% with 10% understaged and 17% overstaged; accuracy for T3 was 89% with 5% understaged and 6% overstaged; and accuracy for T4 was 89% with 11% understaged. A review of the literature shows variation in accuracy with T: 75% to 82% for T1, 64% to 85% for T2, 89% to 94% for T3, and 88% to 100% for T4 (12). The most unreliable of cT EUS determinations is for cT2 (13,14). A metaanalysis of 27 articles demonstrates EUS as being highly effective in the differentiation of T1 and T2 from T3 and T4 cancers (15).

EUS and esophagoscopy are complementary and should be performed together. A malignant stricture that prohibits passage of the examining instrument is highly predictive of an advanced stage cancer (16–18). A tumor length greater than 5 cm is predictive of T3 cancers with 89% sensitivity, 92% specificity, 89% positive predictive value, and 92% negative predictive value (18).

Exclusion of cT4 cancers, demonstrated by the preservation of fat planes between an esophageal cancer and adjacent structures, is the only role of computed tomography (CT) in the determination of cT (Fig. 14.8). Contiguous soft tissues provide radiographic contrast necessary to define the esophagus; however, these planes may be absent in cachectic patients. In normal patients, fat between an esophageal cancer and aorta, trachea, left main bronchus, or pericardium may be absent. Physiologic absence of fat planes complicates the assessment of invasion of adjacent structures. Alternative CT criteria have been proposed to predict T4 status. Aortic invasion is suggested by an arc of contact between the tumor and the aorta greater than 90 degrees, although this is not an absolute confirmation of a T4 tumor. Thickening or indentation of the normally flat or slightly convex posterior membranous wall of the intrathoracic trachea or left main bronchus is suggestive of airway invasion. On occasion, tumor in the airway lumen or a fistula between the esophagus and airway may be visualized; however, bronchoscopic confirmation with biopsy is necessary. Pericardial invasion is suspected if pericardial thickening, pericardial effusion, or indentation of the heart with loss of the pericardial fat plane at the level of the tumor is seen. Magnetic resonance imaging (MRI) offers no significant advantage over CT.

Positron emission tomography (PET) using 2-[^{18}F]fluoro-2-deoxy-D-glucose (FDG) is reported to accumulate in 92% to 100% of esophageal cancers (19,20). FDG PET and other imaging modalities do not provide definition of the esophageal wall or paraesophageal tissue and, therefore, have no value in the determination of cT.

Theoretically, thoracoscopy could exclude a cT4 tumor but requires dissection of the primary tumor and the adjacent structure thought to be invaded. Although mentioned as a possible staging tool for cT4 detection (21,22), only documentation of T4 is the detection of cT4 disease in 14% of patients undergoing thoracoscopy and laparoscopy for regional lymph node staging (23).

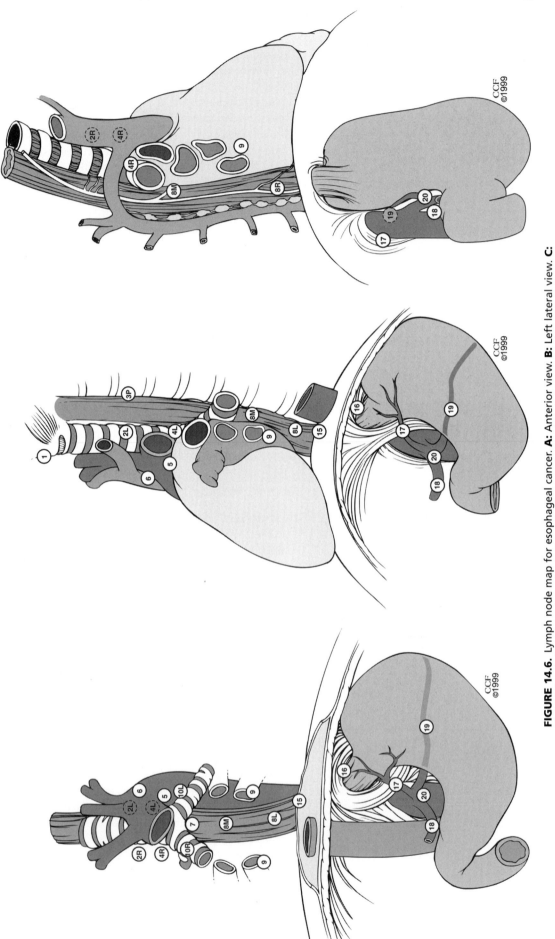

FIGURE 14.6. Lymph node map for esophageal cancer. **A:** Anterior view. **B:** Left lateral view. **C:** Right lateral view. Lymph node stations: 1, supraclavicular; 2R, right paratracheal; 2L, left paratracheal; 3P, posterior mediastinal; 4R, right tracheobronchial angle; 4L, left tracheobronchial; 5, aortopulmonary; 6, anterior mediastinal; 7, subcarinal; 8M, middle paraesophageal; 8L, lower paraesophageal; 9, inferior pulmonary ligament; 10, hilar; 15, diaphragmatic; 16, paracardial; 17, left gastric; 18, common hepatic; 19, splenic; 20, celiac.

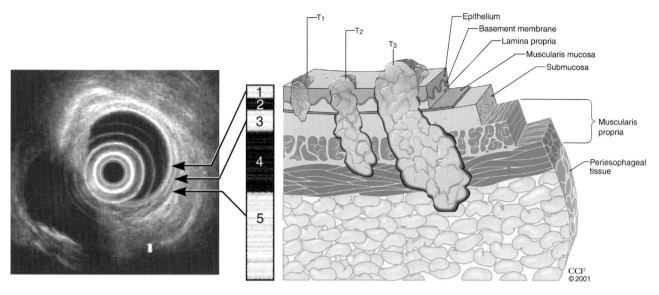

FIGURE 14.7. The esophageal wall is visualized as five alternating layers of differing echogenicity by esophageal ultrasound (EUS). The first layer is hyperechoic (*white*) and represents the superficial mucosa (epithelium and lamina propria). The second layer is hypoechoic (*black*) and represents the deep mucosa (muscularis mucosa). The third layer is hyperechoic and represents the submucosa. The forth ultrasound layer is hypoechoic and represents the muscularis mucosa. This layer (muscularis propria) is critical in differentiating T1, T2, and T3 tumors. The fifth ultrasound layer is hyperechoic and represents the periesophageal tissue. The thickness of the EUS layers is not equal to the actual thickness of anatomic layers.

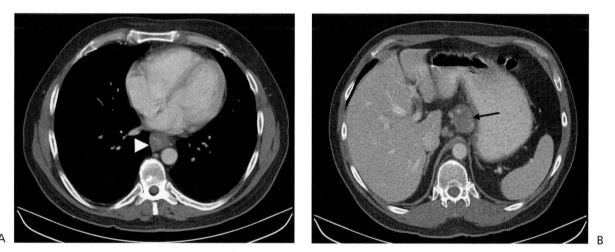

FIGURE 14.8. A: Nonspecific computed tomographic (CT) finding of esophageal cancer (*arrowhead*) is thickening of the esophageal wall. CT does not discriminate between cTis, cT1, cT2, and cT3 tumors. Preservation of periesophageal fat excludes cT4 cancer. In this study, preservation of fat planes excludes invasion of the prevertebral fascia, aorta, and pericardium. **B:** In this same patient, an enlarged celiac axis lymph node (*arrow*) is seen.

Determination of cN (Regional) and cM1 (Nonregional) Lymph Node Status

EUS evaluates nodal size, shape, border, and internal echo characteristics in regional lymph node assessment. In a retrospective review of 100 EUS examinations, determination of N was 89% sensitive, 75% specific, and 84% accurate (24). Positive predictive value of EUS for N1 disease was 86%; negative predictive value was 79%. A metaanalysis of 21 series reported EUS as being 77% accurate for N, 69% for N0, and 89% for N1 (11). EUS FNA further refines clinical staging by adding tissue sampling to endosonography findings. In a multicenter study, 171 patients had EUS FNA of 192 lymph nodes (25). EUS FNA for determination of lymph node status was 92% sensitive, 93% specific, 100% positively predictive, and 86% negatively predictive. Combined EUS and EUS FNA assessment of celiac lymph nodes was 72% sensitive, 97% specific, 95% positively predictive, and 82% negatively predictive (26). FNA confirmed positive EUS M1a disease in 88% of patients. Recent experience of this group reported 98% accuracy of EUS FNA detection of malignant celiac lymph nodes (27).

Surface ultrasound examination of cervical lymph nodes detects nonpalpable metastasis in patients with squamous cell carcinoma (28,29).

An enlarged lymph node by CT suggests nodal metastasis (Fig. 14.8). The short axis of these nodes is easily measured; intrathoracic and abdominal lymph nodes greater than 1 cm are enlarged. Supraclavicular lymph nodes with a short axis greater than 0.5 cm and retrocrural lymph nodes greater than 0.6 cm are pathologic (30). However, the probability is small that cN status can be determined by lymph node size alone (31). Normal-sized nodes that contain metastatic deposits and metastatic nodes in direct contact with the tumor may be indistinguishable from the primary tumor. These result in false-negative examinations and influence the sensitivity and negative predictive value. All enlarged lymph nodes may not be malignant. Inflammatory nodes are the most common cause of a false-positive examination and of lower specificity and positive predictive value. CT assessment of lymph nodes varies with anatomic site; accuracies of 61% to 96%, sensitivities of 8% to 75%, and specificities of 60% to 98% were reported for cervical, mediastinal, and abdominal nodes (32). MRI offers no important advantage over CT.

Physiologic evaluation of esophageal carcinoma provided by FDG PET relies not only on size of the metastatic deposit but also on the intensity of FDG uptake and decay. Theoretically, it is possible to identify microscopic metastases if glucose metabolism is sufficient to concentrate large quantities

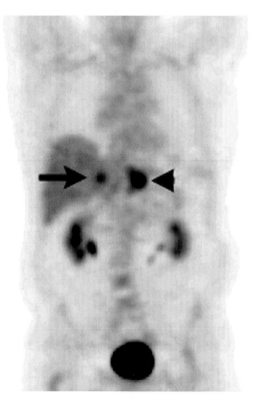
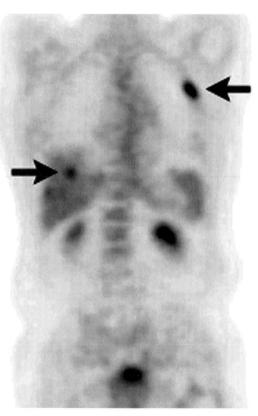

A

B

FIGURE 14.9. Positron emission tomography of a T3N1M1b esophageal cancer. **A:** Primary tumor and regional lymph nodes cannot be differentiated and appear as one large mass (*arrowhead*). **A** and **B:** There are two sites of metastases (*arrows*), two metastases in the liver and one in the left rib. The kidneys excrete and the bladder stores 2-[^{18}F]-fluoro-2-deoxy-D-glucose.

of FDG. FDG PET cannot differentiate adjacent N1 from the primary tumor (19) (Fig. 14.9). FDG PET is least sensitive in assessment of lymph nodes in the mid and lower thoracic esophagus (33). The accuracy of FDG PET in the detection of lymph node metastases from esophageal carcinomas is variable, ranging from 37% to 90% (20,34–37). Compared with detection of lymph node metastases in lung cancer, FDG PET is much less accurate in esophageal carcinoma (38). Because of its high sensitivity, the main role of FDG PET is confirmation of cN0 status (39). The addition of [Methyl-(11)C]choline PET to FDG PET may increase the accuracy of PET cN1 staging (40,41).

Thoracoscopic and laparoscopic staging have been used to evaluate cN and cM1 lymph node status. A combination of thoracoscopic and laparoscopic staging is 94% accurate in detecting lymph node metastases (23). For thoracic lymph nodes, sensitivity, specificity, and positive predictive value are 63%, 100%, and 100%, respectively. For abdominal lymph nodes, sensitivity, specificity, and positive predictive value are 85%, 100%, and 100%, respectively. Of 88 patients entered into the study, thoracoscopy was performed in 82 (93%), laparoscopy in 55 (63%), and both in 49 (57%). Induction chemoradiotherapy was administered to 34 (39%) patients. These procedures are not without serious morbidity (42) and the possibility of port site metastasis (43). Only 47 (53%) patients underwent resection, making comparative pathologic stage available in only 13 (15%) patients. The best operative time and hospital stay reported are 3.6 hours and 1.8 days, respectively (44).

Determination of Nonnodal M1b Status

In patients with recently diagnosed esophageal carcinoma, metastases were found in the liver in 35%, in the lung in 20%, in the bone in 9%, in the adrenal gland in 2%, in the brain in 2%, and 1% each in the pericardium, pleura, soft tissues, stomach, pancreas and spleen (45). Except for the brain,

CT scanning of the esophagus includes all or a portion of all other sites. Contrast-enhanced CT scanning with imaging during the portal venous phases of contrast distribution provides both screening for and diagnosis of masses in these areas.

Hepatic metastases appear as ill-defined, low-density lesions of variable size (Fig. 14.10). Conventional CT imaging (dynamic incremental scanning with intravenous bolus contrast enhancement) is excellent in the detection of hepatic metastases greater than 2 cm (46). Sensitivity is 70% to 80% (30). Although no study is available for esophageal cancer, spiral CT produced similar results to conventional CT in the detection of colorectal liver metastases; sensitivity of 76% and a positive predictive value of 90% have been reported (47). CT frequently does not recognize subcentimeter metastases; they are the main cause of false-negative examinations and the low sensitivity of CT in the detection of liver metastases. To distinguish benign from malignant nodules, ultrasound is used for diagnosis of benign cysts and MRI for hemangiomas. Adrenal metastases cause heterogeneous focal enlargement of the adrenal gland. Contrast-enhanced CT is a sensitive but nonspecific screening tool for adrenal masses. Noncontrast CT, MRI, percutaneous FNA, or laparoscopy may be required to confirm the nature of these nodules.

In a cohort of patients with predominate squamous cell carcinoma of the esophagus, solitary lung metastases were rare at diagnosis of the primary cancer and were likely to be benign nodules or synchronous primary lung cancer (48). Although multiple lung metastases were uncommon at diagnosis, they became more common during the late stages of the disease (Fig. 14.10). Many were not visualized by chest radiograph. CT is very sensitive in the detection of pulmonary nodules; however, histologic confirmation of these abnormalities is required if their presence alone determines therapy.

The presence of ascites, pleural effusion, or nodules in the omentum or pleura suggests metastases to these mesothelial-lined surfaces. Laparoscopy or thoracoscopy confirms these findings.

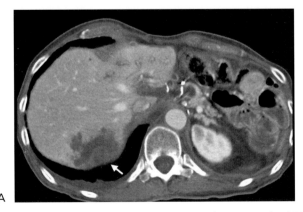
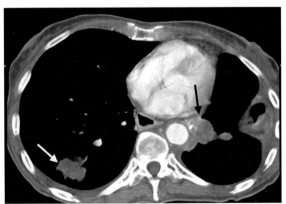

A

B

FIGURE 14.10. A: Computed tomography (CT) of a hepatic metastasis appears as ill-defined, low-density lesion in the posterior portion of the right lobe (*arrow*). **B:** CT of a pulmonary metastasis in the right lower lobe (*white arrow*) and mediastinal lymph nodes (*black arrow*) in the same patient with diffusely metastatic esophageal carcinoma.

Brain metastases are reported in 2% to 4% of patients presenting with esophageal carcinoma (45,49). They tend to occur in patients with large adenocarcinoma of the esophagogastric junction with local invasion or metastases to lymph nodes. Pretreatment CT of the brain may be reasonable in these patients.

Despite improved technology, CT is only 37% to 66% sensitive in screening for distant metastases in patients with esophageal cancer (34,35,38,50). FDG PET is superior to CT in detecting M1b disease. In 91 patients undergoing 100 FDG PET studies, distant metastatic disease was detected in 39 scans at 51 sites (38). Seventy distant metastases were confirmed by biopsy or at resection. The sensitivity of FDG PET was 69%, specificity 93%, and overall accuracy 84%. In this series, the sensitivity of CT was 46%, specificity 74%, and accuracy 63%. FDG PET failed to diagnose distant metastases in the liver in ten patients, pleura in four patients, lung in two patients, and peritoneum in one patient. All metastases were less than 1 cm in diameter. Of 21 false-negative CT scans, FDG PET identified distant metastases in 11 (62%); of 12 false-negative FDG PET scans, CT was accurate in four (33%). These mature results are less favorable than in an earlier report by the same group in which sensitivity of FDG PET in detection of distant metastases was 88%, specificity 93%, and accuracy 91% (36).

Five (71%) of 7 patients with distant metastatic disease were diagnosed by FDG PET (19). A liver metastasis less than 1 cm in diameter was not visualized and a pancreatic metastasis was misinterpreted as a left gastric lymph node metastasis. There were no false-positive examinations in 36 patients. Over a similar time period, the same group reported 17 distant metastases in 59 patients with FDG PET. There were no false-negative examinations; however, transhiatal esophagectomy was commonly used to obtain pathologic stage (34).

FDG PET detects radiographically occult distant metastatic disease in 10% to 20% of patients with esophageal cancer (34–36,38). The combination of FDG PET and CT has a diagnostic accuracy of 80% to 92% (34,35) and avoids unnecessary surgery in 90% (35). FDG PET provides additional staging information in 22% of patients, upstaging 15% and downstaging 7% (39).

Laparoscopy is reported to change therapy in 10% of patients, allowing resection in 2% who are overstaged and avoiding resection in 8% with undetected M1b disease (51). The sensitivities of laparoscopy in detecting peritoneal and liver metastases are 71% and 86%, respectively. Heath and colleagues reported that laparoscopy changed the treatment in 17% (52). Laparoscopic ultrasonography does not improve staging by laparoscopy alone (53,54).

EUS has limited value in screening for distant metastases (M1b). The distant organ must be in direct contact with the upper gastrointestinal tract for EUS to be useful (e.g., the left lateral segment of the liver and retroperitoneum).

Role of Clinical Staging

CT, EUS, EUS FNA, and FDG PET are mainstays in clinical staging of esophageal carcinoma. Results of these studies determine the necessity for invasive staging techniques such as thoracoscopy and laparoscopy and direct their use. Clinical stage is highly predictive of pathologic stage and outcome (Fig. 14.11 and 14.12) and is key in determining therapy. Equally important to decision making is the assessment of the patient.

THE PATIENT

Patient assessment, selection, and preoperative preparation are crucial in reducing postoperative morbidity and mortality and ensuring improved survival following surgery for esophageal cancer.

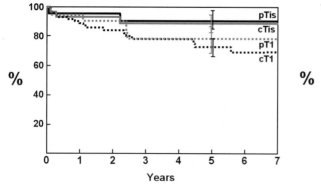
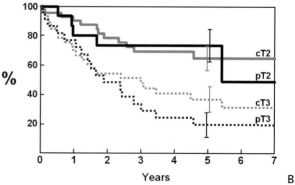

FIGURE 14.11. Kaplan-Meier survival estimates of 153 clinically staged patients undergoing surgery alone for esophageal cancer. **A:** N0M0 cancers confined to the esophageal wall. **B:** N0M0 cancers invading beyond the esophageal wall. cT is clinically determined depth of tumor invasion; pT is pathologic depth of tumor invasion determined by examination of the resected tumor.

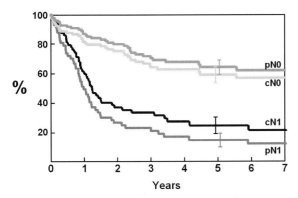

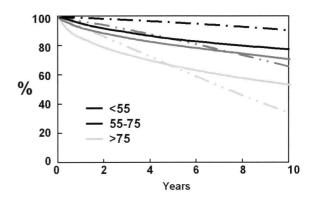

FIGURE 14.12. Kaplan-Meier survival estimates of 230 clinically staged patients undergoing surgery alone for esophageal cancer. cN is clinically determined regional lymph node status; pN is pathologic regional lymph node status determined by examination of the resection specimen.

FIGURE 14.13. Survival within age groups compared with a matched U.S. population. The dot-dash curve is the matched survival among patients younger than 55 years of age. The dash-dot-dot-dash curve is the population life table for patients between the ages of 55 and 75 years. The lowest dash-dot-dot-dash curve is for the matched population more than 75 years of age. (From Rice TW, Blackstone EH, Goldblum JR, et al. Superficial adenocarcinoma of the esophagus. *J Thorac Cardiovasc Surg* 2001;122:1077–1090, with permission.)

General Condition

The patient's overall state of health, although hard to define or quantify, significantly influences outcome. The amalgam of history and physical examination, a surgeon's accumulated experience, clinical acumen, and "feeling" about the patient often form the entire assessment of general health. However, quantification of a patient's general condition by the preoperative Karnofsky index can accurately predict outcome (55). Patients with a score less than 80 are more likely to have a complicated or lethal postoperative course.

Key to successful postoperative recovery is the cooperation of the patient in his or her care. Subtle impairment that affects intellect or cooperation, and which may be overlooked in the preoperative assessment of the elderly or alcoholic patient, may be of prime significance during the postoperative course. A simple grading of the patient's ability to cooperate as either good or poor is predictive of outcome (55). Bartel and colleagues proposed the classification of a patient's general condition as normal (Karnofsky index greater than 80 and "good" cooperation), compromised (Karnofsky index less than 80 or "poor" cooperation), and severely impaired (Karnofsky index less than 80 and "poor" cooperation).

Age

Survival following surgery for esophageal cancer is inversely related to age. The effect of age is best appreciated in patients with superficial adenocarcinoma because the overwhelming effect of esophageal cancer on survival is minimized in early stage cancers (56). In these patients, increasing age is an independent predictor of decreasing survival. However, compared with age-matched cohorts, survival improves with age (Fig. 14.13). Although uncommon, a cancer death in a younger patient with superficial esophageal adenocarcinoma is significant compared to age-matched patients who are unlikely to die of any cause. As patients age, the incidence of death from other causes increases; thus, in the highly selected "good risk" elderly patients chosen for resection of "good prognosis" superficial esophageal adenocarcinoma, survival is similar to their contemporaries without cancer.

Preoperative risk factors, advanced stage cancers, postoperative morbidity and mortality, and late deaths are variably reported to occur more frequently in elderly patients undergoing esophagectomy (57–65). In these reports age is not analyzed as a continuum, but rather as artificially picked cutoffs (e.g., 65, 70, 75, 80 years), making incorporation of these data into practice difficult. However, despite the variable definition of "elderly," comparisons of unmatched but highly selected groups of young and old patients undergoing surgery indicate that similar palliation and survival can be achieved regardless of age. Increasing age is a relative contraindication to surgery. In carefully chosen elderly patients with early stage cancers, surgery with curative intent may be indicated. In high-risk elderly patients or elderly patients with advanced stage cancers, nonsurgical palliation may be optimum.

Histologic Cell Type

In contrast to patients with adenocarcinoma, patients with squamous cell carcinoma have higher alcohol and tobacco consumptions and greater impairment of pulmonary and hepatic functions (66). Patients with adenocarcinoma are generally better educated, are from a higher socioeconomic stratum, and are more likely to be overweight (up to 50% of patients), and suffer cardiovascular impairment. In either cell type, incidence in men predominates. Although these are profiles and do not apply to individual patients, they highlight potential comorbidities and postoperative complications that should be considered when tissue diagnosis of esophageal carcinoma is made.

Pulmonary Function

Pulmonary complications are common following esophagectomy. In a large retrospective series, they occurred in 20% to 35% of patients (67). In a small prospective study of 20 patients, 50% developed pulmonary complications, defined as temperature greater than 38° C and pulmonary infiltrate documented radiography (68). Pulmonary complications, defined by atelectasis, pleural effusion, or pneumothorax on chest radiograph, are a universal occurrence in patients undergoing esophagectomy for cancer (69,70). Increasing age (odds ratio [OR] 1.31; 95% confidence interval, 0.99–1.74; $p = .06$) and impaired pulmonary function, measured by decreased percent forced expiratory volume in 1 second (FEV_1) (OR 1.21; 95% confidence interval, 1.07–1.38; $p = .003$), are identified as independent predictors of major pulmonary complications (67). In addition, Avendano (70) and colleagues found patients receiving preoperative chemoradiotherapy more likely to experience postoperative complications.

Improvement in operative mortality in current esophageal surgery is primarily the result of reducing pulmonary complications (71), which are associated with a 4.5-fold increase in operative mortality (67). Long-term (10 year) survival in patients with superficial esophageal adenocarcinoma decreases exponentially with a decrease in preoperative FEV_1 less than 2 L (56) (Fig. 14.14). Reducing pulmonary complications following thoracic surgery is tantamount to improving outcome.

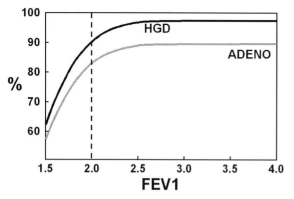

FIGURE 14.14. Ten-year survival of two types of patients, according to forced expiratory volume (FEV). One patient group has high-grade dysplasia (*HGD*) on preoperative biopsy, the other invasive adenocarcinoma (*ADENO*). Both are in a Barrett surveillance program, and both would have a planned transhiatal esophagectomy. Note the evident differences (nonoverlapping lower and upper confidence limits) below FEV_1 of approximately 2 L. (From Rice TW, Blackstone EH, Goldblum JR, et al. Superficial adenocarcinoma of the esophagus. *J Thorac Cardiovasc Surg* 2001;122:1077–1090, with permission.)

Preoperative assessment of all patients considered for esophagectomy should include pulmonary function testing and arterial blood gases. Smoking cessation for a period of 4 to 8 weeks before surgery has been shown to reduce postoperative morbidity in major pulmonary resections (72,73). Reversible airway disease and bronchitis should be aggressively treated. Pulmonary rehabilitation may be beneficial, especially in patients with early stage cancer who have time before surgery for this valuable therapy.

Cardiovascular Function

Dysrhythmias are common following esophagectomy, reported to occur in as many as 60% of patients (74). The prevalence in most series ranges from 10% to 25%. Supraventricular arrhythmias are associated with a significant increase in postoperative morbidity and mortality (57). However, arrhythmias are not the cause of death, but a marker for lethal complications. Predictors of supraventricular arrhythmias are increasing age and poor pulmonary function measured by preoperative theophylline use and a low diffusing capacity for carbon monoxide (57). Maximal oxygen uptake during exercise testing correlates with postoperative pulmonary complications and cardiac dysrhythmias (75). The preoperative maneuvers used to reduce pulmonary complications may have a similar effect on cardiac dysrhythmias.

Coronary artery disease is a common finding in patients with carcinoma of the esophagus (76), although myocardial infarction is uncommon. In octogenarians undergoing esophagectomy, myocardial infarction occurs in only 3% of patients (77). Preoperative predictors of infarction have not been identified. This is most likely due to careful patient selection based on preoperative cardiac evaluation along with preesophagectomy intervention in resectable patients with significant coronary artery disease.

As many as 11% of postoperative deaths are attributed to cardiac causes (71). Simple assessment of cardiac risk by a cardiologist as normal, increased, or high is a strong predictor of postoperative mortality (78).

Other Organ Systems

Cirrhosis is a contraindication to esophagectomy. In a small series of 18 patients with cirrhosis (11 patients were Child A and seven were Child B), operative morbidity was 83% and mortality was 17% (79). Impaired hepatic function assessed by serum albumin, serum bilirubin, partial thromboplastin time, aminopyrine breath test, and the presence or absence of cirrhosis is a predictor of hospital mortality (55,76).

In other surgical series, comorbidities such as diabetes, renal dysfunction, and peripheral vascular disease were not associated with an increase in either morbidity or mortality. However, in individual patients, recognition, assessment, and treatment of comorbidities are essential in improving outcome.

TABLE 14.3. COMPOSITE PREOPERATIVE SCORE

Factor	Score	Weight	Minimum	Maximum
General status	1–3	4	4	12
Cardiac function	1–3	3	3	9
Pulmonary function	1–3	2	2	6
Hepatic function	1–3	2	2	6
Composite score			11	33

Score: 1 normal, 2 compromised, 3 severely impaired.
(From Stein HJ, Brucher BL, Sendler A, et al. Esophageal cancer: patient evaluation and pre-treatment staging. *Surg Oncol* 2001;10:103–111, with permission.)

Preoperative Risk Score

Stein and colleagues developed a composite score for assessing risk of postoperative mortality after esophagectomy (76). Four factors (patient's general status and cardiac, pulmonary, and hepatic functions) are rated as 1 for normal, 2 for compromised, or 3 for severely impaired. These are weighted and summed to produce scores ranging from 11 to 33 (Table 14.3). Scores less than 18 are associated with low mortality and allow patients to be considered for aggressive therapy, including extensive resection or multimodality therapy. Scores greater than 21 are predictive of excessive mortality. Using this tool, the authors excluded 30% of patients with otherwise resectable tumors from surgery. This resulted in a decreased operative mortality from 10% before initiation of this system to 2% after its inception.

THE OPERATION

Operation for cancer of the esophagus and esophagogastric junction requires resection and reconstruction. Because each component influences the other, one cannot be performed separately without consideration of the other.

Resection

Primary Tumor

The extent of resection is determined by characteristics of the primary tumor and details of reconstruction (Fig. 14.15). In 3% of patients, the existence of cancer 10.5 cm proximal to visible tumor led to adoption of a 12 cm proximal margin for esophagectomy (80). A proximal margin less than 5 cm from the primary tumor is associated with a

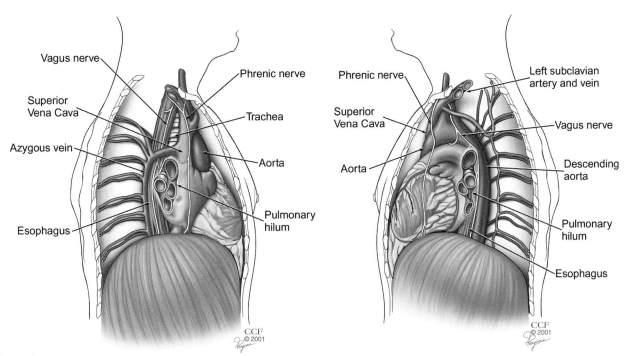

A   B

FIGURE 14.15. Thoracic esophageal resection. **A:** Right mediastinal view. **B:** Left mediastinal view.

20% chance of local recurrence. If the margin is 5 to 10 cm, recurrence is reduced to 8% (81). Mean length from the tumor to the resection margin is 2.7 cm in patients with anastomotic recurrence and 4.4 cm in patients without recurrence (*p* = .007) (82). A recent study recommended a macroscopic margin of 5 cm beyond the primary tumor to achieve a consistently negative distal resection margin (83). Compared with esophagogastrectomy, total thoracic esophagectomy with cervical esophagogastric anastomosis increases the length from the tumor to the proximal resection margin and decreases the incidence of anastomotic recurrence (84).

Accumulated experience with superficial carcinoma provides useful data to guide extent of resection. Subepithelial extension of primary tumor (defined as lymphatic, vascular or ductal permeation, intramural metastases, or direct invasion) is related to depth of tumor invasion (85). Only 4% of patients with tumors limited to the mucosa, 37% with submucosal invasion, and 46% with muscularis propria invasion have subepithelial extension. Risk of a positive resection margin is similarly related to depth of invasion (86). To ensure a less than 5% chance of a positive resection margin, a length from tumor to resection margins greater than 10 mm is required for tumors confined to the esophageal wall and greater than 30 mm for those invading beyond the esophageal wall.

Anastomotic recurrence is reported in 10% of patients with positive margins (R1 resection has microscopic positive margin, R2 resection has macroscopic positive margin) and 5% of patients with negative margins (R0 resection) (*p* = .15). Of 463 patients undergoing esophagectomy, 12 (3%) experienced an anastomotic recurrence (87). Ten anastomotic recurrences were in patients with negative margins. In 16 patients with positive margins, distant metastases developed in 11 and anastomotic recurrence developed in two. Only in patients without regional lymph node metastases or with low burden of regional lymph node metastases (<25% nodes positive) is survival decreased by a positive resection margin (88).

Lateral extent of the resection should include the periesophageal tissue and may include the pleura and pericardium. Preservation of the spleen is recommended, because splenectomy at esophagectomy for cancer is associated with increased septic complications (pneumonia, intraabdominal abscess, postoperative sepsis, and anastomotic leak) and postoperative mortality (36% versus 8%; *p* < .01) (89). Invasion of the trachea, aorta, vertebral bodies, lung, or heart precludes resection (Fig. 14.15).

If stomach is planned for reconstruction, a cervical anastomosis may provide the best long-term functional results. A low intrathoracic esophagogastric anastomosis has long been known to be unsatisfactory, because of excessive gastroesophageal reflux (90). One year after esophagectomy, patients with cervical anastomosis reported less reflux than those with intrathoracic anasto-

mosis (91). Both reflux symptoms (4% vs. 50%; *p* = .0001) and esophagitis (8% vs. 53%; *p* = .0001) are less severe in patients with cervical anastomosis. Although 86% of patients experienced excellent or very good late functional results, only 6% of patients who underwent cervical anastomosis had a Visick score of 3 or 4 versus 23% in patients with an intrathoracic anastomosis. Long-term function and quality of life assessment following esophagectomy identifies cervical anastomosis as a predictor of reduced reflux symptoms (92).

Considerations of resection of the primary tumor and particulars of reconstruction lead most surgeons to perform a thoracic esophagectomy with cervical or high intrathoracic anastomosis for thoracic esophageal cancers and cancers of the esophagogastric junction. For true gastric tumors invading the esophagus, distal esophagectomy and total gastrectomy may produce the best results (93,94). Squamous cell cancers of the cervical esophagus are generally unresectable because of location, but pharyngolaryngoesophagectomy may be considered in select patients. Alternatively, a limited resection with jejunal replacement may be used.

Regional Lymph Nodes

At least 12 regional lymph nodes must be included in the resection specimen and examined microscopically to accurately determine pN status of an esophageal cancer (95). This mandates vigorous sampling of regional lymph nodes or lymphadenectomy (Fig. 14.6). Lymphadenectomy may provide more regional lymph nodes but requires thoracotomy. It is of questionable benefit.

Although extensive lymphadenectomy has been abandoned during resection of most other cancers, its value in esophageal cancer is still debated. There are essentially two options: two-field—abdominal and thoracic—lymphadenectomy and three-field—abdominal, thoracic, and cervical—lymphadenectomy. Cervical exploration is, in essence, a dissection of lymph nodes around the recurrent laryngeal nerves. Proponents of three-field lymphadenectomy report an incidence of metastases to recurrent laryngeal lymph nodes of approximately 30%, even in patients with tumors of the distal esophagus and esophagogastric junction. The addition of a three-field lymphadenectomy upstages 24% of surgical candidates (96).

Survival advantage of three-field lymphadenectomy is not conclusive. A nationwide survey in Japan reports an improved 5-year survival with three-field lymphadenectomy for both N0, (57% vs. 45%) and N1 (33% vs. 29%) cancers (97). Why patients with N0 disease benefit from this procedure is unknown. Two randomized trials, both with selective admission criteria, reported conflicting survival results with three-field lymphadenectomy (98,99). Analyses of multiple reports suggest patients with superficial esophageal cancer or advanced stage cancer (indicated by lymph node metastases in all three fields, more than five lymph node metastases, or lower esophageal cancer with cervical lymph node metastases) may not benefit from three-field lymphadenectomy.

Three-field lymphadenectomy can be perilous. Recurrent laryngeal palsy is reported in as many as 70% of patients (100). In a randomized trial of lymphadenectomy, three-field lymphadenectomy was associated with an increased incidence of phrenic nerve paralysis (13% vs. 0%; $p < .001$) and tracheostomy (53% vs. 10%; $p < .001$) (98). Despite these obvious pulmonary complications, some authors report a similar incidence of pulmonary complications in patients undergoing three-field or two-field lymphadenectomy (19% vs. 17%). Pulmonary complications in the range of at least 30% are reported in most series. Quality of life is severely reduced in patients undergoing three-field lymphadenectomy who experience vocal cord paralysis (101). A significant decrease in vital capacity persists for 3 years following esophagectomy. Ideal body weight is decreased for periods up to 5 years. Decreased performance status and difficulty talking persist in these patients for more than 5 years.

Although practiced commonly in East Asia, three-field lymphadenectomy is rarely used in North America. Most patients in North America have adenocarcinoma of the distal esophagus or esophagogastric junction. Cervical lymph node metastases in these patients are stage IVA (M1a), uncommon in the absence of abdominal or thoracic metastases and usually a marker for other distant metastases. Morbidity and potential mortality from increased pulmonary complications are prohibitive factors in these patients. Cervical recurrence in these patients accounts for 6% of recurrent cancer, suggesting three-field lymphadenectomy unnecessary in the majority of patients in the Western Hemisphere (102).

Reconstruction

The ideal esophageal substitute connects the esophagus to stomach and replicates esophageal function. The stomach, however, is not an esophageal substitute. The esophagus shortened by resection maintains the upper sphincter and an abbreviated but peristaltic esophageal body. Advancing the stomach bridges the gap between the proximal esophagus and stomach. The stomach is freed from its abdominal attachments by dividing the short gastric and left gastric vasculature. The stomach, based on the right gastroepiploic and right gastric arteries, is anastomosed to the esophagus. This represents reconstruction of the gastrointestinal tract and not esophageal replacement. Problems with this reconstruction stem from lack of a physiologic lower esophageal sphincter and a denervated intrathoracic stomach. The stomach may, indeed, lose its reservoir function. These difficulties may be overcome by surgical anastomotic technique, constructing the anastomosis high in the chest or neck and draining the stomach with either a pyloroplasty or pyloromyotomy (103). A change in eating habits, diet modification, and the use of acid suppression and prokinetic medication (104,105) may be useful in dealing with postoperative problems of gastric reconstruction. Use of stomach may result in difficulty with the distal resection margin and completeness of regional and nonregional lymphadenectomy (106). Excessive gastric resection and denervation may limit the reservoir function of the stomach. A side-to-side anastomosis that uses endostapling technology has reduced anastomotic complications (107,108) (Fig. 14.16).

The colon was the first organ used for esophageal replacement. Only recently have long-term results become known. Advantages of colon replacement are few. Adequate length of colon is usually available. Blood supply, although less reliable than for the stomach, is easily assessed and generally adequate. Disadvantages of colon replacement are multiple. Preoperative evaluation and preparation of the colon are more demanding than evaluation or preparation of either the stomach or jejunum because of frequent intrinsic colonic disease and abundant bacterial colonization of the colon. Colon replacement is a more complex operation than either gastric or simple jejunal replacement. Three anastomoses are mandatory to reestablish gastrointestinal continuity in colon and jejunal replacements; only one anastomosis is required in gastric substitution. Early complication of colonic graft necrosis is uniformly lethal if not recognized early and treated by excision of the colon replacement. There is a propensity to late complications, a result of limited acid resistance of the colonic mucosa, and tendency of the colon replacement to dilate and form redundant loops. In the largest series with long-term follow-up of 69 patients with long segment colon interpositions, 10% required anastomotic revision and 25% developed significant colonic redundancy (109).

The colon should be considered for esophageal replacement only in patients in whom the stomach is not available and who have potential for long-term survival with an otherwise functional gastrointestinal tract. The segment of colon used (i.e., right, transverse, or left) and the direction of replacement (i.e., isoperistaltic or antiperistaltic) are determined by the state of the colon and the surgeon's preference and experience.

Jejunum is the replacement of choice following distal esophagectomy and total gastrectomy. The reconstruction may be done as a simple loop with an end-to-side esophagojejunal anastomosis. To protect the esophagus from duodenal reflux, it is best to perform this reconstruction using a Roux-en-Y technique. If the stomach and colon are not available for esophageal reconstruction, then jejunum by default becomes the organ of choice. Mesenteric and not jejunal length is limiting in esophageal reconstruction. The

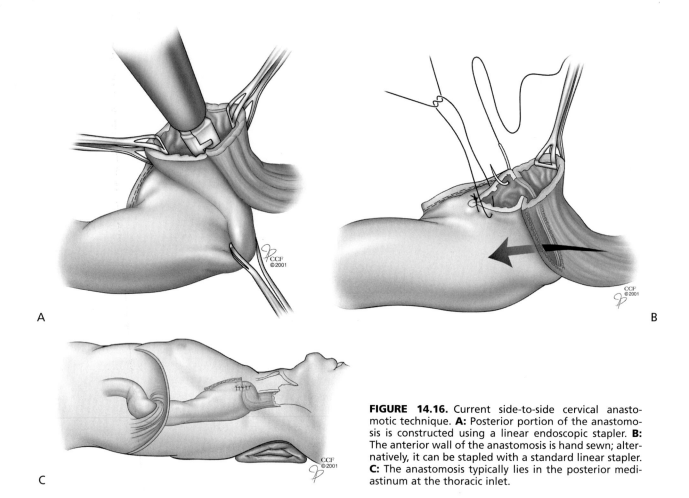

FIGURE 14.16. Current side-to-side cervical anastomotic technique. **A:** Posterior portion of the anastomosis is constructed using a linear endoscopic stapler. **B:** The anterior wall of the anastomosis is hand sewn; alternatively, it can be stapled with a standard linear stapler. **C:** The anastomosis typically lies in the posterior mediastinum at the thoracic inlet.

arc of jejunum is based on a radiating arcade of mesenteric vessels, much like a parachute canopy (jejunum) and shrouds (vessels) (110). Dividing limbs of the vascular arcade may open the semicircular architecture of the vascular arcade. However, this makes the vasculature dependent on the distal limb of the artery and vein, eliminating the multiple channels of the arcade. In excess, this renders the blood supply inadequate, necessitating "supercharging" of the arterial supply and venous drainage with a microvascular anastomosis of the distal jejunal vessels to native vessels at the proximal anastomotic site (111,112). Alternatively, if an adequate length of vascular arcade is chosen, a redundant jejunal reconstruction results, necessitating jejunal resection, with preservation of the arcade in the midportion of the jejunal loop (113).

Route

The route of reconstruction can be posterior mediastinal in the bed of the esophagus, transpleural either anterior or posterior to the pulmonary hilum, substernal, or subcutaneous (Fig. 14.17). The bed of the esophagus is the preferred route. It is the shortest and most direct route (114)

and minimizes angulation of the anastomosis between the esophagus and organ of reconstruction. The thoracic inlet is sufficiently large to accommodate the stomach and colon. It is reported to have a lower incidence of cardiopulmonary and anastomotic complications (115). However, it may not be available because of incomplete (R1 or R2) resection, previous inflammation, or scarring (116).

The substernal route is used when the posterior mediastinum is not available or when postoperative palliative radiation of the esophageal bed is required. This route usually requires excision of a portion of the manubrium, clavicular head, and first rib to prevent vascular compromise of the organ of reconstruction. Previous or planned anterior mediastinal or cardiac surgery may preclude its use. Transpleural and subcutaneous routes of reconstruction are rarely used and only as alternatives if the two principal routes are not available or acceptable.

Approach

Two options exist for open surgery: with thoracotomy (transthoracic) or without (transhiatal) (Fig. 14.18). This presents considerable surgical philosophic controversy:

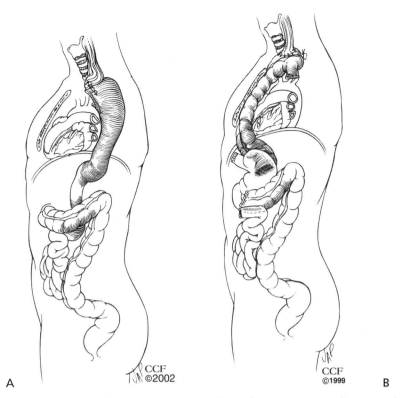

FIGURE 14.17. The routes of reconstruction typically used are posterior mediastinum, depicted here as stomach is placed in the bed of the resected esophagus **(A)**, and substernal, depicted here as the colon is placed in the retrosternal tunnel **(B)**.

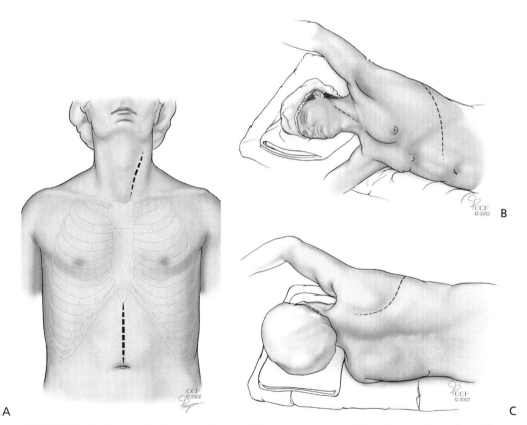

FIGURE 14.18. The surgical approaches are **(A)** esophagectomy without thoracotomy (transhiatal)—a midline laparotomy, and left cervical incisions are used; **(B)** esophagectomy with thoracotomy—thoracoabdominal alone requires a low intra-thoracic anastomosis or with simultaneous cervical incision; or **(C)** right thoracotomy—with laparotomy Ivor-Lewis esophagectomy, with laparotomy and cervical incision McKeown esophagectomy.

should extensive (transthoracic) resection be used to improve long-term survival or should resection be curtailed (transhiatal) to reduce early mortality and morbidity? Thoracotomy allows controlled *en bloc* excision of thoracic esophageal cancers and an intrathoracic lymphadenectomy. Ivor-Lewis (laparotomy and right thoracotomy) or McKeown (laparotomy, right thoracotomy, and cervical incision) approaches are necessary to perform a complete thoracic lymphadenectomy. A left thoracotomy with division of the diaphragm, separate abdominal incision, or as part of a left thoracoabdominal incision, allows excellent exposure of the distal thoracic esophagus and esophagogastric junction. It does, however, limit lymphadenectomy distal to the aortic arch and makes an intrathoracic anastomosis necessary unless a cervical incision is added. A transhiatal esophagectomy requires only an abdominal and thoracic incision. The thoracic esophagus is bluntly dissected through the esophageal hiatus and the cervical incision. This does not permit *en bloc* excision of the cancer or thoracic lymphadenectomy, but a thoracotomy is avoided. Metaanalysis of 24 reports comparing transthoracic and transhiatal esophagectomies shows an increase in pulmonary complications and postoperative mortality with transthoracic esophagectomy. Long-term survival is similar regardless of approach (117). A randomized study of transhiatal esophagectomy and esophagectomy with thoracotomy demonstrated similar hospital mortality and survival (overall, disease-free, and quality adjusted) (118). Operative morbidity was less with a transhiatal approach. However, in patients with superficial esophageal cancer and in whom long-term prognosis is excellent and less dependent on cancer stage, a transhiatal approach is associated with improved survival (56).

Details of minimally invasive esophagectomy are presently being investigated. Although technically feasible, the question of completeness of resection plagues this procedure. There has been no reduction in operative mortality and morbidity with this approach (119). Without an early survival advantage, it will be difficult to impart a survival advantage compared to open surgery. Port site recurrence and intracavitary tumor dissemination with pneumoperitoneum are new problems introduced by this approach (103,120–122).

Results

Morbidity

Complications are common following esophagectomy. In a multiinstitutional study of induction chemoradiotherapy versus surgery, Kelsen and colleagues (123) reported major complications in 26% and minor complications in 31% of 217 patients undergoing surgery alone. Walsh and co-workers (124) reported 50 different complications in 55

patients undergoing resection of esophageal adenocarcinoma. Complications occur during three distinct intervals: intraoperative, postoperative, and late.

Important intraoperative complications include hemorrhage, tracheobronchial injury, hypotension, and arrhythmias. Postoperative complications are dominated by pulmonary morbidity. However, anastomotic leakage, gastric or colonic necrosis, chylothorax, and recurrent laryngeal nerve injury are significant problems that impact outcome. Anastomotic leakage rates as high as 41% have been reported (125). Although an anastomotic leak may be twice as common following cervical anastomosis than intrathoracic anastomosis, mortality is three times greater following an intrathoracic leak (126). Necrosis of the organ of esophageal reconstruction occurs in about 2% of gastric replacements and 10% of colon replacements and is fatal in 90% (127). Chylothorax is infrequent, occurring in less than 1% of patients but carries a 50% mortality (125). Prompt recognition and early surgical intervention with intrathoracic ligation of the thoracic duct are critical to good outcome (128). Limiting the extent of cervical dissection and attention and care during cervical dissection can reduce the incidence of recurrent laryngeal nerve injury. The impact of this single complication on early and long-term outcome is enormous.

Late complications are dominated by gastrointestinal tract dysfunction. Anastomotic stricture occurs in 10% to 15% of patients and is successfully treated with dilation (129,130). An anastomotic leak is the most reliable predictor of an anastomotic stricture. Dumping, delayed gastric emptying, and reflux can be minimized by careful surgical technique. Gastrointestinal dysfunction can be managed successfully with dietary and lifestyle modifications and judicious use of acid suppression and prokinetic medications.

Mortality

Postoperative mortality has decreased to a single digit level; most specialty centers have mortality rates less than 5%. Short-term outcome is greatly improved as volume (131–135) (measured by number of esophagectomies, number of operations, and hospital size) and surgeon's experience increase (136,137). Increasing volume and experience also decrease stays in both the intensive care unit and hospital.

Long-term outcome is a function of stage and completeness of resection. A recent survey of 828 hospitals performing 5,044 esophagectomies for cancer from 1994 to 1995 report 1-year survival rates of 71% for stage I, 57% for stage II, 41% for stage III, and 18% for stage IV (138). More than half these patients received adjuvant therapy. For patients receiving surgery alone, survival is stage dependent (Fig. 14.19).

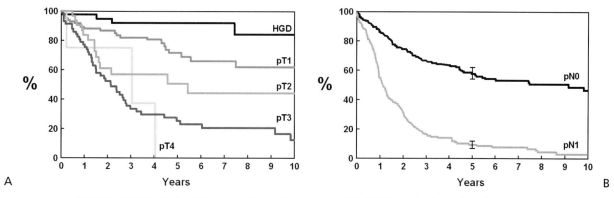

FIGURE 14.19. Kaplan-Meier survival estimates for 252 N0M0 patients undergoing surgery alone stratified by pT **(A)** and for 395 patients undergoing surgery alone stratified by pN **(B)** .

Recurrence

Following transhiatal esophagectomy used indiscriminately and without staging selection, approximately half the patients developed recurrent cancer during follow-up (median 24 to 27 months) (139,140). Median time to recurrence was 11 months (139,140); most were detected by 2 years (139). The prevalence of recurrent carcinoma was similar for adenocarcinoma and squamous cell carcinoma. Recurrences were nearly equal in distribution among locoregional, distant, or both. Cervical lymph node recurrence was seen in only 8% of all patients (140). Distant recurrences were found in the liver in 38%, in the bone in 25%, and in the lung in 18%. Recurrent carcinomas were associated with lymph node metastases, R1 resection, and poorly differentiated histology.

Data for recurrent cancer following two-field lymphadenectomy is remarkably similar. Forty-eight percent of patients, followed up for a mean of 26 months, experienced recurrent cancer (102). Median time to recurrence was 12 months. There were no differences between adenocarcinoma and squamous cell carcinoma. Recurrent carcinoma was locoregional in 27% and distant in 18%.

Quality of Life

Quality of life deteriorates immediately following esophagectomy but improves over time. Six weeks after surgery, patients reported a lessened quality of life compared to that before surgery (141). In patients who survive more than 2 years, quality of life returns to preoperative level by 9 months. For patients surviving less than 2 years, quality of life never returns to preoperative levels. There is a direct relationship between improved quality of life and increased survival (142). As expected, sense of well-being is greater in patients with curative surgery.

Patients undergoing palliative esophagectomy reported an improvement in diet (measured by type and quantity of food eaten) and reduction of diet-related symptoms. This benefit is sometimes offset by a significant problem with pain (143). Quality of life scores are significantly lower in these patients 6 to 9 months after esophagectomy than in patients with curative resections. Younger age, female gender, and intrathoracic anastomosis are all associated with decreased quality of life (92). The negative impact of recurrent nerve paralysis is profound and long lasting (101,144). The effects of patient education along with support of other patients on the improvement of quality of life are incalculable (145).

Compared to radiation, esophagectomy is twice as likely to improve swallowing and offers a survival advantage (146). Although surgery is more costly than palliation, cost per month of survival are similar for both modalities (147).

Adjuvant Therapy

Three randomized phase III trials comparing induction chemotherapy with cisplatin and fluorouracil and surgery versus surgery alone for esophageal cancer (Table 14.4) produced conflicting results. Law and colleagues (148) reported chemotherapy was safe, resulting in significant downstaging (5% complete response, 36% partial response) and increased curative resections (67% versus 35%) in patients with squamous cell carcinoma. Although survival of responders (median, 42.2 months) was superior to the surgical group (median, 13.8 months), there were no survival differences between the randomized treatment groups. Kelsen and colleagues (123) reported that chemotherapy and surgery did not improve survival, resectability, or local control. There were no differences between patients with squamous cell carcinoma or with adenocarcinoma (123). Weight loss was a predictor of poor outcome. The Medical Research Council of England conducted a trial randomizing 802 patients with resectable esophageal cancer (149). Patients receiving induction chemotherapy had an estimated 21% reduction in the risk of death. Median and 2-year survival was better in patients receiving chemotherapy and surgery versus surgery alone, 512 days versus 405 days,

TABLE 14.4. PHASE III TREATMENT TRIALS FOR ESOPHAGEAL CARCINOMA

Author	Cell Type	Rx 1	Rx 2	Survival	Positive Findings
Law et al. (148)	Squ	Surg	Che/Surg	Same	↑ Downstage, Rx 2 ↑ Curative resection, Rx 2
Kelsen et al. (123)	Both	Surg	Che/Surg	Same	
MRC (149)	Both	Surg	Che/Surg	43% vs. 34% (2 years)	↓ T and N Rx 2
Walsh et al. (124)	Adeno	Surg	Che/Rad/Surg	6% vs. 32% (3 years)	↓ N1 and M1, Rx 2
Bosset et al. (150)	Squ	Surg	Che/Rad/Surg	Same	↑ DF survival, Rx 2 ↑ Curative resection, Rx 2
Urba et al. (151)	Both	Surg	Che/Rad/Surg	Same	↑ survival in responders
Ando et al. (152)	Squ	Surg	Surg/Che	Same	
Xiao (153)	Squ	Surg	Surg/Rad	Same	IIA and III, Rx 2

Adeno, adenocarcinoma; Che, chemotherapy; Rad, radiation therapy; Squ, squamous cell carcinoma; Surg, surgery; Rx 1, control treatment; Rx 2, adjuvant treatment; DF, disease-free.

and 43% versus 34%, respectively. This was accomplished without additional adverse events. It is not known whether this survival advantage persists long term.

Three randomized phase III trials compared induction chemoradiotherapy and surgery versus surgery alone for esophageal cancer (Table 14.4). Walsh and colleagues reported patients with adenocarcinoma of the esophagus who received induction chemoradiotherapy (two courses of cisplatin and fluorouracil and 40 Gy of radiation) followed by surgery had an improved survival compared with those who had surgery alone (124). Survival advantage was evident at 3 years (32% versus 6%; *p* = .01). Of patients receiving multimodality therapy, 42% had lymph node or distant metastases at surgery, in contrast to 82% of patients treated with surgery alone who had lymph node or distant metastases. The survival of patients treated with surgery only is much worse than expected from previous experience. Bosset and colleagues (150) treated patients with squamous cell carcinoma of the esophagus with induction chemoradiotherapy (cisplatin and 18.5 Gy) plus surgery and with surgery alone. Although there were no survival differences between the groups, patients receiving induction chemoradiotherapy had longer disease-free survival, longer local disease-free interval, lower rate of cancer-related deaths, and higher rate of curative resections. Multimodality therapy was associated with an increased postoperative mortality. Predictors of reduced survival were weight loss greater than 5% of body weight, tumors located within 25 cm of the mandibular arch, N1 disease, and an incomplete resection. Urba and colleagues (151) did a randomized study of induction chemoradiotherapy using cisplatin, 5-fluorouracil and vinblastine, and 45 Gy of radiotherapy. No survival differences were apparent after a median of 8.2 years of follow-up.

Postoperative adjuvant chemotherapy with cisplatin and vindesine offers no survival advantage over surgery alone in patients with squamous cell carcinoma (152) (Table 14.4). Survival was similar even with stratification of N1 disease. The site of cancer recurrence was similar for both groups. A randomized study of postoperative adjuvant radiotherapy performed in China without patient consent demonstrated no survival advantage for the entire study group as a whole (153). However, in patients with stage IIB and III cancer, a survival improvement was gained with adjuvant radiotherapy.

In all these phase III studies, adjuvant therapy was offered regardless of stage. The conflicting results of these studies are in part the result of nonselective adjuvant therapy.

CLEVELAND CLINIC TREATMENT STRATEGY

A single-treatment strategy for all patients with the spectrum of locoregionally contained esophageal carcinoma is outdated (154,155). A tailored, stage-dependent treatment of esophageal cancer is now possible with detection of cancer at an earlier stage by Barrett's surveillance, accurate clinical staging, advanced surgical techniques, and developments of new treatments. Since esophagectomy

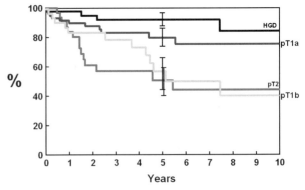

FIGURE 14.20. Kaplan-Meier survival estimates for N0M0 patients with tumor invasion confined to the esophageal wall. HGD is high-grade dysplasia, T1a is intramucosal cancer, T1b is submucosal cancer. (From Rice TW, Blackstone EH, Rybicki LA, et al. Refining esophageal cancer staging. *J Thorac Cardiovasc Surg* 2003;125:1103–1113.)

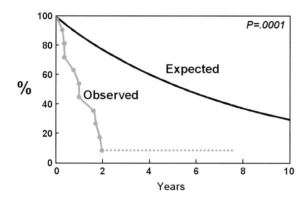

FIGURE 14.21. Observed and expected survival in patients with cT1N0 and cT2N0 carcinoma receiving induction therapy. (From Rice TW, Blackstone EH, Adelstein D, et al. Role of clinically determined depth of tumor invasion in the treatment of esophageal carcinoma. *J Thorac Cardiovasc Surg* 2003;125: 1091–1102, with permission.)

should be offered in the appropriate patient and done only with curative intent, treatment modifications according to stage are mandatory. One operation for all patients is an obsolete philosophy. It denies individual patients the benefits of personalized procedures and exposes them to unnecessary risk. The optimum operation should be chosen only after investigating both the patient and the tumor.

At one end of the cancer spectrum is high-grade dysplasia and intramucosal cancers. Surgery alone offers excellent survival (56) (Fig. 14.20). Regional lymph node metastases do not occur in patients with high-grade dysplasia and are uncommon (<5%) in patients with intramucosal cancer (156). Radical lymphadenectomy, therefore, is not required. In these patients, transhiatal esophagectomy minimizes morbidity and mortality and should be considered if

the tumor can be completely resected through the esophageal hiatus and lymph nodes sampled (56). For these patients, the toxicity of adjuvant therapy outweighs any small survival advantage (13) (Fig. 14.21).

At the opposite end of the cancer spectrum are marginally operable tumors because of either bulky T3 or T4 disease or significant regional lymph node metastases (Fig. 14.19). An incomplete resection (R1 and R2) is likely if surgery is the only treatment option. Surgery alone offers little hope of cure. Induction therapy downstages one third of these patients and subsequent resection offers responders an intermediate survival (157) (Fig. 14.22). Downstaging may also improve resectability. Survival advantage in responders far outweighs the toxicity of treatment. Nonresponders derive no benefit from therapy, however, presently these patients are difficult to identify preoperatively. In nonresponders, identified after induction therapy, surgery might be avoided and the best choice of palliation offered. In the future, preoperative identification of likely responders will further refine this approach.

Esophageal cancers that lie between these two ends of the spectrum affect many patients who have intermediate survival after surgery alone (Figs. 14.19 and 14.20). Once esophageal cancers have invaded the submucosa (T1b) or muscularis propria (T2), esophagectomy with thoracotomy is the procedure of choice for patients clinically staged as T1bN0M0 and T2N0M0. This approach facilitates the resection of these larger tumors and allows lymphadenectomy. The incidence of regional lymph node metastases increases exponentially with increasing depth of tumor invasion, with at least 25% of T1b tumors and 50% of T2 tumors metastasizing to regional lymph nodes (N1) (156). Because EUS accuracy in the determination of N is 80%, lymphadenectomy is mandatory to detect clinically occult N1 disease. The goal of lymphadenec-

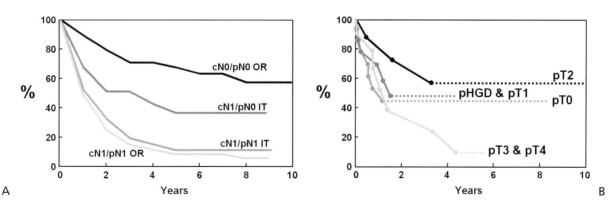

FIGURE 14.22. The effect of induction therapy. **A:** Downstaging (cN1/pN0 IT) produces an intermediate survival compared to pN0 and pN1 patients undergoing surgery alone. Failure to downstage (cN1/pN1 IT) produces similar survival to pN1 patients undergoing surgery alone. **B:** For cN1/pN0 patients, inability to achieve synchronous downstaging (pT3 and pT4) fails to impact survival. Synchronous downstaging of T and N homogenizes survival. (From Rice TW, Blackstone EH, Adelstein DJ, et al. N1 esophageal carcinoma: the importance of staging and downstaging. *J Thorac Cardiovasc Surg* 2001;121:454–464, with permission.)

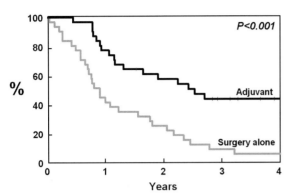

FIGURE 14.23. Survival in matched patients undergoing either surgery followed by adjuvant therapy or surgery alone. For surgery followed by adjuvant therapy, survival estimates, their standard error, and, in parentheses, number of patients remaining at risk at 1, 2, 3, and 4 years were 77 ± 7.5% (24), 58 ± 8.9% (17), 44 ± 9.0% (10), and 44 ± 9.0% (6), respectively. For surgery alone, these same statistics were 42 ± 8.9% (13), 26 ± 7.9% (8), 9.7 ± 5.3% (3), and 6.4 ± 4.4% (2), respectively. (From Rice TW, Adelstein DJ, Chidel MA, et al. Benefit of postoperative adjuvant chemotherapy in locoregionally advanced esophageal carcinoma. *J Thorac Cardiovasc Surg* [*in press*], with permission.)

tomy is accurate pathologic staging; its impact on survival is controversial.

Resection followed by postoperative adjuvant therapy may be considered in the following clinical situations: (a) patients with incorrect clinical staging who have resection and are found to have more advanced disease (T3 or N1 or M1a); (b) patients with T3 or N1 cancers (few regional nodal metastases) who appear technically resectable (R0 resection possible) and are not candidates for induction therapy; and (c) patients with deep submucosal invasion (T1bN0M0) or invasion into the muscularis propria (T2N0M0) without regional nodal metastases. In a propensity-matched study, postoperative adjuvant chemoradiotherapy improved survival in patients with locally advanced esophageal cancer (158) (Fig. 14.23).

SUMMARY

Diagnosis and clinical staging of esophageal carcinoma is afforded by the combination of esophagoscopy and biopsy, EUS FNA, and CT and FDG PET scanning. Patient selection and preparation are critical to minimizing operative morbidity and mortality. Surgery is the mainstay of curative therapy for esophageal carcinoma. Outcome in early stage disease is impacted by surgical approach. In locally advanced cancer, the effect of stage overshadows operative approach. Surgery alone is unlikely to cure patients with locally advanced esophageal cancer. Unfortunately, randomized studies of adjuvant therapy report conflicting results with all modalities and regimens. Regardless, multimodality therapy should be

considered for select patients with locally advanced esophageal cancer.

REFERENCES

1. Levine MS, Chu P, Furth EE, et al. Carcinoma of the esophagus and esophagogastric junction: sensitivity of radiographic diagnosis. *Am J Roentgenol* 1997;168:1423–1426.
2. Faigel DO, Deveney C, Phillips D, et al. Biopsy-negative malignant esophageal stricture: diagnosis by endoscopic ultrasound. *Am J Gastroenterol* 1998;93:2257–2260.
3. Provenzale D, Schmitt C, Wong JB. Barrett's esophagus: a new look at surveillance based on emerging estimates of cancer risk. *Am J Gastroenterol* 1999;94:2043–2053.
4. Streitz JM Jr, Ellis FH Jr, Tilden RL, et al. Endoscopic surveillance of Barrett's esophagus: a cost-effectiveness comparison with mammographic surveillance for breast cancer. *Am J Gastroenterol* 1998;93:911–915.
5. Esophagus. In: Greene FL, ed. *AJCC Cancer Staging Manual*, sixth ed. Philadelphia: Lippincott Williams & Wilkins, 2002:91–98.
6. Rice TW, Blackstone EH, Rybicki LA, et al. Refining esophageal cancer staging. *J Thorac Cardiovasc Surg* 2003;125: 1103–1113.
7. Roder JD, Busch R, Stein HJ, et al. Ratio of invaded to removed lymph nodes as a predictor of survival in squamous cell carcinoma of the oesophagus. *Br J Surg* 1994;81:410–413.
8. Holscher AH, Bollschweiler E, Bumm R, et al. Prognostic factors of resected adenocarcinoma of the esophagus. *Surgery* 1995; 118:845–855.
9. Korst RJ, Rusch VW, Venkatraman E, et al. Proposed revision of the staging classification for esophageal cancer. *J Thorac Cardiovasc Surg* 1998;115:660–669; discussion 669–670.
10. Christie NA, Rice TW, DeCamp MM, et al. M1a/M1b esophageal carcinoma: clinical relevance. *J Thorac Cardiovasc Surg* 1999;118:900–907.
11. Rosch T. Endosonographic staging of esophageal cancer: a review of literature results. *Gastrointest Endosc Clin North Am* 1995;5:537–547.
12. Saunders HS, Wolfman NT, Ott DJ. Esophageal cancer. Radiologic staging. *Radiol Clin North Am* 1997;35:281–294.
13. Rice TW, Blackstone EH, Adelstein DJ, et al. Role of clinically determined depth of tumor invasion in the treatment of esophageal carcinoma. *J Thorac Cardiovasc Surg* 2003;125: 1091–1102.
14. Heidemann J, Schilling MK, Schmassmann A, et al. Accuracy of endoscopic ultrasonography in preoperative staging of esophageal carcinoma. *Dig Surg* 2000;17:219–224.
15. Kelly S, Harris KM, Berry E, et al. A systematic review of the staging performance of endoscopic ultrasound in gastro-oesophageal carcinoma. *Gut* 2001;49:534–539.
16. Van Dam J, Rice TW, Catalano MF, et al. High-grade malignant stricture is predictive of esophageal tumor stage. Risks of endosonographic evaluation. *Cancer* 1993;71:2910–2917.
17. Pfau PR, Ginsberg GG, Lew RJ, et al. Esophageal dilation for endosonographic evaluation of malignant esophageal strictures is safe and effective. *Am J Gastroenterol* 2000;95:2813–2815.
18. Bhutani MS, Barde CJ, Markert RJ, et al. Length of esophageal cancer and degree of luminal stenosis during upper endoscopy predict T stage by endoscopic ultrasound. *Endoscopy* 2002;34: 461–463.
19. Flanagan FL, Dehdashti F, Siegel BA, et al. Staging of esophageal cancer with 18F-fluorodeoxyglucose positron emission tomography. *Am J Roentgenol* 1997;168:417–424.

20. Rankin SC, Taylor H, Cook GJ, et al. Computed tomography and positron emission tomography in the pre-operative staging of oesophageal carcinoma. *Clin Radiol* 1998;53:659–665.

21. Krasna MJ. Minimally invasive staging for esophageal cancer. *Chest* 1997;112:191S–194S.

22. Buenaventura P, Luketich JD. Surgical staging of esophageal cancer. *Chest Surg Clin North Am* 2000;10:487–497.

23. Krasna MJ, Mao YS, Sonett J, et al. The role of thoracoscopic staging of esophageal cancer patients. *Eur J Cardiothorac Surg* 1999;16[Suppl 1]:S31–S33.

24. Catalano MF, Sivak MV Jr, Rice T, et al. Endosonographic features predictive of lymph node metastasis. *Gastrointest Endosc* 1994;40:442–446.

25. Wiersema MJ, Vilmann P, Giovannini M, et al. Endosonography-guided fine-needle aspiration biopsy: diagnostic accuracy and complication assessment. *Gastroenterology* 1997;112: 1087–1095.

26. Reed CE, Mishra G, Sahai AV, et al. Esophageal cancer staging: improved accuracy by endoscopic ultrasound of celiac lymph nodes. *Ann Thorac Surg* 1999;67:319–321; discussion 322.

27. Eloubeidi MA, Wallace MB, Reed CE, et al. The utility of EUS and EUS-guided fine needle aspiration in detecting celiac lymph node metastasis in patients with esophageal cancer: a single-center experience. *Gastrointest Endosc* 2001;54:714–719.

28. Natsugoe S, Yoshinaka H, Shimada M, et al. Assessment of cervical lymph node metastasis in esophageal carcinoma using ultrasonography. *Ann Surg* 1999;229:62–66.

29. Doldi SB, Lattuada E, Zappa MA, et al. Ultrasonographic evaluation of the cervical lymph nodes in preoperative staging of esophageal neoplasms. *Abdom Imaging* 1998;23:275–277.

30. van Overhagen H, Becker CD. Diagnosis and staging of carcinoma of the esophagus and gastroesophageal junction, and detection of postoperative recurrence, by computed tomography. In: Meyers M, ed. *Neoplasms of the digestive tract. Imaging, staging and management.* Philadelphia: Lippincott-Raven, 1998: 31–48.

31. Doi N, Aoyama N, Tokunaga M, et al. Possibility of pre-operative diagnosis of lymph node metastasis based on morphology. *Hepatogastroenterology* 1999;46:977–980.

32. Chandawarkar RY, Kakegawa T, Fujita H, et al. Comparative analysis of imaging modalities in the preoperative assessment of nodal metastasis in esophageal cancer. *J Surg Oncol* 1996;61: 214–217.

33. Kato H, Kuwano H, Nakajima M, et al. Comparison between positron emission tomography and computed tomography in the use of the assessment of esophageal carcinoma. *Cancer* 2002;94:921–928.

34. Block MI, Patterson GA, Sundaresan RS, et al. Improvement in staging of esophageal cancer with the addition of positron emission tomography. *Ann Thorac Surg* 1997;64:770–776; discussion 776–777.

35. Kole AC, Plukker JT, Nieweg OE, et al. Positron emission tomography for staging of oesophageal and gastroesophageal malignancy. *Br J Cancer* 1998;78:521–527.

36. Luketich JD, Schauer PR, Meltzer CC, et al. Role of positron emission tomography in staging esophageal cancer. *Ann Thorac Surg* 1997;64:765–769.

37. Lerut T, Flamen P, Ectors N, et al. Histopathologic validation of lymph node staging with FDG-PET scan in cancer of the esophagus and gastroesophageal junction: a prospective study based on primary surgery with extensive lymphadenectomy. *Ann Surg* 2000;232:743–752.

38. Luketich JD, Friedman DM, Weigel TL, et al. Evaluation of distant metastases in esophageal cancer: 100 consecutive positron emission tomography scans. *Ann Thorac Surg* 1999;68: 1133–1136; discussion 1136–1137.

39. Flamen P, Lerut A, Van Cutsem E, et al. The utility of positron emission tomography for the diagnosis and staging of recurrent esophageal cancer. *J Thorac Cardiovasc Surg* 2000;120: 1085–1092.

40. Jager PL, Que TH, Vaalburg W, et al. Carbon-11 choline or FDG-PET for staging of oesophageal cancer? *Eur J Nucl Med* 2001;28:1845–1849.

41. Kobori O, Kirihara Y, Kosaka N, et al. Positron emission tomography of esophageal carcinoma using (11)C-choline and (18)F-fluorodeoxyglucose: a novel method of preoperative lymph node staging. *Cancer* 1999;86:1638–1648.

42. Gilbert TB, Goodsell CW, Krasna MJ. Bronchial rupture by a double-lumen endobronchial tube during staging thoracoscopy. *Anesth Analg* 1999;88:1252–1253.

43. Freeman RK, Wait MA. Port site metastasis after laparoscopic staging of esophageal carcinoma. *Ann Thorac Surg* 2001;71: 1032–1034.

44. Luketich JD, Schauer P, Landreneau R, et al. Minimally invasive surgical staging is superior to endoscopic ultrasound in detecting lymph node metastases in esophageal cancer. *J Thorac Cardiovasc Surg* 1997;114:817–821; discussion 821–823.

45. Quint LE, Hepburn LM, Francis IR, et al. Incidence and distribution of distant metastases from newly diagnosed esophageal carcinoma. *Cancer* 1995;76:1120–1125.

46. Wernecke K, Rummeny E, Bongartz G, et al. Detection of hepatic masses in patients with carcinoma: comparative sensitivities of sonography, CT, and MR imaging. *Am J Roentgenol* 1991;157:731–739.

47. Valls C, Lopez E, Guma A, et al. Helical CT versus CT arterial portography in the detection of hepatic metastasis of colorectal carcinoma. *Am J Roentgenol* 1998;170:1341–1347.

48. Margolis ML, Howlett P, Bubanj R. Pulmonary nodules in patients with esophageal carcinoma. *J Clin Gastroenterol* 1998; 26:245–248.

49. Gabrielsen TO, Eldevik OP, Orringer MB, et al. Esophageal carcinoma metastatic to the brain: clinical value and cost-effectiveness of routine enhanced head CT before esophagectomy. *AJNR Am J Neuroradiol* 1995;16:1915–1921.

50. O'Brien MG, Fitzgerald EF, Lee G, et al. A prospective comparison of laparoscopy and imaging in the staging of esophagogastric cancer before surgery. *Am J Gastroenterol* 1995;90: 2191–2194.

51. Bonavina L, Incarbone R, Lattuada E, et al. Preoperative laparoscopy in management of patients with carcinoma of the esophagus and of the esophagogastric junction. *J Surg Oncol* 1997;65:171–174.

52. Heath EI, Kaufman HS, Talamini MA, et al. The role of laparoscopy in preoperative staging of esophageal cancer. *Surg Endosc* 2000;14:495–499.

53. Bemelman WA, van Delden OM, van Lanschot JJ, et al. Laparoscopy and laparoscopic ultrasonography in staging of carcinoma of the esophagus and gastric cardia. *J Am Coll Surg* 1995;181:421–425.

54. Romijn MG, van Overhagen H, Spillenaar Bilgen EJ, et al. Laparoscopy and laparoscopic ultrasonography in staging of oesophageal and cardial carcinoma. *Br J Surg* 1998;85: 1010–1012.

55. Bartels H, Stein HJ, Siewert JR. Risk analysis in esophageal surgery. *Recent Results Cancer Res* 2000;155:89–96.

56. Rice TW, Blackstone EH, Goldblum JR, et al. Superficial adenocarcinoma of the esophagus. *J Thorac Cardiovasc Surg* 2001; 122:1077–1090.

57. Amar D, Burt ME, Bains MS, et al. Symptomatic tachydysrhythmias after esophagectomy: incidence and outcome measures. *Ann Thorac Surg* 1996;61:1506–1509.

58. Alexiou C, Beggs D, Salama FD, et al. Surgery for esophageal

cancer in elderly patients: the view from Nottingham. *J Thorac Cardiovasc Surg* 1998;116:545–553.

59. Ellis FH Jr, Williamson WA, Heatley GJ. Cancer of the esophagus and cardia: does age influence treatment selection and surgical outcomes? *J Am Coll Surg* 1998;187:345–351.

60. Kinugasa S, Tachibana M, Yoshimura H, et al. Esophageal resection in elderly esophageal carcinoma patients: improvement in postoperative complications. *Ann Thorac Surg* 2001;71: 414–418.

61. Chino O, Makuuchi H, Machimura T, et al. Treatment of esophageal cancer in patients over 80 years old. *Surg Today* 1997;27:9–16.

62. Fontes PR, Nectoux M, Escobar AG, et al. Is age a risk factor for esophagectomy? *Int Surg* 2001;86:94–96.

63. Sabel MS, Smith JL, Nava HR, et al. Esophageal resection for carcinoma in patients older than 70 years. *Ann Surg Oncol* 2002;9:210–214.

64. Poon RT, Law SY, Chu KM, et al. Esophagectomy for carcinoma of the esophagus in the elderly: results of current surgical management. *Ann Surg* 1998;227:357–364.

65. Thomas P, Doddoli C, Neville P, et al. Esophageal cancer resection in the elderly. *Eur J Cardiothorac Surg* 1996;10:941–946.

66. Bollschweiler E, Schroder W, Holscher AH, et al. Preoperative risk analysis in patients with adenocarcinoma or squamous cell carcinoma of the oesophagus. *Br J Surg* 2000;87:1106–1110.

67. Ferguson MK, Durkin AE. Preoperative prediction of the risk of pulmonary complications after esophagectomy for cancer. *J Thorac Cardiovasc Surg* 2002;123:661–669.

68. Crozier TA, Sydow M, Siewert JR, et al. Postoperative pulmonary complication rate and long-term changes in respiratory function following esophagectomy with esophagogastrostomy. *Acta Anaesthesiol Scand* 1992;36:10–15.

69. Gillinov AM, Heitmiller RF. Strategies to reduce pulmonary complications after transhiatal esophagectomy. *Dis Esophagus* 1998;11:43–47.

70. Avendano CE, Flume PA, Silvestri GA, et al. Pulmonary complications after esophagectomy. *Ann Thorac Surg* 2002;73: 922–926.

71. Whooley BP, Law S, Murthy SC, et al. Analysis of reduced death and complication rates after esophageal resection. *Ann Surg* 2001;233:338–344.

72. Vaporciyan AA, Merriman KW, Ece F, et al. Incidence of major pulmonary morbidity after pneumonectomy: association with timing of smoking cessation. *Ann Thorac Surg* 2002;73: 420–425; discussion 425–426.

73. Nakagawa M, Tanaka H, Tsukuma H, et al. Relationship between the duration of the preoperative smoke-free period and the incidence of postoperative pulmonary complications after pulmonary surgery. *Chest* 2001;120:705–710.

74. Ritchie AJ, Whiteside M, Tolan M, et al. Cardiac dysrhythmia in total thoracic oesophagectomy. A prospective study. *Eur J Cardiothorac Surg* 1993;7:420–422.

75. Nagamatsu Y, Shima I, Yamana H, et al. Preoperative evaluation of cardiopulmonary reserve with the use of expired gas analysis during exercise testing in patients with squamous cell carcinoma of the thoracic esophagus. *J Thorac Cardiovasc Surg* 2001;121: 1064–1068.

76. Stein HJ, Brucher BL, Sendler A, et al. Esophageal cancer: patient evaluation and pre-treatment staging. *Surg Oncol* 2001; 10:103–111.

77. Naunheim KS, Hanosh J, Zwischenberger J, et al. Esophagectomy in the septuagenarian. *Ann Thorac Surg* 1993;56:880-3; discussion 883–884.

78. Bartels H, Stein HJ, Siewert JR. Preoperative risk analysis and postoperative mortality of oesophagectomy for resectable oesophageal cancer. *Br J Surg* 1998;85:840–844.

79. Tachibana M, Kotoh T, Kinugasa S, et al. Esophageal cancer with cirrhosis of the liver: results of esophagectomy in 18 consecutive patients. *Ann Surg Oncol* 2000;7:758–763.

80. Miller C. Carcinoma of thoracic oesophagus and cardia. A review of 405 cases. *Br J Surg* 1962;49:507–522.

81. Tam PC, Siu KF, Cheung HC, et al. Local recurrences after subtotal esophagectomy for squamous cell carcinoma. *Ann Surg* 1987;205:189–194.

82. Law S, Arcilla C, Chu KM, et al. The significance of histologically infiltrated resection margin after esophagectomy for esophageal cancer. *Am J Surg* 1998;176:286–290.

83. Casson AG, Darnton SJ, Subramanian S, et al. What is the optimal distal resection margin for esophageal carcinoma? *Ann Thorac Surg* 2000;69:205–209.

84. McManus K, Anikin V, McGuigan J. Total thoracic oesophagectomy for oesophageal carcinoma: has it been worth it? *Eur J Cardiothorac Surg* 1999;16:261–265.

85. Kuwano H, Masuda N, Kato H, et al. The subepithelial extension of esophageal carcinoma for determining the resection margin during esophagectomy: a serial histopathologic investigation. *Surgery* 2002;131:S14–S21.

86. Tsutsui S, Kuwano H, Watanabe M, et al. Resection margin for squamous cell carcinoma of the esophagus. *Ann Surg* 1995; 222:193–202.

87. Kato H, Tachimori Y, Watanabe H, et al. Anastomotic recurrence of oesophageal squamous cell carcinoma after transthoracic oesophagectomy. *Eur J Surg* 1998;164:759–764.

88. Dexter SP, Sue-Ling H, McMahon MJ, et al. Circumferential resection margin involvement: an independent predictor of survival following surgery for oesophageal cancer. *Gut* 2001;48: 667–670.

89. Kyriazanos ID, Tachibana M, Yoshimura H, et al. Impact of splenectomy on the early outcome after oesophagectomy for squamous cell carcinoma of the oesophagus. *Eur J Surg Oncol* 2002;28:113–119.

90. Jeyasingham K. Long-term results of colon replacement. In: Pearson FG, Cooper JD, Deslauriers J, et al, eds. *Esophageal surgery*, second ed. Philadelphia: Churchill Livingstone, 2002:931–937.

91. De Leyn P, Vansteenkiste J, Deneffe G, et al. Result of induction chemotherapy followed by surgery in patients with stage IIIA N2 NSCLC: importance of pre-treatment mediastinoscopy. *Eur J Cardiothorac Surg* 1999;15:608–614.

92. McLarty AJ, Deschamps C, Trastek VF, et al. Esophageal resection for cancer of the esophagus: long-term function and quality of life. *Ann Thorac Surg* 1997;63:1568–1572.

93. Siewert JR, Stein HJ. Adenocarcinoma of the gastroesophageal junction. Classification, pathology and extent of resection. *Dis Esophagus* 1996;9:173–182.

94. Stein HJ, Feith M, Siewert JR. Individualized surgical strategies for cancer of the esophagogastric junction. *Ann Chir Gynaecol* 2000;89:191–198.

95. Dutkowski P, Hommel G, Bottger T, et al. How many lymph nodes are needed for an accurate pN classification in esophageal cancer? Evidence for a new threshold value. *Hepatogastroenterology* 2002;49:176–180.

96. Altorki N, Lerut T. Three-field lymph node dissection for cancer of the esophagus. In: Pearson FG, Cooper JD, Deslauriers J, et al, eds. *Esophageal surgery*, second ed. Philadelphia: Churchill Livingstone, 2002:866–870.

97. Isono K, Sato H, Nakayama K. Results of a nationwide study on the three-field lymph node dissection of esophageal cancer. *Oncology* 1991;48:411–420.

98. Nishihira T, Hirayama K, Mori S. A prospective randomized trial of extended cervical and superior mediastinal lymphadenectomy for carcinoma of the thoracic esophagus. *Am J Surg* 1998;175:47–51.

99. Kato H, Watanabe H, Tachimori Y, et al. Evaluation of neck lymph node dissection for thoracic esophageal carcinoma. *Ann Thorac Surg* 1991;51:931–935.

100. Fujita H, Kakegawa T, Yamana H, et al. Mortality and morbidity rates, postoperative course, quality of life, and prognosis after extended radical lymphadenectomy for esophageal cancer. Comparison of three-field lymphadenectomy with two-field lymphadenectomy. *Ann Surg* 1995;222:654–662.

101. Baba M, Aikou T, Natsugoe S, et al. Quality of life following esophagectomy with three-field lymphadenectomy for carcinoma, focusing on its relationship to vocal cord palsy. *Dis Esophagus* 1998;11:28–34.

102. Dresner SM, Griffin SM. Pattern of recurrence following radical oesophagectomy with two-field lymphadenectomy. *Br J Surg* 2000;87:1426–1433.

103. Law S, Cheung MC, Fok M, et al. Pyloroplasty and pyloromyotomy in gastric replacement of the esophagus after esophagectomy: a randomized controlled trial. *J Am Coll Surg* 1997;184:630–636.

104. Gutschow CA, Collard JM, Romagnoli R, et al. Bile exposure of the denervated stomach as an esophageal substitute. *Ann Thorac Surg* 2001;71:1786–1791.

105. Nakabayashi T, Mochiki E, Garcia M, et al. Gastropyloric motor activity and the effects of erythromycin given orally after esophagectomy. *Am J Surg* 2002;183:317–323.

106. Schroder W, Baldus SE, Monig SP, et al. Lesser curvature lymph node metastases with esophageal squamous cell carcinoma: implications for gastroplasty. *World J Surg* 2001;25:1125–1128.

107. Singh D, Maley RH, Santucci T, et al. Experience and technique of stapled mechanical cervical esophagogastric anastomosis. *Ann Thorac Surg* 2001;71:419–424.

108. Orringer MB, Marshall B, Iannettoni MD. Eliminating the cervical esophagogastric anastomotic leak with a side-to-side stapled anastomosis. *J Thorac Cardiovasc Surg* 2000;119:277–288.

109. Jeyasingham K, Lerut T, Belsey RH. Revisional surgery after colon interposition for benign oesophageal disease. *Dis Esophagus* 1999;12:7–9.

110. Hiebert CA, Bredenberg CE. Selection and placement of conduits. In: Pearson FG, Cooper JD, Deslauriers J, et al, eds. *Esophageal surgery*, second ed. Philadelphia: Churchill Livingstone, 2002:794–801.

111. Fujita H, Yamana H, Sueyoshi S, et al. Impact on outcome of additional microvascular anastomosis—supercharge—on colon interposition for esophageal replacement: comparative and multivariate analysis. *World J Surg* 1997;21:998–1003.

112. Golshani SD, Lee C, Cass D, et al. Microvascular "supercharged" cervical colon: minimizing ischemia in esophageal reconstruction. *Ann Plast Surg* 1999;43:533–538.

113. Wong J. The use of small bowel for oesophageal replacement following oesophageal resection. In: Jamieson GG, ed. *Surgery of the oesophagus*. New York: Churchill Livingstone, 1988:749–760.

114. Maillard JN, Hay JM. Surgical anatomy of available routes for oesophageal bypass. In: Jamieson GG, ed. *Surgery of the oesophagus*. New York: Churchill Livingstone, 1988:721–726.

115. Urschel JD. Does the interponat affect outcome after esophagectomy for cancer? *Dis Esophagus* 2001;14:124–130.

116. DiPierro FV, Rice TW, DeCamp MM, et al. Esophagectomy and staged reconstruction. *Eur J Cardiothorac Surg* 2000;17:702–709.

117. Hulscher JB, Tijssen JG, Obertop H, et al. Transthoracic versus transhiatal resection for carcinoma of the esophagus: a meta-analysis. *Ann Thorac Surg* 2001;72:306–313.

118. Hulscher JB, van Sandick JW, de Boer AG, et al. Extended transthoracic resection compared with limited transhiatal resection for adenocarcinoma of the esophagus. *N Engl J Med* 2002;347:1662–1669.

119. Law S, Wong J. Use of minimally invasive oesophagectomy for cancer of the oesophagus. *Lancet Oncol* 2002;3:215–222.

120. Segalin A. Parietal seeding of esophageal cancer after thoracoscopic resection. *Dis Esophagus* 1994;7:64–65.

121. Dixit AS, Martin CJ, Flynn P. Port-site recurrence after thoracoscopic resection of oesophageal cancer. *Aust N Z J Surg* 1997;67:148–149.

122. Ziprin P, Ridgway PF, Peck DH, et al. The theories and realities of port-site metastases: a critical appraisal. *J Am Coll Surg* 2002;195:395–408.

123. Kelsen DP, Ginsberg R, Pajak TF, et al. Chemotherapy followed by surgery compared with surgery alone for localized esophageal cancer. *N Engl J Med* 1998;339:1979–1984.

124. Walsh TN, Noonan N, Hollywood D, et al. A comparison of multimodal therapy and surgery for esophageal adenocarcinoma. *N Engl J Med* 1996;335:462–467.

125. Bains MS. Complications of abdominal right-thoracic (Ivor Lewis) esophagectomy. *Chest Surg Clin North Am* 1997;7:587–598; discussion 598–599.

126. Muller JM, Erasmi H, Stelzner M, et al. Surgical therapy of oesophageal carcinoma. *Br J Surg* 1990;77:845–857.

127. Horvath OP, Lukacs L, Cseke L. Complications following esophageal surgery. *Recent Results Cancer Res* 2000;155:161–173.

128. Cerfolio RJ, Allen MS, Deschamps C, et al. Postoperative chylothorax. *J Thorac Cardiovasc Surg* 1996;112:1361–1365; discussion 1365–1366.

129. Gandhi SK, Naunheim KS. Complications of transhiatal esophagectomy. *Chest Surg Clin North Am* 1997;7:601–610; discussion 611–612.

130. Sherry KM. How can we improve the outcome of oesophagectomy? *Br J Anaesth* 2001;86:611–613.

131. Birkmeyer JD, Siewers AE, Finlayson EV, et al. Hospital volume and surgical mortality in the United States. *N Engl J Med* 2002;346:1128–1137.

132. Kuo EY, Chang Y, Wright CD. Impact of hospital volume on clinical and economic outcomes for esophagectomy. *Ann Thorac Surg* 2001;72:1118–1124.

133. Swisher SG, Deford L, Merriman KW, et al. Effect of operative volume on morbidity, mortality, and hospital use after esophagectomy for cancer. *J Thorac Cardiovasc Surg* 2000;119:1126–1132.

134. van Lanschot JJ, Hulscher JB, Buskens CJ, et al. Hospital volume and hospital mortality for esophagectomy. *Cancer* 2001;91:1574–1578.

135. Dimick JB, Pronovost PJ, Cowan JA, et al. Surgical volume and quality of care for esophageal resection: do high-volume hospitals have fewer complications? *Ann Thorac Surg* 2003;75:337–341.

136. Matthews HR, Powell DJ, McConkey CC. Effect of surgical experience on the results of resection for oesophageal carcinoma. *Br J Surg* 1986;73:621–623.

137. Miller JD, Jain MK, de Gara CJ, et al. Effect of surgical experience on results of esophagectomy for esophageal carcinoma. *J Surg Oncol* 1997;65:20–21.

138. Daly JM, Fry WA, Little AG, et al. Esophageal cancer: results of an American College of Surgeons Patient Care Evaluation Study. *J Am Coll Surg* 2000;190:562–572; discussion 572–573.

139. van Sandick JW, van Lanschot JJ, ten Kate FJ, et al. Indicators of prognosis after transhiatal esophageal resection without thoracotomy for cancer. *J Am Coll Surg* 2002;194:28–36.

140. Hulscher JB, van Sandick JW, Tijssen JG, et al. The recurrence pattern of esophageal carcinoma after transhiatal resection. *J Am Coll Surg* 2000;191:143–148.

141. Blazeby JM, Farndon JR, Donovan J, et al. A prospective longitudinal study examining the quality of life of patients with esophageal carcinoma. *Cancer* 2000;88:1781–1787.

142. Blazeby JM, Brookes ST, Alderson D. The prognostic value of quality of life scores during treatment for oesophageal cancer. *Gut* 2001;49:227–230.

143. Branicki FJ, Law SY, Fok M, et al. Quality of life in patients with cancer of the esophagus and gastric cardia: a case for palliative resection. *Arch Surg* 1998;133:316–322.

144. Baba M, Natsugoe S, Shimada M, et al. Does hoarseness of voice from recurrent nerve paralysis after esophagectomy for carcinoma influence patient quality of life? *J Am Coll Surg* 1999;188:231–236.

145. Kirby JD. Quality of life after oesophagectomy: the patients' perspective. *Dis Esophagus* 1999;12:168–171.

146. Badwe RA, Sharma V, Bhansali MS, et al. The quality of swallowing for patients with operable esophageal carcinoma: a randomized trial comparing surgery with radiotherapy. *Cancer* 1999;85:763–768.

147. Farndon MA, Wayman J, Clague MB, et al. Cost-effectiveness in the management of patients with oesophageal cancer. *Br J Surg* 1998;85:1394–1398.

148. Law S, Fok M, Chow S, et al. Preoperative chemotherapy versus surgical therapy alone for squamous cell carcinoma of the esophagus: a prospective randomized trial. *J Thorac Cardiovasc Surg* 1997;114:210–217.

149. Medical Research Council Oesophageal Cancer Working Group. Surgical resection with or without preoperative chemotherapy in oesophageal cancer: a randomised controlled trial. *Lancet* 2002;359:1727–1733.

150. Bosset JF, Gignoux M, Triboulet JP, et al. Chemoradiotherapy followed by surgery compared with surgery alone in squamous-cell cancer of the esophagus. *N Engl J Med* 1997;337:161–167.

151. Urba SG, Orringer MB, Turrisi A, et al. Randomized trial of preoperative chemoradiation versus surgery alone in patients with locoregional esophageal carcinoma. *J Clin Oncol* 2001;19: 305–313.

152. Ando N, Iizuka T, Kakegawa T, et al. A randomized trial of surgery with and without chemotherapy for localized squamous carcinoma of the thoracic esophagus: the Japan Clinical Oncology Group Study. *J Thorac Cardiovasc Surg* 1997;114: 205–209.

153. Xiao ZF, Yang ZY, Liang J, et al. Value of radiotherapy after radical surgery for esophageal carcinoma: a report of 495 patients. *Ann Thorac Surg* 2003;75:331–336; discussion 336.

154. Rice TW, Adelstein DJ. Precise clinical staging allows treatment modification of patients with esophageal carcinoma. *Oncology (Huntingt)* 1997;11:58–62.

155. Kitajima M, Kitagawa Y. Surgical treatment of esophageal cancer—the advent of the era of individualization. *N Engl J Med* 2002;347:1705–1709.

156. Rice TW, Zuccaro G Jr, Adelstein DJ, et al. Esophageal carcinoma: depth of tumor invasion is predictive of regional lymph node status. *Ann Thorac Surg* 1998;65:787–792.

157. Rice TW, Blackstone EH, Adelstein DJ, et al. N1 esophageal carcinoma: the importance of staging and downstaging. *J Thorac Cardiovasc Surg* 2001;121:454–464.

158. Rice T, Adelstein D, Chidel M, et al. Benefit of postoperative adjuvant chemotherapy in locoregionally advanced esophageal carcinoma. *J Thorac Cardiovasc Surg* (*in press*).

ESOPHAGEAL WEBS AND RINGS

DAVID A. KATZKA

Webs and rings of the esophagus constitute a curious and, at times, confusing set of disorders for several reasons. First, other than Schatzki's rings, these disorders are relatively rare. Second, in most cases, the causes of webs and rings have remained elusive; many of the proposed etiologies are given anecdotally by case reports. Third, investigators cannot completely agree on the definitions that separate rings from webs. Indeed, what some esophagologists call rings, others cause webs, and vice versa. This chapter defines their pathogenesis, clinical presentation, and treatment. Further information is also given on some of the emerging etiologies, particularly in the concept of the "ringed" esophagus.

DEFINITIONS

In the last edition of *The Esophagus* (1), a web is defined as a thin, eccentric membrane of tissue occurring anywhere in the esophagus. In contrast, a ring is concentric and most commonly occurs in the distal esophagus. In other textbooks and reports, however, webs are variably defined as occurring in the proximal esophagus, and rings distally, both as thin and potentially concentric narrowings. Histologic differentiation is also unproductive. For example, Schatzki's rings have been described as a mucosal hypertrophy of the cellular lining of the esophagogastric squamocolumnar junction (2), whereas in other studies, biopsies of this type of ring may be normal (3). Just as discordant is the fact that, in the ringed esophagus, multiple histopathologies may be present depending on the specific etiology. Furthermore, the ringed esophagus may occur in any part of or diffusely through the esophagus, making definitions based on esophageal location also unreliable. As a result, in my opinion, attempting to define rings as separate from webs in esophageal disorders is not helpful. They should both be used as a morphologic description only to denote a thin membranous type of narrowing of the esophagus of varying diameter that may be concentric or unilateral. Further definition of a ring or web rests mostly on its specific etiology or syndrome when known. This chapter discusses specific entities that include either ring or web formation without attempt to group them into disorders based on these arbitrary morphologic descriptors. They are discussed moving proximally to distally in the esophagus.

PROXIMAL ESOPHAGEAL WEBS

Prevalence and Etiology

Of all the diseases discussed herein, proximal esophageal webs represent the least understood of the web and ringlike disorders of the esophagus. This is, in part, due to the heterogeneous causes of these webs and that they rarely cause symptoms. The prevalence of these webs has not been well described because there have been no large endoscopic or radiographic prospective studies that specifically examine this question. Webs are commonly found incidentally, suggesting that estimating true prevalence would require study of the normal population rather than only patients with dysphagia. When large series of patients do undergo radiographic or endoscopic evaluation for dysphagia, 5% to 15% of patients are found to have webs (4–6). Even so, the incidental and often subtle nature of these webs calls into question whether they had contributed to the dysphagia that prompted the examination. Similarly, because of the sometimes subtle nature of these webs, they may be missed endoscopically (because this is an area in which the endoscope is often passed through blindly) as well as radiographically (because the most proximal esophagus is not always examined in detail unless specifically requested by the ordering physician).

The cause of upper esophageal rings is also unclear. Most cases are idiopathic at this point, although gastroesophageal reflux has been suggested as a possible cause. In many case reports, a secondary cause has also been suggested (7–23) (Table 15.1). Which of these represents cause and effect is unclear.

D. A. **Katzka:** Department of Gastroenterology, Hospital of the University of Pennsylvania, Philadelphia, Pennsylvania.

TABLE 15.1. CONDITIONS ASSOCIATED WITH UPPER ESOPHAGEAL WEBS

Zenker's Diverticulum (7)
Epidermolysis Bullosa (8–11)
Pemphigus or pemphigoid vulgaris (12,13)
Psoriasis (14)
Heterotopic gastric mucosa (15–17)
Graft vs. host disease (18)
Radiation therapy (personal observation)
Bronchoesophageal fistula with an esophageal web (19)
Laryngeal carcinoma (20)
Esophageal duplication cyst (21)
Zinsser-Engman-Cole-Fanconi disease (22)
Pediatric growth failure (23)

Symptoms and Diagnosis

Most patients complain of solid food or pill-induced dysphagia. Because of the proximal location of these webs, patients may present with the sensation of choking while eating and even a "steakhouse" syndrome rarely with tracheal compression. As with any syndrome in which dysphagia occurs, weight loss has been reported (24). Complaints of additional liquid dysphagia should prompt search for an additional cause of the patient's symptoms.

Diagnosis is best made by barium esophagography. The radiologist must be asked to focus on the area of the proximal esophagus to detect these rings, usually with performance of a video barium swallow. This includes not only cine technique but careful examination of the esophagus just distal to the upper esophageal sphincter (UES) with both anteroposterior and lateral views. Sometimes, challenge with a solid food bolus or pill is helpful in visualizing the web as well as determining possible clinical significance. Webs appear as a thin membranous filling defect just below the UES and are seen best on a lateral view. They may project from one of the walls as a unilateral defect or may appear circumferentially (Fig. 15.1A). In contrast to videoesophagraphy, endoscopic detection, particularly of subtle webs, is not reliable unless the endoscopist methodically performs a careful examination of the proximal esophagus under direct visualization. Sometimes, the diagnosis is made by encountering mild resistance upon esophageal intubation with a small amount of blood seen in the esophagus concordantly. When appreciated endoscopically, an upper esophageal web appears again as a unilateral or circumferential band of bland-appearing esophageal mucosa compromising the esophageal lumen (Fig. 15.1B). Depending on the degree of luminal compromise, these webs may permit passage of the endoscope with mild resistance or may prevent passage of the scope altogether. A secondary cause of the web should be sought, particularly heterotopic gastric mucosa (15–17). Furthermore, a complete examination of the esophagus should be made, searching for another cause of dysphagia as a result of the commonly incidental nature of these webs.

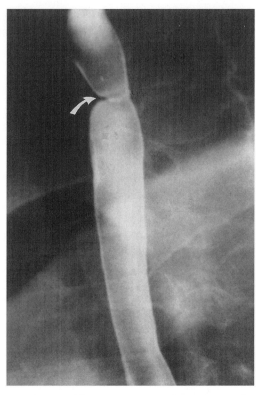

FIGURE 15.1. Double contrast esophagogram of upper esophageal web (*arrow*). (Courtesy of Dr. Marc Levine.)

Treatment

The first question as regards treatment is in determining which patients need treatment. Unlike Schatzki's rings, there is no clear study indicating to what degree the lumen should be occluded for symptoms to be produced. At this time, the clinician must rely on clinical judgment and the exclusion of other causes of dysphagia either independent of the web or as secondary contributors (e.g., ineffective mastication or consumption of large pills). Once treatment is decided upon, a variety of treatments have been used for upper esophageal webs (25–29) (Table 15.2) but the majority are treated by rupture of the webs with passage of the endoscope or with some sort of dilation. The most commonly used technique is Savary dilation over a guidewire. The need for fluoroscopy is operator dependent. Optimal dilator size has not been studied, although, anecdotally, most investigators use 15 mm or above, par-

TABLE 15.2. METHODS OF TREATMENT FOR UPPER ESOPHAGEAL WEBS

Endoscopic biopsy of the web
Guidewire-directed Savary dilation (25,26)
Endoscopic balloon dilation (25,27)
Laser ablation (28,29)
Surgery (25)

ticularly for smaller webs. Although not studied, endoscopic obliteration of the web by biopsy technique may also be tried. For more refractory webs, other techniques may be considered, but I have never resorted to any of these methods in my experience. Webs may persist following effective symptomatic treatment (25). Whether this indicates that complete obliteration of the web is not needed for symptomatic relief, a placebo effect occurred, the patient has adapted, or that another condition (e.g., cricopharyngeal dysfunction) was more effectively treated by the dilation is unknown. Finally, two caveats must be considered before performing the dilation. The first is a report of six patients with upper esophageal webs associated with Zenker's diverticulum (7). The possibility of esophageal perforation during endoscopic evaluation and dilation of the esophagus in the presence of an unsuspected Zenker's diverticulum is well known. Second is that some skin diseases such as epidermolysis bullosa (8–11), or pemphigus or pemphigoid vulgaris (12,13) may be associated with esophageal webs. Endoscopy or dilation of the esophagus involved by these conditions may lead to marked additional bullous and web formation.

PLUMMER-VINSON SYNDROME

This unusual syndrome that originally described the association of iron deficiency anemia and upper esophageal webs has been controversial from its original description. The first controversy starts with its name. It was originally described by Dr. Plummer (30), then by laryngologists Drs. Paterson (31) and Kelly (32), and 3 years later by gastroenterologist Dr. Vinson (33). As a result, this syndrome is commonly referred to as Paterson-Kelly and sometimes Paterson-Brown Kelly (Dr. Kelly's first name) syndrome. The name of Plummer-Vinson seems to predominate, however, in part because the physician who coined the eponym confessed ignorance of the earlier studies from 1919 (34). An even more basic controversy is whether the syndrome even exists, specifically, the association of iron deficiency anemia with upper esophageal webs (35). Given the commonality of iron deficiency throughout the world, some authors have questioned why the formation of upper esophageal webs in response to the anemia should be more restricted to Northern European women or why then isn't web formation more common? Indeed, some investigators have shown that patients with webs are equally likely to be as iron deficient as control subjects (36,37). Evidence that supports the association of iron deficiency with web formation comes from four sources: (a) not only the strong association of iron deficiency with webs (38–40) but also documentation of cases in which the iron deficiency anemia precedes webs (41); (b) experimental evidence suggesting that iron deficiency causes esophageal epithelial change predisposing to web forma-

tion (42); (c) correction of the webs with iron repletion (41–43); (d) a corresponding decreasing incidence of Plummer-Vinson syndrome and iron deficiency anemia in the general population (35,44). There is also some suggestion that web formation in iron deficiency would be more common if the hypopharynx was more carefully studied in these patients given the lack of sensitivity for upper esophageal webs as seen on routine endoscopy or esophagography. Still, review of the evidence has prompted investigators to seek other etiologic factors, including heredity, and other nutritional deficiencies, such as riboflavin (44).

Since its description, several further characteristics have been described. The webs are typically in the hypopharynx or upper esophagus and may be single or multiple. They may also be associated with stricture formation with pathology revealing fibrosis, epithelial atrophy, hyperplasia, and sometimes chronic inflammation (44,45). As discussed, it is most common in middle-aged and elderly white women, but patients of other ethnicities (46), men (43), young adults and adolescents (43,46–48), and even children have been described (49). Furthermore, many other conditions have been associated with this syndrome. These include an increased incidence of hypopharyngeal, oral, and perhaps upper gastrointestinal tract cancer (36,40,44), thyroiditis (50), celiac disease (51,52), glossitis and stomatitis (53), rheumatoid arthritis, Sjögren's syndrome (54), and pernicious anemia (55).

Because of the tenuous association of iron deficiency anemia with esophageal web formation, initial evaluation should be that of ruling out other sources of iron deficiency anemia. Once this has been performed, treatment can then be directed at correction of the iron deficiency anemia not only for possible reversal of the web formation but also for correction of possible esophageal motility abnormalities that may be contributing to the dysphagia in these patients (56). Dilation of the webs or strictures (57) in combination with iron repletion may also be necessary in patients with persistent dysphagia and webs. Patients should also undergo thorough evaluation to rule out concordant oropharyngeal, laryngeal, or upper gastrointestinal tract cancer. Whether they should be enrolled in a screening program following treatment is unclear but has been suggested (58).

THE RINGED ESOPHAGUS

The "ringed" esophagus is usually defined by the finding of multiple ringlike structures seen during endoscopy or barium esophagography. Definition of this concept is strictly morphologic, and it is unknown whether there are single or multiple pathophysiologies and how to precisely define the disease. Answers to these questions are paramount in formulating a treatment plan not only for initial disruption of the rings but also for prevention of recurrence.

TABLE 15.3. CHARACTERISTIC RADIOGRAPHIC OR ENDOSCOPIC APPEARANCE OF RINGED ESOPHAGUS

1. Multiple regular ringlike structures in a smooth tapered stricture ("corrugated" or "tachealized" appearance)
2. Location may be proximal, mid, or distal esophagus
3. Length may vary from short (1.5 cm) to long (20 cm) segment
4. Normal appearing overlying mucosa

Definition and Appearance

Because the ringed esophagus is defined descriptively, its definition is given by its radiographic or endoscopic appearance (Table 15.3, Fig. 15.2, and Color Plate 15.3). In this section, the ringed esophagus is defined (usually radiographically) as a discrete area of the esophagus having the appearance of multiple closely associated rings with a "corrugated" or "trachedalized" appearance. It is typically associated with a stricture in which the luminal diameter in the area of the rings is compromised. There may be associated intramural diverticulosis as well. Variation may occur in length, location, and luminal diameter. The narrowing tends to be concentric. For example, in one study (59), stricture length varied from 1.5 to 20 cm and width varied from 0.8 to 1.7 cm; stricture location could be found in proximal, mid, or distal esophagus. The

mucosa appears normal not only within the area of ring formation but also in the remainder of the esophagus. Hiatal hernia is unusual.

Endoscopic appearance mirrors radiology. There is often a trachealized appearance with multiple closely approximated concentric rings with normal-appearing mucosa. The abnormalities may be obvious or subtle (better appreciated radiologically). There is often moderate resistance in passing the scope through the strictured area. Sometimes, because the location of these strictures is commonly proximal, the endoscopist's first awareness of the ringed esophagus is when resistance is encountered upon intubation of the proximal esophagus. If passage occurs, there may be incidental mild bleeding upon passage of the scope.

Pathologic biopsy may reveal normal overlying mucosa or nonspecific inflammation, or in some cases, a preponderance of eosinophils.

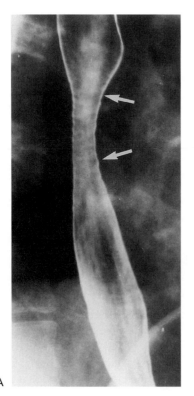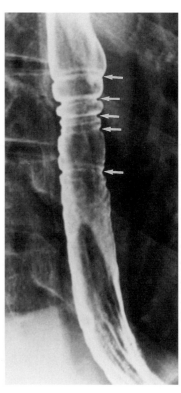

A   B

FIGURE 15.2. Double contrast esophagograms of ringed esophagus. **A:** Smooth, tapered, slightly ringed stricture in mid to distal esophagus (*arrows*). **B:** More prominent corrugated ring appearance to distal esophageal stricture (*multiple arrows*). (Courtesy of Marc Levine, M.D.)

Etiology

One of the challenges of the ringed esophagus is understanding its etiology. Three general causative factors have been proposed (Table 15.4): gastroesophageal reflux, congenital causes, and an eosinophilic or allergic-mediated phenomenon. There are several lines of evidence suggesting that gastroesophageal reflux disease (GERD) may be an important factor in ringed esophagus. The first is that some of these patients may demonstrate histologic or erosive esophagitis on endoscopy (60,61). In case reports and review of ringed esophagus, several patients were found to have ulceration, erythema, or friability of the distal esophagus. All had histologic change of reflux characterized by basal zone hyperplasia and intraepithelial eosinophils; all but one had papillary lengthening (62,63). The second line of evidence, albeit scant, is the finding of abnormal ambulatory pH monitoring in some of these patients (63). In this same series, two of the three patients studied had evidence of prolonged distal acid exposure. There are several difficulties in ascribing ringed esophagus to GERD, however. For example, the finding of abnormal acid exposure has been documented in relatively few patients. In one series, one patient studied did not have abnormal acid exposure (59). Even in the prior series cited, the two abnormal studies were only mildly abnormal (both with total distal acid exposure less than 9%). Similarly, the finding of other associated reflux lesions such as peptic stricture or Barrett's is not found. Additionally, patients have not been shown to have a change in esophageal appearance in response to acid suppressing therapy including proton pump inhibitors. Finally, histologic findings of mild GERD in the absence of gross mucosal injury are nonspecific.

The second proposed etiology is that ringed esophagus represents a congential process or what some have termed congenital esophageal stenosis. The reasons for this association are several. Similar to eosinophilic esophagitis, disease often starts in childhood. In several series, patients frequently remember having dysphagia early in childhood (59,64). The radiographic and endoscopic findings also described are similar to those found in congenital esophageal stenosis in children and infants. Interestingly, the pathology in infants may include a fibromuscular obliteration of the esophageal wall layers in the area of stricture (65) as suggested by finding on endoscopic ultrasound in two adult series (59,66). As in adults, congenital esophageal stenosis is also a rare entity, estimated to occur in 1 in 25,000 to 50,000 births (67,68). Several features, however,

TABLE 15.4. PROPOSED CAUSES OF RINGED ESOPHAGUS

1. Gastroesophageal reflux disease
2. Congenital esophageal stenosis
3. Eosinophilic esophagitis

speak against congenital esophageal stenosis as the cause in most cases. For example, congenital esophageal stenosis in children and infants does not seem to have the same male predominance as is seen in ringed esophagus. It is also hard to explain the onset of symptoms later in life (as opposed to infancy or early childhood once solid food is consumed) although some authors believe that patients may alter eating habits early to adjust to the stricture (66,69). Finally, Langdon (70) described two patients who developed ringed esophagus after previously documented endoscopies without such a finding.

The third possibility and perhaps the most common cause of the ringed esophagus is eosinophilic esophagitis. Several lines of evidence support this. First, most of the patients described are young. In recent series of patients with ringed esophagus, most patients are younger than age 30 years, which is consistent with eosinophilic esophageal disease (71,72). Second, most patients are male, a demographic finding also commonly found in eosinophilic esophagitis (71,72). Third, in several series, increased eosinophils on esophageal biopsy is a common finding (73,74). Fourth, stricture formation in general is well described in eosinophilic esophagitis (71,72). Finally, a recent case report by Siafakas and colleagues (73) documented an 8-year-old boy with multiple esophageal rings and prominent eosinophils on esophageal biopsy who had marked resolution of both rings and histologic findings in response to a food elimination diet. Furthermore, recent data also document many cases of ringed esophagus in association with clear-cut eosinophilic esophagitis (74–76). Although tenable, not all evidence points to ringed esophagus being a form of eosinophilic esophagitis. Despite finding prominent eosinophils on biopsy in many of these patients, it is not clear that greater than 20 eosinophils per high-power field were seen on biopsy (i.e., the reported diagnostic feature of this disease). In one series of ringed esophagus, no patient met this criteria (59). Furthermore, not all patients give clear allergic or asthmatic histories consistent with eosinophilic type disease, although this is not a requirement for this type of esophagitis either. Thus, although eosinophilic esophagitis may turn out to be the dominant cause of ringed esophagus, it is still clear that one etiology may not decisively explain its existence in all patients.

Epidemiology

The prevalence of ringed esophagus is unknown. It is seemingly rare in that only a few cases have been published; the largest series available describes only 11 patients. Isolated case reports are also available. The five patients discussed in our series came from a compilation of three teaching hospitals over 2 years among physicians with a referral practice for esophageal disease, thus also suggesting a very low prevalence. On the other hand, because ringed esophagus is poorly understood and probably misdiagnosed, it may be underreported. Furthermore, with the emerging interest in eosinophilic esophagitis, it may become better recognized as suggested by the marked increase in publications on this topic over the past several years.

Two demographic factors distinguish this disease. First, most patients described are younger than age 30 years, although patients up to the age of 75 years have been well described. Second, most patients with ringed esophagus are male. In compiling data from the four largest series of patients, 28 of 32 (85%) were men (59,60,64,66). There is not enough evidence to analyze whether any race preference exists, although most reported patients were white.

Symptoms

The most prominent symptom is longstanding solid food dysphagia, often remembered since early childhood. In one study of five patients, the average duration of dysphagia was 16 years (59). Patients often underestimate the degree of dysphagia by accommodating to the stenosis. This may be done by such mechanisms as diet adjustment, excessive chewing, and slow eating early in childhood so dysphagia is not readily apparent. As a result, patients with ringed esophagus commonly present with an acute food impaction as their primary and sometimes only symptom, most likely having subconsciously accommodated to their stricture in early childhood but erring with a piece of meat or other solid food material not adequately chewed or eaten too quickly. Chest pain has also been described (66).

Treatment

Treatment for the ringed esophagus revolves first around generalized treatment for the stricture and then therapy directed at one of the proposed causes. Generalized treatment consists of diet modification and dilation. Younes and Johnson (64) specifically outline a "dysphagia diet" for these patients consisting of avoidance of tough meats, fruits and vegetables with skins, and fresh, doughy bread products. Other typical stricture precautions include chewing slowly and carefully, eating slowly, and combining fluids with solids when swallowing. Dilation for ringed esophagus has been performed with both Savary dilators and balloons. Neither has been shown to have superiority in that only small numbers of patients have been studied with short follow-up. Chest pain, sometimes severe, following dilation has been described because the mucosa is torn easily in these patients, often down to the muscularis (70). The long-term efficacy of dilation is unclear, although one series cited no need for repeat dilation in ten patients followed up for a mean of 3 years with patients maintained on the dysphagia diet (64). No data show that treatment with acid-suppressing agents alters the course of ringed esophagus. If reflux is strongly considered, an ambulatory pH study should be performed for evaluation. It is hoped that with doc-

umentation of eosinophilic esophagitis in a significant number of these patients, specific therapy directed at this entity will either help prevent or at least control further ring formation. Recent data demonstrating efficacy of fluticasone for this eosinophilic esophagitis may be helpful in treating the ringed esophagus (72,77). Whether avoidance of allergic type foods, similar to treatment for eosinophilic esophagitis (72,78), will consistently lead to resolution or reduction of ring formation (73) is unclear. Clearly more intense study of treatment of ringed esophagus is needed.

LOWER ESOPHAGEAL RINGS

Before discussing Schatzki's rings, it is important to review the concept of "A," "B," and "C" rings. An "A" ring is a concentrically constricted area commonly seen on barium esophagogram approximately 2 cm proximal to the gastroesophageal junction. It is thought to represent muscular contraction, in my opinion is physiologic, and rarely produces symptoms. A "C" ring represents, again best seen radiographically, the indentation on the esophagus of the diaphragmatic crura. The bulk of this discussion focuses on the "B" ring, otherwise known as Schatzki's ring.

SCHATZKI'S RING

Schatzki's ring was described by two sets of investigators in Boston in 1953: Drs. Schatzki and Gary (79) and Drs. Ingelfinger and Kramer (80). The ring was first described anatomically (as opposed to clinically) as early as 1944 by Templeton (81). Because of his initial and sustained intensive study of the entity, the ring was given Dr. Schatzki's name. This entity is commonly referred to as the *lower esophageal ring*.

Epidemiology, Pathology, and Pathogenesis

The occurrence of Schatzki's rings has not been extensively studied although it appears to be common, particularly in asymptomatic individuals. Studies using barium esophagography have demonstrated a prevalence of 0.2% to 14% in the general population (82–85). The wide variation in prevalence probably reflects the assiduousness with which the radiologist searches out the presence of a ring. The incidence increases with age and occurrence in children is rare (86). Pathologically, these rings are annular membranes composed of mucosa and submucosa occurring in the area of the gastroesophageal junction (85). As a result, they typically are composed of squamous mucosa proximally with underlying gastric columnar mucosa distally. Histologic evidence of chronic inflammation and fibrosis may be seen as well (87–89). In my experience, biopsies of this area, however, usually show normal histology.

Despite the commonality of this problem, the etiology of Schatzki's ring remains enigmatic. Original theories included a congenital etiology in which Steinnon proposed a pleating and infolding of the mucosa secondary to esophageal shortening occurring with contraction (90). The growing tide of data, however, supports gastroesophageal reflux as a likely etiology. Such evidence includes the following:

1. Several studies have noted the finding of chronic inflammatory change on biopsy of the Schatzki ring.
2. Symptoms of reflux, hiatal hernia, and reflux esophagitis are commonly found in patients with Schatzki's rings (89,91).
3. Esophageal rings may be more common in patients with scleroderma, a disease in which reflux is common (92).
4. Recurrence of Schatzki's rings is common, suggesting that there is some continued untreated etiologic factor in some of these patients.
5. Ambulatory pH monitoring has demonstrated abnormal esophageal acid exposure (65%) in patients with rings when studied (93). It may well be that these patients have increased acid exposure limited to the gastroesophageal junction, not detected by conventional testing nor generating typical reflux sequelae but this is speculation.

Presentation and Diagnosis

Schatzki's rings classically present with intermittent solid food dysphagia and are the most common cause of this symptom in some series (94). The interval between the dysphagia episodes may be days to years. Of a more serious nature, food impaction is another common presentation of lower esophageal rings with or without more subtle symptoms of dysphagia or subacute impaction between major episodes. Typically these patients present with meat impactions prompting emergency department visits with inability to keep down secretions or liquids, drooling, and chest pain. Rarely, Schatzki's rings may present with esophageal perforation (95). One of the questions asked early was "How compromised does the esophageal lumen have to be in order for a lower esophageal ring to produce symptoms?" In a follow-up study from his original description, Dr. Schatzki (84) demonstrated that if the luminal diameter is (a) greater than 20 mm, symptoms are rare, (b) between 13 and 20 mm, symptoms may be present, or (c) less than 13 mm, symptoms are almost always present. These parameters are good guidelines but are not absolute. As is typical for disorders with dysphagia, patients often learn adaptive mechanisms such as chewing carefully and eating slowly to minimize symptoms even when tight rings are present. Conversely, one large, poorly chewed, quickly eaten piece of meat may be enough to cause impaction in patients with minimal luminal compromise.

Diagnosis of the lower esophageal ring is best done with barium radiography (Fig. 15.4A and Color Plate 15.4B). It is important to alert the radiologist to the possibility of a ring because the optimal technique used to identify rings is in contrast to current methods of performing barium studies. Specifically, low-volume, double-contrast examinations of the esophagus are much more likely to miss rings than the older methods of large-volume, single-contrast esophagrams with maximal esophageal distention by the barium to accentuate the ring (96). Hang-up of a barium tablet, barium marshmallow, or barium-soaked solid food bolus at the ring during the study is also helpful in determining clinical significance of the ring. Endoscopy is not as sensitive as radiography for detection of the ring, but similar methods used for barium studies such as distention of the distal esophagus (in this case by air insufflation) and asking the patient to perform the Valsalva maneuver can improve sensitivity. The differentiation of a ring from an early annular peptic stricture can be difficult. It is not unusual in my experience to see a Schatzki ring at first endoscopy only to find a more evident peptic stricture upon recurrence of symptoms. Whether this represents a miscall on the initial endoscopy or a harbinger of more serious reflux disease is unclear.

Treatment of Schatzki's Rings

In patients with symptomatic rings, the standard treatment for Schatzki's rings has been some form of bougienage, most likely endoscopy with Savary dilation. Usually a

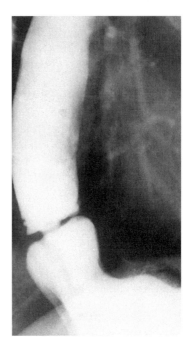

FIGURE 15.4A. Double contrast esophagogram **(A)** and endoscopic photograph **(B)** of Schatzki's ring. See Color Plate 15.4B.

TABLE 15.5. TREATMENT OF SCHATZKI'S RING

1. Single large diameter (>48 French) Savary dilation
2. Endoscopic biopsy obliteration of the ring
3. Electrocautery type techniques (rare)
4. Pneumatic dilation (rare)

large-bore dilator (larger than 48 Fr) is used to rupture the ring as opposed to use of serial dilations, which are used with strictures wherein risk of perforation is higher because of presence of extensive fibrotic tissue. The efficacy of a single dilation has been studied by Eckardt and colleagues (91). In this study of 33 patients undergoing prospective evaluation after single dilation, all were symptom free by 4 weeks. In more long-term follow-up (mean 24.3 months), however, 42% of patients had return of symptoms severe enough to warrant repeat dilation with only 11% expected to remain symptom free at 5 years. One might question whether the recurrence is a result of uncontrolled reflux, but neither ring diameter nor the presence of esophagitis or reflux symptoms determined the need for subsequent dilation in the study. Still, these parameters are not necessarily reliable in evaluating the presence of reflux at the gastroesophageal junction. The question follows, then, whether patients with Schatzki's rings should be treated with acid-suppressing therapies to prevent recurrence. In the absence of other reasons necessitating reflux treatment (erosive esophagitis, chronic reflux symptoms), one might consider an ambulatory pH study to further evaluate for the presence of acid reflux, but no data suggest that such treatment does reduce ring recurrence.

One dictum that may be changing, however, is the concept of never dilating a patient with a Schatzki ring at the time of acute food impaction. A recent study (97) suggested that dilation at presentation is efficacious and safe without increased risk for perforation as previously feared. I believe that close inspection of the esophageal mucosa is advisable, particularly in patients with greater than 12 hours of impaction in whom more underlying, deeper wall injury may exist. Furthermore, forceful passage of the food bolus into the stomach often causes ring rupture. One new and easy method that has been supported is biopsy rupture of the ring rather than dilation. In a recent trial of 26 patients randomized to dilation with 52 French Maloney dilator or four-quadrant biopsy of the ring (98), follow-up at 3 and 12 months showed no difference in dysphagia score between the groups. Furthermore, as expected, the groups undergoing endoscopy and biopsy, found their procedure more tolerable. This is something I do in my practice. Uncommonly used methods of ring ablation that have been described include pneumatic dilation (99), electrocautery (100), and sphincterotome cutting of the ring (101).

REFERENCES

1. Tobin RA. Esophageal rings and webs. In Castell DO, Richter JE, eds. *The esophagus*, third ed. Philadelphia: Lippincott Williams and Wilkins, 1999:295–300.
2. Johnston JH, Griffin JC. Anatomic location of the lower esophageal ring. *Surgery* 1967;61:528–534.
3. MacMahon HE, Schatzki R, Gary JE. Pathology of the lower esophageal ring: report of a case, with autopsy, observed for nine years. *N Engl J Med* 1958;259:1–8.
4. Clements JL, Cox GW, Torres WE, et al. Cervical esophageal webs: a roentgen-anatomic correlation. *Am J Roentgen Radium Ther Nucl Med* 1974;121:221–231.
5. Ekkberg O, Nylander G. Webs and web like formations in the pharynx and cervical esophagus. *Diagn Imaging* 1983;52:10.
6. Webb WA, McDaniel L, Jones L. Endoscopic evaluation of dysphagia in two hundred and ninety-three patients with benign disease. *Surg Gynecol Obstet* 1984;158:152.
7. Low DE, Hill LD. Cervical esophageal web associated with Zenker's diverticulum. *Am J Surg* 1988;156:34–37.
8. Orlando RC, Bozymksi EM, Briggaman RA, et al. Epidermolysis bullosa: gastrointestinal manifestations. *Ann Intern Med* 1974;81:203.
9. Marsden RA, Gowar FJS, MacDonald AF, et al. Epidermolysis bullosa of the esophagus with esophageal web formation. *Thorax* 1974;29:287–295.
10. Hillemeier C, Touloukian R, McCallum R, et al. Esophageal web: a previously unrecognized complication of epidermolysis bullosa. *Pediatrics* 1981;67:678.
11. Sehgal VN, Jain VK, Bhattadcharya SN, et al. Esophageal web in generalized epidermolysis bullosa. *Int J Dermatol* 1991;30: 51–52.
12. Al-Kutoubi MA, Eliot A. Esophageal involvement in benign mucosa membrane pemphigoid. *Clin Radiol* 1984;35:131.
13. Naylor MF, MacCarty RL, Rogers RS. Barium studies in esophageal cicatricial pemphigoid. *Abdom Imaging* 1995;20:97.
14. Harty RF, Boharski MG, Harned RK. Psoriasis, dysphagia and esophageal webs or rings. *Dysphagia* 1988;2:136.
15. Steadman C, Kerlin P, Teague C, et al. High esophageal stricture: a complication of "inlet patch" mucosa. *Gastroenterology* 1988;94:521–524.
16. Buse PE, Zuckerman GR, Balfe DM. Cervical esophageal web associated with a patch of heterotopic gastric mucosa. *Abdom Imaging* 1993;18:227–228.
17. Waring JP, Wo JM. Cervical esophageal web caused caused by an inlet patch of gastric mucosa. *South Med J* 1997;90: 554–555.
18. McDonald GB, Sullivan KM, Plumley TF. Radiographic features of esophageal involvement in chronic graft-vs.-host disease. *Am J Roentgenol* 1984;142:501.
19. Turrentine MW, Kesler KA, Mahomed Y. Bronchoesophageal fistula with an esophageal web. *Ann Thorac Surg* 1990;50: 473–475.
20. Belafsky PC, Postma GN, Koufman JA. Laryngeal carcinoma and a lower esophageal web. *Ear Nose Throat J* 2001;80:788.
21. Snyder Cl, Bickler SW, Gittes GK, et al. Esophageal duplication cyst with esophageal web and tracheoesophageal fistula. *J Pediatr Surg* 1996;31:968.
22. de Roux-Serratrice C, Serratrice J, Escoffier JM, et al. Esophageal web in Zinsser-Engman-Cole-Fanconi disease. *Gastrointest Endosc* 2000;52:561–562.
23. Kumuro H, Makino S, Tsuchiya I, et al. Cervical esophageal web in a 13-year old with growth failure. *Pediatr Int* 1999;41: 568–570.

24. Lesser PB, Moyer P, Andrews PJ, et al. Upper esophageal ring. *Ann Intern Med* 1978;88:657–658.

25. Lindgren S. Endoscopic dilatation and surgical myotomy of symptomatic cervical esophageal webs. *Dysphagia* 1991;6:235.

26. Webb WA, McDaniel L, Jones L. Endoscopic evaluation of dysphagia in two hundred and ninety-three patients with benign disease. *Surg Gynecol Obstet* 1984;158:152.

27. Huynh PT, de Lange EE, Shagger HA. Symptomatic webs of the upper esophagus: treatment with fluoroscopically guided balloon dilation. *Radiology* 1995;196:789.

28. Krevsky B, Pusateri JP. Laser lysis of an esophageal web. *Gastrointest Endosc* 1989;35:451–453.

29. Roy GT, Cohen RC, Williams SJ. Endoscopic laser division of an esophageal web in a child. *J Pediatr Surg* 1996;31:439–440.

30. Plummer HS. Diffuse dilation of the esophagus without anastomotic stenosis (cardiospasm), a report of ninety-nine cases. *JAMA* 1912;34:285–288.

31. Paterson DR. A clinical type of dysphagia. *J Laryngol Rhinol Otol* 1919;34:289.

32. Kelly AB. Spasms at the entrance to the esophagus. *J Laryngol Rhinol Otol* 1919;34:285.

33. Vinson PP. Hysterical dysphagia. *Minn Med* 1922;5:107.

34. Baron JH. The Paterson-Brown Kelly syndrome of sideropenic dysphagia does not exist. *J R Coll Physicans Lond* 1991;25:361.

35. Chen TSN, Chen PSY. Rise and fall of the Plummer-Vinson syndrome. *J Gastroenterol Hepatol* 1994;9:654–658.

36. Elwood PC, Jacobs A, Pitman RG, et al. Epidemiology of the Paterson-Kelly syndrome. *Lancet* 1964;2:716–720.

37. Nosher JL, Campbell WL, Seaman WB. The clinical significance of cervical esophageal and hypopharyngeal webs. *Diagn Radiol* 1975;117:45–47.

38. Jacobs A, Kilpatrick GS. The Paterson-Kelly syndrome. *BMJ* 1964;2:79–82.

39. Chisolm M, Ardran GM, Gallender ST, et al. A follow-up study of patients with post-cricoid webs. *Q J Med* 1971;40:409–420.

40. Chisolm M. The association between webs, iron and post-cricoid carcinoma. *Postgrad Med J* 1974;50:215–219.

41. Bredenkamp JK, Castro DJ, Mickel RA. Importance of iron repletion in the management of Plummer-Vinson syndrome. *Ann Otol Rhinol Laryngol* 1990;99:51–54.

42. Okamura H, Tsutumi S, Inaki S, et al. Esophageal web in Plummer-Vinson syndrome. *Laryngoscope* 1988;98:994–998.

43. Malecki D, Cameron AJ. Plummer-Vinson syndrome associated with chronic blood loss anemia and large diaphragmatic hernia. *Am J Gastroenterol* 2002;97:190–193.

44. Larsson L-G, Sandstom A, Westling P. Relationship of Plummer-Vinson disease to cancer of the upper alimentary tract in Sweden. *Cancer Res* 1975;35:3308–316.

45. Entwhistle CC, Jacobs A. Histologic findings in the Paterson-Kelly syndrome. *J Clin Pathol* 1965;18:408–413.

46. Mansell N, Jani P, Bailey CM. Plummer-Vinson syndrome—a rare presentation in a child. *J Laryngol Otol* 1999;113:475–476.

47. Crawford M, Jacobs A, Murphy B, et al. Paterson-Kelly syndrome in adolescence: a report of five cases. *BMJ* 1965;1:693–695.

48. Beyler AR, Yurdaydin C, Bahar K, et al. Dilation therapy of upper esophageal webs in two cases of Plummer-Vinson syndrome. *Endoscopy* 1996;28:266–267.

49. Anthony R, Sood S, Strachan DR, et al. A case of Plummer-Vinson syndrome in childhood. *J Pediatr Surg* 1999;34:1570–1572.

50. Chisolm M, Ardan GM, Callander ST, et al. Iron deficiency anemia and autoimmunity in post cricoid webs. *Q J Med* 1971;40:421–433.

51. Rashid Z, Kumar A, Komar M. Plummer-Vinson syndrome and postcricoid carcinoma: late complications of unrecognized celiac disease. *Am J Gastroenterol* 1999;94:1991.

52. Dickey W, McConnell B. Celiac disease presenting as the Paterson-Brown Kelly (Plummer-Vinson) syndrome. *Am J Gastroenterol* 1999;94:527–529.

53. Geerlings SE, Statios van Eps LW. Pathogenesis and consequences of Plummer-Vinson syndrome. *Clin Invest* 1992;70:629–630.

54. Dejmkova H, Pavelka K. An unusual clinical manifestation of secondary Sjögren's syndrome and concomitant Paterson-Kelly syndrome. *Clin Rheumatol* 1994;13:305–308.

55. Hoffman RM, Jaffe PE. Plummer-Vinson syndrome. A case report and literature review. *Arch Intern Med* 1995;155:2008–2001.

56. Dantas RO, Villanova MG. Esophageal motility impairment inh Plummer-Vinson syndrome. Correction by iron treatment. *Dig Dis Sci* 1993;38:968–971.

57. Beyler AR, Yurdaydin C, Bahar K, et al. Dilation therapy of upper esophageal webs in two cases of Plummer-Vinson syndrome. *Endoscopy* 1996;28:266–267.

58. Hoffman RM, Jaffe PE. Plummer-Vinson syndrome. A case report and literature review. *Arch Intern Med* 1995;155:2008–2011.

59. Katzka DA, Levine MS, Ginsberg GG, et al. Congenital esophageal stenosis in adults. *Am J Gastroenterol* 2000;95:32–36.

60. Agarwal VP, Marcel BR. Multiple esophageal rings. *Gastrointest Endosc* 1990;36:147.

61. McKinley MJ, Eisner TD, Fisher ML, et al. Multiple rings of the esophagus associated with gastroesophageal reflux. *Am J Gastroenterol* 1996;91:574.

62. Bousvaros A, Antonioli D, Winter HS. Ringed esophagus: an association with esophagitis. *Am J Gastroenterol* 1992;87:1187–1190.

63. Morrow JB, Vargo JJ, Goldblum JR, et al. The ringed esophagus: histological features of GERD. *Am J Gastroenterol* 2001;96:984–989.

64. Younes Z, Johnson DA. Congenital esophageal stenosis: clinical and endoscopic features. 1996;91:1901(abst).

65. Nishima T, Tsuchida Y, Saito S. Congenital esophageal stenosis is due to tracheobronchial remnants and its associated anomolies. *J Pediatr Surg* 1981;16:190–193.

66. McNally PR, Lemon JC, Goff JS, et al. Congenital esophageal stenosis presenting as noncardiac, esophageal chest pain. *Dig Dis Sci* 1993;38:369–373.

67. Wright VM. Chapter 25, part 1. In Walker WA, et al, eds. *Pediatric gastrointestinal disease*. Philadelphia: BC Decker, 1991:369–370.

68. Nihoul-Fekete C, DeBacker A, Lortat-Jacob S, et al. Congenital esophageal stenosis. A review of 20 cases. *Pediatr Surg Int* 1987;2:86–92.

69. McNally PR, Collier EG III, Lopiano MC, et al. Congenital esophageal stenosis. A rare cause of food impaction in the adult. *Dig Dis Sci* 1990;35:263–266.

70. Langdon DE. "Congenital" esophageal stenosis, corrugated ringed esophagus, and eosinophilic esophagitis. *Am J Gastroenterol* 2000;95:2123–2124.

71. Teitelbaum JE, Fox VL, Twarog FJ, et al. Eosinophilic esophagitis in children: immunopathological analysis and response to fluticasone propionate. *Gastroenterology* 2002;122:1216–1225.

72. Spergel JM, Beausoleil JL, Mascarenhas M, et al. The use of skin prick tests and patch tests to identify causative foods in eosinophilic esophagitis. *J Allergy Clin Immunol* 2002;109:363–368.

73. Siafakas CG, Ruyan CK, Brown MR, et al. Multiple esophageal

rings: an association with eosinophilic esophagitis. *Am J Gastroenterol* 2000;95:1572–1575.

74. Vasilopoulos S, Shaker R. Defiant dysphagia: small-caliber esophagus and refractory benign esophageal strictures. *Curr Gastroenterol Rep* 2001;3:225–230.

75. Orenstein S, Shalaby T, Lorenzo CD, et al. The spectrum of pediatric eosinophilic esophagitis beyond infancy: a clinical series of 30 children. *Am J Gastroenterol* 2000;95:1422–1430.

76. Potter JW, Shaker R, Saeian K, et al. Eosinophilic esophagitis in adults: an emerging problem with unique esophageal deformities. *Gastroenterology* 2002;122:A341(abst).

77. Faubion WA, Perrault J, Burgart LJ, et al. Treatment of eosinophilic esophagitis with inhaled corticosteroids. *J Pediatr Gastroenterol Nutr* 1998;27:90–93.

78. Kelly KJ, Lazenby AJ, Rowe PC, et al. Eosinophilic esophagitis attributed to gastroesophageal reflux: improvement with an amino acid-based formula. *Gastroenterology* 1995;109:1503–1512.

79. Schatzki R, Gary JE. Dysphagia due to diaphragm-like narrowing in lower esophagus ("lower esophageal ring"). *Am J Roentgennol Radiat Ther Nucl Med* 1953;70:911–922.

80. Ingelfinger FJ, Kramer P. Dysphagia produced by contractile ring in lower esophagus. *Gastroenterology* 1953;23:419.

81. Templeton FE. X-ray examination of the stomach. In *A description of the roentgenologic anatomoy, physiology and pathology of the esophagus, stomach and duodenum.* Chicago: University of Chicago Press, 1944:94–102.

82. Kramer P. Frequency of the asymptomatic lower esophageal contractile ring. *N Engl J Med* 1956;254:692–694

83. Keyting WJ, Baker G, McCarver RR, Daywitt AL. The lower esophagus. *Am J Roentgenol* 1960;84:1070–1075.

84. Schatzki R. The lower esophageal ring. Long-term follow-up of symptomatic and asymptomatic rings. *Am J Roentgenol* 1963; 90:805–810.

85. Goyal RK, Glancy JJ, Spiro HM. Lower esophageal ring. *N Engl J Med* 1970;282:1298–1305.

86. Keyting WS, Raker GM, McCarver RR. The lower esophagus. *Am J Roentgenol* 1960;84:1070–1075.

87. Postlewait RW, Musser AW. Pathology of the lower esophageal web. *Surg Gynecol Obstet* 1965;120:571.

88. Vansant JH. Surgical significance of the lower esophageal ring. *Ann Surg* 1972;175:733–739.

89. Eastridge CE, Pate JW, Mann JA. Lower esophageal ring: experiences in treatment of 88 patients. *Ann Thorac Surg* 1984;37: 103–107.

90. Steinnon OA. The anatomic basis for the lower esophageal contraction ring: plication theory and its application. *Am J Roentgenol Radiat Ther Nucl Med* 1963;90:811.

91. Eckardt VF, Kanzler G, Willems D. Single dilation of symptomatic Schatzki rings. A prospective evaluation of its effectiveness. *Dig Dis Sci* 1992;37:577–582.

92. Lovy MR, Levine JS, Steigerwald JC. Lower esophageal rings as a cause of dysphagia in progressive systemic sclerosis—coincidence or consequence. *Dig Dis Sci* 1983;28:780–783.

93. Marshall JB, Kretschmar JM, Diaz-Arias AA. Gastroesophageal reflux as a pathogenic factor in the development of lower esophageal rings. *Arch Intern Med* 1990;150: 1669–1672.

94. Ott DJ, Gelfand DW, Wu WC, et al. Esophagogastric region and its rings. *Am J Roentgenol* 1984;142:281–287.

95. Miller S, Hines C, Ochsner JL. Spontaneous perforation of the esophagus associated with a lower esophageal ring. *Am J Gastroenterol* 1988;83:1405–1408.

96. Ott DJ, Chen YM, Wu WC, et al. Radiographic and endoscopic sensitivity in detecting lower esophageal mucosal ring. *Am J Roentgenol* 1986;147:261.

97. Vicari JJ, Johanson JF, Frakes JT. Outcomes of acute esophageal food impaction: success of the push technique. *Gastrointest Endosc* 2001;53(2):178–181.

98. Chotiprasidhi P, Minocha A. Effectiveness of single dilation with Maloney dilator versus endoscopic rupture of Schatzki's ring using biopsy forceps. *Dig Dis Sci* 2000;45:281–284.

99. Arvanitakis C. Lower esophageal ring: endoscopic and therapeutic aspects. *Gastrointest Endosc* 1977;24:17–18.

100. Burdick JS, Venu RP, Hogan WJ. Cutting the defiant lower esophageal ring. *Gastrointest Endosc* 1993;39:616–619.

101. Groskreutz JL, Kim CH. Late results in patients with Schatzki ring treated by endoscopic electrosurgical incision of the ring. *Gastrointest Endosc* 1987;33:96.

ESOPHAGEAL DIVERTICULA

EDGAR ACHKAR

An esophageal diverticulum is a sac that protrudes from the esophageal wall. As in the rest of the gastrointestinal tract, a true diverticulum is one that contains all layers of the wall. A false diverticulum consists of mucosa, submucosa, and a few muscle fibers. Esophageal diverticula can be classified in many ways. They can be divided into congenital and acquired based on origin, into pulsion and traction based on etiology, or into false or true based on histology; but the simplest and most practical way is to classify them according to anatomy, into four categories: Zenker's (hypopharyngeal) diverticula; midesophageal diverticula; epiphrenic diverticula; and intramural pseudodiverticulosis.

Esophageal diverticula have been described in all age groups, but they are most commonly seen in adults. Esophageal diverticula are rare, occurring in less than 1% of upper gastrointestinal roentgenograms and accounting for less than 5% of dysphagia cases (1).

Motor abnormalities of the esophagus are often associated with esophageal diverticula, but the belief that all diverticula are due to a motor disorder of the esophagus is not established with certainty.

ZENKER'S DIVERTICULUM

Zenker's diverticulum, also called *pharyngoesophageal diverticulum*, is described as an esophageal pouch. In fact, this type of diverticulum occurs in a location proximal to the esophagus, above the upper esophageal sphincter (UES), and should be considered as a hypopharyngeal diverticulum. The pharyngeal constrictor muscles form a funnel, and the mouth of the esophagus is like a transverse slit at the bottom of this funnel. At endoscopy, the larynx with its moving vocal cords is in the center, the piriform sinuses are lateral, and the esophageal opening appears as a posterior slit. The fibers of the cricopharyngeus muscle run transversely and form the UES at the esophageal inlet. Above the cricopharyngeus muscle, the walls of the hypopharynx contain oblique fibers of the inferior constrictor muscles. Between the transverse fibers of the cricopharyngeus muscle below and the oblique fibers of the inferior constrictors above, a triangular area containing fewer muscle fibers constitutes a region of relative weakness and is referred to as the triangle of Killian or Killian's dehiscence (Fig. 16.1). The mucosa of the hypopharynx is allowed to bulge posteriorly at Killian's triangle, and with time a pouch may develop, forming a Zenker's diverticulum.

Etiology and Pathogenesis

Several mechanisms have been invoked to explain the pathogenesis of Zenker's diverticulum, but none has been proven. Age may play a role in the development of Zenker's diverticulum. A decrease in tissue elasticity leading to an increased weakness of the triangle of Killian may explain why Zenker's diverticulum is rarely seen in individuals younger than 40 years. Additionally, the prevalence of Zenker's diverticulum increases in the elderly, reaching 50% in the seventh and eight decades of life, particularly in women (2).

The most widely accepted mechanism for Zenker's diverticulum is a functional disturbance of the hypopharynx, such as increased resting pressure of the sphincter, lack of complete sphincter relaxation, or incoordination between the sphincter and the hypopharynx. The UES is formed mainly by the cricopharyngeus muscle, with participation from fibers from the inferior portion of the inferior pharyngeal constrictors and some fibers of the cervical esophagus. The sphincter is shaped like a slit, not a circle, leading to marked radial asymmetry during tonic contractions. Normally, the UES is closed during tonic contraction, and, immediately after a swallow, excitation of the muscle stops transiently and the UES relaxes, allowing passage of the bolus into the upper esophagus. UES function is under the influence of bolus volume as well as the nature of the upper esophageal contents (3,4).

Traditionally, the most frequently proposed mechanism for a hypopharyngeal diverticulum is premature closure of the UES during swallowing, as shown by Ellis and colleagues (5). The concept of *cricopharyngeal achalasia*, that is, failure of the sphincter to relax on time, was accepted for a long time

E. Achkar: Department of Gastroenterology and Hepatology, Cleveland Clinic Foundation, Cleveland, Ohio.

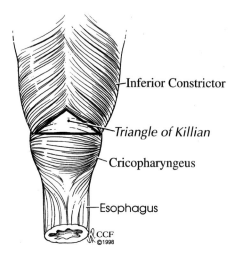

FIGURE 16.1. Triangle of Killian, an area of weakness that allows Zenker's diverticulum to develop.

as the reason for the development of Zenker's diverticula. Achalasia was demonstrated with the help of pharyngography by Asherson in 1950 (6), and other authors, such as Sutherland (7), perpetuated this theory. Nilsson and co-workers (8) studied ten patients with symptomatic hypopharyngeal diverticulum using simultaneous radiography and manometry. Pressures were measured using triple microtransducers, allowing the authors to measure pressures at three levels of the UES, including the level immediately below the neck of the diverticulum. Cineradiography used simultaneously provided a correlation between the pressures generated and the passage of contrast material. Results showed that below the entrance of the diverticulum the sphincter pressure exceeded UES resting pressure as the bolus entered the pharynx. The authors concluded that this phenomenon represented incoordination. They also found within the UES, during swallowing, double pressure peaks, which they called a *split UES.* These results were not found in all patients, and no asymptomatic controls were used. Nevertheless, Nilsson and colleagues (8) explained the pathogenesis of Zenker's diverticulum by pressures on the pharyngeal wall from the bolus forced against a contracted UES. Knuff and co-workers (9) compared nine patients with Zenker's diverticulum and a mean age of 60 years with a control group of 15 patients matched for age. Manometric measurements were obtained using a water-perfused system, which produces less reliable measurements than microtransducers. The tracings were analyzed into four time intervals, and the relationship of pharyngeal contractions to UES relaxation was studied. Using these four parameters, no difference between the two groups was found. However, there was a marked difference in mean UES resting pressure between patients with Zenker's diverticulum and those without. The authors had no explanation for the low resting pressure, but because of the absence of abnormal cricopharyngeal coordination, they questioned the concept that the diverticulum is the result of incomplete relaxation of the UES.

The notion of pharyngoesophageal incoordination or achalasia was contradicted further by Cook and colleagues (10), who studied 14 patients with diverticula and nine healthy, age-matched control subjects using simultaneous videoradiography and manometry. Manometric studies were obtained with a sleeve catheter equipped with metallic markers, allowing exact localization of the recording sites during radiography. There was no difference between patients and control subjects in timing of pharyngeal contractions and sphincter relaxation. However, the authors found a significantly reduced sphincter opening associated with greater intrabolus pressure, suggesting an impairment of UES opening. The authors concluded that Zenker's diverticulum is a disorder of longstanding diminished UES opening with increased hypopharyngeal pressures, eventually causing formation of the diverticulum. They dispelled the notion that UES opening is impaired by pharyngoesophageal incoordination or lack of sphincter relaxation. A histologic study carried out by the same group (11) seems to support the concept of diminished UES opening. Muscle strips were obtained from 14 patients with Zenker's diverticulum during surgical myotomy. Tissue was also obtained from ten control patients without history of dysphagia, nine from autopsy and one from a patient with laryngeal cancer. Of the 14 patients with Zenker's diverticulum, ten showed greater than 50% replacement of cricopharyngeal muscle fibers by fibrous adipose tissue. None of the control subjects showed similar findings. The authors thought that degenerative changes may account for the abnormality observed in patients with Zenker's diverticulum. Muscle degeneration would prevent the sphincter from opening completely because of decreased elasticity, while normally the UES should relax during normal swallowing as a result of external traction and propulsive forces within the sphincter. Lerut and colleagues (12) obtained biopsy specimens from 62 patients with Zenker's diverticulum and compared them with tissue obtained from 15 control subjects. Histologic and immunochemical studies were carried out on most specimens and contractility bath studies on all specimens of cricopharyngeus muscles. Reduced amplitude and lower contractions were found in eight patients with Zenker's diverticulum and not in the control subjects. Neurogenic and myogenic abnormalities were also found on histologic examination.

A study of another condition thought to be due to cricopharyngeal spasm or achalasia may shed some light on the pathogenesis of Zenker's diverticulum. A cricopharyngeal bar, which is detected as a marked indentation on esophagram, was also thought to be due to incoordination. Figure 16.2 illustrates a cricopharyngeal bar.

Dantas and co-workers (13) studied patients with cricopharyngeal bars who had a prominent indentation during radiography but in whom no diverticulum could be elicited. Six patients with bars underwent concurrent fluoroscopic and manometric examination of the pharynx and UES, as did eight volunteers. Patients with bars had smaller openings of the UES during swallowing and increased intra-

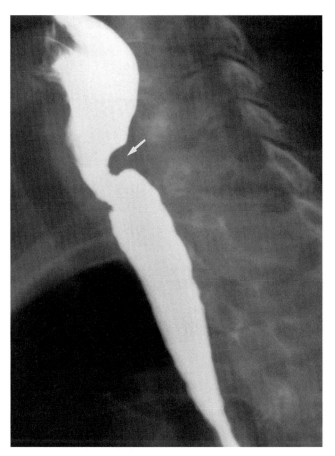

FIGURE 16.2. Cricopharynqeal bar.

further increases in pressure. These findings suggest that the UES acts as a barrier to acid reflux, possibly preventing aspiration. However, Vakil and colleagues (16) found that esophageal acid exposure did not affect UES pressure in normal volunteers or in patients with esophagitis. Although gastroesophageal reflux can result in throat symptoms such as cough, hoarseness, and globus as well as the lesion of posterior laryngitis, it is not known whether anatomic abnormalities such as Zenker's diverticulum can result from chronic gastroesophageal reflux. Hunt and co-workers (15) found a greater resting UES pressure in patients with reflux esophagitis than in control subjects. In five patients with Zenker's diverticulum, the UES pressure was also elevated but there was no evidence of reflux esophagitis. Others have tried using the presence of a hiatal hernia to establish a link between reflux and Zenker's diverticulum. Gage-White (17) showed a 39% occurrence of hiatal hernia in patients with Zenker's diverticulum compared with 16% in control subjects, suggesting that the two disorders may be due to a common pathophysiologic phenomenon. Resouly and colleagues (18) reported an increased occurrence of reflux symptoms in patients with pharyngeal pouches but did not show any objective results. At this point, there is no solid evidence that a direct relationship exists between Zenker's diverticulum and gastroesophageal reflux disease (2,19). Should patients with Zenker's diverticulum exhibit symptoms of heartburn or chest pain, they should be studied for the presence of acid reflux. However, we cannot support aggressive medical or surgical treatment of reflux disease as a way to avoid the development of Zenker's diverticulum.

Clinical Features

Many pharyngoesophageal diverticula are asymptomatic and discovered by chance during radiologic evaluation. In general, symptoms of Zenker's diverticulum depend on the stage of the disease. In the early phase, patients may complain only of a sensation of sticking in the throat or a sensation of vague irritation. They may also report intermittent cough, excessive salivation, and intermittent dysphagia, usually to solid foods. Some patients may present with such minor symptoms that they are dismissed as having "globus." Because of the vagueness of their symptoms, these patients are often labeled as *globus hystericus,* an unfortunate term in that some patients with globus have a significant pathology such as reflux, diverticula, or other disorder of the voluntary phase of swallowing.

When the sac becomes large, more severe symptoms develop. Dysphagia becomes more frequent. Regurgitation of food ingested several hours earlier is reported, and gurgling sounds occur upon swallowing. Patients learn to use special maneuvers to empty the pouch by pressing on the neck or coughing and clearing the throat. In rare cases, the pouch is so large that it obstructs the esophagus, but more frequently a bulging in the left side of the neck takes place. Pulmonary aspiration leading to pneumonia or lung abscess may occur but is infrequent (20).

bolus pressure when compared with control subjects. These findings indicate a reduced muscle compliance, preventing total relaxation of the cricopharyngeus. No evidence of spasm could be found and sphincter relaxation was complete during manometry. Studies such as this one and others performed on patients with Zenker's diverticulum indicate that there are few scientific data to support using the term *cricopharyngeal achalasia* to describe these disorders. Although no single pathogenetic mechanism for the development of Zenker's diverticulum has been established, it appears that reduced UES compliance rather than cricopharyngeal incoordination accounts for the genesis of the pouch. The consistent finding in recent studies is increased intrabolus pressure in patients with Zenker's diverticulum (14).

Gastroesophageal reflux has been implicated in the genesis of Zenker's diverticulum. It was suggested that acid reflux leads to cricopharyngeal spasm and that eventually a pharyngoesophageal diverticulum develops (15). The UES is responsive to infusion of solutions in the esophagus and has been shown to react to the presence of acid. Gerhardt and co-workers (3) studied nine normal subjects, infusing different solutions in the esophagus. When 0.1 normal HCl was infused in the upper esophagus, high UES pressures were produced when compared with infusion of normal saline. Additionally, an increase in the rate of infusion resulted in

Rare complications of Zenker's diverticulum have been described. Hendren and co-workers (21) reported massive bleeding in a diverticulum. Obstruction and tracheodiverticular fistula are rare. Isolated cases of squamous cell carcinoma associated with Zenker's diverticulum have been reported (22,23).

In large series, the occurrence of carcinoma appears to be low; at the Mayo Clinic over a 53-year period, cancer was found in only 0.4% of 1,249 patients (24). The diagnosis of cancer is rarely made clinically and is suspected usually because of a defect seen on x-ray film (22). Most patients with carcinoma report additional symptoms, such as weight loss and increasingly worsening dysphagia. Cancer appears to be more frequent in men and in longstanding cases. Because of the long period of time between the discovery of a diverticulum and the occurrence of a carcinoma, it is speculated that cancer results from chronic irritation and inflammation of the diverticulum as a result of stasis. The frequency of carcinoma arising in Zenker's diverticulum has been less frequent in recent years, perhaps because of earlier diagnosis and treatment. Bowdler and Stell (23) reviewed this issue in 1987, finding only 38 cases in the English literature. Most of the cancers in these reports were squamous cell carcinoma, with an occasional basal cell or spindle cell carcinoma. Bradley and colleagues (25) reviewed 91 cases of Zenker's diverticulum seen over a period of 15 years and found two cases of squamous cell carcinoma and two of carcinoma *in situ*. In three of the cases, the cancer was not found until histologic examination was performed after diverticulectomy. Because the authors believe that malignant transformation results from chronic irritation, they advocate excision of the pouch in patients younger than 65 years in an attempt to avoid progression to cancer. Overall, the frequency of carcinoma arising in Zenker's diverticulum is not high enough to constitute by itself justification for surgery. From a practical standpoint, the decision to treat is based on the severity of symptoms.

Diagnosis

A barium esophagram with special attention to the oropharyngeal phase of swallowing is the best diagnostic test for Zenker's diverticulum. Small diverticula may be missed, but careful evaluation with lateral and oblique views detect even small pouches. The diverticulum protrudes posteriorly, and barium tends to fall into the pouch before progressing into the esophagus *(Fig. 16.3)*. In the case of a very small diverticulum, the sac may be visible only during the phase of UES contraction and not during relaxation. Some authors have tried to classify Zenker's diverticula in stages or categories based on the size and shape of the diverticulum as well as the presence during contraction or relaxation of the UES. Ponette and Coolen (26) reviewed 143 cases of diverticula and attempted to relate the morphology of the pouch to upper sphincter function. These efforts to grade Zenker's diverticula based on shape and size result from the fact that barium studies sometimes reveal a temporary posterior

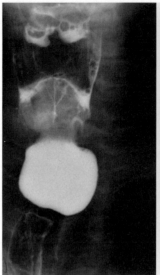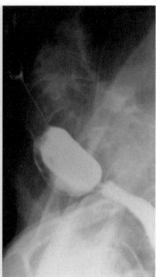

FIGURE 16.3. Zenker's diverticulum, anteroposterior and lateral views.

bulge at the level of or just above the UES. The bulge is not large enough and consistent enough through the study to be referred to as a diverticulum, and terms such as *transient diverticulum* and *early diverticulum* have been used (2). Whether such changes represent a diverticulum or a manifestation of a cricopharyngeal bar that can be seen in association with a diverticulum (Fig. 16.4) or simply a trivial phenomenon is unknown. At any rate, such observations are of limited clinical importance and one must be guided by the patient's complaints. It is doubtful that a transient posterior bulge would cause significant throat symptoms, and if dysphagia is truly present, a more careful evaluation of the entire esophagus must be undertaken.

There is an area of weakness, distinct from Killian's triangle, located just below the cricopharyngeal muscle called the Killian-Jamieson space (27). Protrusions through this area of weakness are rare, but when they occur, they may be confused with a Zenker's diverticulum. However, a Killian-Jamieson diverticulum arises from the lateral wall, below the UES, and tends to be small (Fig. 16.5). Patients with Killian-Jamieson pouches are usually asymptomatic. Rubesin and Levin (28) found that 3 of 16 patients with Killian-Jamieson diverticulum had symptoms; two had dysphagia and one had cough. In contrast, 19 of 26 patients with Zenker's diverticulum had symptoms.

Endoscopy adds little to the evaluation of pharyngoesophageal pouches. If it has to be performed for other reasons, caution should be exercised to not enter the diverticulum and risk a perforation (29). A large diverticulum may make esophageal intubation difficult. Sometimes a guidewire must be passed into the stomach under fluoroscopy with the endoscope then carefully passed over the guidewire.

Manometric testing of UES function has been recently refined, and accurate measurements with analysis of various phases of deglutition are possible (30). However, the tech-

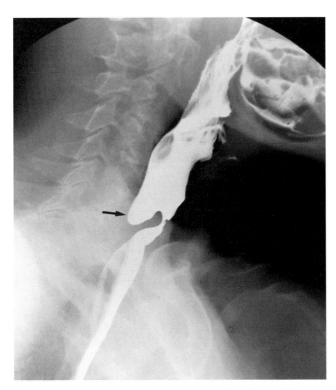

FIGURE 16.4. Marked cricopharyngeal indentation with a posterial bulge *(arrow)*, most likely representing a Zenker's diverticulum.

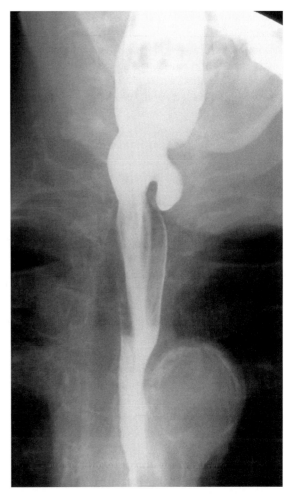

FIGURE 16.5. Killian-Jamieson diverticulum. The pouch arises from the lateral esophageal wall below the upper esophageal sphincter.

nique is of little value in the management of patients. Furthermore, manometry may be difficult to perform because the manometric catheter tends to coil in the diverticulum. There have been reports of low resting pressure of the sphincter (9,31) as well as normal basal pressures (10) in patients with Zenker's diverticulum. The finding of cricopharyngeal incoordination is inconsistent, as discussed in the section on pathogenesis. Manometric testing of the cricopharyngeal area should be reserved for clinical research and is not necessary in evaluating patients with pharyngeal pouches (32).

Treatment

Small Zenker's diverticula discovered by chance do not require any intervention and may be followed by periodic esophagrams. When needed, the only effective treatment of Zenker's diverticulum is surgical. Surgical techniques include, separately or in combination, diverticulopexy, diverticulectomy, and cricopharyngeal myotomy. Endoscopic treatment is emerging as an alternative to open surgery.

In the early 1900s, diverticulopexy became popular because attempts to excise the diverticulum in the 1800s were not encouraging. In diverticulopexy, the fundus of the diverticulum is attached high up in the neck to the prevertebral fascia after being dissected from surrounding tissues. By attaching the fundus of the diverticulum high in the neck, drainage is allowed to occur. A two-stage operation was also developed in which the diverticulum was ligated and an ostomy per-

formed to allow drainage. In a second stage, the diverticulum was then resected. Various modifications to this operation were made to avoid infection and other complications. Today, diverticulopexy alone is rarely performed, whereas it is used sometimes in association with a myotomy. Diverticulectomy and myotomy, separately or together, constitute the most traditional approach to surgical treatment of Zenker's diverticulum (33). At the Mayo Clinic, a one-stage pharyngoesophageal diverticulectomy with or without myotomy produced excellent results with only a 3.6% recurrence rate (34). In an updated report in 1992, Payne (35) described his experience with more than 900 patients treated for Zenker's diverticulum. Mortality was low at 1.2%, morbidity was 8%, and the rate of recurrence was still 3.6%. In the interval between the two reports, however, the surgical technique had varied from simple diverticulectomy to diverticulectomy associated with myotomy and, in some cases, myotomy alone without resection. Additionally, a mechanical stapling device was used in some cases. Therefore, it is difficult to conclude, based on this report, what is the single best technique to treat Zenker's diverticulum. When the diverticulum recurs, reoperation presents major technical difficulties, complications are more frequent, and mortality increases to 3.2% (36).

The open surgical technique involves usually a left cervical incision. The diverticulum once identified is retracted, dissected, and eventually resected and the point of insertion either sutured or stapled. When a myotomy is performed, it is done either before (37) or after (38) the diverticulectomy. Myotomy is extramucosal, dissecting the fibers of the cricopharyngeal muscles away from the mucosa. The incision is extended 3 to 4 cm above the esophagus. Fegiz and colleagues (38) reported 15 patients with Zenker's diverticulum. Twelve were treated by resection only and three by resection and myotomy. The result was good in all three patients treated with a combined procedure. In the 12 treated by resection alone, results were good in eight and fair in three, with recurrence in one. Ellis and Crozier (39) treated ten patients, three of whom had undergone a diverticulotomy earlier. Cricopharyngeal myotomy was performed in all patients, but diverticulectomy was performed in only two and diverticulopexy in one. There were no complications and follow-up showed good results in all patients. Lerut and colleagues (12) justified the need to perform a cricopharyngeal myotomy by the pathophysiologic changes present in patients with Zenker's diverticulum. They asked two questions: Is a myotomy of the cricopharyngeus useful? How long should it be? The finding of abnormal contractility and abnormal histology led them to advocate the use of myotomy, emphasizing that the incision should be no less than 4 to 5 cm long. These authors reported 100 consecutive patients treated by myotomy and in most cases, diverticulopexy. The mean follow-up was 4 years and morbidity was minimal. Schmit and Zuckerbraun (40) performed cricopharyngeal myotomy alone under local anesthesia. Good results occurred in 70% of patients and fair results in 17%. Because of these favorable results, they concluded that the operation under local anesthesia without resecting the diverticulum was safe and effective, even though the size of the diverticulum had a mean of 3.3 cm with a range of 1 to 8 cm. Patient follow-up was conducted by telephone and direct contact was possible in only 63% of patients. Diverticulectomy with cricopharyngeal myotomy achieves good results, but the physiologic consequences of this anatomic disruption have not been rigorously analyzed. A videofluoroscopic study of 15 patients treated surgically showed that the process of swallowing becomes abnormal following surgery (41). Among the changes observed are pooling of contrast material, aspiration, and premature closure of the cricopharyngeus muscle. In this study, seven patients reported absence of symptoms after surgery, whereas six had mild residual dysphagia, one reported no difference, and one believed that the symptoms were worse than preoperatively. There was no significant difference in the number of abnormalities recorded postoperatively between asymptomatic and symptomatic patients. Shaw and co-workers (42) studied eight patients preoperatively and postoperatively and showed that cricopharyngeal myotomy normalized UES opening by reducing hypopha-

ryngeal intrabolus pressure. Zaninotto and colleagues (43) showed a significant decrease in UES resting pressure and pharyngeal intrabolus pressure after myotomy.

Open surgical treatment of Zenker's diverticulum may result in complications such as fistulae, infection, vocal cord paralysis, and aspiration (35,36,40). A technique of inversion of the diverticulum resulting in invagination rather than excision has been advocated to avoid complications (44). This technique is reserved for small diverticula and can be carried out in a short period of time. However, some authors disagree with its usefulness (45). Other technical variations have also been suggested, such as the use of myotomy, diverticulectomy, and cervical esophagostomy with a feeding tube for the ostomy and removal of the feeding tube with closure of the esophagostomy in a second stage. This operation is advocated for severely debilitated patients (46).

Zenker's diverticulum may be treated endoscopically. Reports have originated from non-U.S. centers (47). Endoscopic treatment of pharyngeal pouches was tried without success in the early 1900s. In 1960, a technique using a rigid esophagoscope with a double lip was established. The endoscope is positioned so that it rides over the bridge between the diverticulum and the esophageal lumen. This wall as well as the cricopharyngeus muscle are then transected at the same time, creating a communication between the diverticulum and the esophagus. In other words, rather than resecting or draining the diverticulum, a common cavity is created and the diverticulum drains openly into the esophagus. Van Overbeek and Hoeksema (48) from The Netherlands reported 211 cases in which a satisfactory rate of 91.5% was found with few complications. The technique may be modified by using laser treatment for transection of the ridge rather than electrocoagulation (49,50). Benjamin and Innocenti (51) treated 15 patients with a microsurgical laser procedure. A minor leak occurred in two patients only, and these responded to conservative treatment. Long-term results in this series appeared favorable, although no details were given on follow-up. Wouters and van Overbeek (52) compared their earlier experience with endoscopic electrocoagulation in 323 cases to the microendoscopic CO_2 laser treatment of 184 cases. They found the results to be comparable but thought that the laser technique produced less pain and allowed the patients to eat earlier. Another modification to the endoscopic treatment of Zenker's diverticulum involved the use of staples (53). An endoscopic stapler is used to divide the wall between the diverticulum and the esophagus, sealing the cut mucosal edges and preventing postoperative salivary leaking (54). Results of this technique appear favorable with good symptom relief and patient satisfaction (54,55). Stapling is not possible in all cases because of inability to expose the esophagus and the diverticulum simultaneously (56). Although the operative cost of endoscopic stapling diverticulectomy is comparable to that of the open technique, the overall cost is less and the hospital stay shorter (57).

It is extremely difficult to conclude from reviewing the literature which operation constitutes the best treatment for

Zenker's diverticulum. The inclusion of patients with Zenker's diverticulum as well as cricopharyngeal achalasia, neurologic disorders, and other abnormalities; the variations in technique; the use of historical controls; and the lack of consistent and objectively structured follow-up are some of the reasons for the confusion. At this point, it appears that endoscopic treatment with or without laser or stapling is gaining popularity in the United States (54,56,58). Despite the debate over the need for myotomy, most surgeons continue to perform the procedure while excising the diverticulum unless it is very small. No causal relationship has been established between gastroesophageal reflux and Zenker's diverticulum. Antireflux surgery is therefore only appropriate when reflux is symptomatic (19,59).

MIDESOPHAGEAL DIVERTICULA

Midesophageal diverticula are given this name to distinguish them from epiphrenic diverticula, which occur in the most distal part of the esophagus, and because most diverticula are found in the midportion of the esophagus.

Etiology and Pathogenesis

It is not known whether midesophageal diverticula are congenital. Most appear to develop in young and older adults. The development of esophageal diverticula in general has traditionally been explained by one of two mechanisms: traction or pulsion. This distinction was made in 1840 by Rokitansky (60). A traction diverticulum is characteristically situated in the middle third of the esophagus and is thought to develop as a result of pulling of the esophageal wall by neighboring inflammatory or scar tissue. Therefore, a traction diverticulum is a true one in that all layers of the esophagus are pulled out. A pulsion diverticulum, on the other hand, is thought to occur because of abnormal forces applied to a portion of the esophageal wall, resulting in an outpouching of mucosa through the muscle layer of the esophagus (61). Zenker's diverticulum is an example of pulsion diverticulum and so is epiphrenic diverticulum, which is discussed later. Midesophageal diverticula, based on this classification, could be of the traction or pulsion type.

Cross and co-workers (62) showed that most esophageal diverticula occur because of an area of spasm or lack of sphincter relaxation; they found motor abnormalities even in cases of isolated midthoracic diverticulum. Esophageal diverticula, which may be multiple, have been described in patients with achalasia, diffuse esophageal spasm, and other motor abnormalities (63). Schima and colleagues (64) studied 30 patients with midesophageal diverticula, some of which were considered of the pulsion type and some of the traction type. Dysphagia was present in 22 patients. Esophageal manometry was performed in only 15 patients, but by associating cinefluoroscopy and manometry, the authors found a motor abnormality in 24 of 30 patients. Evander and colleagues (65)

reported on ten patients with motor abnormalities, eight of whom had epiphrenic diverticula. The two patients with midesophageal diverticula had no abnormality in lower esophageal sphincter (LES) function but showed occasional simultaneous or repetitive contractions in the thoracic esophagus. An important study was carried out by Dodds and co-workers (66) in 1975, who attempted to determine the importance of motor abnormalities in the genesis of midesophageal diverticula. The authors purposely chose six patients who had no evidence of esophageal motor disorder by radiology and manometry. Pressures were measured by four recording ports positioned radially around the lumen. In five of six patients, the orifice facing the mouth of the diverticulum recorded a lower pressure than the other three ports. In two patients, bizarre wave forms were seen with abrupt onset or offset of the contraction, and in two others, high peristaltic pressure amplitude greater than 250 mm Hg was found in the distal half of the esophagus. The radial asymmetry at the level of the diverticulum was attributed to the presence of the diverticulum, the bizarre forms were attributed to longitudinal motion of the diverticulum during recording, and the high peristaltic pressure was thought to represent perhaps the reason leading to the diverticulum by forces pushing out the esophageal wall. This study does not prove that weakness at one point of the esophageal wall is the reason for the occurrence of diverticula because the pressure could be the result rather than the cause of the outpouching.

Clinical Features

Most midesophageal diverticula are asymptomatic (Fig. 16.6). Indeed, the diverticulum tends to be small and points upward, making food accumulation rare. In some patients, chest pain and dysphagia are reported, but these are usually present in patients who have an esophageal motor disorder. Figure 16.7 illustrates a midesophageal diverticulum in a patient with diffuse esophageal spasm.

Gastroesophageal reflux is also noted in some patients with midesophageal diverticula (64). Of the 30 patients Schima and colleagues (64) studied, five had gastroesophageal reflux.

Complications are unusual. Spontaneous rupture, exsanguination (67), aspiration (65,68), fistula formation (69), and carcinoma (70) have been reported. These complications are usually seen in patients with motor disorders or when, in the distant past, traction diverticula were associated with pulmonary tuberculosis (61). Inflammatory lymph nodes around the esophagus account for the outpouching of the tissue.

Atypical diverticula of the esophagus have been reported. Herman and McAlister (71) found diverticula in two children whose strictures had developed as a result of unsuspected foreign body ingestion. Diverticula were present above the foreign body. Saccular dilatation was reported in a patient after excision of an asymptomatic congenital cyst (72) and may also be seen postoperatively after repair of an esophageal perforation or laceration. Intraluminal diverticula, which result

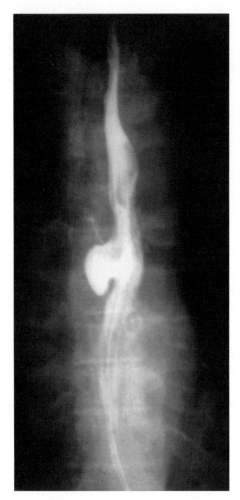

FIGURE 16.6. Small, asymptomatic midesophageal diverticulum.

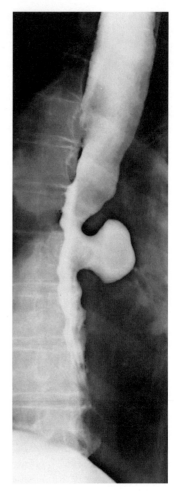

FIGURE 16.7. Midesophageal diverticulum in a patient with diffuse esophageal spasm.

in the appearance of a double esophageal lumen, are difficult to diagnose, may result in dysphagia or esophagitis, and are of unknown origin (73). Finally, in progressive systemic sclerosis, pseudodiverticula of the esophagus may develop. Clements and colleagues (74) reported five cases of unusual diverticula associated with progressive systemic sclerosis and other collagen vascular diseases. Wide-mouthed saccular pouches were seen at various levels of the esophagus. Coggins and co-workers (75) reported a similar case.

Diagnosis

Most midesophageal diverticula are discovered by chance during barium esophagram carried out for other reasons. Diverticula may be of various sizes and can be single or multiple (66,76). Figure 16.8 illustrates a case of multiple diverticula. In case of complication, radiology determines the presence of a fistula. An intraluminal diverticulum may be missed by x-ray study.

Endoscopy with today's flexible instruments is not contraindicated, but the procedure is not necessary for the diagnosis of diverticula.

Treatment

Because most midesophageal diverticula are uncomplicated and cause no symptoms, treatment is not required. If treatment becomes necessary, the procedure of choice is diverticulectomy. It is imperative, however, to rule out an associated esophageal motility disorder before contemplating surgery. If a motor disorder is present, diverticulectomy alone may be followed by a recurrence of the diverticulum and symptoms would not be relieved (77). Altorki and co-workers (68) studied 20 patients with thoracic esophageal diverticula over a 20-year period and found that 45% had dysphagia, 55% regurgitation, and 25% pulmonary symptoms. Seventeen patients agreed to the operation, with successful results. However, 18 of the 20 patients had an associated motor disorder, such as achalasia, diffuse esophageal spasm, Zenker's diverticulum, and other nonspecific disorders.

Surgery is rarely necessary for midesophageal diverticula and, when indicated, is dictated by the presence of a motor abnormality or a complication (70). Diverticulectomy with or without myotomy is the treatment of choice (60,77). Some surgeons add a fundoplication (65,70).

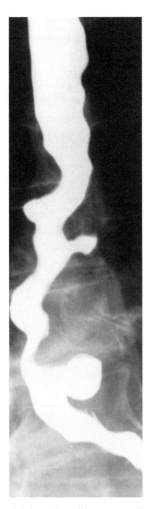

FIGURE 16.8. Multiple mid and lower esophageal diverticula.

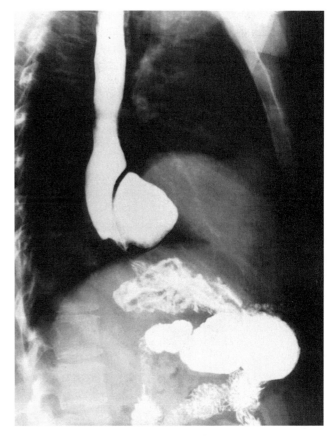

FIGURE 16.9. Epiphrenic diverticulum.

EPIPHRENIC DIVERTICULA

As the name indicates, epiphrenic diverticula arise near the diaphragm *(Fig. 16.9)*. However, the epiphrenic segment of the esophagus has been defined by some as the distal 4 cm, by others as 10 cm, and even by others as the distal one third of the esophagus (78). Most authors reserve the term *epiphrenic diverticulum* for those occurring in the distal 3 to 4 cm of the esophagus.

Etiology and Pathogenesis

The issue of traction and pulsion diverticulum was discussed earlier. For a long time, epiphrenic diverticula were thought to be of the pulsion type and were therefore labeled as pseudodiverticula. Such considerations have little clinical relevance. The important issue is that epiphrenic diverticula are almost always the result of an esophageal motor abnormality, such as incoordination between the distal esophagus and the LES, or a more diffuse abnormality, such as achalasia or diffuse esophageal spasm.

The strong association between epiphrenic diverticula and motor abnormalities of the esophagus was noted even in early reports. Bruggeman and Seaman (78) reported a motor abnormality in 48% of cases. It is probable that the proportion would have been higher had a method other than x-ray study been used. In the same series, all patients with a diverticulum larger than 5 cm were found to have a significant abnormal motility disorder. Debas and co-workers (79) noted an abnormal motility disorder in 50 of 65 patients. This conclusion was reached based on manometry and roentgenology. However, only 36 patients had complete motility studies. In the 15 patients who did not have an abnormal motility disorder, 13 had a hiatal hernia, five of whom had severe esophageal strictures.

Clinical Features

Epiphrenic diverticula occur at all ages. The series of Bruggeman and Seaman (78) included 80 patients whose age ranged from 18 to 88 years, with 75% being between 41 and 70 years old.

Although the exact incidence of epiphrenic diverticula is not known, the condition appears to be infrequent. In 20 years, 160 patients were reported from the Mayo Clinic (80), and 80 patients were seen over a period of 18 years at the Columbia Presbyterian Medical Center (78). The frequency is estimated to be 20% that of Zenker's diverticulum (81).

Patients with epiphrenic diverticula may be totally asymptomatic. Small diverticula may be discovered during an incidental roentgenographic examination. There appears to be no correlation between symptoms and size of the diverticulum. The presence and the severity of symptoms depend on the associated motor abnormality. It is imperative in patients with epiphrenic diverticula to obtain manometric studies to rule out a motility disorder. The most frequent abnormalities are achalasia and diffuse spasm (78,79,82), but other nonspecific abnormalities have been described as well (83). Chest pain and regurgitation may also be presenting symptoms, particularly in giant diverticula (84). Acute esophageal obstruction from food accumulating in the epiphrenic diverticulum has been reported (85). Other complications are similar to those seen in midesophageal diverticula, such as perforation, fistula formation, and a rare case of carcinoma (86,87).

Diagnosis

An epiphrenic diverticulum is easily diagnosed on a barium roentgenogram. Multiple views should be obtained in different positions to evaluate the size of the diverticulum and the site of its mouth. A videoesophagram is helpful in subtle cases for identifying a motor abnormality. In patients with achalasia, the esophagus is tortuous and more than one diverticulum may be seen (Fig. 16.10). On computed tomography, a diverticulum appears as a thin-walled or air-fluid–filled structure if an obstruction or motor disorder exists. The images may be confused with those of an abscess, a tumor, or a hiatal hernia (88).

Endoscopy, although not necessary, is helpful in diagnosing complications and esophageal inflammation. The procedure should be performed cautiously so that the endoscope does not inadvertently enter the cavity of the diverticulum.

Manometric studies are important to establish the presence of an associated motor abnormality. Usually, the area of the diverticulum reveals low, poorly transmitted, or simultaneous contractions. Whether these changes are the result or the cause of the diverticulum is not known. Attention, therefore, should be given to the pressures and relaxation of the LES and abnormalities in peristalsis throughout the entire esophagus.

Treatment

Small, asymptomatic epiphrenic diverticula probably do not require any treatment. However, the search for an associated motor abnormality should be carried out with the same intensity as in a symptomatic patient with a large diverticulum.

The goal of therapy should be to treat the motor disorder with the hope of avoiding further enlargement of the diverticulum (Fig. 16.11). The traditional treatment of an epiphrenic diverticulum consists of diverticulectomy alone or with myotomy (80,81,82,89). Surgical results are

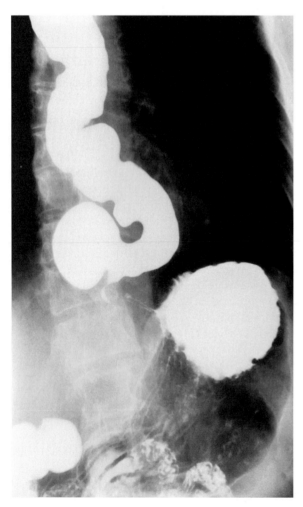

FIGURE 16.10. Epiphrenic diverticulum in a patient with achalasia. The esophagus is dilated and tortuous; other sacculations are seen.

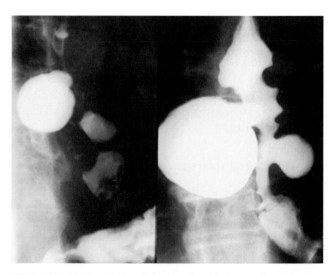

FIGURE 16.11. Multiple epiphrenic diverticula are shown in two barium esophagograms obtained 3 years apart in a 76-year-old man with solid-food dysphagia. The patient refused surgery at the time of the earlier study (*left*). Note the progressive enlargement of the diverticula, which correlated with the patient's worsening symptoms.

reported by most authors to be excellent, but little information is available about long-term follow-up. Hudspeth and co-workers (89) treated nine patients surgically and reported a follow-up of 94%, ranging from 3 months to 12 years, with good to excellent results in all patients as measured by symptom relief, weight gain, and absence of clinical recurrence. No details are given about radiographic appearance. On the other hand, Benacci and colleagues (81) operated on 33 patients, half of whom at least had had an associated motor disorder and had a follow-up in 29 patients ranging from 4 months to 15 years. The long-term results were good, but there were three operative deaths (9%) and an esophageal leak in 18%. All patients who showed an esophageal leak had had a diverticulectomy. In a related editorial, Orringer (90) pointed out the risks associated with surgical treatment of epiphrenic diverticula and discussed the need to perform antireflux surgery in many patients. Diverticulectomy with myotomy in all patients is advocated by Mulder and co-workers (91). Chami and colleagues (92) treated a patient successfully by transhiatal laparoscopic approach.

It is difficult to assess the proper surgical technique for epiphrenic diverticula. Surgical series include a large proportion of patients with esophageal motor abnormalities. Some patients have been studied with manometry and many have not. It is not clear whether a diverticulectomy is necessary. Most authors agree that a diverticulectomy alone would result in a recurrence and advocate a long esophagomyotomy. The choice of operation should be based on the underlying disorder. For instance, in the case of a large, tortuous esophagus with esophageal sacculations resulting from achalasia, the addition of a diverticulectomy to myotomy would make no difference. If myotomy is not successful, esophagectomy should be considered. DeVault (93) treated three elderly patients by injecting botulinum toxin in the area distal to the diverticulum in a manner and with a dose similar to those used in achalasia. All patients reported improvement but follow-up information is given only for one with sustained benefit over 6 months.

Pneumatic dilation for achalasia has been considered dangerous when an epiphrenic diverticulum is present because of a possibly increased risk of perforation. This concern, however, is not based on any evidence. The presence of diverticula should not be a deterrent to pneumatic dilation if the procedure is carried out with the usual precautions and under fluoroscopic control. We have performed pneumatic dilation in a few patients with lower esophageal diverticular deformities without complications.

ESOPHAGEAL INTRAMURAL PSEUDODIVERTICULOSIS

Esophageal intramural pseudodiverticulosis is characterized by numerous minute, flasklike outpouchings along the esophageal wall.

Etiology and Pathogenesis

Mendl and colleagues (94) described the condition as intramural diverticulosis resulting from herniation of the mucosa through gaps in the muscularis as a result of increased pressure. They likened the condition to the gallbladder sinuses of Rokitansky-Aschoff. Later studies using biopsy material and autopsy specimens revealed cystic dilatation of the esophageal gland ducts. The condition was thought to represent multiple mucous cysts of the submucosa, but because these pouches communicate with the lumen, the term *cyst* is not appropriate and the name *intramural pseudodiverticulosis* is accurate (95). Hammon and co-workers (96) thought that the submucosal glands get impacted with inflammatory material secondary to stasis and suggested the term *esophageal adenitis*. Others thought that the pseudocystic dilatations were an exaggeration of normal anatomy, that is, dilated glandular ducts (97). Umlas and Sakhuja (98), studying carefully an esophagus obtained at autopsy, found thickening of the esophageal wall caused by submucosal fibrosis at the level of a stricture, and the diverticular structures represented main excretory ducts of the submucosal glands rather than the glands themselves. Medeiros and colleagues (99), who described two similar cases, proceeded to study 100 esophageal specimens collected during past autopsies as well as 20 cases obtained prospectively, in which sections were collected from various locations. The results of this study showed that, in the random specimens obtained retrospectively, dilated excretory ducts were found in 14% of cases and cysts in 7%. Comparatively, in the prospective study, 55% of specimens revealed dilated ducts and 15% cysts. In both groups, chronic inflammation was found in 65% to 67%. Additionally, cysts were found only in patients older than age 40 years . From these findings, Medeiros and colleagues (99) concluded that the pathogenesis of intramural pseudodiverticulosis is extensive chronic inflammation leading to dilated ducts, which in time develop small cysts and, when the cysts become large enough, possibly decreased inflammation. They also pointed out that early changes of intramural pseudodiverticulosis were more common than described.

The frequent association of strictures in patients with pseudodiverticulosis and the frequent occurrence of pseudodiverticula above the stricture have been used as an argument to attribute the cause of the disorder to motor abnormalities. Various motor abnormalities have been described in these patients. Hammon and colleagues (96) found nonperistaltic contractions in two of three patients, and others have described nonspecific motility abnormalities (100). One patient was reported with changes consistent with nutcracker esophagus (101), but esophageal motility may be normal in some cases (96,97).

Clinical Features

Intramural pseudodiverticulosis is a relatively rare condition. The exact prevalence is not known. In two large radiologic studies, it was present respectively in 0.09% (102) and 0.15% (103) of patients undergoing evaluation for a variety of conditions. Overall, less than 200 cases have been reported in the English literature (104).

The condition is found in both sexes. Most cases are discovered in the sixth and seventh decades, but a few cases have been reported in children and infants (105).

Patients with intramural pseudodiverticulosis present almost always with dysphagia (95,96,106). Dysphagia usually occurs with solid foods and may be abrupt (107). Bleeding from an associated weblike stricture has been reported in one case (108). Spontaneous perforation after vomiting was the presenting manifestation of pseudodiverticulosis with stricture in another one (109).

When a stricture is associated with pseudodiverticulosis, it is most often proximal. In that case, pseudodiverticula occur above the stricture.

Other conditions have been described in association with intramural pseudodiverticulosis. Candidiasis is frequent and present in about 50% of cases. The presence of monilia may be attributed to stasis, which is quite frequent in cases of pseudodiverticulosis and does not seem to be the cause of the disease, even though chronic candidiasis may cause chronic esophageal inflammation (96,100,101).

Kochhar and co-workers (110) studied 59 patients with sequelae of corrosive acid injury and found 14 patients with esophageal intramural pseudodiverticulosis. The association with motor abnormalities is discussed earlier. Pseudodiverticulosis was described in a case of achalasia (111). Plavsic and colleagues (102) reviewed the esophagrams of 245 patients with carcinoma of the esophagus and compared them with 6,400 roentgenograms obtained for other reasons. They found intramural pseudodiverticulosis in 4.5% of patients with cancer compared with 0.09% in the control group. They concluded that there may be an increased risk of carcinoma in pseudodiverticulosis and stated that periodic surveillance for carcinoma may be worthwhile in patients with intramural pseudodiverticulosis. The coexistence of carcinoma and pseudodiverticulosis does not indicate a cause-and-effect relationship. Indeed, it is possible that pseudodiverticulosis is simply the result of stasis caused by obstruction from the carcinoma just as it is observed in benign strictures. There is no evidence that intramural pseudodiverticulosis constitutes a risk for cancer, and surveillance should not be recommended.

Diagnosis

The diagnosis of esophageal intramural pseudodiverticulosis is usually made on a barium esophagram. The pouches are small, varying in length from 1 to 6 mm and usually less than 4 mm wide (110). The neck of each diverticulum rarely measures more than 1 mm. The pouches are best seen when a double air contrast technique is performed (102). Pseudodiverticulosis may be diffuse or segmental (98,107, 112,113) (Figs. 16.12 and 16.13).

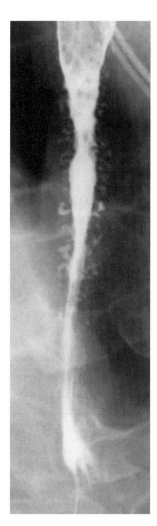

FIGURE 16.12. Segmental intramural pseudodiverticulosis.

Pseudodiverticulosis is not always recognized during endoscopy, but visualization of pinpoint openings in the esophageal wall is easier since the advent of fiberoptic endoscopy (106,114,115).

Pearlberg and colleagues (116) described the computed tomographic (CT) features of esophageal intramural pseudodiverticulosis in one patient. They found marked thickening of the esophageal wall and loss of normal soft tissue planes with small intramural gas collections. The loss of soft tissue planes raised the question of malignancy, leading to a repeat endoscopy and biopsies, which never confirmed the presence of a malignancy.

CT scanning does not seem to contribute to the diagnosis of pseudodiverticulosis and may create confusion in some cases. CT scans have been reported as normal (114) or showing thickening of the esophageal wall (115). Devereaux and Savides (117) recommend the use of endoscopic ultrasound to elucidate the nature of esophageal wall thickening based on experience with one case. Ultrasound revealed thickening of the mucosal and submucosal layers with normal muscular propria and no adenopathy.

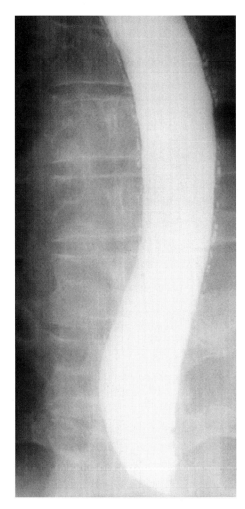

FIGURE 16.13. Diffuse intramural pseudodiverticulosis.

Esophageal manometry is indicated only in cases in which a stricture is not present and when the radiographs suggest other abnormalities in the esophagus.

Treatment

Intramural pseudodiverticulosis responds to esophageal dilatation with relief of symptoms for a few years (1–4,106). Some patients may require periodic dilatations (106).

Medical treatment of candidiasis when present is appropriate and results in improvement (118) but is not always necessary (100). In pseudodiverticulosis, treatment aims at relieving obstructive symptoms.

REFERENCES

1. Ekberg O, Mylander G. Cineradiography of the pharyngeal phase of deglutition in 250 patients with dysphagia. *Br J Radiol* 1982;55:258–262.
2. Watemberg S, Landau O, Avrahami R. Zenker's diverticulum: reappraisal. *Am J Gastroenterol* 1996;91:1494–1498.
3. Gerhardt DC, Shuck TJ, Bordeaux RA, et al. Human upper esophageal sphincter. *Gastroenterology* 1978;75:268–274.
4. Kahrilas PJ, Dodds WJ, Dent J, et al. Upper esophageal sphincter function during deglutition. *Gastroenterology* 1988;95: 52–62.
5. Ellis FH, Schlegel JF, Lynch VP, et al. Cricopharyngeal myotomy for pharyngoesophageal diverticulitis. *Ann Surg* 1969; 170:340–349.
6. Asherson N. Achalasia of the cricopharyngeal sphincter: a record of cases, with profile pharyngograms. *J Laryngol Otol* 1950;64:747–758.
7. Sutherland HD. Cricopharyngeal achalasia. *J Thoracic Cardiovascular Surg* 1962;43:114–126.
8. Nilsson ME, Isberg A, Schiratzki H. The hypopharyngeal diverticulum. *Acta Otolaryngol* 1988;106:314–320.
9. Knuff TE, Benjamin SB, Castell DO. Pharyngoesophageal (Zenker's) diverticulum: a reappraisal. *Gastroenterology* 1982; 82:734–736.
10. Cook IJ, Gabb M, Panagopoulos V, et al. Pharyngeal (Zenker's) diverticulum is a disorder of upper esophageal sphincter opening. *Gastroenterology* 1992;103:1229–1235.
11. Cook IJ, Blumbergs P, Cash K, et al. Structural abnormalities of the cricopharyngeus muscle in patients with pharyngeal (Zenker's) diverticulum. *J Gastroenterol Hepatol* 1992;7: 556–562.
12. Lerut T, van Raemdonck D, Guelinckx P, et al. Zenker's diverticulum: is a myotomy of the cricopharyngeus useful? How long should it be? *Hepatogastroenterology* 1992;39:127–131.
13. Dantas RO, Cook IJ, Dodds WJ, et al. Biomechanics of cricopharyngeal bars. *Gastroenterology* 1990;99:1269–1274.
14. McConnel FMS, Hood D, Jackson K, et al. Analysis of intrabolus forces in patients with Zenker's diverticulum. *Laryngoscope* 1994;104:1571–1581.
15. Hunt PS, Connell AM, Smiley TB. The cricopharyngeal sphincter in gastric reflux. *Gut* 1970;11:303–306.
16. Vakil NB, Kahrilas PJ, Dodds WJ, et al. Absence of an upper esophageal sphincter response to acid reflux. *Am J Gastroenterol* 1989;84:606–610.
17. Gage-White L. Incidence of Zenker's diverticulum with hiatus hernia. *Laryngoscope* 1988;98:527–530.
18. Resouly A, Braat J, Jackson A, et al. Pharyngeal pouch: link with reflux and oesophageal dysmotility. *Clin Otolaryngol* 1994; 19:241–242.
19. Fuessner H, Siewert JR. Zenker's diverticulum and reflux. *Hepatogastroenterology* 1992;39:100–104.
20. Welsh GF, Payne WS. The present status of one-stage pharyngoesophageal diverticulectomy. *Surg Clin North Am* 1973;53: 953–958.
21. Hendren WG, Anderson T, Miller JI. Massive bleeding in a Zenker's diverticulum. *South Med J* 1990;83:362.
22. Johnson JT, Curtin HD. Carcinoma associated with Zenker's diverticulum. *Ann Otol Rhinol Laryngol* 1985;94(3): 324–325.
23. Bowdler DA, Stell PM. Carcinoma arising in posterior pharyngeal pulsion diverticulum (Zenker's diverticulum). *Br J Surg* 1987;74:561–563.
24. Huang B, Unni KK, Payne WS. Long-term survival following diverticulectomy for cancer in pharyngoesophageal (Zenker's) diverticulum. *Ann Thorac Surg* 1984;38:207–210.
25. Bradley PJ, Kochaar A, Quraishi MS. Pharyngeal pouch carcinoma: real or imaginary risks? *Ann Otol Rhinol Laryngol* 1999; 108:1027–1032.
26. Ponette E, Coolen J. Radiological aspects of Zenker's diverticulum. *Hepatogastroenterology* 1992;39:115–122.
27. Rubesin SE, Yousem DM. Structural Abnormalities. In: Gore RM, Levine MS, Laufer I, eds. *Textbook of gastrointestinal radiology*. Philadelphia: WB Saunders, 1994:244–276.

28. Rubesin SE, Levine MS. Killian-Jamieson Diverticula: radiographic findings in 16 patients. *Am J Roentgenol* 2001;177: 85–89.

29. Duranceau A. Oropharyngeal dysphagia and disorders of the upper esophageal sphincter. *Ann Chir Gynaecol* 1995;84: 225–233.

30. Castell JA, Dalton BC, Castell DO. Pharyngeal and upper esophageal sphincter manometry in humans. *Am J Physiol* 1990; 258:G173–G178.

31. Migliore M, Payne H, Jeyasingham K. Pathophysiologic basis for operation on Zenker's diverticulum. *Ann Thorac Surg* 1994; 57:1616–1621.

32. Fulp SR, Castell DO. Manometric aspects of Zenker's diverticulum. *Hepatogastroenterology* 1992;39:123–126.

33. Grégoire J, Duranceau A. Surgical management of Zenker's diverticulum. *Hepatogastroenterology* 1991;39:132–138.

34. Payne WS, Reynolds RR. Surgical treatment of pharyngoesophageal diverticulum (Zenker's diverticulum). *Surg Rounds* 1982;5(6):18–24.

35. Payne WS. The treatment of pharyngoesophageal diverticulum: The simple and complex. *Hepatogastroenterology* 1992;39: 109–114.

36. Huang B, Payne WS, Cameron AJ. Surgical management for recurrent pharyngoesophageal (Zenker's) diverticulum. *Ann Thoracic Surg* 1984;37:189–191.

37. Brouillette D, Martel E, Chen LQ, et al. Pitfalls and complications of cricopharyngeal myotomy. *Chest Surg Clin North Am* 1997;7:457–475.

38. Fegiz G, Paolini A, DeMarchi C, et al. Surgical management of esophageal diverticula. *World J Surg* 1984;8:757–765.

39. Ellis FH, Crozier RE. Cervical esophageal dysphagia: indications for and results of cricopharyngeal myotomy. *Ann Surg* 1981;194:279–289.

40. Schmit PJ, Zuckerbraun L. Treatment of Zenker's diverticula by cricopharyngeus myotomy under local anesthesia. *Am Surg* 1992;58:710–716.

41. Zeitoun H, Widdowson D, Hammad Z, et al. A video-fluoroscopic study of patients treated by diverticulectomy and cricopharyngeal myotomy. *Clin Otolaryngol* 1994;19:301–305.

42. Shaw DW, Cook IJ, Jamieson GG, et al. Influence of surgery on deglutitive upper oesophageal sphincter mechanics in Zenker's diverticulum. *Gut* 1996;38:806–811.

43. Zaninotto M, Costantini M, Boccu C, et al. Functional and morphological study of the cricopharyngeal muscle in patients with Zenker's diverticulum. *Br J Surg* 1996;83:1263–1267.

44. Morton RP, Bartley JRF. Inversion of Zenker's diverticulum: the preferred option. *Head Neck* 1993;15:253–256.

45. Banerjee AJ, Westmore GA. Letter to the editor. Inversion of Zenker's diverticulum. *Head Neck* 1994;16:291–292.

46. Louie HW, Zuckerbraun L. Staged Zenker's diverticulectomy with cervical esophagostomy and secondary esophagostomy closure for treatment of massive diverticulum in severely debilitated patients. *Am Surg* 1993;12:842–845.

47. van Overbeek JJM. Meditation on the pathogenesis of hypopharyngeal (Zenker's) diverticulum and a report of endoscopic treatment in 545 patients. *Ann Otol Rhinol Laryngol* 1994;103:178–185.

48. van Overbeek JJM, Hoeksema PE. Endoscopic treatment of the hypopharyngeal diverticulum: 211 cases. *Laryngoscope* 1982;92: 88–91.

49. Mahieu HF, deBree R, Dagli SA, et al. The pharyngoesophageal segment: endoscopic treatment of Zenker's diverticulum. *Dis Esophagus* 1996;9:12–21.

50. Nyrop M, Svendstrup F, Jorgensen KE. Endoscopic CO_2 laser therapy of Zenker's diverticulum—experience from 61 patients. *Acta Otolaryngol* 2000;(Suppl 543):232–234.

51. Benjamin B, Innocenti M. Laser treatment of pharyngeal pouch. *Aust N Z J Surg* 1991;61:909–913.

52. Wouters B, van Overbeek JJM. Endoscopic treatment of the hypopharyngeal (Zenker's) diverticulum. *Hepatogastroenterology* 1992;39:105–108.

53. Collard JM, Otte JB, Kestens PJ. Endoscopic stapling technique of esophagodiverticulostomy for Zenker's diverticulum. *Ann Thorac Surg* 1993;56:573–576.

54. Scher RL, Richtsmeier WJ. Long-term experience with endoscopic staple-assisted esophagodiverticulostomy for Zenker's diverticulum. *Laryngoscope* 1998;108:200–205.

55. Stoeckli SJ, Schmid S. Endoscopic stapler-assisted diverticuloesophagostomy for Zenker's diverticulum: Patient satisfaction and subjective relief of symptoms. *Surgery* 2002;131:158–162.

56. Thaler ER, Weber RS, Goldberg AN, et al. Feasibility and outcome of endoscopic staple-assisted esophagodiverticulostomy for Zenker's diverticulum. *Laryngoscope* 2001;111: 1506–1508.

57. Smith SR, Genden EM, Urken ML. Endoscopic stapling technique for the treatment of Zenker diverticulum vs standard open-neck technique. *Arch Otolaryngol Head Neck Surg* 2002; 128:141–144.

58. Adams J, Sheppard B, Andersen P, et al. Zenker's diverticulostomy with cricopharyngeal myotomy. *Surg Endosc* 2001;15: 34–37.

59. Duda M, Sery Z, Vojacek K, et al. Etiopathogenesis and classification of esophageal diverticula. *Int Surg* 1985;70:291–295.

60. Harrington SW. The surgical treatment of pulsion diverticula of the thoracic esophagus. *Ann Surg* 1949;129:606–618.

61. Case records of the Massachusetts General Hospital Weekly clinicopathological exercises. Case 7-1977. *N Engl J Med* 1977;296:384–389.

62. Cross FS, Johnson GF, Gerein AN. Esophageal diverticula. Associated neuromuscular changes in the esophagus. *Arch Surg* 1961;83:525–533.

63. Case records of the Massachusetts General Hospital. Weekly clinicopathological exercises. Case 32-1982. *N Engl J Med* 1982;307:426–433.

64. Schima W, Schober E, Stacher G, et al. Association of midoesophageal diverticula with oesophageal motor disorders. *Acta Radiol* 1997;38:108–114.

65. Evander A, Little AG, Ferguson MK, et al. Diverticula of the mid- and lower esophagus: pathogenesis and surgical management. *World J Surg* 1986;10:820–828.

66. Dodds WJ, Stef JJ, Hogan WJ, et al. Radial distribution of esophageal peristaltic pressure in normal subjects and patients with esophageal diverticulum. *Gastroenterology* 1975;69:584–590.

67. Schick A, Yesner R. Traction diverticulum of esophagus with exsanguination: report of a case. *Ann Intern Med* 1953;39: 345–349.

68. Altorki NK, Sunagawa M, Skinner DB. Thoracic esophageal diverticula. Why is operation necessary? *J Thorac Cardiovasc Surg* 1993;105:260–264.

69. Balthazar EJ. Esophagobronchial fistula secondary to ruptured traction diverticulum. *Gastrointest Radiol* 1977;2:119–121.

70. Fekete F, Vonns C. Surgical management of esophageal thoracic diverticula. *Hepatogastroenterology* 1992;39:97–99.

71. Herman TE, McAlister WH. Esophageal diverticula in childhood associated with strictures from unsuspected foreign bodies of the esophagus. *Pediatr Radiol* 1991;21:410–412.

72. Mahajan RJ, Marshall JB. Severe dysphagia, dysmotility, and unusual saccular dilation (diverticulum) of the esophagus following excision of an asymptomatic congenital cyst. *Am J Gastroenterol* 1996;91:1254–1258.

73. Schreiber MH, Davis M. Intraluminal diverticulum of the esophagus. *Am J Roentgenol* 1977;129:595–597.

74. Clements JL, Abernathy J, Weens HS. Atypical esophageal diverticula associated with progressive systemic sclerosis. *Gastrointest Radiol* 1978;3:383–386.

75. Coggins CA, Levine MS, Kesack CD, et al. Wide-mouthed sacculations in the esophagus: a radiographic finding in scleroderma. *Am J Roentgenol* 2001;176:953–954.

76. Jancu J, Marvan H. Multiple diverticula of the esophagus. *Am J Gastroenterol* 1973;60:408–409.

77. Ferraro P, Duranceau A. Esophageal diverticula. *Chest Surg Clin North Am* 1994;4:741–767.

78. Bruggeman LL, Seaman WB. Epiphrenic diverticula. An analysis of 80 cases. *Am J Roentgenol* 1973;119:266–276.

79. Debas HT, Payne WS, Cameron AJ, et al. Physiopathology of lower esophageal diverticulum and its implications for treatment. *Surg Gynecol Obstet* 1980;151:593–600.

80. Allen TH, Clagett OT. Changing concepts in the surgical treatment of pulsion diverticula of the lower esophagus. *J Thorac Cardiovasc Surg* 1965;50:455–462.

81. Benacci JC, Deschamps C, Trastek VF, et al. Epiphrenic diverticulum: results of surgical treatment. *Ann Thorac Surg* 1993;55:1109–1114.

82. Falk G. Regurgitation in a patient with an esophageal diverticulum. *Cleve Clin J Med* 1994;61:409–411.

83. Hurwitz AL, Way LW, Haddad JK. Epiphrenic diverticulum in association with an unusual motility disturbance: report of surgical correction. *Gastroenterology* 1975;68:795–798.

84. Conrad C, Nissen F. Giant epiphrenic diverticula. *Eur J Radiol* 1982;2:48–49.

85. Niv Y, Fraser G, Krugliak P. Gastroesophageal obstruction from food in an epiphrenic esophageal diverticulum. *J Clin Gastroenterol* 1993;16:314–316.

86. Schultz SC, Byrne DM, Cunzol DW, et al. Carcinoma arising within epiphrenic diverticula. A report of two cases and review of the literature. *J Cardiovasc Surg* 1996;37:649–651.

87. Guerra JM, Zull M, García I, et al. Epiphrenic diverticula, esophageal carcinoma and esophagopleural fistula. *Hepatogastroenterology* 2001;48:718–719.

88. Kim KW, Berkmen YM, Auh YH, et al. Diagnosis of epiphrenic esophageal diverticulum by computed tomography. *J Comput Tomogr* 1988;12:25–28.

89. Hudspeth DA, Thorne MT, Conroy R, et al. Management of epiphrenic esophageal diverticula. A fifteen-year experience. *Am Surg* 1993;59:40–42.

90. Orringer MB. Epiphrenic diverticula: fact and fable. *Ann Thorac Surg* 1993;55:1067–1068.

91. Mulder DG, Rosenkranz E, DenBesten L. Management of huge epiphrenic esophageal diverticula. *Am J Surg* 1989;157:303–307.

92. Chami Z, Fabre JM, Navarro F, et al. Abdominal laparoscopic approach for thoracic epiphrenic diverticulum. *Surg Endosc* 1999; 13:164–165.

93. DeVault KR. Dysphagia from esophageal diverticulosis responding to botulinum toxin injection. *Am J Gastroenterol* 1997;92:895–897.

94. Mendl K, McKay JM, Tanner CH. Intramural diverticulosis of the esophagus and Rokitanski-Aschoff sinuses in the gallbladder. *Br J Radiol* 1960;33:496–501.

95. Boyd RM, Bogoch A, Greig JH, et al. Esophageal intramural pseudodiverticulosis. *Radiology* 1974;113:267–270.

96. Hammon JW Jr, Rice RP, Postlethwait RW, et al. Esophageal intramural diverticulosis. *Ann Thorac Surg* 1974;17:260–267.

97. Graham DY, Goyal RK, Sparkman J, et al. Diffuse intramural esophageal diverticulosis. *Gastroenterology* 1975;68:781–785.

98. Umlas J, Sakhuja R. The pathology of esophageal intramural pseudodiverticulosis. *Am J Clin Pathol* 1976;65:314–320.

99. Medeiros LJ, Doos WG, Balogh K. Esophageal intramural pseudodiverticulosis: a report of two cases with analysis of similar, less extensive changes in "normal" autopsy esophagi. *Hum Pathol* 1988;19:928–931.

100. Castillo S, Aburashed A, Kimmelman J, et al. Diffuse intramural esophageal pseudodiverticulosis. New cases and review. *Gastroenterology* 1977;72:541–545.

101. Murney RG, Linne JH, Curtis J. High-amplitude peristaltic contractions in a patient with esophageal intramural pseudodiverticulosis. *Dig Dis Sci* 1983;28:843–847.

102. Plavisc BM, Chen MYM, Gelfand DW, et al. Intramural pseudodiverticulosis of the esophagus detected on barium esophagograms: increased prevalence in patients with esophageal carcinoma. *Am J Roentgenol* 1995;165:1381–1385.

103. Levine MS, Moolten DN, Herlinger H, et al. Esophageal intramural pseudodiverticulosis: a reevaluation. *Am J Roentgenol* 1986;147:1165–1170.

104. Herter B, Dittler HJ, Wuttge-Hannig A, et al. Intramural pseudodiverticulosis of the esophagus: a case series. *Endoscopy* 1997; 29:109–113.

105. Daud AS, O'Connor F. Oesophageal intramural pseudodiverticulosis: a cause of dysphagia in a 10-year-old boy. *Eur J Pediatr* 1997;156:530–532.

106. Mahajan SK, Warshauer DM, Bozymski EM. Esophageal intramural pseudo-diverticulosis: endoscopic and radiologic correlation. *Gastrointest Endosc* 1993;39:565–567.

107. Montgomery RD, Mendl K, Stephenson SF. Intramural diverticulosis of the oesophagus. *Thorax* 1975;30:278–284.

108. Hahne M, Schilling D, Arnold JC, et al. Esophageal intramural pseudodiverticulosis. *J Clin Gastroenterol* 2001;33(5):378–382.

109. Murakami M, Tsuchiya K, Ichikawa H, et al. Esophageal intramural pseudodiverticulosis associated with esophageal perforation. *J Gastroenterol* 2000;35:702–705.

110. Kochhar R, Mehta SK, Nagi B, et al. Corrosive acid-induced esophageal intramural pseudodiverticulosis. *Gastroenterology* 1991;13:371–375.

111. Dua KS, Stewart E, Arndorfer R, et al. Esophageal intramural pseudodiverticulosis associated with achalasia. *Am J Gastroenterol* 1996;91:1859–1860.

112. Flora KD, Gordon MD, Lieberman D, et al. Esophageal intramural pseudodiverticulosis. *Dig Dis* 1997;15:113–119.

113. Canon CL, Levine MS, Cherukuri R, et al. Intramural tracking: a feature of esophageal intramural pseudodiverticulosis. *Am J Roentgenol* 2000;175:371–374.

114. Gillessen A, Konturek J, Roos N, et al. Esophageal intramural pseudodiverticulosis: a characteristically unusual path to diagnosis. *Endoscopy* 1996;28:640.

115. van der Putten ABMM, Loffeld RJLF. Esophageal intramural pseudodiverticulosis. *Dis Esophagus* 1997;10:61–63.

116. Pearlberg JL, Sandler MA, Madrazo BL. Computed tomographic features of esophageal intramural pseudodiverticulosis. *Radiology* 1983;147:189–190.

117. Devereaux CE, Savides TJ. EUS appearance of esophageal pseudodiverticulosis. *Gastrointest Endosc* 2000;51:228–231.

118. Cantor DS, Riley TL. Intramural Pseudodiverticulosis of the esophagus. *Am J Gastroenterol* 1982;77:454–456.

FOREIGN BODIES

STANLEY B. BENJAMIN
E. CHRISTIAN NOGUERA

Foreign bodies are common in the gastrointestinal tract, and the esophagus is the place where they are most likely to cause clinical illness. Although foreign bodies in the esophagus can be iatrogenic for therapeutic indications (stents or clips), nutrition (feeding tubes) or diagnostic (manometry), ingested objects are only considered true foreign bodies when they are associated with certain clinical or radiographic presentations.

The oldest reference to the removal of an esophageal foreign body dates to 500 BC when Aesop told of a crane placing his head in the mouth of a wolf to remove a bone lodged in the wolf's esophagus during rapid consumption of his prey (1). The problem of foreign bodies in the esophagus differs from foreign bodies in other parts of the gastrointestinal tract for several reasons. The lack of a serosal layer increases the likelihood of complications arising from perforation of the esophagus. In addition, its location deep in the thorax can make foreign bodies and their possible complications difficult to identify in some clinical situations. Finally, the close proximity of the esophagus to the respiratory tract can lead to serious respiratory involvement. For all these reasons, perforation and serious complications from a foreign body are more likely to occur in the esophagus than in the rest of the gastrointestinal tract (2).

Although the true incidence of esophageal foreign bodies is not known, a recent estimate of the annual incidence of "food" impaction was 13 episodes per 100,000, making it the third most common nonbiliary endoscopic emergency in gastroenterology (3). Despite significant advances in both diagnostic and therapeutic modalities, foreign bodies continue to cause significant morbidity and mortality, with an estimated 1,500 patients dying every year in the United States (4). The management of patients with acute esophageal foreign bodies has shifted in recent years from the surgical and radiologic fields to that of gastroenterology.

Since the first reported use of a rigid esophagoscope for removing sharp foreign bodies from the esophagus in 1911 (5), perhaps the most significant advance has been the introduction in 1972 of the flexible fiberoptic endoscope for the removal of foreign bodies (6,7). Because of the wide variety of foreign bodies that can be swallowed and the multitude of unique circumstances that even the most experienced gastroenterologist can face, every foreign body should be considered a new challenge. However, the incidence of foreign bodies has declined during the last few years thanks to increased public health awareness, so most gastroenterologists are less often exposed to foreign bodies in the esophagus and therefore have limited training in their management. These changes make the management of foreign bodies one of the most difficult procedures for the endoscopist to perform.

Although 80% to 90% of ingested foreign bodies pass spontaneously and uneventfully once they have reach the stomach, 10% to 20% require endoscopic removal and a small number of patients still require surgical management (8). It is therefore important to consider every foreign body as a medical emergency because the risk of developing severe complications still exists. Some of the most common localized complications are associated with mucosal changes, including tears, ulcers, bleeding, perforation, localized edema, luminal obstruction, and respiratory compromise resulting from airway obstruction or aspirations. Proximal complications are usually considered to be those within the thoracic cavity and are a consequence of the migration of the foreign body from the esophagus, compromising different nearby organs. These include arterioesophageal fistulae (9), aortoesophageal fistulae (10), mediastinitis (11), pericarditis (12), and pericardial effusions (13). More distant complications are usually in areas of the gastrointestinal tract where the lumen narrows significantly, such as the duodenal sweep, ileocecal valve, and sigmoid colon.

The gastroenterologist should seriously consider several factors when confronted with a patient who has ingested a foreign body. These involve not only the patient's clini-

S.B. Benjamin, E.C. Noguera: Department of Gastroenterology, Georgetown University Medical Center, Washington, DC.

cal condition but also the type of foreign body presumed to have been ingested by the patient. It should be emphasized that the ultimate goal is to relieve the obstruction and symptoms without further complications. Some of the "golden rules" physicians should always consider follow:

1. Location of the foreign body
2. Type and nature of the object (blunt, sharp or pointed, toxic or nontoxic, live or dead)
3. Size of ingested material
4. Timing between ingestion and presentation (hours, days, or months)
5. Associated symptoms related either to complete esophageal obstruction (e.g., ability to manage secretions) or airway compromise
6. Number of objects involved: multiple or single
7. Stability of the foreign body: stable and uncomplicated or progressing with ongoing complications (e.g., perforations, fistulae)
8. Previous esophageal pathology or surgical disruption
9. Radiologic evidence and location of foreign body (e.g., radiolucent, already migrated from esophagus)
10. Safe retrievability with available equipment (Table 17.1)

Certainly knowledge of the nature of the ingested object allows the endoscopist to rehearse its removal outside the patient with a similar object, thus increasing the likelihood of success. Anesthesia and surgical backup should always be available, because respiratory compromise is not an infrequent scenario and vascular invasion may require surgical intervention. Postextraction complications should always be considered. These may result from either the extraction maneuver or incomplete removal of the foreign body, and close monitoring or follow-up is mandatory in every patient.

The nature of foreign bodies ingested differs significantly not only by geographic area but also by patient's age and oropharyngeal sensitivity. For example, in one series in which almost 100% of the population was Chinese, a fish-loving people who eat fish in small pieces, 84% of foreign bodies in the esophagus were fish bones (2). Most series from the pediatric population instead have reported a high number of ingested coins (14). In adults, the wearing of dentures is the most commonly associated risk factor because they compromise the tactile sensitivity of the palate and can lead to the swallowing of too large a food bolus or the swallowing of extraneous small items that may be disguised in a food bolus (15).

ANATOMIC AND PATHOPHYSIOLOGIC CONSIDERATIONS

Ingested foreign bodies can be lodged at any level of the gastrointestinal tract but most commonly become impacted in areas with fixed or dynamic narrowing that are physiologically or pathologically smaller than the object involved. This fact may explain why the esophagus is the most common site of foreign body impaction in the gastrointestinal tract, accounting for 75% of all impactions (16). The adult esophagus is a flattened hollow muscular tube with a sphincter at each end that arises proximally at the pharyngoesophageal junction (e.g., C5-6 vertebral interspace) and courses through the posterior mediastinum to end at the gastroesophageal junction (e.g., T11 level). The esophageal lumen can distend to approximately 2 cm in anteroposterior diameter and up to 3 cm in lateral diameter to accommodate a swallowed bolus. Structurally, the esophageal wall is composed of four layers: the innermost mucosa, submucosa, muscularis propria, and outermost adventitia; unlike the remainder of the gastrointestinal tract, the esophagus has no serosa. The length of the adult esophagus is variable but ranges from 18 to 26 cm (17,18). The normal esophagus has five physiologic constriction sites of narrowing: (a) the cricopharyngeal sphincter, the narrowest point of the gastrointestinal tract, which is 14 mm in diameter (C6 vertebral level), (b) the thoracic inlet (T1 vertebral level), (c) the aortic arch, which is between 15 and 17 mm (T4 vertebral level), (d) the tracheal bifurcation or left mainstem bronchus (T6 vertebral level), and (e) the hiatal narrowing or lower esophageal sphincter, which is between 16 and 19

TABLE 17.1. GOLDEN RULES TO CONSIDER BEFORE REMOVING ESOPHAGEAL FOREIGN BODIES

Location of the foreign body
   Type and nature of the object
   Size of ingested material
   Timing between ingestion and presentation
Associated symptoms related either to complete obstruction or airway compromise
   Number of objects involved
   Stability of the foreign body
   Previous esophageal pathology or surgical disruption
   Radiologic evidence and location of the foreign body
   Ability to safely retrieve the foreign body with the available equipment

mm (T10-11 vertebral level) (19,20) (Fig. 17.1). The clinician must know these critical areas of narrowing not only when predicting the areas of possible foreign body impactions but also when removing these objects endoscopically. One rarely sees problems with the ingestion of dimes (17 mm) or pennies (18 mm), rather it is larger coins, like quarters (24 mm), that lodge at the level of the cricopharyngeus or just distal to it (21). This may explain why the cervical portion of the esophagus (at the lower level of the cricopharyngeus muscle) is the most common location of impaction (2,22,23).

Because pathologic narrowing of the esophageal lumen predisposes foreign bodies to become impacted, it should be considered in every patient. Whereas congenital conditions are usually rare even in the pediatric population, acquired disease is common in adults. Webb and colleagues (21) noted that 97% of the adult population with meat impaction have esophageal disease in the distal esophagus (strictures, esophagitis, or hiatal hernia). This is supported by a more recent epidemiologic study from Longstreth and co-workers (3) in which 88% of patients had either a Schatzki's ring or peptic stricture. On the other hand,

because children usually do not have esophageal abnormalities, the use of "blind" bougienage or balloon catheter withdrawal under fluoroscopic guidance is considered by some authorities to be an appropriate option for the management of smooth foreign bodies in this population (24,25).

When considering foreign bodies in the esophagus, the size of the object relative to the lumen plays the most important role, but motility dysfunction should also be considered in patients in whom no mucosal abnormality is present. Motility dysfunction is rarely implicated as a cause of esophageal impaction and only two bezoars of the esophagus have been described in patients with achalasia (26,27).

EPIDEMIOLOGY

The type of foreign body as well as the clinical presentation of patients with esophageal foreign bodies differs significantly between the pediatric and adult populations.

The natural curiosity of children and their lack of knowledge lead them to place many types of foreign bodies inside their mouth. Inevitably some of these objects are accidentally ingested and, as previously noted by Koch and colleagues (28), 80% enter the gastrointestinal tract and only 20% the tracheobronchial tree. This fact was also noted by Webb (21); in his observations, only 7.5% of the objects entered the tracheobronchial tree (21). Children most often ingest coins, toys, safety pins, button batteries, marbles, screws, crayons, and ballpoint pen caps, whereas adults commonly tend to have problems with meat and bones (29). One study in children younger than 12 years old found that most admissions were in the months of July, August, and December, correlating these peak incidences with school vacations in the Northern Hemisphere. No significant differences were noted between gender and race (30). Coins are popular in the pediatric population and are a frequent reason for calls to poison control centers in the United States. The American Association of Poison Control Centers Database reported more than 2,800 cases in 1987 (31), and many coin ingestions are handled at home without advice from a physician or poison control center (32). The size of the coin ingested can be correlated with the age of the child. In one series of 128 pediatric patients, most pennies were ingested by children younger than 2 years of age, the peak incidence of nickel ingestion was at age 2 years, and most quarters were ingested by children 3 years of age or older. Perhaps the youngest case reported in the literature was a baby only 10 days old who had a safety pin and a button lodged in the cervical esophagus (33).

It is clear that the oral cavity plays an important role in adults with foreign bodies in the gastrointestinal tract. Most adults become more vulnerable after their seventh decade, correlating with the use of dentures. In the same study, the researchers reported that the male to female ratio was 1.7:1,

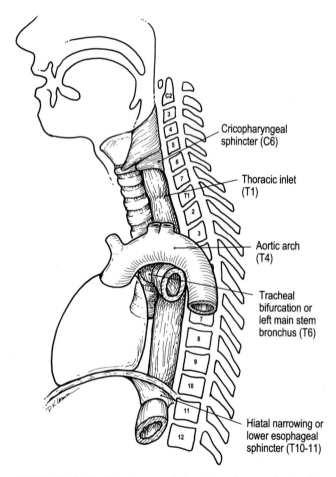

FIGURE 17.1. Physiologic constriction sites of narrowing in the normal esophagus.

and nearly half of the patients for whom body mass index was calculated were overweight, raising the possibility that the eating habits of obese patients predispose them to food impaction (3). Although esophageal impaction prompts individuals to think of esophageal narrowing, in most cases narrowing is not caused by cancer. This has been reported in different studies either documenting benign disease as the cause of impaction in the distal esophagus (3,21) or noting a very low incidence of malignancy in multiple series. In the study from Nandi and Ong (2), for example, in which 2,394 cases were reviewed in a 12-year period, only nine cases of esophageal carcinoma presented with a foreign body. This is especially surprising considering the high incidence of esophageal carcinoma in Hong Kong: their unit, in the same time period, treated about 140 cases of carcinoma of the esophagus each year. Another significant study by Brooks found that, of 200 patients with esophageal foreign bodies treated during a 10-year period, none of the patients had malignant disease (34).

Although less common but more dangerous in adults, nondigestible items are sometimes deliberately swallowed, either for potential benefits (incarcerated, drug smugglers), because of psychiatric or mental impairment (schizophrenia, dementia), or intoxication (drug, alcohol).

CLINICAL PRESENTATION

Patients can present with a wide variety of signs and symptoms. It is clear that children and adults swallow different foreign bodies and show different clinical presentations. Because many adults can give a clear history, their evaluation is usually faster, easier, and more focused toward the type of foreign body and intervention needed. Rarely, the ingestion may be occult or remote. Young children, on the other hand, are usually unable to express or appropriately locate their symptoms, the history is usually not clear and must be obtained from a parent or a caretaker, and the type of ingested body is often unknown. Most adults seek medical attention within the first 6 hours of impaction and almost all within the first 24 hours (35), and symptoms of impaction such as dysphagia, odynophagia, sensation of foreign body, and excessive salivation are common. In children, respiratory symptoms frequently predominate over gastrointestinal symptoms because their soft tracheal rings are easily compressed by the esophageal foreign body, leading to compression of the small-caliber trachea (36). Stridor, persistent cough, drooling, or refusal to take feedings are the usual presentations and physicians must have a high index of suspicion to establish a correct diagnosis in this population (37). Adults more frequently had an underlying esophageal abnormality (peptic stricture, hiatal hernia or Schatzki's ring) before the retention of the foreign body (3,21), and previous endoscopic management or hospitalization for treatment of foreign body impaction is not uncommon (38). Children usually have no esophageal disease, and social risk factors, especially child abuse, must be considered in some situations. One reported case in a 6-year-old girl in which a tooth avulsed and was swallowed causing esophageal perforation with associated retropharyngeal and mediastinal abscess was not initially thought of as a cause of physical abuse until 5 months later when a follow up appointment of her esophageal-cutaneous fistula revealed multiple physical evidences of child abuse (39).

One life-threatening situation associated with meat impaction in the esophagus is the "café coronary" (40). This phrase is used to describe a true medical emergency in which a food bolus impacts at the level of the upper esophageal sphincter and can result in death from asphyxiation as a result of acute airway obstruction. This absolute medical emergency should be rapidly recognized because the Heimlich maneuver can be lifesaving as noted in an 8-year-old child in whom a hard candy obstructing the cervical esophagus was dislodged (41). Even so, the Heimlich maneuver should not be advocated to the general population unless there is unquestionable airway compromise because esophageal rupture has been described in a woman when a bystander attempted to dislodge a bolus of food from her esophagus using this method (42).

A thorough search for physical findings is always necessary but most likely unrewarding. As many as 90% of patients with esophageal impaction have a normal physical examination (43). Pharyngeal erythema or abrasions of the mouth or pharynx may be secondary to a foreign body. Subcutaneous emphysema in the chest or neck is suggestive of esophageal perforation, and fever may indicate mediastinitis or abscess formation

Finally, penetrating esophageal foreign bodies can present with hematemesis and shock resulting from an aortoesophageal fistula. Usually these foreign bodies are sharp (e.g. bones), and patients have a classic history that was first observed by Chiari. He described the "aortoesophageal syndrome" in 1914 as a painful esophageal injury followed by a symptom-free interval then a "signal hemorrhage," followed in hours to days by exsanguinating hemorrhage (44). This has been validated in subsequent reports (45–47), in which the unique features of its clinical presentation permit early recognition and perhaps improve salvage.

EVALUATION

The initial approach to the patient with a foreign body in the esophagus must include (a) a thorough history, (b) the clinical condition, (c) an attempt to localize the exact location of the foreign body, and (d) any associated complications.

Obtaining a careful history, if possible, from the patient, relatives, or witnesses is essential. This may disclose the type and nature of the object (blunt, sharp or pointed, toxic or nontoxic, live or dead); size of ingested material; number of objects involved (multiple or single); the timing between ingestion and presentation (hours, days, or months); and previous esophageal pathology, surgical disruption, or food impactions. When a history of ingestion is lacking, physicians may fail to make the appropriate diagnosis by not considering a foreign body as the etiology of the complaint. This is especially true in children who can swallow different objects inadvertently, possibly delaying diagnosis and leading to inappropriate medical management (48).

The clinical conditions differ significantly between patients with complete esophageal obstruction caused by the foreign body or those with airway compromise and those with mild or subtle symptoms. It is important to distinguish early in the evaluation which patients have an unstable airway or are unable to handle secretions, because invasive and urgent management is required.

Determining the exact location of the foreign body is probably the most critical step in the evaluation of esophageal foreign bodies and is usually associated with the patient's age as well as the type and size of the foreign body. All patients should have as many diagnostic evaluations as needed to localize the foreign body and any associated complications. The oldest and probably the main diagnostic technique used to localize a foreign body is the use of radiographs. Plain films of the neck or chest can easily localize radiopaque objects, and type and size can also be evaluated. They can also demonstrate findings suggesting a complication such as subcutaneous emphysema, widened mediastinum or pneumomediastinum secondary to perforation, and pleural effusion or pulmonary infiltrates secondary to aspiration. Plain films are particularly important when button batteries or meat impaction are the foreign bodies involved. Because a button battery lodged in the esophagus is a true emergency, radiologists and gastroenterologists should distinguish between a coin and a button battery. When viewed in an anteroposterior projection, the latter demonstrates a double-density shadow caused by the bilaminar structure of the battery. On the lateral view, the edges of the battery are round and present a step-off at the junction of the cathode and anode. A coin has a much sharper edge on the lateral view (29). In cases of meat impaction, plain films reveal imbedded bone fragments. As mentioned earlier, the location of entrapment differs with the patient's age (Table 17.2). In children, 63% to 84% of

foreign bodies are entrapped at the level of the cricopharyngeus muscle, 10% to 17% at the level of the aortic crossover, and 5% to 20% at the lower esophageal sphincter. In adults, the majority of esophageal foreign bodies are entrapped at the lower esophageal sphincter (63% to 74%), only 8% to 10% at the aortic crossover, and 24% to 39% are at the upper esophageal sphincter (2,4,37,49).

Furthermore, radiographs determine the size of the foreign body, which influences subsequent treatment. Elongated objects such as bobby pins, open paper clips or safety pins, long, stiff wires, or objects longer than 6 cm in children or 13 cm in adults can easily be visualized. Prompt endoscopic removal of these is necessary because they have a high incidence of penetration, perforation, or entrapment in the small bowel (36). Smaller objects (except sharp objects and button batteries) may be allowed to pass through the digestive tract once they have reach the stomach; their progress can be assessed by checking the stool for the object or by serial radiographs.

Although radiographic evaluation is usually the first step in attempting to localize the foreign body, a negative radiologic examination should not delay or preclude an endoscopic evaluation. This is especially true in patients with probable radiolucent objects, such as wood, aluminum, glass, plastic, and meat or small fish or chicken bones that may not be visible on plain radiographs.

The type of suspected foreign body ingested is essential in the initial evaluation and frequently correlates with the patient's age. Coins seem to be the favorite object for children to swallow and account for the majority of pediatric esophageal foreign bodies (50–53). The clinical spectrum of esophageal coins varies significantly; some children are asymptomatic whereas others have multiple complaints. Therefore, considerable controversy has evolved over recommendations that a child who remains asymptomatic after swallowing a coin should be promptly evaluated and a radiograph performed (37,54–66). In a home-based survey of parents in Maryland, 85% of coins ingested were managed at home without calling a physician or poison control center (32). Hodge and colleagues (56) studied 80 children who presented to the emergency department with a complaint of coin ingestion and found that, in 25 patients (31%), the coin was radiographically visualized in the esophagus, that is, cervical esophagus in 15 patients (18%) and mid-lower esophagus in ten patients (13%). The most striking fact was that 11 (44%) of the patients with positive radiographs were asymptomatic. Schunk and co-workers (37), in a study of 42 patients, reported a similar experience. On the other hand, Caravati and colleagues (67) evaluated 162 children who where recommended by a local poison control center to undergo a routine roentgenography after coin ingestion. Only 66 patients (41%) complied with the recommendation. A coin was visualized in the esophagus of 13 patients (20%), 11 of whom were symptomatic and two of whom were

TABLE 17.2. LEVEL OF ESOPHAGEAL FOREIGN BODIES

Level	Pediatrics (%)	Adults (%)
Cricopharyngeus muscle	63–84	24–39
Aortic crossover	10–17	8–10
Lower esophageal sphincter	5–20	63–74

From Stack LB, Munter DW. Foreign bodies in the gastrointestinal tract. *Emerg Med Clin North Am* 1996;14:493–521, with permission.

asymptomatic at the time of ingestion. No symptoms were reported in 118 patients (73%) at the time of ingestion and all of them remained asymptomatic throughout a 5-day follow-up period. Their conclusions was that children who are asymptomatic at home need not immediately undergo roentgenography as long as they can tolerate oral fluids without difficulty and close follow-up is available. Because of their radiopaque characteristics, coins are easily visualized on plain radiographs. They are usually seen in a coronal alignment (frontal) on anteroposterior films, and sagittally on lateral films when they lodge in the esophagus. Because of the configuration of the tracheal rings, with the cartilage incomplete posteriorly, coins in the trachea are seen in sagittal and coronal orientations on anteroposterior and lateral films, respectively. Both anteroposterior and lateral films are usually needed, because foreign objects noted on the anteroposterior films can appear to be in the esophagus when actually in the pulmonary tree (68). Lateral views are also helpful when radiopaque objects are overlying the spine and may not be apparent on an anterior view. Recently, several studies have shown the utility of handheld metal detectors as an alternative to radiography for localizing coins, with a sensitivity of 93% to 100% and specificity of 100% (69,72).

Because of significant advances in radiologic technology, contrast studies will rarely be needed again for the evaluation of foreign bodies in the gastrointestinal tract, except in rare exceptions. If needed, for radiolucent objects such as those previously described, the choice is usually between barium sulfate and a water-soluble solution such as meglumine diatrizoate (Gastrografin). The major inconvenience of using barium is that the presence of barium in the esophagus complicates removal of the object because it obscures endoscopic visualization. Gastrografin is the contrast agent of choice if perforation is suspected because it is water soluble and readily absorbed from the mediastinum or pleural space. However, if food impaction is suspected, its use is contraindicated because it is extremely hypertonic and causes a severe chemical pneumonitis if aspirated into the lung. Newer nonionic contrast agents, such as metrizamide or iohexol, are probably safer because they have minimal tissue reactivity but are more costly (36,68,73).

Recently, computed tomography (CT) has proven of significant value for evaluating foreign bodies in the cervical esophagus. Using soft tissues and bone windows with 3-mm cuts, thin and slightly calcified foreign bodies in the cervical esophagus can be well visualized even after more conventional radiologic or endoscopic methods are nondiagnostic (74–76). Furthermore, spiral CT was demonstrated a pseudoaneurysm with aortoesophageal fistula in an 18-year-old woman who had swallowed a fish bone 2 weeks earlier and presented with hematemesis and shock. The spiral CT was fast and accurate after the "sentinel hemorrhage" to confirm the diagnosis and to determine the site of the fistula. More importantly, it may hasten lifesaving surgery as well as indicate the correct choice of surgical approach (77). Another important piece of information that a CT scan can provide is the evidence of other damage (abscess, pseudoaneurysm) or secondary inflammatory changes in the neighboring structures of the esophagus that cannot be visualized with either plain or contrast films or with endoscopy (76–78).

Even with this extensive workup, a significant number of patients who complain of foreign body sensation have no specific findings. This has prompted several authors to suggest that the only result of this workup is to delay the definitive intervention, endoscopy (79,80).

There is no question that endoscopy plays a significant role in the early evaluation of esophageal foreign bodies. Endoscopy not only can demonstrate the location, type, and configuration of the object involved, but also can provide fast and appropriate management. It is also useful to evaluate other mucosal changes not previously visualized during the radiographic evaluation that may require additional diagnostic studies or prior management before the extraction of the foreign body. Intubation should be performed under direct visualization not only to evaluate the hypopharynx but also to avoid hitting a foreign body lodged in the cervical esophagus. Occasionally a foreign body escapes detection even on endoscopy because it has become embedded in or has penetrated the mucosal wall (75,76). To prevent this, we strongly believe that diagnostic as well as therapeutic endoscopy should be performed as early as possible in every patient with esophageal foreign bodies.

MANAGEMENT

When facing a patient with an entrapped esophageal foreign body, the most important questions guiding subsequent management are, in order:

1. Is there any evidence of airway compromise or respiratory distress that will require securing the airway before any further intervention?
2. Where is the foreign body located and is there any need to retrieve it?
3. When should the foreign body be removed, urgently or electively?
4. Is the appropriate equipment, team, and experience available for the management of this specific foreign body?

Most foreign bodies do not require any intervention and pass spontaneously and safely through the gastrointestinal tract. On the other hand, patients who come for evaluation are more likely to be those who require further management. Even though most of the information on the management of foreign bodies is based on collected experience or case report series and not clinical trials, this collective experience suggests certain "golden" rules that should be applied. Endoscopic removal is the only safe, nonsurgical way to remove objects that are sharp, such as open safety pins, straight pins, razor blades, nails, or bones (29,36, 68,81,82). When endoscopic removal is attempted, the axiom of Chevalier Jackson "Leading edges perforate, following edges do not" (1) should always be considered (Fig. 17.2). Button batteries lodged in the esophagus should be removed urgently because contact time of as little as 1 hour can result in mucosal injury and within 4 hours full-thickness damage may ensue (83). Finally, in patients who attempt to smuggle illicit drugs contained in swallowed balloons or condom, known as "body packers," endoscopic removal should be avoided because rupture of the packages can result in severe intoxication or even death (84). Early surgical removal of the packages offers the safest and fastest method of removal. The only definite indication for a conservative approach is when the ingested drug is known to be cannabis because no recorded fatality has been published (85).

The appropriate way to manage foreign bodies in the gastrointestinal tract, especially those impacted in the esophagus, has dramatically changed in the last 3 decades, mostly because of the introduction of flexible endoscopy as a successful option with minimal morbidity and mortality. In the following sections, management of specific types of the most common foreign bodies is reviewed. Also discussed are some interesting new techniques that can help with certain unique foreign bodies in clinical practice as well as a few nonendoscopic, pharmacologic methods to remove certain foreign bodies.

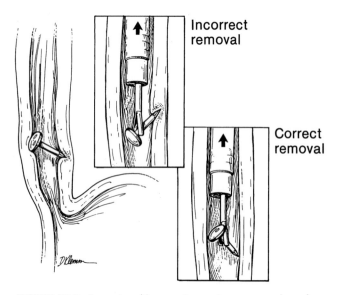

FIGURE 17.2. Correct and incorrect ways to remove a sharp foreign body.

COINS

Coins are popular in the pediatric population and because infants and children have a narrower esophagus, any size coin can become lodged in the esophagus. In children, most coins lodge in the upper end at the level of the cricopharyngeus muscle (53,86–88). The most important thing to remember in managing coins is that those at the level of the cricopharyngeus muscle require a patent airway at all times (29). The mechanism of injury from esophageal coins is most often from direct pressure necrosis that can cause tracheoesophageal fistula or esophageal perforation (89,90). Zinc pennies, which have been manufactured in the United States since 1982 (97.6% zinc, 2.4% copper), are more corrosive when lodged in the esophagus than are the older copper pennies (95% copper, 5% zinc) (29).

Various strategies and techniques have been described to remove a lodged coin in the upper end of the esophagus, including rigid (55,86) or flexible esophagoscopy (91), Foley's catheter dislodgment (25), the "penny pincher" technique (92), and "blind" esophageal bouginage (24). Coins lodged in the distal esophagus usually do not require any intervention and temporization, allowing the coin a chance to pass into the stomach on its own, is probably the best approach (93). Recently, the use of Magill forceps technique in children with coins in the upper end of the esophagus has been described as a quick, easy, and safe technique (94).

Rigid esophagoscopy under general anesthesia is also a safe technique with few complications and several advantages. It provides excellent visualization of the esophagus, airway protection, a variety of types and sizes of extraction instruments, and almost 100% success rate. In addition, the child is in no discomfort and there is greater control over both the patient and the procedure. Coins can be grasped and removed under direct vision and the esophagus can be examined after removal of the foreign body. This method, however requires general anesthesia with its own risks, a chest radiograph to rule out pneumomediastinum after the procedure, and a postoperative observation period in the hospital, all of which increases the cost significantly (93,94).

The use of the Foley's catheter is an interesting technique that was first reported in the medical literature in 1966 (95). It has been used primarily for the extraction of blunt esophageal foreign bodies in children at the level of the upper esophageal end where coins are the most common object extracted (25,88,96). The indications for Foley catheter removal should be carefully reviewed and well known; furthermore, strict inclusion criteria should be enforced. These include duration of the foreign body impaction of less than 72 hours; single, smooth, blunt, and radiopaque characteristics of the object; no prior history of esophageal disease or surgery; and no respiratory distress or evidence of perforation. Because airway compromise can occur while removing the foreign body, resuscitation equipment and advanced airway management skills should always be available. Finally, because Foley catheter removal fails in a small number of cases, endoscopic removal is required and appropriate backup must be prepared in advanced (25,68).

The Foley catheter technique is a simple, cost-saving technique for extraction of blunt esophageal foreign bodies that most radiologists should be familiar with and trained in, especially those working in centers where endoscopy is not always available. The materials required for foreign body removal include a mouth gag, water-soluble contrast material, a 10-mL syringe, and a number 14- or 16-French Foley catheter. Emergency items including a pediatric laryngoscope, blades, and forceps. The oropharynx is sprayed with a small amount of a local anesthetic. Before inserting the Foley catheter, it is essential to inflate the balloon with the contrast agent to evaluate for possible leaks and to ensure that it inflates symmetrically. The foreign body is localized and under fluoroscopic guidance the catheter is inserted orally. Once the tip of the catheter is just beyond the foreign body, the balloon is inflated with the contrast material. Before removing the catheter, the patient is placed into a prone oblique position and the fluoroscopic table is turned into a relatively steep head-down position. The catheter is then withdrawn from the esophagus with moderate and steady traction. By using the oral approach, one ensures that the foreign body is in the oropharynx only a brief moment. The nasal approach should be avoided because it can cause epistaxis, may convert an esophageal foreign body into a nasopharyngeal foreign body, and requires balloon deflation in the hypopharynx with the attendant risk of aspiration of the foreign body. To persist with numerous intubations or the application of forceful traction is unwarranted and contraindicated (25,97).

The success rate of the Foley extraction is 85% to 100% with complication risks from 0% to 2%. The most common complications are nosebleeds, hyperpyrexia, laryngospasm, and hypoxia (25,98,99). Probably the most striking factor that was noticed in one study comparing the Foley catheter technique with endoscopic removal was the significant cost difference between both techniques. In this study, the total hospital charges were 400% higher in the group undergoing endoscopic removal and the success rate was the same (88).

The use of "blind" esophageal bougienage is another inexpensive, fast, and safe method to advance an ingested coin lodged in the esophagus into the stomach in children with acute single coin ingestion. In more than 20 years of experience using this technique, Bonadio and colleagues (24) have managed an estimated 250 cases of ingested coins lodge in the esophagus, but most importantly, no patient required reevaluation by the surgical service for a complication related to its performance. All procedures were performed by a surgeon experienced in the bougienage technique. However, strict inclusion criteria, as in patients who are managed by the Foley catheter technique, must always be respected and fulfilled. These mandatory criteria include the following:

The foreign body must be a coin and should be radiographically located in the esophagus.

There can only be a *single* coin ingested acutely (less than 24 hours).

There can be no marked discrepancy between the coin size and esophageal size.

There can be no previous history of esophageal foreign body, disease process, or surgical procedure previously performed and no respiratory compromise on physical examination.

It cannot be overemphasized that if any contraindication to performing this procedure exists, an alternative method of coin extraction must be used (24,100).

Despite the high success rate and reported safety of these two techniques (Foley catheter dislodgment and blind esophageal bouginage to remove coins from the esophagus), only a few centers have the knowledge and experience to perform them. The major concern is that control of the object is limited and direct visualization of the esophageal mucosa and the object is not feasible. Most importantly, even though the history might have been complete and thorough, some children could have swallowed a second "radiolucent" foreign body, in which case, either of these two "blind" procedures would be contraindicated. Most patients also subsequently require a diagnostic endoscopy for the evaluation of the esophageal mucosa and to rule out an underlying pathology as the cause of foreign body obstruction. Because endoscopy should always be available when these techniques fail to remove the foreign body, there is no need to perform a rushed and blind procedure with the available technology. There is no question that flexible endoscopy is clearly the method of choice to remove foreign bodies and will continue to facilitate the removal of esophageal coins from the esophagus.

A variety of endoscopic accessories are useful in removing coins from the esophagus, for example, the retrieval Dormia basket, polyp grabber, biopsy forceps, foreign-body forceps, and polypectomy snare (101), but the Roth retrieval net may become the easiest and most secure device for removing blunt foreign bodies in the esophagus. Using the Roth retrieval, net we were able to grasp and securely remove a coin that was lodged in the distal esophagus in a man with no evidence of mucosal abnormalities (personal experience) (Color Plate 17.3). Its use has already been validated in a pig animal model, in which it was found to be the best endoscopic device for retrieving smooth objects such as the button disc battery with a 100% success rate and superior to the Dormia basket

(102). The foreign body grasping forceps (rat tooth) are especially useful to grasp the elevated edge of a coin (101), but its security and the risk of accidental dislodgment, especially while retrieving the coin through the oropharynx, can make it dangerous. This is unlikely to happen if the coin is inside a Roth net.

Finally, an unconventional but successful report illustrates the importance of endoscopy as well as physician ingenuity. Two children had a penny removed from the midesophagus that was embedded in the esophageal wall. Neither flexible esophagoscopy through the mouth nor rigid esophagoscopy or laryngoscopy were able to remove the coins and the patients were referred for thoracotomy for coin removal. A surgical gastrostomy was performed and a flexible endoscope was passed through the gastrostomy incision and advanced through the distal esophagus to the level of the coins. With Pelican grasping forceps, the coins were withdrawn through the gastrostomy site. Both children were subsequently treated with intravenous antibiotics, parenteral nutrition, and gastrostomy drainage. They were discharged home on gastrostomy feeding and serial esophageal dilations. The patients were without symptoms of dysphagia after 1 and 2 years. The procedure, "retrograde gastroscopy," obviated the necessity for a thoracotomy and its morbidity, and should be considered when standard flexible and rigid esophagoscopy have been unsuccessful because of technical problems (103).

With any technique used for the removal of esophageal coins, experience and the level of comfort with the available equipment is probably the most important issue. However, flexible endoscopy should be considered the standard of care for patients with esophageal coins.

MEAT IMPACTION

Of the major groups of esophageal foreign bodies (coins, button batteries, sharp objects, and meat), the management of meat impaction is probably the most controversial. This is probably because, for many years, flexible endoscopy was not an option in the armamentarium for patients with food impactions. Since the advent of flexible endoscopy, it has become possible to appropriately evaluate mucosal abnormalities, and these have been found to play an important role in the pathophysiology of food impaction. Most patients have distal esophageal pathology and, in cases of complete obstruction, they are unable to handle secretions. Some nonendoscopic methods used have multiple reported complications and should be discouraged. The following discussion divides the management of meat impaction into nonendoscopic and endoscopic techniques, which should be the standard of care for patients with meat impactions.

NONENDOSCOPIC TECHNIQUES

Several nonendoscopic techniques have been used to either extract a food bolus or promote its passage into the stomach. Most of them have slowly been falling into disuse because of dangerous complications that have developed with their use. Probably the most well-known pharmacologic agent used for this purpose is glucagon, which relaxes the smooth muscle of the lower esophageal sphincter. The first reported cases using glucagon for esophageal food impaction by Ferrucci and colleagues (104) showed a response rate of 50%. Since then, the success rate has ranged from 12% to 50% (36,49,105,106). Its use is not very popular, most likely because glucagon does not affect the diameter of lower esophageal rings or strictures. However, glucagon therapy is safe, does not preclude subsequent endoscopic removal, and a trial before endoscopy is a reasonable approach. The gastroenterologist is usually familiar with the regular use of glucagon and its safety profile because of its regular use in both endoscopic retrograde or endoscopic ultrasound procedures. The most common side effects of nausea, vomiting, and hyperglycemia are minor and easy to manage. However, its use is absolutely contraindicated in patients with insulinoma, pheochromocytoma, Zollinger-Ellison syndrome, or sensitivity to the drug. The dose of glucagon normally used is 1 to 2 mg intravenously in adults and 0.02 to 0.03 mg/kg in children weighing less than 20 kg with a maximum dose of 0.5 mg (68). The patient should be upright and must be given water following the injection. Patients with inadequate airway protective reflexes must be excluded because vomiting may occur. This dose may be repeated after 5 to 10 minutes, but if the first two doses are ineffective, further doses are not indicated (81,106,107). Because the upper third of the esophagus contains striated muscle, glucagon is ineffective for foreign bodies in this area (107). Some authors have used warm water, an effervescent agent, and gas-forming agents in conjunction with glucagon, but the success rate was not improved and one patient had an esophageal perforation (108–110). Other pharmacologic agents that have been used to relax the lower esophageal sphincter such as calcium channel blockers, nitrates, benzodiazepines, anticholinergics, and meperidine offer no significant advantage over glucagon (68,101,107).

The use of a proteolytic enzyme to digest the meat was first describe by Richardson in 1945 (111) and became the treatment of choice for over a decade. Papain (commercially available as Adolf's Meat Tenderizer), an enzyme obtained from a tropical melon tree, can digest approximately 55 times its weight of lean meat (112). In 1959, Andersen and co-workers (113) reported the first fatality in a 27-year-old woman with an impaction in her cervical esophagus. She suffered an esophageal perforation with subsequent erosion into the wall of her common carotid artery on the fourteenth day of her illness. This was subsequently confirmed in 1968 when Holsinger reported another esophageal perforation 8 hours after papain was given to relieve a food impaction. The patient died on the tenth hospital day after a massive hemorrhage from erosion of the descending thoracic aorta (114). Another potential lethal complication of papain is inadvertent aspiration, causing hemorrhagic pulmonary edema (115). It is clear that papain cannot be recommended for the management of meat impaction. Other enzymes, like trypsin and chymotrypsin, have also been tried (112,116), but their use will probably never become popular because of the severe complications from papain and the existence of better ways to manage a meat impaction.

The use of gas-forming agents has also been described in the literature as another option to move the foreign body into the stomach (117–119). This method was first described in 1983 by Rice and colleagues (117) when they reported a 3-year experience with 100% success rate in eight patients with meat impaction. They use an acid-based "cocktail" of tartaric acid and sodium bicarbonate solutions, which upon being mixed form carbon dioxide. With the upper esophageal sphincter closed, the increased pressure distends the walls of the esophagus and exerts downward pressure on the bolus of meat, forcing it into the stomach. Although esophageal disease was present in all patients (i.e., benign strictures, Schatzki's ring, and hiatal hernia) and retching was observed in all of them, no esophageal tears or ruptures occurred. They were careful to quote that "impactions lasting more than 24 hours might be a relative contraindication." Subsequently, Zimmers and co-workers (119) reported their experience in 26 patients using the same "cocktail" of tartaric acid and sodium bicarbonate. The success rate was only 65% and one patient suffered an esophageal mucosal tear. They attributed their complication to the fact that the food bolus was impacted in the esophagus for more than 18 hours, so they recommended the use of these agents to be limited to impactions of less than 6 hours. But an esophageal perforation was reported by Smith and colleagues (109) in 1986 in which glucagon and an effervescent agent (E-Z Gas) were used in a patient with a fixed esophageal stricture. Carbonated beverages also released sufficient amounts of carbon dioxide to distend the esophagus, relax the lower esophageal sphincter, and force the passage of impacted meat and other foreign bodies into the esophagus. Mohammed and colleagues (118) were able to successfully dislodge impacted foreign bodies in the esophagus in 80% of patients using carbonated beverages, but they failed in patients with very narrow strictures because of reflux esophagitis or cancer.

These observations confirmed the previous concerns about the risks of gas-forming agents and esophageal disease in patients with meat impactions, so their use cannot be recommended for the treatment of patients with food obstructions.

Finally, a modified gastric lavage tube has also been used successfully to extract a meat bolus from the esophagus (120). In using this technique, the distal 8 cm of a 34-French lavage tube is cut off and advanced under fluoroscopic guidance to the level of impaction. While applying negative pressure with a 120-mL syringe, the food bolus is withdrawn from the esophagus. To avoid dropping the meat in the oropharynx, an overtube can also be used to protect the airway.

ENDOSCOPIC TECHNIQUES

Since the first successful report of removal of foreign bodies from the esophagus in 1972 using a flexible endoscope, the scientific literature has been replete with anecdotal case reports using flexible endoscopes to remove food impactions. Endoscopy not only allows the physician to manipulate the food bolus under direct visualization but also immediately evaluate the underlying mucosa and appropriately treat any underlying pathology in one session. Rigid endoscopy under general anesthesia is also used, but should only be reserved for those few meat impactions in which flexible endoscopy has not been successful. Although no prospective, randomized trials comparing these two endoscopic techniques have been published, there is a strong preference for flexible endoscopy as the method of choice to remove meat impactions from the esophagus. When Shaffer and Klug (121) retrospectively compared their institution's experience between rigid and flexible endoscopy in meat bolus obstructions, the success rates were 88% and 92%, respectively. It is well accepted that the forward-viewing flexible endoscope is the instrument of choice because of the greater patient comfort and acceptance, because there is no need for general anesthesia (thus eliminating the associated risks and significant costs), and because there is greater visualization and maneuverability (29). Successful removal depends mostly on proper preparation, as well as the gastroenterologist's training, experience, dexterity, and ingenuity. The patient must be well sedated and in the left lateral decubitus position. Secretions should be managed appropriately. The endoscope should be introduced under direct visualization and an assistant must be available exclusively to help the endoscopist. Surgical backup must be readily available. If any of these "essential" steps cannot be accomplished and the intervention is not urgent, endoscopy should be postponed to a reasonably convenient time, because most food impactions often pass spontaneously. However, endoscopic intervention should not be delayed beyond 24 hours from presentation, because the risk of complications may increase (30). In addition, as time passes, the meat softens significantly and extraction in one single piece becomes more difficult. Once the meat has softened, multiple attempts are usually necessary to extract it in small pieces. This is safer and better accomplished by using an overtube, which is left in place in the hypopharynx while the endoscope is inserted and withdrawn multiple times, avoiding trauma and the possibility of dropping fragments in the hypopharynx, with potential pulmonary aspiration in a patient with conscious sedation and no gag reflex (122,123). A variety of snares, graspers, baskets, retrieval nets, and forceps can be passed through the 2.8-mm biopsy channel of a diagnostic upper endoscope and the meat bolus can usually be removed whole or in a piecemeal fashion. If the anatomy of the distal esophagus is known or the endoscope (easier with a smaller pediatric endoscope) can be advanced around the impacted meat to evaluate the distal esophagus (Fig. 17.4C), the endoscope can then be pulled back proximally to the bolus, which can be gently and carefully pushed into the stomach (3,123). If the endoscope cannot be passed beyond the meat bolus, gentle pushing in some cases can be safely performed as long as a careful history has been taken to rule out prior dysphagia (122,123). A hiatal hernia is usually present and the esophagogastric junction usually takes a left turn as it enters the hernia. Therefore, it is important to push from the right side of the meat bolus rather than straight on (Fig. 17.4A–B) (29).

Finally, physician inventiveness and resourceful utilization of the entire spectrum of endoscopic equipment can sometimes resolve easily and successfully a meat impaction in the esophagus. The Nd:YAG laser was used once in an elderly man with a bolus of steak impacted in the distal esophagus that was unsuccessfully removed after several measures were taken, including prolonged endoscopic manipulation. Using the laser, the center of the meat was cooked, shrank rapidly, and cavitated inwardly. After repeated lasering of the center, the meat fell into the stomach (125).

Despite the availability of several methods of treatment, it is the endoscopist who is best able to endeavor a simple, safe, efficient, and cost-effective technique for the relief of food bolus obstruction in the presence or absence of organic strictures of the esophagus.

COMPLICATIONS

Although the true complication rate related to ingested foreign bodies in the esophagus will never be known, most large studies report a 1% to 4% of cases (126). They include aspiration, airway obstruction, pneumonia, penetration, perforation, bleeding, mucosal abrasions or tears, esophageal necrosis, retropharyngeal abscess, fistulae, mediastinitis, pleural effusions, pneumothorax, pneumomediastinum, pericarditis, pericardial effusions and tamponade, and vascular injuries, among others complications not always reported in the medical literature. Latent complications include chronic respiratory problems, esophageal strictures, and even failure to thrive in some children.

CONCLUSION

Because the swallowing of foreign bodies is a problem that will never be eliminated and technology continues to advance, it should be of great interest to develop standard devices and techniques that provide an easy and fast solution to the problem. This should be facilitated by the use of flexible endoscopes and the eagerness of the gastroenterologist to establish a "standard of care" for the management of esophageal foreign bodies. In the meantime, making the correct decision for their management can be difficult and should be individualized to each patient's circumstances. However, endoscopic removal should virtually always prevail before other more invasive, controversial, or risky methods are attempted.

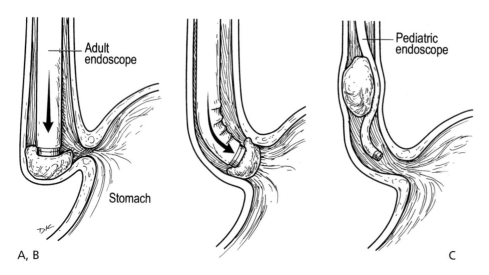

FIGURE 17.4. Meat impacted in the distal esophagus—endoscopic evaluation and management. **A:** Pushing "straight" can perforate the distal esophagus. **B:** It is easier to push from the "right side" to advance it into the stomach. **C:** It is always better and safer to evaluate the distal esophagus before pushing blindly.

REFERENCES

1. Jackson CL. Ancient foreign body cases. *Laryngoscope* 1917;27: 583–584.
2. Nandi P, Ong GB. Foreign body in the esophagus: review of 2394 cases. *Br J Surg* 1978;65:5–9.
3. Longstreth GF, Longstreth KJ, Yao JF. Esophageal food impaction: epidemiology and therapy. A retrospective, observational study. *Gastrointest Endosc* 2001;53:193–198.
4. Schwartz GF, Polsky HS. Ingested foreign bodies of the gastrointestinal tract. *Am Surg* 1976;42:236–238.
5. Lerche W. The esophagoscope in removing sharp foreign bodies from the esophagus. *JAMA* 1911;56:634–637.
6. Rösch W, Classen M. Fiberendoscopic foreign body removal from the gastrointestinal tract. *Endoscopy* 1972;4:193.
7. Morrissey JF. Progress in gastroenterology. *Gastroenterology* 1972;62:1241–1268.
8. Perelman H. Toothpick perforation of the gastrointestinal tract. *J Abdom Surg* 1962;4:51–53.
9. Mok CK, Chiu CSW, Cheung HHC. Left subclavian arterioesophageal fistula induced by a foreign body. *Ann Thorac Surg* 1989;47:458–460.
10. Sloop RD, Thompson JC. Aorto-esophageal fistula: report of a case and review of literature. *Gastroenterology* 1967;53:768.
11. Janik JS, Bailey WC, Burrington JD. Occult coin perforation of the esophagus. *J Pediatr Surg* 1986;21:794–797.
12. Bozer AY, Saylam A, Ersoy U. Purulent pericarditis due to perforation of esophagus with foreign body. *J Thorac Cardiovasc Surg* 1974;67:590–592.
13. Welch TG, White TR, Lewis RP, et al. Esophagopericardial fistula presenting as cardiac tamponade. *Chest* 1972;62:728.
14. Erbes J, Babbitt DP. Foreign bodies in the alimentary tract of infants and children. *Appl Ther* 1965;7:1103–1109.
15. Dick ET. Cocktail stick perforation of the large bowel. *N Z Med J* 1966;65:986.
16. Webb WA. Management of foreign bodies of the upper gastrointestinal tract: update. *Gastrointest Endosc* 1995;41:39–51.
17. Long JD, Orlando RC. Anatomy and developmental and acquired anomalies of the esophagus. In: Feldman M, Scharschmidt BF, Sleisenger MH, eds. *Sleisenger and Fordtran's gastrointestinal and liver disease*. Philadelphia: WB Saunders, 1998:457–554.
18. Meyer GW, Austin RM, Brady CE, et al. Muscle anatomy of the human esophagus. *J Clin Gastroenterol* 1986;8:131–134.
19. Zwischenberger JB, Alpard SK, Orringer MB. Esophagus. In: Twonsend CM Jr, Beauchamp RD, Evers BM, eds. *Sabiston textbook of surgery*. New York: WB Saunders, 2001;709–768.
20. Flett RL. Esophageal foreign bodies and their complications. *J Laryngol Otol* 1945;1:1–15.
21. Webb WA, McDaniel L, Jones L. Foreign bodies of the upper gastrointestinal tract: current management. *South Med J* 1984; 77:1083–1086.
22. Goff WF. What to do when foreign bodies are inhaled or ingested. *Postgrad Med* 1968;44:135–138.
23. Holinger PH, Johnston KC, Greengard J. Congenital anomalies of the esophagus related to esophageal foreign bodies. *Am J Dis Child* 1949;78:467–476.
24. Bonadio WA, Jona JZ, Glicklich M, et al. Esophageal bougienage technique for coin ingestion in children. *J Pediatr Surg* 1988;23:917–918.
25. Campbell JB, Quattromani FL, Foley LC. Foley catheter removal of blunt esophageal foreign bodies. Experience with 100 consecutive children. *Pediatr Radiol* 1983;13:116–119.
26. Mamel JJ. Bezoar of the esophagus occurring in achalasia. *Gastrointest Endosc* 1984;30:317–318.
27. Shah SWH, Khan AA, Alam A, et al. Esophageal bezoar in achalasia: a rare condition. *J Clin Gastroenterol* 1997;25: 395–396.
28. Koch H. Operative endoscopy. *Gastrointest Endosc* 1977;24: 65–68.
29. Webb WA. Management of foreign bodies of the upper gastrointestinal tract. *Gastroenterology* 1988;94:204–216.
30. Chaikhouni A, Kratz JM, Crawford FA. Foreign bodies of the esophagus. *Am Surg* 1985;51:173–179.
31. Litovitz TL, Schmitz BF, Matyunas N, et al. 1987 annual report of the American Association of Poison Control Centers National Data Collection System. *Am J Emerg Med* 1988;6: 479–515.
32. Conners GP, Chamberlain JM, Weiner PR. Pediatric coin ingestion: a home-based survey. *Am J Emerg Med* 1995;13:638–640.
33. Jackson CL. Foreign Bodies in the esophagus. *Am J Surg* 1957;93:308–312.
34. Brooks JW. Foreign bodies in the air and food passages. *Ann Surg* 1972;175:720–732.
35. Herranz-Gonzalez J, Martinez-Vidal J, Garcia-Sarandeses A, et al. Esophageal foreign bodies in adults. *Otolaryngol Head Neck Surg* 1991;105:649–654.
36. Brady PG. Esophageal foreign bodies. *Gastroenterol Clin North Am* 1991;20:691–701.
37. Schunk JE, Corneli H, Bolte R. Pediatric coin ingestions. A prospective study of coin location and symptoms. *Am J Dis Child* 1989;143:546–548.
38. Tibbling L, Stenquist M. Foreign bodies in the esophagus. A study of causative factors. *Dysphagia* 1991;6:224–227.
39. Ablin DS, Reinhart MA. Esophageal perforation by a tooth in child abuse. *Pediatr Radiol* 1992;22:339–341.
40. Haugen RK. The café coronary. *JAMA* 1963;186:142–143.
41. Nelson KR. Heimlich maneuver for esophageal obstruction. *N Engl J Med* 1989;320:1016.
42. Meredith MJ, Liebowitz R. Rupture of the esophagus caused by the Heimlich maneuver. *Ann Emerg Med* 1986;15:106–107.
43. Chaikhouni A, Kratz JM, Crawford FA. Foreign bodies of the esophagus. *Am Surg* 1985;51:173–179.
44. Chiari H. Üeber Fremdkorperverletzung des Oesophagus mit Aortenperforation. *Berlin Klin Wschr.* 1914;51:7–9.
45. Sloop RD, Thompson JC. Aorto-esophageal fistula: report of a case and review of literature. *Gastroenterology* 1967;53:768–777.
46. Laforet EG. Aorto-esophageal fistula due to foreign body: report of two cases. *Mil Med* 1975;278–280.
47. Ctercteko G, Mok CK. Aorta-esophageal fistula induced by a foreign body. The first recorded survival. *J Thorac Cardiovasc Surg* 1980;80:233–235.
48. Savitt DL, Wason S. Delayed diagnosis of coin ingestion in children. *Am J Emerg Med* 1988;6:378–381.
49. Blair SR, Graeber GM, Cruzzavala JL, et al. Current management of esophageal impactions. *Chest* 1993;104:1205–1209.
50. Binder L, Anderson WA. Pediatric gastrointestinal foreign body ingestions. *Ann Emerg Med* 1993;13:112–117.
51. Baraka A, Bikhazi G. Oesophageal foreign bodies. *BMJ* 1975; 51:561–563.
52. Crysdale WS, Sendi KS, Yoo J. Esophageal foreign bodies in children: 15-year review of 484 cases. *Ann Otol Rhinol Laryngol* 1991;100:320–324.
53. Hawkins DB. Removal of blunt foreign bodies from the esophagus. *Ann Otol Rhinol Laryngol* 1990;99:935–940.
54. Boothroyd AE, Carty HML, Robson WJ. "Hunt the thimble": A study of the radiology of ingested foreign bodies. *Arch Emerg Med* 1987;4:33–38.
55. Paul RI, Christoffel KK, Binns HJ, et al. Foreign body ingestions in children: risk of complications varies with site of initial health care contact. *Pediatrics* 1993;91:121–127.

56. Hodge D III, Tecklenburg F, Fleischer G. Coin ingestion: does every child need a radiograph? *Ann Emerg Med* 1985;14: 443–446.

57. Fulginiti VA. Is standard practice in pediatrics "standard"? A potential lesson for experts and practitioners. *Am J Dis Child* 1989;143:529–530.

58. Bader M. Is standard practice "standard" in community pediatrics? *Am J Dis Child* 1990;144:11.

59. Jessee RA. Is standard practice "standard" in community pediatrics? *Am J Dis Child* 1990;144:11.

60. Jones JE. Is standard practice "standard" in community pediatrics? *Am J Dis Child* 1990;144:13.

61. Preston EN. Is standard practice "standard" in community pediatrics? *Am J Dis Child* 1990;144:12–13.

62. Toll D. Is standard practice "standard" in community pediatrics? *Am J Dis Child* 1990;144:11–12.

63. Joseph PR. Management of coin ingestion. *Am J Dis Child* 1990;144:449–450.

64. Stringer MD, Capps SNJ. Rationalizing the management of swallowed coins in children. *BMJ* 1991;302:1321–1322.

65. Cooke MW, Glucksman EE. Swallowed coins. *BMJ* 1991;302: 1607.

66. Savitt DL, Wason S. Delayed diagnosis of coin ingestion in children. *Am J Emerg Med* 1988;6:378–381.

67. Caravati EM, Bennett DL, McElwee NE. Pediatric coin ingestion: a prospective study on the utility of routine roentgenograms. *Am J Dis Child* 1989;143:549–551.

68. Stack LB, Munter DW. Foreign bodies in the gastrointestinal tract. *Emerg Med Clin North Am* 1996;14:493–521.

69. Ros SP, Cetta F. Successful use of a metal detector in locating coins ingested by children. *J Pediatr* 1992;120:752–753.

70. Biehler JL, Tuggle D, Stacy T. Use of the transmitter-receiver metal detector in the evaluation of pediatric coin ingestion. *Pediatr Emerg Care* 1993;9:208–210.

71. Sachetti A, Carraccio C, Lichenstein R. Hand-held metal detector identification of ingested foreign bodies. *Pediatr Emerg Care* 1994;10:204–207.

72. Basset KE, Schunk JE, Logan L. Localizing ingested coins with a metal detector. *Am J Emerg Med* 1999;17:338–341.

73. Gelfand DW. Complications of gastrointestinal radiologic procedures: complications of routine fluoroscopic procedures. *Gastrointest Radiol* 1980;5:293.

74. Braverman I, Gomori JM, Polv O, et al. The role of CT imaging in the evaluation of cervical esophageal foreign bodies. *J Otolaryngol* 1993;22:311–314.

75. Douglas M, Sistrom CL. Chicken bone lodged in the upper esophagus: CT findings. *Gastrointest Radiol* 1991;16:11–12.

76. Gamba JL, Heaston DK, Ling D, et al. CT diagnosis of an esophageal foreign body. *Am J Roentgenol* 1983;140:289–290.

77. Lim CCT, Cheah FK, Tan JCH. Spiral computed tomography demonstration of aorto-oesophageal fistula from fish bone. *Clinical Radiol* 2000;55:976–977.

78. Nakshabendi IM, Maldonado ME, Brady PG. Chest pain: overlooked manifestation of unsuspected esophageal foreign body. *South Med J* 2001;94:333–335.

79. Hess GP. An approach to throat complaints: foreign body sensation difficulty swallowing and hoarseness. *Emerg Med Clin North Am* 1987;5:313–334.

80. Sundgren PC, Burnett A, Maly PV. Value of radiography in the management of possible fishbone ingestion. *Ann Otol Rhinol Laryngol* 1994;103:628–631.

81. Lyons MF, Tsuchida AM. Foreign bodies of the gastrointestinal tract. *Med Clin North Am* 1993;77:1101–1114.

82. Ricote GC, Torre LR, De Ayala VP, et al. Fiberendoscopic removal of foreign bodies of the upper gastrointestinal tract. *Surg Gynecol Obstet* 1985;160:499–504.

83. Byrne WJ. Foreign bodies, bezoars, and caustic ingestion. *Gastrointest Endosc Clin North Am* 1994;4:99–119.

84. Suarez CA, Arango A, Lester JL III. Cocaine-condom ingestion, surgical treatment. *JAMA* 1977;238:1391–1392.

85. Dunne JW. Drug smuggling by internal bodily concealment. *Med J Aust* 1983;2:436–439.

86. McPherson RI, Hill JG, Othersen HB, et al. Esophageal foreign bodies in children: diagnosis, treatment and complications. *Am J Roentgenol* 1996;166:919–924.

87. Calkins CM, Christians KK, Sell LL. Cost analysis in the management of esophageal coins, endoscopy versus bougienage. *J Pediatr Surg* 1999;34:412–414.

88. Kelly JE, Leech MH, Carr MG. A safe and cost effective protocol for the management of esophageal coins in children. *J Pediatr Surg* 1993;28:898–900.

89. Obiako MN. Tracheoesophageal fistula: a complication of foreign body. *Ann Otol Rhinol Laryngol* 1982;91:325–327.

90. Nahman BJ, Mueller CF. Asymptomatic esophageal perforation by a coin in a child. *Ann Emerg Med* 1984;13:627–629.

91. Bendig DW. Removal of blunt esophageal foreign bodies by flexible endoscopy without general anesthesia. *Am J Dis Child* 1986;40:789–790.

92. Gauderer MW, DeCou JM, Abrams RJ, et al. The "penny pincher": a new technique for fast and safe removal of esophageal coins. *J Pediatr Surg* 2000;35:276–278.

93. McGahren ED. Esophageal foreign bodies. *Pediatr Rev* 1999; 20:129–133.

94. Connors GP. A literature based comparison of three method of pediatric esophageal coin removal. *Pediatr Emerg Care* 1997; 13:154–157.

95. Bigler FC. The use of a Foley catheter for removal of blunt foreign bodies from the esophagus. *J Thorac Cardiovasc Surg* 1966; 51:759–760.

96. Berggreen PJ, Harrison ME, Sanowski RA, et al. Techniques and complications of esophageal foreign body extraction in children and adults. *Gastrointest Endosc* 1993;39:626–630.

97. Mariani PJ, Wagner DK. Foley catheter extraction of blunt esophageal foreign bodies. *J Emerg Med* 1986;4:301–306.

98. McGuirt WF. Use of Foley catheter for removal of esophageal foreign bodies: a survey. *Ann Otol Rhinol Laryngol* 1982;91: 599–601.

99. Schunk JE, Harrison AM, Corneli HM, et al. Fluoroscopic Foley catheter removal of esophageal foreign bodies in children: experience with 415 episodes. *Pediatrics* 1994;94:709–714.

100. Jona JZ, Glicklich M, Cohen RD. The contraindications for blind esophageal bougienage for coin ingestion in children. *J Pediatr Surg* 1988;23:328–330.

101. Yoshida CM, Peura DA. Foreign bodies. In: Castell DO, ed. *The esophagus.* New York, Little Brown, 1995:379–394.

102. Faigel DO, Stotland BR, Kochman ML, et al. Device choice and experience level in endoscopic foreign body retrieval: an *in vivo* study. *Gastrointest Endosc* 1997;45:490–492.

103. Winkler AR, McClenathan DT, Borger JA, et al. Retrograde esophagoscopy for foreign body removal. *J Pediatr Gastroenterol Nutr* 1989;8:536–540.

104. Ferrucci JT Jr, Long JA Jr. Radiologic treatment of esophageal food impaction using intravenous glucagon. *Radiology* 1977; 125:25–28.

105. Trenkner SW, Maglinte DT, Lehman G, et al. Esophageal food impaction: treatment with glucagon. *Radiology* 1983;149: 401–403.

106. Giordano A, Adams G, Boies L Jr, et al. Current management of esophageal foreign bodies. *Arch Otolaryngol* 1981;107: 249–251.

107. Taylor RB. Esophageal foreign bodies. *Emerg Med Clin North Am* 1987;5:301–311.

108. Robbins MI, Shortsleeve MJ. Treatment of acute esophageal food impaction with glucagon, an effervescent agent, and water. *Am J Roentgenol* 1994;162:325–328.

109. Smith JC, Janower ML, Geiger AH. Use of glucagon and gas-forming agents in acute esophageal food impaction. *Radiology* 1986;159:567–568.

110. Kaszar-Seibert DJ, Korn WT, Bindman DJ, et al. Treatment of acute esophageal food impaction with a combination of glucagon, effervescent agent and water. *Am J Roentgenol* 1990;154:533–534.

111. Richardson JR. A new treatment for esophageal obstruction due to meat impaction. *Ann Otol Rhino Laryngol* 1945;54:328–348.

112. Robinson AS. Meat impaction in the esophagus treated by enzymatic digestion. *JAMA* 1962;181:1142–1143.

113. Andersen HA, Bernatz PE, Gridlay JH. Perforation of the esophagus after use of a digestant agent: report of a case and experimental study. *Ann Otol* 1959;68:890–896.

114. Holsinger JW, Fuson RL, Sealy WC. Esophageal perforation following meat impaction and papain ingestion. *JAMA* 1968;204:734–735.

115. Hall ML, Huseby JS. Hemorrhagic pulmonary edema associated with meat tenderizer treatment for esophageal meat impaction. *Chest* 1988;94:640–642.

116. Nighbert E, Dorton H, Griffin WO. Enzymatic relief of the steakhouse syndrome. *Am J Surg* 1968;116:467–469.

117. Rice BT, Speigel PK, Dombrowski PJ. Acute esophageal food impaction treated by gas-forming agents. *Radiology* 1983;146:299–301.

118. Mohammed SH, Hegedus V. Dislodgement of impacted oesophageal foreign bodies with carbonated beverages. *Clin Radiol* 1986;37:589–592.

119. Zimmers TE, Chan SB, Kouchoukos PL, et al. Use of gas-forming agents in esophageal food impactions. *Ann Emerg Med* 1988;17:693–695.

120. Kozarek RA, Sanowski RA. Esophageal food impaction: description of a new method for bolus removal. *Dig Dis Sci* 1980;25:100–103.

121. Schaffer RD, Klug T. A comparative study of techniques for esophageal foreign body removal with special emphasis on meat bolus obstruction. *Wis Med J* 1981;80:33–36.

122. Garrido J, Barkin JS. Endoscopic modifications for safe foreign body removal. *Am J Gastroenterol* 1985;80:957–958.

123. Henderson CT, Engel J, Schlesinger P. Foreign body ingestion: review and suggested guidelines for management. *Endoscopy* 1987;19:68–71.

124. Vicari JJ, Johnson JF, Frakes JT. Outcomes of acute esophageal food impactions: success of the push technique. *Gastrointest Endosc* 2001;53:178–181.

125. Klein I. Resourceful management of esophageal food impaction. *Gastrointest Endosc* 1990;36:80.

126. Quinn PG, Connors PJ. The role of upper gastrointestinal endoscopy in foreign body removal. *Gastrointest Endosc Clin North Am* 1994;4:571–593.

18

SURGERY FOR ESOPHAGEAL MOTOR DISORDERS

BRANT K. OELSCHLAGER
THOMAS R. EUBANKS
CARLOS A. PELLEGRINI

Esophageal motor disorders may be divided into two simple categories: disorders of increased muscular activity and disorders of decreased muscular activity. Similarly, surgical intervention for motor disorders of the esophagus is based on two simple concepts: when the muscular activity is too great, the surgical treatment is based on transecting the appropriate muscle; if the muscular activity is insufficient, the only surgical treatment is esophageal resection.

Despite the limited surgical options available, a large body of literature has been generated on the surgical management of esophageal motor dysfunction. The controversies regarding motor disorders are rooted in areas such as indication, technique, and outcome of the various operations.

The motor disorders of the esophagus are discussed in relation to their anatomic location, starting from the upper esophageal sphincter (UES) and working toward the gastroesophageal junction. A summary of each disease is presented, followed by the assessment and surgical treatment. The controversial issues for each topic are discussed at the end of each section.

UPPER ESOPHAGEAL SPHINCTER

Swallowing consists of oral, pharyngeal, and esophageal phases. The UES plays a role in the pharyngeal phase and in the transition from the pharyngeal to the esophageal phase. Pharyngoesophageal diverticulum (Zenker's diverticulum) and cricopharyngeal bar, also referred to as cricopharyngeal achalasia, have been identified as pathologic entities of the UES. Understanding the anatomy and function of the UES is essential to planning an operation to treat these maladies.

The pharynx meets the esophagus where the inferior pharyngeal constrictor joins the cricopharyngeus muscle. The inferior constrictor takes origin from the thyroid and cricoid cartilage, and its fibers run obliquely and horizontally to insert on the median raphe (posterior aspect) of the pharynx. The cricopharyngeus muscle arises from the cricoid cartilage, passes posteriorly to the pharyngoesophageal junction, and inserts on the contralateral side of the cricoid cartilage. Some anatomists view the cricopharyngeal muscle as simply the most inferior segment of the inferior constrictor, differing from the other muscle fibers in that they do not insert into the median raphe (1). However, the structures are seen as distinctly separate in the surgical approach to the UES. The interlacing of muscle fibers at the posterior aspect of the pharynx leaves areas of potential weakness where herniation of the mucosa may occur, especially when intraluminal pressures are elevated. The triangle of Killian is one of these areas and is found between the inferior constrictor and the cricopharyngeus muscle (2,3). Two additional areas where the relative paucity of muscle fibers creates a relative weakness in the pharyngeal wall are the Killian-Jamieson's area, between the fibers of the cricopharyngeus, and Laimer's triangle between the junction of the cricopharyngeus and the first circular fibers of the esophagus (4) (Fig. 18.1). The purpose of the inferior constrictor is to compress the pharynx during swallowing, displacing the food bolus downward. The cricopharyngeus muscle maintains tonic contraction, closing the inlet to the esophagus between swallows, and relaxes during swallowing to allow bolus entry into the esophagus. The cricopharyngeus muscle generates most of the pressure at the manometrically identified UES, because the physiologic high-pressure zone is often found to be of greater length than the anatomically identified muscle fibers. The function of the UES is to prevent the entrance of air into the esophagus and more recently has been recognized for its role in preventing high gastroesophageal reflux from entering the larynx (5).

B. K. Oelschlager, T. R. Eubanks, C. A. Pellegrini: Department of Surgery, University of Washington, Seattle, Washington.

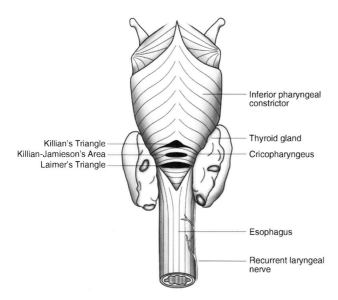

FIGURE 18.1. Schematic drawing of the posterior aspect of the pharyngoesophageal junction with areas of weakness identified.

Labels in figure:
Inferior pharyngeal constrictor
Killian's Triangle
Killian-Jamieson's Area
Laimer's Triangle
Thyroid gland
Cricopharyngeus
Esophagus
Recurrent laryngeal nerve

When a swallow is initiated, the UES relaxes while the oral and pharyngeal phases of deglutition proceed. As the tongue propels the bolus posteriorly, the larynx is elevated and compressed to prevent the bolus from entering the trachea. The bolus passes into the pharynx and the constrictors then contract to propel the bolus into the esophagus. The tonic contraction of the UES is inhibited and the bolus proceeds into the esophagus. This is a conceptually simple interpretation of deglutition. However, extensive study of the physiology of the UES and the pathophysiology of the diseases that affect the UES have revealed the complexity of the UES activity. A more concise description may be found elsewhere in this book.

PHARYNGOESOPHAGEAL DIVERTICULUM (ZENKER'S)

Since all reported cases of pharyngoesophageal diverticulum have occurred in elderly patients, it is assumed to be an acquired disease. The diverticulum is not a true one, in that it consists of only mucosa, which escapes the pharynx between the areas of weakness in the muscle fibers described earlier. It is classified as a pulsion diverticulum because it is thought to arise from increased pressure within the pharynx. The reason for this increase in intraluminal pressure within the pharynx is not known, but at least four hypotheses have been advanced as an explanation (6). The early explanation was that the UES was maintaining tonic contraction during swallowing in response to lower esophageal disease, such as gastroesophageal reflux. Then, the concept of achalasia of the UES, a failure to relax, was put forward as the explanation for the high resistance at the pharyngo-

esophageal junction. As manometric evaluation of the UES became available, it was found that the UES was capable of relaxing, but that lack of coordination between bolus propagation and sphincter relaxation was the primary cause of the increased pressure in the pharynx. Finally, evidence suggests that the muscles of the cricopharyngeus and the proximal esophagus are fibrosed and therefore do not function as they normally would.

The last two theories have the greatest support, and both contribute conceptually to understanding the dysfunction of the UES. Manometry of the UES shows some degree of incoordination in more than two thirds of patients (7). The dysfunction occurs most frequently during the UES closure after relaxation and the initiation of the proximal esophageal peristalsis (8). The precise nature of the dysfunction can be difficult to assess with stationary manometry because the UES is relatively narrow compared with the vertical distance it moves during normal deglutition. The combination of manometry with simultaneous fluoroscopy has helped resolve this problem. By ensuring proper placement of the manometry catheter at the UES, it was found that the sphincter was not relaxing completely and that its baseline pressure was also decreased (9). Further investigation of the sphincter muscles showed that they were replaced by fibrotic tissue, which explained the abnormal response of the sphincter to swallowing (10–12). It is not known whether the fibrosis is a cause or effect of the disease.

Clinical Evaluation

Pharyngoesophageal diverticulum usually occurs in the seventh or eighth decade of life. Cervical esophageal dysphagia and regurgitation are the most common complaints. Dysphagia may occur as a result of the dysfunctional UES. It may also be due to displacement or obstruction of the pharyngoesophageal junction caused by a large diverticulum and its contents. As the diverticulum enlarges, regurgitation of undigested food particularly during recumbency becomes more prevalent. Aspiration, halitosis, excessive salivation, and a fullness in the neck may also occur. The physical examination is usually not helpful but may reveal a palpable mass, most commonly on the left side of the neck, and a foul odor may be detected on the breath.

A contrast esophagogram should be obtained. It usually reveals the diverticulum and helps exclude a high esophageal tumor (Fig. 18.2). Although a videoesophagram also demonstrates abnormal movement of the contrast during deglutition, it is probably not necessary to obtain one. Other studies that can confirm the diagnosis include esophagoscopy and manometry. A 24-hour pH study has been used to determine whether there is associated gastroesophageal reflux, which is believed by some to contribute to the pathogenesis of the disease. None of the last three tests is likely to alter the therapy, and they are probably not nec-

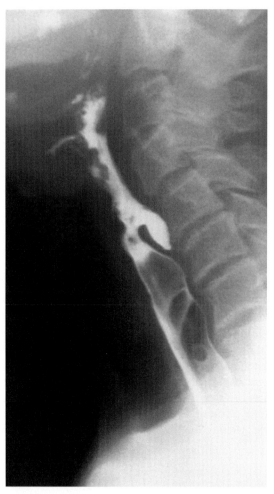

FIGURE 18.2. Lateral view of an esophagogram demonstrating a Zenker's diverticulum projecting downward posterior to the cricopharyngeus muscle.

essary in the average patient with a pharyngoesophageal diverticulum.

Treatment

Before operative treatment of the diverticulum, the patient should be on a liquid diet for 1 or 2 days to minimize the amount of retained food particles in the diverticulum. Although the preoperative contrast study helps decide which side of the neck will provide the best exposure for the procedure, the left side is usually preferred. Most diverticula originate in the posterior aspect of the pharynx. As they grow, about 25% project to the left side and 10% project to the right side; thus, the left side is used in 90% of cases. The approach from the left is easier from an anatomic standpoint. The tracheoesophageal groove and the recurrent laryngeal nerve are more accessible because of the slight rightward shift of the trachea relative to the esophagus in the neck.

Access to the area is gained through a low cervical incision along the anterior border of the sternocleidomastoid muscle. The dissection proceeds along the avascular plane anterior to the sternocleidomastoid muscle, which is retracted laterally. The carotid sheath is retracted laterally as well, and the thyroid gland medially. Often, the middle thyroid vein is ligated and transected, as is the omohyoid muscle to improve exposure. As the tracheoesophageal groove is approached, care must be taken to avoid injuring the recurrent laryngeal nerve. With the posterolateral aspect of the esophagus exposed, a bougie may be carefully passed into the esophagus. The surgeon should guide the bougie to prevent it from entering the diverticulum. With the bougie in place, a circumferential dissection of the esophagus is performed. The esophagus is then dissected cephalad along the posterior midline toward its junction with the pharynx. During this dissection, the diverticulum is encountered (Fig. 18.3).

The diverticulum is grasped with a Babcock forceps, dissected free from adjacent structures, and elevated into the wound (Fig. 18.4). The neck of the diverticulum is cleared of the surrounding tissues. This should reveal the triangle of Killian. At this point, a myotomy is performed. The cricopharyngeus muscle and the proximal few centimeters of the longitudinal and circular muscle of the esophagus are also transected, so that the mucosa protrudes through the myotomy site (Fig. 18.5). The diverticulum should be excised whenever possible to reduce the amount of redun-

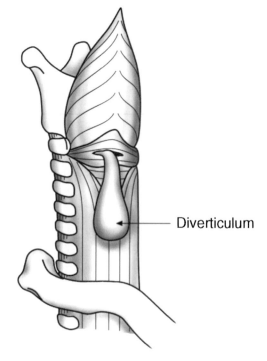

FIGURE 18.3. Drawing of a diverticulum relative to the surgical landmarks of the posterior pharynx.

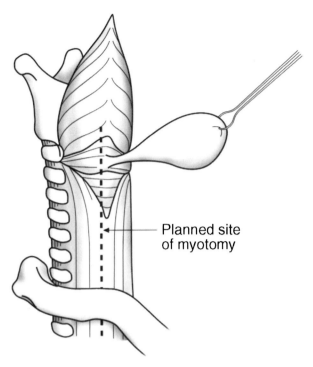

FIGURE 18.4. Diverticulum elevated from the dissection site. The site of the planned myotomy is marked by the dotted line.

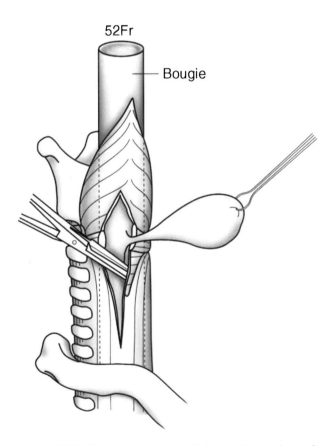

FIGURE 18.5. The myotomy is extended onto the esophagus for several centimeters.

dant mucosa at the pharyngoesophageal junction. To accomplish this, a linear stapler is placed across the neck of the diverticulum with a bougie inside the esophagus to prevent narrowing of the lumen (Fig. 18.6). The platysma is closed loosely and the skin is approximated. Drainage of the wound is not necessary. The patient is allowed a liquid diet on the first postoperative day, and if no evidence of a leak is present, the diet may be advanced.

Outcome

Resolution of dysphagia and regurgitation may be expected and has been reported in 82% to 100% of patients treated with this approach (7,13,14). Despite the symptomatic improvement, the mechanism of deglutition is not entirely restored to normal. For example, postoperative video contrast studies show abnormalities in pharyngeal peristalsis, a visible cricopharyngeus, premature closure of the cricopharyngeus, and, occasionally, a residual diverticulum (15).

Complications

Mortality from this procedure should be less than 1%. The most disturbing complication, esophagocutaneous fistula, occurs in 6% to 20% of cases but heals spontaneously (14). Other potential complications include soft tissue infection, mediastinitis, recurrent laryngeal nerve

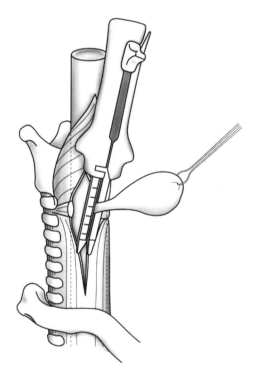

FIGURE 18.6. The stapling and cutting device is placed across the neck of the diverticulum. Note that the bougie is in place before transecting the diverticulum.

injury, hematoma, and late stenosis. The frequency of these complications ranges between 1% and 6% (10). Some authors feel that mucosal injury and recurrent laryngeal nerve injury may be reduced by operating with loupe magnification (16). Recurrence rates are low, and if the diverticulum is excised while a bougie is in the esophagus, postoperative stenosis is rare.

Controversies in Treatment

All patients with pharyngoesophageal diverticula who are able to tolerate an operation should probably be treated, because the natural history of the disease is one of progression leading to complications (6). No medical therapy has been shown to be effective at treating these diverticula. Several elements of the surgical treatment have been topics of debate.

Peroral or Endoscopic Approach

The approach described previously has been the mainstay of surgical treatment in North America for several decades (17–21). By contrast, many European surgeons prefer some variant of the peroral approach to treating pharyngoesophageal diverticula (2,3,22–28). More recently, there has been some crossover in the approaches (13,16,29–31). There have been no prospective, randomized trials comparing the transcervical and peroral approaches for treating pharyngoesophageal diverticula.

Most peroral methods of treating diverticula are variations of Dohlman's modification of Mosher's first description in 1917 (23). Rigid endoscopy is used to gain exposure to the pharynx while the patient is under general anesthesia. The esophageal lumen and the diverticular neck are thus identified. The intervening muscle between the lumen of the esophagus and the pouch of the diverticulum is divided. The diverticulum is no longer a blind-ended pouch, in that the anterior wall of the diverticulum communicates with the esophageal lumen. Most surgeons who use this technique use cautery or laser technology to divide the muscles between the diverticulum and the esophagus. One of the problems with this technique is that it allows communication between the lumen of the esophagus and the deep tissue planes of the neck. Although the potential complications of deep tissue infection and mediastinitis are concerns, they occurred in only 12 of 544 patients treated in one of the largest studies (3).

Another method of transecting the tissue between the two structures is to use a commercially available automatic stapling and cutting device (24). This gained significant popularity in the last few years. One arm of the device is placed into the lumen of the esophagus and the other into the diverticulum. Four rows of staples are then fired into the tissue bridge, and a blade cuts between the inner two rows of staples (Fig. 18.7). Thus, the tissue is stapled and divided, theoretically preventing the escape of esophageal contents from the cut edges. Several series have shown this to be a safe and effective procedure with satisfaction rates in the 90% range (34–36).

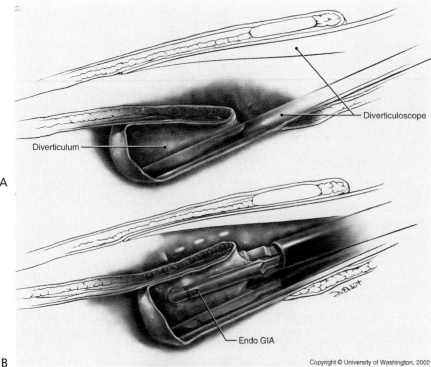

Copyright © University of Washington, 2002

FIGURE 18.7. A: Exposure of the esophagus and diverticulum is gained with a diverticuloscope placed perorally. **B:** The linear stapler is across the cricopharyngeus muscle by placing a blade in the esophagus and the diverticulum. (From University of Washington, Seattle, WA, with permission.)

Limitations and contraindications to the procedure include restrictions in exposure (small oral cavity, prominent dentition, or cervical spine disease) and a very small diverticulum (<3 cm). Endoscopic stapling may not be adequate for extremely large diverticulum, in that there is often persistent bolus pooling in the diverticulum. The most serious complication is esophageal or pharyngeal perforation, which occurs up to 10% of the time in some series (34). Inadequate cricopharyngeal transection may also occur, leading to persistent or recurrent symptoms and requiring surgical revision. The advantage is that it takes less time to complete, does not require an incision, and therefore may have less morbidity. This is an important consideration because this disease most commonly presents in the seventh and eighth decade of life.

There are few comparison trials between endoscopic and open treatment of Zenker's diverticulum. Smith and colleagues showed in a retrospective analysis that the endoscopic stapling technique took less operative time (26 vs. 88 minutes), but because of the equipment costs of the stapling technique the operative charges were equivalent ($5,178 vs. $5,113) (37). The mean length of stay, however, was much shorter for the endoscopic procedure (1.3 days vs. 5.2 days), thus the inpatient hospital charges were less for this procedure ($3,589 vs. $11,439). For patients with significant comorbidities and anatomy amenable to this approach, endoscopic stapling provides a reasonable alternative to the traditional transcervical approach. Long-term results and better comparative studies are needed, however, before endoscopic stapling should be considered as the standard operation.

Diverticulectomy versus Diverticulopexy

In an effort to decrease the incidence of soft tissue infection and mediastinitis, the diverticulum may be sutured to the precervical fascia so that the apex is cephalad to the neck (Fig. 18.8). By not breaching the esophageal mucosa, the incidence of infection would theoretically be decreased. In a nonrandomized study of 43 patients approached by a transcervical route, all patients had myotomies performed; 14 had diverticulectomy, and 29 had diverticulopexy (16). Neck infection developed in two patients in both groups, and mediastinitis developed in one patient in the diverticulectomy group. There was no statistical difference in the incidence of wound infection or mediastinitis between the two groups. It may be argued that the study did not have enough patients to detect a difference in infectious complications. This may obscure the theoretical benefit of the diverticulopexy procedure. However, diverticulopexy was the procedure of choice in the most recent patients, in that the authors discarded the use of diverticulectomy for treatment. Thus, no known difference exists between the two procedures with respect to outcome or complications.

Although in the past some advocated diverticulectomy alone, the incidence of recurrence was so high that it is now

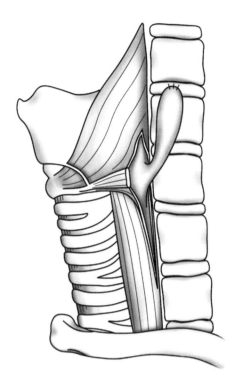

FIGURE 18.8. Drawing of a diverticulopexy. The apex of the diverticulum is sutured to the precervical fascia.

inadvisable to treat the diverticulum without performing a myotomy (17).

Treating Associated Foregut Pathology

Other abnormalities of esophageal and gastric function may be found in up to 60% of patients with pharyngoesophageal diverticula (31). The most common finding is gastroesophageal reflux disease. As with cricopharyngeal bar (discussed later), the association between the two is thought to stem from an attempt by the UES to prevent gastric contents from reaching the pharynx. The issue of addressing both entities simultaneously has waxed and waned for the past 30 years depending on the accepted explanation of the pathophysiology of pharyngoesophageal diverticulum (38). Some surgeons believe that, if abnormal gastroesophageal reflux is demonstrated preoperatively, it should be treated surgically during the same procedure as the pharyngoesophageal diverticulum. The rationale behind this approach is the assumption that once the cricopharyngeal myotomy is performed, the refluxed contents from the stomach may more easily enter the larynx, causing laryngitis, hoarseness, and even aspiration. However, not all patients with Zenker's diverticulum have concomitant foregut pathology. The best approach is to address each pathologic entity based on its severity and the discomfort it creates for the patient. If heartburn, regurgitation of digested food, and esophagitis are the predominant findings in a patient who has a small Zenker's diverticulum on a contrast study, the reflux should be treated first, because some relief from both may be gained (5). Similarly, if the patient has cervical dysphagia, regurgitation of undigested food, and a mildly abnormal 24-hour pH study, the pharyngoesophageal diverticulum should be treated alone.

Conclusion

Zenker's diverticula are the result of a dysfunctional UES and a weakness in the posterior muscular fibers of the pharyngoesophageal junction. Regurgitation and cervical dysphagia are the most common symptoms. Diagnostic workup may be limited to a contrast study of the pharynx and the esophagus. Concurrent foregut pathology should be addressed on its own merit. No medical therapy is effective in the treatment of pharyngoesophageal diverticula. Surgical treatment, including resection of the diverticulum and cricopharyngeal myotomy, relieves symptoms and has excellent results.

CRICOPHARYNGEAL BAR (UPPER ESOPHAGEAL SPHINCTER ACHALASIA)

A cricopharyngeal bar is identified radiographically by a persistent posterior indentation of contrast in the pharyngoesophageal segment. This is seen on a lateral view during a videoesophagram or barium swallow (Fig. 18.9). In addition, residual contrast may be seen above the cricopharyn-

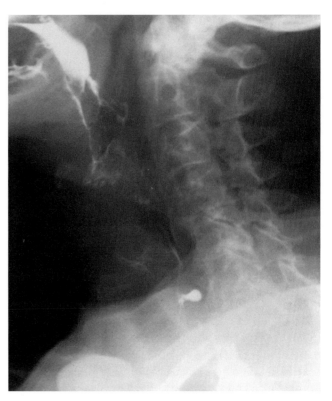

FIGURE 18.10. The same patient at a later phase of swallowing, showing the persistent contrast above the cricopharyngeus muscle. Note how the relative position of the cricopharyngeus muscle has descended back toward the clavicle.

geus well after the UES has closed (Fig. 18.10). Despite the presence of such a finding, no consistent clinical symptoms have been identified in these patients. In fact, the etiology and the significance of a cricopharyngeal bar are unknown.

Based on the concept that the UES relaxes during swallowing, the persistent indentation has been described as either a failure to relax (thus the term UES achalasia) or incoordination of the constrictors and the cricopharyngeus muscle. Dantas and colleagues examined six patients with cricopharyngeal bars and eight control subjects without this finding on barium swallow (39). The subjects were assessed using videofluoroscopy and UES manometry. The patients were found to have normal contraction of the pharynx, UES pressure, and bolus flow rate. When compared with control subjects, the patients with cricopharyngeal bars had reduced UES relaxation during swallowing and increased upstream bolus pressures. From these data, it appears that cricopharyngeal bars arise as a result of failure of the muscle to completely relax. Others have found that resting, relaxation, and contraction pressures are normal in patients with cricopharyngeal bar (40). In fact, these authors claim that the cricopharyngeal muscle is the only normal portion of the pharyngoesophageal segment and that the inferior constrictor and the proximal esophagus are abnormally dilated.

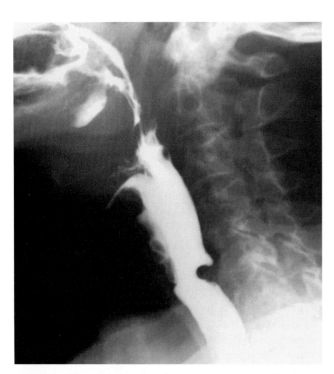

FIGURE 18.9. Lateral view of an esophagogram showing a cricopharyngeal bar. The persistent indentation posteriorly is caused by the cricopharyngeus muscle.

Even when a cricopharyngeal bar can be demonstrated, the clinical significance of this finding is difficult to discern. Patients who are asymptomatic may have the same degree of narrowing as patients being evaluated for cervical esophageal dysphagia (39). Furthermore, cricopharyngeal bar is seen in greater than 50% of patients with gastroesophageal reflux (41). Because of the ambiguity of the finding and the lack of symptoms attributable to this dysfunction, surgical intervention for cricopharyngeal bar is only appropriate for selected patients. The patients should not have a medical condition known to affect motility (myopathy, Parkinson's disease, or myasthenia gravis), neoplasia must be excluded, and gastroesophageal reflux should be eliminated as a cause of the cricopharyngeal bar (42). If these requirements are satisfied and the patient has symptoms referable to the cervical esophagus, a cricopharyngeal myotomy may provide some relief.

ACHALASIA

Achalasia is the most common esophageal motor disorder that warrants surgical intervention. This disease is characterized by incomplete lower esophageal sphincter (LES) relaxation and absent esophageal peristalsis. As a consequence, esophageal emptying is impaired, which causes progressive dilation and lengthening of the organ. Both medical and surgical treatments are geared toward decreasing resistance to flow through the gastroesophageal junction. Although this improves emptying and relieves symptoms of the disease, it does not directly affect the underlying etiology of the pathologic process.

Despite multiple attempts at defining the pathophysiology of achalasia, little is known about the etiology of the disease. Chagas disease does provide some insight into achalasia, because the symptoms, the anatomic findings, and the physiologic aspects of the two diseases are similar. In Chagas disease, *Trypanosoma cruzi* destroys the myenteric plexus of the esophagus, which is thought to be the cause of altered motor dysfunction and LES relaxation. Patients with achalasia also have a decreased number of neural cells in their myenteric plexus.

Because most cases occur between the fourth and sixth decades of life, there is little suspicion of a congenital cause. However, familial achalasia has been reported in up to six siblings in a single family (43). Robertson and colleagues (44) reported finding varicella zoster virus DNA in the esophageal muscular wall of 33% of patients with achalasia. Other investigators have reported no correlation between viral infections and the incidence of achalasia (45).

The one pathologic finding that is agreed upon in achalasia is the relative paucity of the myenteric plexus in the esophageal wall. Whether this is a cause or an effect of achalasia is unknown. The lack of LES relaxation is thought to be related to impaired nonadrenergic, noncholinergic inhibitory control and the lack of nitric oxide synthase (46). Despite the lack of nitric oxide, the LES is still sensitive to other enteric hormones such as secretin (47). More investigation is needed to determine the etiology of achalasia and, therefore, for the chance to halt progression or prevent the disease. For now, palliation of the symptoms is all physicians have to offer.

Clinical Evaluation

Achalasia usually presents with symptoms of progressive dysphagia and regurgitation of undigested food. Other symptoms may include substernal chest pain, heartburn, and, rarely, abdominal pain. As the esophagus becomes more dilated, patients tend to complain less about dysphagia and more about regurgitation. Weight loss is common, and, occasionally, patients are malnourished. Dysphagia is primarily related to the ingestion of solid food. Most patients relate a "need to push food down with liquids" and frequent episodes of complete occlusion of the esophagus leading to "vomiting." Because progression of the disease is insidious, most patients do not seek medical attention for quite some time. The average length of time between the onset of symptoms and operative intervention is 60 months (48).

Whenever a patient presents with these complaints, other etiologies must be considered, such as tumors of the gastroesophageal junction, neurologic diseases, and connective tissue disorders. Pseudoachalasia, also called secondary achalasia, may be caused by neoplasms, paraneoplastic syndromes, pseudocysts, and postoperative obstruction of the gastroesophageal junction after a perihiatal operation (49,50). These patients present with manometric and radiologic signs of achalasia and may be difficult to distinguish from patients with achalasia. A careful history and physical examination often aids in identifying patients with pseudoachalasia. Tumors generally occur in older patients, and the progression of dysphagia and weight loss is more rapid. Thus, the physician should be wary when the diagnosis of achalasia is entertained in a patient older than age 70 years, particularly when the duration of symptoms is less than 6 months and the weight loss is greater than 20 lb. These patients should be carefully examined in search of palpable supraclavicular lymphadenopathy and other signs of a neoplastic process. In addition, their diagnostic evaluation should include an accurate assessment of the morphology of the esophageal wall. The test of choice is a transesophageal endoscopic ultrasound. If this is not available, a computed tomography scan may provide useful information.

Achalasia is rare in children, and a timely diagnosis is difficult. The time lapse between symptoms and correct diagnosis is between 6 months and 9 years. Children may manifest the disease by recurrent episodes of pneumonia, failure to thrive, coughing, and hoarseness (51). Some teenagers have even been given a diagnosis of anorexia nervosa (52).

Diagnostic Tests

Evaluation of patients suspected of having achalasia should include manometry, an esophagogram, and upper endoscopy. If possible, a 24-hour pH study should also be performed.

Manometry

Manometry is the gold standard for diagnosing achalasia. The criteria for diagnosis are (a) aperistalsis of the esophageal body, (b) incomplete relaxation of the LES, and (c) normal or hypertonic LES pressure (see Chapter 11). Disorganized contractions of the esophageal body usually have normal or less than normal amplitudes. The waves are not propagated throughout the length of the esophagus and are often simultaneous. The LES pressure fails to drop to the gastric baseline as it does in the normal state.

In some patients, chest pain is a predominant symptom. Many patients have high-amplitude contractions. In this variant of the disease, called *vigorous achalasia*, the high-amplitude waves are thought to cause pain. Thus, dilation or myotomy limited to the gastroesophageal junction, although enough to relieve dysphagia, may not be adequate to relieve pain in these patients. Parrilla and colleagues (53), however, reported excellent pain relief following a standard myotomy in patients with vigorous achalasia. To help understand the origin of these high-amplitude contractions, Stuart and colleagues (54) performed manometry on 13 patients with achalasia while they were consuming a standard meal. Elevated baseline esophageal pressures developed and peak contractile pressures ranged from 65 to 120 mm Hg in all patients (54). Although none of these patients had a diagnosis of vigorous achalasia on stationary manometry, all developed high contractile pressures when their esophagus became distended. The results of this study question the diagnosis of vigorous achalasia on stationary manometry alone.

The LES may also be assessed using vector volume analysis. This is performed with four or eight radially placed pressure transducers at the distal end of the probe. The probe is slowly pulled past the LES, and measurements are recorded from each transducer. A three-dimensional image is produced from the forces generated by the LES (55). The benefit of this technique over routine manometry has not been established.

Assessment of the esophagus can also be performed with ambulatory 24-hour manometry. Two transducers are placed in the body of the esophagus, neither at the LES. It may be performed in patients when the stationary manometry is equivocal. The need for preoperative manometry when contemplating a functional procedure on the esophagus is unquestionable. It is necessary to prevent performing an improper operation, such as a total fundoplication on untreated achalasia (56).

Esophagogram

The esophagogram defines the anatomy of the esophageal body and may help exclude tumor. The esophageal body is dilated and the lumen is smooth without evidence of peristaltic waves. Often, an air-fluid level is visible. A discrete narrowing at the gastroesophageal junction is noted (Fig. 18.11). The tapering of the distal esophagus should be concentric, without evidence of a mass effect. Advanced disease often reveals a tortuous esophagus or a "sigmoid esophagus" (Fig. 18.12). A diverticulum may be an associated finding.

Some have used contrast studies to evaluate the degree of esophageal dilation and the height of the contrast column before and after intervention (57). Although improvement in these measures can be seen after treatment of achalasia, the correlation with clinical outcome is not clear.

Endoscopy

Upper endoscopy is essential in patients with dysphagia to exclude intraluminal esophageal neoplastic processes. It may also identify other pathology in the stomach and duodenum. The expected findings in a patient with achalasia are a dilated proximal esophagus, retained food or liquid,

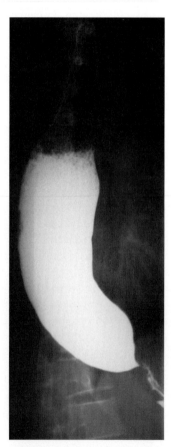

FIGURE 18.11. Esophagogram demonstrating achalasia. The patient has a smooth, abrupt tapering of the distal esophagus and an air-fluid level proximally.

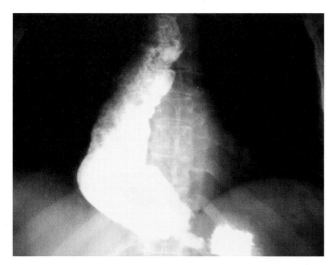

FIGURE 18.12. A patient with more advanced achalasia demonstrating a sigmoid esophagus.

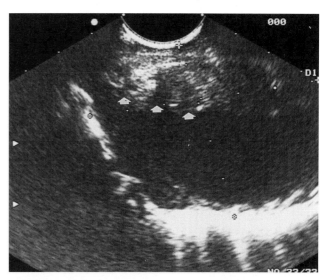

FIGURE 18.14. Endoscopic ultrasound of the same patient as in Figure 18.12. *Arrows* show the tumor of the distal esophagus disrupting the normal tissue planes.

and no evidence of esophagitis. The endoscope should pass the LES with minimal effort in patients with achalasia; if stubborn resistance is met, other causes of esophageal obstruction must be suspected. Endoscopic ultrasound is useful in these situations, because it provides a detailed view of the entire wall and may help identify tumors at the gastroesophageal junction (Figs. 18.13 and 18.14). It can also

identify the proximal extent of hypertrophic muscle in the esophageal wall.

24-Hour pH Monitoring

The pH study usually shows little, if any, reflux in classic achalasia. The pH in both the proximal and distal channels should remain greater than 4. If, however, gastroesophageal reflux does occur, it cannot be cleared by the aperistaltic esophagus. For this reason, preoperative episodes of gastroesophageal reflux are important to document.

Interpreting the pH data may be difficult and requires some degree of experience with achalasia. A computer program that receives the data directly from a digital recording device often analyzes the data. The automated analysis can be misleading because achalasia patients may have an acidic environment (pH <4.0) without any reflux. This phenomenon has been demonstrated by Crookes and colleagues (58), who showed that fermentation of bland food can generate a pH less than 4.0 when mixed with saliva. Careful inspection of the graphic tracing reveals a gradual decrease in pH over several hours as opposed to the rapid decline in pH seen with episodes of reflux (Fig. 18.15). The distinction is important for clinical assessment in both preoperative and postoperative studies (59).

Other Studies

Stationary manometry may not be possible in some patients because the gastroesophageal junction cannot be negotiated by the catheter. In this case, esophageal function may be determined using radionuclide transit and videofluoroscopic studies. Using manometry as the standard, these studies have a sensitivity of 68% and 41%, respectively (60).

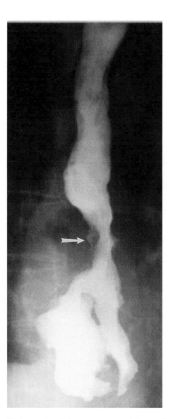

FIGURE 18.13. This patient has a ragged tapering of the distal esophagus, which is suspicious for malignancy.

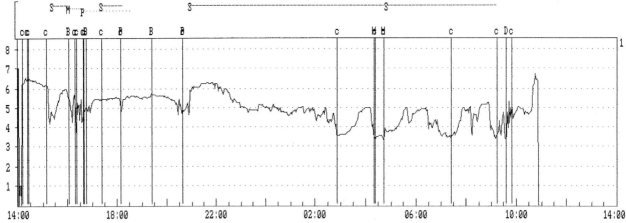

FIGURE 18.15. A 24-hour pH monitor tracing of a patient with achalasia. Between the times of 22:00 and 04:00, there is a gradual decrease in the pH consistent with fermentation.

Surgical Treatment

The aim of treatment is to decrease LES pressure and improve esophageal emptying. Both medical and surgical approaches are available. The decision to proceed with one or the other is discussed later. The standard surgical treatment is a myotomy with or without an antireflux procedure. The myotomy should be extended onto the cardia because 45% of the LES pressure is maintained by the stomach (61). The principles of operative therapy are to transect completely the longitudinal and circular muscle fibers of the esophagus and the sling fibers of the cardia. The cut edges of the muscle must be separated widely and prevented from reapproximating. The length of the myotomy should be great enough to extend onto the stomach for 2 to 3 cm and to extend up the esophagus until normal muscle thickness is encountered.

Minimally invasive surgery techniques provide an excellent approach to this operation. Both laparoscopic and thoracoscopic approaches may be used (62–65). For the average patient with achalasia, an abdominal approach is recommended because there is less pain, better access to the gastroesophageal junction, no need to collapse the lung during the operation, and better results. The preparation and operation are carried out as described in the following paragraphs.

Preparation

The patient should be restricted to a liquid diet for at least 2 days before the operation. This helps clear solid material from the dilated body of the esophagus and prevents aspi-

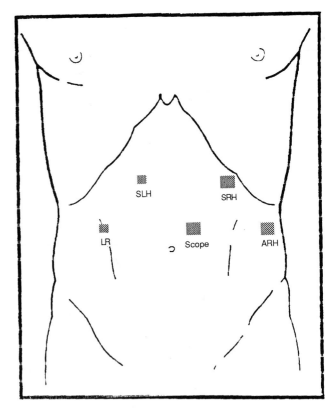

FIGURE 18.16 Diagram showing the port placement for a laparoscopic Heller-Toupet procedure. *SLH* and *SRH* mark the ports for the surgeon's left and right hands, respectively. *Scope* and *ARH* mark the ports for the assistant's left and right hands, respectively. *LR* marks the port for the liver retractor.

ration of food into the airway at the time of intubation. Use of a lighted bougie dilator and esophagoscopy should be available during the operation to facilitate transection of the muscle fibers and to determine the adequacy of the myotomy (66).

Operation

The patient is placed in a low lithotomy position with the surgeon standing between the patient's legs and the assistant standing on the patient's left. A laparoscope holder may be used to secure the instrument, which retracts the liver. Five trocars are used during the procedure. The assistant operates the laparoscope with the left hand and provides retraction with the right (Fig. 18.16).

After retracting the left lobe of the liver anteriorly, the peritoneum overlying the left crus is divided. The short gastric vessels are divided and the phrenoesophageal membrane is opened anteriorly. The right crus is then dissected so that the lateral and anterior attachments of the abdominal esophagus are freed. Posterior mobilization of the esophagus is required only when a Toupet fundoplication is

planned after completion of the myotomy. The anterior aspect of the esophagus should be dissected well into the mediastinum. At this time, the lighted bougie (number 52 French) is introduced into the esophagus transorally. The fat overlying the gastroesophageal junction should be removed, and the anterior vagus dissected free from the esophageal wall. The cardiomyotomy site is marked with cautery in a straight line along the anterior portion of the esophagus and the stomach (Fig. 18.17). The distal esophageal muscle fibers are usually the most difficult to dissect, especially if previous dilation or botulinum toxin injection has been performed (67). For this reason, the initial dissection is started on the stomach or an area of less-fibrosed esophagus. Cautery is used to divide the muscle fibers down to the submucosa (Fig. 18.18). When the proper plane is identified, the cardiomyotomy is extended cephalad until normal esophageal muscle is identified and caudad until the sling fibers of the cardia are divided (Fig. 18.19). Intraoperative endoscopy may be performed to identify the gastroesophageal junction and to ensure the myotomy is of sufficient length. This may be confirmed by

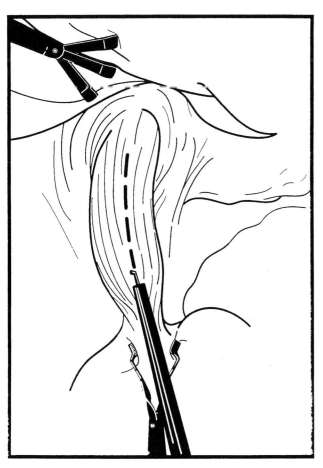

FIGURE 18.17. The planned myotomy site is marked along the anterior surface of the esophagus with electrocautery.

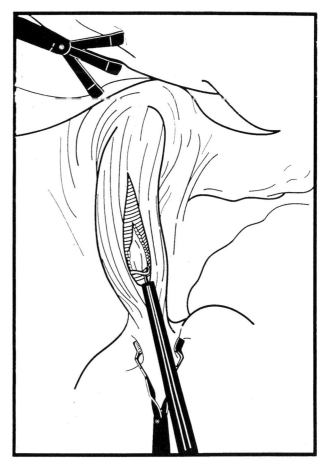

FIGURE 18.18. The longitudinal and circular muscle fibers are transected with a combination of electrocautery and blunt dissection.

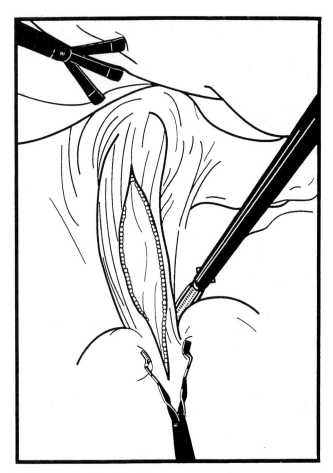

FIGURE 18.19. Completed myotomy extending onto the stomach.

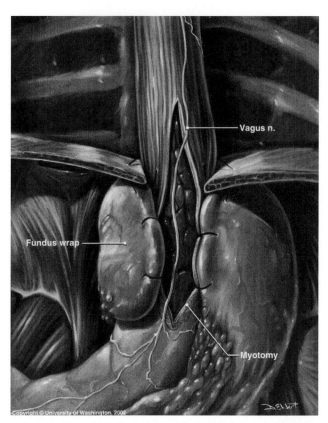

FIGURE 18.20. The posterior fundoplication (Toupet) is performed suturing the fundus to the cut edges of the myotomy and securing the stomach to the diaphragm. (From University of Washington, Seattle, WA, with permission.)

adequate distention of the esophagus with insufflation. Since we began extending our myotomy 3 cm onto the stomach, we have no concern about insufficient length.

Once the cardiomyotomy is sufficient, a partial posterior fundoplication (Toupet) is performed (Fig. 18.20). The posterior fundus is placed around the esophagus, and the top is fixated to the esophagus and diaphragm. The leading edge of the stomach is sutured to the edge of the myotomy and is separately secured to the right crus. The same is done with the anterior fundus on the left side. Alternatively, an anterior fundoplication (Dor) may be performed (Fig. 18.21), and is recommended to buttress an intraoperative perforation if it occurs. With the bougie or the flexible endoscope in the esophagus, the fundus of the stomach is positioned anterior to the myotomy. Sutures are placed to anchor the fundus to the right and left crura as well as to the transected edges of the esophageal muscle. When the wrap is completed, the liver retractor is removed, and the incisions are closed.

A nasogastric tube is not used postoperatively. The patient is allowed a liquid diet on the night of the operation and begins a graduated solid diet the next morning. Most

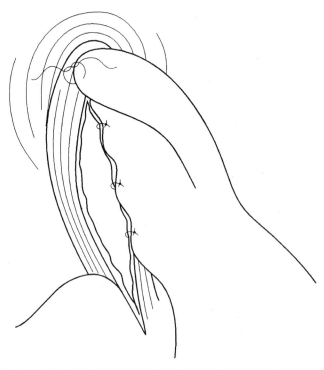

FIGURE 18.21. The anterior hemifundoplication (Dor) is performed suturing the fundus to the cut edges of the myotomy site.

patients may be discharged from the hospital within 2 days. All patients are strongly encouraged to have manometry and pH studies 6 to 8 weeks after surgery.

Postoperative evaluation of the esophagus is important because the most common cause for late failure is likely to be gastroesophageal reflux disease. As discussed later in this section, it is often asymptomatic, so patients do not seek treatment. If pathologic reflux is present on the 24-hour pH study, the patients should be treated to help prevent peptic stricture formation at a later date.

Outcome

At the University of Washington, we converted from a thoracoscopic approach to a laparoscopic Heller myotomy in 1994. The impetus for this was the recognition that a limited gastric myotomy did not protect the patient from gastroesophageal reflux and that many patients required an extension of the myotomy for relief of their dysphagia. The laparoscopic approach still allowed for a long esophageal myotomy, but it could be extended onto the stomach (1.5 to 2.0 cm). We could then add a Dor fundoplication decrease the amount of gastroesophageal reflux disease (GERD). Over the next 4 years, 52 patients were operated on using this approach, with the majority having excellent improvement in their dysphagia (over 90%). Still there was the occasional patient who had inadequate relief or recurrence of dysphagia, some of whom improved with reoperation to extend the myotomy. Therefore, in 1998 we changed our approach, extending the myotomy 3 cm on the gastric side. We also began performing a Toupet fundoplication rather than a Dor, both because an anterior fundoplication was difficult to do with such a long myotomy and the hope that a Toupet might provide better control of reflux. A comparison of the two approaches confirmed that an extended myotomy with Toupet (EM/Toupet) more effectively obliterated the LES than the shorter myotomy with Dor fundoplication (SM/Dor) as evidenced by the residual LES pressure (9.5 vs. 15.8 mm Hg). This translated into improved clinical outcomes, in that dysphagia was both less frequent (once a month vs. once a week on average) and less severe (3.2 vs. 5.3 on a 10-point visual analog scale) in the EM/Toupet group. This improvement in the EM/Toupet approach was not at the expense of more reflux, in that the mean distal esophageal acid exposure was equivalent (EM/Toupet 6.0% vs. SM/Dor 5.9%).

These results are similar to those reported by others. Relief from dysphagia is between 85% and 95% at 5 years, weight gain is common, and overall satisfaction with the operation is high (58,68,69). Because the obstruction to flow is relieved, regurgitation is reduced. Relief from chest pain may occur in 60% to 75% of patients who had the symptom preoperatively.

Improved esophageal motility has been demonstrated after cardiomyotomy for achalasia (70). Proximal peristalsis can be demonstrated in up to 50% of patients, midesophageal peristalsis in 25%, and distal in up to 9% (71). This finding implies that LES contributes to the esophageal body dysfunction, but is not solely responsible for the disorganized peristalsis. Others argue that this finding does not represent an intrinsic change in the motility of the esophagus but is an artifact of manometry and that an apparent improvement in peristalsis is only a function of the decreased caliber of the esophagus after surgery (11).

Complications

Complications of the procedure are uncommon. In our experience at the University of Washington, perforations occur in less than 5% of cases. Perforations are more common when patients are treated with one or more botulinum toxin injections. The overall complication rate is around 5%, and we have experienced no mortality.

Esophageal perforation is repaired intraoperatively. The mucosa is closed primarily, then buttressed with the serosa of the stomach by performing an anterior partial fundoplication (Dor). Initially, mucosal laceration was considered a reason for converting to an open procedure. However, if the surgeon is comfortable with videoendoscopic suturing, the procedure does not need to be converted.

Pneumothorax, bleeding, wound infection, and intraabdominal abscess are other complications that have been reported in less than 3% of cases (72). Most early complications can be avoided by careful dissection. However, previous operations or botulinum toxin injections distort the natural tissue planes and thus increase the likelihood of one of these complications.

Late complications of myotomy are related mostly to the recurrence of the initial symptoms, particularly dysphagia.

Postoperative dysphagia may be caused by several discrete entities: incomplete myotomy, perihiatal scarring, progressive dysmotility of the esophagus, peptic stricture, and tumor. Some clinical clues may help distinguish among these, but physiologic and anatomic information must be obtained to confirm the diagnosis.

In 129 patients followed up for an average of 12 years, 40 were identified as having postoperative dysphagia (73). Symptoms of incomplete myotomy occurred early and rarely caused dysphagia after 3 years. Postoperative scarring caused dysphagia 1 to 2 years after surgery. Gastroesophageal reflux caused dysphagia after 6 years. The authors were 100% accurate in diagnosing the cause of dysphagia using esophagogram, endoscopy, and manometry in the 12 patients whose diagnosis was confirmed by reoperation.

Incomplete myotomy may be prevented by extending the incision onto the stomach to ensure transection of the sling fibers. The cut edges of the myotomy must be separated by at least 30% of the esophageal circumference. Perihiatal scarring may be prevented by minimizing the amount of electrocautery injury to the crura.

Pathologic gastroesophageal reflux may be detected in up to 40% of patients if 24-hour pH studies are performed (74). This study assessed reflux after a limited thoracoscopic myotomy without the addition of an antireflux procedure. Most authors believe that the incidence of abnormal gastroesophageal reflux in a patient undergoing a myotomy and an antireflux procedure to be about 10% (68). In the patients treated at the University of Washington, 19% of patients had symptoms of heartburn more frequently than once per week after a laparoscopic Heller-Dor or Heller-Toupet procedure. Of the patients who had postoperative 24-hour pH studies, 35% had abnormal acid exposure. Although it seems that adding an antireflux procedure to the myotomy would help prevent abnormal gastroesophageal reflux, this has not been demonstrated in a randomized study.

The tradeoff between relieving dysphagia and limiting reflux is clear—the greater the improvement of dysphagia, the higher is the incidence of reflux. This is clearly shown in a study by Pandolfo and co-workers (69). In 11 patients, the authors used intraoperative manometry to assess the extent of LES relaxation during an open cardiomyotomy and anterior hemifundoplication via an abdominal approach. Manometric readings of the LES pressure were performed before and after the myotomy was completed. The myotomy was not considered complete until the LES pressure was less than 5 mm Hg. The results were compared with 16 patients who underwent the same procedure without the intraoperative study. Patients with intraoperative manometry had a 0% dysphagia rate but an 18.2% reflux rate. This compared with a 21.5% dysphagia rate and a 7.3% reflux rate in those who did not have intraoperative manometry. A more thorough myotomy leads to less dysphagia but more reflux.

Besides peptic stricture, postoperative reflux may lead to other complications including esophagitis and Barrett's esophagus. Although some patients have pathologic reflux, many do not have symptoms. Jaakkola and colleagues (75) found that Barrett's esophagus developed in 4 of 46 patients after cardiomyotomy after an average follow-up of 13 years. Others found dysplasia and intramucosal adenocarcinoma in patients with reflux after myotomy (73). In a series of 100 patients undergoing myotomy, cancer developed in three (70). This stresses two points: the need to know which patients have reflux after the operation and the importance of following these patients with endoscopy.

The management of patients with postoperative dysphagia is not well defined. An attempt at conservative treatment using dilation is appropriate as long as no evidence of tumor is present. Parkman and colleagues successfully managed six patients with peptic stricture using multiple dilations (average 3.6 per patient) and acid suppression (76). Conservative management is a reasonable strategy, in that reoperation for dysphagia has a lower success rate than the initial operation (77).

Recurrent Achalasia

Recurrence after operative treatment is reported to range from 8% to 13% (78,79). Late recurrence must be assessed carefully, because dysphagia may develop from other causes mentioned earlier. The diagnosis of recurrence must be confirmed by manometry, which should show a normal or elevated LES pressure and incomplete relaxation. Manometry may also reveal another motor disorder, which may explain the symptoms and affect the treatment. Endoscopy and a contrast esophagogram should also be obtained to exclude other diseases such as a tumor or paraesophageal hernia. If recurrence is confirmed, there are several options available depending on the findings, the overall health of the patient, and the available expertise. Some patients may be treated with dilation. The endoscopist must be skilled in the use of pneumatic dilation because only the mucosa stands between the balloon and the mediastinum or the peritoneal cavity. If dilation is not available or if it fails to resolve the symptoms, a repeat myotomy may be considered. Between 70% and 80% of patients respond to a repeat operation for recurrent or persistent achalasia (80,81) and most of these patients can be approached laparoscopically (82). If the preoperative manometry reveals a diffuse esophageal abnormality, then a thoracic approach may be beneficial, especially if the first approach was by way of the abdomen. Otherwise, there is little evidence to support one approach over the other. If repeat myotomy is not helpful, then esophageal resection may be the only surgical alternative. The patient must be informed that this is a more extensive procedure and has a mortality rate between 2% and 8% (79,83). If esophageal resection is performed, the results can be expected to be good to excellent in 78% to 90% of patients (50,79). The choice of conduit for the operation is discussed later in this chapter.

Emergent Operation after Perforation

Esophageal perforation may occur after pneumatic dilation in the treatment of achalasia. The management of the perforation depends on clinical assessment and the interpretation of the esophagogram. In a stable patient, a small contained perforation that does not communicate with other mediastinal structures or the pleural space may be treated with antibiotics and cessation of oral intake. If the patient has clinical manifestations or if radiographic studies show free communication with either the pleural cavity or the mediastinum (Fig. 18.22), then urgent operative intervention is indicated. Regardless of the initial management plan, a surgical evaluation should be obtained as soon as a perforation is expected.

The principles of operative intervention include debridement and irrigation to remove injured and necrotic tissue, closure of the perforation site, and myotomy. A posterolateral thoracic approach through the seventh intercostal space

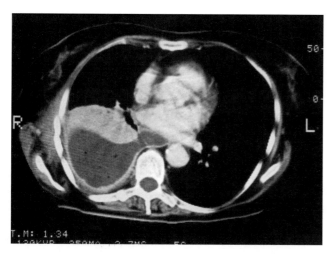

FIGURE 18.22. Computed tomography scan showing communication of esophageal perforation with right pleural space.

is used. The mediastinum is exposed and cleansed of all esophageal contamination. After the perforation is debrided, a two-layered closure is used. The mucosa is sutured with an absorbable polyglyconate-based 3-0 suture, and the muscularis is closed with a permanent suture. A myotomy should be performed on the opposite side of the perforation. Occasionally, the diaphragm may be enlarged and the cardia of the stomach used to place a serosal patch over the repair. In general, this is not feasible or advisable, because it creates a hiatal hernia. Two chest tubes are placed for drainage, and the incision is closed.

If the degree of soiling is extensive or if delay to operative intervention is prolonged, Schwartz and co-workers (84) recommend diversion. This would consist of esophagostomy, gastrostomy, and interruption of the gastroesophageal continuity. Rarely is it necessary to divert a patient, because esophageal resection or wide drainage of the perforated area can be safely performed in such situations (85). Although a myotomy is usually performed during the emergent operation, one group has reported six patients in whom they simply repaired the perforation without performing a myotomy (86). They found that none of their patients had recurrent symptoms of dysphagia after an average follow-up of 5 years. Others have approached perforation after dilation using minimally invasive surgery. These authors performed a primary repair using videoendoscopy and then drained the thorax with chest tubes (87).

The outcome of emergent surgery for perforation is often said to be the same as elective surgery. Ferguson and colleagues reported six patients treated emergently for perforation and compared them with 54 patients undergoing elective treatment for achalasia (88). They found all six patients had good or excellent results based on symptoms scoring, whereas 88% of the elective cases had the same score. Postoperative endoscopy, pH studies, and manome-

try were not reported for either group. In another study, seven patients with perforation were compared with five undergoing elective procedures (84). These authors found that the length of the operation, stay in the intensive care unit, and length of hospitalization were the same. Again, no postoperative studies were reported. Although there was no difference in the outcomes measured, these parameters may not be applicable today. For example, the average length of hospitalization was 11 days, and the intensive care unit stay was 1 day for the elective cases. Currently, the average length of stay is 2 days, and the patients rarely, if ever, go to the intensive care unit. Although it is often stated that the outcomes are no different in patients operated on for perforation, the issue may need to be revisited with the advent of minimally invasive procedures.

Controversies in Achalasia

The approach to surgical management of achalasia may appear to be straightforward, but many issues in the management of this disease process are topics of current debate.

Medical Versus Surgical Treatment

Medical therapy with calcium channel blockers or nitrates is clinically ineffective and has been relegated to a role as a temporizing measure before or a supplemental treatment after definitive therapy (89–92). A more recent therapeutic modality involves injecting botulinum toxin into the LES. The effect of this treatment is also temporary, with only 66% of patients experiencing symptomatic relief at 6 months (91). Although this may be appropriate therapy for patients who are at risk for operative intervention because of age or comorbid conditions, its long-term efficacy is unproved.

The two types of definitive therapy include pneumatic dilation and surgical transection of the esophageal muscle. Each approach has advantages and disadvantages. When the two are compared, the following issues arise: symptom resolution, immediate morbidity, degree of reflux as a result of therapy, and cost. Although several studies have been performed in an attempt to resolve the quandary, a consensus has not been reached. Retrospective studies comparing the results of surgery and forceful dilation are inconclusive because of selection bias, use of historical controls, and small sample size (93–95).

Only one study has prospectively randomized patients to either pneumatic dilation or surgery (80,96). In this study, 39 patients were treated by dilation and 42 by surgery. After 5 years of follow-up, excellent or good results were present in 65% of patients undergoing dilation and 95% of patients treated surgically. Interestingly, the authors of this paper performed both surgery and dilation on their study patients. The surgical procedure performed was an open abdominal cardiomyotomy extending onto the stomach for

5 to 10 mm and an anterior (Dor) fundoplication. Pneumatic dilation was accomplished using a Mosher bag inflated to 12 to 15 psi for 10 to 20 seconds. Two patients underwent emergency surgery for perforation of the esophagus after dilation. Postprocedure "acid reflux tests" were performed in both groups, and reflux was documented in 8% of the dilation patients and 28% of the surgery patients. The authors concluded that surgery offered better clinical results than did dilation.

Their conclusion was questioned for several reasons (97). The technical complaint was that the study only had a 65% response to pneumatic dilation because the duration and pressure of dilation were not sufficient. Others have reported a response rate of between 75% and 85% using more aggressive techniques (89,92,98,99). The degree of postoperative gastroesophageal reflux in the patients who underwent operation was criticized as being too high. Furthermore, because surgery required a longer inpatient and outpatient recovery, this facet of treatment should not have been ignored when assessing the appropriateness of the intervention. Indeed, the cost of surgical treatment was 2.4 times higher in a study comparing open operations to pneumatic dilations (100).

Gastroesophageal reflux has been thought to occur less frequently after dilation than surgical myotomy (89,93). However, studies that are cited to support this contention assess only symptoms of reflux. One study compared 24-hour pH monitoring on consecutive patients undergoing surgical and pneumatic dilation for achalasia (74). Reflux was documented in 6 of 17 patients after dilation and in 6 of 15 after surgery. Only 33% of patients with objective evidence of reflux had symptoms. The authors concluded that the amount of reflux is similar between the two modes of treatment and that the absence of symptoms does not exclude pathologic reflux.

The analysis of cost differences is valid, but the conclusions were drawn before surgeons used minimally invasive approaches. Comparing dilation to open operative procedures generated the data that supports nonsurgical therapy. Patients required 7 to 10 days of hospital care and several weeks of recuperation at home (93,96,100). With minimally invasive techniques, the inpatient stay averages 2 days, and depending on lifestyle, patients may return to work in 1 week (101–104). Just as operative intervention evolved, so did pneumatic dilation. This procedure is now being performed on an outpatient basis and thus should lower the cost of this procedure as well (105,106).

The question of the optimal initial treatment for achalasia remains unanswered. Aggressive pneumatic dilation may be able to attain similar results as operative therapy. However, because it is an uncontrolled disruption of the LES, the number of perforations is proportional to the aggressiveness of the dilation technique. Furthermore, as greater success is obtained with dilation, the incidence of reflux will approach that of surgical intervention without an antireflux

procedure. Further evaluation of the two interventions is needed to resolve these issues. Certainly, young individuals with achalasia who are fit for an operation benefit from having a surgical myotomy as the first approach.

Operative Approach

The first operative treatment of achalasia was described in 1913 by the procedure's namesake, Ernest Heller. His approach was via a laparotomy and consisted of a double myotomy. The open thoracic approach was championed in the United States by F. Henry Ellis in the 1950s. These two approaches were the only methods available to the surgeon until 1991, when Cuschieri and co-workers (65) first described a successful laparoscopic myotomy. Shortly after that, Pellegrini and colleagues (63) described a thoracoscopic approach for achalasia and reported their experience with 17 patients. Since then, many authors have addressed the issues of open and videoendoscopic surgery.

The outcomes with the open and videoendoscopic abdominal approach appear to be similar (107–110). The benefits of minimally invasive surgery for the patient are to be found in the decreased hospital stay and recuperation.

Cuschieri and co-workers (65) were the first to point out the potential advantages of reduced trauma and quicker recovery using a videoendoscopic technique. Others supported their observation by demonstrating decreased recovery time, less pain, and improved aesthetic appearance of the incisions with laparoscopic myotomy (111). In one study, the authors compared a matched group of laparotomy and laparoscopy Heller-Dor procedures (112). Seventeen patients in each group were analyzed retrospectively for operative time, hospital stay, and return to normal activity. Although the operative time was greater for the minimally invasive group (178 vs. 125 minutes), the patients were discharged from the hospital earlier (4 vs. 10 days) and returned to normal activity earlier (14 vs. 30 days). Based on charges at the authors' institution, the cost of a laparoscopic myotomy compared with that of an open myotomy was about $400 lower. The largest component of cost in the laparoscopic procedure was the surgical supplies, and the largest component of cost in the open procedure was the length of stay. As experience has evolved, it has become clear that the use of an imaging system that allows for substantial magnification of the images and the excellent view of the field inherent in a videoendoscopic approach probably enhances the ability of surgeons to perform the operations with greater accuracy.

Chest Versus Abdomen

As videoendoscopic procedures replaced the open techniques, the issue of whether the myotomy should be performed through the chest or the abdomen was raised. The same question existed during the era of open surgery, wherein the discussion focused on outcome—response to treatment, postoperative gastroesophageal reflux, and recurrence. Those who employ the thoracic approach point out that the esophagus and the gastroesophageal junction are more accessible from the chest. They also note that less mobilization of the structures that support the competency of the cardia is necessary, and, therefore, an antireflux procedure is not needed (113,114). The laparoscopic approach, although requiring a larger mobilization of the cardioesophageal junction, allows instruments to be parallel to the axis of the esophagus, as opposed to being perpendicular during thoracoscopy. Also, the majority of the LES is intraabdominal and thus easier to approach laparoscopically (101). The anesthetic management is simplified because there is no need to use single-lung ventilation and there is no need to use a chest tube postoperatively. Finally, another advantage of the abdominal approach is the ease of adding an antireflux procedure. Thus, most surgeons who treat achalasia using minimally invasive techniques use this approach (101,103, 115–117).

Adding an Antireflux Procedure

The issue of adding an antireflux procedure to a cardiomyotomy is controversial. It was reasoned in the past that if the cardiomyotomy extends too far onto the stomach, it may disrupt all the physiologic and anatomic contributions to the lower esophageal sphincter, thereby allowing gastroesophageal reflux to occur. If the cardiomyotomy does not extend too far onto the stomach, then no reflux occurs; however, the results of the operation may be inferior in terms of relieving dysphagia. In an attempt to solve both problems, the cardiomyotomy may be extended onto the stomach for a distance and then the LES mechanism may be reconstructed with an antireflux procedure.

As previously noted, clinical assessment of reflux status underestimates the amount of reflux when compared with 24-hour pH studies in patients treated for achalasia. This holds true for patients treated operatively or by pneumatic dilation (74). Therefore, all patients who undergo a myotomy should be evaluated postoperatively by 24-hour pH monitoring to determine objectively whether pathologic reflux is occurring. Whether subclinical reflux causes late failure in the treatment of achalasia is not known.

If the myotomy is performed through the chest, a partial wrap can be constructed using the fundus of the stomach. Advocates of the thoracic approach believe that their procedure can usually be performed without the addition of an antireflux procedure, because they extend the myotomy onto the stomach for only a few millimeters (113,114,118). The indications for adding an antireflux procedure are presence of a hiatal hernia, evidence of preoperative reflux, or gastric stasis. The reported rate of gastroesophageal reflux in patients undergoing myotomy by

way of the thoracic approach without an antireflux procedure is between 5% and 62% (48,77,119). The variability in the incidence of reflux is due to the manner in which reflux was measured. If the diagnosis is made clinically, then the rate is low (5% to 16%) (77,119); however, if patients are subjected to pH studies, the rates are higher (35% to 62%) (48,74). Because gastroesophageal reflux was identified so frequently after thoracic myotomy, many surgeons moved to an abdominal approach where it is easier (and necessary) to perform some type of antireflux procedure.

Two types of fundal wraps are available to the surgeon using an abdominal approach to the esophagus: a complete wrap (Nissen) or some variation of a partial wrap (Dor or Toupet). Most surgeons perform a partial fundoplication because a total fundoplication causes to much resistance and more commonly results in dysphagia. There is controversy, however, regarding which type of fundoplication should be used. An anterior fundoplication (Dor) eliminates the need to perform a posterior esophageal dissection, preserving some attachment of the esophagus to the hiatus, and helps to maintain an intraabdominal segment of distal esophagus. The second advantage of the Dor is that it allows the wall of the stomach to buttress the myotomy site. The cardia helps seal any injury to the esophageal mucosa, prevents adhesion of the esophagus to the left lobe of the liver, and allows the myotomy edges to be sutured in an open position. A posterior fundoplication (Toupet), on the other hand, may provide better control of reflux. In addition, it naturally separates the edges of the myotomy, theoretically keeping it from joining and causing recurrent dysphagia.

The amount of gastroesophageal reflux is less with the addition of an antireflux procedure. Peracchia and colleagues (64) reported only an 8% pathologic gastroesophageal reflux rate based on pH studies after laparoscopic Heller-Dor procedures. Similarly, Parrilla and co-workers (57) reported a 12% reflux rate after open Heller-Toupet procedures using 24-hour pH studies (57). Another study reported no gastroesophageal reflux by pH studies in patients undergoing laparoscopic myotomies with partial fundoplications (103). Although no randomized study has been performed comparing myotomy without fundoplication to myotomy with fundoplication, it appears that the addition of an antireflux procedure may reduce the likelihood of reflux and thus may improve long-term results by avoiding complications associated with reflux. Which fundoplication is more efficacious, though, is also in doubt and needs comparative investigation.

Conclusion

The symptoms of achalasia may be effectively treated by operative therapy. The principles of the operation include sufficient length of the myotomy, adequate separation of the transected muscle, and a plan to prevent postoperative gastroesophageal reflux. The operation may be performed using minimally invasive techniques. Postoperative assessment of gastroesophageal reflux should be performed in all patients to prevent late failure resulting from peptic stricture.

SPASTIC DYSMOTILITY

The use of stationary and ambulatory esophageal manometry in the evaluation of patients with noncardiac chest pain has led to the identification of several uncommon esophageal dysmotility syndromes. Although criteria have been developed to aid in the diagnosis of these syndromes, the relative paucity of cases has hindered the development of standard treatment. All are considered together in this section because the experience with each is limited and the surgical treatments are similar.

Diffuse esophageal spasm (DES) is characterized by simultaneous contractions and intermittent normal peristalsis on manometry. Repetitive contractions, prolonged wave duration, high-amplitude contractions, spontaneous contractions, and an elevated LES pressure may also be observed (Fig. 18.23). *Nutcracker esophagus* (NE) is diagnosed in patients who have a distal esophageal contraction

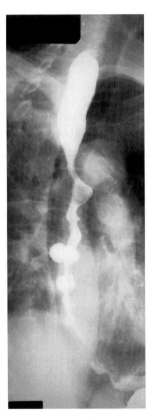

FIGURE 18.23. Esophagogram showing diffuse esophageal spasm.

amplitude greater than 180 mm Hg. An elevated LES pressure and prolonged wave duration may also be encountered but are not necessary for the diagnosis. In essence, this condition appears to be an "exaggeration" in the amplitude and duration of otherwise normal peristaltic waves. *Hypertensive lower esophageal sphincter* (HLES) is a condition diagnosed when the LES pressure is greater than 40 mm Hg and there is an absence of any other disorders of the esophageal body, which may account for the elevated sphincter pressure. More than 50% of patients with elevated LES pressures have other disorders of peristalsis (120). *Nonspecific esophageal dysmotility* (NED) is a catchall category for patients with abnormal manometric findings that do not conform to the criteria of the other dysmotility syndromes. This category has been essentially replaced by *ineffective esophageal motility* (see Chapter 12).

Epiphrenic diverticula are considered in this section because they are associated with some type of esophageal dysmotility in about 60% of patients (121). When an operation is indicated, treatment of the disease is similar to the treatment of other motility disorders.

Clinical Evaluation

Most patients present with the complaint of dysphagia and chest pain. Some may also complain of heartburn and regurgitation, especially if a diverticulum is present. Most often, the patients have undergone some form of cardiac evaluation for their chest pain. If this is not the case, the patient should be evaluated by the appropriate clinician to ensure this more common, life-threatening etiology is not the cause of the chest pain.

The clinical evaluation of a patient with noncardiac chest pain is similar to that of achalasia, which is described in the previous section. It should include manometry, a contrast study of the esophagus, and upper endoscopy. Manometry is necessary to define the type of motility disorder. The esophagogram and endoscopy are necessary to exclude other etiologies of abnormal motility such as benign and malignant neoplasms.

Gastroesophageal reflux should always be considered when evaluating patients with spastic dysmotility, because it has been hypothesized to be a contributing factor to different esophageal disorders, such as HLES and high-amplitude peristaltic contractile disorders such as NE (120). Therefore, 24-hour pH monitoring is an essential test for anyone with such a disorder. Traditional surgical management for spastic dysmotility included an esophageal myotomy, but for some patients gastroesophageal reflux may be the primary disorder and the spastic dysmotility secondary. In such cases, therapy directed toward reflux may be more appropriate. We recently reported successfully treating patients with GERD and various hypercontractile esophageal motility disorders (such as HLES and NE) with a Nissen fundoplication (122). Thus, GERD should be investigated in all patients with dysphagia or chest pain. A hypercontractile esophagus in patients with GERD should not be considered a contraindication to antireflux therapy; instead it may be the treatment of choice rather than esophageal myotomy in such situations.

Another consideration in the preoperative evaluation of patients with spastic dysmotility is the indication for 24-hour manometry. Although experience with this technique is limited to a few centers, the information gained may be helpful in guiding therapy and predicting prognosis (123). Ambulatory manometry is particularly useful in patients with daily symptoms who have been diagnosed with NE and NED on stationary manometry, because it may change the diagnosis in up to 30% of cases (124). Ambulatory manometry allows the physician to correlate symptoms as reported by the patient in an event diary with the manometric measurements. Although the diagnosis may change with NE and NED, ambulatory manometry disagrees less often with stationary manometry when the diagnosis is DES. In this case, 24-hour manometry need not be performed. In difficult situations, endoscopic ultrasonography may define the area of the esophagus that is most affected, because the thickness of the muscularis can be accurately estimated by this study.

Occasionally, an epiphrenic diverticulum is found on a patient who has an upper gastrointestinal contrast study for an unrelated problem (Fig. 18.24). If the patient is clearly asymptomatic, then he or she may not need an operation. A follow-up esophagogram in 1 to 2 years helps gauge the progression of the diverticulum and reveal associated disease. Most of the asymptomatic diverticula do not progress into clinical problems (121). If, however, the patient has symptoms referable to the diverticulum, operative treatment is recommended. In this case, it is imperative to have a reliable manometric evaluation before operation because it affects the surgical approach and the procedure.

Treatment

Spastic dysmotility disorders of the esophagus have been infrequently treated by surgical therapy. The reason for this is based partly on the fact that some reports have shown an 80% response to medical therapy (120) and partly on the reluctance of physicians to eliminate all peristaltic activity in the body of the esophagus with an operation. As with achalasia, spastic disorders are well suited to a minimally invasive operative approach. The procedure performed in most cases consists of a myotomy with or without an antireflux procedure. If a diverticulum is present, a diverticulectomy is also performed. The laparoscopic approach to a myotomy is described in the previous section; the thoracoscopic approach is described here. This approach is usually used when treating spastic motility disorders because a longer esophageal myotomy is needed to treat the symptoms of disease.

Two principles of operative therapy are important in treating spastic dysmotility. The first is that the site and extent of the myotomy must be directed by the findings of the manometry study. For example, if manometry shows the entire thoracic esophagus to be involved in the pathologic process, then the myotomy must span the length of the thoracic esophagus. The second issue is ablating the LES. Even if the LES pressure is normal, it should be transected. After an extensive myotomy of the esophageal body, the ability to transmit a bolus of food normally is lost. Even a normal LES pressure presents a challenge to a myotomized esophagus.

The patient should be placed on a liquid diet for 2 days before the operation if esophageal emptying is inhibited. This decreases the amount of solid debris in the lumen of the esophagus. A bougie, preferably lighted, is needed for the operation. The bougie should be placed under direct vision during the operation, especially if a diverticulum is present. This prevents injury to the esophagus. A double-lumen endotracheal tube is necessary to allow single-lung ventilation.

A lateral decubitus position is used. Access to the lower esophagus, cardioesophageal junction, and upper stomach can only be achieved through a left-sided approach. Because most pathologic processes described earlier require ablation of the LES, the majority of myotomies are performed from the left. The right-sided approach is best if the patient needs

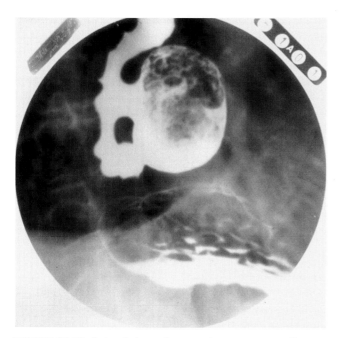

FIGURE 18.24. Lateral view of an esophagogram revealing an anterior esophageal diverticulum.

a myotomy of the entire esophagus, except its most inferior aspect. This approach is also useful for a midesophageal diverticulum located on the right side. An antireflux procedure cannot be performed easily from this approach. The working ports are placed to allow maximum vision of the inferior thoracic esophagus and the superior esophagus if needed. The ports are placed in an equilateral triangle, notably much closer than what is normally done in the abdomen, with the videoendoscope located in the fifth intercostal space, just inferior to the scapular tip. The working ports should be located in the posterior axillary line. A fourth port in the anterior axillary line is used by the assistant to retract the lung (Fig. 18.25). Both the surgeon and the assistant stand on the same side of the operating table, which is the ipsilateral side of chosen approach. Thus, both are standing at the patient's back, while the video cart monitor is in front of the patient. Carbon dioxide insufflation is not necessary for the procedure, because single-lung ventilation usually suffices.

The lung is retracted anteriorly after it is deflated (Fig. 18.26). The inferior pulmonary ligament is divided with cautery and blunt dissection, avoiding the inferior pulmonary vein. Once this is accomplished, the pleural reflection over the esophagus is taken down with cautery dissection so that the longitudinal muscle fibers of the esophagus may be identified (Fig. 18.27). At this point, the lighted bougie is passed into the esophagus by the anesthesiologist. By splaying the muscle fibers of the esophagus over the bougie with one instrument, cautery dissection down to the submucosa is performed. A combination of blunt dissection, spreading, and cauterization is used to divide the muscular layers of the esophagus for the length of the myotomy (Figs. 18.28 and 18.29). Flexible endoscopy should be used

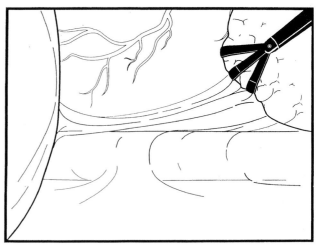

FIGURE 18.26. The lung is retracted anteriorly, exposing the pleural reflection over the esophagus.

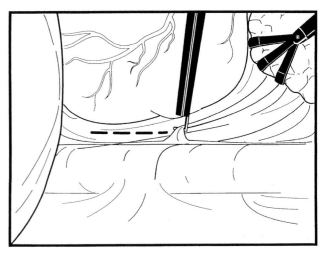

FIGURE 18.27. The pleura is incised to expose the esophagus.

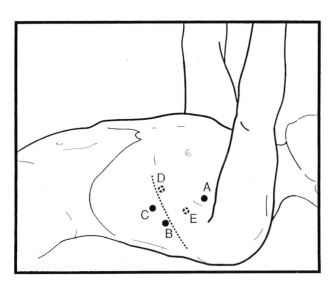

FIGURE 18.25. Port placement for a thoracoscopic myotomy. **A:** Optional lung retraction port. **B:** Scope port. **C:** Surgeon's left hand. **D:** Lung retractor. **E:** Surgeon's right hand.

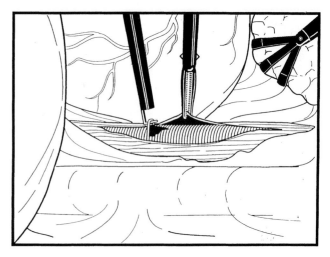

FIGURE 18.28. The longitudinal and circular muscle fibers are transected.

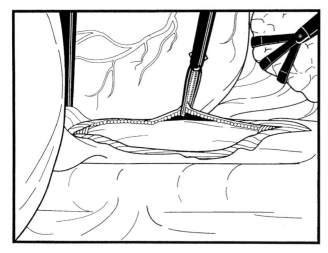

FIGURE 18.29. Completed myotomy.

to verify the adequacy of the myotomy (Fig. 18.30). The vagus nerves should be avoided during this dissection. If a left-sided approach is used, a partial wrap (Dor or Belsey) may be added. If the right-sided approach is used, then the antireflux procedure is not possible. If a diverticulum is present, it may be dissected to its neck and transected by an automatic stapling and cutting device.

Two chest tubes are placed through trocar sites, and the remaining sites are closed. The patient is allowed to consume a liquid diet on the day of the operation, unless a diverticulum was resected, in which case the diet is started on the third postoperative day. Hospital stay varies, but patients are usually discharged within 2 days of starting a diet.

The length of the myotomy varies with each of the disease processes and with the findings of the preoperative evaluation. If HLES without concomitant esophageal body

dysmotility is being treated, the myotomy is confined to the distal esophagus, LES, and cardia. If NE is being treated and preoperative manometry revealed high-amplitude contractions in the proximal esophagus, an extended myotomy should be performed, perhaps through a right thoracoscopic approach.

Outcome

The surgical approach to patients with spastic motility disorders is based mostly on transferred principles from achalasia. Because the number of patients with these disorders is so small, and even fewer of them come to surgical therapy, only limited experience is available. Most information comes from case reports and technique articles (125–127). Although no prospective, randomized studies are available comparing medical with surgical therapy, one article prospectively compared the outcome of the two treatments in patients with esophageal motility disorders (128). In this study, patients with achalasia, DES, and NE were treated by medical therapy, including dilation, or operative therapy based on the request of the referring physician. The operation was performed via left thoracoscopy. Eight of 10 patients with DES or NE had good or excellent relief with surgical treatment. Only 8 of 30 patients had the same level of relief with medical therapy. Although this study was not randomized, it did show the benefits of operative therapy over medical therapy. No long-term studies are available to assess the outcome of surgically treated patients.

Complications

The operative complications are similar to those of myotomy performed for achalasia, except if a diverticulectomy is added. In this case, additional morbidity may be expected from opening the esophageal mucosa. Esophageal leak rates have been reported to be as high as 18% using an open technique (121). Not enough data are available from videoendoscopic procedures to assess the incidence of esophageal leak.

Conclusion

Operative intervention for spastic motility is not common. The myotomy should be tailored to the manometric findings. The thoracoscopic approach allows for a longer myotomy if necessary. After surgical intervention, dysphagia improves more often than pain.

ESOPHAGEAL RESECTION

Resection of the esophagus is usually performed for malignant disease; however, this procedure is contemplated in esophageal motility disorders when certain conditions exist.

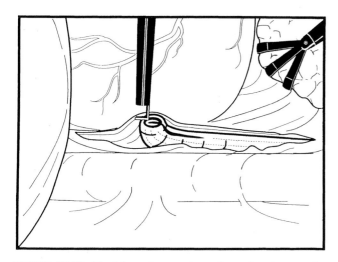

FIGURE 18.30. Flexible endoscopy is performed to inspect the myotomy.

If the esophagus is severely dilated and elongated after years of untreated disease, some authors have recommended resection as an initial therapy. Benign stricture, occurring as a result of previous intervention or as a natural sequelae of untreated disease, which cannot be treated by dilation is another indication for esophageal resection. Failure of previous operative therapy to relieve symptoms associated with motility disorders is another. Indeed after two or three operations on the esophagus to treat a stricture, esophagectomy is the best alternative. Some have used esophageal resection as treatment for a perforation occurring after dilation, particularly when the esophagus has other underlying pathology.

Patients must be aware of the technical challenge the operation poses. They should be aware of the significant morbidity (20% to 30%) and mortality (2% to 8%) accompanying the operation. Given the information, they may decide their symptoms are more acceptable than the risk of the procedure.

The principles of esophageal resection center on safe, effective removal of the esophagus and replacement using a conduit that allows for adequate nutritional intake. The most common approach to this procedure is a transhiatal approach from the abdomen, using the stomach as the conduit to anastomose to the cervical esophagus.

Operative Approach

Patients requiring esophagectomy for esophageal motor disorders are often nutritionally depleted. If preoperative nutritional supplementation is possible with high-calorie, high-protein liquids, some advantage in postoperative healing may be gained. The patients should be on a liquid diet 2 days before the operation to minimize the amount of solid debris present in the esophagus.

The patient is placed in the supine position on the operating table with the head turned to the right. A roll is usually placed across the lumbar area elevating the costal margin. This position facilitates exposure to the cervical esophagus, the abdomen, and the distal thoracic esophagus. The abdominal portion of the operation is performed first.

Generous mobilization of the duodenum is performed, elevating the second and third portions to the patient's left. The stomach is then mobilized along the greater curvature taking care to preserve the gastroepiploic artery. All short gastric vessels are ligated and transected to free the cardia. Division of the lesser omentum and the left gastric artery is performed next. The right gastric artery is carefully preserved. This frees the lesser curvature down to the previously mobilized duodenum. Any posterior attachments of the stomach are freed at this time.

Dissection of the lower esophagus requires a 2- to 3-cm opening of the hiatus. This is performed anteriorly after incising the phrenoesophageal ligament. After the anterior and lateral hiatal attachments are freed, circumferential dis-section of the esophagus is completed. The gastroesophageal junction and the distal 5 cm of the esophagus can be dissected sharply from the abdomen.

Posterior mediastinal dissection of the esophagus is performed bluntly. The plane of dissection is along the longitudinal muscle fibers of the esophagus. The pleura should not be violated. Blunt dissection can be performed to the thoracic outlet. During the blunt dissection of the esophagus, a second team (if available) may perform the neck dissection. Otherwise, the transhiatal dissection should proceed as far as possible before starting the neck dissection. Dissection of the esophagus is greatly facilitated if a bougie (number 38 to 48 French) is placed and left in the lumen.

The approach to the cervical esophagus is similar to that of a pharyngoesophageal diverticulum. The longitudinal incision along the sternocleidomastoid muscle is extended to the suprasternal notch. The incision is developed through the avascular plane anterior to the sternocleidomastoid muscle. The carotid sheath is retracted laterally, the thyroid medially. Often, the middle thyroid vein is ligated and transected, as is the omohyoid muscle, to improve exposure. As the tracheoesophageal groove is approached, care must be taken to avoid injuring the recurrent laryngeal nerve. A bougie may be used to identify the extent of the esophageal diameter. Circumferential dissection of the esophagus is completed and a small Penrose drain is passed around the esophagus. The esophagus is then mobilized by a combination of blunt and sharp dissection toward the thoracic outlet. A sponge stick may be used to mobilize the inferior cervical esophagus. Simultaneous transhiatal and cervical dissection is done to facilitate esophageal mobilization. When the esophagus has been completely mobilized, a pyloroplasty is performed.

The stomach is then transected with an automatic stapling and cutting device so that a tube of stomach is created along the greater curvature. The stapler is placed at a point on the greater curvature 5 cm to the left of the gastroesophageal junction and angled toward the incisura on the lesser curvature. Two loads of the automatic stapling and cutting device may be necessary. The portion of stomach attached to the esophagus is then sutured to a short segment of surgical tubing. The tubing is sutured to the tubular stomach. The esophagus is then delivered from the cervical incision, carrying the replacement conduit behind. The stomach should be guided into the chest to prevent torsion and undue pressure on the sutures.

Once the stomach is in the neck, the surgical tubing is removed. The stomach should reach the planned site of the anastomosis easily. Any tension increases the likelihood of an anastomotic leak postoperatively. If too much tension is present, the stomach must either be mobilized more, or an alternative conduit should be considered A point on the cervical esophagus is chosen for the anastomosis. A double-layered hand-sewn or stapled anastomosis is performed. When the anastomosis is completed, the incisions are closed. The neck incision is drained with closed suction to allow egress of luminal contents in case a leak occurs.

Patients are admitted to the intensive care unit for cardiopulmonary support and monitoring for postoperative bleeding. If the patient progresses well after the first day, he or she may be transferred out of the intensive care unit. A liquid diet is started on the third postoperative day. If an anastomotic leak is suspected, a barium contrast study is performed before the initiation of a diet. Patients are instructed to eat small meals in an upright position to limit gastric distention in the chest and facilitate transit to the abdominal portion of the stomach.

Outcome

Using the stomach as conduit, 78% of patients are able to swallow well and require no further intervention (129). Although they will not have normal transit, they are able to maintain their weight and nutritional status. Less than 5% of patients have regurgitation that requires lifestyle modification consisting mostly of head elevation while supine. Overall, long-term follow-up 5 years after operative therapy shows good to excellent results in 68% of patients when all aspects of quality of life are considered (129). Others have reported good results in 90% of patients undergoing esophageal resection for recurrent achalasia (79).

Complications

Perioperative mortality ranges from 2% to 8% (129–131). Intraoperative death usually occurs from bleeding, which occurs during the blunt dissection in the mediastinum. Postoperative deaths occur as a result of nosocomial infections or an exacerbation of preexisting conditions (130).

In a review of 23 papers reporting transhiatal esophagectomy in 1,353 patients, the most common complications after surgery were found to be anastomotic leak (15%) and anastomotic stricture (14%) (132). Most leaks may be treated without further operative intervention. Maintaining nutritional support and drainage of the wound via the closed suction catheter are all that is required. Anastomotic stricture is thought to occur as a result of a narrow anastomosis and the occurrence of a postoperative leak (133). Other complications include hoarseness resulting from recurrent laryngeal nerve injury, symptomatic gastroesophageal reflux, and infection. Perioperative cardiac dysrhythmia has been reported in nearly 50% of patients but can be controlled medically (134).

Controversies

The conduit used for esophageal replacement and the surgical approach to replacement are the main controversies in esophageal replacement. Of the conduits available, the stomach and the colon are the most common. The advan-

tages of using the stomach are that only one anastomosis is performed as opposed to three, the blood supply to the stomach is better than that of the colon, and the plasticity of the stomach allows for easier lengthening (129–131). Those who favor the colon as a conduit state that a longer segment may be replaced by the colon with less tension and long-term function is better (135,136). Furthermore, the likelihood of regurgitation and anastomotic stricture as a result of acid exposure is less with colonic interposition. Still, most gastrointestinal surgeons continue to use the stomach as the conduit of choice.

The surgical approach to a total esophagectomy for benign disease is accomplished efficiently through a transhiatal approach. The benefit is that the patient need not have a thoracotomy, with its inherent morbidity of the incision and single lung-ventilation. Although the procedure can be accomplished via a combined thoracoabdominal approach, this is generally not necessary for benign disease (131,137). A discussion of esophagectomy for malignancy is found elsewhere in this book.

Conclusion

The esophagus can be safely resected and replaced with the stomach. The patient should fully understand the risks of the operation, especially if it is being considered for benign disease. Operative principles include preservation of the blood supply of the stomach, careful mediastinal dissection, and a tension-free anastomosis. Patients have a good functional outcome in 78% to 90% of cases. Benign stricture and anastomotic leak are the most common technical complications of the procedure.

REFERENCES

1. Agur A. *Grant's atlas of anatomy.* Baltimore: Williams and Wilkins, 1991:650.
2. Fremling C, Raivio M, Karppinen I. Endoscopic discision of Zenker's diverticulum. *Ann Chir Gynaecol* 1995;84:169.
3. van Overbeek JJ. Meditation on the pathogenesis of hypopharyngeal (Zenker's) diverticulum and a report of endoscopic treatment in 545 patients. *Ann Otolrhinolaryngol* 1994;103:178.
4. Westrin KM, Ergun S, Carlsoo B. Zenker's diverticulum—a historical review and trends in therapy. *Acta Otolaryngol* 1996;116:351.
5. Cote DN, Miller RH. The association of gastroesophageal reflux and otolaryngologic disorders. *Comprehens Ther* 1995;21:80.
6. Ellis FH Jr. Pharyngoesophageal (Zenker's) diverticulum. *Adv Surg* 1995;28:171.
7. D'Ugo D, Cardillo G, Granone P, et al. Esophageal diverticula. Physiopathological basis for surgical management. *Eur J Card Thorac Surg* 1992;6:330.
8. Migliore M, Payne H, Jeyasingham K. Pathophysiologic basis for operation on Zenker's diverticulum. *Ann Thorac Surg* 1994;57:1616; discussion 1620.

9. McConnel FM, Hood D, Jackson K, et al. Analysis of intrabolus forces in patients with Zenker's diverticulum. *Laryngoscope* 1994;104:571.

10. Lerut T, van Raemdonck D, Guelinckx P, et al. Zenker's diverticulum: is a myotomy of the cricopharyngeus useful? How long should it be? *Hepatogastroenterology* 1992;39:127.

11. Zaninotto G, Costantini M, Anselmino M, et al. Onset of oesophageal peristalsis after surgery for idiopathic achalasia. *Br J Surg* 1995;82:1532.

12. Venturi M, Bonavina L, Colombo L, et al. Biochemical markers of upper esophageal sphincter compliance in patients with Zenker's diverticulum. *J Surg Res* 1997;70:46.

13. Barthlen W, Feussner H, Hannig C, et al. Surgical therapy of Zenker's diverticulum: low risk and high efficiency. *Dysphagia* 1990;5:13.

14. Laing MR, Murthy P, Ah SKW, et al. Surgery for pharyngeal pouch: audit of management with short- and long-term follow-up. *J R Coll Surg Edinb* 1995;40:315.

15. Zeitoun H, Widdowson D, Hammad Z, et al. A video-fluoroscopic study of patients treated by diverticulectomy and cricopharyngeal myotomy. *Clin Otolaryngol* 1994;19:301.

16. Laccourreye O, Menard M, Cauchois R, et al. Esophageal diverticulum: diverticulopexy versus diverticulectomy. *Laryngoscope* 1994;104:889.

17. Gregoire J, Duranceau A. Surgical management of Zenker's diverticulum. *Hepatogastroenterology* 1992;39:132.

18. Louie HW, Zuckerbraun L. Staged Zenker's diverticulectomy with cervical esophagostomy and secondary esophagostomy closure for treatment of massive diverticulum in severely debilitated patients. *Am Surg* 1993;59:842.

19. Nguyen HC, Urquhart AC. Zenker's diverticulum. *Laryngoscope* 1997;107:1436.

20. Schmit PJ, Zuckerbraun L. Treatment of Zenker's diverticula by cricopharyngeus myotomy under local anesthesia. *Am Surg* 1992;58:710.

21. Spiro SA, Berg HM. Applying the endoscopic stapler in excision of Zenker's diverticulum: a solution for two intraoperative problems. *Otolaryngol Head Neck Surg* 1994;110:603.

22. Benjamin B, Innocenti M. Laser treatment of pharyngeal pouch. *Aust N Z J Surg* 1991;61:909.

23. Bradwell RA, Bieger AK, Strachan DR, et al. Endoscopic laser myotomy in the treatment of pharyngeal diverticula. *J Laryngol Otol* 1997;111:627.

24. Collard JM, Otte JB, Kestens PJ. Endoscopic stapling technique of esophagodiverticulostomy for Zenker's diverticulum. *Ann Thorac Surg* 1993;56:573.

25. Ishioka S, Sakai P, Maluf FF, et al. Endoscopic incision of Zenker's diverticula. *Endoscopy* 1995;27:433.

26. Wouters B, van Overbeek JJ. Pathogenesis and endoscopic treatment of the hypopharyngeal (Zenker's) diverticulum. *Acta Gastroenterol Belg* 1990;53:323.

27. Wouters B, van Overbeek JJ. Endoscopic treatment of the hypopharyngeal (Zenker's) diverticulum. *Hepatogastroenterology* 1992;39:105.

28. van Overbeek JJ. Microendoscopic CO_2 laser surgery of the hypopharyngeal (Zenker's) diverticulum. Adv *Otorhinolaryngol* 1995;49:140.

29. Engel JJ, Panje WR. Endoscopic laser Zenker's diverticulotomy. *Gastrointest Endosc* 1995;42:368.

30. Holinger PH, Johnston KC. Endoscopic surgery of Zenker's diverticula. Experience with the Dohlman technique. *Ann Otolrhinolaryngol* 1995;104:751.

31. Lerut T, Van Raemdonck D, Guelinckx P, et al. Pharyngo-oesophageal diverticulum (Zenker's). Clinical, therapeutic and morphological aspects. *Acta Gastroenterol Belg* 1990;53:330.

32. Scher RL, Richtsmeier WJ. Endoscopic staple-assisted esophagodiverticulostomy for Zenker's diverticulum. *Laryngoscope* 1996;106:951.

33. von Doersten PG, Byl FM. Endoscopic Zenker's diverticulotomy (Dohlman procedure): forty cases reviewed. *Otolaryngol Head Neck Surg* 1997;116:209.

34. Counter PR, Hilton ML, Baldwin DL. Long-term follow-up of endoscopic stapled diverticulotomy. *Ann R Coll Surg Engl* 2002; 84:89.

35. Narne S, Cutrone C, Bonavina L, et al. Endoscopic diverticulotomy for the treatment of Zenker's diverticulum: results in 102 patients with staple-assisted endoscopy. *Ann Otolrhinolaryngol* 1999;108:810–815.

36. Stoeckli SJ, Schmid S. Endoscopic stapler-assisted diverticuloesophagostomy for Zenker's diverticulum: patient satisfaction and subjective relief of symptoms. *Surgery* 2002;131:158.

37. Smith SR, Genden EM, Urken ML. Endoscopic stapling technique for the treatment of Zenker diverticulum vs standard open-neck technique. *Otolaryngol Head Neck Surg* 2002;128: 141–144.

38. Watemberg S, Landau O, Avrahami R. Zenker's diverticulum: reappraisal. *Am J Gastroenterol* 1996;91:1494.

39. Dantas RO, Cook IJ, Dodds WJ, et al. Biomechanics of cricopharyngeal bars. *Gastroenterology* 1990;99:1269.

40. Ekberg O. Cricopharyngeal bar: myth and reality. *Abdom Imaging* 1995;20:179.

41. Brady AP, Stevenson GW, Somers S, et al. Premature contraction of the cricopharyngeus: a new sign of gastroesophageal reflux disease. *Abdom Imaging* 1995;20:225.

42. Herberhold C, Walther EK. Endoscopic laser myotomy in cricopharyngeal achalasia. *Adv Oto Rhino Laryngol* 1995;49: 144.

43. Monnig PJ. Familial achalasia in children. *Ann Thorac Surg* 1990;49:1019.

44. Robertson CS, Martin BA, Atkinson M. Varicella-zoster virus DNA in the oesophageal myenteric plexus in achalasia. *Gut* 1993;34:299.

45. Niwamoto H, Okamoto E, Fujimoto J, et al. Are human herpes viruses or measles virus associated with esophageal achalasia? *Dig Dis Sci* 1995;40:859.

46. Mearin F, Mourelle M, Guarner F, et al. Patients with achalasia lack nitric oxide synthase in the gastro-oesophageal junction. *Eur J Clin Invest* 1993;23:724.

47. Miyata M, Sakamoto T, Hashimoto T, et al. Effect of secretin on lower esophageal sphincter pressure in patients with esophageal achalasia. *Gastroenterol Jpn* 1991;26:712.

48. Pellegrini CA, Leichter R, Patti M, et al. Thoracoscopic esophageal myotomy in the treatment of achalasia. *Ann Thorac Surg* 1993;56:680.

49. Ellingson TL, Kozarek RA, Gelfand MD, et al. Iatrogenic achalasia. A case series. *J Clin Gastroenterol* 1995;20:96.

50. Parrilla P, Aguayo JL, Martinez DHL, et al. Reversible achalasia-like motor pattern of esophageal body secondary to postoperative stricture of gastroesophageal junction. *Dig Dis Sci* 1992; 37:1781.

51. Myers NA, Jolley SG, Taylor R. Achalasia of the cardia in children: a worldwide survey. *J Pediatr Surg* 1994;29:1375.

52. Illi OE, Stauffer UG. Achalasia in childhood and adolescence. *Eur J Pediatr Surg* 1994;4:214.

53. Parrilla PP, Martinez DHLF, Ortiz EA, et al. Short myotomy for vigorous achalasia. *Br J Surg* 1993;80:1540.

54. Stuart RC, Byrne PJ, Lawlor P, et al. Meal area index: a new technique for quantitative assessment in achalasia by ambulatory manometry during eating. *Br J Surg* 1992;79:1162.

55. Stein HJ, Korn O, Liebermann MD. Manometric vector volume analysis to assess lower esophageal sphincter function. *Ann Chir Gynaecol* 1995;84:151.

56. Mattox HE, Albertson DA, Castell DO, et al. Dysphagia following fundoplication: "slipped" fundoplication versus achalasia complicated by fundoplication. *Am J Gastroenterol* 1990;85: 1468.

57. Parrilla PP, Martinez DHL, Ortiz A, et al. Achalasia of the cardia: long-term results of oesophagomyotomy and posterior partial fundoplication. *Br J Surg* 1990;77:1371.

58. Crookes PF, Corkill S, DeMeester TR. Gastroesophageal reflux in achalasia. When is reflux really reflux? *Dig Dis Sci* 1997;42: 1354.

59. Shoenut JP, Micflikier AB, Yaffe CS, et al. Reflux in untreated achalasia patients. *J Clin Gastroenterol* 1995;20:6.

60. Stacher G, Schima W, Bergmann H, et al. Sensitivity of radionuclide bolus transport and videofluoroscopic studies compared with manometry in the detection of achalasia. *Am J Gastroenterol* 1994;89:1484.

61. Mattioli S, Pilotti V, Felice V, et al. Intraoperative study on the relationship between the lower esophageal sphincter pressure and the muscular components of the gastro-esophageal junction in achalasic patients. *Ann Surg* 1993;218:635.

62. Delgado F, et al. Laparoscopic treatment of esophageal achalasia. *Surg Laparosc Endosc* 1996;6:83.

63. Pellegrini C, et al. Thoracoscopic esophagomyotomy. Initial experience with a new approach for the treatment of achalasia. *Ann Surg* 1992;216:291; discussion 296.

64. Peracchia A, Rosati R, Bona S, et al. Laparoscopic treatment of functional diseases of the esophagus. *Int Surg* 1995;80:336.

65. Shimi S, Nathanson LK, Cuschieri A. Laparoscopic cardiomyotomy for achalasia. *J R Coll Surg Edinb* 1991;36:152.

66. Patti MG, Pellegrini CA. Endoscopic surgical treatment of primary oesophageal motility disorders. *J R Coll Surg Edinb* 1996; 41:137.

67. Horgan SHK, Eubanks TR, Pellegrini CA. Does Botox injection make esophagomyotomy a more difficult operation? Presented at SAGES Scientific Session, Seattle, WA, April 1–4, 1998.

68. Bonavina L, Nosadini A, Bardini R, et al. Primary treatment of esophageal achalasia. Long-term results of myotomy and Dor fundoplication. *Arch Surg* 1992;127:222; discussion.

69. Pandolfo N, Bortolotti M, Spigno L, et al. Manometric assessment of Heller-Dor operation for esophageal achalasia. *Hepatogastroenterology* 1996;43:160.

70. Csendes A, Braghetto I, Mascaro J, et al. Late subjective and objective evaluation of the results of esophagomyotomy in 100 patients with achalasia of the esophagus. *Surgery* 1988;104:469.

71. Parrilla P, Martinez DHLF, Ortiz A, et al. Factors involved in the return of peristalsis in patients with achalasia of the cardia after Heller's myotomy. *Am J Gastroenterol* 1995;90:713.

72. Martins P, Morais BB, Cunha MJR. Postoperative complications in the treatment of chagasic megaesophagus. *Int Surg* 1993;78:99.

73. Di SMP, et al. Onset timing of delayed complications and criteria of follow-up after operation for esophageal achalasia. *Ann Thorac Surg* 1996;61:1106; discussion 1110.

74. Shoenut JP, Duerksen D, Yaffe CS. A prospective assessment of gastroesophageal reflux before and after treatment of achalasia patients: pneumatic dilation versus transthoracic limited myotomy. *Am J Gastroenterol* 1997;92:1109.

75. Jaakkola A, Reinikainen P, Ovaska J, et al. Barrett's esophagus after cardiomyotomy for esophageal achalasia. *Am J Gastroenterol* 1994;89:165.

76. Parkman HP, Ogorek CP, Harris AD, et al. Nonoperative management of esophageal strictures following esophagomyotomy for achalasia. *Dig Dis Sci* 1994;39:2102.

77. Ellis FH. Esophagomyotomy by the thoracic approach for esophageal achalasia. *Hepatogastroenterology* 1991;38:498.

78. Johnson O. Achalasia of the cardia: experience of extramucosal cardiomyotomy during a ten-year period. *Ethiop Med J* 1994; 32:89.

79. Miller DL, Allen MS, Trastek VF, et al. Esophageal resection for recurrent achalasia. *Ann Thorac Surg* 1995;60:922; discussion 925.

80. Csendes A, Braghetto I, Henriquez A, et al. Late results of a prospective randomised study comparing forceful dilatation and oesophagomyotomy in patients with achalasia. *Gut* 1989; 30:299.

81. Gayet B, Fekete F. Surgical management of failed esophagomyotomy (Heller's operation). *Hepatogastroenterology* 1991;38:488.

82. Gorecki PJ, Hinder RA, Libbey JS, et al. Redo laparoscopic surgery for achalasia. *Surg Endosc* 2002;16:772.

83. Ximenes MR. Esophageal resection for recurrent achalasia. *Ann Thorac Surg* 1996;62:322.

84. Schwartz HM, Cahow CE, Traube M. Outcome after perforation sustained during pneumatic dilatation for achalasia. *Dig Dis Sci* 1993;38:1409.

85. Flynn AE, Verrier ED, Way LW, et al. Esophageal perforation. *Arch Surg* 1989;124:1211; discussion 1214.

86. Pricolo VE, Park CS, Thompson WR. Surgical repair of esophageal perforation due to pneumatic dilatation for achalasia. Is myotomy really necessary? *Arch Surg* 1993;128:540; discussion 543.

87. Nathanson LK, Gotley D, Smithers M, et al. Videothoracoscopic primary repair of early distal oesophageal perforation. *Aust N Z J Surg* 1993;63:399.

88. Ferguson MK, Reeder LB, Olak J. Results of myotomy and partial fundoplication after pneumatic dilation for achalasia. *Ann Thorac Surg* 1996;62:327.

89. Bourgeois N, Coffernils M, Sznajer Y, et al. Non-surgical management of achalasia. *Acta Gastroenterol Belg* 1992;55:260.

90. Efrati Y, Horne T, Livshitz G, et al. Radionuclide esophageal emptying and long-acting nitrates (Nitroderm) in childhood achalasia. *J Pediatr Gastroenterol Nutr* 1996;23:312.

91. Pasricha PJ, Kalloo AN. Recent advances in the treatment of achalasia. *Gastrointest Endosc Clin North Am* 1997;7:191.

92. Tack J, Janssens J, Vantrappen G. Non-surgical treatment of achalasia. *Hepatogastroenterology* 1991;38:493.

93. Abid S, Champion G, Richter JE, et al. Treatment of achalasia: the best of both worlds. *Am J Gastroenterol* 1994;89:979.

94. Anselmino M, et al. Heller myotomy is superior to dilatation for the treatment of early achalasia. *Arch Surg* 1997;132:233.

95. Makela J, Kiviniemi H, Laitinen S. Heller's cardiomyotomy compared with pneumatic dilatation for treatment of oesophageal achalasia. *Eur J Surg* 1991;157:411.

96. Csendes A, Velasco N, Braghetto I, et al. A prospective randomized study comparing forceful dilatation and esophagomyotomy in patients with achalasia of the esophagus. *Gastroenterology* 1981;80:789.

97. Richter JE. Surgery or pneumatic dilatation for achalasia: a head-to-head comparison. Now are all the questions answered? *Gastroenterology* 1989;97:1340.

98. McJunkin B, McMillan WO Jr, Duncan HE Jr, et al. Assessment of dilation methods in achalasia: large diameter mercury bougienage followed by pneumatic dilation as needed. *Gastrointest Endosc* 1991;37:18.

99. Supe AN, Samsi AB, Bapat RD, et al. Pneumatic dilatation in achalasia cardia results and follow-up. *J Postgrad Med* 1990;36: 181.

100. Parkman HP, Reynolds JC, Ouyang A, et al. Pneumatic dilatation or esophagomyotomy treatment for idiopathic achalasia: clinical outcomes and cost analysis. *Dig Dis Sci* 1993;38:75.

101. Holzman MD, Sharp KW, Ladipo JK, et al. Laparoscopic surgical treatment of achalasia. *Am J Surg* 1997;173:308.

102. Jorgensen JO, Hunt DR. Laparoscopic management of pneumatic dilatation resistant achalasia. *Aust N Z J Surg* 1993;63:386.

103. Raiser F, et al. Heller myotomy via minimal-access surgery. An evaluation of antireflux procedures. *Arch Surg* 1996;131:593; discussion 597.

104. Xynos E, Tzovaras G, Petrakis I, et al. Laparoscopic Heller's cardiomyotomy and Dor's fundoplication for esophageal achalasia. *J Laparoendosc Surg* 1996;6:253.

105. Barkin JS, Guelrud M, Reiner DK, et al. Forceful balloon dilation: an outpatient procedure for achalasia. *Gastrointest Endosc* 1990;36:123.

106. Ciarolla DA, Traube M. Achalasia. Short-term clinical monitoring after pneumatic dilation. *Dig Dis Sci* 1993;38:1905.

107. Ancona E, Peracchia A, Zaninotto G, et al. Heller laparoscopic cardiomyotomy with antireflux anterior fundoplication (Dor) in the treatment of esophageal achalasia. *Surg Endosc* 1993;7:459.

108. Collard JM, Romagnoli R, Lengele B, et al. Heller-Dor procedure for achalasia: from conventional to video-endoscopic surgery. *Acta Chir Belg* 1996;96:62.

109. Graham AJ, Finley RJ, Worsley DF, et al. Laparoscopic esophageal myotomy and anterior partial fundoplication for the treatment of achalasia. *Ann Thorac Surg* 1997;64:785.

110. Morino M, Rebecchi F, Festa V, et al. Laparoscopic Heller cardiomyotomy with intraoperative manometry in the management of oesophageal achalasia. *Int Surg* 1995;80:332.

111. Vara TC, Herrainz R. Esophageal achalasia: laparoscopic Heller cardiomyotomy. *Int Surg* 1995;80:376.

112. Ancona E, et al. Esophageal achalasia: laparoscopic versus conventional open Heller-Dor operation. *Am J Surg* 1995;170:265.

113. Ellis FH Jr. Invited letter concerning: technique for prevention of gastroesophageal reflux after transthoracic Heller's operation. *J Thorac Cardiovasc Surg* 1993;105:555.

114. Gatzinsky P, Dernevik L, Bjork S, et al. Technique for prevention of gastroesophageal reflux after transthoracic Heller's operation. *J Thorac Cardiovasc Surg* 1993;105:553.

115. Hunter JG, Trus TL, Branum GD, et al. Laparoscopic Heller myotomy and fundoplication for achalasia. *Ann Surg* 1997;225:655; discussion 664.

116. Patti MG, Arcerito M, Pellegrini CA. Thoracoscopic and laparoscopic Heller's myotomy in the treatment of esophageal achalasia. *Ann Chir Gynaecol* 1995;84:159.

117. Slim K, Pezet D, Chipponi J, Boulant J, et al. Laparoscopic myotomy for primary esophageal achalasia: prospective evaluation. *Hepatogastroenterology* 1997;44:11.

118. Ellis FH Jr, Watkins E Jr, Gibb SP, et al. Ten to 20-year clinical results after short esophagomyotomy without an antireflux procedure (modified Heller operation) for esophageal achalasia. *Eur J Card Thorac Surg* 1992;6:86; discussion 90.

119. Cade RJ, Martin CJ. Thoracoscopic cardiomyotomy for achalasia. *Aust N Z J Surg* 1996;66:107.

120. Katada N, et al. The hypertensive lower esophageal sphincter. *Am J Surg* 1996;172:439; discussion 442.

121. Benacci JC, Deschamps C, Trastek VF, et al. Epiphrenic diverticulum: results of surgical treatment. *Ann Thorac Surg* 1993;55:1109; discussion 1114.

122. Barreca M, Oelschlager BK, Pellegrini CA. Outcomes of laparoscopic Nissen fundoplication in patients with the "hypercontractile esophagus." *Arch Surg* 2002;137:724.

123. Eypasch EP, Stein HJ, DeMeester TR, et al. A new technique to define and clarify esophageal motor disorders. *Am J Surg* 1990;159:144; discussion 151.

124. Stein HJ, DeMeester TR, Eypasch EP, et al. Ambulatory 24-hour esophageal manometry in the evaluation of esophageal motor disorders and noncardiac chest pain. *Surgery* 1991;110:753; discussion 761.

125. Filipi CJ, Hinder RA. Thoracoscopic esophageal myotomy—a surgical technique for achalasia diffuse esophageal spasm and "nutcracker esophagus." *Surg Endosc* 1994;8:921; discussion 925.

126. McBride PJ, et al. Surgical treatment of spastic conditions of the esophagus. *Int Surg* 1997;82:113.

127. Shimi SM, Nathanson LK, Cuschieri A. Thoracoscopic long oesophageal myotomy for nutcracker oesophagus: initial experience of a new surgical approach. *Br J Surg* 1992;79:533.

128. Patti MG, et al. Comparison of medical and minimally invasive surgical therapy for primary esophageal motility disorders. *Arch Surg* 1995;130:609; discussion 615.

129. Orringer MB, Marshall B, Stirling MC. Transhiatal esophagectomy for benign and malignant disease. *J Thorac Cardiovasc Surg* 1993;105:265; discussion 276.

130. Daniel TM, Fleischer KJ, Flanagan TL, et al. Transhiatal esophagectomy: a safe alternative for selected patients. *Ann Thorac Surg* 1992;54:686; discussion 689.

131. Davis EA, Heitmiller RF. Esophagectomy for benign disease: trends in surgical results and management. *Ann Thorac Surg* 1996;62:369.

132. Katariya K, Harvey JC, Pina E, et al. Complications of transhiatal esophagectomy. *J Surg Oncol* 1994;57:157.

133. Honkoop P, et al. Benign anastomotic strictures after transhiatal esophagectomy and cervical esophagogastrostomy: risk factors and management. *J Thorac Cardiovasc Surg* 1996;111:1141; discussion 1147.

134. Patti MG, Wiener KJP, Way LW, et al. Impact of transhiatal esophagectomy on cardiac and respiratory function. *Am J Surg* 1991;162:563; discussion 566.

135. Mansour KA, Bryan FC, Carlson GW. Bowel interposition for esophageal replacement: twenty-five-year experience. *Ann Thorac Surg* 1997;64:752.

136. Gupta NM, Goenka MK, Behera A, et al. Transhiatal oesophagectomy for benign obstructive conditions of the oesophagus. *Br J Surg* 1997;84:262

137. Watson TJ, Peters JH, DeMeester TR. Esophageal replacement for end-stage benign esophageal disease. *Surg Clin North Am* 1997;77:1099.

19

CLINICAL SPECTRUM AND DIAGNOSIS OF GASTROESOPHAGEAL REFLUX DISEASE

ROBERT C. HEADING
DONALD O. CASTELL

CLINICAL SPECTRUM

Thirty years ago, most patients who complained of heartburn, regurgitation, and water brash were given a diagnosis of "hiatal hernia" (1), despite evidence then emerging that a hernia is not found in all patients with these symptoms (2). Twenty years ago, the diagnosis offered for the same symptoms would probably have been esophagitis, even though endoscopy sometimes showed a normal esophagus. Today, the acronym *GERD* has gained favor to denote the clinical manifestations of gastroesophageal reflux disease, being used as a diagnostic term that embraces the whole variety of symptoms and types of tissue damage that may be caused by reflux of gastric contents into the esophagus. GERD denotes abnormality and so should not be confused with the gastroesophageal reflux that occurs in healthy subjects, (*physiologic reflux*), which does not cause symptoms or esophageal mucosal injury.

Clinical presentations of GERD vary considerably but can be logically placed into three categories: typical symptoms, atypical symptoms, and complications. These comprise the spectrum of GERD (Fig. 19.1).

Typical Symptoms

Heartburn and regurgitation are the typical symptoms of GERD. When they are a patient's only symptoms, or predominant symptoms, they are specific but not sensitive as a basis for diagnosis (3). Many patients with GERD have a less specific presentation, however, such as epigastric pain or other dyspepsia together with some retrosternal heartburn.

R. C. Heading: Centre for Liver and Digestive Disorders, Royal Infirmary, Edinburgh, Scotland.

D. O. Castell: Department of Medicine, Medical University of South Carolina, Charleston, South Carolina.

Reliable diagnosis on the basis of symptoms is not then possible. Less than 50% of patients with GERD have endoscopic evidence of esophagitis and neither the pattern nor the severity of symptoms predict its presence or absence (1,4–6).

Heartburn and regurgitation are characteristically worsened after eating, by bending or stooping, and by lying down in bed at night, especially by lying on the right side rather than the left. Heartburn and regurgitation may also be experienced during sexual intercourse (*reflux dyspareunia*)—a manifestation of reflux disease that is not commonly discussed. In one series of 100 women with chronic reflux symptoms, 77% complained of troubling heartburn during intercourse (7).

Atypical Symptoms

Angina-like chest pain, sometimes including an exertional component, is one of the less typical symptoms of GERD. Ambulatory recordings of intraesophageal pH have been used to document directly the relationship of chest pain episodes to reflux. Findings of such studies indicate that previously unrecognized GERD is a major cause of noncardiac chest pain (8–13).

Reflux also may be present as chronic hoarseness or other voice abnormalities associated with posterior inflammation of the larynx and vocal cords, a manifestation often referred to as *reflux laryngitis*. When studied with prolonged pH monitoring, more than 75% of such patients have been shown to have abnormal reflux, and acid exposure in the hypopharynx can be documented occasionally (14–16). It has even been suggested that chronic reflux injury may promote malignant change. Ward and Hanson (17) reported the occurrence of laryngeal cancer in 19 of 138 patients with moderate or severe reflux during a 10-year period. None of these patients smoked or consumed alcohol, activ-

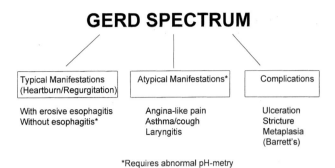

FIGURE 19.1. Demonstration of the various manifestations comprising the clinical spectrum of gastroesophageal reflux disease.

ities usually expected to be associated with laryngeal malignancies.

Various pulmonary symptoms may be associated with GERD. Nocturnal episodes of nonallergic asthma, particularly when preceded by a history of chronic reflux symptoms, are highly suggestive of reflux disease. Intraesophageal pH monitoring studies have demonstrated abnormal amounts of reflux in more than 20% of patients with chronic cough (18) and in more than 80% of unselected patients with chronic asthma (19). Although pH monitoring may show that pulmonary symptoms occur after a reflux episode, often they may occur during reflux or even before it, making it hard to ascertain whether reflux is causing coughing or coughing is causing reflux (20).

Protracted hiccups also have been observed in reflux patients. In one such case, hiccups resolved in response to treatment with cimetidine and recurred on esophageal exposure to acid during a Bernstein test (21). A specific causal relationship has been questioned, however, in that changes in esophageal pressures during hiccups are likely to cause reflux (22). A variety of other atypical symptoms of GERD have been suggested. These include globus sensation, erosion of dental enamel, ear pain, night sweats, and intermittent torticollis or peculiar posturing in children (Sandifer's syndrome).

Complications

GERD can also present with the complications of reflux, such as erosive or ulcerative esophagitis, which may cause bleeding and anemia, or peptic stricture, which may cause dysphagia. However, intermittent dysphagia may be a feature of GERD even when no stricture is present (23). Presumably it then occurs as a consequence of impaired bolus propulsion resulting from suboptimal esophageal body peristalsis (24). Severe chronic reflux may also induce metaplastic change of the squamous epithelium of the lower esophagus to a glandular (columnar) epithelium, referred to as *Barrett's esophagus*. This is of particular concern because it carries an increased risk of esophageal adenocarcinoma. In one study, 12% of unselected patients with chronic symptoms of heartburn and regurgitation had endoscopic and histologic changes in the esophageal epithelium consistent with Barrett's esophagus (6). Recent epidemiologic evidence has given further strong support to the belief that longstanding reflux symptoms are associated with an enhanced risk of developing esophageal adenocarcinoma (25).

PREVALENCE

Quantitative estimates of the actual prevalence of GERD in the United States are difficult to obtain because of the sparsity of epidemiologic studies and because many individuals do not seek medical care for their symptoms. One often cited study provided information on the prevalence of heartburn from a questionnaire survey of 1,004 individuals (26). Included in the study population were 335 normal control subjects, 200 surgical inpatients, 246 medical inpatients, 121 patients attending a gastrointestinal clinic, and 102 pregnant patients attending an obstetrics clinic (Table 19.1). Overall, 11% of the entire study group reported daily heartburn, and an additional 12% and 15% described weekly and monthly heartburn, respectively, resulting in a total prevalence of 38% for heartburn in this sample of U.S. adults. The substantially higher prevalence of daily heartburn (25%) described by pregnant women in the obstetrics

TABLE 19.1. ESTIMATED HEARTBURN PREVALENCE IN THE UNITED STATES

Study Group	No. of Patients	Percentage Experiencing Heartburn			
		Daily	Weekly	Monthly	Total
Controls	335	7	14	15	36
Surgical inpatients	200	6	12	19	37
Medical inpatients	246	14	12	14	40
Gastrointestinal clinic patients	121	15	12	13	40
Obstetrics clinic patients	102	25	10	17	52
Total	1,004	11	12	15	38

From Nebel OT, Fornes MF, Castell DO. Symptomatic gastroesophageal reflux: incidence and precipitating factors. *Am J Dig Dis* 1976;21:953, with permission.

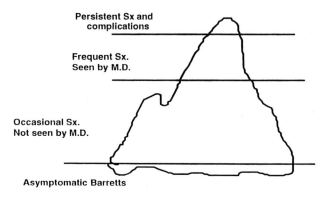

FIGURE 19.2. The gastroesophageal reflux disease iceberg displays the clinical presentations of typical manifestations. Details are provided in text. *Sx*, symptoms.

clinic as compared with subjects in the other four groups reflects the well-known association between heartburn and pregnancy. The popular concepts that heartburn occurs daily in approximately 10% of U.S. adults and that more than one third of that population have occasional heartburn had their genesis in these data.

The concept of the GERD iceberg, shown in Figure 19.2, was developed to demonstrate the clinical presentation of typical GERD symptoms. Most of patients with heartburn and regurgitation have intermittent symptoms for which they do not consult their physicians and for which they frequently take over-the-counter medications. Those with more persistent symptoms are more likely to see a physician for advice, with a small percentage of symptomatic individuals (probably 10% or less) represented by that group with complicated GERD seen by the gastroenterologist. Community-based studies suggest that the prevalence of reflux symptoms is much the same in adults of all ages but that the proportion of individuals who seek medical help for the symptoms increases with age (27,28). One disturbing element in the clinical scenario is the group of patients who have Barrett's esophagus and who experience minimal reflux symptoms. They have little reason to consult a physician and consequently their increased risk of esophageal adenocarcinoma goes unrecognized. In one study, 28% of patients presenting with symptomatic adenocarcinoma in a Barrett's esophagus had no preceding history of reflux symptoms (29).

INFLUENCE OF FOOD ON REFLUX SYMPTOMS

Although the pathophysiology of GERD is complex and the effects of eating on reflux are part of the complexity, there are some clear relationships between symptoms and certain foods. An early study of intolerance to 39 different types of food in 25 patients with daily heartburn and 25 patients with only monthly symptoms found an inverse

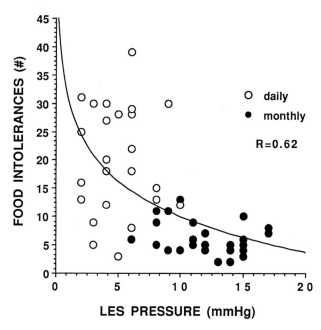

FIGURE 19.3. Relationship between 39 foods causing heartburn and resting lower esophageal sphincter (*LES*) pressure in 25 patients with daily and 25 patients with monthly reflux symptoms.

correlation between the number of food intolerances and resting tonic lower esophageal sphincter (LES) pressure (30) (Fig. 19.3). Individuals with a normal LES pressure reported heartburn only after eating certain foods, including fried foods, spicy foods, and hot dogs, whereas those with very low LES pressures experienced reflux symptoms after eating almost all types of food surveyed. Moreover, LES pressures were lower in the patients with daily heartburn than in the patients with less frequent symptoms. All the patients with daily symptoms had a resting LES pressure of less than 10 mm Hg (Fig. 19.4), indicating that patients with poor sphincter function tend to experience symptoms regardless of the type of food consumed.

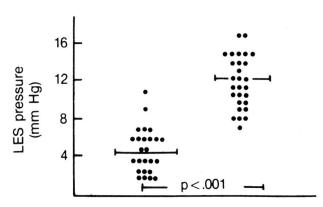

FIGURE 19.4. Resting lower esophageal sphincter pressures for 25 patients with daily heartburn (**left**) and 25 patients with monthly heartburn (**right**).

Transient lower esophageal sphincter relaxations (TLESRs) are the dominant mechanism responsible for the occurrence of reflux episodes in normal subjects and in individuals with relatively mild reflux disease, whereas other mechanisms, notably sphincteric incompetence, make a progressively greater contribution as the severity of reflux disease increases (see Chapter 21). This difference explains, at least in part, some of the effects of meals in general and of specific foods in particular on reflux symptoms: the well-known relationship between fat ingestion and reflux can be examined against this background. Resting LES pressure in healthy volunteers is reduced by fat (30) and fat also increases the frequency of TLESRs (31). Thus, when TLESRs are the main mechanism of reflux, meals with a high fat content may be expected to have a relatively specific effect, predisposing to symptoms. However, in comparison with the fasting state, TLESR frequency is also somewhat increased by distention of the gastric fundus, so any meal that distends the stomach, regardless of its chemical composition, promotes reflux to some degree via this mechanism. In individuals with incompetence of the LES, the liability to postprandial reflux occurs regardless of meal composition because the ineffectiveness of the LES barrier function has little to do with the nature of gastric contents. The patients with an incompetent sphincter are more likely to experience provocation of symptoms by bending down, by stooping, and by recumbency, however, because these maneuvers expose the incompetence of the sphincter.

One study illustrating these relationships compared the effect of high-fat (61% by calorie) and low-fat (16%) meals on esophageal acid exposure, determined by pH monitoring (32). In normal subjects maintaining an upright posture postprandially, increased esophageal acid exposure occurred after the high-fat compared with the low-fat meal, particularly during the second and third hours after food ingestion. The fat content of the meal had little influence, however, on the acid exposure in reflux patients in the upright position, who experienced reflux after both the high-fat and the low-fat meals (Table 19.2). When normal subjects and reflux

patients were studied in the recumbent position after eating, increased exposure of the esophagus to acid was observed in both groups after both high-fat and low-fat meals.

Many other observations illustrate the singular importance of dietary fat in predisposing to reflux. The effects of fat and of meals on tonic LES pressures, on TLESRs, and on gastric fundic distention and relaxation account for many of the observations, but an additional effect derives from the fact that gastric emptying takes longer with large meals than small meals, and with meals of high rather than low caloric density. When compared with a small meal of low nutrient content, a large meal of high caloric density (such as one containing much fat) therefore causes the stomach to be in its postprandial mode—when TLESRs occur at postprandial frequency and facilitate reflux—for a longer period of time.

The risk of developing GERD may well be related in part to habits of the modern Western world. As discussed in subsequent chapters, these include a diet that is characterized by fatty and large meals, by obesity, smoking, and chocolate consumption, and, possibly, by long-term use of certain drugs.

DIAGNOSTIC EVALUATION

The diagnostic approach to the patient with possible GERD is multilayered, depending on the presentation. Because the symptoms are believed to be due to chronic reflux, the evaluation should attempt to document this abnormality. This patient who presents with typical heartburn and regurgitation with the usual positional and postprandial relationships requires little, if any, additional information to establish a presumptive diagnosis and initiate therapy. The patient whose symptoms are less clear or include atypical manifestations usually needs additional diagnostic testing. The variety of tests and procedures available to evaluate the patient with possible GERD can cause diagnostic confusion if not used appropriately. It is preferable to begin the diagnostic approach by defining the question to be answered in the individual patient. In Table 19.3, the variety of diagnostic tests that has been advocated for the patient with possible reflux is categorized according to the question being asked.

Is Abnormal Reflux Present?

The critical question often is whether the patient has abnormal reflux, particularly in the patient with an atypical symptom pattern. Simply confirming that abnormal reflux is present is often satisfactory to support the clinical impression.

Traditionally, the first test performed to evaluate possible reflux, particularly by the primary care physician, has been

TABLE 19.2. AVERAGE UPRIGHT ESOPHAGEAL ACID EXPOSURE (% TIME) AFTER HIGH-FAT VERSUS LOW-FAT MEALS IN NORMALS AND REFLUX PATIENTS[a]

Normals	Low-Fat Meals	High-Fat Meals
First hour	1.8	7.4
Second hour	2.1	8.1
Third hour	0.5	2.9
Reflux patients		
First hour	19.5	25.8
Second hour	22.3	27.2
Third hour	26.1	9.8

[a]The fat content, by calories, of the low-fat and high-fat meals was 16% and 61%, respectively.

TABLE 19.3. DIAGNOSTIC TESTS FOR GASTROESOPHAGEAL REFLUX DISEASE CATEGORIZED ACCORDING TO SPECIFIC QUESTIONS

Is abnormal reflux present?
  Barium upper gastrointestinal series
  Gastroesophageal radionuclide scan
  Standard acid reflux test
Is abnormal acid reflux present?
  Ambulatory pH monitoring
Is there mucosal injury?
  Endoscopy
  Barium upper gastrointestinal (air contrast) study
  Mucosal biopsy
Are symptoms due to acid reflux?
  Ambulatory pH monitoring (with symptom index)
  Bernstein test
  PPI treatment response
Can prognostic or useful preoperative information be obtained?
  Esophageal motility evaluation
  Ambulatory pH monitoring

PPI, proton pump inhibitor.

an upper gastrointestinal series. Despite being supplanted in recent years by upper gastrointestinal endoscopy, it is worth noting that endoscopy cannot answer the question "is abnormal reflux present?" Radiology can effectively rule out complications of GERD (ulcer, stricture) or other structural abnormalities of the esophagus, stomach, or duodenum, and can demonstrate reflux—the flow of barium from the stomach into the esophagus either spontaneously or induced by various maneuvers. However, radiographic reflux has limited diagnostic value. Reflux is dependent on the state of competence of the antireflux mechanism at a particular moment and has been demonstrated radiographically in as few as 60% of severely symptomatic patients or in as many as 25% of patients having no reflux symptoms. Thus, its reliability is questionable, with both poor specificity and sensitivity (33,34). Air contrast techniques provide more information (see Chapter 3). Because normal individuals have brief intermittent episodes of reflux (so-called physiologic reflux), particularly on those occasions when the LES spontaneously relaxes (35), observing the occurrence of reflux during a radiographic study does not itself imply abnormality.

Radionuclide scans have been advocated to document reflux and to provide quantitation of the amount of reflux. The gastroesophageal scan uses a radioisotope (technetium-99m sulfur colloid) as a marker for reflux. Graded abdominal compression is used to unmask incompetence of the reflux barrier. Although originally proposed as a sensitive test of reflux (36), its reliability is doubtful (37) and is no longer favored.

The use of an intraesophageal pH electrode to detect reflux was initially reported by Tuttle and Grossman in 1958 (38). Subsequently, the standard acid reflux test was developed to stress the antireflux barrier in the laboratory while measuring reflux with a pH probe placed 5 cm above the LES. Following instillation of 300 mL of 0.1N hydrochloric acid into the stomach, the patient performs four maneuvers—deep breathing, Valsalva, Müller (inspiration against a closed glottis), and cough—repeated in the supine and right and left lateral decubitus positions and with the head down 20 degrees. Overall, 16 possibilities for acid reflux occur. A decrease in esophageal pH to less than 4 on at least three occasions is considered evidence of abnormal reflux. This test has relatively good overall sensitivity and specificity but is cumbersome and time-consuming in practice, so it is rarely used (34).

Prolonged ambulatory intraesophageal pH monitoring is considered the procedure of choice to demonstrate the occurrence of abnormal acid reflux (see Chapter 6). Patients record the time that they experience reflux symptoms during monitoring, thus allowing correlation of intraesophageal pH and subjective symptoms. A symptom index (SI) often helps clarify the association of specific symptoms with episodes of reflux, using the following equation (39):

$$SI = \frac{\text{No. of symptoms occurring with pH} < 4.0 \times 100}{\text{Total no. of symptoms}}$$

This test is of no value if the patient is incapable of gastric acid production. Clinical indications include difficult diagnostic problems or atypical reflux symptoms (chest pain, cough, hoarseness), nonresponse to therapy, and preoperative and postoperative evaluation of antireflux surgery.

Is There Evidence of Mucosal Injury?

Esophagitis is the *sine qua non* of GERD. This can occasionally be documented by careful air contrast barium esophagram showing mucosal lesions (erosions, ulcers) or stricture. Direct comparison of this technique with endoscopy has revealed that the finding of esophageal injury on air contrast esophagram is highly specific, although not very sensitive (40).

Endoscopy is the diagnostic approach most frequently used to document esophageal injury. Erosions or ulcerations of the mucosa visualized through the endoscope are indications of reflux injury. The findings are definitive when unequivocally present but may be subtle or absent, and it is important that clinicians appreciate that many patients with GERD do not have esophagitis (4). Only 34% of patients with chronic heartburn evaluated in one study had esophagitis apparent on endoscopy (6). Moreover, many published studies of reflux and esophagitis have failed to address the problems of interpretation arising from interobserver variation in recognition of the milder degrees of esophagitis (41). The Los Angeles system of grading esophagitis has been validated in this respect (42).

Potentially, esophageal mucosal biopsy should be a more sensitive test of the presence of reflux injury because histologic abnormalities may be present even when careful endoscopic examination indicates a normal-appearing esophagus. The most reliable criterion for esophagitis on endoscopic biopsy is the presence of acute inflammatory cells (polymorphonuclear leukocytes or eosinophils). These are present in esophageal biopsy specimens of only 20% of patients with reflux symptoms, however, and other epithelial changes have been proposed as providing better diagnostic criteria. Increased papillary extension and basal zone hyperplasia have been thought to be more sensitive findings occurring secondary to chronic gastroesophageal reflux (43). However, there is no good evidence that these or other findings on biopsy are helpful in the context of ordinary clinical practice. Indeed, there is persuasive evidence that conventional endoscopic pinch biopsies are of little value (44,45). Suction biopsies may be no better unless many samples are obtained (46).

Are Symptoms Due to Gastroesophageal Reflux Disease?

In many patients, a key question is whether their symptoms are clearly related to acid exposure and sensitivity of the esophageal mucosa to chronic reflux. The acid perfusion (Bernstein) test was used for many years as a test of acid sensitivity, with a reported specificity and sensitivity of approximately 80% in GERD (34). If the patient's symptoms are reproduced during perfusion of the esophagus with dilute hydrochloric acid and resolve following saline perfusion, it is appropriate to conclude that chronic acid reflux is the cause of spontaneously occurring symptoms. This test is purely qualitative in character and provides no information on the magnitude of reflux.

If the SI is calculated as described earlier, 24-hour pH monitoring can define the relationship between specific symptoms and reflux. This test is limited by the requirement that the patient's symptoms must occur during the test period. With this limitation, it is nonetheless considered by many investigators to represent an endogenous Bernstein test (16).

The opposite approach to acid reflux testing is the use of a proton pump inhibitor (omeprazole, 20 mg twice daily, or lansoprazole, 30 mg twice daily) as a diagnostic tool. The disappearance of symptoms by strong acid inhibition, given for at least 1 week, is a simple and inexpensive approach to the diagnosis of GERD and has the advantage of avoiding the day-to-day variation in magnitude of reflux that limits the reliability of 24-hour pH monitoring (47). However, systematic evaluation of this "proton pump inhibitor test" indicates it is perhaps less specific than might initially be supposed (48,49).

Can Prognostic Information Be Obtained?

Measurement of tonic LES pressure was previously suggested as a possible means to diagnose reflux disease. The importance of the LES as a major barrier to reflux is well established. Although an LES pressure of less than 10 mm Hg has been considered an indication of an incompetent esophagogastric junction, there is much variation in this value. Many patients with well-documented esophagitis have an LES pressure greater than 10 mm Hg, and some asymptomatic subjects have pressures less than this value. Consequently, LES pressure in a given patient is often too imprecise to identify a potential for reflux and its variability severely limits the sensitivity and specificity of LES pressure measurement as a diagnostic test. Nevertheless, a pressure of less than 6 mm Hg correlates well with abnormal reflux on pH testing and very low LES pressures in this range are predictive of a more severe degree of reflux and a worse prognosis (50). The barrier function of the LES depends on the length of the sphincter as well as its pressure, and there is an inverse relationship between the length of the sphincter and the severity of GERD (51,52).

In addition to LES pressure measurements, assessment of peristaltic activity in the esophageal body may be informative in the evaluating reflux disease and assessing its prognosis (53,54). Until recently, these measurements have also been thought important in the preoperative assessment of GERD patients to inform the surgeon of potentially defective peristalsis that might constitute a risk for troublesome dysphagia after fundoplication. It seems that the occurrence of postoperative dysphagia correlates poorly with impaired peristalsis preoperatively (55).

Ambulatory pH monitoring can also provide important information about the severity of reflux disease and the reflux pattern present in a particular patient. That is, does the patient have reflux predominantly at night, or is upright, postprandial reflux more prevalent?

What Is the Importance of a Hiatal Hernia?

Although once considered to be of major importance in the production of GERD, the finding of a hiatal hernia either radiographically or endoscopically has little value in predicting whether a patient's symptoms are secondary to reflux. When carefully sought, a sliding hiatal hernia can be found in a high percentage of persons, most of whom are asymptomatic. In a review of more than 1,000 patients in 1968, Palmer (1) estimated that only 9% of those with a radiographically demonstrated hiatal hernia had typical reflux symptoms. Other careful studies have likewise indicated no consistent cause-and-effect relationship between the presence of symptomatic reflux and the finding of a hiatal hernia (56). Nevertheless, it is clear that contraction of the crural diaphragm enhances pressure in the normally located LES (57). Apart from any diminution of the LES barrier function resulting from hiatal hernia, there may also be a contribution to the severity of GERD by "trapping" acid in the hernial sac, which thus becomes more available to reflux during LES relaxation. This mechanism may prolong acid exposure and delay its clearance from the esophageal mucosa (5,58). Most patients undergoing endoscopy for upper GI symptoms do not have esophagitis if they do not have a hiatal hernia, whereas a hiatal hernia is found in most patients with severe esophagitis (56).

REFERENCES

1. Palmer ED. The hiatus hernia–esophagitis–esophageal stricture complex. Twenty year prospective study. *Am J Med* 1968;44:566.
2. Ellis FH. Esophageal hiatal hernia. *N Engl J Med* 1972;287:646.
3. Klauser AG, Schindlbeck NE, Muller-Lissner SA. Symptoms in gastro-esophageal reflux disease. *Lancet* 1990;335:205.
4. Johnsson F, Joelsson B, Gudmundsson K, et al. Symptoms and endoscopic findings in the diagnosis of gastroesophageal efflux disease. *Scand J Gastroenterol* 1987;22:714.
5. Sloan S, Kahrilas PJ. Impairment of esophageal emptying with hiatal hernia. *Gastroenterology* 1991;100:596.
6. Winters C, Spurling TJ, Chobanian SJ. Barrett's esophagus. A prevalent, occult complication of gastroesophageal reflux disease. *Gastroenterology* 1987;92:118.
7. Kirk AJ. Reflux dyspareunia. *Thorax* 1986;41:215.
8. Breumelhof R, et al. Analysis of 24-hour esophageal pressure and pH data in unselected patients with noncardiac chest pain. *Gastroenterology* 1990;99:1257.
9. Cherian P, et al. Esophageal tests in the evaluation of non-cardiac chest pain. *Dis Esophagus* 1995;8:129.
10. DeCaestecker JS, et al. The oesophagus as a cause of recurrent chest pain: which patients should be investigated and which tests should be used? *Lancet* 1985;2:1143.
11. DeMeester TR, et al. Esophageal function in patients with angina-type chest pain and normal coronary angiograms. *Ann Surg* 1982;196:488.
12. Hewson EG, et al. Twenty-four hour esophageal pH monitoring: the most useful test for evaluating noncardiac chest pain. *Am J Med* 1991;90:576.
13. Schofield PM, et al. Exertional gastroesophageal reflux: a mechanism for symptoms in patients with angina pectoris and normal coronary angiograms. *BMJ* 1987;294:1459.
14. Katz PO. Ambulatory esophageal and hypopharyngeal pH monitoring in patients with hoarseness. *Am J Gastroenterol* 1989;85: 38.
15. Shaker R, et al. Esophagopharyngeal distribution of refluxed gastric acid in patients with reflux laryngitis. *Gastroenterology* 1995; 109:1575.
16. Wiener GJ, et al. The symptom index: a clinically important parameter of ambulatory 24-hour esophageal pH monitoring. *Am J Gastroenterol* 1988;83:358.
17. Ward PH, Hanson DG. Reflux as an etiological factor of carcinoma of the laryngopharynx. *Laryngoscope* 1988;98:1195.
18. Irwin RS, Curley FJ, French CL. Chronic cough. The spectrum and frequency of causes, key components of the diagnostic evaluation, and outcome of specific therapy. *Am Rev Respir Dis* 1990; 141:640.
19. Sontag SJ, et al. Most asthmatics have gastroesophageal reflux with or without bronchodilator therapy. *Gastroenterology* 1990; 99:613.
20. Hetzel DJ, Heddle R. Gastroesophageal reflux disease, pH monitoring, and treatment. *Curr Opin Gastroenterol* 1993;9:629.
21. Gluck M, Pope CE. Chronic hiccups and gastroesophageal reflux disease. *Ann Intern Med* 1986;105:291.
22. Marshall JB, Landreneau RJ, Beyer KL. Hiccups: esophageal manometric features and relationship to gastroesophageal reflux. *Am J Gastroenterol* 1990;85:1172.
23. Dakkak M, et al. Oesophagitis is as important as oesophageal stricture diameter in determining dysphagia. *Gut* 1993;34:152.
24. Williams D, et al. Diminished traction forces with swallowing in gastro-oesophageal reflux disease and in functional dysphagia. *Gut* 1994;35:165.
25. Lagergren J, et al. Symptomatic gastroesophageal reflux as a risk factor for esophageal adenocarcinoma. *N Engl J Med* 1999;340: 825.
26. Nebel OT, Fornes MF, Castell DO. Symptomatic gastroesophageal reflux: incidence and precipitating factors. *Am J Dig Dis* 1976;21:953.
27. Kennedy T, Jones R. Gastro-oesophageal reflux symptoms in the community. *Aliment Pharmacol Ther* 2000;14:1589.
28. Locke GR, et al. Prevalence and clinical spectrum of gastroesophageal reflux: a population based study in Olmstead County, Minnesota. *Gastroenterology* 1997;112:1448.
29. Cameron AJ, Ott BJ, Payne WS. The incidence of adenocarcinoma in columnar-lined (Barrett's) esophagus. *N Engl J Med* 1985;313:857.
30. Nebel OT, Castell DO. Lower esophageal sphincter pressure changes after food ingestion. *Gastroenterology* 1972;63:778.
31. Holloway RH, et al. Effect of intraduodenal fat on lower oesophageal sphincter function and gastro-oesophageal reflux. *Gut* 1997;40:449.
32. Becker DJ, et al. A comparison of high and low fat meals on postprandial esophageal acid exposure. *Am J Gastroenterol* 1989;84:782.
33. Johnston BT, et al. Comparison of barium radiography with esophageal pH monitoring in the diagnosis of gastroesophageal reflux disease. *Am J Gastroenterol* 1996;91:1181.
34. Richter JE, Castell DO. Gastroesophageal reflux. Pathogenesis, diagnosis, and therapy. *Ann Intern Med* 1982;97:93.
35. Dodds WJ, et al. Mechanisms of gastroesophageal reflux in patients with reflux esophagitis. *N Engl J Med* 1982;307:1547.
36. Fisher RS, et al. Gastroesophageal (GE) scintiscanning to detect and quantitate GE reflux. *Gastroenterology* 1976;70:301.
37. Jenkins AF, Cowan RJ, Richter JE. Gastroesophageal scintigraphy: is it a sensitive test for gastroesophageal reflux disease? *J Clin Gastroenterol* 1985;7:127.
38. Tuttle SG, Grossman MI. Detection of gastroesophageal reflux by simultaneous measurements of intraluminal pressure and pH. *Proc Soc Exp Biol Med* 1958;93:225.
39. Wiener G, et al. Chronic hoarseness secondary to gastroesophageal reflux disease. *Am J Gastroenterol* 1989;12:1503.
40. Ott DJ, Gelfand DW, Wu WC. Reflux esophagitis: radiographic and endoscopic correlation. *Radiology* 1979;130:583.
41. Bytzer P, Havelund T, Hansen JM. Interobserver variation in the endoscopic diagnosis of reflux esophagitis. *Scand J Gastroenterol* 1993;28:119.
42. Lundell LR, et al. Endoscopic assessment of oesophagitis: clinical and functional correlates and further validation of the Los Angeles classification. *Gut* 1999;45:172–180.
43. Ismail-Beigi F, Horton PF, Pope CE. Histological consequences of gastroesophageal reflux in man. *Gastroenterology* 1970;58:163.
44. Knuff TE, et al. Histological evaluation of chronic gastroesophageal reflux. *Dig Dis Sci* 1984;29:194.
45. Schindlbeck NE, et al. Diagnostic value of histology in non-erosive gastro-oesophageal reflux disease. *Gut* 1996;39:151.
46. Collins BJ, et al. Oesophageal histology in reflux oesophagitis. *J Clin Pathol* 1985;38:1265.

47. Schenk BE, et al. Omeprazole as a diagnostic tool in gastroesophageal reflux disease. *Am J Gastroenterol* 1997;92:1997.

48. Johnsson F, et al. One-week omeprazole treatment in the diagnosis of gastro-oesophageal reflux disease. *Scand J Gastroenterol* 1998; 33:15.

49. Juul-Hansen P, et al. High dose proton pump inhibitors as a diagnostic test of gastro-oesophageal reflux disease in endoscopic-negative patients. *Scand J Gastroenterol* 2001;36:806.

50. Lieberman DA. Medical therapy for chronic reflux esophagitis: long-term follow-up. *Arch Intern Med* 1987;147:1717.

51. DeMeester TR, et al. Relationship of a hiatal hernia to the function of the body of the esophagus and the gastroesophageal junction. *J Thorac Cardiovasc Surg* 1981;82:547.

52. Fein M, et al. Role of the lower esophageal sphincter and hiatal hernia in the pathogenesis of gastroesophageal reflux disease. *J Gastrointest Surg* 1999;3:405.

53. Kahrilas PJ, et al. Esophageal peristaltic dysfunction in peptic esophagitis. *Gastroenterology* 1986;91:897.

54. Leite LP, et al. Ineffective esophageal motility (IEM): the primary finding in patients with non-specific esophageal motility disorder. *Dig Dis Sci* 1997;42:1853.

55. Fibbe C, et al. Esophageal motility in reflux disease before and after fundoplication: a prospective, randomized, clinical and manometric study. *Gastroenterology* 2001;121:5.

56. Kaul B, et al. Hiatus hernia in gastroesophageal reflux disease. *Scand J Gastroenterol* 1986;21:31.

57. Mittal RK. The crural diaphragm, an external lower esophageal sphincter: a definitive study. *Gastroenterology* 1993; 105:1565.

58. Mittal RK, Lange RC, McCallum RW. Identification and mechanism of delayed esophageal acid clearance in subjects with hiatus hernia. *Gastroenterology* 1987;92:130.

HIATUS HERNIA

PETER J. KAHRILAS
JOHN E. PANDOLFINO

Although hiatus hernia was occasionally noted as a congenital anomaly or a consequence of abdominal trauma in the preradiographic literature, the prevalence of this condition was not appreciated until the evolution of imaging technology. Illustrative of this, Bowditch (1) presented a treatise on diaphragmatic hernia to the Boston Society for Medical Observation in 1847 and commented that "especially as the disease is so rare that no person would be likely to have more than one or two opportunities for operation during his whole lifetime." The irony of this quotation in the introduction of a modern treatise by Skinner, "Surgical Management of Esophageal Reflux and Hiatus Hernia. Long-Term Results with 1,030 Patients," is apparent (2). Also illustrating the dependence on radiography for the detection of hiatus hernia, the first description of a paraesophageal hernia was at postmortem examination in 1903 (3).

With the maturation of imaging technology, especially barium contrast radiography, it became reasonably easy to detect hiatus hernia antemortem. In 1926, Akerlund reported that hiatal hernia was found in 2.3% of all upper gastrointestinal x-ray studies (4). With the improvement of radiographic techniques and a more systematic approach to their detection, more hernias were identified, such that by 1955 the reported incidence was 15% (5). When provocative maneuvers were employed to accentuate herniation during fluoroscopy, the frequency increased more dramatically; of 955 patients subject to abdominal compression during an upper gastrointestinal x-ray series, hiatus hernia was diagnosed in 55% (6). Coincident with this evolution in imaging, the clinical understanding of reflux disease also evolved. Our present concept of peptic esophagitis dates back to 1935 when Winkelstein first suggested that gastric secretions were the cause of the mucosal damage observed in peptic esophagitis (7). The term "reflux esophagitis" was

later introduced in 1946 by Allison, thereby acknowledging that irritant gastric juices were refluxed from the stomach to the esophagus (8). Since then, there has been considerable controversy regarding the relationship between esophagitis, heartburn, hiatal hernia, and the physiology of the lower esophagus. Recognizing this controversy and the fact that the main significance of hiatus hernia is in its relationship to reflux disease, it is impossible to discuss hiatus hernia without some discussion of reflux disease. Thus, this chapter first focuses on the relevant anatomy and classification of hiatus hernia and then examines current understanding of the relationship between these anatomic variables and the pathophysiology of reflux disease.

ANATOMY AND PHYSIOLOGY OF THE GASTROESOPHAGEAL JUNCTION

The hiatal orifice is an elliptically shaped opening through the diaphragm with its long axis in the sagittal plane through which the esophagus and vagus nerves gain access to the abdomen. Although there is some anatomic variability with partial contribution from the left crus, the most common anatomy is for the hiatus to be formed by elements of the right diaphragmatic crus (9). The crura arise from tendinous fibers emerging from the anterior longitudinal ligament over the upper lumbar vertebrae; the left crus is usually attached to two lumbar vertebrae and the right to three. Additionally, accessory tendons may arise from the fascia over the psoas muscles and from the medial arcuate ligaments but, for the most part these fibers eventually fan out laterally to insert into the central tendon of the diaphragm, away from the hiatal limbs. The crura pass upward in close contact with the vertebral bodies for most of their course and only incline forward as they arch around the esophagus (9).

Once muscle fibers emerge from the tendinous origin of the right crus, they form two overlying ribbon-like bundles separated from each other by connective tissue. The dorsal bundle forms the left limb of the right crus (thoracic aspect)

P. J. Kahrilas: Division of Gastroenterology, Department of Medicine, Feinberg School of Medicine, Chicago, Illinois.

J. E. Pandolfino: Division of Gastroenterology and Hepatology, Deptartment of Medicine, Northwestern University Medical School, Chicago, Illinois.

and the ventral bundle becomes the right limb (abdominal aspect) of the right crus. As they approach the hiatus, the muscle bands diverge and cross each other in a scissors-like fashion with the ventral bundle passing upward and to the right and the dorsal bundle passing upward and to the left. The lateral fibers of each hiatal limb insert directly into the central tendon of the diaphragm but the medial fibers, which form the hiatal margins, incline toward the midline and decussate with each other in a trellis-like fashion in front of the esophagus (9). Although there are variations of this standard pattern, the basic organization of two flattened muscle bundles first diverging like a scissors and then merging anterior to the esophagus is common to all arrangements (Fig. 20.1). Normally there is about a centimeter of muscle separating the anterior rim of the hiatus from the central tendon of the diaphragm.

Under normal circumstances, the esophagus is anchored to the diaphragm and the stomach cannot be displaced through the hiatus into the mediastinum. The main restraining structures are the phrenoesophageal ligaments, alternatively referred to as the phrenoesophageal membrane, and an aggregation of posterior structures including the vagus nerve and radicles of the left gastric vein and artery (10,11). The phrenoesophageal membrane is formed from the fascia transversalis on the under surface of the diaphragm and, to a lesser degree, fused elements of the endothoracic fascia. This elastic membrane inserts circum-

ferentially into the esophageal musculature, close to the squamocolumnar junction, and extends for about a centimeter above the gastroesophageal junction, at which point it thins and merges with the perivisceral fascia of the esophagus (12). Thus, the axial position of the squamocolumnar junction is normally within or slightly distal to the diaphragmatic hiatus (13).

The anatomic relationship of the distal esophagus, hiatus, and stomach is transiently altered during swallow-initiated peristalsis. Physiologically, peristalsis is a sequenced contraction of both the longitudinal and circular muscle of the esophageal wall that is responsible for bolus propulsion through the esophagus (14). In particular, with contraction of the esophageal longitudinal muscle, the esophagus shortens and the phrenoesophageal membrane is stretched; relaxation of the longitudinal muscle along with the elastic recoil of the phrenoesophageal membrane is then responsible for pulling the squamocolumnar junction back to its normal position at the termination of the peristaltic sequence. This is, in effect, "physiologic herniation," since the gastric cardia tents through the diaphragmatic hiatus with each swallow (13) (Fig. 20.2). This paradox has led to a confusing array of terminology summarized in Figure 20.3. The globular structure seen radiographically that forms above the diaphragm, beneath the tubular esophagus, during deglutition is termed the *phrenic ampulla*, which is bounded from above by the distal esophagus and from below by the crural diaphragm. Emptying of the ampulla occurs between inspirations in conjunction with re-lengthening of the esophagus (15). As becomes apparent in the discussion of sliding hiatus hernia, a type I hiatus hernia is an exaggeration of the normal phrenic ampulla, the estimated prevalence of which varies widely at least in part because of inconsistent conventions of measurement. Not all of the structures illustrated in Figure 20.3 are always evident radiographically. Commonly, only an A ring is evident (Fig. 20.4), in which case the limits of the measurement defining hiatus hernia becomes arbitrary. In such cases, the demonstration of rugal folds traversing the diaphragm is often used as a defining criterion. Alternatively, a B ring but not an A ring may be evident radiographically as in Figure 20.5, in which case the B ring is of such prominence (luminal diameter < 13 mm) as to be termed a Schatzki's ring. In such a case, it is easy to apply the ≥2 cm between the B ring and the hiatus criterion for defining a sliding hiatus hernia (16).

Aside from its antegrade propulsive function discussed earlier, the gastroesophageal junction also minimizes gastroesophageal reflux. This is accomplished by a complex valvular mechanism, the function of which is partly attributable to the esophagus, partly to the stomach, and partly to the crural diaphragm. The esophageal element has been extensively analyzed and consists of the lower esophageal sphincter (LES), which is a 2-cm segment of tonically contracted smooth muscle. The proximal margin of the LES extends up to and a short distance proximal to the squamo-

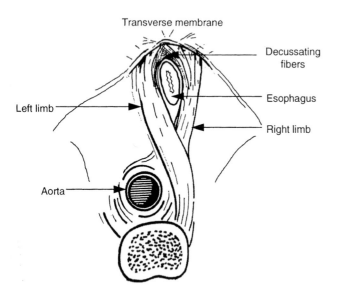

FIGURE 20.1. The most common anatomy of the diaphragmatic hiatus in which the muscular elements of the crural diaphragm derive from the right diaphragmatic crus. The right crus arises from the anterior longitudinal ligament overlying the lumbar vertebrae. Once muscular elements emerge from the tendon, two flat muscular bands form, which cross each other in scissors-like fashion, form the walls of the hiatus, and decussate with each other anterior to the esophagus. (Modified from Marchand P. The anatomy of esophageal hiatus of the diaphragm and the pathogenesis of hiatus herniation. *Thorac Surg* 1959;37:81–92.)

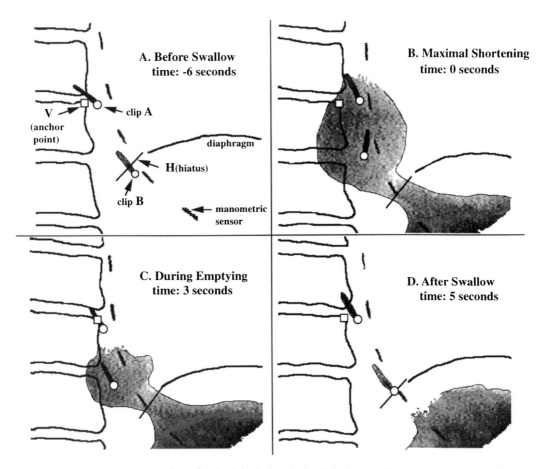

FIGURE 20.2. Demonstration of "physiologic herniation" during swallow using endoscopically placed mucosal clips. **A:** Before swallow. Clip B marks the position of the squamocolumnar junction 0.4 cm distal to the hiatus and 3.5 cm distal to the anchor point on the vertebral body (V). Clip A is affixed to the esophageal mucosa 3.1 cm proximally. Clip movements are referenced to point V on the vertebral column. **B:** At the time of maximal esophageal shortening, with clip B 1.8 cm proximal to the hiatus and 2.0 cm distal to point V. The distance between clips A and B is reduced to 2.2 cm, indicative of 29% shortening. **C:** As elongation proceeds, first both clips descend, after which clip B descends, stretching the A-B segment back to its initial length. **D:** After swallow, clip B is again at the level of the hiatus. (From Kahrilas PJ, Wu S, Lin S, et al. Attenuation of esophageal shortening during peristalsis with hiatus hernia. *Gastroenterology* 1995;109:1818, with permission.)

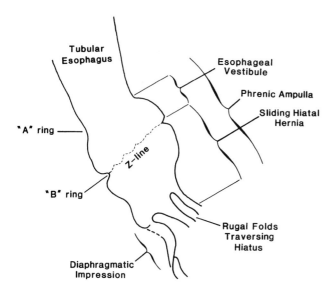

FIGURE 20.3. Anatomic features of a sliding hiatus hernia viewed radiographically during swallowing. The A ring is a muscular ring visible during swallowing, which demarcates the superior margin of the lower esophageal sphincter. The B ring at the squamocolumnar junction is present in only about 15% of individuals and allows for accurate division of the phrenic ampulla into the esophageal vestibule (A ring to B ring) and the sliding hiatus hernia (B ring to the subdiaphragmatic stomach). By convention, the distinction between normal and hiatus hernia is a ≥2-cm separation between the B ring and the hiatus. Rugal folds traversing the hiatus support the conviction that a portion of the stomach is supradiaphragmatic. (From Kahrilas PJ. Hiatus hernia causes reflux: fact or fiction? *Gullet* 1993;3(Suppl):21, with permission.)

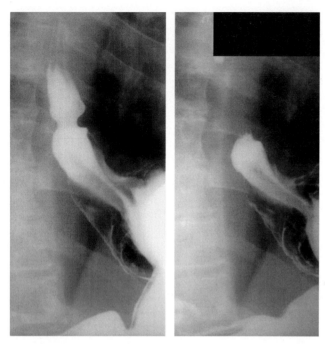

FIGURE 20.4. Radiograph of a patient with a small axial hiatal hernia, a well-developed A ring, and no B ring evident. In such cases, the criterion for defining hiatus hernia is the appearance of rugal folds traversing the diaphragmatic hiatus. The A ring has no anatomic correlate but physiologically corresponds to the superior aspect of the lower esophageal sphincter.

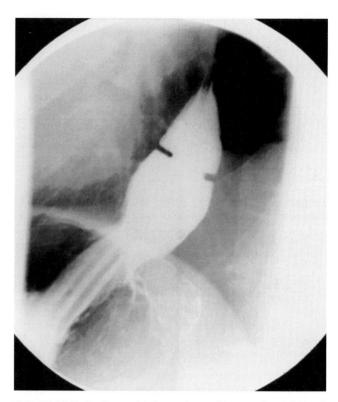

FIGURE 20.5. Radiograph of a patient with a small axial hiatal hernia, a prominent B ring, and no A ring evident. The B ring occurs at the squamocolumnar junction and, when subtle, is referred to as the transverse mucosal fold. In instances such as this where there is marked compromise of the esophageal lumen, the B ring is referred to as a Schatzki's ring and is a frequent cause of episodic solid food dysphagia. When a B ring is evident, the criterion for defining hiatus hernia is a separation of ≥2 cm between the B ring and the diaphragmatic hiatus.

columnar junction. The distal margin of the LES is more difficult to define but careful anatomic studies suggest that it is, in fact, composed of elements of the gastric musculature, and the opposing clasp and sling fibers are composed of the gastric cardia (17). Finally, surrounding the LES at the level of the squamocolumnar junction is the crural diaphragm, composed mainly of the right diaphragmatic crus (18). However, in other instances, the left crus is dominant, both crura provide equal contributions, or a band from the left crus crosses to the right (band of Low) (12). Elegant physiologic studies have clearly demonstrated that diaphragmatic contraction augments gastroesophageal junction pressure, in essence serving as an external sphincter (19). Furthermore, if the esophagogastric junction is defined as either the end of the LES or the point at which the tubular esophagus joins the saccular stomach, there are normally about 2 cm of tubular esophagus distal to the squamocolumnar junction within the abdomen (13).

TYPES OF HIATAL HERNIA

In general terms, hiatus hernia refers to herniation of elements of the abdominal cavity through the esophageal hiatus of the diaphragm. The most comprehensive classification scheme recognizes four types of hiatal hernia as enumerated here.

With *type I or sliding hiatal hernia*, there is a widening of the muscular hiatal tunnel and circumferential laxity of the phrenoesophageal membrane, allowing a portion of the gastric cardia to herniate upward. Largely because of the inherent subjectivity in defining type I hiatal hernia, estimates of prevalence vary enormously, from 10% to 80% of the adult population in North America (18). In all probability, most type I hiatal hernias are asymptomatic and, even with larger type I hernias, the main clinical implication is the propensity to develop reflux disease, the likelihood of which increases with increasing hernia size. With a well-developed hernia, the esophageal hiatus abuts directly on the transverse membrane of the central tendon of the diaphragm and the anterior hiatal muscles are absent or reduced to a few atrophic strands (9). The hiatus itself is no longer a sagittal slit but a rounded opening whose transverse diameter approximates the sagittal diameter in size (Fig. 20.6). This change in caliber of the hiatus is most apparent during distention (20). Associated with the widening of the hiatal orifice, the phrenoesophageal membrane becomes attenuated and inconspicuous in comparison to its normal prominence. However, although thinned, the phrenoesophageal

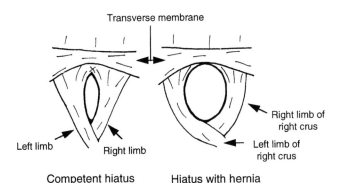

Competent hiatus   Hiatus with hernia

FIGURE 20.6. Alteration of the hiatal anatomy associated with sliding hiatal hernia. Note that the main change is a widening of the hiatal canal. Associated with this there can be substantial atrophy of the abutting muscular elements, thinning and elongation of the phrenoesophageal membrane, and axial displacement of the gastric cardia. (Modified from Marchand P. The anatomy of esophageal hiatus of the diaphragm and the pathogenesis of hiatus herniation. *Thorac Surg* 1959;37:81–92.)

membrane remains intact and the associated herniated gastric cardia is contained within the posterior mediastinum (18) (Fig. 20.7). In marginal instances, type I hiatal hernia is simply an exaggeration of the normal phrenic ampulla making its identification dependent on measurement technique. However, when a sliding hiatal hernia enlarges further, such that more than 3 cm of gastric pouch is herniated upward, its presence is obvious regardless of technique because gastric folds are evident traversing the diaphragm both during swallow-induced shortening and at rest (Fig. 20.8). The progression from normal anatomy to obvious type I hernia is well illustrated in a recent analysis of the endoscopic appearance of the cardia, viewed in retroflexion (21) (Fig. 20.9).

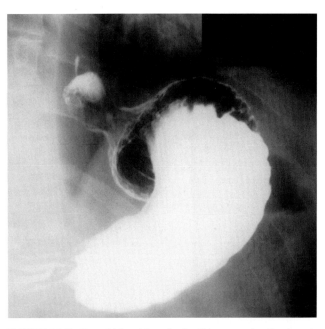

FIGURE 20.8. Type I hiatal hernia. In this example, the herniated gastric cardia is evident at rest, after completion of esophageal emptying. Note the rugal folds traversing the diaphragmatic hiatus.

Although there are instances in which trauma, congenital malformation, and iatrogeny can be clearly implicated, a variety of lines of evidence suggest that type I hiatus hernia is usually an acquired condition. Allison (22) observed that the typical age of onset was in the fifth decade of life. Pregnancy has long been suspected to be an inciting factor (23). Conceptually, Marchand argues that the compounded stresses of age-related degeneration, pregnancy, and obesity take their toll on a relative weak point of the anatomy. The positive peritoneopleural pressure gradient acts to extrude the abdominal contents into the chest and, although this extrusion is opposed by the entire surface of the diaphragm, of the openings through the diaphragm, only the esophageal hiatus is vulnerable to visceral herniation because it faces directly into the abdominal cavity. Furthermore, because the esophagus does not tightly fill the hiatus, the integrity of this opening depends on its intrinsic structures, especially the phrenoesophageal membrane, which are designed to achieve a fine balance of mobility and stability (24). Add to this vulnerability the repetitive stresses of deep inspiration—Valsalva, vomiting, the physiologic herniation accompanying swallowing, and postural change—and then compound the stress by packing the abdominal cavity with adipose tissue or a gravid uterus and eventually the integrity of the hiatus is gradually compromised. Another potential source of stress on the phrenoesophageal membrane is tonic contraction of the esophageal longitudinal muscle induced by gastroesophageal reflux and mucosal acidification (25).

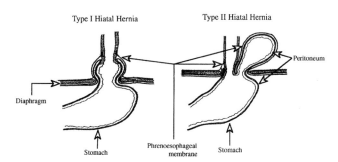

FIGURE 20.7. Sliding versus paraesophageal hiatal hernia. With sliding or axial hiatal hernia, there is thinning and elongation of the phrenoesophageal membrane leading to herniation of the stomach into the posterior mediastinum. As such, there is no potential for incarceration or strangulation. With paraesophageal herniation, visceral elements herniate through a focal weakness in the phrenoesophageal membrane with the potential to lead to the usual array of complications associated with visceral herniation through a constricted aperture. (Modified from Skinner DB. Hernias [hiatal, traumatic, and congenital]. In: Berk JE, ed. *Gastroenterology.* Philadelphia: WB Saunders, 1985:705.)

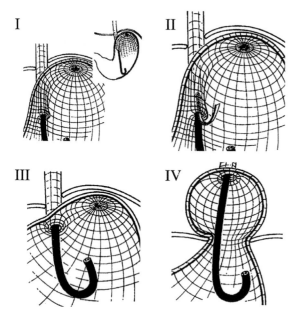

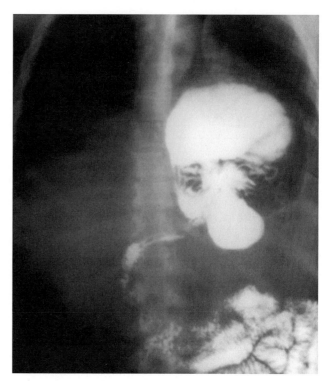

FIGURE 20.9. Three-dimensional representation of the progressive anatomic disruption of the gastroesophageal junction as occurs with development of a type I hiatus hernia. In the grade I configuration (*upper left*), a ridge of muscular tissue is closely approximated to the shaft of the retroflexed endoscope. With a grade II configuration (*upper right*), the ridge of tissue is slightly less well defined and there has been slight orad displacement of the squamocolumnar junction along with widening of the angle of His. In the grade III appearance (*lower left*), the ridge of tissue at the gastric entryway is barely present and there is often incomplete luminal closure around the endoscope. Grade III deformity is nearly always accompanied by an obvious hiatal hernia. With grade IV deformity (*lower right*), no muscular ridge is present at the gastric entry. The gastroesophageal area stays open all the time, and squamous epithelium of the distal esophagus can be seen from the retroflexed endoscopic view. A hiatus hernia is always present. (Modified from Hill LD, Kraemer SJM, Aye RW, et al. Laparoscopic Hill repair. *Contemp Surg* 1994;44:1.)

FIGURE 20.10. Type II paraesophageal hiatal hernia. In this example, the entire stomach has herniated into the chest, leading to an "upside down stomach." Because the gastroesophageal junction remains within the hiatus, there is no element of type I herniation in this example. See also Figure 20.23 for an image of the resultant gastric configuration.

The *type I*, or "sliding," hiatal hernia described earlier accounts for most hiatal hernias. The less common types, *types II, III, and IV* are varieties of *"paraesophageal hernias."* Taken together, these account for, at most, 5% to 15% of all hiatal hernias (26–28). Although these hernias may also be associated with significant gastroesophageal reflux, their main clinical significance lies in the potential for mechanical complications. A type II hernia results from a localized defect in the phrenoesophageal membrane, whereas the gastroesophageal junction remains fixed to the preaortic fascia and the median arcuate ligament (18) (Fig. 20.7). The gastric fundus then serves as the leading point of herniation. The natural history of a type II hernia is progressive enlargement so that the entire stomach eventually herniates, with the pylorus juxtaposed to the gastric cardia, forming an upside-down, intrathoracic stomach (Fig. 20.10). Either as cause or effect, paraesophageal hernias are associated with abnormal laxity of structures normally preventing displacement of the stomach: the gastrosplenic and gastrocolic liga-

ments. As the hernia enlarges, the greater curvature of the stomach rolls up into the thorax. Because the stomach is fixed at the gastroesophageal junction, the herniated stomach tends to rotate around its longitudinal axis, resulting in an organoaxial volvulus (29) (Fig. 20.11). Infrequently, rotation may alternatively occur around the transverse axis, resulting in a mesenteroaxial volvulus (29) (Fig. 20.12).

Types III and IV hiatal hernias are variants of the type II (purely paraesophageal) hernia described previously. Type III hernias have elements of both types I and II hernias. With progressive enlargement of the hernia through the

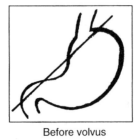
Before volvus

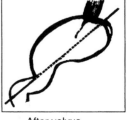
After volvus

FIGURE 20.11. Organoaxial volvulus. The axis of rotation is the long axis of the stomach. (Modified from Peridikis G, Hinder RA. Paraesophageal hiatal hernia. In: Nyhus LM, Condon RE, eds. *Hernia*. Philadelphia: JB Lippincott, 1995:544.)

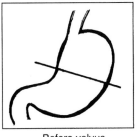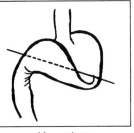

Before volvus   After volvus

FIGURE 20.12. Mesenteroaxial volvulus. The axis of rotation is along the mesenteric attachment much the same as is seen with sigmoid colon volvulus. (Modified from Peridikis G, Hinder RA. Paraesophageal hiatal hernia. In: Nyhus LM, Condon RE, eds. *Hernia*. Philadelphia: JB Lippincott, 1995:544.)

hiatus, the phrenoesophageal membrane stretches, displacing the gastroesophageal junction above the diaphragm, thereby adding a sliding element to the type II hernia (Fig. 20.13). Type IV hiatus hernia is associated with a large defect in the phrenoesophageal membrane, allowing other organs, such as colon, spleen, pancreas, and small intestine to enter the hernia sac (Fig. 20.14).

Although their etiology is usually unclear, paraesophageal hernias are a recognized complication of surgical dissection of the hiatus as during antireflux procedures, esophagomyotomy, or partial gastrectomy. Many patients with a type II hernia are either asymptomatic or have only vague, intermittent symptoms. When present, symptoms are generally related to ischemia or either partial or complete obstruction. The most common symptoms are epigastric or substernal pain, postprandial fullness, substernal fullness, nausea, and retching. An upright radiograph of the thorax may be diagnostic, revealing a retrocardiac air-fluid level within a paraesophageal hernia or intrathoracic stomach. Barium contrast studies are almost always diagnostic and attention should focus on the position of the esophagogastric junction (EGJ) in order to differentiate type II and III hernias. Upper endoscopy is also useful in the diagnosis and evaluation of patients with paraesophageal hernias. A type II paraesophageal hernia is noted on retroflexion by observing a distinct opening adjacent to the EGJ with gastric folds extending into the opening. Type III paraesophageal hernias can be identified by visualizing a gastric pouch above the crural impression with the EGJ located in the proximal portion of the herniated pouch. Gastric volvulus and partial prolapse of the intrathoracic stomach through the hiatus are associated with difficulty passing the scope through the EGJ and may

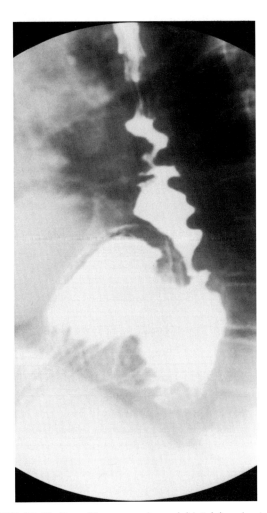

FIGURE 20.13. Type III paraesophageal hiatal hernia. In this example, much of the stomach has herniated into the chest, but the leading edge of the herniating stomach has additionally herniated through a weakening of the phrenoesophageal membrane contributing a paraesophageal component to the hernia. Because the gastroesophageal junction is well above the diaphragmatic hiatus, this is a mixed, or type III paraesophageal hernia.

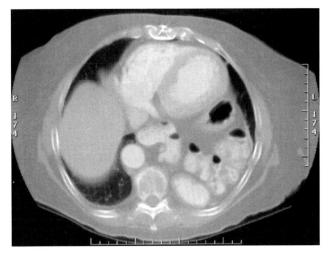

FIGURE 20.14. Computed tomography image through the chest showing a type IV paraesophageal hiatal hernia. In this example, the sigmoid colon (containing contrast) is clearly evident adjacent to the heart (also contrast enhanced). Lower cuts show the patient to be postsplenectomy consistent with the observation that paraesophageal herniation occurs most commonly after surgical dissection in the area of the hiatus.

lead to triple obstruction at the esophageal, midgastric, and duodenal levels.

Most complications of a type II hernia are reflective of the mechanical problem caused by the hernia. Dysphagia may occur as a result of compression of the esophagus within the hiatus by the herniated portion of the stomach or by gastric volvulus. Vomiting is usually intermittent and associated with retching without emesis. Postprandial bloating and early satiety are related to mechanical compression of the proximal stomach while postcibal pain is usually related to gastric torsion. Bleeding, although infrequent, occurs from gastric ulceration or gastritis within the incarcerated hernia pouch (18). Respiratory complications such as dyspnea and recurrent pneumonia result from mechanical compression of the lung by a large hernia or other organs herniating through the hiatus. Paraesophageal hernias may present with life-threatening complications, warranting emergent intervention. Gastric volvulus may lead to acute gastric obstruction, incarceration, and perforation. Consequently, symptomatic patients with a history of surgical manipulation of the diaphragmatic hiatus should be evaluated for this potential complication. The triad of epigastric pain, inability to vomit, and inability to pass a nasogastric tube may herald impending gangrene and should prompt immediate intervention (30).

ASSOCIATION OF TYPE I HIATUS HERNIA WITH REFLUX DISEASE

Endoscopic and radiographic studies suggest that 50% to 94% of patients with gastroesophageal reflux disease (GERD) have a type I hiatal hernia while the corresponding prevalence in control subjects ranges from 13% to 59% (16,29,31,32). Most patients with severe esophagitis have a hiatus hernia (33,34) and 96% of patients with Barrett's esophagus have a hiatus hernia of 2 cm or greater (35). However, the importance of a type I hiatus hernia is obscured by the misconception that this is an "all-or-none" phenomenon. It is more useful to view type I hiatus hernia as a continuum of progressive disruption of the gastroesophageal junction, as illustrated in Figure 20.9. Type I hiatus hernia impacts on reflux both by affecting the competence of the gastroesophageal junction in preventing reflux and in compromising the process of esophageal acid clearance once reflux has occurred.

Pathogenesis

Symptomatic GERD results when the balance between aggressive forces (acid reflux, potency of refluxate) and defensive forces (esophageal acid clearance, mucosal resistance) tilts in favor of the aggressive forces. The intermittent nature of symptoms in some individuals with GERD suggests that the aggressive and defensive forces are part of a delicately balanced system. Significant aberration in any one of these pathophysiologic influences can result in tipping the balance of forces acting on the esophageal mucosa from a compensated condition to a decompensated condition (i.e., heartburn, esophagitis). Although GERD is multifactorial in etiology with potentially important modifying roles played by mucosal defensive factors and differences in the potency of refluxate, the key events in the pathogenesis of GERD are reflux of acid and pepsin from the stomach into the esophagus and the effectiveness of esophageal acid clearance.

The complexity of the gastroesophageal junction as an antireflux barrier has led to three dominant theories of pathogenesis of gastroesophageal junction incompetence: (a) transient LES relaxations, (b) hypotensive LES, and (c) anatomic disruption of the gastroesophageal junction associated with a hiatal hernia. Which reflux mechanism dominates seems to depend on a number of factors including the anatomy of the EGJ. Transient LES relaxations account for the overwhelming majority of reflux events in normal individuals and GERD patients without hiatus hernia. Transient LES relaxations (TLESR) appear without fixed temporal relation to an antecedent pharyngeal contraction, are unaccompanied by esophageal peristalsis, and persist for longer periods (>10 seconds) than do swallow-induced LES relaxations (36). The likelihood of reflux occurring during a TLESR is influenced by both the circumstances of the recording and the temporal proximity to a meal, with reflux during as many as 93% or as few as 9% (37,38).

Whereas TLESRs typically account for up to 90% of reflux events in normal subjects or in GERD patients without hiatus hernia, patients with hiatus hernia have a more heterogeneous mechanistic profile with reflux episodes, frequently occurring in the context of low LES pressure, straining, and swallow-associated LES relaxation (39). These observations support the concept that the functional integrity of the EGJ is dependent on both the intrinsic LES and extrinsic sphincteric function of the diaphragmatic hiatus. In essence, gastroesophageal reflux requires "two hits" to the EGJ. Patients with a normal EGJ require inhibition of both the intrinsic LES and extrinsic crural diaphragm for reflux to occur: physiologically this occurs only in the setting of a TLESR. In contrast, patients with hiatal hernia may exhibit preexisting compromise of the hiatal sphincter. In that setting, reflux can occur with only relaxation of the intrinsic LES, as may occur during periods of LES hypotension or even deglutitive relaxation.

Once the esophageal mucosa has been acidified by reflux of gastric juice across the gastroesophageal junction, the normal process of esophageal acid clearance (defined as restoration of esophageal pH to a value of 4) requires both effective esophageal emptying and normal salivation (40). Esophageal emptying is defined as elimination of fluid from the esophagus. Thus, the two major potential causes of prolonged esophageal acid clearance are impaired esophageal emptying and impaired salivary function. Reduced salivary rate results in diminished salivary neutralizing capacity. Diminished salivation during sleep explains why reflux events during sleep or immediately before sleep are associated with markedly prolonged acid clearance times (41). However, in the only large-scale analysis of salivary function in GERD, no difference was found between the resting salivary function of the patients with esophagitis, young control subjects, or age-matched control subjects (42).

Impaired esophageal emptying in reflux disease was inferred by the observation that patients with abnormal acid clearance times were improved by an upright posture or by head of bed elevation, suggesting that gravity could improve abnormal clearing (43). Two mechanisms of impaired volume clearance have been identified: (a) peristaltic dysfunction and (b) "re-reflux" secondary to hiatal hernia. Significant findings of peristaltic dysfunction include the occurrence of failed peristaltic contractions and hypotensive (<30 mm Hg) peristaltic contractions that incompletely empty the esophagus (44). Hiatal hernia and esophageal emptying are discussed in following sections.

HIATUS HERNIA AND THE DIAPHRAGMATIC SPHINCTER

Theories of the mechanism of gastroesophageal junction competence have seesawed between strictly anatomic explanations, focusing on type I hiatus hernia, and physiologic explanations focusing on the vigor of LES contraction while ignoring the significance of anatomic factors. As detailed later, current thinking recognizes contributions from both sphincteric components. However, before discussing recent experimentation, it is instructive to read the work of Allison who, except for his ignorance with respect to the existence of the intrinsic lower esophageal sphincter, exhibited masterful understanding of the gastroesophageal junction (22):

> And that the position of the stomach in relationship to the diaphragm is only important in so far as the diaphragm acts as a sphincter....When the right crus of the diaphragm contracts, its action on the cardia is twofold: first, it compresses the walls of the esophagus from side to side, and second, it pulls down and increases the angulation of the esophagus.

Allison also understood the analogy between the gastroesophageal junction and the anal sphincters:

> The alimentary canal passes through two diaphragms, the thoracoabdominal and the pelvic. In each of these nature has adopted the same device to achieve continence. In each the canal is made to take a fairly abrupt bend, and at the bend is supported by an intrinsic and an extrinsic muscular mechanism [Fig. 20.15]. At the anorectal junction the internal sphincter is relatively well developed, but the main factor for continence is the puborectalis muscle which forms a lasso round the bend and hitches it forward to the back of the pubic

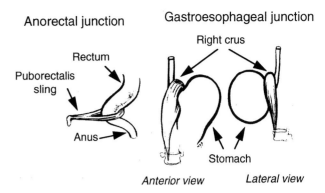

FIGURE 20.15. The "pinchcock" action of the pelvic and crural diaphragms on the alimentary canal as it enters and exits the abdominal cavity. **A:** The puborectalis sling around the anorectal junction. **B:** Anterior view of the right crus of the diaphragm forming a sling around the gastroesophageal junction. **C:** Lateral view of the crural sling. In each case, contraction of the diaphragm increases the angulation of the visceral tube, pinching it off and bolstering continence. (From Allison PR. Reflux esophagitis, sliding hiatal hernia, and the anatomy of repair. *Surg Gynecol Obstet* 1951;92:419–431, with permission.)

bone. At the esophagogastric junction there is no thickening of the circular muscle fibers of the esophagus to form a sphincter, but the canal takes a bend forward and to the left, and this bend is lassoed and maintained by the right crus of the diaphragm which hitches it down to the lumbar spine.

Since the time of Allison's writings, the intrinsic sphincter of the gastroesophageal junction (the LES) was described and much of his elegant conjecture forgotten. However, recent physiologic investigations have again advanced the "two sphincter hypothesis" of gastroesophageal junction competence, suggesting that both the intrinsic LES sphincter and the crural diaphragm encircling the LES serve a sphincteric function (45–48).

Evidence supporting a specialized sphincteric role of the crural diaphragm comes from the observation that the actions of the costal and crural parts of the diaphragm function independently during certain gastrointestinal functions. During esophageal distention, vomiting, and eructation, electrical activity of the crural fibers was reportedly silent at the same time as the dome of the diaphragm was entirely active, suggesting that the crural diaphragm participates in LES relaxation (49,50). In addition, swallow-induced LES relaxation is associated with minimal crural inhibition, whereas TLESRs are accompanied by significant inhibition of the crural diaphragm (51).

Crural diaphragmatic dysfunction may promote gastroesophageal reflux by three mechanisms: (a) disrupting the "pinchcock effect" of crural contraction, (b) altering the morphology and pressure of the LES, and (c) increasing compliance at the EGJ, creating wider opening diameters during LES relaxation. The diaphragm augments the LES by a "pinchcock effect" of crural contraction as illustrated in Figure 20.15. Thus, crural contraction augments the antireflux barrier during transient periods of increased intraabdominal pressure such as occur during inspiration, coughing, or abdominal straining. As evident by the data in Figure 20.16, the susceptibility to reflux under these circumstances of abrupt increases of intraabdominal pressure depends on both the instantaneous LES pressure and the integrity of the diaphragmatic sphincter (52). Statistical modeling of the data in Figure 20.16 suggests that the susceptibility to this mode of reflux is proportional to the size of a type I hernia (52) (Fig. 20.17). The implication is that patients with hiatal hernia exhibit progressive disruption of the diaphragmatic sphincter proportional to the extent of axial herniation. Therefore, although neither hiatus hernia nor a hypotensive LES alone results in severe gastroesophageal junction incompetence, the two conditions interact with each other as evidenced by the statistical modeling in Figure 20.17. This conclusion is consistent with the clin-

ical experience that exercise, tight-fitting garments, and activities involving bending at the waist exacerbate heartburn in GERD patients (most of whom have hiatal hernias), especially after having consumed meals that reduce LES pressure.

Another hypothesis regarding the interrelationship between hiatal hernia and the LES is that type I hiatus hernia in and of itself may diminish LES pressure, a hypothesis consistent with observations made both in both humans and animals. Klein and co-workers (53) studied the thoracoabdominal junction of ten patients after oncologically motivated resection of the gastroesophageal junction removing the entire intrinsic lower esophageal sphincter. Subsequent manometric analysis revealed an end-expiratory intraluminal pressure of 6 ± 1 mm Hg within the "sphincterless" gastroesophageal junction, a value similar to the 3 ± 0.2 mm Hg observed within the hiatal canal of hernia sub-

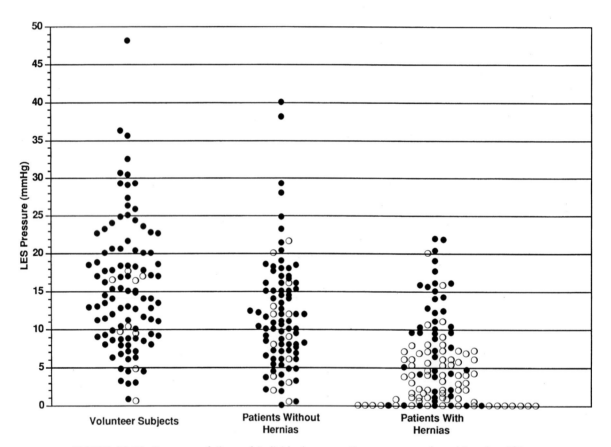

FIGURE 20.16. Success or failure of individual provocative maneuvers (coughing, leg lifting, abdominal compression, Valsalva) at eliciting gastroesophageal reflux as a function of lower esophageal sphincter (LES) pressure among groups of normal control subjects, patients without hiatus hernia, and patients with radiographically defined hiatus hernia. Lower esophageal sphincter pressure values were determined immediately before the onset of the maneuver. *Open circles* indicate individual trials of provocative maneuvers associated with gastroesophageal reflux and *solid circles* indicate trials in which reflux did not occur. Reflux by the stress mechanism was much more easily elicited among the hiatus hernia patients. (From Sloan S, Rademaker AW, Kahrilas PJ. Determinants of gastroesophageal junction incompetence: hiatal hernia, lower esophageal sphincter, or both? *Ann Intern Med* 1992;117:977, with permission.)

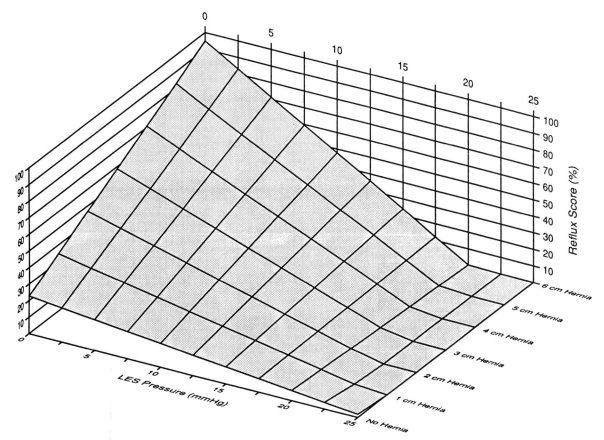

FIGURE 20.17. Model of the relationship among lower esophageal sphincter pressure (LES) (x-axis), size of hernia (y-axis), and the susceptibility to gastroesophageal reflux induced by provocative maneuvers that increase abdominal pressure as reflected by the reflux score (z-axis). The statistical model was created by stepwise regression analysis of the data in Figure 20.16. The overall equation for the model is as follows: reflux score = 22.64 + 12.05 (hernia size) – 0.83 (LES pressure) – 0.65 (LES pressure hernia size). The multiple correlation coefficient of this equation for the 50-subject data set was 0.86 (R^2 = 0.75), indicating that 75% of the observed variance in susceptibility to stress reflux among individuals was accounted for by the size of hiatus hernia and the instantaneous value of LES pressure. (From Sloan S, Rademaker AW, Kahrilas PJ. Determinants of gastroesophageal junction incompetence: hiatal hernia, lower esophageal sphincter, or both? *Ann Intern Med* 1992;117:977, with permission.)

jects (54). Relevant animal data come from experimentally severing the phrenoesophageal ligament in dogs, analogous to the effect of axial hiatus hernia in which the ligament is stretched and its diaphragmatic attachments loosened (13,55). Severing the ligament substantially reduced peak gastroesophageal junction pressure, which was then restored with reanastomosis (56). In the case of the hiatus hernia patients, reducing the hernia is the equivalent of reanastomosing the phrenoesophageal ligament, and doing so in effect increases the LES pressure by causing the hiatal canal pressure to be superimposed on the intrinsic LES pressure (57). Perhaps the only contradictory data are from diaphragmatic electromyographic (EMG) recordings, which strongly support the notion of a phasic, but not tonic, diaphragmatic contribution to gastroesophageal junction pressure (45–48). However, relying on EMG

recordings to completely represent the diaphragmatic contribution to gastroesophageal junction pressure ignores the possible contribution of passive forces such as diaphragmatic and arcuate ligament elasticity to intraluminal pressure. In the case of the upper esophageal sphincter, such passive forces contribute an intraluminal pressure of similar magnitude after experimental abolition of the myogenic tone (58).

Another interesting observation pertains to the effect of hiatus hernia on the morphology of the LES high-pressure zone. Not only does the peak pressure within the LES high-pressure zone negatively correlate with the presence of hiatal hernia, but also the overall length of the high-pressure zone can be significantly reduced in patients with large hiatal hernias, principally because of loss of the segment distal to the squamocolumnar junction (13) (Fig.

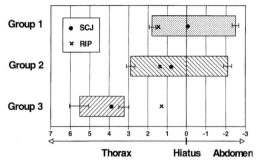

FIGURE 20.18. Length and position of gastroesophageal junction high-pressure zone relative to the diaphragmatic hiatus among groups of normal subjects (group 1), subjects in whom the squamocolumnar junction was 0 to 2 cm above the diaphragm at rest (group 2), and subjects in whom the squamocolumnar junction was greater than 2 cm above the diaphragm at rest (group 3). Subject groups were defined by radiographically imaging an endoscopically placed metal mucosal clip. The horizontal bars depict the average limits of the high-pressure zone within each subject group (mean ± SE cm). The position of the respiratory inversion point (RIP) is constant among subject groups whereas the position of the squamocolumnar junction is progressively more cephalic in groups 2 and 3. Similar to the type IV patients in Figure 20.9, the group 3 subjects in this investigation had a patulous hiatus and no detectable high-pressure zone at the diaphragmatic hiatus. Thus, the net effect was of shortening the high-pressure zone and positioning the squamocolumnar junction relatively distally within the high-pressure zone such that it likely would be visible endoscopically from a retroflexed view. (From Kahrilas PJ, Wu S, Lin S, et al. Attenuation of esophageal shortening during peristalsis with hiatus hernia. *Gastroenterology* 1995;109:1818, with permission.)

20.18). This distal segment of the LES may be attributable to the sling fibers and clasp fibers of the gastric cardia, also referred to as the intraabdominal segment of the esophagus (17,59). This is probably the most confusing segment of esophageal anatomy, referred to by Ingelfinger as an anatomic and functional "no man's land" (60). Highlighting this confusion, Wolf remarked that "it is indeed strange that, when normally located below the hiatus, the 'submerged segment' resembles the esophagus while, when displaced above the hiatus, it resembles stomach. In fact, when a large hiatal hernia is present, the original submerged segment is incorporated into the hernia sac (61)." Liebermann-Meffert and colleagues (17) described a "fold transition line" evident in postmortem specimens that appears analogous to the intragastric margin of the gastroesophageal junction as imaged endoscopically and related to the angle of His as identified externally. The squamocolumnar junction was 10.5 ± 4.4 mm proximal to the fold transition line when measured along the greater curvature. Although the relevance of this distal sphincter segment is controversial, Hill and colleagues (21) found the integrity of this "flap valve" (Fig. 20.9) to correlate with gastroesophageal junction competence against an antegrade pressure gradient in postmortem experiments. With progressive proximal displacement of the squamocolumnar junction above the hiatus, this distal segment

eventually becomes disrupted and splays open, creating a radiographically evident saccular structure identifiable as a nonreducing hiatal hernia (55). These observations suggest that the observed shortening of the LES high-pressure zone commented on by surgeons as indicative of a mechanically defective sphincter is probably largely a manometric correlate of a large nonreducing hiatal hernia (59,62).

A recent study evaluating the mechanistic profile for reflux in GERD patients with and without hiatus hernia provided some additional insight into the role of EGJ competence in GERD (39). In these ambulatory manometry experiments, 90% of reflux events in normal subjects and GERD patients without hiatus hernia were attributable to TLESRs. In contrast, patients with hiatus hernia had a more heterogeneous mechanistic profile with reflux episodes frequently occurring in the context of low LES pressure, straining, and swallow-associated LES relaxation. In contemplating this difference in mechanistic profile, it is necessary to explore mechanical variables of the system that may account for a relaxed EGJ remaining closed in one case and open in another; one such mechanical variable is sphincter compliance or distensibility.

Acquired anatomic changes attributable to hiatus hernia may alter the compliance at the relaxed EGJ, thereby decreasing the resistance to gastroesophageal flow. Recent physiologic studies exploring the role of compliance in GERD reported that GERD patients with hiatus hernia had increased compliance at the EGJ compared with compliance in normal subjects (63) or in patients having undergone fundoplication (64). These experiments used a combination of barostat-controlled distention, manometry, and fluoroscopy to quantify EGJ compliance. Several parameters of EGJ compliance were shown to be increased in hiatus hernia patients with GERD: (a) the EGJ opened at lower distention pressure, (b) when relaxed, the EGJ opened at distention pressures that were at or near resting intragastric pressure, and (c) for a given distention pressure, the EGJ opened approximately 0.5 cm wider (63). These alterations of EGJ mechanics are likely secondary to a disrupted, distensible crural aperture and likely contribute to the physiologic aberrations associated with hiatus hernia and GERD. Other potential anatomic manifestations of dilatation of the diaphragmatic hiatus include hiatus hernia and disruption of the gastroesophageal flap valve, both of which are strongly associated with reflux disease. Once the hiatus is physiologically disrupted, it is no longer protective in preventing gastroesophageal reflux. In that setting, reflux no longer requires "two hits" because the extrinsic sphincteric mechanism is already disrupted and the only prerequisite for reflux becomes LES relaxation, be that in the setting of swallow-induced relaxation, TLESR, or a period of prolonged LES hypotension.

Increased compliance may also help explain why GERD patients are more likely to sustain acid reflux in association with TLESRs compared with asymptomatic subjects. In an experiment that sought to quantify this difference, normal subjects exhibited acid reflux with 40% to 50% of TLESRs compared with 60% to 70% in patients with GERD (65). This difference may be attributable to increased EGJ compliance and its effect on trans-EGJ flow. This hypothesis is based on an equation modeling flow across the EGJ:

$$flow = \frac{\Delta P \times R^4}{C \times L \times \eta}$$

In the flow equation, flow is directly proportional to EGJ diameter to the fourth power and inversely proportional to the length of the narrowed segment and the viscosity of the gas or liquid traversing the segment. If TLESRs occur in the context of an EGJ with increased compliance, wider opening diameters occur under a given set of circumstances and therefore trans-EGJ flow increases. Patients without obvious hiatus hernia may still have increased compliance secondary to more subtle defects at the EGJ not readily evident using current radiographic or endoscopic methods of evaluation. These defects may be more akin to minor anatomic variants of the EGJ such as a class 2 gastroesophageal flap valve illustrated in Figure 20.9.

In addition to affecting the opening diameter of the EGJ during TLESRs, hiatus hernia may also increase the frequency of TLESRs. A study examining the effects of gastric distention on TLESR frequency in normal subjects and GERD patients with and without hiatus hernia revealed that continuous air infusion was a potent stimulus for TLESRs and acid reflux in all subject groups (66). An interesting finding was that the degree of augmentation of TLESR frequency was directly proportional to axial separation between the squamocolumnar junction (SCJ) and hiatal canal. Thus, increased sensitivity to distention-induced TLESR is yet another mechanism by which altered EGJ anatomy may predispose to GERD.

COMPROMISE OF ESOPHAGEAL EMPTYING RELATED TO HIATUS HERNIA

The defining abnormality with esophagitis is excessive mucosal acid exposure, which, in turn, is dependent on both the frequency of reflux events and the time required to achieve acid clearance for each event. Prolongation of acid clearance among patients with reflux disease has long been recognized, especially with type I hiatus hernia while recumbent (67). A recent study evaluating the characteristics of esophageal acid exposure in asymptomatic control subjects and GERD patients with and without esophagitis provided further support of the importance of hiatus hernia

in the development of esophagitis (68). This study reported that the esophagitis patients have significantly greater esophageal acid exposure compared with that in normal control subjects and nonerosive GERD patients and that the increased acid exposure was attributable to impaired acid clearance. The variable associated with the greatest impairment of esophageal acid clearance was hiatus hernia. In fact, there was a direct correlation between axial hiatus hernia size and total esophageal acid exposure.

The mechanisms by which hiatus hernia compromises fluid emptying from the distal esophagus have been explored (69,70). Sloan and Kahrilas analyzed the impact of hiatal hernia on esophageal emptying using simultaneous videofluoroscopy and manometry in patients with axial hiatal hernias compared with that in normal subjects (70). Subjects were divided into three groups: (a) volunteers with a phrenic ampulla of less than 2 cm in length, (b) patients or volunteers with maximal ampullary or hiatal hernia length greater than 2 cm that reduced between swallows (reducing hernia group), and (c) patients with hernias that did not reduce between swallows (nonreducing hiatus hernia). Each subject performed ten barium swallows and the outcome of each in terms of esophageal emptying was noted. Possible outcomes were of complete clearance, minimal clearance because of failed peristalsis, late retrograde flow of barium from the ampulla backup the tubular esophagus (Fig. 20.19), or early retrograde flow from the ampulla occurring coincident with LES relaxation (Fig. 20.20). As shown in Figure 20.21, the overall efficacy of esophageal emptying was significantly impaired in both hiatus hernia groups, but it was especially poor in the group with nonreducing hernias. The group with nonreducing hernias had complete emptying in only one third of test swallows and exhibited early retrograde flow, a phenomenon unique to this group, in almost half.

This work corroborated findings by Mittal and co-workers (69) who used concurrent pH recording and scintiscanning to examine the efficacy of fluid emptying and acid clearance in patients with hiatal hernia and compared those findings with those in a group of esophagitis patients without hernias. Regardless of the presence of esophagitis, the hernia groups had impaired acid clearance because there was *re-reflux* from the hernia sac during swallowing (Fig. 20.22). Re-reflux occurs predominantly during inspiration and can be attributed to loss of the normal one-way valve function of the crural diaphragm. By pinching off the distal esophagus, the crural diaphragm prevents backward flow from the stomach during each inspiration when it would be favored by a positive abdominal-thoracic pressure gradient. This one-way valve function of the crural diaphragm is grossly impaired with large type I hernias because a gastric pouch persists above the diaphragm as seen in Sloan's patients with nonreducing hernias (70).

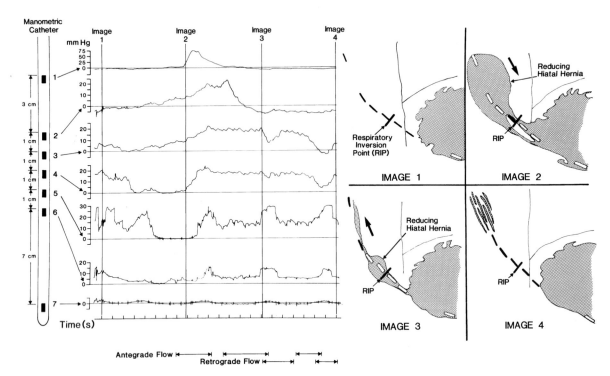

FIGURE 20.19. Concurrent manometric and videofluorographic recording of a 10-mL barium swallow in a subject with a reducing hiatal hernia characterized by late retrograde flow. The tracings from the video images on the right correspond to the four selected times from the swallowing sequence indicated by the numbers at the top of the vertical lines intersecting the manometric record. The schematic diagram to the left indicates the relative spacing of the pressure sensing ports (side holes located proximal to the markers in the fluoroscopic images). The lines at the bottom of the tracing indicate the timing and direction of barium flow. Image 1 depicts the instant of swallowing when barium was visible only in the stomach. Image 2 depicts the instant the stripping wave was at the level of the most proximal sensor; the hiatal hernia had formed and sensors 2, 3, and 4 were in a common cavity within the hernia. Image 3 depicts when retrograde flow began, at which point sensors 2 and 3 were above the hernia, sensor 4 was measuring intrahernial pressure, sensors 5 and 6 were at the level of the diaphragm, and sensor 7 remained within the stomach. Image 4 shows residual barium in the distal esophagus and no hiatal hernia with sensors 3, 4, 5, and 6 straddling the high-pressure zone comprised of the LES and diaphragm. (From Sloan S, Kahrilas PJ. Impairment of esophageal emptying with hiatal hernia. *Gastroenterology* 1991;100:596, with permission.)

Conclusion

The gastroesophageal junction is anatomically and physiologically complex, making it vulnerable to dysfunction by several mechanisms. GERD has several potential causes, the unifying theme being increased esophageal acid exposure. A variety of lines of evidence suggest that hiatal hernia is a significant pathophysiologic factor in approximately 50% of instances. The importance of hiatal hernia is obscured by imprecise use of the term and the misconception that hiatal hernia is an all-or-none phenomenon. It is more accurate to view hiatal hernia as a continuum of progressive disruption of the gastroesophageal junction, with larger hernias being of greater significance. The dynamic anatomy of the gastroesophageal junction outlined herein highlights the difficulty of defining hiatal hernia and elucidating the rela-

tionship between hiatal hernia, the diaphragmatic hiatus, the lower esophageal sphincter, and gastroesophageal reflux disease. Hence, although it is clear that hiatal hernia is a contributing factor in the pathogenesis of gastroesophageal reflux disease, it is equally clear that GERD is a multifactorial process that defies overly reductionist explanation.

TREATMENT

Repair of an isolated, asymptomatic type I hiatal hernia is rarely indicated. If symptoms of GERD occur in association with a large hiatus hernia, either medical or surgical treatment is indicated to control the reflux as discussed extensively elsewhere in this volume. Conversely, enlarging types

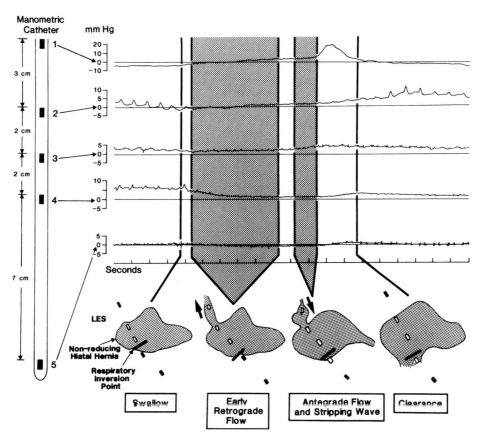

FIGURE 20.20. Concurrent manometric and video recording of a 10-mL barium swallow characterized by early retrograde flow in a subject with a nonreducing hiatal hernia. Tracings from the video images are below the manometric record and correspond to the times on the manometric tracings intersected by the vertical lines. The schematic diagram to the left depicts the relative spacing of the pressure sensors whose tracings are depicted. The arrows next to the video image indicate the direction of barium flow. The first video image to the far left shows a barium filled hiatal hernia at the time the swallow is initiated with sensor 1 in the distal esophagus, sensor 2 in the lower esophageal sphincter (LES), sensor 3 within the hernia, sensor 4 measuring crural contractile activity, and sensor 5 within the abdominal stomach. The second image was obtained about 1 second after the swallow and depicts the onset of retrograde flow; intrahernial pressure was 2 mm Hg and LES pressure was 0 mm Hg. Retrograde flow continued for 5 seconds until the peristaltic contraction reached the distal esophagus. The third image depicts antegrade flow with the stripping wave progressing down the esophagus and LES pressure increasing to equal intrahernial pressure (approximately 4 mm Hg). The final image to the far right shows barium cleared from the esophagus with the LES pressure exceeding intrahernial pressure. (From Sloan S, Kahrilas PJ. Impairment of esophageal emptying with hiatal hernia. *Gastroenterology* 1991;100:596, with permission.)

II, III, and IV hernias pose a risk of serious complications similar to complications of viscera herniated through an aperture elsewhere in the body (2). Skinner and co-workers reported that 6 of 21 patients with paraesophageal hernia treated medically died of complications of incarceration, perforation, and bleeding. More recent studies, however, suggest that these catastrophic complications are less common than initially reported. Allen and colleagues (71) followed up 23 patients for a median of 78 months and found that only four patients had progression of symptoms with only three cases of gastric strangulation in 735 patient-years. In addition, there was only one death in that series resulting from aspiration during an esophagram. Despite these more recent data, most experts still recommend that elective repair be treatment of choice in patients able to tolerate surgery. These hernias never regress and progressively

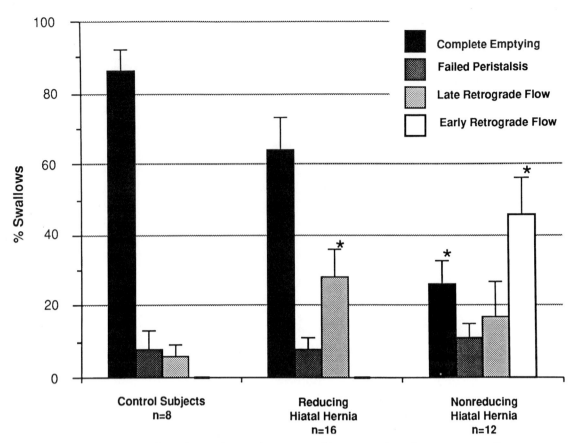

FIGURE 20.21. Esophageal emptying results among subject groups based on ten test swallows. Control subjects had complete esophageal emptying without retrograde flow in 86% ± 6% of test swallows compared with 61% ± 9% in the reducing hernia group and 31% ± 8% in the nonreducing hernia group ($p < .05$ vs. control subjects). The distinction between reducing hernia and nonreducing hernia was the radiographic observation of persistent rugal folds traversing the diaphragmatic hiatus in the nonreducing hernia group. The reducing hernia group exhibited significantly more instances of late retrograde flow (Fig. 20.19) ($p < .05$ vs. control subjects) and the nonreducing hernia group were the only individuals to exhibit early retrograde flow (Fig. 20.20) ($p < .001$ vs. other groups). (From Sloan, S, Kahrilas, PJ. Impairment of esophageal emptying with hiatal hernia. *Gastroenterology* 1991;100:596, with permission.)

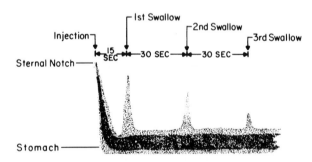

FIGURE 20.22. Radionuclide acid clearance study in a subject with a hiatus hernia. Fifteen seconds after the injection of a 15-mL bolus of 0.1N HCl labeled with 200 μCi of ^{99m}Tc-sulfur colloid, subjects swallowed every 30 seconds. The vertical axis represents the region from the sternal notch to the stomach. The horizontal axis is the time scale. The radioactivity is represented by the black area and no radioactivity is represented by the absence of black color. Soon after injection, the radioactivity appears in the stomach. However, note the biphasic response, that is, an initial reflux of isotope into the esophagus followed by clearance of the isotope during the first three swallows. (From Mittal RK, Lange RC, McCallum RW. Identification and mechanism of delayed esophageal acid clearance in subjects with hiatus hernia. *Gastroenterology* 1987;92:130, with permission.)

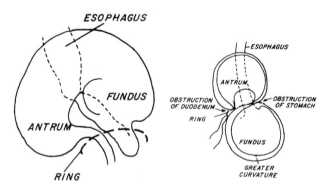

FIGURE 20.23. Obstruction and entrapment as a complication of type II paraesophageal hernia with an upside down stomach. The drawing on the left shows the hernia before obstruction with the gastroesophageal junction still fixed at the hiatus. This drawing is analogous to the radiograph in Figure 20.10. With distention and filling of the fundus, it has the potential to form an organoaxial volvulus (Fig. 20.11) and reherniate through the hiatus. Obstruction then develops at the duodenum and at the midportion of the stomach. Mortality of this condition is substantial. (From Hill LD. Incarcerated paraesophageal hernia: a surgical emergency. *Am J Surg* 1973;126:286–291, with permission.)

enlarge. If left untreated, the paraesophageal hernia may eventually reach the stage of the giant intrathoracic stomach. At this point, the patient may have substernal pain and pressure, or a gastric ulcer may develop in the poorly draining stomach (72). More problematic, when the fundus becomes distended and prolapses out of the posterior mediastinum through the esophageal opening into the abdomen, obstruction occurs at the esophageal, midgastric, and duodenal levels (Fig. 20.23). If this is not relieved promptly, incarceration may become irreducible. Among a group of ten such patients with strangulated and incarcerated hiatal hernias, Hill reported a 50% mortality rate. Conversely, among 19 patients in whom preoperative preparation and decompression was possible, there were no deaths (72). Thus, once a paraesophageal hernia is identified, it should be treated surgically, even in the absence of symptoms.

Surgical approaches to type II hiatal hernias can be divided into five components, not all of which are required in each case (73): (a) reduction of the herniated stomach into the abdomen, (b) herniotomy (excision of the hernia sac), (c) herniorrhaphy (closure of the hiatal defect), (d) antireflux procedure, and (e) gastropexy (attachment of the stomach subdiaphragmatically to prevent rehernation. The operation can be approached via a transthoracic or transabdominal route with each approach having its advantages and disadvantages. Thoracotomy provides excellent exposure of the esophagus and hernia sac, facilitating dissection of sufficient esophageal length and possible creation of a gastroplasty to lengthen the esophagus if needed to ensure a tension-free repair. The transabdominal approach facilitates the reduction of gastric volvulus and occasionally a thoracotomy is converted to a thoracolaparotomy for giant hernias with herniation of abdominal contents into the chest (74).

Opinion varies as to whether or not an antireflux procedure is necessary if concomitant pathologic reflux has not been demonstrated. The most common procedure done is a Nissen fundoplication. Gastropexy is used if the stomach is unusually mobile after reduction. Following surgical repair of a type II hiatal hernia, the prognosis is excellent. The recurrence rate for type II hernias is higher than that for type I hernias, presumably because the tissues of the hiatus are more compromised (18).

In an effort to reduce the morbidity associated with open procedures, a laparoscopic approach has been developed. Although similar to laparoscopic antireflux surgery, laparoscopic paraesophageal hernia repair is a more challenging procedure. Initial experience has revealed shorter hospital stays and reduced major and minor complications (75). However, mortality is still significant, and has been reported to be as high as 5% in some series (74,76). In addition, laparoscopic repair is also associated with higher recurrence rates compared with open procedures (30). Thus, the decision of whether to pursue laparoscopic versus open repair remains controversial.

However, because paraesophageal hernias are more common with advancing age, many patients who present with paraesophageal hernias have significant comorbidities. In this patient population, the risks of surgery may be substantial and therefore less invasive techniques may be more appropriate. Kercher and co-workers (77) described a technique combining endoscopic reduction of the hernia with percutaneous endoscopic gastrostomy (PEG). This technique was performed in 11 ASA (American Society of Anesthesiology) III patients who presented with symptomatic paraesophageal hernia. Laparoscopic assistance was required in nine subjects for reduction and gastropexy with a mean operative time of 61 minutes and hospital stay of 2.8 days. Three major complications (atrial fibrillation, transient ischemic event, one reoperation for an internal hernia) and one minor complication (PEG site infection) occurred. This technique may represent a valuable alternative management for symptomatic patients with severe comorbidity.

In conclusion, paraesophageal hernia represents a potentially catastrophic condition that warrants immediate attention in all patients and urgent intervention in symptomatic individuals. Subjects deemed to be good surgical risks should be offered surgical correction before complications occur because emergent surgery in the setting of incarceration has an extremely high mortality. However, the choice of operative approach is controversial and all techniques have acceptable long-term results. Patients with severe comorbidity may benefit from a less invasive technique that focuses on reduction of the hernia and prevention of gastric volvulus.

REFERENCES

1. Bowditch HI. *Treatise on diaphragmatic hernia.* Buffalo, NY: Hewett, Thomas, 1853.
2. Skinner DB, Belsey RH. Surgical management of esophageal reflux and hiatus hernia. Long-term results with 1,030 patients. *J Thorac Cardiovasc Surg* 1967;53:33–54.
3. Andrew LT. The height of the diaphragm in relation to certain abdominal viscera. *Lancet* 1903;1:790.
4. Akerlund A. Hernia diaphragmatica hernia oesopagei, von anatomischen unt rontgenologischen Gesichtspunct. *Acta Radiol* 1926;6:3.
5. Serpanti M. The results of systematic search for hiatal hernia in the course of 480 upper gastrointestinal X-ray series. *J Radiol* 1955;36:919.
6. Stilson WJ. Hiatal hernia and gastroesophageal reflux. *Radiology* 1969;93:1323.
7. Winkelstein A. Peptic esophagitis. A new clinical entity. *JAMA* 1935;104:906–909.
8. Allison PR. Peptic ulcer of the esophagus. *J Thorac Surg* 1946; 15:308–317.
9. Marchand P. The anatomy of the esophageal hiatus of the diaphragm and the pathogenesis of hiatus herniation. *Thorac Surg* 1959;37:81–92.
10. Barrett NR. Discussion on hiatus hernia. *Proc R Soc Med* 1932; 122:736–796.
11. Schatzki R. Die hernien des hiatus oesophageus. *Deutsches Arch F Klin Med* 1932;173:85–103.

12. Low A. A note on the crura of the diaphragm and the muscle of Treitz. *J Anatomy Lond* 1907;42:93–96.
13. Kahrilas PJ, Wu S, Lin S, et al. Attenuation of esophageal shortening during peristalsis with hiatus hernia. *Gastroenterology* 1995;109:1818–1825.
14. Pouderoux P, Lin S, Kahrilas PJ. Timing, propagation, coordination, and effect of esophageal shortening during peristalsis. *Gastroenterology* 1997;112:1147–1154.
15. Lin S, Brasseur JG, Pouderoux P, et al. The phrenic ampulla: distal esophagus or potential hiatal hernia? *Am J Physiol* 1995;268:G320–G327.
16. Ott DJ, Gelfand DW, Wu WC, et al. Esophagogastric region and its rings. *Am J Roentgenol* 1984;142:281–287.
17. Liebermann-Meffert D, Allgower M, Schmid P, et al. Muscular equivalent of the lower esophageal sphincter. *Gastroenterology* 1979;76:31–38.
18. Skinner DB. Hernias (hiatal, traumatic and congenital). In: Berk JE, ed. *Gastronterology*, fourth ed. Philadelphia: WB Saunders, 1985:705–716.
19. Mittal RK, Rochester DF, McCallum RW. Sphincteric action of the diaphragm during a relaxed lower esophageal sphincter in humans. *Am J Physio* 1989;256:G139–G144.
20. Pandolfino JE, Shi G, Cisler J, et al. Opening characteristics of the relaxed EGJ during low pressure distention in normal subjects and hiatus hernia patients. *Gastroenterology* 2002;122:430:A450.
21. Hill LD, Kozarek RA, Kraemer SJ, et al. The gastroesophageal flap valve: *in vitro* and *in vivo* observations. *Gastrointest Endosc* 1996;44:541–547.
22. Allison PR. Reflux esophagitis, sliding hiatal hernia and the anatomy of repair. *Surg Gynecol Obstet* 1951;92:419–431.
23. Rigler LG, Eneboe JB. Incidence of hiatus hernia in pregnant women and its significance. *J Thorac Surg* 1935;4:262–268.
24. Marchand P. A study of the forces productive of gastroesophageal regurgitation through the diaphragmatic hiatus. *Thorax* 1957;12:189–202.
25. Paterson WG, Kolyn DM. Esophageal shortening induced by short-term intraluminal acid perfusion in opossum: a cause for hiatus hernia? *Gastroenterology* 1994;107:1736–1740.
26. Kahrilas PJ. Hiatus hernia: fact or fiction? *Gullet* 1993;3[Suppl]:21.
27. Perdikis G, Hinder RA. Paraesophageal hernia. In: Nyhus LM, Condon RE, eds. *Hernia*. Philadelphia: JB Lippincott, 1995:544.
28. Postlethwait RW. *Surgery of the esophagus*. Norwalk: Appleton Century-Crofts, 1979.
29. Wright RA. Relationship of hiatal hernia in endoscopically proved reflux esophagitis. *Dig Dis Sci* 1979;24:311–313.
30. Hashemi M, Sillin LF, Peters JH. Current concepts in the management of paraesophageal hiatal hernia. *J Clin Gastroenterol* 1999;29:8–13.
31. Berstad A, Weberg R, Froyshov Larsen I, et al. Relationship of hiatus hernia to reflux oesophagitis. A prospective study of coincidence, using endoscopy. *Scand J Gastroenterol* 1986;21:55–58.
32. Petersen H, Johannessen T, Sandvik AK, et al. Relationship between endoscopic hiatus hernia and gastroesophageal reflux symptoms. *Scand J Gastroenterol* 1991;26:921–926.
33. Jones MP, Sloan SS, Rabine JC, et al. Hiatal hernia size is the dominant determinant of esophagitis presence and severity in gastroesophageal reflux disease. *Am J Gastroenterol* 2001;96:1711–1717.
34. Sontag SJ, Schnell TG, Miller TQ, et al. The importance of hiatal hernia in reflux esophagitis compared with lower esophageal sphincter pressure or smoking. *J Clin Gastroenterol* 1991;13:628–643.
35. Cameron AJ. Barrett's esophagus: prevalence and size of hiatal hernia. *Am J Gastroenterol* 1999;94:2054–2059.
36. Holloway RH, Penagini R, Ireland AC. Criteria for objective definition of transient lower esophageal sphincter relaxation. *Am J Physiol* 1995;268:G128–G133.
37. Kahrilas PJ, Gupta RR. Mechanisms of acid reflux associated with cigarette smoking. *Gut* 1990;31:4–10.
38. Mittal RK, Holloway RH, Penagini R, et al. Transient lower esophageal sphincter relaxation. *Gastroenterology* 1995;109:601–610.
39. van Herwaarden MA, Samsom M, Smout AJ. Excess gastroesophageal reflux in patients with hiatus hernia is caused by mechanisms other than transient LES relaxations. *Gastroenterology* 2000;119:1439–1446.
40. Helm JF. Role of saliva in esophageal function and disease. *Dysphagia* 1989;4:76–84.
41. Orr WC, Lackey C, Robinson MG, et al. Esophageal acid clearance during sleep in patients with Barrett's esophagus. *Dig Dis Sci* 1988;33:654–659.
42. Sonnenberg A, Massey BT, Jacobsen SJ. Hospital discharges resulting from esophagitis among Medicare beneficiaries. *Dig Dis Sci* 1994;39:183–188.
43. Stanciu C, Bennett JR. Oesophageal acid clearing: one factor in the production of reflux oesophagitis. *Gut* 1974;15:852–857.
44. Kahrilas PJ, Dodds WJ, Hogan WJ. Effect of peristaltic dysfunction on esophageal volume clearance. *Gastroenterology* 1988;94:73–80.
45. Boyle JT, Altschuler SM, Nixon TE, et al. Responses of feline gastroesophageal junction to changes in abdominal pressure. *Am J Physiol* 1987;253:G315–G322.
46. Boyle JT, Altschuler SM, Nixon TE, et al. Role of the diaphragm in the genesis of lower esophageal sphincter pressure in the cat. *Gastroenterology* 1985;88:723–730.
47. Mittal RK, Fisher M, McCallum RW, et al. Human lower esophageal sphincter pressure response to increased intra-abdominal pressure. *Am J Physiol* 1990;258:G624–G630.
48. Mittal RK, Rochester DF, McCallum RW. Electrical and mechanical activity in the human lower esophageal sphincter during diaphragmatic contraction. *J Clin Invest* 1988;81:1182–1189.
49. Altschuler SM, Boyle JT, Nixon TE, et al. Simultaneous reflex inhibition of lower esophageal sphincter and crural diaphragm in cats. *Am J Physiol* 1985;249:G586–G591.
50. Monges H, Salducci J, Naudy B. Dissociation between the electrical activity of the diaphragmatic dome and crura muscular fibers during esophageal distension, vomiting and eructation. An electromyographic study in the dog. *J Physiol (Paris)* 1978;74:541–554.
51. Mittal RK, Fisher MJ. Electrical and mechanical inhibition of the crural diaphragm during transient relaxation of the lower esophageal sphincter. *Gastroenterology* 1990;99:1265–1268.
52. Sloan S, Rademaker AW, Kahrilas PJ. Determinants of gastroesophageal junction incompetence: hiatal hernia, lower esophageal sphincter, or both? *Ann Intern Med* 1992;117:977–982.
53. Klein WA, Parkman HP, Dempsey DT, et al. Sphincterlike thoracoabdominal high pressure zone after esophagogastrectomy. *Gastroenterology* 1993;105:1362–1369.
54. Lin S, Chen J, Manka M, et al. The LES and hiatal sphincter: in unity there is strength. *Gastroenterology* 1997;112:A199.
55. Friedland GW. Historical review of the changing concepts of the lower esophageal anatomy: 430 BC–1977. *Am J Roentgenol* 1978;131:373–388.
56. Michelson E, Siegel C. The role of the phrenico-esophageal ligament in the lower esophageal sphincter. *Surg Gynecol Obstet* 1964;118:1291–1294.
57. Kahrilas PJ, Lin S, Chen J, et al. The effect of hiatus hernia on gastro-oesophageal junction pressure. *Gut* 1999;44:476–482.
58. Asoh R, Goyal RK. Electrical activity of the opossum lower

esophageal sphincter *in vivo*. Its role in the basal sphincter pressure. *Gastroenterology* 1978;74:835–840.

59. Zaninotto G, DeMeester TR, Schwizer W, et al. The lower esophageal sphincter in health and disease. *Am J Surg* 1988;155: 104–111.

60. Ingelfinger FJ. Esophageal motility. *Physiol Rev* 1958;38: 533–584.

61. Wolf BS. Sliding hiatal hernia: the need for redefinition. *Am J Roentgenol* 1973;117:231–247.

62. Stein HJ, DeMeester TR, Naspetti R, et al. Three-dimensional imaging of the lower esophageal sphincter in gastroesophageal reflux disease. *Ann Surg* 1991;214:374–383; discussion 383–384.

63. Pandolfino JE, Shi G, Curry J, et al. Esophagogastric junction distensibility: a factor contributing to sphincter incompetence. *Am J Physiol Gastrointest Liver Physiol* 2002;282:G1052–1058.

64. Curry J, Shi G, Pandolfino JE, et al. Mechanical characteristics of the EGJ after fundoplication compared to normal subjects and GERD patients. *Gastroenterology* 2001;120:A112.

65. Sifrim D, Tack J, Lerut T, et al. Transient lower esophageal sphincter relaxations and esophageal body muscular contractile response in reflux esophagitis. *Dig Dis Sci* 2000;45:1293–1300.

66. Kahrilas PJ, Shi G, Manka M, et al. Increased frequency of transient lower esophageal sphincter relaxation induced by gastric distention in reflux patients with hiatal hernia. *Gastroenterology* 2000;118:688–695.

67. Johnson LF. 24-Hour pH monitoring in the study of gastroesophageal reflux. *J Clin Gastroenterol* 1980;2:387–399.

68. Jones MP, Sloan SS, Jovanovic B, et al. Impaired egress rather than increased access: an important independent predictor of erosive esophagitis. *Neurogastroenterol Motil* 2002;14:625–631.

69. Mittal RK, Lange RC, McCallum RW. Identification and mechanism of delayed esophageal acid clearance in subjects with hiatus hernia. *Gastroenterology* 1987;92:130–135.

70. Sloan S, Kahrilas PJ. Impairment of esophageal emptying with hiatal hernia. *Gastroenterology* 1991;100:596–605.

71. Allen MS, Trastek VF, Deschamps C, et al. Intrathoracic stomach. Presentation and results of operation. *J Thorac Cardiovasc Surg* 1993;105:253–258; discussion 258–259.

72. Hill LD. Incarcerated paraesophageal hernia. A surgical emergency. *Am J Surg* 1973;126:286–291.

73. Menguy R. Surgical management of large paraesophageal hernia with complete intrathoracic stomach. *World J Surg* 1988;12: 415–422.

74. Rogers ML, Duffy JP, Beggs FD, et al. Surgical treatment of para-oesophageal hiatal hernia. *Ann R Coll Surg Engl* 2001;83:394–398.

75. Schauer PR, Ikramuddin S, McLaughlin RH, et al. Comparison of laparoscopic versus open repair of paraesophageal hernia. *Am J Surg* 1998;176:659–665.

76. Wu JS, Dunnegan DL, Soper NJ. Clinical and radiologic assessment of laparoscopic paraesophageal hernia repair. *Surg Endosc* 1999;13:497–502.

77. Kercher KW, Matthews BD, Ponsky JL, et al. Minimally invasive management of paraesophageal herniation in the high-risk surgical patient. *Am J Surg* 2001;182:510–514.

PATHOPHYSIOLOGY OF GASTROESOPHAGEAL REFLUX DISEASE: MOTILITY FACTORS

RAVINDER K. MITTAL

Is gastroesophageal reflux disease an acid or motility disorder of the esophagus? Indeed, gastric acid is the major offender and is primarily responsible for the esophageal mucosal damage in reflux diseases. However, the gastric acid secretion in the majority if not all patients with reflux disease is normal. The reason that gastric acid reaches the esophagus is due to the motility abnormality of the lower esophageal sphincter (LES). Deranged esophageal peristalsis, when present, allows acid and possibly other noxious agents to remain in the esophagus for extended periods of time and induce esophageal mucosal damage. Therefore, even though the major noxious agent in reflux disease is gastric acid, the motility abnormalities of the LES and esophagus are primary etiologic factors and fundamental to the understanding of reflux disease.

LOWER ESOPHAGEAL SPHINCTER

Historical Perspective

A person can stand upside down after eating a large hearty meal, yet no food refluxes into the mouth or the esophagus. It is intuitively clear that there must be a valvular or sphincter mechanism at the lower end of the esophagus. In a 1958 review article, Ingelfinger (1) stated that the pinchcock action of the diaphragm was important in the prevention of gastroesophageal reflux. Fyke and Code (2) were the first to record an intraluminal high-pressure zone between the esophagus and the stomach; they suggested that intrinsic muscles of the lower end of the esophagus were entirely responsible for maintaining this pressure. It was not until 1985 that the diaphragmatic hiatus was proven to play a role in the valvular mechanism at the esophagogastric junction (EGJ) (3). Studies conducted during the last several years convincingly show that there is not one, but two LESs. The dual-sphincter mechanism at the EGJ is composed of intrin-

sic smooth muscles of the LES and extrinsic skeletal muscles of the diaphragmatic hiatus. In humans, under normal conditions, the LES is approximately 4 cm in length and the crural diaphragm, which forms the esophageal hiatus, is about 2 cm in length. The crural diaphragm encircles the proximal 2 cm of the LES (4). Therefore, a portion of the LES is intra-abdominal and a portion is located in the hiatus itself (Fig. 21.1). The intra-abdominal portion of the LES is frequently termed the submerged segment of the esophagus (5). The lower end of the esophagus has also been referred to as the phrenic ampulla by radiologists because it has a bulbar shape on barium swallow (6). The anatomic structure of the phrenic ampulla, however, is poorly characterized.

Recent studies using ultrasound technique (7) demonstrate that the muscles of the LES are thicker than those of the adjacent esophagus. However, the muscle thickness in the LES region is not fixed; it changes with changes in LES pressure and there is a direct relationship between LES pressure and muscle thickness (8). The LES has a rich nerve supply but the location of the neurons in the LES differs from the rest of the esophagus (9). Within the LES, the myenteric plexus lies in several muscle planes, in contrast to the body of the esophagus, where the major plexus lies between the longitudinal and the circular muscle layers.

Intrinsic muscles of the stomach may also contribute to the antireflux barrier. The sling or oblique fibers of the stomach are located below the high-pressure zone. These fibers are arranged in a C-shaped fashion with the closed end of the C located on the greater curvature and the open end oriented toward the lesser curvature (10). The exact function of these fibers is not clear; they may be responsible for the flap-valve mechanism considered to be important in the prevention of gastroesophageal reflux (11).

The respiratory diaphragm, which is the major organ for the ventilatory function of the lung, also has a LES function. The diaphragm is composed of a costal part, arising from the ribs, and a crural part, which originates from the vertebral column. The two parts of the diaphragm have separate embryologic origins. The crural diaphragm develops from

R. K. Mittal: Department of Gastroenterology, School of Medicine University of California, San Diego; Gastroenterology Section, Medical Service, Department of Veterans Affairs Medical Center, La Jolla, California.

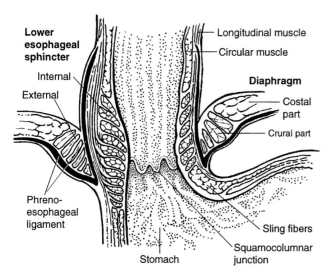

FIGURE 21.1. Schematic of the anatomy of the esophagogastric junction. The smooth muscles of the lower end of the esophagus and the crural diaphragm are the two sphincteric mechanisms at the esophagogastric junction. The two sphincters are anatomically superimposed and anchored to each other by the phrenoesophageal ligament. (From Mittal RK, Balaban DH, Mechanisms of disease: the esophagogastric junction, *N Engl Med* 1997;336: 924, with permission.)

the dorsal mesentery of the esophagus, and the costal diaphragm from myoblasts originating in the lateral body wall (12). The crural diaphragm, which forms the esophageal hiatus and constitutes the "extrinsic sphincter mechanism," is actually shaped like a canal. In humans, this canal is formed primarily by the right crus of the diaphragm (13). The fibers in this canal are oriented in a cranial to caudal direction toward the outer aspect and obliquely toward the inner aspect. The LES and crural diaphragm are anchored to each other by the phrenoesophageal ligament, a condensation of the loose areolar tissue. This ligament extends from the undersurface of the diaphragm and attaches to the esophagus approximately at the upper border of the LES.

Esophagogastric Junction Pressure under Various Physiologic Conditions

The intraluminal pressure at the EGJ is a measure of the strength of the antireflux barrier. There are convincing data in both animals and humans that the two anatomic structures— i.e., the LES and crural diaphragm—contribute to the EGJ pressure. Electrical stimulation of the crural diaphragm increases the EGJ pressure in cats (14). Furthermore, the crural diaphragm is capable of maintaining a high-pressure zone at the abdomino-thoracic junction in patients who have undergone surgical resection of the smooth muscle LES (15).

To avoid confusion, the intraluminal pressure at the lower end of the esophagus shall be referred to as the EGJ pressure in this chapter. The pressure generated from the contraction of LES smooth muscle is referred to as the LES pressure, and pressure due to contraction of the crural diaphragm is termed

as the crural diaphragm pressure. Distinguishing these two pressures is important because it emphasizes the individual contributions of each structure to the EGJ pressure.

The LES or EGJ pressure is measured in reference to the intragastric pressure. Prolonged continuous pressure monitoring reveals that the EGJ pressure varies over time. These variations are either due to LES or crural diaphragm contractions. The LES pressure varies from minute to minute, and these pressure fluctuations are usually of small amplitude, ranging from 5 to 10 mm Hg. However, large LES pressure fluctuations coupled with the migrating motor complex (MMC) activity of the stomach may also occur. The frequency of these phasic pressure fluctuations is the same as that of MMC, usually three per minute. The LES pressure may exceed 80 mm Hg during phase III of the MMC, and typically peaks prior to the onset of gastric contraction (16).

The second type of variation in the EGJ pressure is related to the crural diaphragm contraction, which is linked with respiration. With each inspiration, as the crural diaphragm contracts, there is an increase in the EGJ pressure (17). The amplitude of the inspiratory pressure increase is directly proportional to the force of crural diaphragmatic contraction. During tidal inspiration, the EGJ pressure increase is 10 to 20 mm Hg, and with deep inspiration the pressure increase ranges from 100 to 150 mm Hg. The crural diaphragm also contributes to the EGJ pressure during nonrespiratory physical activities such as straight leg raising and abdominal compression. These activities can induce sustained or tonic contractions of the crural diaphragm (18). The crural diaphragm reflexively contracts during coughing, Valsalva maneuver, and any physical condition that increases intra-abdominal pressure.

Neural Control of the Lower Esophageal Sphincter and Crural Diaphragm

The tone in the LES muscle is the result of myogenic and neurogenic mechanisms. The relative contribution of these two mechanisms varies among different species. In humans, the LES tone is comprised of both neurogenic and myogenic components. A significant percentage of the LES tone in humans is due to cholinergic innervation (19). Myogenic tone is due to shifts of intracellular calcium stores within the LES muscle (20).

There are a large number of excitatory and inhibitory neurotransmitters within LES muscle; however, their physiologic significance remains unclear. The modulation of LES tone that occurs with MMC activity is largely mediated through the vagus nerve (21,22). The swallow-associated LES relaxation is mediated through the central nervous system (dorsomotor nucleus of the vagus nerve). The efferents travel to the LES via the vagus nerve and the myenteric plexus. The synapse between the vagal fibers and myenteric neurons employs a cholinergic mechanism, and the postsynaptic neurotransmitter is noncholinergic and nonadrenergic (23). Several studies confirm that nitric oxide is the noncholinergic, nonadrenergic neurotransmitter (24), but vasoactive intestinal peptide may also play a role.

The crural diaphragm, like the remainder of the diaphragm, is controlled through the phrenic nerves. Although the diaphragmatic hiatus is composed of muscles mainly from the right crus, it is innervated through the left and right phrenic nerves. Spontaneous inspiratory activity of the crural diaphragm is due to the activity of inspiratory neurons located in the syncytium of the brain stem (25). This activity is transmitted to the phrenic nerve nucleus located in the cervical spinal cord. Voluntary control of the diaphragm originates within the cortical neurons. The crural diaphragm contracts a fraction of a second earlier than the costal diaphragm, and this may have physiologic significance in relationship to its antireflux barrier function (26).

Esophageal sensory mechanisms can mediate reflex relaxation of the crural diaphragm. Esophageal distension and a swallow induce selective inhibition of the crural diaphragm muscle (27). Transient relaxation of the LES—a major mechanism of gastroesophageal reflux, belching, and vomiting—is also accompanied by simultaneous relaxation of the LES and crural diaphragm (28,29).

Physiologic Significance of Two Lower Esophageal Sphincters

Why do we need two lower esophageal sphincters? The answer to this question rests on the physical principle that the intraluminal EGJ pressure determines the strength of the antireflux barrier, and the pressure gradient between the esophagus and stomach (PGES) is the driving force for gastroesophageal reflux. Under normal situations, the EGJ pressure is constantly adapting to changes in the PGES that occur during various physiologic circumstances. The changes in PGES are related either to muscular contractions of the esophagus and stomach or to pressure changes within the intrathoracic and intrabdominal cavities. Contraction of the esophagus is protective with respect to reflux. On the other hand, gastric contraction increases the pressure gradient in favor of reflux. Therefore, LES contraction is coupled with gastric contraction during MMC activity of the stomach, thus preventing reflux. Contraction of the inspiratory muscles of respiration produces negative intrathoracic and intraesophageal pressure, thus increasing the PGES. Similarly, contraction of the abdominal wall and diaphragm increases the stomach pressure and PGES. All of the maneuvers accompanied by contraction of the inspiratory and the abdominal wall muscles that increase PGES are accompanied by contraction of the crural diaphragm and a protective increase in EGJ pressure. The rapid changes in PGES caused by skeletal muscle contraction of the chest and abdomen are thus counteracted by the rapidly contracting skeletal sphincter muscle of the crural diaphragm.

Mechanisms of Reflux

Based on an understanding of the two lower esophageal sphincters, one would intuitively think that weakness of either the LES or crural diaphragm is the cause of gastroesophageal reflux. Indeed, some patients with reflux disease have a weak LES, some have a weak crural diaphragm, and some have both. However, in mild to moderate nonerosive reflux disease, the LES (30) and crural diaphragm pressures (31) are normal. In fact, a number of patients with mild to moderate disease have a hypertensive LES (32). The incidence of low LES pressure increases with the severity of esophagitis (30), and spontaneous inspiratory crural diaphragm pressure is low in 50% of patients with endoscopic reflux disease (31). A large body of information indicates that transient relaxation of the LES and crural diaphragm (TLESR) is the major mechanism of reflux in normal subjects and patients with reflux disease (33).

TRANSIENT LOWER ESOPHAGEAL SPHINCTER RELAXATION

McNally et al. (34) first observed non–swallow-related LES relaxation as a mechanism of belching in 1964. However, it was not until 1980 that the phenomenon of TLESR and its relationship to gastroesophageal reflux was described in detail (35). Overall, TLESR is the single most common mechanism underlying gastroesophageal reflux. In normal subjects, the majority of reflux episodes occur during TLESRs, with almost all the remainder occurring during swallow-induced LES relaxation associated with failed or incomplete primary peristalsis. This pattern of reflux mechanism is remarkably consistent among subjects, both supine and ambulant (36). Most studies have shown that TLESR is also the most common mechanism of reflux in patients with reflux disease and accounts for between 63% and 74% of reflux episodes (37–39). Similar findings have also been reported in children with reflux disease (40,41).

Mechanisms of reflux in patients with reflux disease are less homogeneous than in normal subjects. While more than 50% of patients, usually those without endoscopic evidence of esophagitis, reflux exclusively through TLESR, many patients have a mixed picture in which a significant number of reflux episodes occur during swallow-induced LES relaxation, persistently absent basal LES pressure, straining by deep inspiration, and increased intra-abdominal pressure. The proportion of reflux episodes that can be ascribed to TLESRs varies inversely with the severity of reflux disease (28), presumably because of the increasing prevalence of defective basal LES pressure as the severity of esophagitis increases (30). The presence or absence of esophagitis does not seem to influence the rate of TLESRs (42,43).

Characteristics of Transient Lower Esophageal Sphincter Relaxation

Transient LES relaxations are abrupt falls in LES pressure to the level of intragastric pressure that are not triggered by swallowing, as manifested by the distinctive pattern of pharyngeal or mylohyoid muscle contraction (Fig. 21.2). In

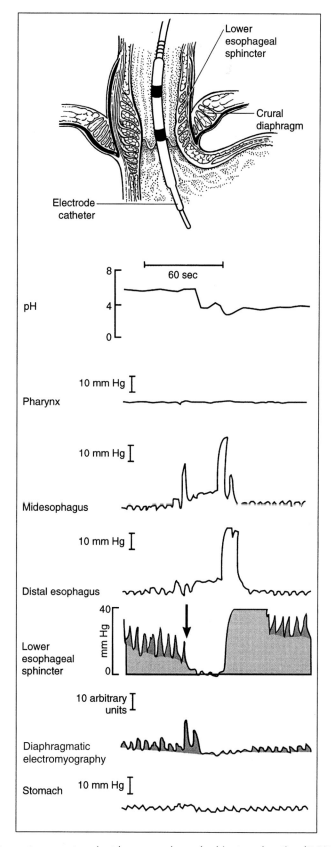

FIGURE 21.2. A spontaneous, transient lower esophageal sphincter relaxation (TLESR). The onset of TLESR is indicated by the *vertical arrow*. Relaxation occurs in the absence of a swallow as manifested by the absence of a pharyngeal pressure wave. The LES relaxation is complete to the level of the intragastric pressure (horizontal line at the bottom of the LES tracing) and is sustained for more than 20 seconds. TLESR is associated with inhibition of the crural diaphragm as indicated by the loss of inspiratory LES pressure oscillations and inspiratory diaphragmatic electromyography. Reflux (drop in esophageal pH) occurs following complete LES and crural diaphragm relaxation and is associated with an increase in intraesophageal pressure. (From Mittal RK, Balaban DH, Mechanisms of disease: the esophagogastric junction. *N Engl J Med* 1997;336:924, with permission.)

most studies, a fall in LES pressure of 5 mm Hg has been regarded as minimum. Transient LES relaxations are typically of longer duration than swallow-induced LES relaxation, lasting from 10 to 45 seconds. The criteria that have proved optimal for the definition of TLESRs are (a) the absence of a pharyngeal swallow signal for 4 seconds before to 2 seconds after the onset of LES relaxation, or a mylohyoid EMG complex for 3 seconds before the onset of LES relaxation; (b) an LES pressure fall of >1 mm Hg/second; (c) a time from the onset to complete relaxation of <10 seconds; and (d) a nadir pressure of <2 mm Hg. Excluding LES relaxations associated with multiple rapid swallows, LES pressure drops to 2 mm Hg, which have a duration of >10 seconds can also be classified as TLESRs (44). A number of events in the esophagus, stomach, and crural diaphragm have been identified that accompany TLESRs. Contractions in the pharynx and mylohyoid muscle have been reported to occur at the onset of 20% to 45% of TLESRs, respectively (45), although these pharyngeal and mylohyoid complexes are much smaller (approximately 50%) than those associated with swallowing and can be interpreted as partial or incomplete swallows. Distal esophageal pressure waves, clearly unrelated to swallowing, often occur at the onset of TLESRs and, when recorded at more than one site, usually have a synchronous onset. During the period of LES inhibition, there is also inhibition of the esophageal body, which is manifested by inhibition of primary peristalsis during prolonged relaxations (46). The gastric fundus also shows changes consistent with active inhibition during TLESRs. A small drop in intragastric pressure, usually in the range of 2 to 4 mm Hg, occurs during TLESRs. In addition to the events in the upper gastrointestinal smooth muscle, there is also selective and complete inhibition of the crural diaphragm despite continued activity of the costal diaphragm during TLESRs (47). Thus, TLESR is not a response localized to the LES. Rather, it appears to be part of a more generalized inhibition of a number of structures within and outside of the upper gastrointestinal tract that influence flow across the gastroesophageal junction. These structures are either innervated by the vagus nerve or are linked to the brain stem, or both. This pattern of inhibition is consistent with a coordinated pattern of activity designed to facilitate the retrograde flow of gastric contents during belching and vomiting.

Stimuli that Trigger Transient Lower Esophageal Sphincter Relaxations

Gastric Distension

Gastric distension is a potent stimulus for TLESR. This is not surprising given the fact that TLESR is the mechanism by which gas is vented from the stomach during belching. Approximately 15 ml of air is delivered to the stomach with each swallow (48) and without an built-in venting mecha-

nism, uncontrolled gastrointestinal bloating would occur. Studies in which the stomach has been partitioned surgically have revealed that the subcardiac region of the stomach is primarily responsible for triggering TLESR (49). Reduction of the compliance of this region by buttressing it with mesh reinforcement substantially reduces TLESR in dogs. Although distension of other parts of the stomach can increase the rate of TLESR, the threshold for distension is substantially higher in these regions and the response less marked. In humans, a volume of 750 to 1,000 ml causes a fourfold increase in the rate of TLESRs within the first 10 minutes. In some studies, a similar effect has been reported after meals (50,51). Meals are also associated with a significant increase in the proportion of TLESRs associated with reflux, and it is possible that this effect rather than an increase in the rate of TLESRs is responsible for the postprandial increase in reflux.

Pharyngeal Mechanisms

Pharyngeal intubation increases the rate of TLESRs. In fasted patients in whom LES pressure was monitored via a gastrostomy tube, pharyngeal intubation for 1 hour increased the rate of TLESRs threefold, from two to six per hour during the period of intubation (52). Pharyngeal stimulation is usually associated with full expression of the oral, pharyngeal, and esophageal phases of deglutition (53). LES relaxation without swallowing can be induced by instillation of minute amounts of liquid into the hypopharynx in humans (54) and light stroking of the pharynx or low-frequency stimulation of the superior laryngeal nerve in the opossum (55). This reflex depends on the afferent nerve fibers from the pharynx or larynx (56) traveling in the superior laryngeal branch of the vagus and the glossopharyngeal nerves; both nerves project to the nucleus tractus solitarii (NTS). The occurrence of small mylohyoid and pharyngeal complexes at the onset of some TLESRs may be an evidence of subthreshold or incomplete swallowing. The LES relaxation caused by stimulation of pharynx with small amounts of water can last up to 60 seconds or longer. Interaction among stimuli is a real possibility; thus, pharyngeal stimulation may either trigger TLESRs directly or lower the threshold for triggering by gastric distension.

Factors Modulating the Rate of Transient Lower Esophageal Sphincter Relaxations are Posture, Sleep, Anesthesia, and Stress

In both healthy humans and dogs, the stimulation of TLESRs produced by gaseous gastric distension is almost totally suppressed in the supine posture (57–59). In patients with reflux disease, TLESRs occur significantly less frequently in the supine (60) and lateral recumbent positions compared to sitting. TLESRs do not occur during stable sleep (61); reflux episodes that do occur during the nighttime sleep periods are totally confined to periods of arousal during sleep that may last for only 10 seconds.

Spontaneous TLESRs are also completely suppressed in dogs by even light general anesthesia (62). Cold stress has also been shown to reduce the frequency of TLESRs (63).

Neural Pathways Mediating Transient Lower Esophageal Sphincter Relaxation: Vagal Control Mechanisms

The vagus mediates swallow-induced LES relaxation (64,65) and inhibition of gastric tone or receptive relaxation during swallowing (66) (Fig. 21.3). The efferent pathway for TLESRs is also presumably in the vagus nerve; in dogs, TLESRs are completely abolished by cooling of the cervical vagus (67), and eructation is substantially inhibited by truncal vagotomy 5 cm above the diaphragm (68). The absence of TLESRs in patients with achalasia suggests that TLESRs share a final common pathway with swallow-induced LES relaxation (69). Gastric distension probably triggers TLESRs through stimulation of tension receptors in the proximal stomach (70,71); particularly the gastric cardia. Afferent fibers, which signal gastric distension, are known to project to the NTS (72) and to the dorsal motor nucleus of the vagus (DMV), either directly or via interneurons (73). The DMV contains the cell bodies of vagal efferent neurons that project to the LES. Gastric mechanoreceptors have been postulated to serve as the afferent pathway for a number of vagal reflexes including reflex relaxation of the gastric corpus. Such a neural pathway could therefore potentially mediate TLESRs. In the opossum, LES relaxation can also be induced by intrinsic gastric nerves independently of extrinsic nerves (74). Whether such a pathway mediates TLESRs is not known, but it cannot be involved in the associated inhibition of the crural diaphragm during TLESRs. The complete abolition of TLESRs by cervical vagal cooling (67) also argues against a dominant role for a local intramural pathway in mediating TLESRs.

The selective inhibition of the crural diaphragm that is characteristic of TLESRs also occurs during vomiting (29) and esophageal distension (27) and to a partial degree during swallowing. Presumably, this inhibition is coordinated in the brain stem, although the precise site at which this occurs is unclear. Rhythmic respiration is controlled mainly by premotor neurons in the dorsal respiratory group within the NTS and the adjacent reticular formation (75), which in turn activate diaphragmatic motor neurons in the ventral horn of the cervical spinal cord. The NTS is also the destination for afferent input from the vagus and glossopharyngeal nerves and has been suggested as a potential site for the integrated neural control of inhibition of respiration during swallowing. However, inhibition of the crural diaphragm by esophageal distension and, by implication, during TLESRs does not appear to be through inhibition of the medullary

premotor inspiratory neurons of the respiratory center, but via a separate, as-yet-unidentified pathway (76).

TLESR is a long period (10 to 60 seconds) of simultaneous LES and crural diaphragm relaxation. Relaxations of both the LES and crural diaphragm during TLESR are essential for the occurrence of reflux in normal subjects (77). Based on the available information, it is possible to construct a hypothetical pathway for the triggering of TLESRs (Fig. 21.3). The basic element is a vagal reflex pathway triggered by gastric distension or pharyngeal stimulation and integrated in the brain stem. The threshold for triggering is lowered by concurrent stimulation of the pharynx (and possibly larynx) and increased potentially by supine posture, sleep, and anesthesia. The efferent vagal output is controlled by a pattern generator in the brain stem and mediates the esophageal, LES, gastric, and diaphragmatic events during TLESR. Under usual circumstances, the pharyngeal components of deglutition are bypassed, but these can be partly activated on occasion causing the small pharyngeal and mylohyoid complexes that occur with some TLESRs.

Gastroesophageal reflux disease is characterized by a higher frequency of reflux episodes. This has been attributed to both a higher frequency of TLESRs and a higher incidence of reflux during TLESRs. Probably the unresolved discrepancy in the frequency of TLESRs is due to the definitions of TLESR that vary according to study. An early study reported that TLESRs occurred at a frequency of about three per hour in patients with reflux disease compared with two per hour in normal subjects, although this study included swallow-associated LES relaxations associated with failed primary peristalsis in the definition of TLESR (78). Since then, several other studies have reported frequencies of TLESRs of three to eight per hour in patients with reflux disease and two to six per hour in normal subjects (79). The size of the meal, posture, and sleep status are some of the variables that influence the frequency of TLESRs and may vary among studies. The presence of a hiatal hernia also increases the frequency of TLESR (80).

The nature of afferent and/or efferent dysfunction that leads to more frequent episodes of TLESR in patients with reflux disease is not clear. More agreement exists about the higher incidence of reflux during TLESRs in patients compared to normal subjects. In normal subjects about 40% to 50% of TLESRs are accompanied by acid reflux compared with 60% to 70% in patients with reflux disease (37,38,54). The factors that determine whether reflux occurs during TLESRs have not been studied systematically. Possibilities include abdominal straining, the presence of hiatal hernia, the degree of esophageal shortening, and duration of TLESRs. Abdominal straining occurs with 15% to 20% of TLESRs and increases the likelihood of reflux from 30% to 60%. However, the prevalence of straining during reflux episodes does not seem to be different between normal subjects and patients with reflux

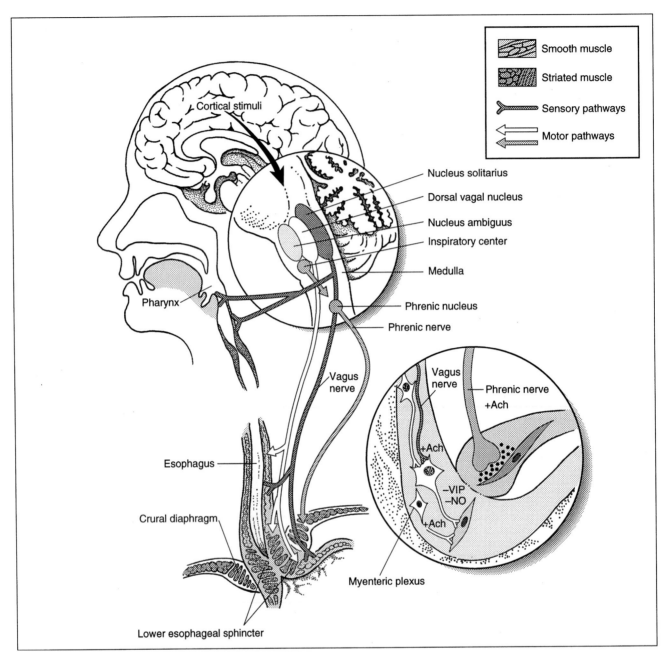

FIGURE 21.3. Schematic of the neural pathway to the lower esophageal sphincter (LES) and crural diaphragm. Swallow-induced esophageal peristalsis and LES relaxation result from excitation of receptors located in the pharynx. The afferent stimulus travels to the sensory nucleus (nucleus tractus solita rius, NTS). A programmed set of events from the dorsomotor nucleus of the vagus and nucleus ambiguus mediate esophageal peristalsis and LES relaxation. The vagal fibers communicate with myenteric neurons, which in turn mediate LES relaxation. The postganglionic transmitter is nitric oxide (NO) and vasoactive intestinal peptide (VIP). Transient LES relaxation (TLESR, the major mechanism of reflux) appears to share the same neural pathway. The afferent signals for TLESR may originate in the pharynx, larynx, and stomach. The efferent pathway is in the vagus nerve, and nitric oxide is the postganglionic neurotransmitter. Crural diaphragm contraction is controlled by the inspiratory center in the brain stem, which communicates with the phrenic nerve nucleus. The crural diaphragm is innervated by right and left phrenic nerves through motor end plates and nicotinic cholinergic receptors. Ach, acetylcholine; +, excitatory; −, inhibitory. (From Mittal RK, Balaban DH. Mechanisms of disease: the esophagogastric junction. *N Engl J Med* 1997;336:924, with permission.)

disease. Hiatal hernia is associated with an increased prevalence of reflux during swallow-induced LES relaxation presumably because of pooling of acid in the herniated gastric pouch (81). A similar mechanism could increase the likelihood of reflux during TLESRs, although this has not been formally examined.

Although not available for clinical use, pharmacologic suppression of TLESR is possible and a desirable form of therapy in reflux disease. Triggering of TLESRs by gastric distension can be inhibited by cholecystokinin (CCK)-A receptor and nitric oxide antagonist (82). This effect of CCK-A antagonist appears to be mediated through a peripheral rather than a central mechanism. Infusion of CCK-A increases the frequency of TLESRs and this increase can be abolished by administration of a nitric oxide antagonist. These observations suggest that CCK-A released after meals may contribute to the provocation of TLESRs by meals, and that nitric oxide is the neurotransmitter released at the postganglionic site in the vagal pathway that is responsible for mediating TLESRs. Even in the absence of CCK-A stimulation, nitric oxide antagonists can block TLESR. However, nitric oxide is important in swallow-induced LES relaxation and its blockade can result in dysphagia and "achalasia-like condition." Atropine also reduces the frequency of TLESRs and reflux after a meal, and the mechanism of its action appears to be at the level of the central nervous system (77,83). Morphine in small doses decreases TLESR frequency in normal subjects through an unknown mechanism (84). Cannabinoid receptor stimulation also inhibits gastric distension–induced TLESR in the dog model (85). The therapeutic potential, however, for most of pharmacologic agents that inhibit TLESR is limited because of the anticipated side effects of these agents. More recently, GABA β-agonist baclofen has been found to reduce TLESR and GER in dogs, ferrets, and humans (86–89). Balcofen significantly reduces the frequency of gastric distension–induced as well as spontaneous TLESR. A single dose of baclofen, 40 mg by mouth, reduced GER as well as TLESR by 50% in normal subjects as well as in patients with GER disease (88,89). It is possible that GABA agonist-like compounds may be useful in treating mild to moderate GER disease.

EFFECT OF ANTIREFLUX THERAPY ON TRANSIENT LOWER ESOPHAGEAL SPHINCTER RELAXATION

The effect of medical therapy for reflux disease on TLESRs has received little attention. In patients with reflux disease, the presence or absence of endoscopically visible esophagitis does not influence the rate of TLESRs after meals. However, the effect of healing of esophagitis with acid suppressants on the rate of TLESRs is controversial; omeprazole has been reported to have no effect (43), while H2 antagonists

have been reported to decrease the rate of TLESRs (42). At standard doses, cisapride does not appear to influence the rate of TLESRs up to 3 hours after a meal (50). The failure of therapy to influence the cause of reflux presumably explains why reflux disease relapses so promptly when medical therapy is terminated. Although a plethora of studies have investigated the effect of antireflux surgery on LES function, only one has examined the effect on TLESRs (90). This study showed that fundoplication has two major effects: a 50% reduction in the rate of TLESRs, and a reduction in the proportion of TLESRs that were accompanied by reflux from 47% to 17%. The mechanisms underlying these effects include (a) the creation of an artificial high-pressure zone around the LES by fundoplication that persists during both transient and swallow-induced LES relaxation (91); and (b) possibly a reduction in the degree of distension of the gastric cardia by the gastric wrap, which may reduce the gastric distension–induced stimulation of TLESRs.

LOWER ESOPHAGEAL SPHINCTER HYPOTENSION IN REFLUX DISEASE

Even though TLESR is the major mechanism of reflux, a low LES pressure is an important mechanism of reflux in patients with reflux disease (92). In the presence of a low LES pressure, reflux is thought to occur either freely from the stomach into the esophagus (free reflux) or during periods of abdominal strain (contraction of abdominal wall, which increases intragastric pressure). Swallow-induced reflux and reflux episodes in which the mechanism cannot be clearly determined also occur in the setting of low LES pressure (38). However, it is interesting that a low LES pressure induced by atropine in normal subjects does not cause reflux episode (77). All the straining maneuvers—that is, coughing, abdominal straining, straight leg raising, and so on—do not induce reflux during LES hypotension induced by atropine. The contraction of the crural diaphragm during these maneuvers is a protective antireflux barrier and is probably sufficient to guard against the occurrence of reflux during periods of increased intra-abdominal pressure. How low LES pressure causes reflux is not entirely clear. One possibility is that both low pressure and hiatal hernia are required for the occurrence of erosive esophagitis. A low LES pressure may allow movement of acid from the herniated pouch into the esophagus across a hypotensive LES. Alternatively, in the presence of a hernia, the diaphragmatic hiatus is incompetent and allows the stomach contents to move freely from the stomach below the diaphragm into the herniated sac and then into the esophagus. Along those lines, the severity of esophagitis appears to correlate directly with the size of hiatal hernia and indirectly with the magnitude of the LES pressure (93,94). The larger the hernia, the wider the esophageal hiatus, and the more likely it is that the crural diaphragm component of the sphincter is incompetent. The hiatal hernia may play an important role in the pathophysiology of reflux from several other aspects (80,95,96) as well (see Chapter 20).

Patients with erosive esophagitis usually have low LES pressure. The degree of endoscopic esophagitis seems to correspond directly with LES pressure. A low LES pressure is the hallmark in patients with scleroderma of the esophagus and is considered to be the primary etiologic factor. Patients with scleroderma have the most severe form of the reflux esophagitis. A low LES pressure in scleroderma is due to the replacement of the LES muscle by connective tissue (97). The reason for low LES pressure in the more common variety of reflux disease is not entirely clear. An anatomical separation between the LES and crural diaphragm, as occurs in hiatal hernia, may contribute to low LES pressure (95). It is possible that low LES pressure is due to primary myogenic or neurogenic failure of the LES muscle. Even though there are no data to prove the matter one way or the other, it is entirely possible that low LES pressure is secondary to acid-induced damage to the LES muscle. Animal experiments reveal that instillation of acid into the cat esophagus results in the reduction of LES pressure (98). However, healing of esophagitis with omeprazole does not improve LES pressure in patients with erosive disease. The reason for the latter may be that acid-induced damage

causes permanent and irreversible alterations in the contractile apparatus of the LES muscle.

It is possible to propose a unifying hypothesis that incorporates TLESR, low LES pressure, and hiatal hernia in the pathogenesis of reflux disease. The initial pathologic event in reflux disease is most likely frequent TLESRs and acid reflux episodes. Acid in the esophagus causes esophagitis, which leads to low LES pressure and esophageal hypotension (98). Furthermore, esophagitis induces esophageal shortening through acid-induced contraction of the longitudinal muscles (99). Subsequently, fibrosis develops, which results in a hiatal hernia. The hiatal hernia, in turn, enlarges the esophageal hiatus, thus impairing the sphincter function of the crural diaphragm. The appearance of a hiatal hernia and a weak diaphragmatic sphincter introduces additional mechanisms of reflux, thus exacerbating the esophagitis. Although plausible, definite proof of this hypothesis awaits further investigation.

ROLE OF ESOPHAGEAL PERISTALSIS IN REFLUX DISEASE

Esophageal peristalsis plays a key role in the clearance of refluxed material from the esophagus. Esophageal acid clearance is a two-step process comprised of bolus clearance and acid neutralization (100,101). If a ≤15-ml bolus of acid

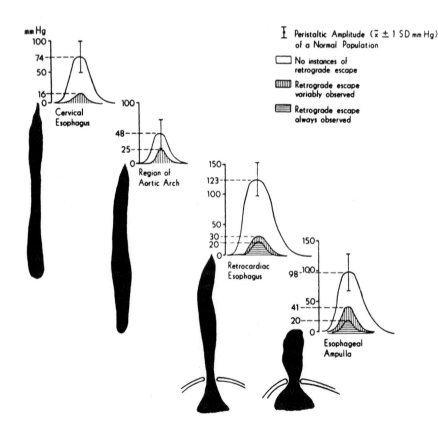

FIGURE 21.4. Data on impaired esophageal volume clearance categorized by esophageal region. The necessary peristaltic amplitude increases progressively with increasingly distal esophageal locations. Upper curves indicate the mean peristaltic amplitude of normal subjects in each esophageal region. Vertically hatched areas indicate peristaltic amplitudes variably associated with impaired esophageal bolus clearance, and horizontal hatched areas indicate amplitudes invariably associated with impaired volume clearance. (From Kahrilas PJ, The anatomy and physiology of dysphagia. In: Gelfand DW, Richter JE, eds. *Dysphagia, diagnosis and treatment.* New York: Igaku-shoin, 1989, with permission.)

is instilled into the esophagus, the majority of the acid can be cleared from the esophagus into the stomach by a peristaltic contraction of the esophagus. The remainder of the acid lining the esophageal mucosa is neutralized by saliva traversing the esophagus during subsequent swallow-induced peristaltic contractions. It takes seven to ten swallows following esophageal acidification for the restoration of the normal esophageal pH of 5 to 7.

How strong of an esophageal peristaltic contraction does one need for an efficient bolus clearance? An esophageal contraction of >30 mm Hg is usually sufficient in the supine position for bolus clearance (102) (Fig. 21.4). However, depending upon the viscosity of the bolus, a contraction of even <30 mm Hg may be able to clear the esophagus efficiently. A subgroup of patients, usually with severe reflux disease, have low esophageal contraction amplitude (termed "ineffective esophageal motility"; see Chapter 11), which could result in an impaired ability to clear an acid

bolus from the esophagus following a reflux episode (103). The prevalence of peristaltic dysfunction increases with the increasing severity of esophagitis. The study by Kahrilas et al. (102) reported that 25% of individuals with mild esophagitis and 50% of patients with severe esophagitis had severe peristaltic dysfunction. The definition of abnormal peristalsis, based on studies in normal subjects, was that 50% of tested peristaltic sequences had to have a demonstrable abnormality (Fig. 21.5). Whether esophageal peristaltic dysfunction is a primary defect or results secondarily from acid-induced esophagitis is not clear. There is good experimental evidence to indicate that acid injury to the esophagus can impair esophageal contraction. However, healing of esophagitis in patients with low contraction amplitudes does not revert the contraction amplitudes back to normal. Patients with scleroderma and mixed connective disorders have a similar defect in peristalsis due to the replacement of the esophageal muscles with fibrous connective tissue (97).

SUMMARY

The smooth-muscle LES and crural diaphragm are two main components of the antireflux barrier. Gastroesophageal reflux occurs primarily due to an incompetent LES. Transient relaxation of the lower esophageal sphincter and crural diaphragm is the major mechanism of reflux in patients with reflux disease. The nature of afferent dysfunction that causes frequent TLESRs is not known. Other reflux mechanisms are a hypotensive LES and the presence of hiatal hernia. Severity of esophagitis correlates directly with hernia size and indirectly with LES pressure. Ineffective esophageal motility found in patients with moderate to severe reflux disease impairs bolus clearance of the acid and thus increases acid contact time with the esophageal mucosa. Future studies need to address the nature of neural dysfunction that leads to frequent TLESRs and the mechanism by which hiatus hernia develops and contributes to the pathogenesis of reflux disease. Novel pharmacologic therapies that inhibit TLESRs are definitely an important avenue that requires further investigation and exploration.

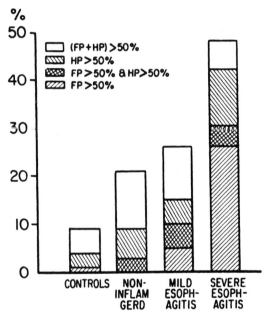

FIGURE 21.5. Bar graph indicating the prevelance of peristaltic dysfunction in patient and control groups. The control group was composed of 31 normal volunteers and 48 patients who were having manometry for reasons other than reflux disease and major motor disorders. Patients with reflux disease (n=33) had a positive Bernstein test, but no demonstrable esophagitis by endoscopy or histology. Patients with mild esophagitis (n=38) had either histologically demonstrable esophagitis or endoscopically evident exudative esophagitis. Patients with severe esophagitis (n=27) had either esophageal ulcerations or strictures. The criteria for abnormality was the occurrence of either failed primary (FP) or regional hypotensive peristalsis (27 mm Hg) in the distal esophagus (HP) with more than half of the test swallows. Overall, 9% of the controls, 21% of patients with mild esophagitis, and 48% of patients with severe esophagitis had abnormal peristaltic function by these criteria. (From Ireland AC, Dent J, Holloway RH. The role of head position in the postural control of transient lower oesophageal sphincter relaxations and belching. *Gullet* 1992;2:81, with permission.)

REFERENCES

1. Ingelfinger FJ. Esophageal motility. *Physiol Rev* 1958;38:533.
2. Fyke FE, Code CF. Gastroesophageal sphincter in healthy human beings. *Gastroenterologia (Basel)* 1956;86:135.
3. Boyle JT, Altschuler SM, Nixon TE, et al. Role of the diaphragm in the genesis of lower esophageal sphincter pressure in the cat. *Gastroenterology* 1985;88:723.
4. Heine KJ, Dent J, Mittal RK. Anatomical relationship between the crural diaphragm and the lower esophageal sphincter: an electrophysiologic study. *J Gastrointest Motil* 1993;5:89.
5. Ott DJ, Gelfand DW, Wu WC, et al. Esophagogastric region and its rings. *AJR Am J Roentgenol* 1984;142:281.

6. Shezhang L, Brasseur JG, Pouderoux P, et al. The phrenic ampulla: distal esophagus or potential hiatal hernia. *Am J Physiol* 1995;268:G320.

7. Liu JB, Miller LS, Goldberg BB, et al. Transnasal ultrasound of the esophagus: preliminary morphologic and function studies. *Radiology* 1992;184:721.

8. Liu J, Parashar V, Mittal RK. Asymmetry of the lower esophageal sphincter: is it related to the muscle thickness or shape of the lower esophageal sphincter? *Am J Physiol* 1997;272:G1509.

9. Sengupta A, Paterson WG, Goyal RK. Atypical localization of myenteric neurons in the opossum lower esophageal sphincter. *Am J Anat* 1987;180:352.

10. Liebermann-Meffert M, Allgower M, Schmidt P, et al. Muscular equivalent of the lower esophageal sphincter. *Gastroenterology* 1979;76:31.

11. Thor K, Hill LD, Mercer CD, et al. Reappraisal of the flap valve mechanism: a study of a new valvuloplasty procedure in cadavers. *Acta Chir Scand* 1987;153:25.

12. Langman J. *Medical embryology*, 3d ed. Baltimore: Williams & Wilkins, 1975.

13. Delattre JF, Palot JP, Ducasse A, et al. The crura of the diaphragm and diaphragmatic passage. *Anat Clin* 1985;4:271.

14. Altschuler SM, Boyle JT, Nixon TE, et al. Disassociation of costal and crural contractile effects on the gastroesophageal high pressure zone. *Gastroenterology* 1985;88:1305.

15. Klein WA, Parkman HP, Williams L, et al. Sphincter-like thoraco-abdominal high pressure zone after esophagogastrectomy. *Gastroenterology* 1993;105:1362.

16. Dent J, Wylie J, Dodds J, et al. Interdigestive phasic contractions of the human lower esophageal sphincter. *Gastroenterology* 1983;84:453.

17. Mittal RK, Rochester DF, McCallum RW. Electrical and mechanical activity in the human lower esophageal sphincter during diaphragmatic contraction. *J Clin Invest* 1988;81:1182.

18. Mittal RK, Fisher M, Rochester DF, et al. Human lower esophageal sphincter response to increased abdominal pressure. *Am J Physiol* 1990;258:624.

19. Dodds WJ, Dent J, Hogan WF, et al. Effect of atropine on esophageal motor function in humans. *Am J Physiol* 1989;240:G290.

20. Biancani P, Hillemeier C, Bitar KN, et al. Contraction mediated by Ca^{2+} influx in esophageal muscle and by Ca^{2+} release in the LES. *Am J Physiol* 1987;253:G760.

21. Chung SA, Diamant NE. Small intestinal motility in fasted and postprandial states: effects of transient vagosympathetic blockade. *Am J Physiol* 1987;252:G301.

22. Collman PI, Tremblay L, Diamant NE. The central vagal efferent supply to the esophagus and lower esophageal sphincter of the cat. *Gastroenterology* 1993;104:1430.

23. Goyal RK, Rattan S. Nature of vagal inhibitory innervation to the lower esophageal sphincter. *J Clin Invest* 1975;55:1119.

24. Yamato S, Saha JK, Goyal RK. Role of nitric oxide in lower esophageal sphincter relaxation to swallowing. *Life Sci* 1992;50:1263.

25. Roussos C, Macklem PT. The respiratory muscle. *N Engl J Med* 1982;307:786.

26. Darian GB, DiMarco AF, Kelsen SG, et al. Effects of progressive hypoxia on parasternal, costal and crural diaphragm activation. *J Appl Physiol* 1989;66:2579.

27. Altschuler SM, Boyle JT, Nixon TE, et al. Simultaneous reflex inhibition of lower esophageal sphincter and crural diaphragm in cats. *Am J Physiol* 1985;249:G586.

28. Martin C, Dodds W, Liem H, et al. Diaphragmatic contribution to gastroesophageal competence and reflux in dogs. *Am J Physiol* 1992;263:G551.

29. Monges H. Dissociation between the electrical activity of the diaphragmatic dome and crura muscular fibers during esophageal distension, vomiting and eructation: an electromyographic study in the dog. *J Physiol Paris* 1978;74:541.

30. Dent J, Holloway RH, Toouli J, et al. Mechanisms of lower esophageal sphincter incompetence in patients with symptomatic gastroesophageal reflux. *Gut* 1988;29:1020.

31. Mittal RK, Chowdhry NK, Liu J. Is the sphincter function of crural diaphragm impaired in patients with reflux esophagitis? *Gastroenterology* 1995;108:A169.

32. Katzka DA, Sidhu M, Castell DO. Hypertensive lower esophageal sphincter pressures and gastroesophageal reflux disease: an apparent paradox that is not unusual. *Am J Gastroenterol* 1995;90:280.

33. Mittal RK, Holloway RH, Penagini R, et al. Transient lower esophageal sphincter relaxation. *Gastroenterology* 1995;109:601.

34. McNally EF, Kelly JE, Ingelfinger FJ. Mechanism of belching: effects of gastric distention with air. *Gastroenterology* 1964;46:254.

35. Dent J, Dodds WJ, Friedman RH, et al. Mechanism of gastroesophageal reflux in recumbent asymptomatic human subjects. *J Clin Invest* 1980;65:256.

36. Schoeman MN, Akkermans LMA, Tippett MD, et al. Mechanisms of gastroesophageal reflux in ambulant healthy human subjects. *Gastroenterology* 1995;109:1315.

37. Dodds WJ, Kahrilas PJ, Dent J, et al. Analysis of spontaneous gastroesophageal reflux and esophageal acid clearance in patients with reflux esophagitis. *J Gastrointest Motil* 1990;2:79.

38. Mittal RK, McCallum RW. Characteristics and frequency of transient relaxations of the lower esophageal sphincter on patients with reflux esophagitis. *Gastroenterology* 1988;95:593.

39. Penagini R, Schoeman M, Holloway R, et al. Mechanisms of reflux in ambulant patients with reflux esophagitis. *Gastroenterology* 1994;A159:106(abst).

40. Cucchiara S, Staiano A, Di Lorenzo C, et al. Pathophysiology of gastroesophageal reflux and distal esophageal motility in children with gastroesophageal reflux disease. *J Pediatr Gastroenterol Nutr* 1988;7:830.

41. Werlin SL, Dodds WJ, Hogan WJ, et al. Mechanisms of gastroesophageal reflux in children. *J Pediatr* 1980;97:244.

42. Baldi F, Longanesi A, Frrarini F, et al. Oesophageal motor function and outcome of treatment with H2-blockers in erosive oesophagitis. *J Gastrointest Motil* 1992;4:165.

43. Downton J, Dent J, Heddle R, et al. Elevation of gastric pH heals peptic oesophagitis—a role for omeprazole. *J Gastroenterol Hepatol* 1987;2:317.

44. Holloway RH, Penagini R. Criteria for the objective definition of transient lower esophageal sphincter relaxation. *Am J Physiol* 1994;268:G183.

45. Mittal RK, McCallum RW. Characteristics of transient lower esophageal sphincter relaxation in humans. *Am J Physiol* 1987;252:G636.

46. Sifrim D, Janssens J, Vantrappen G, et al. Is the esophageal body inhibited during inappropriate LES relaxations? *Gastroenterology* 1992;102:A514(abst).

47. Mittal RK, Fisher MJ. Electrical and mechanical inhibition of the crural diaphragm during transient relaxation of the lower esophageal sphincter. *Gastroenterology* 1990;99:1265.

48. Ergun G, Kahrilas P, Lin S, et al. Shape, volume, and content of the deglutitive pharyngeal chamber imaged by ultrafast computerised tomography. *Gastroenterology* 1993;105:1396.

49. Franzi S, Martin C, Cox M, et al. Response of canine lower esophageal sphincter to gastric distension. *Am J Physiol* 1990;259:G380.

50. Holloway RH, Downton J, Mitchell BE, et al. Effect of cis-

apride on postprandial gastrooesophageal reflux. *Gut* 1989;30: 1187.

51. Penagini R, Bartesaghi B, Conte D, et al. Rate of transient lower oesophageal sphincter relaxations of healthy humans after eating a mixed nutrient meal: time course and comparison with fasting. *Eur J Gastroenterol Hepatol* 1992;4:35.

52. Mittal RK, Stewart WR, Schirmer BD. Effect of a catheter in the pharynx on the frequency of transient lower esophageal relaxations. *Gastroenterology* 1992;103:1236.

53. Miller AJ. Neurophysiological basis of swallowing. *Dysphagia* 1986;1:91.

54. Mittal RK, Chiareli C, Liu J, et al. Characteristics of LES relaxation induced stimulation of the pharynx with minute amounts of water. *Gastroenterology* 1996;111:378.

55. Paterson WG, Rattan S, Goyal RK. Experimental induction of isolated lower esophageal sphincter relaxation in anesthetized opossums. *J Clin Invest* 1986;77:1187.

56. Storey AT. Laryngeal initiation of swallowing. *Exp Neurol* 1968; 20:359.

57. Ireland AC, Dent J, Holloway RH. Preservation of postural suppression of belching in patients with reflux esophagitis. *Gastroenterology* 1992;102:A87(abst).

58. Ireland AC, Dent J, Holloway RH. The role of head position in the postural control of transient lower oesophageal sphincter relaxations and belching. *Gullet* 1992;2:81.

59. Little A, Cox M, Martin C, et al. Influence of posture on transient lower oesophageal sphincter relaxation and gastrooesophageal reflux in dogs. *J Gastroenterol Hepatol* 1989;4:49.

60. Freidin N, Mittal RK, McCallum RW. Does body posture affect the incidence and mechanism of gastro-oesophageal reflux? *Gut* 1991;32:133.

61. Freidin N, Fisher MJ, Taylor W, et al. Sleep and nocturnal acid reflux in normal subjects and patients with reflux esophagitis. *Gut* 1991;32:1275.

62. Cox M, Martin C, Dent J, et al. Effect of general anaesthesia on transient lower oesophageal sphincter relaxations in the dog. *Aust NZ J Surg* 1988;58:825.

63. Penagini R, Bartesaghi B, Bianchi PA. Effect of cold stress on postprandial lower esophageal sphincter competence and gastroesophageal reflux in healthy subjects. *Dig Dis Sci* 1992;37: 1200.

64. Reynolds RPE, El-Sharkawy TY, Diamant NE. Lower esophageal sphincter function in the cat: role of central innervation assessed by transient vagal blockade. *Am J Physiol* 1984; 246:G666.

65. Ryan JP, Snape WJ, Cohen S. Influence of vagal cooling on esophageal function. *Am J Physiol* 1977;232:E159.

66. Cannon WB, Lieb CW. The receptive relaxation of the stomach. *Am J Physiol* 1912;29:267.

67. Martin CJ, Patrikios J, Dent J. Abolition of gas reflux and transient lower esophageal sphincter relaxation by vagal blockage in the dog. *Gastroenterology* 1986;91:890.

68. Strombeck D, Harrold D, Ferrier W. Eructation of gas through the gastroesophageal sphincter before and after truncal vagotomy in dogs. *Am J Vet Res* 1987;48:207.

69. Holloway RH, Wyman JB, Dent J. Failure of transient lower oesphageal sphincter relaxation in response to gastric distention in patients with achalasia: evidence for neural mediation of transient lower oesophageal sphincter relaxations. *Gut* 1989;30:762.

70. Andrews PLR, Grundy D, Scratcherd T. Vagal afferent discharge from mechanoreceptors in different regions of the ferret stomach. *J Physiol* 1980;298:513.

71. Blackshaw L, Grundy D, Scratcherd T. Vagal afferent discharge from gastric mechanoreceptors during contraction and relaxation of the ferret corpus. *J Auton Nerv Sys* 1987;18:19.

72. Rinaman L, Card JP, Schwaber JS, et al. Ultrastructural demonstration of a gastric monosynaptic vagal circuit in the nucleus of the solitary tract in rat. *J Neurosci* 1989;9:1985.

73. Kalia M, Mesulam MM. Brainstem projections of sensory and motor components of the vagus complex in the cat. II. Laryngeal, tracheobronchial, pulmonary, cardiac, and gastrointestinal branches. *J Comp Neurol* 1980;193:467.

74. Schulze-Delrieu K, Percy WH, Ren J, et al. Evidence for inhibition of opossum LES through intrinsic gastric nerves. *Am J Physiol* 1989;256:G198.

75. Berger AJ, Mitchell RA, Severingham SW. Regulation of respiration I. *N Engl J Med* 1977;297:134.

76. Altschuler SM, Davies RO, Pack AI. Role of medullary inspiratory neurones in the control of the diaphragm during oesophageal stimulation in the cats. *J Physiol* 1987;391:289.

77. Mittal RK, Holloway R, Dent J. Effect of atropine on the frequency of transient lower esophageal sphincter relaxation and acid reflux in normal subjects. *Gastroenterology* 1995;109:1547.

78. Dodds WJ, Dent J, Hogan WJ, et al. Mechanism of gastroesophageal reflux in patients with reflux esophagitis. *N Engl J Med* 1982;307:1547.

79. Sifrim D, Holloway R. Transient lower esophageal sphincter relaxations: how many or how harmful? *Am J Gastroenterol* 2001;96:2529.

80. Kahrilas PJ, Shi G, Manka M, et al. Increased frequency of transient lower esophageal sphincter relaxation induced by gastric distention in reflux patients with hiatal hernia. *Gastroenterology* 2000;118:688.

81. Mittal RK, Lange RC, McCallum RW. Identification and mechanism of delayed esophageal acid clearance in subjects with hiatus hernia. *Gastroenterology* 1987;92:130.

82. Boulant J, Fioramonti J, Dpoigny M, et al. Cholecystokinin and nitric oxide in transient lower esophageal sphincter relaxation to gastric distension in dogs. *Gastroenterology* 1994;107:1059.

83. Fang JC, Sarosiek I, Arora T, et al. Cholinergic blockade inhibits gastroesophageal reflux and transient lower esophageal sphincter relaxation through a central mechanism. *Am J Gastroenterol* 1997;9:1590.

84. Penagini R, Picone A, Bianchi P. Morphine reduces gastroesophageal reflux in reflux disease though a decrease in the rate of transient lower esophageal sphincter relaxation. *Gastroenterology* 1996;110:A227.

85. Lehmann A, Blackshaw LA, Branden L, et al. Cannabinoid receptor agonism inhibits transient lower esophageal sphincter relaxations and reflux in dogs. *Gastroenterology* 2002;123: 1129–1134. Erratum in: *Gastroenterology* 2002 Dec;123(6): 2162–2163.

86. Blackshaw LA, Staunton E, Lehmann A, et al. Inhibition of transient LES relaxations and reflux in ferrets by GABA receptor agonists. *Am J Physiol* 1999;277:867–874.

87. Lehmann A, Antonsson M, Bremner-Danielsen M, et al. Activation of the GABA(B) receptor inhibits transient lower esophageal sphincter relaxations in dogs. *Gastroenterology* 1999; 117:1147.

88. Lidums I, Lehmann A, Checklin H, et al. Control of transient lower esophageal sphincter relaxations and reflux by the GABA(B) agonist baclofen in normal subjects. *Gastroenterology* 2000;118:7–13.

89. Zhang Q, Lehmann A, Rigda R, et al. Control of transient lower oesophageal sphincter relaxations and reflux by the GABA$_B$ agonist baclofen in patients with gastro-oesophageal reflux disease. *Gut* 2001;50:19.

90. Ireland AC, Holloway RH, Toouli J, et al. Mechanisms underlying the antireflux action of fundoplication. *Gut* 1993;34:303.

91. Kiroff GK, Maddern GJ, Jamieson GG. A study of factors responsible for the efficacy of fundoplication in the treatment of gastro-oesophageal reflux. *Aust NZ J Surg* 1984;54:109.

92. Holloway RH, Dent J. Pathophysiology of gastroesophageal reflux: lower esophageal dysfunction in reflux disease. *Gastorenterol Clin North Am* 1990;19:517.

93. Jones MP, Sloan SS, Rabine JC, et al. Hiatal hernia size is the dominant determinant of esophagitis presence and severity in gastroesophageal reflux disease. *Am J Gastroenterol* 2001;96:1711.

94. Sloan S, Rademaker AW, Kahrilas PJ. Determinants of gastroesophageal junction incompetence: hiatal hernia, lower esophageal sphincter, or both? *Ann Intern Med* 1992;117:977.

95. Kahrilas PJ, Lin S, Chen J, et al. The effect of hiatus hernia on gastro-oesophageal junction pressure. *Gut* 1999;44:476.

96. Pandolfino JE, Shi G, Curry J, et al. Esophagogastric junction distensibility: a factor contributing to sphincter incompetence. *Am J Physiol Gastrointest Liver Physiol* 2002;282:1052.

97. Miller LS, Liu JB, Klenn PJ, et al. Endoluminal ultrasonography of the distal esophagus in systemic sclerosis. *Gastroenterology* 1993;105:31.

98. Eastwood GL, Castell DO, Higgs RH. Experimental esophagitis in cats impairs lower esophageal sphincter pressure. *Gastroenterology* 1975;69:14.

99. Paterson WG, Kolyn DM. Esophageal shortening induced by short-term intraluminal acid perfusion in opossum: a cause for hiatus hernia? *Gastroenterology* 1994;107:1738.

100. Helm JF, Dodds WJ, Riedel DR, et al. Determinants of esophageal acid clearance in normal subjects. *Gastroenterology* 1983;85:607.

101. Helm JF, Dodds WJ, Pelc LR, et al. Effect of esophageal emptying and saliva on clearance of acid from the esophagus. *N Engl J Med* 1984;310:284.

102. Kahrilas PJ, Dodds WJ, Hogan WJ. Effect of peristaltic dysfunction on esophageal volume clearance. *Gastroenterology* 1988;94:73.

103. Kahrilas PJ, Dodds WJ, Hogan WJ, et al. Esophageal peristaltic dysfunction in peptic esophagitis. *Gastroenterology* 1986;91:897.

PATHOPHYSIOLOGY OF GASTROESOPHAGEAL REFLUX DISEASE: ESOPHAGEAL EPITHELIAL RESISTANCE

ROY C. ORLANDO

Twenty-four-hour intraesophageal pH monitoring reveals that the phenomenon of gastroesophageal (acid) reflux is for the most part a benign physiologic process that occurs in everyone every day, and is especially common following meals (1,2). This indicates that the antireflux barriers—as constituted by the lower esophageal sphincter (LES), diaphragm, acute angle of His, phrenoesophageal ligament, mucosal rosette, and other structures—are functionally imperfect by design. The reasons for this are to some extent apparent in as much as there is the regular need to vent gas (belch) from the stomach, especially postprandially, and, at times, vomiting is required to more rapidly and completely empty the stomach. Yet, and presumably as an unintended consequence of gas venting, which activates transient LES relaxations, acid as well as gas escapes from the stomach and into the esophagus. Moreover, esophageal exposure to highly acidic gastric contents even occurs postprandially despite the buffering of the majority of the gastric luminal contents by the meal. This results from the presence of an "acid pocket" in the upper stomach that enables unbuffered gastric juice to escape into the esophagus during transient LES relaxations triggered by meal-induced gastric (fundic) distension (3). Nonetheless, while repeated daily contact of the esophageal epithelium with acidic gastric contents is universal, reflux-induced damage to esophageal epithelium is not.

The reason for the lack of correlation between reflux frequency per se and reflux damage to the esophageal epithelium is due to the existence of two additional esophageal defenses: (a) the luminal clearance mechanisms; and (b) esophageal epithelial (tissue) resistance. The luminal clearance mechanisms can be viewed as the second major defense against acid injury to the esophagus. They come into play after an episode of reflux occurs and consist of gravity and peristalsis for removal of the refluxed bolus and swallowed salivary secretions and esophageal submucosal gland secretions for dilution and neutralization of any residual esophageal acidity. Consequently, acid reflux alone appears relatively inconsequential as long as the clearance mechanisms are operative, which limit the contact time between acidic gastric juice and the esophagus in healthy subjects to a few minutes (3 to 5) per episode and a total of 1 to 2 hours of acidity per day. Nonetheless, as is apparent by the cited contact times, acid clearance is not immediate and neither is it uniform, with episodes even more prolonged at night when most clearance mechanisms are inoperative (4–6). Therefore, it becomes apparent that the final arbiter between health and disease is tissue resistance, the third and last esophageal defense. Specifically, it is the intrinsic resistance of the esophageal epithelium that ultimately determines whether the rate and degree of acid clearance are sufficient to prevent injury. Moreover, and perhaps surprising to some, the intrinsic resistance of the esophageal epithelium to acid injury is considerable, effectively providing a wide margin of protection in both animals and humans. This is amply illustrated, for example, by the *in vivo* observations that even 3.5 hours of continuous perfusion of the rabbit esophagus with hydrochloric (HCl) acid, pH 2, or 30 minutes of continuous perfusion of the human esophagus with HCl, pH 1.1 (Bernstein test), are inadequate to produce damage to the epithelium or (in humans) elicit the symptom of heartburn (7–12). "Tissue resistance," or what makes the esophagus relatively invulnerable to these levels of acidity, is the subject of this chapter.

For the sake of discussion, the components of "tissue resistance" can be separated into three categories based on their anatomic relationship to the epithelium proper: pre-epithelial, epithelial, and postepithelial factors as listed in

R. C. Orlando: Section of Gastroenterology and Hepatology, Center for Esophageal and Swallowing Disorders, Tulane University School of Medicine, New Orleans, Louisiana.

TABLE 22.1. FACTORS CONTRIBUTING TO ESOPHAGEAL MUCOSAL RESISTANCE AGAINST INJURY BY LUMINAL ACID

Pre-epithelial defense
   Mucous layer
   Unstirred water layer
   Surface bicarbonate ion concentration
Epithelial defense
Structures
   Cell membranes
   Intercellular junctional complexes (tight junctions,
      glycoconjugates/lipid)
Functions
   Epithelial transport (Na^+/H^+ exchanger, Na^+-dependent
      Cl^-/HCO_3^- exchanger)
   Intracellular and extracellular buffers
   Cell restitution
   Cell replication
Postepithelial defense
   Blood flow
   Tissue acid-base status

Modified from Orlando RC. Esophageal epithelial defenses against acid injury. *Am J Gastroenterol* 1994;89;S48, with permission.

Table 22.1. Since acid and pepsin are the major injurious factors in reflux esophagitis, tissue resistance will be described as it relates to the defense against these agents. Moreover, the approach taken is based on the generally accepted concept that reflux esophagitis results from the luminal attack of acid and pepsin and that cell injury and death are the result of cytosolic acidification.

PRE-EPITHELIAL DEFENSES

The pre-epithelial components of tissue resistance are listed in Table 22.1; they include mucus, surface bicar-bonate, and the unstirred water layer. Since these factors are situated on the luminal side of the epithelium, they are the last hurdles before acidic luminal content can access the epithelium proper. This is particularly well illustrated in the stomach and duodenum, which, like the esophagus, also must withstand high levels of luminal acidity. In the stomach and duodenum, there is a pronounced viscoelastic surface mucus layer that is the product of secretions from mucus cells located along the gastric and duodenal surface. Mucus itself is composed of high-molecular-weight glycoproteins and water and serves as a lubricant and protective barrier against mechanical and chemical injury. Mucus, for example, can prevent large protein molecules, such as pepsin, from accessing the underlying epithelium (13), although it has only limited capacity to impede the diffusion of hydrogen ions (H^+) (14,15). Nonetheless, the aqueous environment within mucus contributes to and expands the area of low turbulence adjacent to the epithelium known as the unstirred water layer (16–18). Moreover, the unstirred water layer acts as a sink for bicarbonate ions (HCO_3^-) that are secreted by gastric and duodenal surface cells (15,19). Consequently, the unstirred water layer (including the mucus component) represents a bicarbonate-rich microenvironment adjacent to the epithelial surface and one capable of neutralizing significant amounts of H^+ as they back-diffuse from lumen toward the epithelium (20–22). Indeed, studies using pH micro- or macro-electrodes have shown that the preepithelial defense in stomach and duodenum is sufficiently developed to maintain a surface pH of 5.0 to 7.0 even at a luminal pH as low as 2.0 (Fig. 22.1).

In contrast to the stomach and duodenum, the buffering capacity of the pre-epithelial defense in both human and animal (rabbits, opossums) esophagus is poor to nonexistent. For example, when acid perfusion lowers the luminal

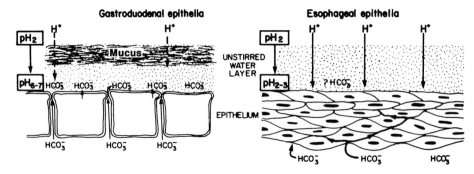

FIGURE 22.1. Pre-epithelial defense. In gastric and duodenal epithelia, H^+ must cross the mucus-unstirred water layer–bicarbonate barrier before contact can be made with the surface of the epithelium. Diffusion of pepsin, but not H^+ is blocked by mucus; however, H^+ can be neutralized by HCO_3^- residing in the unstirred water layer. In contrast to gastric and duodenal epithelia, the preepithelial defense in the esophagus is poorly developed, having an ineffective mucus–HCO_3^- barrier to buffer backdiffusing H^+. (From Orlando RC. Esophageal epithelial defense against acid injury. *J Clin Gastroenterol* 1991;13(suppl 2):S1–S5, with permission.)

pH to 2.0, surface pH in the esophagus falls to 2.0 to 3.0 (21) (Fig. 22.1). And one major reason for this deficiency may be that the esophagus lacks a definable surface mucus layer (23). The lack of a mucus layer is to some degree surprising given that the esophagus is regularly bathed by swallowed salivary secretions containing mucins and, in some species such as humans, by mucins that are secreted from the esophageal submucosal glands (24–27). Presumably, these mucins remain in soluble form due to a lack of appropriate characteristics to form a viscoelastic gel or to be bound to the esophageal surface. In either case lack of a surface mucus layer would impair the preepithelial defense by allowing ready access of refluxed pepsin to the epithelium and by reducing the magnitude of the unstirred water layer with its bicarbonate-rich environment. Moreover, the amount of bicarbonate trapped within the unstirred water layer may be even further reduced by the inability of surface squamous cells to secrete HCO_3^- (27) and the limited permeability across the paracellular route in squamous epithelium for passive diffusion of bicarbonate from blood to lumen (28). Regardless of cause, however, the lack of protection by the preepithelial defense in the esophagus places the major burden for protection against refluxed gastric acid and pepsin squarely on the epithelium proper.

EPITHELIAL DEFENSES

The epithelial defenses are intrinsic properties of the esophageal-stratified squamous epithelium. They come into play when acidic gastric contents enter the esophageal lumen and remain there even for a brief period because of the inadequacy of the buffering capacity of the pre-epithelial defense. For discussion purposes the epithelial defenses within stratified squamous epithelium can be dissected into structural or functional elements, with the best defined listed in Table 22.1.

Esophageal Epithelium: Structure

Structurally, the esophageal epithelium in humans is a partially keratinized, stratified squamous epithelium (24,29). In this respect it is dissimilar to the simple columnar-lined stomach and duodenum, resembling more closely the lining of the oropharynx, larynx, skin, cervix and, in other species, rumen and frog skin. The esophageal-stratified squamous epithelium can be divided into three layers: stratum corneum, stratum spinosum, and stratum germinativum. Occasionally there is a fourth layer known as the stratum granulosum. The stratum granulosum can be identified by the presence in the cytoplasm of keratohyalin granules. The stratum corneum consists of multiple layers of flattened cells lining the luminal surface, with the uppermost cells facing the lumen the oldest and in varying stages of desquamation (29). Consequently, these cells principally provide

mechanical protection against luminal contents but little in the way of barrier function against the permeation of H^+—the latter residing in the remaining, more viable, cell layers of stratum corneum (30–32). Given the inadequacy of the preepithelial defense, the stratum corneum can be viewed as the true first line of (epithelial) defense against back-diffusing H^+.

The structures within the stratum corneum that subserve barrier function are the lipid bilayers of the cell membranes and the intercellular junctional complexes. The junctional complexes regulate (paracellular) permeability between the cells and consist of tight junctions in series with an intercellular matrix composed of glycoconjugates (mostly glycoproteins). Together the apical cell membranes (the section of membrane on the luminal side of the tight junctional proteins) and tight junctions form a planar sheet that serve as a resistor to the permeation of ions and molecules through the cell or through the junctions, respectively. Further, since esophageal epithelium is stratified squamous, planar sheets of squamous epithelial cells and adjacent junctional complexes exist at multiple levels extending the length of the stratum corneum and to some extent into the stratum spinosum below. Moreover, between these planar sheets, sandwich style, is the intercellular matrix of glycoproteins so that together these structures form a series of resistors that impart to the overall epithelial structure a high electrical resistance (30–31) (Fig. 22.2). For example, the transepithelial electrical resistance of esophageal epithelium ranges from 1,000 to 2,500 ohms.cm^2 for human and rabbit esophageal epithelium (9,26,33,34). Electrical resistances of this magnitude indicate the presence of a "tight" epithelium with a low rate of transepithelial ion diffusion. In contrast ion-permeable "leaky" epithelia, such as that of the gallbladder and small intestine, have electrical resistances that are <500 ohms.cm^2 (28,35). Additionally, circuit analysis performed on healthy (rabbit) esophageal epithelium indicates that the transcellular route across apical and basolateral membranes has a resistance that is twice that of the resistance across the paracellular pathway and that the paracellular pathway permits diffusion of small molecules such as mannitol (molecular weight [MW] 182), but not dextrans of 4,000 MW, across the epithelium (36). Moreover, the regulation of the paracellular pathway is in part controlled by e-cadherin, a transmembrane protein that is part of the junctional complex known as the zonula adherens (37). Also, investigations by J. Mullin at Lankenau Institute for Medical Research (unpublished data, Wynnewood, PA, 2003) indicate that the esophagus contains occludin and claudins (isotypes 1 and 2), which are typically found as transmembrane protein components of the tight junction). However, the role of these proteins in the regulation of junctional permeability in esophagus has yet to be clarified.

Tight junctions (zonula occludens and zonula adherens) formed by the interaction of integral membrane proteins

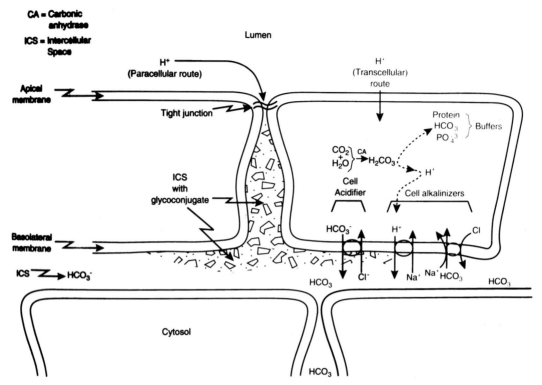

FIGURE 22.2. Epithelial defense. Some of the recognized epithelial defenses against acid injury are illustrated. Structural barriers to H$^+$ diffusion include the cell membrane and intercellular junctional complex. Functional components include intracellular buffering by negatively charged proteins and HCO$_3^-$ and H$^+$ extrusion processes (Na$^+$/H$^+$ exchange and Na$^+$-dependent Cl$^-$/HCO$_3^-$ exchange) for regulation of intracellular pH. (Modified from Orlando RC, Esophageal epithelial defense. In: Castell DO, Wu WC, Ott DJ, eds. *Gastroesophageal reflux disease: pathogenesis, diagnosis, therapy.* Mount Kisco, NY: Futura, 1985:55, with permission.)

from adjacent cell membranes encircle the cells of the layer and seal off the lumen from the intercellular space, much as the plastic wrapping around a six-pack of canned beverages seals off the space above and below the plane of the cans' surface (35). Thus, tight junctions act as a barrier to molecules passing between the cells from lumen to blood and vice versa. Tight junctions, however, are neither impermeable nor equally permeable to all ions; that is, the junction exhibits permselectivity in the rates at which different ionic species pass through it (28,35). Since most tissues have negatively charged ions (e.g., carboxyl, phosphate, and sulfate groups) lining the junctions, they are usually more permeable to cations than to anions. However, as H$^+$ enters the junction, it can titrate the negatively charged ions and so change its permselectivity from cation selective to anion selective (28,35,38). This change in permselectivity then acts to slow the rate of H$^+$ entry into the tissue.

The esophageal epithelium of rabbit and mouse contains an intercellular material that appears to contribute to its barrier function. In this regard, the esophageal epithelium more closely resembles human skin, a dry, stratified squamous epithelium in which spot welds (maculae occlu-

dentes) are supported in their function by the presence of an intercellular lamellar-lipid material. This material is apparently secreted into the intercellular space from membrane-coating granules localized within the lower layers of epidermis (30,39,40). Notably, it is this lamellar-lipid material that appears to create the barrier to diffusion through the intercellular space of human skin and mouse esophagus (30). However, an intercellular glycoprotein, rather than a lipid, appears to subserve a similar barrier function in rabbit esophageal epithelium (31), and, presumably human esophageal epithelium (41).

Esophageal Epithelium: Function

To appreciate the means by which the esophageal epithelium functions to protect itself against acid injury, it is instructive to review what is known about its ion transport capability. *In vivo* esophageal-stratified squamous epithelium has a lumen negative potential difference (PD) of approximately −30 mV in rabbit and −15 mV in humans (42). *In vitro* Ussing chamber studies show that this PD in humans (9) and rabbits (33) is primarily due to the active transport of Na$^+$ from lumen to blood and that this transport is inhibited by serosal application of ouabain (33). Based on Na⁺ transport across frog skin, another moist stratified squamous epithelium (43), luminal Na⁺ passively enters the surface cells down its concentration gradient through apical membrane Na⁺ channels. Na⁺ then diffuses to adjacent cells through cell-to-cell connections called gap junctions and exits across the basolateral membrane to the intercellular spaces by the action of the sodium pump, that is, NaK,ATPase. Since the junctional complex limits Na⁺ diffusion toward the lumen, it diffuses predominantly to the serosal surface of the tissue and into the blood stream. Further, the net movement of Na⁺ from lumen to serosa is relatively rapid while diffusion of its accompanying anion, usually Cl⁻, along its electrochemical gradient is relatively slow. Consequently, there is a net separation of charges in space that creates the measurable PD noted above. With the understanding that the factors which determine PD are of more than theoretical interest, the transmural PD has been used to study the pathogenesis of acid injury to the esophageal epithelium (29,44,45) and for identifying patients with reflux esophagitis and Barrett's esophagus (46,47).

Since the *in vivo* measurement of esophageal PD in healthy animals reflects the structural and functional integrity of the tissue, it is not surprising that the PD is altered in acid-injured epithelia (47–50). However, such alterations are not unidimensional in that PD may rise or fall as a result of changes in epithelial ion permeability and/or transport as well as from nonepithelial factors, such as liquid junction potentials—the latter reflecting differences in ion composition between the luminal solution and recording electrode (45,47,51). For this reason, the observed changes in the *in vivo* PD should be interpreted cautiously and further validated using *in vitro* techniques where variables can be better controlled.

Animal Model of Acid Injury to Esophageal Epithelium

Experimental acid perfusion of the rabbit esophagus *in vivo* results in a biphasic pattern in the esophageal PD (29,44,45). Initially, PD increases and then declines progressively until it reaches zero at 60 minutes (Fig. 22.3). A biphasic PD pattern also can be discerned in humans during acid-perfusion (Bernstein) tests (9) and the abolition of PD demonstrated in those with severe esophagitis (47). From studies of rabbit esophageal epithelium in the Ussing chamber, the initial increase in PD was shown to result from H⁺ diffusion from lumen to blood (45). Indeed, investigators have used the luminal disappearance of H⁺ as a marker of epithelial permeability and damage (11,48,49, 52,53,54).

The path that H⁺ takes across the tissue may be via the cell membranes (transcellular route) and/or the intercellu-

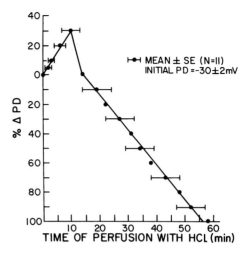

FIGURE 22.3. The percent change in rabbit esophageal transmural potential difference (delta PD) plotted against the time of exposure to 80 mmol HCl–80 mmol NaCl. A transient increase in PD occurs during the first 10 minutes. This is followed by a progressive decline in PD until it reaches zero at 1 hour. Values are means ± standard error, N = 11. PD = –30 mV ± 2 mV. (From Orlando RC, Powell DW, Carney CN. Pathophysiology of acute acid injury in rabbit esophageal epithelium. *J Clin Invest* 1981; 68:286, with permission.)

lar junctions (paracellular route) (45,55). The potential for H⁺ to travel through the apical membrane Na⁺ channel was reported previously by Palmer (56) in toad bladders; and an effect of luminal acidity on apical membrane Na channels was suggested for esophageal epithelium by the fact that Na⁺ absorption decreased in the presence of luminal acid and increased upon its removal (45). However, when surface squamous cells within intact esophageal epithelium were impaled with pH-sensitive microelectrodes, it was evident that this was not the case since the apical cell membranes were found to be highly impermeant to H⁺ even at luminal pH 2.0. Also, more recent studies by Tobey et al. (57) indicate that luminal acid can regulate the activity of the Na⁺ channel, making it less and less permeable to cations (both Na⁺ and H⁺) as the lumen becomes more and more acidic, thereby providing an effective defense against direct cell acidification. The potential for H⁺ to traverse the intercellular junctions was suggested by the observation that rabbit esophageal PD can be lowered by 50% during acid perfusion without histologic evidence of cell damage but in association with a substantial increase in mannitol flux (44). Further, although cell damage was absent, the increase in mannitol flux across the junctions was associated with "dilated intercellular spaces" on transmission electron microscopy. Notably, "dilated intercellular spaces" have subsequently been identified in humans with nonerosive as well as erosive (reflux) esophagitis (58–62) (Fig. 22.4). In acid-exposed frog skins, separation of the epithelial tight junc-

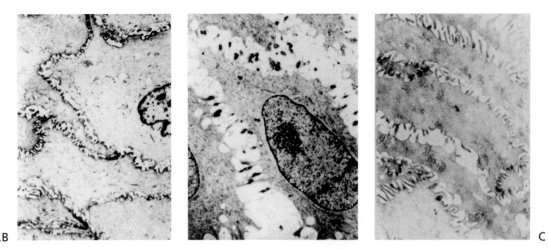

A,B   C

FIGURE 22.4. Transmission electron photomicrographs of an esophageal mucosal biopsy from a (control) subject without esophageal disease **(A)**, a subject with heartburn and erosive esophagitis **(B)**, and a subject with heartburn and nonerosive esophagitis on endoscopy **(C)**. Note the widened intercellular spaces in the two subjects with heartburn. Original magnification ×3,000. (Adapted from Tobey NA, Carson JL, Alkiek RA, et al. Dilated intercellular spaces: a morphological feature of acid reflux—damaged human esophageal epithelium. *Gastroenterology* 1996;111: 1200, with permission.)

tions has been identified as one explanation for these observations (63); however, neither transmission electron microscopy nor freeze fracture showed junctional abnormalities in the acid-treated esophageal epithelium (R.C. Orlando, unpublished data, Tulane University School of Medicine, New Orleans, LA, 2003). Nonetheless, the presence of dilated intercellular spaces in the absence of cell necrosis in patients with reflux disease supports, as in acid-damaged rabbit esophagus, an increase in junctional permeability. Moreover, since there is evidence that sensory neurons in esophageal epithelium can extend to within three cell layers of the lumen, an increase in junctional permeability would increase H^+ access to neurons and provide a reasonable explanation for development of heartburn in patients with nonerosive reflux disease (64,65) (Fig. 22.5). Although the presence of heartburn—or as a surrogate marker in rabbits a decline in esophageal PD by 50%—signals in most (but not necessarily all instances since a leaky barrier permits other nonacidic, yet noxious, luminal content access to the sensory nerves) instances acid permeation into the tissue, cell necrosis is not a preordained outcome (44). This indicates the existence of additional "functional" mechanisms that assist the "structural" mechanisms for protection of the epithelium against irreversible cell damage and necrosis.

Esophageal Epithelial Functions

The functional elements that comprise the epithelial defense against luminal HCl are shown in Table 22.1. These include intracellular and extracellular buffers for

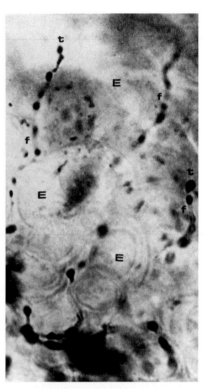

FIGURE 22.5. Photomicrograph showing the nerve fibers (*f*) traversing the intercellular spaces of esophageal epithelium. Macaque, OsO_4–ZnI_2 solution, ×320. (From Rodrigo J, Hernandez DJ, Vidal MA, et al. Vegetative innervation of the esophagus. III. Intraepithelial endings. *Acta Anat (Basel)* 1975;92:242, with permission.)

H+, intracellular pH (pH$_i$) regulation, and mechanisms for tissue repair. Buffers for the neutralization of back-diffusing H+ both within the cytosol and within the intercellular space include phosphates, proteins, and HCO$_3^-$. HCO$_3^-$ is a critical element since its removal from the bathing solution of acid-exposed Ussing-chambered esophageal epithelium leads more readily to cell necrosis than in its presence (66). This buffer is derived from two major sources: one is through the action of carbonic anhydrase, an enzyme within esophageal epithelium (67), and the other through the passive diffusion from blood into the intercellular space of the epithelium (Fig. 22.6). As with all defensive systems, however, the buffering capacity within the esophageal epithelium has limits, especially when the junctional barrier is breached and excessive amounts of luminal H+ diffuse down their concentration gradient from lumen (refluxate pHs in humans as low as 1.0) through the intercellular space toward blood (pH 7.4). Indeed, preservation of a neutral intercellular pH is vital since acidification of the intercellular space is readily translated into acidification of the cell cytosol (66,68). The reason for this is that the basolateral

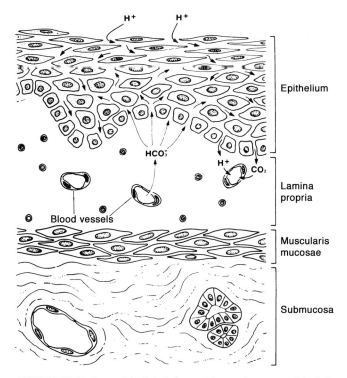

FIGURE 22.6. Postepithelial defense. The major postepithelial defense against acid injury is an adequate blood supply. In addition to providing essential nutrients and oxygen for cell metabolism, the blood supply maintains tissue acid–base balance, a defense dependent on blood delivery of HCO$_3^-$ and removal of H+ and CO$_2$. (From Orlando RC. Reflux esophagitis. In: Yamada T, Alpers DH, Owyang C, et al., eds. *Textbook of gastroenterology.* Philadelphia: JB Lippincott Co, 1991:1123, with permission.)

cell membrane of esophageal epithelial cells—in contrast to the apical cell membrane—is more acid permeable, and a major factor for this feature is the presence within the basolateral membrane of a DIDS-sensitive, (Na-independent) Cl$^-$/HCO$_3^-$ exchanger (66,68). This exchanger is involved in the regulation of pH$_i$ and it does so by preventing the cell from becoming too alkaline by the activity of its acid-extruding mechanisms (see below). The way the exchanger operates to keep pH$_i$ within a neutral range is by extruding HCO$_3^-$ in exchange for extracellular Cl$^-$, an action that is tantamount to the absorption of HCl since cell loss of HCO$_3^-$ from cytosolic H$_2$CO$_3$ is equivalent to cytosolic gain of H+ (see Fig. 22.2). Notably, this gradient-driven operation is beneficial to the cell as long as the intercellular pH—the pH to which it is adjusting cytosolic pH—is neutral. Consequently, when intercellular pH becomes acidic, the gradient favors acid absorption into the cell cytosol through the action of the basolateral membrane Cl$^-$/HCO$_3^-$ exchanger (69). In effect, cell acidification occurs and is deemed appropriate since the Cl$^-$/HCO$_3^-$ exchanger is regulating pH$_i$ to reflect the pH of the intercellular environment. The validity of this model as a modus for cell necrosis in acid-exposed esophageal epithelium has been demonstrated in Ussing chamber studies by documenting the ability of serosal DIDS/SITS to prevent cell necrosis upon exposure of the epithelium to serosal (guaranteeing intercellular) acidity (66,68). Moreover, and both establishing the Cl$^-$ dependence of the process and inability of sulfate to substitute for Cl$^-$ as the exchanged anion on the transporter, similar degrees of serosal acidification with sulfuric acid did not result in cell necrosis. In contrast, serosal acidification with nitric acid (indicating that nitrate can substitute for Cl$^-$ on the exchanger) produced cell necrosis to a similar degree that serosal HCl did in tissues not pretreated with DIDS/SITS.

As described above, cell acidification following intercellular acidification is a prerequisite for cell necrosis. However, all episodes of cell acidification do not result in cell death. This is because esophageal cells also possess two acid-extruding mechanisms that are designed to keep pH$_i$ from falling to and/or remaining at levels of acidity that are destructive to the cell. These mechanisms are an amiloride-sensitive Na+/H+ exchanger (NHE-1 isotype), and a DIDS-sensitive, Na+-dependent Cl$^-$/HCO$_3^-$ exchanger (70–73) (Fig. 22.2). Both are driven by the gradient for Na+ entry into the cytosol that is created by the lowering of intracellular Na by the action of the sodium pump (Na,K,ATPase). Indeed, these two mechanisms work well under normal physiologic conditions in which the ion composition of the fluid within the intercellular space is in equilibrium with blood whose pH is 7.4 and having >30 mM bicarbonate. Consequently, when cellular metabolism produces acidic by-products, these are readily buffered within the cell or within the intercellular space following their removal from the cytosol by the acid-extruding transporters. However, when intercellular acidity is lowered to acidic levels—as a result of luminal acid diffusion across reflux-damaged junctional structures—restoration of pHi to neutrality is delayed due to loss of extracellular buffer (bicarbonate) for acid-extrusion by the Na-dependent Cl^-/HCO_3^- exchanger and the continued influx of acid via the Na-independent Cl^-/HCO_3^- exchanger. Under these conditions, then, the restoration of pHi to neutrality awaits effective luminal acid clearance to reduce the influx of H^+ into the tissue and return of intercellular pH to neutrality. Intercellular pH returns to neutrality by the re-generation of HCO_3^- by carbonic anhydrase and by the renewed influx of HCO_3^- from the blood (see below).

POSTEPITHELIAL DEFENSES

The postepithelial factors that contribute to esophageal protection against acid injury are products of the blood supply (Fig. 22.6). The blood supply delivers nutrients and oxygen for normal cell functions, including cell repair, and removes potentially noxious metabolic by-products, including CO_2 and acids. In regard to the latter, it is important to recognize that the blood supply is critical for preservation of normal tissue acid–base balance, especially because it supplies HCO_3^- to the intercellular space for the buffering of extracellular H^+. The importance of tissue acid–base balance in protecting gastric mucosa against injury has been well documented (74–76). However, the mechanism for this protection may be different than described above for the esophagus in that one report suggests that the mechanism for HCO_3^- protection against acid injury was by the buffering of H^+ intracellularly rather than within the intercellular space (75). It is also important to recognize that protection of the esophagus against acid injury by the blood supply is not a static process, but rather one with adaptive properties. For instance, it has been shown in a number of animal models that esophageal blood flow increases in response to luminal acid perfusion, and in the opossum that the mediators of this change include the release of histamine, nitric oxide and calcitonin gene-related peptide (CGRP) (77–80). These data are in agreement with what has recently been shown for the effects of luminal acidity on gastric blood flow in which back-diffusion of gastric acid leads to protective vasodilation through activation of both sensory neurons with the release of CGRP and mast cells through the release of histamine (H1 and H3 receptors). Moreover, mast cell histamine release in the gastric blood flow model is mediated in part through CGRP release from sensory neurons (81).

EPITHELIAL CELL INJURY

When luminal acid exposure is prolonged, the preepithelial, epithelial, and postepithelial defenses can all be overwhelmed, leading to a decline in pHi and irreversible cell injury. This is evident *in vivo* when acid perfusion in rabbit esophagus has reduced the PD by 80% to 100% of initial value (i.e., approaches zero) (Fig. 22.3). Functionally, net Na^+ transport and NaK,ATPase activity are inhibited (44,45), and morphologically, cell edema and cell necrosis are evident. It is tempting to attribute cell injury and death to the observed H^+ inhibition of NaK,ATPase activity, with its consequent ability to impair both cellular pHi and volume regulation. However, this appears not to be the case, since cell necrosis does not accompany inhibition of NaK,ATPase activity by ouabain (82,83). This lack of cell injury by ouabain may reflect the presence of feedback mechanisms that reduce Na^+ entry across the apical cell membranes in response to decreased Na^+ exit (84). One such mechanism may involve stimulation of a Na^+/Ca^{2+} exchanger, with the resultant increase in intracellular Ca^{2+} reducing the permeability of the apical membrane Na^+ channels (85). An increase in intracellular Ca^{2+}, however, is a two-edged sword since acidification appears to activate via a calcium-dependent mechanism, a membrane NaK2Cl cotransporter. This protein then transports large numbers of ions into the cell, and at a time when the cell has little ability to extrude ions. Consequently, an osmotic gradient is created that favors excessive water entry and thus cell edema (86,87). Since one effect of cell edema is to reduce the concentration of H^+ and raise pH_i, one might speculate that under such circumstances the cell sacrifices volume regulation in favor of pHi regulation. Finally, whether the cell dies a volume-regulatory death is unclear since cell acidity may produce necrosis by other processes working in parallel with those that produce cell edema. Prominent among the other processes identified and defined in other injury models that may contribute to cell necrosis are (a) activation of endonucleases, proteases, and phospholipases by the acid-induced elevation in intracellular calcium (88)—with the endonucleases damaging nuclear chromatin, phospholipases and proteases damaging the cell membrane, and ATPases depleting energy stores critical for cell metabolism, repair and transport; and (b) activation of the mitochondrial permeability transition (MPT) (89). The MPT is activated either by cell acidification or elevation in cytosolic calcium and results from the opening of high-conductance pores in the inner mitochondrial membrane. The consequence of the change in pore conductance is mitochondrial depolarization, uncoupling of oxidative phosphorylation and mitochondrial swelling. Cell death subsequently ensues either by cell necrosis or apoptosis, with the choice of pathway dependent upon the level of cytosolic ATP. Activation of the MPT leads to cell necrosis when ATP is depleted and to apoptosis when ATP is present (89).

EPITHELIAL INFLAMMATION AND REPAIR

Erosive esophagitis develops when the degree of cell necrosis from acid exposure is not offset by the mechanisms designed for epithelial repair. For epithelial repair to take place normally, there must be preservation of the stratum germinativum, the latter being the only cells within the tissue capable of replication and restitution (90–96). Although not experimentally proved, the destruction of the stratum germinativum or its basement membrane would appear to be a necessary step for the development of the most serious complication of reflux esophagitis, that is, replacement of the squamous lining with the metaplastic specialized columnar epithelium, well known as Barrett's esophagus (97).

Although the mechanisms controlling the rate of cell replication in the esophagus are unknown, there is experimental evidence that cell replication increases after acute acid exposure and clinical evidence that it increases during prolonged acid injury. Thus, DeBacker and colleagues (98) reported that a single, 30-minute exposure to HCl stimulates cell replication in dog esophagus within 20 to 34 hours of exposure, and Livstone and co-workers (99) found an increase in tritiated thymidine uptake, a marker of epithelial turnover, in esophageal biopsies from patients with severe esophagitis. Basal cell hyperplasia, which is considered one of the biopsy hallmarks of reflux esophagitis, represents the morphologic correlate of this increased rate of

cell replication (100) (Fig. 22.7). Moreover, recent experimental data suggest that one stimulus for repair of acid-damaged esophagus is increased epithelial permeability to epidermal growth factor—the latter derived from swallowed salivary secretions (101). Based on studies in mice and humans, a normal turnover rate for the esophageal epithelium appears to be 5 to 8 days (91,102). Since the rate of replication increases with HCl injury, it would seem possible for the epithelium to regenerate in as little as 2 to 4 days. From a therapeutic standpoint, this suggests that complete epithelial protection from H^+ for even short periods of time might be sufficient for recovery, although clinically this does not appear to be entirely borne out.

In gastric and duodenal epithelium, another important reparative defense after injury is epithelial restitution (103). Epithelial restitution is of importance because it occurs rapidly (as little as 30 minutes). This is the case because it does not require DNA synthesis and cell replication, only the migration of adjacent viable cells over basement membrane denuded of injured and necrotic cells. There is some evidence that suggests that in acid-injured esophagus, epithelial restitution for the repair of breaks in epithelial barrier function either does not occur or occurs at far slower rates than in gastroduodenal epithelia (86). Epithelial restitution, however, has been demonstrated in injured rabbit esophageal epithelial cells growing in primary culture (94–96). Further, this mechanism for repair can be stimulated by growth factors including hepatocyte growth factor, epidermal growth factor, and insulin-like growth factor, but not prostaglandins. However, this mechanism is also exquisitely acid sensitive, being inhibited to an increasing degree as bathing solution pH is lowered from 6.5 to 3.0.

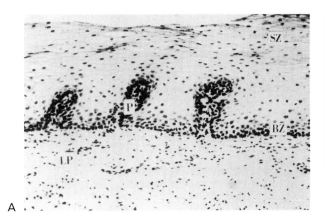 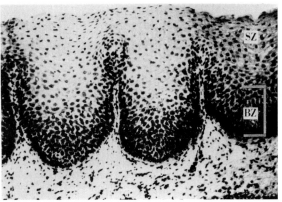

FIGURE 22.7. A: Normal esophageal suction biopsy from a healthy subject without esophagitis. Basal zone thickness is approximately 10% of total epithelial thickness; papillae extend approximately one-half the distance to the epithelial surface. **B:** Abnormal suction biopsy from a subject with symptomatic reflux. Basal zone thickness is approximately 35% of total epithelial thickness; papillae extend over two-thirds of the distance to the epithelial surface. BZ, basal zone, SZ, stratified zone; P, papillae; LP, lamina propria. Hematoxylin and eosin ×170. (From Ismail-Beigi F, Horton PF, Pope CE 2nd. Histological consequences of gastroesophageal reflux in man. *Gastroenterology* 1970;58:163, with permission.)

This suggests that restitution may play a beneficial role in esophageal repair when the level of injury extends to the basement membrane where a suitable scaffold for cell migration is present. Yet, it is also evident that for this process to function optimally, luminal acidity must be well controlled—this perhaps accounts to some extent for the requirement for proton pump inhibitor therapy in patients with erosive esophagitis (94).

A key component of erosive esophagitis is inflammation. Recent preliminary data in patients with erosive esophagitis indicate that the mediators of this process include the proinflammatory cytokines, interleukin (IL)-1β, IL-6, and IL-8, and that the source of the IL-6 and IL-8 is the damaged squamous epithelium (104). In addition, Naya et al. (105), Lanas et al. (106), and Soteras et al. (107) have described a rabbit model of erosive esophagitis secondary to acid-pepsin perfusion. In this model the recruitment of inflammatory cells to the area of injury increased the extent of tissue necrosis, with the added damage mediated by inflammatory cell-derived free radicals, especially superoxide anion. This is evident in that inhibition of inflammatory cell migration with ketotifen or antibodies to CD11 and treatment with superoxide dismutase, a scavenger of superoxide anions, protected against the development of erosive esophagitis. In addition, and contributing to tissue damage in this model, was the formation of peroxynitrites, a potent cytotoxin produced by the reaction of superoxide anion with nitric oxide (107,108). Notably, since some of the above interleukins and the peroxynitrites and their more stable end products (e.g., sodium nitrite) are capable of relaxing smooth muscle, inflammation itself may have a significant and detrimental impact on esophageal motor function—that is, impairing LES and/or peristaltic function and so increasing esophageal exposure to high levels of luminal acidity. In effect, the development of esophageal inflammation may be one factor responsible for the progression of reflux disease from nonerosive to erosive forms in some patients.

EFFECT OF BILE AND OTHER AGENTS ON THE EPITHELIUM

Although the major focus of this chapter is on acid injury, the esophageal epithelium can be damaged by other factors derived either from ingested material or present in the refluxate. These include conjugated bile salts, alcohol, pepsin, heat, hypertonicity, and tobacco products (8, 10–12,109–115). Yet, these factors appear relatively innocuous in the absence of an acidic environment—acid being necessary to either potentiate the action of the agent (e.g., pepsin), or to take advantage of mild injury produced by the agent (e.g., hypertonicity or heat). For this reason, these factors may be viewed as primary means for impairing epithelial defense against acid. Moreover, the

mechanism(s) by which specific agents alter barrier function are highly variable. For example, bile salts enhance transcellular H^+ entry in both gastric and esophageal mucosa by micellar dissolution of cell membrane lipids (12,19), whereas the proteolytic enzyme pepsin appears to enhance paracellular H^+ entry by digestion of intercellular proteins in the esophagus (12). Further, tobacco products inhibit active $Na+$ transport and so can impair pHi and cell volume regulation under acidic conditions while alcohol can act by enhancing H^+ entry through both transcellular and paracellular pathways (109,113,115,116), the former by increasing cell membrane fluidity and the latter through its junctional damaging effects. Hypertonic solutions have also been shown to increase paracellular permeability in stratified squamous epithelium including that of the esophagus (117,118). Moreover, experimentally, esophageal sensitivity to acid injury occurs in rabbit esophagus that has been pretreated with a hypertonic solution even for as little as 10 minutes and with otherwise innocuous levels of acidity, such as pH 2 (119). A parallel of this in humans is that hypertonic solutions can induce heartburn in subjects known to have an acid-sensitive esophagus (120). It is unknown, however, whether the symptoms result from stimulation of nerve endings by the hypertonic environment or by concomitant exposure to refluxed acid during the procedure. Nonetheless, regardless of specific mechanism, the common denominator by which these agents operate is through enhancement of H^+ entry. H^+ entry is the factor that ultimately transforms what would be a minor insult to the tissue into one that is clinically significant. Such a crucial role for acid has recently been supported by the dramatic success of the proton pump inhibitors in reflux esophagitis, the drugs acting by potent and selective inhibition of the gastric parietal cell's acid-secretory mechanism (121,122).

REFERENCES

1. DeMeester TR, Johnson LF, Joseph GJ, et al. Patterns of gastroesophageal reflux in health and disease. *Ann Surg* 1976;184:459.
2. Johnson LF, DeMeester TR. Twenty-four hour pH monitoring of the distal esophagus. *Am J Gastroenterol* 1974;62:325.
3. Fletcher J, Wirz A, Young J, et al. Unbuffered highly acidic gastric juice exists at the gastroesophageal junction after a meal. *Gastroenterology* 2001;121:775.
4. Dent J, Dodds WJ, Friedman RH, et al. Mechanism of gastroesophageal reflux in recumbent asymptomatic subjects. *J Clin Invest* 1980;65:256.
5. Lichter I, Muir RC. The pattern of swallowing during sleep. *Electroencephalogr Clin Neurophysiol* 1975;38:427.
6. Schneyer LH, et al. Rate of flow of human parotid, sublingual and submaxillary secretions during steep. *J Dent Res* 1956;35:109.
7. Bateson MC, Hopwood D, Milne G, et al. Oesophageal epithelial ultrastructure after incubation with gastrointestinal fluids and their components. *J Pathol* 1981;133:33.

8. Lillemoe KD, Johnson LF, Harmon JW. Role of the components of the gastroduodenal contents in experimental acid esophagitis. *Surgery* 1982;92:276.

9. Orlando RC, Powell DW. Studies of esophageal epithelial electrolyte transport and potential difference in man. In: Allen A, Flemström G, Garner A, et al., eds. *Mechanisms of mucosal protection in the upper gastrointestinal tract*. New York: Raven Press, 1984:75.

10. Redo SF, Bames WA, de la Sierra CA. Perfusion of the canine esophagus with secretions of upper gastrointestinal tract. *Ann Surg* 1959;149:556.

11. Salo J, Kivilaakso E. Role of luminal H⁺ in the pathogenesis of experimental esophagitis. *Surgery* 1982;92:61.

12. Salo JA, Lehto VP, Kivilaakso E. Morphologic alterations in experimental esophagitis: light microscopic and scanning and transmission electron microscopic study. *Dig Dis Sci* 1983;28:440.

13. Allen A, Phil D. The structure and function of gastrointestinal mucus. In: Harmon JW, ed. *Basic mechanisms of gastrointestinal mucosal cell injury and protection*. Baltimore: Williams & Wilkins, 1981:351.

14. Pfeiffer CJ. Experimental analysis of hydrogen ion diffusion in gastrointestinal mucus glycoprotein. *Am J Physiol* 1981;240:G176.

15. Williams SE, Turnberg LA. Studies of the "protective" properties of gastric mucus: evidence for mucus bicarbonate barrier. *Gut* 1979;20:A922.

16. Mantle M, Mantle D, Allen A. Polymeric structure of pig small-intestinal mucus glycoprotein. *Biochem J* 1981;195:277.

17. Thomson ABR. Unstirred water layers: a basic mechanism of gastrointestinal mucosal cell cytoprotection. In: Harmon JW, ed. *Basic mechanisms of gastrointestinal mucosal cell injury and protection*. Baltimore: Williams & Wilkins, 1981:327.

18. Thomson ABR. Unstirred water layers: possible adaptive and cytoprotective function. In: Allen A, Flemström G, Garner A, et al., eds. *Mechanisms of mucosal protection in the upper gastrointestinal tract*. New York: Raven Press, 1984:233.

19. Duane WC, Weigand DM. Mechanism by which bile salt disrupts the gastric mucosal barrier in the dog. *J Clin Invest* 1980;66:1044.

20. Kivilaakso E, Flemstrom G. HCO₃⁻ secretion and pH gradient across the surface mucus gel in rat duodenum. *Gastroenterology* 1982;82:1101A.

21. Quigley EMM, Turnberg LA. pH of the microclimate lining the human gastric and duodenal mucosa in vivo—studies in control subjects and in duodenal ulcer patients. *Gastroenterology* 1987;92:1876.

22. Williams SE, Turnberg LA. The demonstration of a pH gradient across mucus adherent to rabbit gastric mucosa: evidence for a mucus–bicarbonate barrier. *Gut* 1981;22:94.

23. Dixon J, Strugala V, Griffin SM, et al. Esophageal mucin: an adherent mucus gel barrier is absent in the normal esophagus but present in Barrett's esophagus. *Am J Gastroenterol* 2001;96:2575.

24. Al Yassin T, Toner PG. Fine structure of squamous epithelium and submucosal glands of human esophagus. *J Anat* 1977;123:705.

25. Hafez ESE. Functional anatomy of mucus-secreting cells. In: Elstein M, Parke DV, eds. *Mucus in health and disease*. New York: Plenum Publishing, 1977:19.

26. Boyd DD, Carney CN, Powell DW. Neurohumoral control of esophageal epithelial electrolyte transport. *Am J Physiol* 1980;239:G5.

27. Hamilton BH, Orlando RC. In vivo alkaline secretion by mammalian esophagus. *Gastroenterology* 1989;97:640.

28. Powell DW. Barrier function of epithelia. *Am J Physiol* 1981;241:G275.

29. Carney CN, Orlando RC, Powell DW, et al. Morphologic alterations in early acid-induced epithelial injury of the rabbit esophagus. *Lab Invest* 1981;45:198.

30. Elias PM, McNutt NS, Friend DS. Membrane alterations during codification of mammalian squamous epithelia: a freeze-fracture, tracer and thin-section study. *Anat Rec* 1977;189:577.

31. Lacy ER, Tobey NA, Cowart K, et al. The esophageal mucosal barrier: structural correlates. *Gastroenterology* 1989;96:A281.

32. Martinez-Palomo A, Erlij D, Bracho H. Localization of permeability barriers in the frog skin epithelium. *J Cell Biol* 1971;50:277.

33. Powell DW, Morris SM, Boyd DD. Water and electrolyte transport by rabbit esophagus. *Am J Physiol* 1975;229:438.

34. Powell DW, Orlando RC, Carney CN. Acid injury of the esophageal epithelium. In: Harmon JW, ed. *Basic mechanisms of gastrointestinal mucosal cell injury and protection*. Baltimore: Williams & Wilkins, 1981:155.

35. Diamond JM. Channels in epithelial cell membranes and junctions. *Fed Proc* 1978;37:2639.

36. Tobey NA, Caymaz-Bor C, Hosseini SS, et al. Circuit analysis of cell membrane and junctional resistances in healthy and acid-damaged rabbit esophageal epithelium. *Gastroenterology* 1999;116:A334.

37. Tobey NA, Hosseini SS, Orlando RC. E-Cadherin is important in the regulation of paracellular permeability in rabbit esophageal epithelium. *Gastroenterology* 2002;122:A518.

38. Moreno JH, Diamond JM. Discrimination of monovalent inorganic cations by "tight" junctions of gallbladder epithelium. *J Membr Biol* 1974;15:277.

39. Elias PM, Friend DS. The permeability barrier in mammalian epidermis. *J Cell Biol* 1975;65:180.

40. Elias PM, Goerke J, Friend DS. Mammalian epidermal barrier layer lipids: composition and influence on structure. *J Invest Dermatol* 1977;69:535.

41. Hopwood D, Logan KR, Coghill G, et al. Histochemical studies of mucosubstances and lipids in normal human oesophageal epithelium. *Histochem J* 1977;9:153.

42. Turner KS, Powell DW, Carney CN, et al. Transmural electrical potential difference in the mammalian esophagus in vivo. *Gastroenterology* 1978;75:286.

43. Mills JW, Ernst SA, DiBona DR. Localization of Na-pump sites in frog skin. *J Cell Biol* 1977;73:88.

44. Orlando RC, Powell DW, Carney CN. Pathophysiology of acute acid injury in rabbit esophageal epithelium. *J Clin Invest* 1981;68:286.

45. Orlando RC, Bryson JC, Powell DW. Mechanisms of HCl injury in rabbit esophageal epithelium. *Am J Physiol* 1984;246:G718.

46. Herlihy KJ, Orlando RC, Bryson JC, et al. Barrett's esophagus: clinical, endoscopic, histologic, manometric and electrical potential difference characteristics. *Gastroenterology* 1984;86:436.

47. Orlando RC, Powell DW, Bryson JC, et al. Esophageal potential difference measurements in esophageal disease. *Gastroenterology* 1982;83:1026.

48. Eckardt VF, Adami B. Esophageal transmural potential difference in patients with symptomatic gastroesophageal reflux. *Klin Wochenschr* 1980;58:293.

49. Khamis B, Kennedy C, Finucane J, et al. Transmural potential difference: diagnostic value in gastro-oesophageal reflux. *Gut* 1978;19:396.

50. Vidins EI, Fox JET, Beck IT. Transmural potential difference (PD) in the body of the esophagus in patients with esophagitis, Barrett's epithelium and carcinoma of the esophagus. *Am J Dig Dis* 1971;16:991.

51. Read NW, Fordtran JS. The role of intraluminal junction

potentials in the generation of the gastric potential difference in man. *Gastroenterology* 1979;76:932.

52. Chung RSK, Magri J, DenBesten L. Hydrogen ion transport in the rabbit esophagus. *Am J Physiol* 1975;229:496.

53. Harmon JW, Johnson LF, Maydonovitch CL. Effects of acid and bile salts on the rabbit esophageal mucosa. *Dig Dis Sci* 1981;87:280.

54. Kivilaakso E, Fromm D, Silen W. Effect of bile salts and related compounds on isolated esophageal mucosa. *Surgery* 1980;87:280.

55. Powell DW. Physiological concept of epithelial barriers. In: Allen A, Flemström G, Garner A, et al., eds. *Mechanisms of mucosal protection in the upper gastrointestinal tract.* New York: Raven Press, 1984:1.

56. Palmer LG. Ion selectivity of the apical membrane Na channel in the toad urinary bladder. *J Membr Biol* 1982;67:91.

57. Tobey NA, Hosseini SS, Caymaz-Bor C, et al. Effect of luminal acidity on the apical membrane Na channel in rabbit esophageal epithelium. *Gastroenterology* 2000;118:A883.

58. Hopwood D, Milne G, Logan KR. Electron microscopic changes in human oesophageal epithelium in oesophagitis. *J Pathol* 1979;129:161.

59. Pope CE II. Gastroesophageal reflux disease (reflux esophagitis). In: Sleisenger MH, Fordtran JS, eds. *Gastrointestinal disease: pathophysiology, diagnosis, management,* vol. 1, 2d ed. Philadelphia: WB Saunders, 1978:541.

60. Tobey NA, Carson JL, Alkiek RA, et al. Dilated intercellular spaces: a morphological feature of acid reflux-damaged human esophageal epithelium. *Gastroenterology* 1996;111:1200.

61. Solcia E, Villani L, Liunetti O, et al. Altered intercellular glycoconjugates and dilated intercellular spaces of esophageal epithelium in reflux disease. *Virchows Arch* 2000;436:207.

62. Villanacci V, Grigolato PG, Cestari R, et al. Dilated intercellular spaces as markers of reflux disease: histology, semiquantitative score and morphometry upon light microscopy. *Digestion* 2001;64:1.

63. Ferreira KG, Hill BS. The effect of low external pH on properties of the paracellular pathway and junctional structure in frog skin. *J Physiol* 1982;332:59.

64. Robles-Chillida EM, Rodrigo J, et al. Ultrastructure of freeending nerve fibers in oesophageal epithelium. *J Anat* 1981;133:227.

65. Rodrigo J, Hernandez DJ, Vidal MA, et al. Vegetative innervation of the esophagus III. Intraepithelial endings. *Acta Anat* 1975;92:242.

66. Tobey NA, Powell DW, Schreiner VJ, et al. Serosal bicarbonate protects against acid injury to rabbit esophagus. *Gastroenterology* 1989;96:1466.

67. Christie KN, Thomson C, Xue L, et al. Carbonic anhydrase isoenzymes I, II, III, and IV are present in human esophageal epithelium. *J Histochem Cytochem* 1997;45:35.

68. Khalbuss WE, Marousis CG, Subramanyam M, et al. Effect of HCl on transmembrane potentials and intracellular pH in rabbit esophageal epithelium. *Gastroenterology* 1995;108:662.

69. Tobey NA, Reddy SP, Keku TO, et al. Mechanisms of HCl-induced lowering of intracellular pH in rabbit esophageal epithelial cells. *Gastroenterology* 1993;105:1035.

70. Layden TJ, Schmidt L, Agnone L, et al. Rabbit esophageal cell cytoplasmic pH regulation: role of Na^+-H^+ antiport and Na^+-dependent HCO_3^- transport systems. *Am J Physiol* 1992;263:G407.

71. Tobey NA, Reddy SP, Khalbuss WE, et al. Na^+-dependent and -independent Cl^-/HCO_3^- exchangers in cultured rabbit esophageal epithelial cells. *Gastroenterology* 1993;104:185.

72. Tobey NA, Reddy SP, Keku TO, et al. Studies of pHi in rabbit esophageal basal and squamous epithelial cells in culture. *Gastroenterology* 1992;103:830.

73. Tobey NA, Koves G, Orlando RC. Human esophageal epithelial cells possess an $Na+/H^+$ exchanger for H^+ extrusion. *Am J Gastroenterol* 1998;93:2075.

74. Kivilaakso E. High plasma HCO_3^- protects gastric mucosa against acute ulceration in the rat. *Gastroenterology* 1981;81:921.

75. Kivilaakso E, Barzilai A, Schiessel R, et al. Ulceration of isolated amphibian gastric mucosa. *Gastroenterology* 1979;77:31.

76. Schiessel R, Merhav A, Matthews J, et al. Role of nutrient HCO_3^- in the protection of amphibian gastric mucosa. *Am J Physiol* 1980;239:G536.

77. Bass BL, Schweitzer EJ, Harmon JW, et al. HCl back diffusion interferes with intrinsic reactive regulation of esophageal mucosal blood flow. *Surgery* 1984;96:404.

78. Hollwarth ME, Smith M, Kvietys PR, et al. Esophageal blood flow in the cat. *Gastroenterology* 1986;90:622.

79. Feldman MJ, Morris GP, Paterson WG. Role of substance P and calcitonin gene-related peptide in acid-induced augmentation of opossum esophageal blood flow. *Dig Dis Sci* 2001;46:1194.

80. Feldman MJ, Morris GP, Dinda PK, et al. Mast cells mediate acid-induced augmentation of opossum esophageal blood flow via histamine and nitric oxide. *Gastroenterology* 1996;110:121.

81. Rydning A, Lyng O, Falkmer S, et al. Histamine release is involved in gastric vasodilation during acid back diffusion via activation of sensory neurons. *Am J Physiol Gastrointest Liver Physiol* 2002;283:G603.

82. MacKnight ADC, Leaf A. Regulation of cellular volume. *Physiol Rev* 1977;57:510.

83. Orlando RC, Tobey NA. Comparative sensitivity of rabbit esophageal epithelium to serosal versus mucosal acid. *Gastroenterology* 1989;96:A512.

84. Cuthbert AW, Shum WK. Does intracellular sodium modify membrane permeability to sodium ions? *Nature* 1977;266:468.

85. Taylor A, Windhager EE. Possible role of cytosolic calcium and Na–Ca exchange in regulation of transepithelial sodium transport. *Am J Physiol* 1979;236:F505.

86. Tobey NA, Cragoe EJ Jr, Orlando RC. HCl-induced cell edema in rabbit esophageal epithelium: a bumetanide-sensitive process. *Gastroenterology* 1995;109:414.

87. Tobey NA, Koves G, Orlando RC. HCl-induced cell edema in primary cultured rabbit esophageal epithelium. *Gastroenterology* 1997;112:847.

88. Cotran R, Vinay K, Robbins S, et al. *Pathologic basis of disease,* 5th ed. Philadelphia: WB Saunders, 1994:1.

89. Lemasters JJ. Mechanisms of hepatic toxicity V. Necrapoptosis and the mitochondrial permeability transition: shared pathways to necrosis and apoptosis. *Am J Physiol Gastrointest Liver Physiol* 1999;276:G1.

90. Eastwood GL. Gastrointestinal epithelial renewal. *Gastroenterology* 1977;72:962.

91. Leblond CP, Greuiich RC, Pereira JPM. Relationship of cell formation and cell migration in the renewal of stratified squamous epithelia. In: Montagna W, Billingham RE, eds. *Wound healing,* vol. 5 of *Advances in biology of skin.* New York: Pergamon Press, 1974:39.

92. Marques-Pereira JP, Leblond CP. Mitosis and differentiation in the stratified-squamous epithelium of the rat esophagus. *Am J Anat* 1965;117:73.

93. Messier B, Leblond CP. Cell proliferation and migration as revealed by radioautography after injection of thymidine-H^3 into rats and mice. *Am J Anat* 1960;106:247.

94. Jimenez P, Lanas A, Piazuelo E, et al. Effects of extracellular pH on restitution and proliferation of rabbit oesophageal epithelial cells. *Aliment Pharmacol Ther* 1999;13:545.

95. Jimenez P, Lanas A, Piazuelo E, et al. Effect of growth factors and prostaglandin E2 on restitution and proliferation of rabbit esophageal epithelial cells. *Dig Dis Sci* 1998;43:2309.

96. Takahashi M, Ota S, Ogura K, et al. Hepatocyte growth factor stimulates wound repair of the rabbit esophageal epithelial cells in primary culture. *Biochem Biophys Res Commun* 1995;216:298.

97. Orlando RC. Pathology of reflux oesophagitis and its complications. In: Jamieson GG, ed. *Surgery of the oesophagus.* New York: Churchill Livingstone, 1988:189.

98. DeBacker A, Haentjens P, Willems G. Hydrochloric acid: a trigger of cell proliferation in the esophagus of dogs. *Dig Dis Sci* 1985;30:884.

99. Livstone EM, Sheahan DG, Behar J. Studies of esophageal epithelial cell proliferation in patients with reflux esophagitis. *Gastroenterology* 1977;73:1315.

100. Ismail-Beigi F, Horton PF, Pope CE II. Histological consequences of gastroesophageal reflux in man. *Gastroenterology* 1970;58:163.

101. Tobey NA, Hosseini SS, Raibstein SR, et al. Nonerosive acid injury increases esophageal permeability to salivary epidermal growth factor. *Gastroenterology* 2000;118:A4885.

102. Bell B, Almy TP, Lipkin M. Cell proliferation kinetics in the gastrointestinal tract of man: III. Cell renewal in esophagus, stomach and jejunum of a patient with treated pernicious anemia. *J Natl Cancer Inst* 1967;38:615.

103. Silen W. Gastric mucosal defense and repair. In: Johnson LR, ed. *Physiology of the gastrointestinal tract*, vol. 2, 2d ed. New York: Raven Press, 1987:1055.

104. Rieder F, Phillips H, West GA, et al. Production of the pro-inflammatory cytokines IL-1B, IL-6 and IL-8 in active esophagitis. *Gastroenterology* 2002;122:A420.

105. Naya MJ, Pereboom D, Ortego J, et al. Superoxide anion produced by inflammatory cells play an important part in the pathogenesis of acid and pepsin induced esophagitis in rabbits. *Gut* 1997;40:175.

106. Lanas A, Soteras F, Jimenez P, et al. Superoxide anion and nitric oxide in high-grade esophagitis induced by acid and pepsin in rabbits. *Dig Dis Sci* 2001;46:2733.

107. Soteras F, Lanas A, Fiteni I, et al. Nitric oxide and superoxide anion in low-grade esophagitis induced by acid and pepsin in rabbits. *Dig Dis Sci* 2000;45:1802.

108. Uc A, Murray J, Kooy N, et al. Effect of peroxynitrite on motor function of the opossum esophagus. *Dig Dis Sci* 2001;46:30.

109. Bor S, Bor-Caymaz C, Tobey NA, et al. Esophageal exposure to ethanol increases the risk of acid damage in rabbit esophagus. *Dig Dis Sci* 1999;44:290.

110. Chung RSK, Johnson GM, DenBesten L. Effect of Na taurocholate and ethanol on hydrogen ion absorption in rabbit esophagus. *Am J Dig Dis* 1975;20:582.

111. Lillemoe KD, Johnson LF, Harmon JW. Alkaline esophagitis: a comparison of the ability of components of gastroduodenal contents to injure the rabbit esophagus. *Gastroenterology* 1983;85:621.

112. Long JD, Marten E, Tobey NA, et al. Effects of luminal hypertonicity on rabbit esophageal epithelium. *Am J Physiol* 1997;273:G647.

113. Safaie-Shirazi S, DenBesten L, Zike WL. Effect of bile salts on the ionic permeability of the esophageal mucosa and their role in the production of esophagitis. *Gastroenterology* 1975;68:728.

114. Sikka D, Marten E, Tobey NA, et al. Effect of heat on the barrier and transport functions of rabbit esophageal epithelium. *Gastroenterology* 1996;110:A258.

115. Orlando RC, Bryson JC, Powell DW. Effect of cigarette smoke on esophageal epithelium of the rabbit. *Gastroenterology* 1986;91:1536.

116. Shirazi SS, Platz CD. Effect of alcohol on canine esophageal mucosa. *J Surg Res* 1978;25:373.

117. Erlij D, Martinez-Palomo A. Opening of tight junctions in frog skin by hypertonic urea solutions. *J Membr Biol* 1972;9:229.

118. Fischbarg J, Whittembury G. The effect of external pH on osmotic permeability, ion and fluid transport across isolated frog skin. *J Physiol* 1978;275:403.

119. Long JD, Marten E, Tobey NA, et al. The relationship between esophageal epithelial paracellular permeability and susceptibility to injury by luminal HCl. *Gastroenterology* 1996;110:A179.

120. Lloyd DA, Borda IT. Food-induced heartburn: effect of osmolality. *Gastroenterology* 1981;80:740.

121. Hetzel DI, Dent J, Reed WD, et al. Healing and relapse of severe peptic esophagitis after treatment with omeprazole. *Gastroenterology* 1988;95:903.

122. Schulman MI, Orlando RC. Treatment of gastroesophageal reflux: the role of proton pump inhibitors. In: Schrier RW, Baxter JD, Abboud F, et al., eds. *Advances in internal medicine*, vol. 40. St. Louis: Mosby–Year Book, 1995:273.

DUODENOGASTROESOPHAGEAL REFLUX

MICHAEL F. VAEZI

Gastroesophageal reflux disease (GERD) represents retrograde flow of gastric contents into the esophagus with or without associated histological changes. Most healthy individuals intermittently reflux gastric contents into the esophagus. These episodes occur most commonly postprandially, are short-lived, and rarely cause symptoms or esophageal mucosal injury. However, excessive gastroesophageal reflux may produce symptoms, and nearly 50% of these patients have complications of GERD, including esophagitis, strictures, or Barrett's esophagus at endoscopy (1).

The noxious agents responsible for injuring the esophageal mucosa originate from both gastric and duodenal sources. Hydrochloric acid and pepsin are the important gastric agents predisposing to the development of esophageal symptoms and mucosal injury (2–5). Additionally, gastric juice may intermix with duodenal contents by transpyloric reflux of bile and pancreatic secretions. Regurgitation of duodenal contents into the stomach is normal occurring most commonly at nights and postprandially (6–9). However, when excessive, it may be associated with gastritis, gastric ulcers, postcholecystectomy syndrome, dyspepsia, and esophageal mucosal damage (10–22). The term duodenogastroensophageal reflux (DGER) refers to regurgitation of duodenal contents through the pylorus into the stomach, with subsequent reflux into the esophagus. Previously, the term "bile reflux" and "alkaline reflux" were used to describe this process. However, duodenal contents contain more than just bile, and recent studies show that the term "alkaline reflux" is a misnomer since pH >7 does not correlate with reflux of duodenal contents (23).

The importance of DGER relates to findings in both animal and human studies that factors other than acid, namely bile and pancreatic enzymes, may play a significant role in mucosal injury and symptoms in patients with GERD. However, the relative importance of acid or DGER

to the development of esophageal mucosal injury is controversial. In the past, the main difficulty has been extrapolating the findings in animal studies to humans. However, studies using state-of-the-art methods for detecting esophageal reflux of both acid and duodenal contents are helping to unravel the role of these potentially injurious agents in producing esophageal mucosal injury. This chapter reviews important animal and human studies that clarify the role of gastric and duodenal contents in causing esophageal symptoms and mucosal damage. Second, the available tests for identifying DGER are discussed and their advantages and disadvantages reviewed. Finally, the medical and surgical therapies for DGER are discussed.

IMPORTANCE OF ACID AND PEPSIN

Animal Studies

Substantial experimental and clinical evidence strongly supports the importance of acid and pepsin in causing esophageal mucosal injury. Using the canine esophagus, Redo et al. (2) investigated the role of acid alone and in combination with various pepsin concentrations by infusing pepsin at concentrations up to 10% and at pH values of <2 and >2. They reported no esophageal damage with HCl infusion alone, while acid in combination with low concentrations of pepsin at pH<2 caused the most severe esophagitis. Meanwhile, Goldberg et al. (5) demonstrated esophageal mucosal damage in the intact feline esophagus, with either very high concentrations of acid (pH 1.0 to 1.3) or lower acid concentrations (pH 1.6 to 2.0) in the presence of pepsin. Using a perfused rabbit esophagus model, Lillemoe et al. (24) confirmed that acid infusion alone did not produce mucosal damage or increase esophageal mucosal permeability as measured by the net flux of H^+, K, glucose, and Hgb. However, the addition of pepsin to the infusate, in a dose-dependent manner, was associated with increased degrees of gross esophageal mucosal injury and changes in esophageal mucosal permeability. Thus, animal studies suggest that the esophageal mucosa is relatively resistant to

---

M. F. Vaezi: Department of Gastroenterology and Hepatology, Center for Swallowing and Esophageal Disorders, The Cleveland Clinic Foundation, Cleveland, Ohio.

reflux of acid alone unless it occurs at very high concentrations (pH 1.0 to 1.3). On the other hand, the combination of acid and even small concentrations of pepsin results in macroscopic as well as microscopic esophageal mucosal injury (Fig. 23.1).

Human Studies

Studies by Aylwin (25) were the first scientific evidence identifying the importance of acid and pepsin in the development of heartburn and esophageal mucosal injury. Using continuous esophageal aspiration in patients with hiatal hernia and esophagitis, they found that patients with esophagitis had aspirates of lower pH and higher pepsin concentration than those without esophagitis. Later, Tuttle et al. (26,27) measured the pH of the distal esophagus, finding that the reflux of pH<4 material coincided with the onset of heartburn, while a rise to a more neutral pH coincided with relief of symptoms.

Subsequently, a series of studies showed that patients with various grades of esophagitis, including Barrett's esophagus, have increased frequency and duration of esophageal exposure to pH<4 refluxate (28–32). Iascone et al. (33) reported a direct relationship between the severity of esophageal mucosal injury and the degree and frequency of mucosal exposure to acid reflux. Later, studies by DeMeester et al. (1)

found that 90% of patients with esophagitis had increased amounts of acid reflux by 24-hour pH monitoring. The same group (34) reported that patients with Barrett's esophagus had significantly higher exposure times to pH<4 than patients with esophagitis, who had higher exposure times than healthy controls. Later, Stein et al. (35) reported that patients with Barrett's esophagus had greater exposure times to more caustic gastric acid concentrations (pH<3 or 2), suggesting a significant role for acid reflux in the development of esophagitis and Barrett's esophagus.

Separating the role of pepsin from acid in the production of esophagitis is difficult, since the optimum pH for the enzymatic activity of pepsin is <3. Studies show a positive correlation between the degree of abnormal acid and pepsin exposure and the severity of esophagitis. Bremner et al. (36) observed that patients with increased esophageal exposure to pH 1 to 2, corresponding to the known pKa of pepsin, had the most significant degrees of esophagitis. In a recent study, Gotley et al. (11) found that esophageal aspirates from patients with esophagitis had significantly higher concentrations of acid and pepsin than the aspirates from healthy controls. Furthermore, patients with Zollinger-Ellison syndrome, where the basal acid output is high and gastric pH favors optimum acidity for pepsin activity, have a 40% to 60% incidence of esophagitis despite normal or increased lower esophageal sphincter (LES) pressures (37).

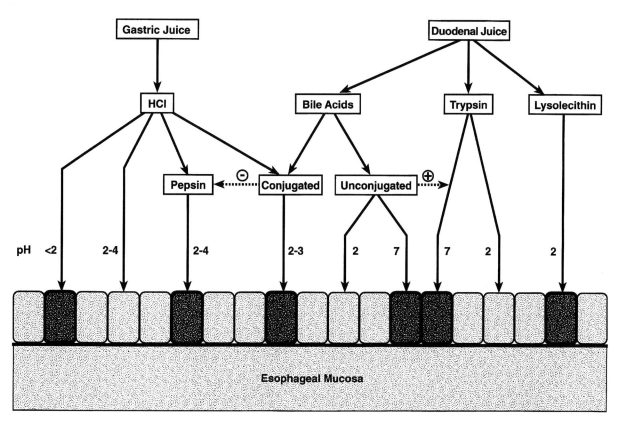

FIGURE 23.1. Proposed agents responsible for esophageal mucosal injury.

It is important to note that the frequency and duration of esophageal acid exposure is not always predictive of the degree of esophageal mucosal injury. This suggests the importance of other factors, including DGER, the inherent resistance of esophageal mucosa to acid injury, and the role of saliva and bicarbonate-producing submucosal glands in the distal esophagus to neutralize refluxed acid (38–41).

ROLE OF DUODENAL CONTENTS

Animal Studies

The role of duodenal contents, specifically bile acids and the pancreatic enzyme trypsin, in the development of esophageal mucosal injury is controversial and the subject of many *in vitro* animal studies (42–46). Early studies by Cross and Wangensteen (42) suggested a role for bile and its constituents, namely bile acids, in esophageal mucosal damage. Using a dog model with biliary diversion and a jejunal conduit anastomosing directly to the esophagus, Moffat and Berkas (43) showed that canine bile was capable of producing various degrees of erosive esophagitis, thereby confirming earlier studies by Cross and Wangensteen (42).

More recent studies show that esophageal mucosal damage by bile acids is dependent on the conjugation state of the bile acids and the pH of the refluxate (Fig. 23.1). Using net acid flux (NAF) across the esophageal lumen as an index of mucosal injury, Harmon et al. (44) showed that taurine-conjugated bile salts, taurodeoxycholate and taurocholate (both with pKa of 1.9), increased NAF at pH 2, while the unconjugated forms increased NAF at pH 7, but not at pH 2. Hence, conjugated bile acids are more injurious to the esophageal mucosa at acidic pH, while unconjugated bile acids are more harmful at pH 5 to 8. Using rabbit esophageal perfusion studies, Kivilaakso et al. (45) confirmed the pH-dependent damage caused by conjugated and unconjugated bile acids, and additionally showed the injurious effect of trypsin on the esophageal mucosa at pH 7.0. Therefore, they concluded that "alkaline" reflux esophagitis was caused by both unconjugated bile acids and trypsin at neutral pH values.

Since the reflux of gastroduodenal contents usually occurs intermixed with the acidic contents of the stomach, several investigators have studied the synergistic and inhibitory interactions of HCl with pepsin, trypsin, and bile acids (24,47–49). Lillemoe et al. (24) compared the injurious effects of the various duodenal components on rabbit esophageal mucosa at pH 2. At this acidic pH, trypsin had no effect on net flux of ions across the esophageal mucosa, since the enzyme is inactive at pH values <4. Meanwhile, taurocholate produced no esophageal mucosal damage at a neutral pH, but in an acidic medium (pH 1.2) there was esophageal mucosal disruption as mea-

sured by net ion permeability. Similarly, Salo and Kivilaakso (47) found that both taurocholate and lysolecithin, the latter a normal constituent of duodenal juice formed by pancreatic phospholipase A hydrolysis of lecithin in bile, causes histological damage and alteration of the rabbit esophageal transmucosal potential difference in the presence of HCl, but there was no effect in the absence of HCl.

Bile acids, depending on their conjugated states, also have both synergistic and inhibitory interactions with trypsin and pepsin. In perfusion studies of the rabbit esophagus, Salo and Kivilaakso (48) found that the unconjugated bile acid cholate significantly increased mucosal damage caused by trypsin at pH 7.0. On the other hand, Lillemoe et al. (49) found that the degree of esophageal mucosal injury and permeability decreased in a dose-dependent manner when increasing concentrations of the conjugated bile acid taurodeoxycholate were added to pepsin.

Therefore, as shown in Fig. 23.1, there is evidence in the animal model for synergism between HCl and pepsin as well as HCl and conjugated bile acids and lysolecithin in causing esophageal mucosal damage. Similarly, unconjugated bile acids seem to augment the damaging effect of trypsin at pH 7. HCl is inhibitory to the damaging effects of trypsin and unconjugated bile acids, whereas conjugated bile acids decrease the damaging effect of pepsin at acidic pH.

Mechanism of Injury

The mechanism of esophageal mucosal damage by pepsin and trypsin are clearly related to the proteolytic properties of these enzymes. Both promote detachment of the surface cells from the epithelium, presumably by digesting the intercellular substances and surface structures that contribute to the maintenance of cohesion between cells (50,51). Each agent causes the most damage at its optimal pH activity range: pH 2 to 3 for pepsin, and pH 5 to 8 for trypsin.

The mechanism for mucosal damage by HCl is more complicated and depends on a series of events. Based on experimental works by Orlando, Powell, and coworkers (52–55) in the rabbit esophagus, H^+ impairs cell volume regulation causing cell death by inactivation of the Na^+/K^+-ATPase pump located in the basolateral cell wall in the stratum spinosum of the mucosa. Inhibition of Na^+/K^+-ATPase occurs at the same time that an amiloride-sensitive Na^+ pump is activated causing increased entry and accumulation of Na^+ intracellularly resulting in excess intracellular volume and subsequent cell death. Snow et al. (56) have proposed an alternative mechanism by which acid-induced esophageal mucosal injury may inhibit normal cell volume-regulatory mechanisms. Using isolated rabbit esophageal mucosal basal cells, these investigators found pH-dependent alteration in K^+ and/or Cl^- conductance.

The mechanism by which bile acids cause mucosal damage is not fully understood. Studies suggest two hypotheses. The first is that bile acids damage mucosal cells by their detergent property and solubilization of the mucosal lipid membranes. This theory is supported by studies in gastric mucosa where bile acid–induced mucosal injury was correlated with the release of phospholipids and cholesterol into the lumen (57–59). However, studies with rabbit esophageal mucosa (60,61) show significant mucosal barrier disruption occurring at bile acid concentrations below the level where phospholipids are solubilized. Therefore, this mechanism is less likely to explain the esophageal mucosal disruption caused by bile acids.

Alternatively, the second and more favored hypothesis suggests that bile acids gain entrance across the mucosa because of their lipophilic state causing intramucosal damage primarily by disorganizing membrane structure or interfering with cellular function. Support for this model comes from several experimental studies. Batzri et al. (62) found that bile acids, once penetrating the mucosal barrier, are trapped inside the cells by intracellular ionization, explaining the several fold increase in intracellular concentrations of bile acids (63). Furthermore, studies by Schweitzer et al. (60,61) have correlated bile acid entry and mucosal accumulation with bile acid mediated mucosal

damage. These findings explain the previous observations of increased mucosal injury by conjugated bile acids at pH 2, and unconjugated bile acids at pH 7. The unionized forms predominate at more acidic pH for conjugated bile acids (pKa 1.9), and at more neutral pH for unconjugated bile acids (pKa 5.1). The unionized forms of the bile acids are more lipophilic, allowing access through the esophageal mucosal barrier into the intracellular compartment where they are trapped by ionization and subsequently cause mucosal damage.

Human Studies

The clinical evidence for the possible damaging effects of DGER on the esophageal mucosa remains controversial. This may be because there is no "gold standard" for detecting DGER. Various direct and indirect methodologies are employed for measuring DGER, including endoscopy, aspiration studies (both gastric and esophageal), scintigraphy, ambulatory pH monitoring, ambulatory bilirubin monitoring, and most recently multichannel intraluminal impedance (MII). As summarized in Table 23.1, these tests have their strengths and shortcomings; however, reviewing the human studies using these tests can help us better appreciate the role of DGER in causing esophageal symptoms and mucosal injury.

TABLE 23.1. ADVANTAGES AND DISADVANTAGES OF THE CURRENTLY AVAILABLE METHODS FOR DETECTING DUODENOGASTROESOPHAGEAL REFLUX

Method	Advantages	Disadvantages
Endoscopy	Easy visualization of bile	Poor sensitivity/specificity/positive predictive value Requires sedation High cost
Aspiration studies	Less invasive than endoscopy No sedation Low cost	Short duration of study Requires familiarity with enzymatic assay for BA
Scintigraphy	Noninvasive	Semiquantitative at best Radiation exposure High cost
pH monitoring	Easy to perform Relatively noninvasive Prolonged monitoring Ambulatory	pH >7 not a marker for DGER Not specific for DGER
Bilirubin monitoring (Bilitec)	Easy to perform Relatively noninvasive Prolonged monitoring Ambulatory gastric BA concentrations	Current design underestimates DGER by about 30% in acidic medium (pH <3.5) Requires modified diet
Multichannel intraluminal impedance (MII)	Easy to perform Relatively noninvasive Prolonged monitoring Ambulatory Measures acidic and nonacidic gas and liquid reflux (combined with pH)	Does not directly show DGER No correlation studies with BA concentrations Not yet widely available

BA, bile acid; DGER, duodenogastroesophageal reflux.

TESTS FOR DGER

Endoscopy

Bile is frequently seen in the esophagus and stomach of patients during endoscopy; however, the clinical significance of these observations is unclear. Recently, Nasrallah et al. (64) evaluated 110 patients with bile-stained gastric mucosa at endoscopy by measuring gastric bile acids and scintigraphic quantitation of bile reflux. They found no correlation between the gastric bile acid concentrations, degree of histologic injury, or severity of endoscopic changes, suggesting that there was little clinical importance to bile-stained mucosa at endoscopy. Similarly, using scintigraphy and gastric pH monitoring to assess DGER, Stein et al. (65) found poor sensitivity (37%), specificity (70%), and positive predictive value (55%) for endoscopy in the diagnosis of excessive DGER.

Aspiration Studies

Stomach

One of the earliest methods used for evaluating DGER was the aspiration of gastric contents with fluid analysis for bile acids. Using this technique, Kaye and Showalter (66) found no significant difference between *fasting* gastric bile acid concentrations of patients with esophagitis (0.057 mg/ml) compared to controls (0.039 mg/ml), while *postprandially* esophagitis patients had higher gastric bile acid concentrations (0.89 mg/ml vs. 0.21 mg/ml). Similarly, Gillen et al. (67) found no difference in the *fasting* bile acid concentrations of patients with complicated (strictures, ulcers, dysplasia, adenocarcinoma) (0.025 mM) or uncomplicated (0 mM) Barrett's esophagus compared to patients with esophagitis (0 mM) or normal controls (0 mM). However, they reported significantly higher *postprandial* bile acid concentrations in patients with complicated Barrett's esophagus (0.19 mM) compared to the other groups (0.017 to 0.040 mM). The studies finding increased postprandial bile acid concentrations have been criticized because they all employed the 3-α-hydroxysteroid dehydrogenase enzymatic assay, which has recently been reported to have low specificity and accuracy in detecting bile acids in the postprandial but not the fasting state (68).

Recent studies by Vaezi and Richter (69) of patients with complicated and uncomplicated Barrett's esophagus found that the mean *fasting* bile acid concentrations were higher in complicated (0.5 mM) compared to uncomplicated (0.24 mM) Barrett's patients, with both concentrations being higher than controls (0.02 mM) (Fig. 23.2). These investigators also found that the increased fasting bile acid concentrations in Barrett's patients was accompanied by greater amounts of acid and bile reflux, suggesting that both components may be synergistically involved in producing esophageal mucosal damage.

A limitation of gastric aspiration studies is the presumption that the presence of bile acids in the stomach is a good indicator of esophageal exposure to duodenal contents and therefore DGER. This is supported by the observations that only half of DGER episodes into the antrum reach the fundus of the stomach and then all that is present in the fundus may not reflux into the esophagus (41).

Esophagus

Continuous and intermittent esophageal aspiration studies have assessed the role of bile acids in esophageal mucosal damage. Unlike studies of gastric aspirates, studies with esophageal aspiration technique are quite variable and are technique dependent. Two independent investigations, Smith et al. (70) and Johnsson et al. (71), found only small concentrations of bile acids (2.5 to 64 μM) in the esophageal aspirate of patients with gastroesophageal reflux disease (GERD). Mittal et al. (68), in a 3-hour postprandial bile aspiration study, found no bile acids in either the fasting or postprandial esophageal aspirates of patients with GERD. The above studies differed with respect to esophageal aspiration period, ranging from 3 hours in studies by Mittal et al. (68) to 15 hours in studies Smith et al. (70) and 24 hours in studies by Johnsson et al. (71).

On the other hand, Gotley et al. (10), studying 45 patients with esophagitis and 10 controls using continuous collection of esophageal aspiration over 16 hours, found increased amounts of conjugated bile acids, measured by high-performance liquid chromatography, in the majority (87%) of aspirates. Most bile acid reflux occurred at night with only 7% of samples having bile acids concentrations above 1.0 mM, the toxic concentration producing esophageal mucosal damage. Interestingly, acid reflux episodes measured by 24-hour pH monitoring occurred concomitantly with reflux of conjugated bile acids. Similarly, a recent study by Kauer et al. (72) using 17-hour continuous esophageal aspiration in 43 normal subjects and 37 patients with reflux disease found significantly ($p<.003$) higher bile acids in reflux patients (86%) than controls (58%). Furthermore, they found that the mean bile salt concentration was higher in patients during the postprandial and supine periods. However, they did not report the pH of the collected esophageal refluxate.

Scintigraphy

Radionucleotide techniques offer a noninvasive method for studying DGER. Tolin et al. (73) compared DGER measured by phenol red aspiration and external scintigraphy measuring 99mTc-HIDA, finding a good correlation between DGER and scintigraphy. Similarly, other investigators (74,75) have compared intragastric bile acid concentrations and scintigraphy, finding a significant correlation between both free and total gastric bile acids and the degree of bile reflux.

Scintigraphic studies find that DGER is a common phenomenon in normal individuals postprandially (6,7),

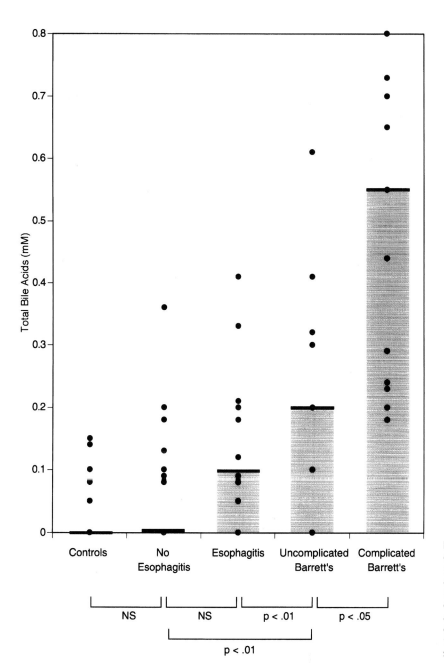

FIGURE 23.2. Individual and median fasting gastric bile acid concentration for five study populations: controls, acid reflux patients with and without esophagitis, and patients with uncomplicated and complicated Barrett's esophagus. (From Vaezi MF, Richter JE. Role of acid and duodenogastroesophageal reflux in gastroesophageal reflux disease. *Gastroenterology* 1996;111:1192–1199, with permission.)

requiring that the evaluation of abnormal DGER be quantitative. Matikainen et al. (76) found no difference in the scintigraphic amount of DGER into the esophagus between 40 patients with esophagitis (10% scintigraphic reflux) and 150 healthy controls (14% scintigraphic reflux). Likewise, Krog et al. (77) found no evidence of DGER in 15 patients with hiatal hernia and esophagitis. However, Waring et al. (78) reported that patients with Barrett's esophagus, especially those with complicated Barrett's, had more frequent DGER detected by 99mTc DISIDA scintigraphy than healthy volunteers. A more recent study by Liron et al. (79) using 99mTc HIDA scanning confirms the above results, finding higher

DGER in patients with Barrett's esophagus than GERD patients without Barrett's or healthy controls.

Although less invasive than other methods for detecting DGER, the reliability and accuracy of scintigraphy have been challenged. Drane et al. (80) observed that scintigraphy was, at best, a semiquantitative measure of bile reflux, finding that several technical problems may compromise the accuracy of this technique for measuring DGER. The most common problem was the overlap of the small bowel and stomach occurring in 36% of patients, which is not correctable. Other problems included overlap of the left lobe of the liver and stomach, patient movement, and the intermittent nature of bile reflux.

Ambulatory pH Monitoring

Prolonged pH monitoring offers a unique opportunity for studying acid and possibly DGER in the ambulatory state throughout the circadian cycle. Stein et al. (81) reported that gastric monitoring of pH>7 was superior to DISIDA radionucleotide scintigraphy in detecting DGER in patients with foregut symptoms. Similarly, Brown et al. (82) observed a good correlation (R=0.36, p<0.001) between gastric bile acid concentrations and ambulatory gastric pH monitoring.

Using 24-hour esophageal pH monitoring, Pellegrini et al. (83) were the first to study the relationship between acid and "alkaline" reflux in patients with gastroesophageal reflux disease. Acid reflux was defined as pH<4 in the lower esophagus, while "alkaline" reflux, an indirect marker of DGER, was defined as pH>7. Normal values were defined as the mean and two standard deviations of values obtained during 24-hour pH studies in 15 healthy volunteers. Com-

pared to patients with acid reflux, alkaline refluxers had less heartburn, but more frequent and severe regurgitation and a higher rate of esophageal strictures. Additionally, there were no pure "alkaline" refluxers, as all patient without prior gastric surgery also had episodes of acid reflux. Later, the same group (84,85) found that patients with esophagitis had less "alkaline" reflux and more acid reflux than patients without esophagitis. In contrast, Schmid et al. (86), studying patients with various degrees of esophagitis, reported significantly higher amounts of both acid and "alkaline" reflux in patients with complicated esophagitis compared to healthy subjects. Their results, similar to the findings in gastric aspiration studies, suggested a synergistic role for acid and bile in esophagitis.

At the same time, Atwood et al. (87–90) reported that "alkaline" reflux was greater in patients with Barrett's esophagus when compared to patients with esophagitis or normal controls. Furthermore, they found that pH>7 was signifi-

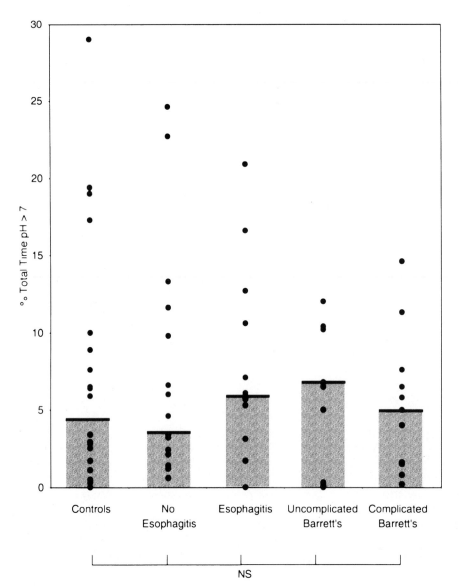

FIGURE 23.3. "Alkaline" reflux (percent of total time pH>7) for five study populations: controls, acid reflux patients with and without esophagitis, and patients with uncomplicated and complicated Barrett's esophagus. Individual data and group median shown. (From Vaezi MF, Richter JE. Role of acid and duodenogastroesophageal reflux in gastroesophageal reflux disease. *Gastroenterology* 1996;111: 1192–1199, with permission.)

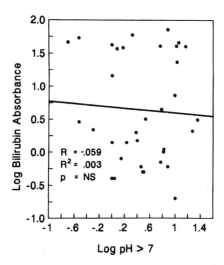

FIGURE 23.4. Relationship between percentage of time that bilirubin absorbance is ≥0.14 as a marker of bile reflux and esophageal pH >7 in a group of healthy controls, patients with GERD, and those with Barrett's esophagus. (From Champion G, Richter JE, Vaezi MF, et al. Duodenogastroesophageal reflux: relationship to pH and importance in Barrett's esophagus. *Gastroenterology* 1994;107:747–754, with permission.)

cantly higher in complicated Barrett's patients (stricture, ulcer, dysplasia) than Barrett's patients without complications, while pH<4 did not distinguish between the two groups. These authors went on to suggest that prolonged exposure to duodenal contents alone may promote the development of complicated Barrett's esophagus and even adenocarcinoma. However, the investigators did not attempt to resolve the physiological paradox of patients with marked amount of acid reflux also refluxing, independently, large amounts of "alkaline" material.

The measurement of esophageal pH>7 as a marker of DGER is confounded by several problems. Precautions must be taken to use only glass electrodes, dietary restriction of foods with pH<7, inspection of patients for periodontal disease, and dilation of strictures to avoid pooling of saliva. Therefore, it is not surprising that several authors (39–41,91) have questioned the accuracy of "alkaline" pH as a parameter for monitoring duodenal reflux into the esophagus. Gotley et al. (91) found no relationship between "alkaline" exposure time and esophageal bile acids or trypsin. Similarly, Mattioli et al. (39), using a triple-probe pH monitor placed in the distal esophagus, fundus, and antrum, found that "alkaline" reflux, defined as a rise in pH>7 from the antrum to esophagus, was extremely uncommon (0.75%) in 279 patients. Therefore, these authors suggested that increases of esophageal pH>7 were most likely due to other reasons (saliva, food, oral infection, obstructed esophagus) rather than reflux of duodenal contents. This speculation was substantiated by studies from Singh et al. (40) and DeVault et al. (41), who found that increased saliva production or bicarbonate production by the esophageal submucosal glands were the most common cause of esophageal pH>7, while DGER was rare in patients with an intact stomach. Using an ambulatory bilirubin monitoring device combined with pH monitoring, Vaezi and Richter (92) reported no difference in the percent of total time that pH>7 among controls, patients with GERD, and those with Barrett's esophagus (Fig. 23.3). Furthermore, Champion et al. (23), as well as other recent studies (93,94), found no correlation between pH>7 and bile reflux into the esophageal lumen (Fig. 23.4), suggesting that the term "alkaline" reflux was a misnomer and should not be used when referring to DGER. Finally, Just et al. (95) found a poor correlation (R=0.26) between intragastric pH ("alkaline shift") and intragastric bilirubin absorbance, concluding that the measurement of "alkaline reflux" in the esophagus or stomach with ambulatory pH monitoring alone is "an outdated technique."

Ambulatory Bilirubin Monitoring (Bilitec 2000)

A fiberoptic spectrophotometer (Bilitec 2000, Synectics, Stockholm, Sweden) detects DGER in an ambulatory setting, independent of pH (96). This instrument utilizes the optical properties of bilirubin, the most common bile pigment. Bilirubin has a characteristic spectrophotometric absorption band at 450 nm. The basic working principle of this instrument is that absorption near this wavelength implies the presence of bilirubin and, therefore, represents DGER (Fig. 23.5).

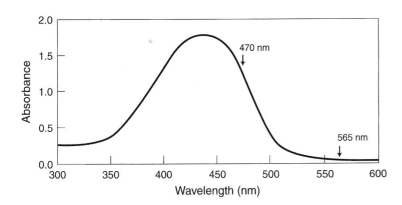

FIGURE 23.5. Spectrophotometric absorbance property of bilirubin. The arrows indicate the two wavelengths used by the Bilitec for detecting DGER. Detection of DGER depends on the difference in absorbance between 470 nm and 565 nm, suggesting reflux of bilirubin.

This system, resembling a standard ambulatory pH unit, consists of a miniaturized fiberoptic probe, which carries light signals into the tip and back to the optoelectronic system via a plastic fiberoptic bundle. The Teflon probe head is 9.5 mm in length and 4 mm in diameter. There is a 2.0-mm open groove in the probe across which two wavelengths of light are emitted and material sampled. Two light-emitting diodes at 470 and 565 nm represent the sources for the measurement of bilirubin and the reference signals, respectively. The portable photodiode system converts the light into an electrical signal. After amplification, the signals are processed by an integrated microcomputer, and the difference in absorption between the two diodes is calculated, representing absorption in the samples of DGER (Fig. 23.5). The period between two successive pulses from the same source, representing sampling time, is 8 seconds. In addition, the software averages between the absorbances are calculated over two successive samplings in order to decrease the noise of the measurements. A total of 5,400 sample recordings may be stored during a 24-hour period.

DGER data are usually measured as percent of time that bilirubin absorbance was >0.14, and can be analyzed separately for total, upright, and supine periods (Fig. 23.6). Percent bilirubin absorbance >0.14 is commonly chosen as a cutoff because studies show that values below this number represent scatter due to suspended particles and mucus present in gastric contents (96). In a recent study (92) using 20 healthy controls, the 95th percentile values for percent total, upright, and supine times that bilirubin was >0.14 were 1.8%, 2.2%, and 1.6%, respectively (Fig. 23.7).

Several reports have indicated a good correlation between Bilitec readings and bile acid concentration measured by duodenogastric aspiration studies: R=0.71, *p*<0.01 (96), and R=0.82, *p*<0.001 (97). Furthermore, our studies show that Bilitec readings correspond to bile acid concentrations in the range of 0.01 to 0.60 mM, which are more representative of bile acid concentrations found in the human stomach (0.1 to 1.0 mM). Additionally, a recent study by Stipa et al. (98) found a good correlation (R=0.7) between Bilitec readings and concentrations of pancreatic enzymes in aspirated esophageal fluid samples from patients with esophagitis. Most recently, Barrett et al. (99) conducted an *in vivo* validation of this device, and showed that although total bile acid and total bilirubin concentrations correlated strongly with Bilitec measurements *in vitro* (r=0.83 and r=0.82, respectively), the correlation was less strong *in vivo* (r=0.64). However, given its overall accuracy, they concurred with the previous studies that this device is a good measure of DGER. Therefore, this spectrophotometric technique is an important advancement in the assessment of DGER permitting more accurate studies of patients with syndromes associated with DGER. Additionally, it should be used concomitantly with pH monitoring to measure the esophageal exposure to both acid and DGER, since both are usually refluxed together in patients with no prior gastric surgery.

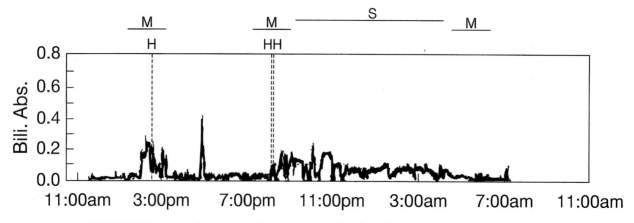

HIGH EPISODE		Total	Upright	Supine	Meal	PostP	Heartburn
Duration	(HH:MM)	19:54	12:54	07:00	00:20	06:00	00:12
Number of episodes	(#)	30	28	2	0	21	1
Number of episodes longer than 30.0 min	(#)	0	0	0	0	0	0
Longest episode	(min)	28	23	28	0	23	4
Total time Absorbance above 0.14	(min)	181	128	53	0	97	4
Fraction time Absorbance above 0.14	(%)	15.2	16.2	12.7	0.0	26.8	33.3
Median Absorbance value		---	---	---	---	---	---

S = Supine   C = Chest pain   M = Meal
H = Heartburn   P = PostP

FIGURE 23.6. A typical tracing and data generated by the Bilitec in measuring DGER. Data are typically reported in percent of time that bilirubin absorbance is >0.14 (total, upright, or supine).

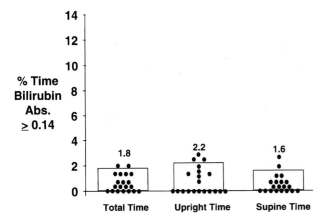

FIGURE 23.7. Percent of total, upright, and supine times that bilirubin absorbance is >0.14 in 20 normal subjects. Values within the boxed-in area represent the 95th percentile of the normal range.

Due to limitations inherent to the current Bilitec model, it is only a semiquantitative means of detecting DGER. Validation studies by Vaezi et al. (97) found that this instrument underestimates bile reflux by least 30% in an acidic medium (pH<3.5). In solutions with pH<3.5, bilirubin undergoes monomer to dimer isomerization, which is reflected by the shift in the absorption wavelength from 453 nm to 400 nm. Since Bilitec readings are based on the detection of absorption at 470 nm, this shift results in underestimation of the degree of DGER. Therefore, Bilitec measurements of DGER must always be accompanied by the simultaneous measurement of esophageal acid exposure using prolonged pH monitoring. Furthermore, a variety of substances may result in false positive readings by the Bilitec, since it indiscriminately records any substance absorbing around 470 nm. This necessitates use of a modified diet to avoid interference and false readings (96,97). Also, it is important to remember that Bilitec measures reflux of bilirubin and not bile acids or pancreatic enzymes; thus, it is presumed that the presence of bilirubin in the refluxate is accompanied by other duodenal contents. Although this is true in most cases, a few medical conditions (Gilbert's and Dubin–Johnson syndromes) may result in disproportionate secretion of bilirubin as compared to other duodenal contents, especially bile acids (100).

Despite its limitations, Bilitec is an important advancement in the assessment of DGER in the clinical arena. Several studies using this device provided important insights into the role of DGER in causing esophageal mucosal injury in humans. In a preliminary report, DeMeester's group (101) found no significant difference in esophageal bilirubin exposure in patients with esophagitis compared to healthy controls; however, patients with Barrett's esophagus had significantly more bilirubin and acid reflux than controls. On the other hand, Champion et al. (23) found a significant but graded increase in *both* acid and DGER from

controls to esophagitis patients, with the highest values observed in patients with Barrett's esophagus (Fig. 23.8). Furthermore, DGER had a strong correlation with acid reflux (R=0.78) but had a poor association with pH>7 (R= −0.06). Further support for the graduated increase in *both* acid and DGER came from studies by Vaezi and Richter (69) of patients with and without complications of Barrett's esophagus. They found that both groups of Barrett's patients refluxed significantly greater quantities of bile and acid into their lower esophagus than controls. More importantly, reflux of acid paralleled DGER and both were significantly higher in patients with complicated Barrett's than the uncomplicated group. The results of these studies were recently confirmed by other investigators (72,92,93). Marshall et al. (93) studied 55 patients with GERD, finding a good correlation between the degree of acid and DGER (R=0.55). Furthermore, expanded studies by Vaezi and Richter (92) found that simultaneous esophageal exposure to both acid and DGER was the most prevalent reflux pattern occurring in 95% of patients with Barrett's esophagus and 79% of GERD patients (Fig. 23.9). In fact, they found a strong correlation (R=0.73) between acid and DGER in controls, reflux patients, and those with Barrett's esophagus (Fig. 23.10). Thus, these studies support the earlier findings in animals that suggested a possible synergy between acid and DGER in the development of esophagitis and Barrett's esophagus.

Recently published epidemiologic studies find conflicting roles for DGER and esophageal adenocarcinoma (102–104). For example, Freedman et al. (102) conducted a population-based study based on the Swedish Cancer Registry finding that chloecystectomized patients had an increased risk of esophageal adenocarcinoma compared to those who did not have cholecystectomy. The implication from this study was that cholecystectomy results in increased DGER, which in turn might increase the risk of esophageal adenocarcinoma. However, these findings were countered by Avidan et al. (103), who found no difference in the rate of gastric surgery in 650 patients with short-segment or 366 patients with long-segment Barrett's esophagus compared to 3,046 controls. Similar conclusions were reached by Birgisson et al. (104) in their retrospective review of 325 patients with esophageal adenocarcinoma and 117 patients with esophageal squamous cell carcinoma, finding no difference in the rate of gastric surgery among the groups. This suggested no association between the potential risk of DGER and the development of esophageal adenocarcinoma. In the latter two studies (103,104), gastric surgery was used as an *in vivo* surrogate marker for DGER and its damaging potential in Barrett's metaplasia. Finally, recent *ex vivo* experiments using biopsies from Barrett's patients suggest an increase in cellular proliferation and decrease in cellular differentiation with exposure to either pulses of acid or bile (105–110). This effect was reduced by acid suppressive therapy (106). However, in contrast to the

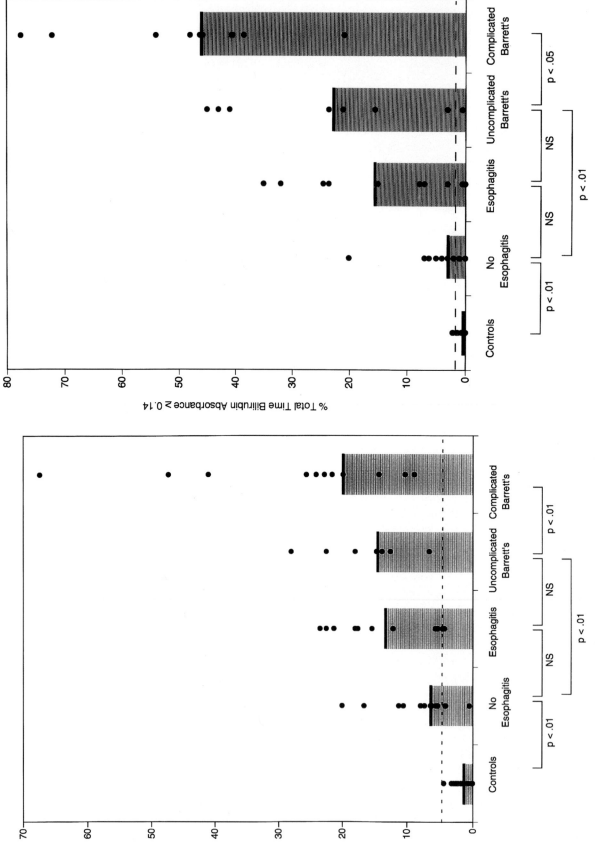

FIGURE 23.8. Group median **(A)** acid reflux and **(B)** DGER for five study populations: controls, acid reflux patients with and without esophagitis, and patients with uncomplicated and complicated Barrett's esophagus. (From Vaezi MF, Richter JE. Role of acid and duodenogastroesophageal reflux in gastroesophageal reflux disease. *Gastroenterology* 1996;111:1192–1199, with permission.)

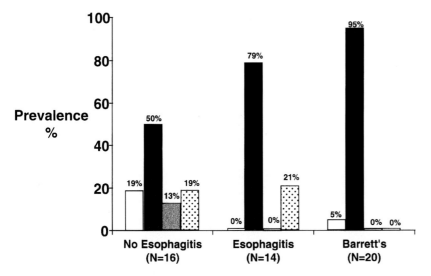

FIGURE 23.9. Prevalence of esophageal exposure to acid and DGER in the GERD subgroups. Esophageal exposure to acid and DGER occurred in 50% of patients without esophagitis, 79% of patients with esophagitis, and 95% of patients with Barrett's esophagus. *Open bar*, acid only; *solid bar*, acid+/DGER+; *shaded bar*, DGER only; *dotted bar*, acid–/DGER–. (From Vaezi MF, Richter JE. Role of acid and duodenogastroesophageal reflux in gastroesophageal reflux disease. *Gastroenterology* 1996;111:1192–1199, with permission.)

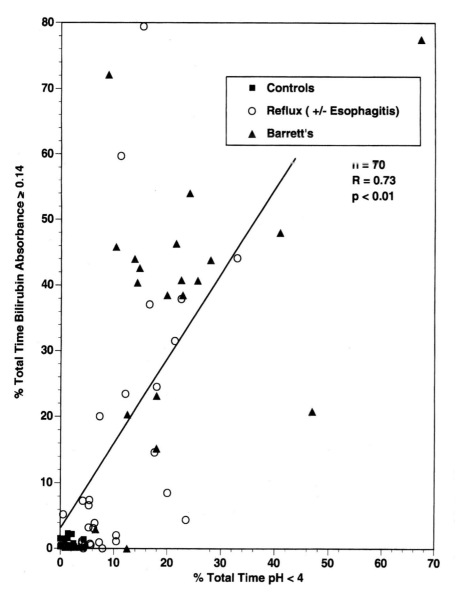

FIGURE 23.10. Relationship between acid reflux (percent of time that pH<4) and DGER (percent of time that bilirubin absorbance ≥0.14) in normal healthy controls, patients with GERD, and patients with Barrett's esophagus. (From Vaezi MF, Richter JE. Role of acid and duodenogastroesophageal reflux in gastroesophageal reflux disease. *Gastroenterology* 1996;111: 1192–1199, with permission.)

clinical data with the Bilitec finding possible synergy between acid and DGER in esophagitis and Barrett's esophagus, these *ex vivo* data suggest inhibition in the damaging potential of acid pulses when combined with bile. These conflicting data await future clarification based on *in vivo* and *ex vivo* trials (107).

The role of DGER in producing esophageal mucosal injury, in the absence of acid reflux, was not clarified until recently. Studies by Marshall et al. (93) using prolonged pH and bilirubin monitoring in 38 patients with GERD found that DGER in the absence of acid reflux was a rare event (7%) in patients without prior gastric surgery. Additionally, Sears et al. (111) studied 13 partial gastrectomy patients with reflux symptoms and found increased DGER by Bilitec monitoring in 77% of patients. This patient population represents an excellent human model for increased DGER because of the incompetent pylorus and free regurgitation of duodenal contents into the stomach, resulting in gastric bile acids concentrations (0.5 to 3.0 mM) known to cause esophageal mucosal injury in the animal model (>1mM). Endoscopic esophagitis, however, was present only in those who had concomitant acid reflux. Subsequently, Vaezi and Richter (112) confirmed these observations and found that only 24% of upper gastrointestinal symptoms reported by partial gastrectomy patients were due to DGER in the absence of acid reflux. These studies show that DGER without excessive acid reflux can cause reflux symptoms but does not usually produce esophagitis.

Multichannel Intraluminal Impedance

MII is an exciting new device that has the potential to measure both acidic as well as nonacidic refluxates of liquid or gas consistencies (113). This device is capable of measuring characteristics of gastroesophageal reflux that are not detectable by the current gold standard, the pH probe. Impedance is a measure of the total resistance to current flow between adjacent electrodes and is capable of differentiating between liquid and gas refluxates based on their inherent current and resistance properties. This device has been studied in a short-term stationary manner in patients with GERD and controls, and the prolonged ambulatory version of MII is currently under validation studies. The experimental and clinical data on this device are not reviewed here since they are covered elsewhere in this book.

MEDICAL AND SURGICAL TREATMENT OF DGER

It is well known that aggressive medical therapy to suppress acid secretion will heal most cases of esophagitis. Recently, some groups (30,87–90) have suggested that prolonged acid suppression in patients with severe esophagitis or Barrett's esophagus may promote DGER causing further mucosal injury with progression to Barrett's esophagus or even adenocarcinoma. This claim is based on isolated animal studies (114,115) and a handful of clinical reports, mainly from the same laboratory (29,87–90). The clinical relevance of these reports is questionable since the association between DGER and complicated Barrett's esophagus or adenocarcinoma was defined by esophageal pH monitoring (i.e., pH>7), which has since been shown to be an unreliable parameter for detecting DGER. More importantly, a careful review of the literature shows that the overwhelming majority of studies do not support this concept.

Both animal and human studies indicate that DGER in the absence of acid reflux is usually not damaging to the esophageal mucosa. Furthermore, recent studies by Champion et al. (23) in nine patients with severe GERD (three with esophagitis, and six with Barrett's esophagus) found that aggressive acid suppression with omeprazole (20 mg BID) dramatically decreased *both* acid and DGER (Fig. 23.11). The above findings have recently been reproduced

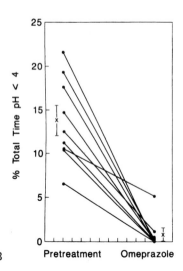
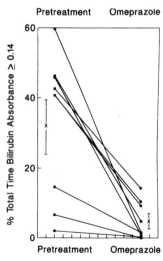

A,B

FIGURE 23.11. Influence of marked acid suppression with omeprazole (20 mg twice daily) on acid reflux (*A*) and DGER (*B*) in nine patients with GERD. (From Champion G, Richter JE, Vaezi MF, et al. Duodenogastroesophageal reflux: relationship to pH and importance in Barrett's esophagus. *Gastroenterology* 1994;107:747–754, with permission.)

by two other independent groups of investigators. Gut et al. (116) found that esophageal acid and DGER were both significantly (*p*<.02) reduced after 28 days of treatment with pantoprazole (40 mg qd) compared to pretreatment values in seven patients with endoscopic evidence of GERD. Similarly, Marshall et al. (117) studied esophageal and gastric bile reflux in 23 patients with Barrett's esophagus finding a significant (*p*<.005) reduction in both esophageal and gastric acid (pH monitoring) and bile (Bilitec) reflux after 6 to 10 weeks of treatment with omeprazole (20 mg bid). The studies by Champion et al. (23) and Marshall et al. (117) suggest that the decrease in DGER measured after proton pump inhibitors may be due to their inhibition of both gastric acidity and volume, making less gastric contents available to reflux into the esophagus despite even a low LES pressure. In support of this proposed mechanism are previous studies showing about 40% reduction in gastric volume by 40 mg of omeprazole (118,119). Therefore, medical therapy with aggressive acid suppression may not only protect the esophageal mucosa from the damaging effects of acid and eliminate the synergy between acid, pepsin, and bile, but also it decreases the volume of both acid and bile refluxing into the esophagus.

Recent studies in patients with Barrett's esophagus using *ex vivo* methodologies suggest that overexpression of COX-2 may affect progression of Barrett's epithelium by increasing proliferation, reducing apoptosis, promoting angiogenesis, and increasing invasiveness and metastatic potential of Barrett's metaplasia (108–110). This *ex vivo* response was eliminated by the addition of cyclooxygenase (COX)-2 inhibitors (120). Hence, some suggest that clinically the addition of COX-2 inhibition using aspirin, nonsteroidal antiinflammatory drugs, or the more selective COX-2 inhibitors to acid suppression with proton pump inhibitors, might enhance the therapeutic benefit. However, there will be no current recommendation in this area until more data are published.

Previously, several agents were used to treat bile gastritis and symptoms associated with DGER, including antacids, namely aluminum hydroxide, sucralfate, prostaglandin E2, cimetidine, ranitidine, cholestyramine, metoclopramide, and ursodeoxycholic acid (121). Although these agents showed efficacy for mild to moderate "bile gastritis," the results were less than promising for "alkaline reflux esophagitis," thereby limiting their use in DGER. Prior to the findings by Champion et al. (23), the best therapy for decreasing DGER into the esophagus was thought to be an antireflux operation, correcting the defective LES. Therefore, the findings by Champion et al. (23) have important implications for treating patients with both acid and bile reflux. This study suggests that medical therapy with proton pump inhibitors may decrease both acid and DGER to a similar degree as antireflux surgery. Medical therapy has the advantage of avoiding a surgical procedure and its associated complications, an important consideration in the

elderly and those with contraindications to surgery. However, in younger patients in whom long-term medical therapy is anticipated, antireflux surgery may be a more suitable and cost-effective alternative.

In partial gastrectomy patients having mild upper GI symptoms due to nonacidic DGER, previous studies found that administration of aluminum hydroxide containing antacids (30cc qid), cholestyramine (1.0 gm qid), or ursodeoxycholic acid may improve symptoms (121). In a recent randomized, double-blind, crossover study (122), cisparide (20 mg qid) was found to significantly reduce both DGER measured by the Bilitec and associated upper GI symptoms (i.e., abdominal pain, bloating, belching, regurgitation, nausea, and vomiting) in patients after vagotomy and antrectomy or pyloromyotomy for chronic ulcer disease. Thus, medical therapy with promotility drugs is an alternative to surgical Roux-en-Y diversion. Medical options are important since a recent study by McAlhany et al. (123) found that up to 36% of patients undergoing Roux-en-Y diversion for bile reflux failed within 6 months of the operation and were unsatisfied with the results of surgery. Nevertheless, patients unresponsive to aggressive medical therapy for well-documented, nonacid DGER should be considered for bile diversion operations such as Roux-en-Y or Henley isoperistaltic jejunal interposition as the best surgical options for this difficult-to-manage problem.

CONCLUSION

Both animal and human studies strongly suggest that acid is the key factor in causing esophageal injury and Barrett's esophagus in patients with GERD. Studies using advanced techniques to identify DGER spectrophotometrically and independent of pH (Bilitec), however, suggest that duodenal contents often are present in the esophageal refluxate. The degree of esophageal exposure to acid and DGER showed a graded and similar increase from controls to esophagitis patients, with the highest value observed in patients with Barrett's esophagus. This close relationship raises the possibility that synergistic actions of acid, pepsin, and conjugated bile acids may be contributing to the development of Barrett's metaplasia and possibly even adenocarcinoma. Human studies show that DGER in a nonacidic environment (i.e., partial gastrectomy patients) may cause symptoms, but does not cause esophageal mucosal injury. Despite suggestions to the contrary by some surgical groups, aggressive acid suppression with proton pump inhibitors decreases both acid and DGER, perhaps by decreasing the volume of gastric contents available to reflux into the esophagus. Furthermore, the high intragastric and intraesophageal pH environment produced by proton pump inhibitors inactivates conjugated bile acids, the main DGER ingredients implicated in causing esophagitis. Thus, the proton pump inhibitors effectively heal esophagitis even in cases of severe reflux and Barrett's esophagus.

REFERENCES

1. DeMeester TR, Wernly JA, Little AG, et al. Technique, indications, and clinical use of 24 hour esophageal pH monitoring. *J Thorac Cardiovasc Surg* 1980;79:656–670.

2. Redo SF, Barnes WA, de la Sierra AO. Perfusion of the canine esophagus with secretions of the upper gastro-intestinal tract. *Ann Surg* 1959;149:556–564.

3. Ferguson DJ, Sanchez-Palomera E, Sako Y, et al. Studies on experimental esophagitis. *Surgery* 1950;28:1022–1039.

4. Kiriluk LB, Merendino KA. Compariative sensitivity of mucosa of various segments of alimentary tract in dog to acid-peptic action. *Surgery* 1954;35:547–556.

5. Goldberg HI, Dodds WJ, Gee S, et al. Role of acid and pepsin in acute experimental esophagitis. *Gastroenterology* 1969;56: 223–230.

6. Mackie C, Hulks G, Cuschieri A. Enterogastric reflux and gastric clearance of refluxate in patients with and without bile vomiting following peptic ulcer surgery. *Ann Surg* 1986;204: 537–542.

7. Muller-Lissner SA, Fimmel CJ, Sonnenberg A. Novel approach to quantify duodenogastric reflux in healthy volunteers and in patients with type I gastric ulcer. *Gut* 1983;24:510–518.

8. Schidlbeck NE, Heinrich C, Stellard F, et al. Healthy controls have as much bile reflux as gastric ulcer patients. *Gut* 1987;28: 1577–1583.

9. King PM, Pryde A, Heading RC. Transpyloric fluid movement and antroduodenal motility in patients with gastroesophageal reflux. *Gut* 1987;28:545–548.

10. Gotley DC, Morgan AP, Cooper MJ. Bile acid concentrations in the refluxate of patients with reflux oesophagitis. *Br J Surg* 1988;75:587–590.

11. Gotley DC, Morgan AP, Ball D, et al. Composition of gastro-oesophageal refluxate. *Gut* 1991;32:1093–1099.

12. Burden WR, Hodges RP, Hsu M, et al. Alkaline reflux gastritis. *Surg Clin North Am* 199171:33–44.

13. Dixon MF. Progress in pathology of gastritis and duodenitis. In: Williams GT, ed. *Current topics in pathology.* New York: Springer-Verlag, 1990:1–39.

14. DuPlessis DJ. Pathogenesis of gastric ulceration. *Lancet* 1965;1: 974–978.

15. Ritchie WP. Alkaline reflux gastritis: a critical reappraisal. *Gut* 1984;25:975–987.

16. Harmon JW, Bass BL, Batzri S. Alkaline reflux gastritis. In: Nyhus LL, ed. *Problems in general surgery.* Philadelphia: Lippincott, 1993:201–206.

17. Hopewood D, Bateson MC, Milner G, et al. Effects of bile acids and hydrogen ion on the fine structure of oesophageal epithelium. *Gut* 1981;22:306–311.

18. Hubens A, Van de Kelft E, Roland J. The influence of cholecystectomy on the duodenogastric reflux of bile. *Hepatogastroenterology* 1989;36:384–386.

19. Kalima TV. Reflux gastritis unrelated to gastric surgery. *Scand J Gastroenterol* 1982;17(suppl 79):66–71.

20. Muller-Lissner SA, Schindlbeck NE, Heinrich C. Bile salt reflux after cholecystectomy. *Scand J Gastroenterol* 1987;22(suppl 139):20–24.

21. Nano M, Palmas F, Giaccone M, et al. Biliary reflux after cholecystectomy: a prospective study. *Hepatogastroenterology* 1990; 37:233–234.

22. Stoker DL, Williams JG. Alkaline reflux oesophagitis. *Gut* 1991;32:1090–1092.

23. Champion G, Richter JE, Vaezi MF, et al. Duodenogastroesophageal reflux: Relationship to pH and importance in Barrett's esophagus. *Gastroenterology* 1994;107:747–754.

24. Lillemoe KD, Johnson LF, Harmon JW. Role of the components of the gastroduodenal contents in experimental acid esophagitis. *Surgery* 1982;92:276–284.

25. Aylwin JA. The physiological basis of reflux esophagitis in sliding distal diaphragmatic hernia. *Thorax* 1953;8:38–45.

26. Tuttle SG, Bettarello A, Gossman MI. Esophageal acid perfusion test and a gastroesophageal reflux in patients with esophagitis. *Gastroenterology* 1960;38:861–872.

27. Tuttle SG, Rufin F, Bettarello A. The physiology of heartburn. *Ann Int Med* 1961;55:292–300.

28. Zamost BJ, Hirschberg J, Ippoliti AF. Esophagitis in scleroderma: Prevalence and risk factors. *Gastroenterology* 1987;92: 421–428.

29. Stein HJ, Barlow AP, DeMeester TR, et al. Complications of gastroesophageal reflux disease. *Ann Surg* 1992;216:35–43.

30. Hennessy TPJ. Barrett's esophagus. *Br J Surg* 1985;72:336–340.

31. Gillen P, Keeling P, Byrne PJ, et al. Barrett's esophagus: pH profile. *Br J Surg* 1987;74:774–776.

32. Stein HJ, Siewert JR. Barrett's esophagus: Pathogenesis, epidemiology, functional abnormalities, malignant degeneration, and surgical management. *Dysphagia* 1993;8:276–288.

33. Iascone C, DeMeester TR, Little AG, et al. Barrett's esophagus: functional assessment, proposed pathogenesis, and surgical therapy. *Arch Surg* 1983;118:543.

34. Stein HJ, Hoeft S, DeMeester TR. Reflux and motility pattern in Barrett's esophagus. *Dis Esophagus* 1992;5:21–28.

35. Stein HJ, Hoeft S, DeMeester TR. Functional foregut abnormalities in Barrett's esophagus. *J Thorac Cardiovasc Surg* 1993; 105:107–111.

36. Bremner RM, Crookes PF, DeMeester TR, et al. Concentration of refluxed acid and esophageal mucosal injury. *Am J Surg* 1992; 164:522–527.

37. Miller LS, Fruacht H, Saeed ZA, et al. Esophageal involvement in the Zollinger Ellison syndrome (ZES). *Gastroenterology* 1990; 98:341–345.

38. Hamilton BH, Orlado RC. In vivo alkaline secretion by mammalian esophagus. *Gastroenterology* 1989;97:640–648.

39. Mattioli S, Pilotti V, Felice V, et al. Ambulatory 24 hour pH monitoring of the esophagus, fundus and antrum. *Dig Dis Sci* 1990;35:929–38.

40. Singh S, Bradley LA, Richter JE. Determinants of oesophageal "alkaline" pH environment in controls and patients with gastro-oesophageal reflux disease. *Gut* 1993;34: 309–316.

41. DeVault KR, Georgeson S, Castell DO. Salivary stimulation mimics esophageal exposure to refluxed duodenal contents. *Am J Gastroenterol* 1993;88:1040–1043.

42. Cross FS, Wangensteen OH. Role of bile and pancreatic juice in the production of esophageal erosions and anemia. *Proc Soc Exp Biol Med* 1961;77:862–866.

43. Moffat RC, Berkas EM. Bile esophagitis. *Arch Surg* 1965;91: 963–966.

44. Harmon JW, Johnson LF, Maydonovitch CL. Effects of acid and bile salts on the rabbit esophageal mucosa. *Dig Dis Sci* 1981;26:65–72.

45. Kivilaakso E, Fromm D, Silen W. Effect of bile salts and related compounds on isolated esophageal mucosa. *Surgery* 1980;87: 280–285.

46. Gillison EW, DeCastro VAM, Nyhus LM, et al. The significance of bile in reflux esophagitis. *Surg Gyn Obstet* 1972;134: 419–424.

47. Salo J, Kivilaakso E. Role of luminal H+ in the pathogenesis of experimental esophagitis. *Surgery* 1982;92:61–68.

48. Salo JA, Kivilaakso E. Contribution of trypsin and cholate to the pathogenesis of experimental alkaline reflux esophagitis. *Scand J Gastroenterol* 1984;19:875–881.

49. Lillemoe KD, Johnson LF, Harmon JW. Taurodeoxycholate modulates the effects of pepsin and trypsin in experimental esophagitis. *Surgery* 1985;97:662–667.

50. Salo JA, Lehto VP, Kivilaakso E. Morphological alteration in experimental esophagitis. *Dig Dis Sci* 1983;28:440–448.

51. Shimono M, Clementi F. Intercellular junction of oral epithelium. *J Ultrastruct Res* 1977;59:101–112.

52. Carney CN, Orlando RC, Powell DW. Morphologic alterations in early acid induced epithelial injury of he rabbit esophagus. *Lab Invest* 1981;45:198–208.

53. Orlando RC, Bryson JC, Powell DW. Mechanism of H+ injury in rabbit esophageal epithelium. *Am J Physiol* 1984;9: G718–G724.

54. Orlando RC, Powell DW, Carney CN. Pathophysiology of acute acid injury in rabbit esophageal epithelium. *J Clin Invest* 1981;68:286–293.

55. Powell DW, Orlando RC, Carney CN. Acid injury of the esophageal epithelium. In: Harmon JW, ed. *Basic mechanism of gastrointestinal mucosal cell injury and protection.* Baltimore: Williams & Wilkins, 1981:55.

56. Snow JC, Goldstein JL, Schmidt LN, et al. Rabbit esophageal cells show regulatory volume decrease: ionic basis and effect of pH. *Gastroenterology* 1993;105:102–110.

57. Duane WC, Wiegand DM. Mechanism by which bile salt disrupts the gastric mucosal barrier in the dog. *J Clin Invest* 1980; 66:1044–1049.

58. Thomas AJ, Nahrwold DL, Rose RC. Detergent action of sodium taurocholate on rat gastric mucosa. *Biochim Biophys Acta* 1972;282:210–213.

59. Tanaka K, Fromm F. Effect of bile acid and salicylate on isolated surface and glandular cells of rabbit stomach. *Surgery* 1983;93: 660–663.

60. Schweitzer EJ, Harmon JW, Bass BL, et al. Bile acid efflux precedes mucosal barrier disruption in the rabbit esophagus. *Am J Physiol* 1984;10:G480–G485.

61. Schweitzer EJ, Bass BL, Batzri S, et al. Lipid solubilization during bile salt-induced esophageal mucosal barrier disruption in the rabbit. *J Lab Clin Med* 1987;110:172–179.

62. Batzri S, Harmon JW, Schweitzer EJ, et al. Bile acid accumulation in gastric mucosal cells. *Proc Soc Exp Biol Med* 1991;197: 393–399.

63. Schweitzer EJ, Bass BL, Batzri S, et al. Bile acid accumulation by rabbit esophageal mucosa. *Dig Dis Sci* 1986;31:1105–1113.

64. Nasrallah SM, Johnston GS, Gadacz TR, et al. The significance of gastric bile reflux seen at endoscopy. *J Clin Gastroenterol* 1987;9:514–517.

65. Stein HJ, Smyrk TC, DeMeester TR, et al. Clinical value of endoscopy and histology in the diagnosis of duodenogastric reflux disease. *Surgery* 1992;112:796–804.

66. Kaye MD, Showalter JP. Pyloric incompetence in patients with symptomatic gastroesophageal reflux. *J Lab Clin Med* 1974;83:198–206.

67. Gillen P, Keeling P, Byrne PJ, et al. Importance of duodenogastric reflux in the pathogenesis of Barrett's oesophagus. *Br J Surg* 1988;75:540–543.

68. Mittal RK, Reuben A, Whitney JO, et al. Do bile acids reflux into the esophagus? A study in normal subject and patients with GERD. *Gastroenterology* 1987;92:371–375.

69. Vaezi MF, Richter JE. Synergism of acid and duodenogastroesophageal reflux in complicated Barrett's esophagus. *Surgery* 1995;117:699–704.

70. Smith MR, Buckton GK, Bennett JR. Bile acid levels in stomach and oesophagus of patients with acid gastroesophageal reflux. *Gut* 1984;25:A556.

71. Johnsson F, Joelsson B, Floren CH, et al. Bile salts in the esophagus of patients with esophagitis. *Scand J Gastroenterol* 1988; 712–716.

72. Kauer WKH, Peters JH, DeMeester TR, et al. Composition and concentration of bile acid reflux into the esophagus of patients with gastroesophageal reflux disease. *Surgery* 1997;122: 874–881.

73. Tolin RD, Malmud LS, Stelzer F, et al. Enterogastric reflux in normal subjects and patients with Bilroth II gastroenterostomy. Measurement of enterogastric reflux. *Gastroenterology* 1979;77: 1027–1033.

74. Eriksson B, Emas S, Jacobsson H, et al. Comparison of gastric aspiration and HIDA scintigraphy in detecting fasting duodenogastric bile reflux. *Scand J Gastroenterol* 1988;23:607–610.

75. Houghton PWJ, Mortensen NJ, Thomas WEG, et al. Intragastric bile acids and scintigraphy in the assessment of duodenogastric reflux. *Br J Surg* 1986;73:292–294.

76. Matikainen M, Taavitsainen M, Kalima TV. Duodenogastric reflux in patients with heartburn and esophagitis. *Scand J Gastroenterol* 1981;16:253–255.

77. Krog M, Gustavsson S, Jung B. Studies on oesophagitis—No evidence for pyloric incompetence as a primary etiological factor. A scintigraphic study with 99Tcm-Solco-HIDA. *Acta Chir Scand* 1982;148:439–442.

78. Warring JP, Legrand J, Chinichian A, et al. Duodenogastric reflux in patients with Barrett's esophagus. *Dig Dis Sci* 1990; 35:759–762.

79. Liron R, Parrilla P, de Haro M, et al. Quantification of duodenogastric reflux in Barrett's esophagus. *Am J Gastroenterol* 1997;92:32–36.

80. Drane WE, Karvelis K, Johnson DA, et al. Scintigraphic evaluation of duodenogastric reflux. Problems, pitfalls, and technical review. *Clin Nucl Med* 1987;12:377–384.

81. Stein HJ, Hinder RA, DeMeester TR, et al. Clinical use of 24-hour gastric monitoring vs o-diisopropyl iminodiacetic acid (DISIDA) scanning in the diagnosis of pathologic duodenogastric reflux. *Arch Surg* 1990;125:966–971.

82. Brown TH, Holbrook I, King RFG, et al. 24-hour intragastric pH measurement in the assessment of duodenogastric reflux. *World J Surg* 1992;16:995–1000.

83. Pellegrini CA, DeMeester TR, Wernly JA, et al. Alkaline gastroesophageal reflux. *Am J Surg* 1978;75:177–184.

84. Little AG, DeMeester TR, Kirchner PT, et al. Pathogenesis of esophagitis in patients with gastroesophageal reflux. *Surgery* 1980;88:101–107.

85. Little AG, Martinez EI, DeMeester TR, et al. Duodenogastric reflux and reflux esophagitis. *Surgery* 1984;96:447–454.

86. Schmid B, DeTarnowsky G, Layden T. Alkaline gastroesophageal reflux: role in esophageal injury. *Gastroenterology* 1981;80:A1275.

87. Attwood SEA, DeMeester TR, Bemner CG, et al. Alkaline gastroesophageal reflux: implications in the development of complications in Barrett's columnar-lined lower esophagus. *Surgery* 1989;106:764–776.

88. Atwood SEA, Barlow AP, Norris TL, et al. Barrett's esophagus: effect of antireflux surgery on symptom control and development of complications. *Br J Surg* 1992;79:1050–1053.

89. Attwood SEA, Ball CS, Barlow AP, et al. Role of intragastric and intraoesophageal alkalinization in the genesis of complications in Barrett's columnar lined lower oesophagus. *Gut* 1993;34: 11–15.

90. Attwood SEA. New advances in the understanding of Barrett's esophagus. *Surg Ann* 1993;25:151–175.

91. Gotley DC, Appleton GVN, Cooper MJ. Bile acids and trypsin are unimportant in alkaline esophageal reflux. *J Clin Gastroenterol* 1992;14:2–7.

92. Vaezi MF, Richter JE. Role of acid and duodenogastrosophageal reflux in gastroesophageal reflux disease. *Gastroenterology* 1996;111:1192–1199.

93. Marshall REK, Anggiansah A, Owen WA, et al. The relationship between acid and bile reflux and symptoms in gastroesophageal reflux disease. *Gut* 1997;40:182–187.

94. Iftikhar SY, Ledingham S, Evans DF, et al. Alkaline gastroesophageal reflux: dual probe pH monitoring. *Gut* 1995;37:465–570.

95. Just RJ, Leite LP, Castell DO. Changes in overnight fasting intragastric pH show poor correlation with duodenogastric bile relux in normal subjects. *Am J Gastroenterol* 1996;91:1567–1570.

96. Bechi P, Paucciani F, Baldini F, et al. Long-term ambulatory enterogastric reflux monitoring. Validation of a new fiberoptic technique. *Dig Dis Sci* 1993;38:1297–1306.

97. Vaezi MF, LaCamera RG, Richter JE. Bilitec 2000 ambulatory duodenogastric reflux monitoring system. Studies on its validation and limitations. *Am J Physiol* 1994;267:G1050–G1057.

98. Stipa F, Stein HJ, Feussner H, et al. Assessment of non-acid esophageal reflux: comparison between long-term reflux aspiration test and fiberoptic bilirubin monitoring. *Dis Esophagus* 1997;10:24–28.

99. Barrett MW, Myers JC, Watson DI, et al. Detection of bile reflux: in vivo validation of the Bilitec fiberoptic system. *Dis Esophagus* 2000;13:44–55.

100. Lumeng L, O'Connor KW. Differential diagnosis of jaundice. In: Ostrow JD, ed. *Bile pigments and jaundice.* New York: Marcel Dekker Inc, 1986:475–538.

101. Kauer WK, Burdiles P, Ireland AP, et al. Does duodenal juice reflux into the esophagus of patients with complicated GERD? Evaluation of a fiber optic sensor for bilirubin. *Am J Surg* 1995;169:98–103.

102. Freedman J, Ye W, Naslund E, et al. Association between cholecystectomy and adenocarcinoma of the esophagus. *Gastroenterology* 2001;121:548–553.

103. Avidan B, Sonnenberg A, Schnell TG, et al. Gastric surgery is not a risk factor for Barrett's esophagus or esophageal adenocarcinoma. *Gastroenterology* 2001;121:1281–1285.

104. Birgisson S, Rice TW, Easley KA, et al. The lack of association between adenocarcinoma of the esophagus and gastric surgery: a retrospective study. *Am J Gastroenterol* 1997;97:216–221.

105. Fitzgerald RC, Omary MB, Triadafilopoulos G. Dynamic effects of acid on Barrett's esophagus. An ex-vivo proliferation and differentiation model. *J Clin Invest* 1996;98:212–218.

106. Quatu-Lascar R, Fitzgerald RC, Triadafilopoulos G. Differentiation and proliferation in Barrett's esophagus and the effect of acid suppression. *Gastroenterology* 1999;224:358–371.

107. Kaur BS, Quatu-Lascar R, Omary MB, et al. Bile salts induce or blunt cell proliferation in Barrett's esophagus in an acid-dependent fashion. *Am J Physiol Gastrointest Liver Physiol* 2000;278:G1000–G1009.

108. Shirvani VN, Quatu-Lascar R, Omary MB, et al. Cyclooxygenase 2 expression in Barrett's esophagus and adenocarcinoma: Ex vivo induction by bile salts and acid exposure. *Gastroenterology* 2000;118:487–496.

109. Kaur BS, Omary MB, Triadafilopoulos G. Bile salts induced PGE2 and COX-2 expression, parallel the increased cell proliferation in an ex-vivo model of Barrett's esophagus. *Gastroenterology* 2000;118:A224.

110. Kaur BS, Triadafilopoulos G. Acid and bile-induced PGE2 release and hyperproliferation in Barrett's esophagus are COX-2 and PKC-e dependent. *Am J Physiol Gastrointest Liver Physiol* 2002;283:G327–G334.

111. Sears RJ, Champion G, Richter JE. Characteristics of partial gastrectomy (PG) patients with esophageal symptoms of duodenogastric reflux. *Am J Gastroenterol* 1995;90:211–215.

112. Vaezi MF, Richter JE. Contribution of acid and duodenogastroesophageal reflux to esophgeal mucosal injury and symptoms in partial gastrectomy patients. *Gut* 1997;41:297–302.

113. Vaezi MF, Shay SS. New techniques in measuring non-acidic esophageal reflux. *Semin Thorac Cardiovasc Surg* 2001;13:255–264.

114. Attwood SEA, Smyrk TC, DeMeester TR, et al. Duodenoesophageal reflux and the development of esophageal adeno-carcinoma in rats. *Surgery* 1992;111:503–510.

115. Pera M, Trastek VF, Carpenter HA, et al. Influence of pancreatic and biliary reflux on the development of esophageal carcinoma. *Ann Thorac Surg* 1993;55:1386–1393.

116. Gut A, Gaia C, Netzer P, et al. Reduction of esophageal bile and acid reflux by pantoprazole in patients with reflux esophagitis. *Gastroenterology* 1997;112:A135.

117. Marshall REK, Anggiansah A, Owen WA, et al. Reduction of gastroesophageal bile reflux by omeprazole in Barrett's esophagus: an initial experience. *Gut* 1996;39:T115.

118. Festen HPN, Tuynman HARE, Defize J, et al. Effect of single and repeated doses of oral omeprazole on gastric acid and pepsin secretion and fasting serum pepsinogen I levels. *Dig Dis Sci* 1986;31:561–566.

119. Lind T, Cederberg C, Ekenved G, et al. Effect of omeprazole-a gastric proton pump inhibitor-on pentagastrin stimulated acid secretion in man. *Gut* 1983;24:270–276.

120. Patrono C, Patrignani P, Garcia-Rodriguez LA. Cyclooxygenase selective inhibition of prostanoid formation: translating biochemical selectivity into clinical read-outs. *J Clin Invest* 2001;108:7–13.

121. Nath BJ, Warshaw AL. Alkaline reflux gastritis and esophagitis. *Ann Rev Med* 1984;35:383–396.

122. Vaezi MF, Sears R, Richter JE. Double-blind placebo-controlled cross-over trial of cisapride in postgastrectomy patients with duodenogastric reflux. *Dig Dis Sci* 1996;41:754–763.

123. McAlhany JC, Hanover TM, Taylor SM, et al. Long-term follow-up of patients with Roux-en-Y gastrojejunostomy for gastric disease. *Ann Surg* 1994;219:451–457.

ROLE OF *HELICOBACTER PYLORI* IN GERD

GARY W. FALK

A variety of abnormalities contribute to the development of gastroesophageal reflux disease (GERD), including transient lower esophageal sphincter (LES) relaxation, low LES pressure, presence of a hiatal hernia, diminished esophageal clearance of refluxed gastric contents, and alterations in esophageal mucosal resistance. *Helicobacter pylori* infection clearly plays a role in the pathogenesis of peptic ulcer disease and mucosa-associated lymphoid tissue (MALT) lymphoma of the stomach and is a definite risk factor for distal gastric cancer. The role of *H. pylori* infection in gastroesophageal reflux disease remains controversial and incompletely understood. While *H. pylori* infection does not cause reflux disease, circumstantial evidence suggests that it may protect against the development of GERD and its complications in some patients. The most likely mechanism whereby *H. pylori* infection protects against GERD is by decreasing the potency of the gastric refluxate in patients with corpus predominant gastritis. There are a variety of implications of *H. pylori* infection on GERD treatment, including the risk of gastric atrophy while on proton pump inhibitor therapy and the efficacy of proton pump inhibitors before and after eradication of *H. pylori*. This chapter will put into perspective our current understanding of the complex, incompletely understood relationship between *H. pylori* infection and GERD.

Epidemiology of *H. pylori* and GERD

H. pylori infection is on the decline in the Western world (1). At the same time, hospitalization and mortality rates for duodenal ulcer disease, gastric ulcer disease, and cancer of the gastric antrum and corpus, all clearly *H. pylori* related diseases, declined markedly between 1970 and 1995 (2). However, hospitalization and mortality rates for both gastroesophageal reflux disease and esophageal adenocarcinoma have increased during that same time interval. Given the clear link between *H. pylori* infection and peptic ulcer disease as well as distal gastric cancer, it has been hypothesized that the decline in *H. pylori* infection may explain these two opposing time trends (2). Furthermore, white subjects have higher rates of reflux disease and esophageal adenocarcinoma and lower rates of gastric cancer compared to nonwhite subjects (2). Since nonwhites in the United States tend to have higher *H. pylori* infection rates, this hypothesis is strengthened still further.

There is clearly no causal relationship between *H. pylori* infection and GERD (3–11). However, some studies suggest that *H. pylori* infection may be less common in patients with GERD (8,10,11). Furthermore, the severity of esophagitis in *H. pylori*–infected patients is either no different or less severe than in GERD patients not infected with *H. pylori* (7,9,12). This has led to the concept that *H. pylori* infection may actually protect against the development of GERD. These observations are especially intriguing in Asia, where the background prevalence of *H. pylori* infection is much higher than in the West and GERD is less common. In a case control study from China, the prevalence of *H. pylori* infection was 31% in GERD patients compared to 61% in age-matched asymptomatic controls (10). Similar findings were seen in Japan, where 41% of patients with esophagitis were infected with *H. pylori* compared to 76% of age-matched asymptomatic controls undergoing screening for gastric cancer (11).

Epidemiology of *H. pylori* and Barrett's Esophagus

The situation described above in GERD is comparable in Barrett's esophagus and esophageal adenocarcinoma. *H. pylori* infection is either no more common or less common in Barrett's esophagus and esophageal adenocarcinoma than in control populations (3–5,13–16). *H. pylori* rarely colonizes Barrett's epithelium, and when it does, it is found

G. W. Falk: Center for Swallowing and Esophageal Disorders, Department of Gastroenterology & Hepatology, The Cleveland Clinic Foundation, Cleveland, Ohio.

exclusively in gastric cardia and fundic type mucosa, not in intestinal metaplasia (13,15,17).

Several studies suggest that infection with *H. pylori*, especially *cagA+* strains, may protect against the development of Barrett's esophagus and its associated dysplasia and adenocarcinoma (4,14,18,19). Chow et al. (18) found that infection with *cagA+* strains of *H. pylori* was associated with a 60% decrease in the risk of esophageal and cardia carcinoma compared to a control population. When compared to a control population (42%), Vicari et al. (4) found that the prevalence of *cagA+* strains of *H. pylori* decreased in patients with more severe complications of GERD (nonerosive GERD, 41.2%; erosive GERD, 30.8%; Barrett's esophagus 13.3%; and adenocarcinoma or dysplasia, 0%). These observations were extended recently by Vaezi et al. (19), who found that colonization with *cagA+* strains of *H. pylori* was less common in both long and short segment Barrett's esophagus than in controls and patients with GERD.

However, these findings remain controversial due to two factors. First, studies to date have involved a relatively small number of patients. Second, these findings have led some to question the need to aggressively diagnose and treat *H. pylori*. This has created confusion among clinicians when *H. pylori* is diagnosed. Does treatment protect against some diseases (peptic ulcer disease, gastric cancer, MALT lymphoma) while enhancing the risk of developing other diseases (GERD, Barrett's esophagus, esophageal adenocarcinoma)? Most experts continue to believe that once *H. pylori* is diagnosed, treatment should ensue.

The Effect of *H. pylori* Eradication on GERD

There continues to be considerable confusion about the effect of *H. pylori* eradication on the *de novo* development of GERD. This issue was first raised by a study in Germany by Labenz et al. (20), in which duodenal ulcer patients successfully cured of *H. pylori* infection developed new onset erosive esophagitis more frequently (26%) than duodenal ulcer patients who remained infected (13%) during three years of follow-up (Fig. 24.1). Esophagitis was low grade in all but one of the patients. Similarly, Fallone et al. (21) found new onset reflux symptoms or esophagitis in 37% of duodenal ulcer patients successfully cured of *H. pylori* infection compared to 13% with ongoing infection at 1 year of follow-up. However, closer reading of that study of only 87 patients indicates that while there was a significant difference in new GERD symptoms in the eradicated (29%) versus the failed eradication group (8%), there was no significant difference in new onset esophagitis between the two groups. Comparable findings have been described in a study of 286 patients from Japan with gastritis alone, duodenal ulcers, gastric ulcers, and both gastric and duodenal ulcers, where 18% of the eradication group developed reflux esophagitis within 3 years compared to 0.3% of a

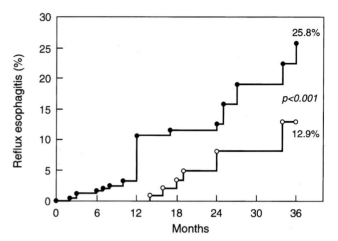

FIGURE 24.1. Incidence of reflux esophagitis in patients with duodenal ulcer cured of *H. pylori* infection (*filled-in circle*) and in patients with duodenal ulcer still infected with *H. pylori* (*hollow circle*). (From Labenz J, Blum AL, Bayerdorffer E, et al. Curing *Helicobacter pylori* infection in patients with duodenal ulcer disease may provoke reflux esophagitis. *Gastroenterology* 112: 1442–1447, 1997, with permission.)

control group who received no treatment for *H. pylori* (22). Importantly, 35 of 36 cases of reflux esophagitis that developed were mild and classified as Los Angeles (LA) A or B. New onset GERD symptoms after *H. pylori* eradication have also been described in approximately one third of duodenal ulcer patients in Greece and Italy (23,24).

In contrast, other studies of peptic ulcer disease patients treated for *H. pylori* infection found no increase in GERD symptoms or endoscopic esophagitis. In a randomized controlled trial of *H. pylori* eradication in 165 patients with active duodenal ulcer in Sweden, there was no difference in the development of heartburn between those in whom *H. pylori* was eradicated compared to those in whom it had not been (25). Furthermore, erosive esophagitis developed in 10% of patients in whom *H. pylori* was eradicated compared to 8% of those with persistent infection. Other studies also suggest that GERD is not increased in duodenal ulcer patients who have undergone eradication of *H. pylori* (26,27).

How does one reconcile these differences? Each of these studies was designed differently. Most studies examined only a small number of patients and follow-up duration varied. Furthermore, erosive esophagitis may be encountered in approximately 22% to 33% of patients with peptic ulcer disease (7,28) and 43% of patients with Zollinger–Ellison syndrome (29). Other possible reasons for GERD to develop after cure of *H. pylori* infection in duodenal ulcer patients include elimination of antisecretory agents used to treat ulcer symptoms, weight gain, alteration of diet, and failure to recognize GERD symptoms or endoscopic signs prior to treatment (24,30). Finally, even if GERD does develop after cure of *H. pylori* infection in duodenal ulcer patients, esophagitis appears to be mild, regardless of which grading system is used.

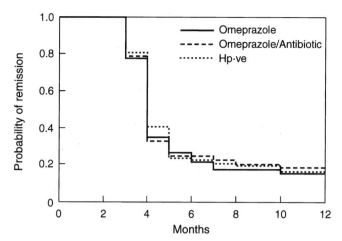

FIGURE 24.2. GERD relapse rates for *H. pylori*⁺ patients treated with omeprazole and antibiotics (*dotted line*); *H. pylori*⁺ patients treated with omeprazole alone (*solid line*); and *H. pylori*⁻ patients treated with omeprazole alone (*dashed line*). All groups received omeprazole therapy for 8 weeks prior to cessation of therapy. There is no difference in relapse rates among the three groups. (From Moayyedi P, Bardhan C, Young L, et al. *Helicobacter pylori* eradication does not exacerbate reflux symptoms in gastroesophageal reflux disease. *Gastroenterology* 2001; 121:1120–1126, with permission.)

Perhaps a more important question to address is the effect of *H. pylori* eradication on reflux esophagitis and symptoms in patients with a prior diagnosis of GERD. In a study of 232 GERD patients, all of whom were treated with proton pump inhibitors for 8 weeks, Moayeddi et al. found no difference in the relapse rate between *H. pylori*⁺ patients treated with antibiotics, *H. pylori*⁺ patients treated with placebo, and *H. pylori*⁻ patients (31) (Fig. 24.2). Each group had an identical relapse rate of 83% at 1 year. Others have found no worsening of esophagitis after *H. pylori* eradication therapy (32).

In summary, GERD may develop in a subset of patients after *H. pylori* eradication. If it develops, esophagitis is typically low grade. In patients with GERD who undergo *H. pylori* eradication, treatment does not seem to be affected.

Mechanisms of a Potential Protective Effect of *H. pylori*

Gastroesophageal reflux develops when the normal barrier between the stomach and esophagus is impaired either transiently or permanently. Factors critical to the development of symptoms of gastroesophageal reflux or mucosal damage include transient LES relaxation, hypotensive LES pressure, a hiatal hernia, inadequate esophageal clearance of refluxed contents, and potency of the refluxate. *H. pylori* infection does not influence the frequency of transient LES relaxations in response to gastric distention (33). Similarly, *H. pylori* infection is unlikely to play a role in basal LES pressure, the presence of a hiatal hernia, or esophageal dys-

motility. The most likely mechanism of any potential protective effect of *H. pylori* infection is by influencing the potency of the gastric refluxate.

Patterns of Gastritis and Gastric Acid Secretion

It is hypothesized that the distribution and severity of *H. pylori*–related gastritis rather than the presence or absence of *H. pylori* infection may affect the potency of the gastric refluxate (Fig. 24.3). Antral predominant gastritis, as typically seen in duodenal ulcer patients, is associated with elevated levels of gastrin, which stimulates parietal cells in an intact corpus thereby causing increased acid secretion (34). Acid secretion subsequently normalizes after cure of the infection (34,35). In contrast, corpus predominant gastritis, often accompanied by gastric atrophy, as typically seen in gastric ulcer patients, is associated with decreased acid secretion, which subsequently increases with cure of infection (34,36–38). The majority of *H. pylori*–infected patients, with no disease outcome, have a mixed pattern of gastritis involving both the antrum and corpus, whereby the elevated gastrin resulting from antral inflammation fails to cause gastric acid hypersecretion due to inflammation of the corpus (34). It remains unclear why different patterns of gastritis develop in different patients, although some interaction of host defenses, virulence factors and environmental influences presumably play a role (34).

A number of studies suggest that the severity of corpus gastritis may protect against the development of GERD. Labenz et al. (20) found that the severity of corpus gastritis in duodenal ulcer patients prior to *H. pylori* eradication was

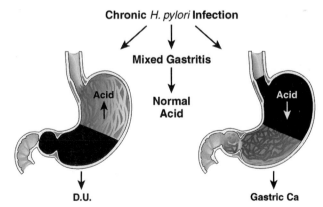

FIGURE 24.3. Divergent patterns of gastritis in response to *H. pylori* infection. In antral predominant gastritis (*left*) acid secretion increases and duodenal ulcers are often the result. In corpus predominant gastritis (*right*) there is a decrease in gastric acid secretion. This pattern is associated with gastric ulcers and gastric cancer. A mixed pattern of gastritis (*middle*) results in no change in acid secretion. (Modified from McColl KE, El-Omar E, Gillen D. Interactions between *H. pylori* infection, gastric acid secretion and anti-secretory therapy. *Br Med Bull* 1998;54: 121–138, with permission.)

a risk factor for the development of posttherapy reflux esophagitis. Similarly, El-Serag et al. (39) found that acute or chronic corpus gastritis was less common in patients with reflux esophagitis or Barrett's esophagus than those without esophagitis. Others have confirmed these findings (11).

Gastric acid hyposecretion has been described in a subgroup of *H. pylori*–infected patients with corpus predominant gastritis and increased gastric atrophy accompanied by intestinal metaplasia (36). This suppression of acid secretion seen with atrophic gastritis is partially reversible after *H. pylori* eradication (36,38). Six of 16 hypochlorhydric subjects described by El-Omar et al. (36) developed new onset heartburn in conjunction with return of acid secretion after *H. pylori* eradication and one individual developed esophagitis. Corpus atrophy is also less common in GERD patients than in control patients without GERD (11,40). Taken together, these findings provide circumstantial evidence that the distribution and severity of gastritis caused by *H. pylori* infection may be a factor in the development of GERD in some patients.

In theory, at-risk individuals—that is those with a hiatal hernia or some degree of LES dysfunction—may develop GERD after *H. pylori* eradication in the setting of corpus predominant gastritis or atrophy. Is there any supportive evidence for this? In a case control study of Japanese patients undergoing *H. pylori* eradication, mild reflux esophagitis (primarily LA class A or B) developed in 18% of patients after eradication therapy compared to 0.3% without therapy (22). Interestingly, patients who developed reflux esophagitis after therapy had a greater prevalence of hiatal hernia and more severe corpus gastritis before therapy (Fig. 24.4). Similarly, Koike et al. (41) found that reflux esophagitis developed in 20% of patients with a hiatal hernia after eradication of *H. pylori* compared to none of the patients without a hiatal hernia.

H. pylori infection may also cause a functional impairment of gastric acid secretion by a number of different mechanisms: inflammation-related loss of M3 muscarinic receptors, increased concentrations of growth factors, and increased production of inflammatory cytokines such as interleukin 1β, a potent inhibitor of acid secretion (34, 42–44). *H. pylori* also produces large amounts of ammonia that could buffer intragastric acid and theoretically decrease the potency of gastric refluxate into the esophagus. Gastric juice ammonia levels decrease markedly after cure of *H. pylori* infection, which could potentially alter the ability to neutralize gastric acid (45).

Virulence Factors

While carriage of *H. pylori* infection causes chronic gastritis in all infected individuals, most patients do not develop peptic ulcer disease, distal gastric cancer, or MALT lymphoma. The ultimate outcome of infection is a result of a complex interplay between host defenses, environmental factors, and *H. pylori* strain differences. One of the most-studied virulence markers is expression of the *cagA* gene. The importance of *cagA* status is most likely as a marker of the *cag* pathogenicity island, a group of genes located in close proximity that enhance the pathogenicity of *H. pylori* (46,47).

Infection with *cagA*⁺ strains of *H. pylori* is associated with higher grades of gastric inflammation, and an increased propensity to develop gastric atrophy and intestinal metaplasia (48–51). Heightened inflammation in the gastric corpus may result in a decrease in acid secretion by parietal cells. Patients harboring *cagA*⁺ strains of *H. pylori* are more likely to develop peptic ulcer disease and distal gastric cancer than are individuals infected with *cagA*⁻ strains (46,47,52). A number of studies suggest that individuals infected with *cagA*⁺ strains

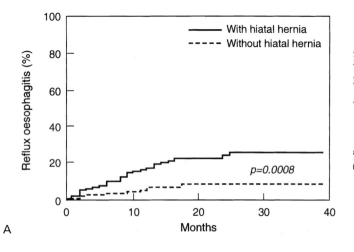

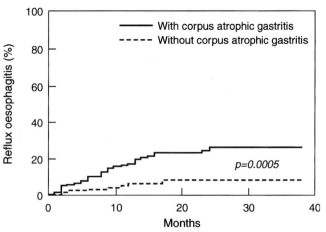

FIGURE 24.4. A: Time to occurrence of reflux esophagitis after *H. pylori* eradication in patients with a hiatal hernia. **B:** Time to occurrence of reflux esophagitis after *H. pylori* eradication in patients with corpus atrophic gastritis. (From Hamada H, Haruma K, Mihara M, et al. High incidence of reflux oesophagitis after eradication therapy for *Helicobacter pylori*: impacts of hiatal hernia and corpus gastritis. *Aliment Pharmacol Ther* 2000;14:729–735, with permission.)

of *H. pylori* are less likely to develop GERD, Barrett's esophagus, and esophageal adenocarcinoma (4,18,53–56). Further provocative information suggesting a protective role of *cagA+* strains of *H. pylori* comes from a study that examined the influence of *cagA* status on risk of esophagitis after successful treatment of *H. pylori* infection (57). In 50 *H. pylori*–infected patients without symptoms or endoscopic findings of GERD prior to treatment, erosive esophagitis developed in 50% of the *cagA+* patients compared to 2.8% of the *cagA–* patients 24 months after eradication (57).

Esophageal Acid Exposure and *H. pylori* Infection

A number of studies demonstrate very little effect of *H. pylori* infection on esophageal acid exposure either before or after eradication. Twenty-four–hour pH monitoring studies done in 58 patients with Barrett's esophagus revealed no difference in esophageal acid exposure between *H. pylori+* and *H. pylori–* patients: the mean time pH <4 was 15.8% in *H. pylori+* patients and 16.1% in *H. pylori–* patients (58). Similar findings are encountered in uncomplicated GERD patients: *H. pylori* status does not influence esophageal acid exposure time (59,60).

What happens to esophageal acid exposure after eradication of *H. pylori*? In a study of asymptomatic individuals before and after eradication of *H. pylori*, Feldman et al. (61) found that esophageal acid exposure as measured by 24-hour pH monitoring, increased almost threefold from a mean of 1.9% before treatment to 5.6% after successful treatment, whereas it was unchanged in subjects with persistent infection. However, while acid reflux increased in seven of the nine individuals after eradication of *H. pylori*, it was in the pathologic range in only three of the nine subjects. Others have found no change in 24-hour acid exposure in asymptomatic patients before or after *H. pylori* eradication (62). In a study of 23 *H. pylori*–infected patients with low-grade reflux esophagitis, Tefera et al. (63) found that the median 24-hour acid exposure was no different before (9.4%) or after (9.6%) *H. pylori* eradication. However, nine patients had increased total acid exposure whereas 14 patients had decreased acid exposure after eradication. Thus, studies to date suggest that the presence or absence of *H. pylori* infection does not appear to be a major factor in esophageal acid exposure in either GERD patients or asymptomatic individuals.

THE INTERACTION OF *H. PYLORI* INFECTION AND PROTON PUMP INHIBITOR THERAPY IN GERD

Most patients with severe GERD require either chronic antisecretory therapy with a proton pump inhibitor or antireflux surgery. We know that proton pump inhibitors are effective and safe when administered chronically to these patients (64). However, questions persist regarding the interaction of proton pump inhibitors and *H. pylori* infection with respect to the efficacy of proton pump inhibitors and the development of atrophic gastritis.

Studies in healthy volunteers and duodenal ulcer patients indicate that *H. pylori* infection enhances the ability of proton pump inhibitors to raise intragastric pH compared to *H. pylori* uninfected subjects (65–67). Furthermore, this effect can be reversed by eradicating the organism (67,68). It is unclear exactly how *H. pylori* infection augments the efficacy of proton pump inhibitors. Postulated mechanisms include presence of a higher content of acid-neutralizing substances such as ammonia in the infected gastric mucosa; increased levels of cytokines such as interleukin 1β, which inhibit gastric acid secretion; and exposure of parietal cells to acid inhibitory substances released by *H. pylori* (69). Recently, Beil et al. (69) demonstrated that *H. pylori* may interact with proton pump inhibitors to augment the antisecretory effect of these drugs at the level of the parietal cell membrane.

Do these observations translate into any clinically meaningful results? Work by Holtmann et al. (70) suggested that this was indeed the case. Healing rates of reflux esophagitis with pantoprazole 40 mg daily (Savary-Miller grades II and III) were superior at both 4 weeks (86.6% vs. 76.3%) and 8 weeks (96.4% vs. 91.8%) in *H. pylori+* compared to *H. pylori–* patients (Fig. 24.5). Relief of heartburn and regurgitation was superior at 4 weeks in the *H. pylori+* patients, but at 8 weeks, there was no significant difference in the *H. pylori+* and *H. pylori–* patients.

Does this finding translate into any meaningful effect on the long-term therapy of GERD? The maintenance dose of

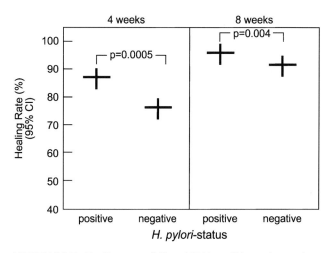

FIGURE 24.5. Healing rates (%) and 95% confidence intervals at 4 and 8 weeks for pantoprazole 40 mg daily in *H. pylori+* and *H. pylori–* patients with GERD. (From Holtmann G, Cain C, Malfertheiner P. Gastric *Helicobacter pylori* infection accelerates healing of reflux esophagitis during treatment with the proton pump inhibitor pantoprazole. *Gastroenterology* 1999;117:11–16, with permission.)

omeprazole needed to keep GERD patients in endoscopic and symptomatic remission does not differ between *H. pylori*⁺ and *H. pylori*⁻ patients (64,71) (Fig. 24.6). In 230 patients followed for a mean period of 6.5 years, there was no difference in either relapse rate or dosage requirements for *H. pylori*⁺ and *H. pylori*⁻ patients (64). Thus, there is very little evidence that *H. pylori* infection has any significant bearing on the efficacy of chronic proton pump inhibitor therapy of GERD.

A more confusing issue is the effect of long-term proton pump inhibitor therapy on gastric histology in *H. pylori*–infected patients. Short-term omeprazole therapy clearly influences the distribution and severity of gastritis in *H. pylori*–infected subjects: it decreases inflammation in the antrum and increases inflammation in the corpus (72). This is accompanied by migration of the organism from the antrum to the proximal stomach (73). This may lead to the accelerated development of atrophic gastritis. Kuipers et al. (74) found that in *H. pylori*–infected GERD patients treated with omeprazole for an average of 5 years, 31% developed gastric atrophy compared to none at baseline. The risk of developing gastric atrophy was associated with significantly higher gastritis scores at 1 year. Furthermore, while only 1.7% had intestinal metaplasia at baseline, it was found in 5.1% at follow-up. In contrast, none of the *H. pylori*–infected GERD patients treated with fundoplication developed gastric atrophy. *H. pylori*–infected GERD patients treated with omeprazole were also far more likely to develop worsening corpus gastritis than the surgery group (74). However, the findings of this study have been criticized because of differences in the patient groups studied: the surgery group was from Sweden whereas the omeprazole group was from the Netherlands;

and the omeprazole group was >10 years older. Studies show that the prevalence of gastric mucosal atrophy is higher in older patients (75). However, similar findings of increased corpus inflammation and glandular atrophy have also been described in *H. pylori*–infected GERD patients treated chronically with lansoprazole (76,77). The long-term omeprazole treatment trial by Klinkenberg-Knol et al. (64) that followed GERD patients who received maintenance therapy with >20 mg omeprazole for a mean of 6.5 years found corpus atrophy in 12% at baseline and 39% at follow-up in *H. pylori*⁺ patients compared to 1.5% and 6.1% in *H. pylori*⁻ patients (64). The annual incidence of atrophy was 0.7% in *H. pylori*⁻ patients and 4.7% in *H. pylori*⁺ patients. However, intestinal metaplasia was rare, and there was no dysplasia or neoplasia detected. Since gastric atrophy is a risk factor for the development of gastric cancer, these findings have led to the recommendation by these authors (74) to test for *H. pylori* and treat it in patients opting for long-term proton pump inhibitor therapy of GERD, an approach that was subsequently endorsed by the European Maastricht consensus conference (78) and others (79).

Further circumstantial support for these recommendations comes from a recent study that randomized GERD patients infected with *H. pylori* to eradication therapy or placebo prior to commencing 12 months of omeprazole for GERD (80). In patients who remained infected with *H. pylori*, the expected changes of decreased antral gastritis and increased corpus gastritis occurred. However, in patients cured of *H. pylori* infection, the severity of both corpus and antral gastritis decreased. No significant changes in atrophy scores were noted in either group. As in all of the above studies, no increase in intestinal metaplasia was encountered.

However, other studies call into question some of the above findings. Twelve months of therapy with either lansoprazole or omeprazole in 111 GERD patients infected with *H. pylori* resulted in no increase in gastric atrophy or intestinal metaplasia (81). A randomized controlled trial that examined antireflux surgery versus omeprazole therapy for treatment of chronic GERD in Scandinavia could find no difference in the development of atrophy between the two age-matched study groups during 3 years of therapy (82). Interestingly, there was a slow progression of glandular atrophy in the *H. pylori*–infected patients in both groups, but only the minority of all patients were infected—34% in the surgery group and 26% in the omeprazole group. However, this study has been criticized because some patients in the surgery group eventually received omeprazole and some also underwent vagotomy. In the United States, neither the Food and Drug Administration nor the American College of Gastroenterology guidelines recommend a "test and treat strategy" prior to long-term therapy with proton pump inhibitors in GERD (83,84).

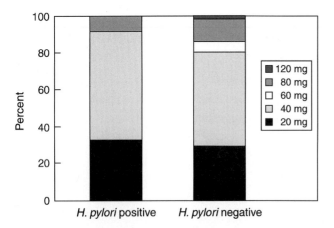

FIGURE 24.6. Maintenance dose of omeprazole required for symptomatic and endoscopic remission in *H. pylori*⁺ and *H. pylori*⁻ patients with GERD. There was no difference in dose requirements between the two groups. (From Schenk BE, Kuipers EJ, Klinkenberg-Knol EC, et al. *Helicobacter pylori* and the efficacy of omeprazole therapy for gastroesophageal reflux disease. *Am J Gastroenterol* 1999;94:884–887, with permission.)

The issue of how best to handle testing and treating GERD patients receiving long-term proton pump inhibitor therapy remains unresolved. Chronic corpus gastritis clearly increases with proton pump inhibitor therapy. This may increase the risk of gastric atrophy, but there are no data demonstrating an increase in the development of intestinal metaplasia. Both of these lesions are known precursors of gastric cancer. As such, it is tempting to test and treat these patients to prevent the theoretical risk of gastric cancer. However, it is important to keep in mind that no studies demonstrate an increase in intestinal metaplasia in these patients. Others would argue that this approach is not evidence based, incurs additional costs of testing and treatment, and encourages increased antimicrobial resistance, and hence should be avoided. Emerging information suggests that serological testing is no longer accurate for determining *H. pylori* status (85). This will make testing more complex, thereby requiring either a urea breath test or stool antigen detection. Perhaps the best approach is a middle ground advocated by Labenz (86). In a young patient facing a lifetime of proton pump inhibitor therapy, it may be advisable to go with the test-and-treat strategy, whereas in the older patient, a "don't look, don't tell" approach may make the most sense.

SUMMARY

The relationship between *H. pylori* infection and GERD remains confusing. GERD is a common problem and the presence or absence of *H. pylori* is most likely unimportant in most patients. However, circumstantial evidence suggests that corpus predominant gastritis caused by *H. pylori* infection may protect patients susceptible to GERD (hiatal hernia, LES dysfunction, esophageal dysmotility) from developing the disease by decreasing the potency of the gastric refluxate. Cure of infection in at-risk individuals may increase the potency of the gastric refluxate and contribute to the development of GERD. It remains unclear if GERD patients requiring long-term proton pump inhibitor therapy should be tested for *H. pylori* and treated if positive, unless other indications for testing exist, such as a prior history of peptic ulcer disease. There are risks as well as benefits of treatment that need to be considered in such patients. Resolution of this dilemma is essential given the widespread use of proton pump inhibitors today and the potential for many decades of therapy in responsive patients.

REFERENCES

1. Banatvala N, Mayo K, Megraud F, et al. The cohort effect and Helicobacter pylori. *J Infect Dis* 1993;68:219–221.
2. El-Serag HB, Sonnenberg A. Opposing time trends of peptic ulcer and reflux disease. *Gut* 1998;43:327–333.
3. O'Connor HJ. Helicobacter pylori and gastro-oesophageal reflux disease—clinical implications and management. *Aliment Pharmacol Ther* 1999;13:117–127.
4. Vicari JJ, Peek RM, Falk GW, et al. The seroprevalence of cagA positive Helicobacter pylori strains in the spectrum of gastroesophageal reflux disease. *Gastroenterology* 1998;115:50–57.
5. Csendes A, Smok G, Cerda G, et al. Prevalence of Helicobacter pylori infection in 190 control subjects and in 236 patients with gastroesophageal reflux, erosive esophagitis or Barrett's esophagus. *Dis Esophagus* 1997;10:38–42.
6. Newton M, Bryan R, Burnham WR, et al. Evaluation of Helicobacter pylori in reflux oesophagitis and Barrett's oesophagus. *Gut* 1997;40:9–13.
7. Hackelsberger A, Schultze V, Gunther T, et al. The prevalence of Helicobacter pylori gastritis in patients with reflux oesophagitis: a case–control study. *Eur J Gastroenterol Hepatol* 1998;10:465–468.
8. Varanasi RV, Fantry GT, Wilson KT. Decreased prevalence of H. pylori infection in gastroesophageal reflux disease. *Helicobacter* 1998;3:188–194.
9. Werdmuller BF, Loffeld RJ. Helicobacter pylori infection has no role in the pathogenesis of reflux esophagitis. *Dig Dis Sci* 1997; 42:103–105.
10. Wu JC, Sung JJ, Ng EK, et al. Prevalence and distribution of Helicobacter pylori in gastroesophageal reflux disease: a study from the East. *Am J Gastroenterol* 1999;94:1790–1794.
11. Haruma K, Hamada H, Mihara M, et al. Negative association between Helicobacter pylori infection and reflux esophagitis in older patients: case control study in Japan. *Helicobacter* 2000;5:24–29.
12. Wu JC, Sung JJ, Chan FK. Helicobacter pylori infection is associated with milder gastro-oesophageal reflux disease. *Aliment Pharmacol Ther* 2000;14:427–432.
13. Lord RV, Frommer DJ, Inder S, et al. Prevalence of Helicobacter pylori infection in 160 patients with Barrett's oesophagus or Barrett's adenocarcinoma. *Aust NZ J Surg* 2000;70:26–33.
14. Weston AP, Badr AS, Topalovski M, et al. Prospective evaluation of the prevalence of gastric Helicobacter pylori infection in patients with GERD, Barrett's esophagus, Barrett's dysplasia, and Barrett's adenocarcinoma. *Am J Gastroenterol* 2000;95:387–394.
15. Paull G, Yardley JH. Gastric and esophageal Campylobacter pylori in patients with Barrett's esophagus. *Gastroenterology* 1988; 95:216–218.
16. Blaser MJ, Perez-Perez GI, Lindenbaum J, et al. Association of infection due to Helicobacter pylori with specific upper gastrointestinal pathology. *Rev Infect Dis* 1991;13(suppl 8):S704–708.
17. Henihan RD, Stuart RC, Nolan N, et al. Barrett's esophagus and the prevalence of Helicobacter pylori. *Am J Gastroenterol* 1998; 193:542–546.
18. Chow WH, Blaser MJ, Blot WJ, et al. An inverse relation between cagA+ strains of Helicobacter pylori infection and risk of esophageal and gastric cardia adenocarcinoma. *Cancer Res* 1998; 58:588–590.
19. Vaezi MF, Falk GW, Peek RM, et al. CagA− positive strains of Helicobacter pylori may protect against Barrett's esophagus. *Am J Gastroenterol* 2000;95:2206–2211.
20. Labenz J, Blum AL, Bayerdorffer E, et al. Curing Helicobacter pylori infection in patients with duodenal ulcer disease may provoke reflux esophagitis. *Gastroenterology* 1997;112:1442–1447.
21. Fallone CA, Barkun AN, Friedman G, et al. Is Helicobacter pylori eradication associated with gastroesophageal reflux disease? *Am J Gastroenterol* 2000;95;914–920.
22. Hamada H, Haruma K, Mihara M, et al. High incidence of reflux oesophagitis after eradication therapy for Helicobacter pylori: impacts of hiatal hernia and corpus gastritis. *Aliment Pharmacol Ther* 2000;14:729–735.

23. Rokkas T, Ladas SD, Liatsos C, et al. Effectiveness of acid suppression in preventing gastroesophageal reflux disease (GERD) after successful treatment of Helicobacter pylori infection. *Dig Dis Sci* 2001;46:1567–1572.

24. Manes G, Mosca S, De Nucci C, et al. High prevalence of reflux symptoms in duodenal ulcer patients who develop gastro-oesophageal reflux disease after curing Helicobacter pylori infection. *Dig Liver Dis* 2001;33:665–670.

25. Befrits R, Sjpstedt S, Odman B, et al. Curing Helicobacter pylori infection in patients with duodenal ulcer does not provoke gastroesophageal reflux disease. *Helicobacter* 2000;5:202–205.

26. Vakil N, Hahn B, McSorley D. Recurrent symptoms and gastro-oesophageal reflux disease in patients with duodenal ulcer treated for Helicobacter pylori infection. *Aliment Pharmacol Ther* 2000; 14:45–51.

27. McColl KE, Dickson A, El-Nujumi A, et al. Symptomatic benefit 1–3 years after H. pylori eradication in ulcer disease: impact of gastroesophageal reflux disease. *Am J Gastroenterol* 2000;95: 101–105.

28. Boyd EJ. The prevalence of esophagitis in patients with duodenal ulcer or ulcer-like dyspepsia. *Am J Gastroenterol* 1996;91: 1539–1543.

29. Miller LS, Vinayek R, Frucht H, et al. Reflux esophagitis in patients with Zollinger–Ellison syndrome. *Gastroenterology* 1990; 98:341–346.

30. Xia HH, Talley NJ. Helicobacter pylori infection, reflux esophagitis and atrophic gastritis: an unexplored triangle. *Am J Gastroenterol* 1998;93:394–400.

31. Moayyedi P, Bardhan C, Young L, et al. Helicobacter pylori eradication does not exacerbate reflux symptoms in gastroesophageal reflux disease. *Gastroenterology* 2001;121:1120–1126.

32. O'Connor HJ, McGee C, Ghabash NM, et al. Prevalence of esophagitis in H. pylori⁻ positive peptic ulcer disease and the impact of eradication therapy. *Hepatogastroenterology* 2001;48: 1064–1068.

33. Zerbbib F, Bicheler V, Leray V, et al. H. pylori and transient lower esophageal sphincter relaxation induced by gastric distention in healthy humans. *Am J Physiol* 2001;281:G350–G356.

34. McColl KE, El-Omar E, Gillen D. Interactions between H. pylori infection, gastric acid secretion and anti-secretory therapy. *Br Med Bull* 1998;54:121–138.

35. El-Omar EM, Penman ID, Ardill JE, et al. Helicobacter pylori infection and abnormalities of acid secretion in patients with duodenal ulcer disease. *Gastroenterology* 1991;109:681–691.

36. El-Omar EM, Oien K, El-Nujumi A, et al. Helicobacter pylori infection and chronic gastric acid hyposecretion. *Gastroenterology* 1997;113:15–24.

37. Gutierrez O, Melo M, Segura AM, et al. Cure of Helicobacter pylori infection improves gastric acid secretion in patients with corpus gastritis. *Scand J Gastroenterol* 1997;32:664–668.

38. Haruma K, Mihara M, Okamoto E, et al. Eradication of Helicobacter pylori increases gastric acidity in patients with atrophic gastritis of the corpus-evaluation of 24-h pH monitoring. *Aliment Pharmacol Ther* 1999;13:155–162.

39. El-Serag HB, Sonnenberg A, Jamal MM, et al. Corpus gastritis is protective against reflux oesophagitis. *Gut* 1999;45:181–185.

40. Koike T, Ohara S, Sekine H, et al. Helicobacter pylori inhibits reflux esophagitis by inducing atrophic gastritis. *Am J Gastroenterol* 1999;94:3468–3472.

41. Koike T, Ohara S, Sekine H, et al. Increased gastric acid secretion after Helicobacter pylori eradication may be a factor for developing reflux oesophagitis. *Aliment Pharmacol Ther* 2001;15: 813–820.

42. Cave DR, Vargas M. Effect of Campylobacter pylori protein on acid secretion by parietal cells. *Lancet* 1989;2:187–189.

43. Wallace JL, Cucala M, Mugridge K, et al. Secretagogue-specific effects of interleukin-1 on gastric acid secretion. *Am J Physiol* 1991;261:G559–G564.

44. Noach LA, Bosma NB, Jansen J, et al. Mucosal tumor necrosis factor-alpha, interleukin-1B, and interleukin-8 production in patients with Helicobacter pylori infection. *Scand J Gastroenterol* 1994;29:425–429.

45. Bercik P, Verdu E, Armstrong D, et al. The effect of ammonia on omeprazole-induced reduction of gastric acidity in subjects with Helicobacter pylori infection. *Am J Gastroenterol* 2000;95: 947–955.

46. Atherton JC. CagA, the cag pathogenicity island and Helicobacter pylori infection. *Gut* 1999;44:307–308.

47. Perez-Perez GI, Peek RM, Legath AJ, et al. The role of CagA status in gastric and extragastric complications of Helicobacter pylori. *J Physiol Pharmacol* 1999;50:833–845.

48. Kuipers EJ, Perez-Perez GI, Meuwisssen SG, et al. Helicobacter pylori and atrophic gastritis: importance of the cagA status. *J Natl Cancer Inst* 1995;87:1777–1780.

49. Peek RM, Miller GG, Perez-Perez GI, et al. Heightened inflammatory response and cytokine expression in vivo to cagA⁺ Helicobacter pylori strains. *Lab Invest* 1995;71:760–770.

50. Van Der Hulst RW, Van Der Ende A, Dekker FW, et al. Effect of Helicobacter pylori eradication on gastritis in relation to cagA: a prospective 1-year follow-up study. *Gastroenterology* 1997;113: 25–30.

51. Maaroos HI, Vorobjova T, Sipponen P, et al. An 18-year follow-up study of chronic gastritis and Helicobacter pylori: association of CagA positivity and development of atrophy and activity of gastritis. *Scand J Gastroenterol* 1999;34:864–869.

52. Van Doorn LJ, Figueiredo C, Sanna R, et al. Clinical relevance of the cagA, vacA, and iceA status of Helicobacter pylori. *Gastroenterology* 1998;115:58–66.

53. Fallone CA, Barkun AN, Gottke MU, et al. Association of Helicobacter pylori genotype with gastroesophageal reflux disease and other upper gastrointestinal diseases. *Am J Gastroenterol* 2000;95: 659–669.

54. Grimley CE, Holder RL, Loft DE, et al. Helicobacter pylori⁻ associated antibodies in patients with duodenal ulcer, gastric and oesophageal adenocarcinoma. *Eur J Gastroenterol Hepatol* 1999; 11:503–509.

55. Loffeld RJ, Werdmuller BF, Kuster JG, et al. Colonization with cagA⁻ positive Helicobacter pylori strains inversely associated with reflux esophagitis and Barrett's esophagus. *Digestion* 2000; 62:95–99.

56. Arents NL, Van Zwet AA, Thijs JC, et al. The importance of vacA, cagA, and iceA genotypes of Helicobacter pylori infection in peptic ulcer disease and gastroesophageal reflux disease. *Am J Gastroenterol* 2001;96:2603–2608.

57. Rokkas T, Ladas SD, Triantafyllou K, et al. The association between CagA status and the development of esophagitis after the eradication of Helicobacter pylori. *Am J Med* 2001;110: 703–707.

58. Peters FT, Kuipers EJ, Ganesh S, et al. The influence of Helicobacter pylori on esophageal acid exposure in GERD during acid suppressive therapy. *Aliment Pharmacol Ther* 1999;13: 921–926.

59. Manes G, Esposito P, Lioniello M, et al. Manometric and pH-metric features in gastro-oesophageal reflux disease patients with and without Helicobacter pylori infection. *Digest Liver Dis* 2000; 32:372–377.

60. Gisbert JP, de Pedro A, Losa C, et al. Helicobacter pylori and gastroesophageal reflux disease. *J Clin Gastroenterol* 2001;32: 210–214.

61. Feldman M, Cryer B, Sammer D, et al. Influence of H. pylori infection on meal-stimulated gastric acid secretion and gastroesophageal acid reflux. *Am J Physiol* 1999;277:G1159–1164.

62. Manifold DK, Anggiansah A, Rowe I, et al. Gastro-oesophageal reflux and duodenogastric reflux before and eradication in Helicobacter pylori gastritis. *Eur J Gastroenterol Hepatol* 2001;13: 535–539.

63. Tefera S, Hatlebakk JG, Berstad A. The effect of Helicobacter pylori eradication on gastro-oesophageal reflux. *Aliment Pharmacol Ther* 1999;13:915–920.

64. Klinkenberg-Knol EC, Nelis F, Dent J, et al. Long-term omeprazole treatment in resistant gastroesophageal reflux disease: efficacy, safety, and influence on gastric mucosa. *Gastroenterology* 2000;118:661–669.

65. Gillen D, Wirz AA, Neithercut WD, et al. Helicobacter pylori infection potentiates the inhibition of gastric acid secretion by omeprazole. *Gut* 1999;44:468–475.

66. Verdu EF, Armstrong D, Fraser R, et al. Effect of Helicobacter pylori status on intragastric pH during treatment with omeprazole. *Gut* 1995;36:539–545.

67. Labenz J, Tillenburg B, Peitz U, et al. Helicobacter pylori augments the pH-increasing effect of omeprazole in patients with duodenal ulcer. *Gastroenterology* 1996;110:725–732.

68. Verdu EF, Armstrong D, Idstrom JP, et al. Intragastric pH during treatment with omeprazole: role of Helicobacter pylori-associated gastritis. *Scand J Gastroenterol* 1996;31:1151–1156.

69. Beil W, Sewing KF, Busche R, et al. Helicobacter pylori augments the acid inhibitory effect of omeprazole on parietal cells and gastric H$^+$/K$^+$-ATPase. *Gut* 2001;48:157–162.

70. Holtmann G, Cain C, Malfertheiner P. Gastric Helicobacter pylori infection accelerates healing of reflux esophagitis during treatment with the proton pump inhibitor pantoprazole. *Gastroenterology* 1999;117:11–16.

71. Schenk BE, Kuipers EJ, Klinkenberg-Knol EC, et al. Helicobacter pylori and the efficacy of omeprazole therapy for gastroesophageal reflux disease. *Am J Gastroenterol* 1999;94:884–887.

72. Kuipers EJ, Uyterlinde AM, Pena AS, et al. Increase of Helicobacter pylori associated corpus gastritis during acid suppressive therapy: implications for long-term safety. *Am J Gastroenterol* 1995;90:1401–1406.

73. Logan RP, Walker MM, Misiewicz JJ, et al. Changes in the intragastric distribution of Helicobacter pylori during treatment with omeprazole. *Gut* 1995;36:12–16.

74. Kuipers EJ, Lundell L, Klinkenberg-Knol EC, et al. Atrophic gastritis and Helicobacter pylori infection in patients with reflux esophagitis treated with omeprazole or fundoplication. *N Engl J Med* 1996;334:1018–1012.

75. Hackelsberger A, Gunther T, Schultze V, et al. Role of aging in the expression of Helicobacter pylori gastritis in the antrum, fundus, corpus, and cardia. *Scand J Gastroenterol* 1999;34:138–143.

76. Berstad AE, Hatlebakk JG, Maartmann-Moe H, et al. Helicobacter pylori gastritis and epithelial cell proliferation in patients with reflux oesophagitis after treatment with lansoprazole. *Gut* 1997;41:740–747.

77. Eissele R, Brunner G, Simon B, et al. Gastric mucosa during treatment with lansoprazole: Helicobacter pylori is a risk factor for argyrophil cell hyperplasia. *Gastroenterology* 1997;112: 707–717.

78. Bazzoli F. Key points from the revised Maastricht consensus report: the impact on general practice. *Eur J Gastroenterol Hepatol* 2001;13(suppl 2):S3–S7.

79. Graham DY. Therapy of Helicobacter pylori: current status and issues. *Gastroenterology* 2000;(suppl)118:S2–S8.

80. Schenk BE, Kuipers EJ, Nelis GF. Effect of Helicobacter pylori eradication on chronic gastritis during omeprazole therapy. *Gut* 2000;46:615–621.

81. Stolte M, Meining A, Schmitz JM, et al. Changes in Helicobacter pylori$^-$ induced gastritis in the antrum and the corpus during 12 months of treatment with omeprazole and lansoprazole in patients with gastro-esophageal reflux disease. *Aliment Pharmacol Ther* 1998;12:247–253.

82. Lundell L, Miettinen P, Myrvold HE, et al. Lack of effect of acid suppression therapy on gastric atrophy. *Gastroenterology* 1999; 117:319–326.

83. Anonymous. Proton pump inhibitors relabeling for cancer risk not warranted. *F-D-C Rep* 1996;58:1–2.

84. Howden CW, Hunt RH. Guidelines for the management of Helicobacter pylori infection. *Am J Gastroenterol* 1998;93: 2330–2338.

85. Vaira D, Vakil N. Blood, urine, stool, breath, money, and Helicobacter pylori. *Gut* 2001;48:287–289.

86. Labenz J. Does Helicobacter pylori affect the management of gastroesophageal reflux disease? *Am J Gastroenterol* 1999;94;867–869.

MEDICAL MANAGEMENT OF GERD

PHILIP O. KATZ

The medical therapy of gastroesophageal reflux disease (GERD) is based on knowledge of the pathophysiology of the disease and a defined set of goals based on symptom presentation and organ damage, and must be individualized to obtain optimal results for the patient. The idealized medical therapy would augment lower esophageal sphincter (LES) pressure and/or reduce the number of transient lower esophageal sphincter relaxations (TLESRs), augment the ability of the esophagus to clear refluxed gastric contents, accelerate gastric emptying, augment mucosal resistance, and neutralize gastric acidity. While conceptually this is possible with many of the agents currently available, we are at present short of the ideal one-size-fits-all therapy. Therefore, the clinician should be prepared to utilize the available agents either alone or in combination in an attempt to achieve complete symptom relief and improvement of quality of life, to heal mucosal lesions should they exist, and to prevent complications. Hopefully, we will soon be able to delay progression to malignancy in the patient with Barrett's esophagus.

Available interventions include lifestyle modifications, antacids, mucosal protectants, prokinetic (promotility) agents, H_2 receptor antagonists (H_2RAs), and the agents of choice at present, proton pump inhibitors (PPIs). In this chapter, I review each of these agents and modalities, discuss a general approach to acute and long-term therapy, and highlight specific clinical situations in which treatment may be modified, including nonerosive GERD, unexplained chest pain, extraesophageal manifestations of GERD, pregnancy, and the medically refractory patient.

LIFESTYLE MODIFICATIONS

Numerous dietary and lifestyle modifications have been advocated to be important in GERD therapy. Prior to the

P. O. Katz: Department of Medicine, Division of Gastroenterology, Graduate Hospital, Philadelphia, Pennsylvania.

availability of antisecretory therapy, these interventions formed the backbone of medical therapy for this disease. However, although sound in their intent and in many cases based on solid laboratory research, these lifestyle changes (Table 25.1) can today be considered only adjuncts to pharmacologic therapy. It is important to educate the patient about these interventions, outlining their rationale so that patients can choose for themselves how to integrate these into their treatment plan. In fact, some patients with mild disease will find them extremely helpful while others with severe disease will find them of minimal benefit. In general, they are of low "cost," although they do require some effort on the part of the patient. The clinician should be aware that many patients have already attempted their own lifestyle changes based on their own evidence of which dietary indiscretions and lifestyles exacerbate their disease.

Sleep Issues

It has been recommended that patients elevate the head of the bed 6 to 8 inches either on bed blocks or with a foam rubber wedge designed to elevate the shoulders and body angle in order to use gravity to aid in clearance of a reflux episode during the sleeping period. This is based on studies using prolonged pH monitoring that have shown an acceleration of esophageal clearance when the head of the bed is elevated compared to sleeping flat (1,2). Unfortunately, there are no clinical outcome studies to suggest that this individual recommendation will affect symptom relief or healing. Several studies suggest that sleeping position might be of equal or greater importance than elevation of the head of the bed. A recent study (3) used a sleep monitor coupled with overnight pH monitoring in patients with GERD and showed that reflux frequency as well as total time that esophageal pH was <4 was decreased in the left side down position, compared to right side down, prone, and supine. This study, done in adults, augments another similar study in children, with similar findings (4). This sleep study confirms other data showing an increase in esophageal acid exposure in the

TABLE 25.1. EFFECTS OF FOODS AND OTHER SUBSTANCES ON GERD SYMPTOMS

Decreases LES Pressure	Mucosal Irritant
Food	Food and drink
Fats	Citrus products
Chocolate	Tomato products
Onions	Spicy foods
Carminatives	Coffee, colas, tea, beer
Alcohol	Medications
Smoking	Aspirin
Medications	NSAIDs
Progesterone	Tetracycline
Theophylline	Quinidine
Anticholinergic agents	Potassium tablets
Adrenergic agonists	Iron salts
Adrenergic antagonists	Alendronate
Diazepam	Zidovudine
Meperidine	
Nitrates	
Calcium channel blockers	

GERD, gastroesophageal reflux disease; LES, lower esophageal sphincter; NSAID, nonsteroidal antiinflammatory drug.

postprandial period when right side down compared to left side down (5), likely due to a decrease in TLESRs when comparing left side down to right side down (6). Unfortunately, there is no currently available commercial device that allows the patient to sleep left side down so this can only be suggested. In addition to these sleeping position recommendations, it is often recommended that the patient refrain from eating within 2 to 3 hours of going to sleep. This suggestion is based on the premise that a full stomach produces gastric distention, an increase in TLESRs and, therefore, an increase in GER. While the lifestyle of many people precludes this change, its recommendation is sound.

Food

Acidic liquid such as colas and teas, and citrus products such as orange, grapefruit, and tomato juice are direct esophageal irritants and will exacerbate symptoms in the GERD patient (7). A variety of foods can decrease LESP (8–11) (Table 25.1). Coffee can decrease LESP, and has been shown to augment acid production and to exacerbate reflux (12). Some studies have shown that the effect of coffee on GER can be reduced if one uses a decaffeinated beverage (12). Studies have clearly shown that a high-fat meal will increase reflux frequency in both normals and patients with GERD (13,14); however, it is not clear whether this is based purely on the presence of fat or on meal size. Fat does delay gastric emptying, which may increase the risk of reflux. While there is reason to recommend a decrease in fat for other health reasons, good outcome studies in GERD patients are again lacking. Choco-

late can also decrease LES due to its high xanthine content (15), but it increases esophageal acid exposure (16) and is on the list of foods to avoid.

Obesity and GERD

Ample debate exists as to the value of weight loss, which is often recommended to the GERD patient, as an effective way of reducing reflux. Recent case control data have suggested that body mass index (BMI) has no effect on the frequency or severity of GERD symptoms and it has been difficult to demonstrate that weight loss itself has a direct effect on reduction of GERD and/or its symptoms (17). However, an increase in BMI is a clear risk for the development of adenocarcinoma in patients with Barrett's esophagus (18) and a BMI of >30 is a clear risk for failure of antireflux surgery (19), suggesting that there is some link between obesity and GERD. Ultimately, weight reduction is of clear value for a patient who needs it for other health reasons; however, it is not a strong argument for reducing GERD.

Alcohol

Alcohol is a smooth muscle relaxant and reduces LESP. One study determined that 4 ounces of whiskey consumed 3 hours before the evening meal increased nocturnal acid reflux in healthy subjects. No participants experienced reflux on the night that they did not drink alcohol (20). The effects of white and red wine on LESP and esophageal pH were assessed in a comparison study (21). Although both types of wine increased the amount of time that esophageal pH was <4, the effect of white wine was more pronounced than red wine, and in another study, the effect of beer was more pronounced than both types of wine. The results of this study suggest that patients with GERD should avoid white wine; however, some epidemiologic data suggest that drinking wine, as opposed to beer and other liquors, is associated with a reduced risk for esophageal adenocarcinoma (22).

Medications

Drugs have the potential to decrease LESP, which may increase esophageal acid exposure in patients with GERD. Other agents have been reported to cause pill-induced esophageal changes and may increase risk of esophageal damage in patients with GERD (23) (Table 25.1). The difficulty in making strong recommendations about any of these drugs in the GERD patient comes from the lack of good clinical trials showing a change in symptoms when these medications are avoided or discontinued. Awareness of the potential for esophageal injury and techniques for avoiding it, along with prudent use of these agents, is the best approach.

Summary

Guidelines from the American College of Gastroenterology recommend lifestyle changes as adjuncts to treatment (24). However, other experts have suggested that they play minimal to no role in the treatment of GERD today. Educating patients about the potential values of sleeping on their left side, going to bed on an empty stomach, and making them aware of the overall potential of these lifestyle modifications to reduce symptoms takes little time and ultimately will help. Unfortunately, in the absence of "hard data," it is difficult to push these interventions in patients who choose not to implement them.

PHARMACOLOGIC THERAPY

When one thinks of pharmacologic therapy, one immediately considers antisecretory therapy with H2RAs or PPIs. Today, these antisecretory options are clearly the agents of choice for medical therapy for this disease. The clinician needs, however, to be familiar with the active mechanisms and of efficacy data on antacids, sucralfate, and prokinetic agents, as they may be of use in patient management. Each of the classes of pharmacologic agents is reviewed, including active ingredient/mechanism, safety, and overall effectiveness in the treatment of GERD. Healing rates of the available agents as a class are presented in Fig. 25.1.

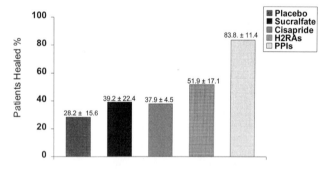

Adapted from Chiba et al. *Gastroenterology.* 1997;112:1798-1810.

FIGURE 25.1. Results of a meta-analysis of multiple clinical trials showing 4- to 12-week healing rates of erosive esophagitis with the major classes of pharmacologic agents used to treat GERD. A, placebo; B, sucralfate; C, cisapride; D, H2RAs; E, PPIs. (Adapted from Chiba N, De Gara CJ, Wilkinson JM, et al. Speed of healing and symptom relief in grade II to IV gastroesophageal reflux disease: a meta-analysis. *Gastroenterology* 1997;112: 1798–1810, with permission.)

Antacids

These agents are perhaps the most widely used agent for treating this disease, as patients with mild heartburn often self-medicate with over-the-counter antacids and never seek treatment for their symptoms. Available evidence suggests that many patients will use antacids to supplement other antisecretory therapy. Both antacids and alginic acid have been shown to be more effective than placebos in the relief of heartburn, and combined antacid and alginic acid therapy may be superior to antacids alone in the control of symptoms. In general, studies assessing the efficacy of antacids have found that even in high doses their effect on healing erosive esophagitis is no greater than placebos (25,26). This may underestimate the efficacy of these agents in patients with milder forms of the disease. A 4-week, randomized, double-blind, placebo-controlled trial compared 7 ounces of liquid antacid, 15 minutes and 1 hour after meals, to 300 mg of cimetidine four times daily using endoscopic and symptom endpoints. Patients in the cimetidine group experienced reduction in frequency and severity of heartburn; the antacid group showed no change compared to the placebo group (27).

Clinicians often minimize the side effects of antacids, which is appropriate when they are used intermittently. However, with chronic use, magnesium-containing antacids may cause diarrhea, and should be avoided in the patient with heart failure, renal insufficiency, and in late trimester pregnancy. Aluminum-containing antacids may cause constipation.

Alginic acid, an alternative to antacids, provides a floating layer on top of the gastric pool, minimizing contact between gastric contents and the esophageal mucosa (23). When given in combination with an antacid, this provides two potential mechanisms for relief of symptoms. Alginic acid alone is comparable to antacids while some studies have demonstrated that the combination may be superior (25,26). Overall, no improvement in the healing of erosive esophagitis can be conclusively demonstrated with either of these therapies, so they should be considered as indicated for symptomatic relief for infrequent heartburn. As primary agents, they are of little use, except perhaps in pregnancy.

Sucralfate

This mucosal protective agent binds to inflamed tissue, perhaps protecting the esophageal mucosa by blocking diffusion of gastric acid and pepsin across the mucosal barrier. Sucralfate may inhibit the erosive action of pepsin and bile (28). Although rarely used in the GERD patient because of the need to administer the drug four times daily, there is value to this agent in special populations such as pregnant women (see below) (29). Little systemic absorption of the agent has been demonstrated, so it is likely safe for this population. When compared to H$_2$RAs head to head, equivalent healing of erosive esophagitis is demonstrated although overall healing rates are not as high (30,31) (Fig. 25.1). Constipation is seen in 2% of patients. This compound is rarely used in modern medical therapy for GERD, with the exception of pregnant patients.

Promotility Therapy

Conceptually, a "promotility or motility-altering agent" might present the ideal agent to treat GERD. Addressing the underlying pathophysiologic defects, thus improving the strength and competence of the LES and augmenting esophageal clearance to shorten the time the esophageal mucosa is exposed to a pH<4 and to improve gastric emptying, would constitute the ideal therapy. Unfortunately, the most commonly prescribed promotility agent, cisapride, has been withdrawn from the market due to side effects (mainly cardiac), and metoclopramide—the remaining agent available in this country—has limited therapeutic efficacy and an unfavorable side effect profile. Thus, this class of agents is currently not a strong competitor in the treatment arena. A brief review of these agents is presented, with the understanding that their usefulness is currently limited.

Metoclopramide is a dopamine antagonist; the precise mechanism of action is unclear. Most commonly, it is reported to sensitize tissues to the action of acetylcholine and has been shown in some studies to increase the amplitude of gastric and esophageal contractions, increase LES pressure (LESP), and accelerate gastric emptying (32). Because it crosses the blood–brain barrier and interacts with dopamine receptors, it produces clinically important central nervous system side effects, such as drowsiness and confusion (32), which preclude its widespread use. When studied head to head with H$_2$RAs, principally cimetidine, clinical trials have found equivalent efficacy of metoclopramide compared to H$_2$RAs in relieving heartburn and other GERD symptoms (33–35). When compared to placebos, 10 mg of metoclopramide three times daily showed little symptom improvement. When the dose was increased to 10 mg four times daily, it is more effective than placebos in improving symptoms (36,37). No study has shown the agent to be more effective than placebos in promoting healing of erosive esophagitis. Because of its centrally acting effects, antidopaminergic side effects are observed in 20% to 30% of patients. Anxiety, agitation, confusion, motor restlessness, hallucinations, and drowsiness are the most common side effects; depression and tardive dyskinesia (potentially irreversible) are the most serious side effects. Side effects appear to be dose related and perhaps higher in children and the elderly.

Cisapride (no longer available in the United States) acts locally and seems to facilitate the release of acetylcholine from postganglionic neurons in the myenteric plexus. There is some evidence that the drug influences the activity of other mediators of gut function, perhaps the serotonin 5-HT4 receptor in the myenteric plexus. There are data supporting its ability to increase smooth muscle contractility, and thus LESP, and to enhance the clearance of esophageal acid (38). Before its removal from the United States, the drug was indicated for treatment of nocturnal heartburn and was clearly the most widely prescribed and effective promotility agent available for the treatment of GERD. It is consistently better than placebos in improving symptoms and may promote healing of lower-grade erosive esophagitis. Ten mg four times daily is likely required for healing, while 10 mg three times daily is adequate for symptom relief. As is the case with metoclopramide, when cisapride was compared to H$_2$RAs, similar efficacy in healing of erosive esophagitis was always found (38). Unfortunately, the drug was withdrawn from the U.S. market due to the potential for cardiac QT prolongation, including ventricular arrhythmias.

Bethanechol, a direct-acting muscarinic receptor agent, has been used in the past as a promotility agent (off-label) for treating GERD. It has been shown to increase LESP and improve esophageal peristaltic clearance (38). However, bethanechol has rarely been used, mainly because of its side effect profile and the availability of cisapride. Abdominal cramps, blurred vision, fatigue, and increased urinary frequency occur in 10% to 15% of patients, and more commonly in the elderly. Numerous contraindications preclude its use as an antireflux agent (38).

Domperidone, a dopamine antagonist that stimulates esophageal peristalsis, increases LESP, and accelerates gastric emptying (38), is available outside the United States and in several U.S. pharmacies that compound the drug (38). Unlike metoclopramide, it does not cross the blood–brain barrier, so has few of the central dopaminergic side effects of that drug. It should not be administered with antisecretory agents or antacids because reduced gastric acidity may impair its absorption. The few available studies are based on small samples and often lack controls. The efficacy studies suggest similarity to H$_2$RAs (ranitidine and famotidine) in symptom relief and in promotion of esophageal healing, and in one combination study with an H$_2$RA, the combination was not significantly better than each administered alone (38,39). Hyperprolactinemia, nipple tenderness, galactorrhea, and amenorrhea are the most common side effects of this agent, which is unlikely to be approved for distribution in the United States.

Tegaserod, a selective partial 5HT4 agonist, has recently been approved for constipation-predominant irritable bowel syndrome in the United States. Its promotility effects suggest a reason to study this agent in disorders of gastric emptying and, perhaps, GERD, although to date no substantial clinical trials have been produced (40).

Ultimately, this class of agents has historically fallen short of expectations. The use of metoclopramide should be undertaken with care, and in the era of potent antisecretory therapy should play a very small role in managing the patient with GERD.

Combination Therapy (H₂RAs and Promotility Agents)

Prior to the availability of PPIs, the combination of an H₂RA and prokinetic was popularized as the management strategy to treat the difficult patient. This is presented here for historical information. While some studies have suggested that a combination of these two agents is more efficacious than either alone, the data are conflicting (35,41). The best study—a maintenance trial comparing ranitidine 150 tid, cisapride 10 mg tid, and a combination of ranitidine and cisapride, as part of a larger study including a PPI and combination of a PPI and cisapride—showed an advantage of combination therapy over H₂ blocker or cisapride alone (42). This study showed a numeric, but not statistical advantage for the combination of the prokinetic and PPI over a PPI alone. In general, the use of combination therapy with an antisecretory agent and a prokinetic should be discouraged as the therapeutic benefit, at best, is small and rarely results in improvement over an increase in the dose of antisecretory therapy. Combination therapy with an H₂RA and a PPI is discussed below.

Acid-Suppressive Therapy

Antisecretory agents are medications of choice for pharmacologic therapy of GERD. Two classes of acid suppressive agents are used today: H₂RAs and PPIs. Understanding of their active mechanisms and efficacy is crucial to optimal use of these agents alone or in combination. A brief review of acid production and active mechanism precedes the review of their overall efficacy.

Acid Production

Parietal cells are located within the mucosa, predominantly in the body of the stomach. They produce an average of 2 liters of gastric acid per day. There are three different types of receptors on the basal lateral membrane of the parietal cell, each of which when stimulated will effect the production of acid. Gastrin, present in the G cells in the gastric antrum, is stimulated by food in the stomach (gastric phase), reaching the parietal cell through the blood. Acetylcholine is released from the vagus nerve and is predominantly stimulated by the cephalic phase—the sight, sound, smell, and taste of food. Release of either of

these two ligands stimulates the enterochromaffin-like (ECL) cell to release histamine, which then binds to its receptor on the parietal cell. Activation of these receptors stimulates protein phosphokinases, principally cyclic adenosine 3′, 5′ monophosphate (cAMP), which then acts as a secondary messenger to stimulate the proton pump, which is in a resting state in the tubulovesicle of the parietal cell. Stimulation of the pump configures it into its active form at the secretory canaliculi where it will exchange a hydrogen for a potassium ion through the hydrogen potassium ATPase enzyme (the so-called proton pump), the final common path of acid secretion. Inhibition of any of the three receptors on the basal lateral membrane will inhibit acid production to some degree, while inhibition of the proton pump inhibits the final common pathway, thus creating the opportunity for superior acid suppression. There are no agents approved for use in GERD that inhibit the gastrin or acetylcholine receptor.

Both classes of agents, histamine receptor H₂ antagonists and PPIs, inhibit gastric secretion and raise intragastric pH. The number of hours of the day in which these agents raise intragastric pH to >4 is an indirect measure of efficacy of symptom relief, correlates with healing of erosive esophagitis, and is important in understanding the overall efficacy data of these agents. When gastric pH is <4, pepsinogen is activated to pepsin, which can exacerbate the esophageal mucosal damage caused by acid. A meta-analysis has linked healing of erosive esophagitis to the duration of time (over 24 hours) that the intragastric pH is <4 (43) (Fig. 25.2). Healing of erosive esophagitis by acid-suppressive agents is thus felt to be directly related to the duration of gastric acid suppression over a 24-hour period. Thus, agents that inhibit gastric acid

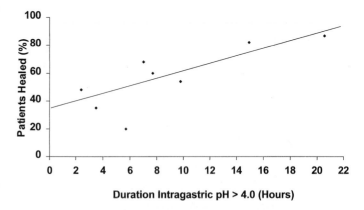

FIGURE 25.2. Results of meta-analysis of treatment trials of endoscopically assessed erosive esophagitis healing at 8 weeks by antisecretory agents. The dots clustered at *lower left* are antacids, in the *middle* H2 receptor antagonists, and the two at the *right* proton pump inhibitors. (From Bell NJ, Burget D, Howden CW, et al. Appropriate acid suppression for the management of gastro-oesophageal reflux disease. *Digestion* 1992;51 (suppl 1):59–67, with permission.)

secretion and potentially raise intragastric pH to >4 for the longest duration, have the greatest potential to provide symptom relief and mucosal healing in GERD.

H₂ Receptor Antagonists

Prior to the availability of PPIs, H2RAs formed the mainstay of GERD therapy. The four available agents—cimetidine, ranitidine, famotidine, and nizatidine—derive their efficacy in GERD exclusively by inhibiting acid secretion. They do not affect LESP, TLESRs, esophageal clearance, nor gastric emptying in humans. H2RAs only block one receptor, and thus have limited effect on acid reduction, and are relatively weak inhibitors of meal-stimulated acid secretion, reducing acid secretion by almost 60% to 70% (44). In general, the antisecretory capabilities of H2RAs are best at night, with duration of acid inhibition longer when the drug is taken in the evening or before bedtime. Equally potent doses of H2RAs equally inhibit acid secretion and as such provide reason for similar efficacy in GERD (Table 25.2). H2RAs were made available as over-the-counter agents in 1995.

Symptom relief has been variable, ranging from 32% to 82% of patients, while endoscopic resolution ranges from 0% to 82% (45). In a later meta-analysis, endoscopic improvement was demonstrated in 31% to 88% of patients, with healing in 27% to 45% of primarily grade 1 or 2 lesions (46). The differences seen in these trials can be accounted for by various symptom endpoints as well as the variability in erosive esophagitis baselines. This underscores the importance of carefully evaluating clinical trials in extrapolating clinical efficacy to specific patient populations.

Higher doses of H2RAs given twice or four times a day may increase efficacy. Some comparative studies have produced 12-week healing rates as high as 70% with ranitidine at 150 mg two to four times daily (47,48,52), 8-week healing rates of up 77% at 800 mg of cimetidine twice daily (48) and famotidine 40 mg twice daily, these high healing rates are unusual in practice and when higher grades of erosive esophagitis are treated (51,52). Although commonly recommended in step-up algorithms, the data above indicate that expectations for efficacy of higher doses may be overestimated in patients with severe disease who require greater acid suppression.

GERD is a chronic disease and, therefore, relapse is common when therapy is discontinued. Maintenance of symptom relief and healing with H2RAs are variable and parallel data from acute healing studies. One well-done study (53) examined symptom relapse over 4 weeks in 423 patients

TABLE 25.2. EQUIPOTENT DOSES OF H₂RAs

Cimetidine	Ranitidine	Famotidine	Nizatidine
600 mg	150 mg	20 mg	150 mg

with GERD symptoms, randomized to either a placebo or 150 mg ranitidine twice or four times daily. Approximately two thirds had a normal-appearing esophagus endoscopically; 28%, grade-1 erosive esophagitis; and only 4.5%, grades 2 to 4 erosive esophagitis. Patients were randomized to receive 150 mg ranitidine twice daily or a placebo for 2 weeks. If patients were satisfied with their treatment (improved or complete relief), they continued with that therapy. If patients were not satisfied, they were re-randomized to receive 150 mg twice or four times daily for another 2 weeks. If symptoms did not respond after 4 weeks, they were removed from follow-up. After 4 weeks, all were taken off therapy, followed for an additional 20 weeks, and evaluated for overall symptom relapse. After 24 weeks, 52% who had nonerosive disease and 67% with erosive disease experienced relapse, resulting in an overall relapse rate of 59%. In general, dosage was unrelated to symptom relapse rate (30). In the Vignieri et al. study (54), which compared cisapride, ranitidine, and omeprazole, ranitidine 150 mg tid maintained remission in 49% at 1 year (54).

Overall, as a class the H2RAs are extremely safe with overall side effects seen in ≤4% of patients. Typically, minor GI side effects of clinical concern include nausea, abdominal pain, and bloating. There have been concerns about drug interactions with these agents, particularly interactions with agents affecting the cytochrome P450 system and, in particular, with cimetidine. Serum concentrations of phenytoin, procainamide, theophylline, and warfarin have been altered after administration of cimetidine, and to a lesser degree ranitidine; these effects are not seen with famotidine and/or nizatidine (55,56). However, the clinical consequences of these interactions are minimal and rarely result in a clinically important interaction. Nevertheless, awareness of these potential complications needs to be considered if H2RAs are prescribed. Some concern about mental confusion, particularly with the intravenous use of these agents, must be considered if they are used in the hospital setting.

Proton Pump Inhibitors

PPIs are clearly the most effective medical regimen available for treatment of GERD at the present time. They provide superior control of intragastric pH over a 24-hour period compared to H2RAs and effect greater symptom relief and healing. By inhibiting the hydrogen potassium ATPase, the final common pathway of acid secretion, these agents suppress daytime, nighttime, and meal-stimulated acid secretion to a significantly greater degree than H2RAs (57). Five available PPIs are omeprazole, lansoprazole, rabeprazole, pantoprazole, and the newest esomeprazole, the S-isomer of omeprazole. PPIs are weak bases that concentrate in the secretory canaliculi at pH <4. They are highly selective and can concentrate up to 1,000-fold in the acidic environment of the canaliculi. It is here that the inactive benzimidazole of the PPI is converted to a cationic sulfonamide, which binds to cysteines on the proton pump and therefore blocks acid-producing capabilities (58,59). The onset of inhibition may be delayed because PPIs need time to accumulate in the canaliculi and initiate activation of the acid production cycle. All available PPIs bind covalently and irreversibly to proton pumps; therefore, the degree of inhibition is related to AUC, not plasma concentration. PPIs block 70% to 80% of active pumps; therefore, for acid secretion to resume, new hydrogen potassium ATPase molecules must be synthesized, a process that takes 36 to 96 hours. Although each of the agents has subtly different binding capabilities, the class in general provides maximal efficacy in control of intragastric pH when taken immediately or longer before a meal, as the drugs bind to actively secreting pumps. It is for this reason that the drugs are administered before the first meal of the day, or when a second dose is needed, before the evening meal, rather than at bedtime. As not all pumps are active at any given time, a single dose of a PPI does not inhibit all pumps and, therefore, does not "completely" inhibit all acid secretion. Acid inhibition is never complete because of the continued synthesis of new pumps and a steady state is required in order to maintain continuous acid control (60). When PPIs are administered twice daily, more active pumps are exposed to the drug and the steady-state inhibition of gastric acid is more rapidly achieved and will be more complete.

PPIs are metabolized in the liver by two enzymes in the cytochrome P450 system: CYP2C19, which forms an inactive 5-hydroxy and 5-O-desmethylmetabolite, and CYP3A4, which forms an inactive sulfone metabolite (59). The subtle differences in how each PPI is metabolized within this system are responsible for subtle differences in plasma concentration and drug interactions (Table 25.3). While rarely a clinical problem, the absorption of other orally administered (acid-dependent) drugs may be affected (Table 25.4). With the exception of esomeprazole, the differences in clinical pharmacology among the available PPIs do not appear to result in dramatic differences in clinical efficacy.

TABLE 25.4. POSSIBLE EFFECTS OF INCREASED INTRAGASTRIC PH ON DRUG ABSORPTION

Absorption Increased	Absorption Decreased
Aspirin	Ketoconazole
Benzylpenicillin	Itraconazole
Didanosine	Cefpodoxime proxetil
Nifedipine	Enoxacin
Midazolam	Indomethacin
Furosemide	Protein-bound cobalamin
Digoxin	

Clinical Efficacy

The increase in pH control over a 24-hour period accounts for the superiority of PPIs over the H₂RA. Omeprazole, lansoprazole, pantoprazole, and rabeprazole are similar in their control of intragastric pH as demonstrated in several studies and highlighted in a comparison study shown in Fig. 25.3. Esomeprazole appears to provide a longer duration of pH control when the 40-mg dose is compared to other doses of PPIs (Table 25.5)

Ultimately, the success of a drug is measured by its ability to relieve symptoms and to effectively provide healing of erosive esophagitis. The PPIs are clearly superior to H₂RAs in this arena. Overall, a once-daily morning dose of a PPI relieves symptoms in slightly less than 90% of patients with GERD, and heals erosive esophagitis in 78% to 95% (61) (Fig. 25.1). The efficacy data are usually achieved after only 4 to 8 weeks of therapy, and as with H₂RAs correlate with severity of erosive esophagitis with all five PPIs. A summary of the results is provided below, with highlights of key comparative clinical trials.

Although all PPIs provide a high level of symptom improvement and are essentially equivalents, there are some variations in PPI performance when compared head to

TABLE 25.3. POSSIBLE DRUG INTERACTIONS WITH PPI THERAPY

PPI	Interactions
Omeprazole	Inhibits metabolism of phenytoin, diazepam, antipyrine, aminopyrine, and the R-isomer of warfarin
	Does not inhibit metabolism of propranolol, theophylline, and the S-isomer of warfarin
Lansoprazole	No clinically significant interactions with most drugs metabolized through the cytochrome P450 system
	Causes 10% increase in metabolism rate of theophylline
Pantoprazole	No clinically significant interactions with drugs metabolized through the cytochrome P450 system
	No interactions with oral contraceptives
Rabeprazole	No clinically significant interactions with drugs metabolized through the cytochrome P450 system
Esomeprazole	No clinically significant interactions with drugs metabolized through the cytochrome P450 system

PPI, proton pump inhibitor.

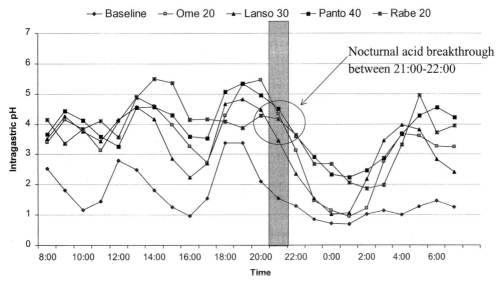

FIGURE 25.3. Studies depicting time curves for intragastric pH control comparing proton pump inhibitors omeprazole, lansoprazole, pantoprazole, and rabeprazole in FDA-approved doses given once daily on control of intragastric pH compared to control in the baseline state without drug. The *gray bar* illustrates the drop in pH to <4 (termed nocturnal acid breakthrough) seen before midnight in comparison to after midnight on twice-daily proton pump inhibitors.

TABLE 25.5. PERCENTAGE OF PATIENTS WITH INTRAGASTRIC PH >4.0 FOR >12 HOURS AND >16 HOURS AFTER 5 DAYS OF THERAPY

	Patients with Intragastric pH >4.0 (%)	
Study/Agent	>12 Hours	>16 Hours
Lind et al.[a]		
Omeprazole 20 mg	45	14
Esomeprazole 20 mg	54	24
Esomeprazole 40 mg	92	56
Röhss et al.[b]		
Omeprazole 40 mg	75	44
Esomeprazole 40 mg	88	55
Röhss et al.[c]		
Lansoprazole 30 mg	57	5
Esomeprazole 40 mg	90	38
Wilder-Smith et al.[d]		
Rabeprazole 20 mg	36	5
Esomeprazole 40 mg	77	32
Wilder-Smith et al.[e]		
Pantoprazole 40 mg	30	10
Esomeprazole 40 mg	90	50

[a]Lind T, Rydberg L, Kyleback A, et al. Esomeprazole provides improved acid control vs. omeprazole in patients with symptoms of gastro-oesophageal reflux disease. *Aliment Pharmacol Ther* 2000;14:861–867.
[b]Röhss K, Lundin C, Rydholm H, et al. Esomeprazole 40 mg provides more effective acid control than omeprazole 40 mg. *Gastroenterology* 2000;95:2432.
[c]Röhss K, Claar-Nilsson C, Rydholm H, et al. Esomeprazole 40 mg provides more effective acid control than lansoprazole 30 mg. *Gastroenterology* 2000;118:A20.
[d]Wilder-Smith C, Röhss K, Claar-Nilson C, et al. Esomeprazole 40 mg provides more effective acid control than rabeprazole 20 mg. *Gut* 2000;47:A63.
[e]Wilder-Smith C, Röhss K, Lundin C, et al. Esomeprazole 40 mg provides more effective acid control than pantoprazole 40 mg. *Gastroenterology* 2000;118:A22.

head. Castell et al. (62) compared efficacy and safety of lansoprazole at 15 and 30 mg once daily, omeprazole at 20 mg daily, and a placebo, in nearly 1,300 patients with grades 2 to 4 endoscopically confirmed erosive esophagitis. Daytime and nighttime relief of heartburn for the two drugs were statistically superior to the placebo; the 30-mg dose of lansoprazole was slightly more effective than 20 mg of omeprazole in speed of heartburn relief. After 8 weeks of therapy, patients who received omeprazole reported heartburn on 12% of days and 9% of nights compared to 9% of days and 6.5% of nights ($p<0.05$) on 30 mg of lansoprazole (62).

In a large comparison study of omeprazole at 20 mg/day versus lansoprazole at 30 mg/day, Richter et al. (63) demonstrated the superiority of lansoprazole in sustained resolution of heartburn (84% vs. 83%, $p<0.05$) after 8 weeks of treatment. In contrast, in a comparison study of symptom relief comparing pantoprazole at 40 mg/day versus omeprazole at 20 mg/day, Mossner et al. (66) found no statistical difference in symptom relief when the two drugs were compared (94% vs. 90%). Subsequently, Dekkers et al. (64) compared rabeprazole at 20 mg/day to omeprazole at 20 mg/day in terms of symptom relief. The difference in improvement in heartburn at 8 weeks between rabeprazole and omeprazole (87% vs. 82%) was not statistically significant.

In a large study (65), the newest PPI, esomeprazole at 40 mg/day, was compared to lansoprazole at 30 mg/day for heartburn relief (n=5,241). At the end of 4 weeks, superiority was demonstrated for esomeprazole (62.9 vs. 60.2%, $p<0.05$). Richter et al. (63) compared esomeprazole at 40 mg/day to omeprazole at 20 mg/day for patients who assessed sustained resolution of heartburn, defined as 7 consecutive days with no heartburn (n=2,375), and found statistical superiority for esomeprazole over omeprazole at any given time point ($p=0.001$).

The overall clinical importance of these small differences among individual patients is unknown. Because of the differences in endpoints, cross-study comparisons are extremely difficult. Consequently, a determination of whether the increase in symptom relief with esomeprazole is clinically important awaits long-term use.

Healing of Erosive Esophagitis

Ultimately, a more objective measure of efficacy in drug–drug comparisons is in healing erosive esophagitis, which is discussed below. An overall summary of healing rates of erosive esophagitis for all classes for pooled data is shown in Fig. 25.1. In general, PPIs produce a healing rate of approximately 11.7% per week, superior to H₂RAs (5.9%), and placebos (2.9%) (61). The comparison studies discussed above related to symptom relief show no difference in healing of erosive esophagitis when lansoprazole, pantoprazole, and rabeprazole are compared to omeprazole (62,64,66) (Fig. 25.4).

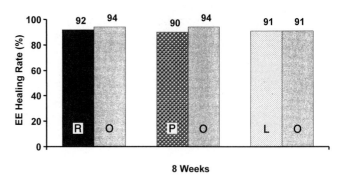

FIGURE 25.4. A comparison of erosive esophagitis healing rates (Y axis) of studies evaluating healing rates of erosive esophagitis at 8 weeks and proton pump inhibitors compared to omeprazole. In each set of two bars, omeprazole (*O*) is seen on the *right* and the comparative proton pump inhibitor (*R*, rabeprazole; *P*, pantoprazole; *L*, lansoprazole) on the *left* set of bars as outlined. *P*, not statistically significant.

Esomeprazole, the S-isomer of omeprazole, is the first PPI to show a statistical advantage over treatment with omeprazole. The first study to demonstrate this, by Kahrilas et al. (67), was a randomized, double-blind, controlled trial (n=1,960), which compared erosive esophagitis healing rates and symptom relief with 20 mg/day of omeprazole compared to 20 mg/day and 40 mg/day of esomeprazole for 8 weeks. Healing rates were statistically superior for esomeprazole compared to omeprazole at both 4 and 8 weeks (Fig. 25.5). A second study by Richter et al. (63) in 2,425 patients confirmed these findings (Fig. 25.5). Of particular interest is the confirmation that the healing rate of erosive esophagitis decreases as the grade of erosive esophagitis increases. The decrement in healing seen with omeprazole was greater than that seen with esomeprazole at 40 mg/day. A large clinical trial compared esomeprazole at 40 mg/day to lansoprazole (65). In this study (n=5,241), healing rates were statistically superior for esomeprazole at 40 mg/day compared to lansoprazole at 30 mg/day (Fig. 25.6), with the difference again most demonstrable at the higher grades of erosive esophagitis (Fig. 25.7). The magnitude of the difference was smaller than in the omeprazole trials. The reason for this difference is not clear. This overall 4% to 8% superiority in healing appears to be greatest in those with "more severe erosive esophagitis," which underscores the importance of intragastric pH control in overall GERD efficacy.

Maintenance Therapy

Healing of mucosal injury or achievement of symptom control alone is not sufficient to alter the natural history of GERD, and almost all patients require some form of maintenance therapy. Individuals with endoscopically documented erosive esophagitis have shown recurrence rates ranging from 75% to 92% following discontinuation of

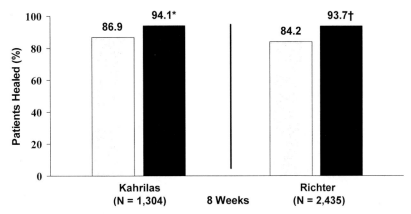

FIGURE 25.5. Healing rates of erosive esophagitis (*Y axis*) in two pivotal trials submitted to the FDA comparing esomeprazole 40 mg to omeprazole 20 mg showing statistical superiority of esomeprazole to omeprazole in given doses. *White bars*, omeprazole 20 mg q.d.; *black bars*, esomeprazole 40 mg q.d. * $P \leq 0.05$; ₊ $P < 0.001$ vs. omeprazole. (Data from Kahrilas PJ, Falk GW, Johnson DA, et al. Esomeprazole improves healing and symptom resolution as compared with omeprazole in reflux oesophagitis patients: a randomized controlled trial. The Esomeprazole Study Investigators. *Aliment Pharmacol Ther* 2000;14:1249–1258, with permission; Richter JE, Kahrilas PJ, Johanson J, et al. Efficacy and safety of esomeprazole compared with omeprazole in GERD patients with erosive esophagitis: a randomized controlled trial. *Am J Gastroenterol* 2001;96:656–665, with permission.)

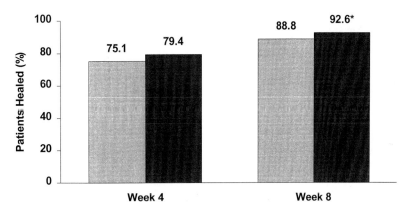

FIGURE 25.6. Healing rates of erosive esophagitis at weeks 4 and 8 comparing esomeprazole 40 and lansoprazole 30 across grades A through D (Los Angeles grades) erosive esophagitis. *P*, 0.0001 vs. lansoprazole. *Light bars*, lansoprazole 30 mg q.d. (n = 2,617); *dark bars*, esomeprazole 40 mg q.d. (n = 2,624). (From Meier-Ewert HK, Van Herwaarden MA, Gideon RM, et al. Effect of age on differences in upper esophageal sphincter and pharynx pressures between patients with dysphagia and control subjects. *Am J Gastroenterol* 2001;96:35–40, with permission.)

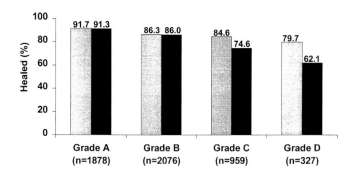

FIGURE 25.7. Healing rates by grade of erosive esophagitis from the previous study cited in Fig. 25.6. The study illustrates the decrement in healing rates as one proceeds from grade A through D. This decrement is less for esomeprazole (*light bars*) compared to lansoprazole (*dark bars*).

PPIs (68). In addition, if a patient has a recurrence and is brought back into remission with a PPI, there is a 90% chance that the patient will have another recurrence if the PPI is discontinued again. In a landmark study comparing five maintenance regimens for patients with healed esophagitis, Vignieri et al. (42) showed significantly higher remission rates with PPI therapy than with H$_2$RAs or prokinetics. A number of attempts to use low-dose PPI maintenance therapies for reasons of cost have met with only varying success, as most patients relapse within a few months. Recently, Ladas et al. (69) reported that when using gastric pH monitoring after healing, one can predict which patients are more likely to remain in remission with low-dose omeprazole therapy.

Dose Response

Increasing the dose of PPIs if symptoms are not relieved is common in practice. Whether this will effectively increase healing of erosive esophagitis—that is, whether a dose response is demonstrable with these agents—is difficult to prove at higher doses when tested in clinical trials. In the comparison study by Castell et al. (65), 15 mg of lansoprazole daily resulted in a healing rate 79% lower than the healing rates for 30 mg of lansoprazole (91%). A similar dose-dependent pattern was demonstrable in a study by Lundell et al. (70), who compared 10-mg and 20-mg doses of omeprazole in healing Los Angeles (LA) grades A to C of erosive esophagitis. With the lower dose of omeprazole, efficacy in healing correlated with the grade of esophagitis (77% of grade A healed, 50% of B, and 20% of C). This correlation of efficacy with grade did not occur with the 20-mg dosage, which healed equivalent percentages of grades A and B (80%), and 40% of grade C. This constitutes higher healing rates than seen with the lower dose and suggests that there is a dose response with antisecretory therapy with PPIs. However, Sontag et al. (71) compared 20- and 40-mg daily doses of omeprazole to placebo in 230 patients with erosive esophagitis grades 2 to 4. At week 8, there was no difference in healing overall between the 20- and 40-mg groups (73.5% and 74.7%, respectively). The 40-mg dose resulted in faster symptom relief; however, no difference in overall symptom relief was observed at the end of 8 weeks. In a long-term observational study, Klinkenberg-Knol et al. (72) showed that by increasing omeprazole dose as needed, almost all patients refractory to ranitidine could be effectively healed.

OPTIMIZATION OF MEDICAL THERAPY IN GERD

All available PPIs are approved for once daily dosing in the morning. Although each affects the bioavailability of each molecule differently, it is recommended that all PPIs be given before meals. This is based on concepts previously discussed and results of an intragastric pH study addressing this issue (73). This two-armed crossover study treated normal subjects with 20 mg of omeprazole or 30 mg of lansoprazole at 8 A.M. daily for 7 days, followed by intragastric pH monitoring performed with the dose given 15 to 30 minutes before the breakfast meal and when given on an empty stomach with no food until lunchtime. A significant superiority in daytime pH control (time intragastric pH>4) was found when the PPI was taken before breakfast compared to an empty stomach (73). Although optimal timing has not been determined, PPIs should be given on an empty stomach and followed by a meal. About 90% of patients will respond to this once-daily dosing with any of the PPIs, achieving effective healing of erosive esophagitis and symptom relief.

However, some patients such as these with extraesophageal symptoms (e.g., asthma, cough, laryngitis, and chest pain) and Barrett's esophagus are often treated with more than a single daily dose of PPI. In this case, splitting the dose and giving a PPI twice daily before breakfast and dinner, provides superior intragastric pH control, particularly at night, when compared to a double dose given once daily.

This observation was first made by a study in 19 normal subjects randomized to receive 40 mg of omeprazole before breakfast, 40 mg before dinner (P.M.), or 20 mg twice daily (before breakfast and dinner) (74). Each was crossed over to all three regimens with a 1-week washout period between 24-hour intragastric pH studies. The most important observation made from these data was the statistical superiority of the 20-mg twice-daily dose in control of 24-hour intragastric pH compared to 40 mg in a single dose. A subsequent three-way crossover study confirmed these observations by evaluating overnight pH control in subjects treated with 40 mg of omeprazole before breakfast, before dinner, or twice daily. Control in daytime pH was similar regardless of regimen; however, nocturnal pH control was significantly improved with the twice-daily regimen compared to double dose once daily (75).

Another observation from intragastric pH studies is the finding of wide intersubject variability in intragastric pH control despite similar dosing regimens. This wide variability is illustrated by a recent study (76) comparing 24-hour intragastric pH control in normal subjects treated with omeprazole at 20 mg and lansoprazole at 30 mg twice daily for 7 days. Both inter- and intra-subject variability in pH response were observed (76). This intrasubject variability in intragastric pH control is uncommon and not easy to explain but may account for the occasional patient who responds to a switch from one PPI to another after one seemingly fails. The intersubject variability in intragastric pH response may be lower with esomeprazole and rabeprazole compared to other PPIs.

Step Therapy

As our understanding of the physiology of acid production, pathogenesis of heartburn, action mechanism of acid suppression, and drug safety profiles have changed over time, so has the therapy of choice. The once-dominant strategy involving lifestyle modifications and over-the-counter antacids is currently used as a first step in treatment, followed by prescription H$_2$RAs, and then introduction of PPIs. This practice of a so-called step-up approach to GERD therapy, which is often emphasized in treatment algorithms, may not be optimal.

This strategy was extensively evaluated in a study by Howden et al. (77) in 593 patients randomly selected into the following treatment groups: (a) ranitidine 150 mg bid for 8 weeks followed by lansoprazole 30 mg q d for 12 weeks; (b) lansoprazole 30 mg qd for 8 weeks followed by ranitidine 150 mg bid for 12 weeks; (c) continuous ranitidine 150 mg bid; and (d) continuous lansoprazole 30 mg q d. The percentage of heartburn-free days at the end of 20 weeks was assessed, with continuous lansoprazole showing the best results over any other strategy. The second-best strategy was step-down therapy (Fig. 25.8).

The question of step-up therapy was addressed in trial comparing high-dose and standard-dose ranitidine therapy in patients initially unresponsive to 6 weeks of therapy with ranitidine at 150 mg twice daily. A total of 481 patients with GERD symptoms initially received a 6-week course of 150 mg twice daily. Sixty percent remained symptomatic and were re-randomized to receive either 150 mg or 300 mg of ranitidine twice daily.

After 8 additional weeks of therapy, 45% of these patients on the lower dose of ranitidine and a similar number (44.8% on the higher dose) had mild or no heartburn. This study underscores key points; there appears to be a peak in efficacy of H$_2$RA therapy regardless of dose and duration of therapy (67).

Step-down therapy has been advocated by some, although data are conflicting. A recent study by Inadomi et al. (78) examined the feasibility of step-down therapy in patients with nonerosive symptomatic GERD who were asymptomatic with PPIs. After baseline demographic and quality-of-life information were obtained, the patients were withdrawn from PPIs in a stepwise fashion. Fifty-eight percent of patients were asymptomatic following discontinuation of treatment after 1 year of follow-up. Thirty-four percent required H$_2$RAs, 7% required prokinetic agents, 1% required both, and 15% remained asymptomatic without medication. Although quality of life was not significantly different, management costs decreased by 37%. Younger age and heartburn were the predominant factors predicting unsuccessful PPI step-down management, suggesting that individuals with "true GERD" require full-dose maintenance therapy.

Nocturnal Gastric Acid Breakthrough on PPIs: A Pharmacologic Phenomenon of Potential but Clinically Variable Importance

Careful studies using continuous intragastric pH monitoring have found that 70% of subjects continue to secrete acid and intragastric pH declines to <4 for at least 1 continuous hour in the overnight monitoring period (10 P.M. to 6 A.M.) even when taking PPIs twice daily (79). This drop in pH, a pharmacologic phenomenon termed nocturnal gastric acid breakthrough (NAB), begins about 6 to 7 hours after the evening dose of a PPI (79) (Fig. 25.9). When PPIs are given as a once-daily dose before breakfast, this nocturnal gastric acid recovery occurs earlier in the evening, beginning around 11 P.M. (80). This NAB appears to be a class effect, and can be demonstrated in normal subjects, and subjects with uncomplicated GERD, Barrett's esophagus, and scleroderma (81). Over 100 normal subjects and patients on omeprazole, lansoprazole, rabeprazole, and pantoprazole at once and twice-daily dosages have been studied, documenting a consistent frequency of gastric acid recovery regardless of PPI. Preliminary study of esomeprazole suggests a decrease in the frequency of nocturnal gastric acid recovery, but more detailed and comprehensive studies are necessary (82).

The clinical importance of this common intragastric finding to appears to have been overestimated, as esophageal reflux occurs during nocturnal breakthrough of

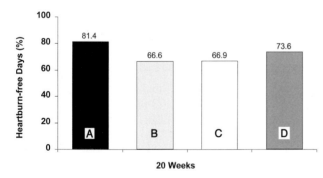

FIGURE 25.8. A clinical trial comparing four strategies for management of heartburn in patients with gastroesophageal reflux disease. Study demonstrating a superiority in heartburn free days (Y axis) in the continuous PPI strategy compared to the other four. *A,* continuous lansoprazole 30 mg q.d. (*P* <0.01); *B,* continuous ranitidine 150 mg q.d.; *C,* step-up therapy (Ranitidine 150 mg b.i.d for 8 weeks, followed by lansoprazole 30 mg q.d. for 12 weeks); *D,* step-down therapy (Lansoprazole 30 mg q.d. for 8 weeks, followed by ranitidine 150 mg b.i.d. for 12 weeks). N=593. (From Howden CW, Henning JM, Huang B, et al. Management of heartburn in a large, randomized, community-based study: comparison of four therapeutic strategies. *Am J Gastroenterol* 2001;96:1704–1710, with permission.)

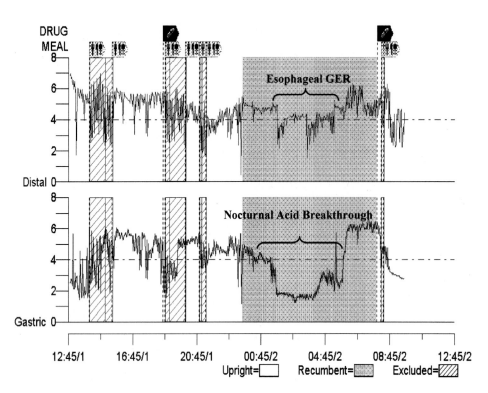

FIGURE 25.9. Dual channel intragastric and intraesophageal pH study illustrating the phenomenon of nocturnal gastric acid breakthrough at approximately 1:00 A.M. in a patient on twice daily proton pump inhibitor. The upper tracing demonstrates simultaneous esophageal reflux (drop in pH to <4) during the period of nocturnal acid breakthrough.

intragastric pH in only 5% of normal subjects and about 15% of patients with uncomplicated GERD (81). This is consistent with the observation from clinical trials that nocturnal heartburn is infrequent (10% to 15%) on once-a-day PPIs. Symptoms during these nocturnal gastric pH drops have not been systematically studied but appear to be uncommon. Overnight gastric acid recovery may be of clinical importance in patients with severe GERD and those with Barrett's esophagus. Up to 50% of patients with Barrett's esophagus or scleroderma and GERD will have increased overnight esophageal acid exposure during NAB (83,84).

Nocturnal gastric acid breakthrough is not the result of PPI resistance, which in fact is an extremely rare phenomenon. Some patients appear resistant to PPIs because of the intersubject variability outlined above. These patients are not truly resistant to the drugs, as intragastric pH control can be improved by increasing the PPI dose. In one study, six of seven patients who appeared to be omeprazole resistant had improved intragastric pH control when the dosage was increased, reinforcing the observation that true PPI resistance is extremely rare (85).

Combination Therapy: PPIs and H₂RAs

While most patients experience little or no reflux during this period of NAB, the few who do (primarily patients with Barrett's esophagus, scleroderma [76], and perhaps those with extraesophageal symptoms) may be at risk for nocturnal symptoms or esophageal damage. The use of

nocturnal H₂RAs has been popularized as a way of controlling NAB. A hierarchy of intragastric pH control is outlined in Table 25.6. Most data are based principally on short-term studies. Two recent papers (86,87) report the results of longer-term use of nocturnal H₂RAs, evaluate the control of intragastric pH in the subjects and patients, and raise important issues regarding long-term efficacy.

Fackler et al. (86) prospectively evaluated 23 healthy volunteers and 20 patients with GERD initially treated with omeprazole at 20 mg bid (before breakfast and dinner) followed by the addition of an H₂RA (ranitidine 300 mg qhs) at bedtime for 28 days. Patients were studied with prolonged ambulatory pH monitoring after 2 weeks of omeprazole bid followed by pH testing after days 1, 7, and 28 of continuous H₂RAs at bedtime.

The median time that pH was <4 for the supine period was similar for GERD patients and normal volunteers. Four

TABLE 25.6. HIERARCHY OF INTRAGASTRIC PH CONTROL

PPI once a day
PPI plus H₂ HS (OTC probably acceptable)[a]
PPI bid[a]
PPI bid plus H₂ HS[a]

[a]These regimens have never been tested head to head in clinical trials.
bid, twice daily; HS, *hora somni* (at bedtime); OTC, over the counter; PPI, proton pump inhibitor.

general patterns of gastric pH response were found. The first subgroup experienced the decreasing effect of H2RA over time (tolerance). A second subgroup (21% of 43 subjects) exhibited a sustained response to H2RA therapy (no tolerance). A third subgroup consisted of three healthy subjects had no NAB on the twice-daily PPI regime, and NAB did not develop when H2RA was added. All three in this group were *H. pylori* positive. The fourth subgroup was marked by an unpredictable response (26% of 43 subjects). This group showed variable outcomes at different time points in the study.

Katz et al. (87) reviewed prolonged ambulatory pH monitoring studies in GERD patients. Group 1 (n=60) took either 20 mg of omeprazole or 30 mg of lansoprazole twice a day. Group 2 (n=45) received a PPI twice a day (omeprazole 20 mg or lansoprazole 30 mg) plus an H2 blocker at bedtime (ranitidine 300 mg, famotidine 40 mg, or nizatidine 300 mg) for >28 days. Group 3 (n=11) patients were evaluated for response to both regimens. The authors evaluated percent time that nocturnal and daytime intragastric pH was >4 and percent of patients with NAB for all groups.

Overall, 27% of patients spent 100% of the recumbent period with intragastric pH>4, and 32% spent >90% of the recumbent period with pH>4. Ten percent spent >50% of the night with pH<4. In contrast, 50% of patients on PPI bid experienced a pH<4 over 50% of the recumbent period; 20% experienced pH>4 during more than 90% of the recumbent period (p<0.001). For patients tested on both regimens (n=11), the median percentage time that intragastric pH was >4 overnight increased from 54.6% without H2RA to 96.5% with H2RA (*p*=0.001).

These two studies (86,87) come to different conclusions. In Fackler et al. (86), there is essentially no overall sustained control of intragastric pH over time with the addition of an H2RA (i.e., tolerance develops). In Katz et al. (87), there is a substantial benefit to the long-term use of these agents at bedtime. However, these differences do not appear to be dramatic upon close examination. In Fackler et al. (86), 21% had a sustained response, with elimination of NAB, which is remarkably similar to the 27% in Katz et al. (87). The absence of a statistical improvement in the Fackler et al. (86) study (*p*=0.06 at 1 week, *p*=0.08 at 1 month) may represent a type II error. Both studies identify a substantial number of patients who do have a sustained effect and many who do not. The studies agree that achieving total acid control (100% of the time that intragastric pH>4) is extremely difficult to achieve with modern pharmacology. Whether the newest PPI, esomeprazole, at 40 mg twice daily, will make this control possible awaits further study. Fortunately, this high degree of pharmacologic control is rarely necessary. Overall, it is fair to say that tolerance to H2RAs at bedtime in addition to a PPI twice a day is real but rel-

ative, and that a sustained response may be seen in a large number of patients. The studies underscore the importance of prolonged ambulatory pH monitoring as a means of documenting this acid control regimen, and the need to avoid using H2RA at bedtime in difficult-to-treat patients.

SELECTED CLINICAL SITUATIONS

Nonerosive GERD (Symptomatic GERD with Normal Upper Endoscopy)

Patients with GERD and normal endoscopy have been believed to have less severe disease than patients with erosive esophagitis. However, clinical trials have suggested an interesting paradox: patients with GERD and a normal endoscopy may not respond as well. Lind et al. (88) compared 10- and 20-mg doses of omeprazole with a placebo in 509 patients with symptoms and normal endoscopy. After 4 weeks of therapy, only 46% of patients on the 20-mg dose reported the complete absence of heartburn. Although superior to the placebo (13% with complete relief), this complete relief is inferior to that seen in erosive esophagitis trials. Bate et al. (89) found similar results in 209 patients comparing 20 mg of omeprazole to placebo. After 4 weeks, 57% were heartburn free and 43% completely asymptomatic (including no regurgitation), and thus superior to the placebo; however, once again these results represent a decrease in efficacy compared to standard erosive esophagitis trials. A study by Carlsson et al. (90) highlights this seeming paradox. The authors conducted a 4-week comparison of the efficacy of omeprazole in 277 patients with, and 261 patients without, erosive esophagitis. A 20-mg dose of omeprazole achieved complete symptom relief in 48% of those with erosions compared to only 29% of those without. While the outcome differences in these studies cannot be easily explained, the study by Lind et al. (88) suggested that patients with an abnormal pH monitoring study were more likely to respond to omeprazole than those with a normal pH. This underscores the difficulty in determining the etiology of symptoms in patients with so-called nonerosive GERD.

Unexplained Chest Pain (Noncardiac Chest Pain)

It is very clear from a large body of research that many patients with unexplained chest pain in whom cardiac disease has been ruled out will have GERD as the proximate cause of their symptoms. When attempting to treat these and other patients with extraesophageal disease, the clinician should keep in mind that for the most part these patients require more aggressive antisecretory therapy for longer periods of time than the typical patient for heartburn. There are few well-designed studies in this patient population, and all are short term. Therefore, long-term treatment of these patients, which is usually required, is based on extrapolation of data from maintenance trials of heartburn and erosive esophagitis.

Pharmacologic therapy for GERD-related chest pain begins with a PPI. The only randomized, double-blind, placebo-controlled treatment trial with PPIs compared omeprazole to placebo in 36 patients with noncardiac chest pain and GERD documented by 24-hour ambulatory pH testing (91). Patients were treated with 20 mg of omeprazole twice daily or a placebo for 8 weeks and kept a daily diary of chest pain frequency and severity. Omeprazole produced a significant decrease in the fraction of chest pain days (39% ±7.2% vs. 10% ±6.9%, p=0.006) and pain severity (40.7 ±8.1 vs. 14.8 ±8.2, p=0.03). Fifteen of 18 (81%) patients receiving omeprazole reported symptomatic improvement, in contrast to only one of 18 (6%) in the placebo group.

A trial of antireflux therapy with a PPI is often recommended as initial therapy for suspected GERD. A recently published randomized, double-blind, placebo-controlled trial evaluated 1 week of high-dose omeprazole as a diagnostic test for GERD in 37 patients with noncardiac chest pain (92). All patients had chest pain at least 3 times a week. Endoscopy and 24-hour ambulatory esophageal pH monitoring were performed in all, and a daily diary of the frequency and severity of chest pain was maintained. Patients were randomly assigned to receive either the placebo or omeprazole (40 mg in the morning and 20 mg in the evening) for 7 days with a crossover to the other arm after a 2-week washout period and repeat baseline symptom assessment. Twenty-three patients (62.2%) were GERD positive and 14 GERD negative, based on the presence of erosive esophagitis or abnormal 24-hour pH monitoring.

The so-called "omeprazole test" was diagnostic of GERD if chest pain scores improved >50% after treatment. Eighteen GERD-positive patients (78%), and two GERD-negative patients (14%) had positive test results, yielding a sensitivity of 78.3% (95% CI [confidence interval], 61.4 to 95.1) and specificity of 85.7% (95% CI, 67.4 to 100), compared with endoscopy and ambulatory pH monitoring for the diagnosis of GERD. Subsequent economic analysis has estimated that this approach would save $573 per patient with chest pain, if a full workshop, including endoscopy, esophageal manometry, and 24-hour ambulatory pH monitoring is done in every patient.

This study supports the clinical experience that a therapeutic trial is effective if properly selected patients are treated. In the more typical patient with less-frequent pain (often less than once a week), this short pharmacologic trial may not be sufficient to evaluate improvement. Treatment after the "omeprazole test" can be a dilemma. How should treatment be continued? Thus, this approach seems most useful for patients with frequent pain. In general, a 4- to 8-week trial of therapy seems more practical.

Extraesophageal Disease

There have been few clinical trials of treatment involving patients with extraesophageal manifestations of GERD, specifically asthma, cough, and voice changes. Most are uncontrolled and do not address long-term maintenance. Treatment is based on the principles advocated for treating patients with heartburn and erosive esophagitis, and observations derive from available clinical trials and clinical experience. While relief of symptoms, healing of mucosal injury, and maintenance of remission remain the primary goals, assessing these endpoints is somewhat more difficult as the "gold standard" for diagnosis is not always clear.

Only one study examined the effect of lifestyle modifications, including raising the head of the bed 6 inches, eliminating meals before bedtime, and using antacids in the treatment of patients with respiratory symptoms and GERD. Outcomes were compared to using no antireflux measures for 2-month periods. In this study, both esophageal and respiratory symptoms improved; however, there were no objective changes noted in pulmonary function (93). This suggests that the addition of the conservative measures outlined in Table 25.1 may be useful in management, especially for patients with postprandial reflux (94).

There are several trials using H$_2$RAs to treat patients with supraesophageal GERD, all in patients with asthma or chronic cough. Larrain et al. (95) randomized patients with mild GERD and abnormal pH studies to placebo, cimetidine at 300 mg four times a day, or antireflux surgery in a 6-month treatment trial. Pulmonary and esophageal symptoms were improved in the cimetidine and surgery group compared to the placebo. This study was the first to show that the clinical response was slower than that seen in patients with heartburn, with many patients achieving optimal response only after 4 to 6 months of therapy (95). Several other short-term studies using H$_2$RAs in doses from 150 mg of ranitidine at bedtime and up to 150 mg three times a day for periods of 1 to 8 weeks have consistently demonstrated improvement in heartburn, but limited improvement in objective changes of pulmonary function and symptoms (96–98). A clear history of reflux-associated asthma appears to be the only predictive factor for improvement in respiratory symptoms. Clinical experience confirms these findings.

Cimetidine has been used successfully in unblinded and uncontrolled trials of patients with chronic cough associated with GER. Improvement of cough has been reported in 70% to 100% of patients (99–102). Time to symptom improvement appears quite prolonged, usually about 161 to 179 days. Despite reports of clinical improvement, no correlation between symptom response and reduction in esophageal acid exposure by poststudy prolonged pH monitoring was observed. With the availability of PPIs and their superior gastric acid control, we now use H$_2$ blockers only in patients who are unable to tolerate these agents (see below). If they are to be used, we believe that high-dose therapy is required, that is, at least the equivalent of ranitidine 150 mg qid.

Improvement of cough in children was seen in two uncontrolled studies of prokinetic agents alone or in combination therapy with H$_2$RAs. Other uncontrolled studies in children have shown efficacy in apnea (103,104).

A recent preliminary report by Khoury et al. (105) compared cisapride at 10 mg four times a day with the placebo. This double-blind controlled trial of 16 adult patients with pulmonary symptoms and abnormal GER by ambulatory pH monitoring, showed significant improvement in FEV1 and FVC in patients on cisapride compared to the placebo. However, no change in esophageal acid exposure by ambulatory pH monitoring nor esophageal symptoms was seen in this small group of patients.

Several clinical trials have been conducted using PPIs in patients with asthma and laryngitis. One trial of omeprazole at 20 mg once a day for 4 weeks (106), and another at 20 mg twice daily for 6 weeks (107), showed an improvement in pulmonary function tests on omeprazole compared to the placebo. Little change in bronchodilator use or asthma scores was demonstrated. The latter study (107), in which 20 mg omeprazole twice daily was studied, found that 6 of 11 patients who failed to improve on omeprazole also did not heal their esophagitis. This suggests that acid suppression was inadequate in these patients. The patients who had control of their asthma also had healed their esophagitis, reinforcing the fact that adequate acid control is required to decrease pulmonary symptoms. A randomized double-blind controlled trial by Boree et al. (108) in 36 patients, comparing omeprazole at 40 mg twice daily to the placebo for 3 months, showed a reduction in nocturnal cough during treatment with omeprazole. Objective changes in FEV$_1$ and other pulmonary function tests could not be demonstrated.

Important insights into treatment of patients with supraesophageal GERD can be gleaned from a well-designed study by Harding et al. (109) in which 30 patients with documented asthma and GER proven by prolonged pH monitoring were treated with increasing doses of omeprazole. Starting at 20 mg/day, the medication was increased by 20 mg after each 4-week treatment period for 3 months, or until esophageal acid exposure was reduced to "normal." Normalization of esophageal acid exposure resulted in improvement in pulmonary symptoms in 70% of patients. Several observations emerged from this trial: eight patients (28%) needed >20 mg/day of omeprazole to normalize esophageal acid exposure; many patients required the entire 3-month period of treatment to achieve optimal symptom relief, with improvement progressing continu-

ously over the 3-month period, confirming the observations of Larrain et al. (95); and a favorable response to omeprazole was seen in patients who presented with frequent regurgitation (more than once a week) and those with abnormal proximal acid exposure demonstrated by ambulatory pH monitoring. This study emphasizes the importance of adequate esophageal acid control to achieve improvement in patients with extraesophageal symptoms. Additional studies are needed to determine the optimal reduction in esophageal exposure required for successful treatment, as simple "normalization" of acid control may not be sufficient. Complete elimination of esophageal acid exposure may be needed in patients with supraesophageal disease to obtain adequate symptom control.

Kamal et al. (110) evaluated 16 patients with posterior laryngitis with omeprazole at 40 mg/day. Laryngeal and esophageal symptom scores improved significantly at the end of 6 weeks, but relapsed within 6 weeks after therapy was stopped. Poorer response was seen in patients with abnormal proximal esophageal acid exposure on ambulatory pH monitoring.

Hanson et al. (111) studied 182 patients with posterior laryngitis and at least one of the following symptoms: post nasal drip, persistent or recurrent sore throat, or cough or hoarseness. Patients were treated sequentially with conservative lifestyle modifications for an initial period of 6 to 12 weeks followed by famotidine at 20 mg at bedtime for 6 weeks. Omeprazole 20 mg at bedtime was given to non-responders. Omeprazole was then increased in 20 mg increments every 6 weeks until 80 mg a day was reached. Laryngitis was characterized as mild if posterior laryngeal erythema was seen; moderate if marked erythema, secretions, and mucosal granularity were present; and severe if ulceration, granulation tissue, or hyperkeratosis were seen. Patients with mild symptoms and minimal laryngeal changes responded to conservative measures or famotidine, while patients with severe laryngitis required PPIs. These studies emphasize variability in response of patients with this manifestation of GERD, the need to treat for longer periods before seeing a response when disease is severe, the need for higher doses of PPIs, and the rapid relapse of symptoms when therapy is discontinued, emphasizing that long-term treatment is often needed in these patients.

A recent study by El-Serag et al. (112) compared lansoprazole at 30 mg twice daily with a placebo for 3 months in 20 patients with posterior laryngitis, abnormal laryngeal examination, and abnormal pH monitoring study. Complete relief of symptoms was seen in 50% in the PPI arm compared to 10% in the placebo arm ($p<0.05$). Unfortunately, there were no predictive factors, either in laryngeal examination or on pH monitoring for improvement. These data provide the "best" evidence for the efficacy of gastric acid suppression in treatment of chronic laryngitis. More trials are clearly needed.

SUMMARY

The optimal treatment for patients with unexplained chest pain and other extraesophageal manifestations of GERD is not clear. Clinical experience suggests that a majority of these patients will respond to a twice-daily dosage of a PPI for 8 to 16 weeks. A suggested approach is to begin empirical therapy with twice daily PPI before breakfast and dinner for 2 to 3 months. If patients do not respond to a trial of antireflux therapy, an evaluation with prolonged ambulatory pH monitoring performed with dual esophageal and gastric pH electrodes while continuing therapy is the procedure of choice (113). This allows assessment of pH control and symptom correlation. In the event that pH control is incomplete—especially when overnight (79) esophageal acid exposure continues (81), and/or symptoms continue in association with continued reflux—higher-dose PPI therapy, or a combination of twice daily PPI plus an H₂RA at bedtime can be considered (79,114). Patients without heartburn or regurgitation (or other symptoms to suggest GERD) should be evaluated earlier with pH monitoring. Patients successfully treated with acid suppression should be considered for long-term maintenance with PPI therapy, although no study has specifically addressed this issue.

GERD in Pregnancy

The frequency of GERD symptoms in pregnant woman varies, with some estimating a prevalence of approximately 66% with others ranging from 45% to 80% (115). Management of the pregnant patient with GERD presents a clinical challenge because of lack of data on the efficacy of traditional medical therapy and concerns about the risk of diagnostic studies. In general, endoscopy in the third trimester is safe, although should rarely be needed. The treatment approach most often recommended is to begin with lifestyle and dietary modifications as the first step using antacids alone or in combination with alginic acid for symptom relief. If this is not sufficient, sucralfate, a mucosal protectant with little or no systemic absorption, may be considered as a second-line agent. In fact, when this agent was given in doses of 1 gm four times a day, greater relief of heartburn (90% vs. 30%) and regurgitation (83% vs. 27%) compared to lifestyle and dietary modifications alone was demonstrated in one randomized study of 66 pregnant patients (115). The clinician should be aware that this agent has been associated with the development of constipation, an important potential problem in pregnancy. The H₂RAs have been designated as Food and Drug Administration pregnancy class B (with exception of nizatidine, which is classified as C because of animal studies demonstrating spontaneous abortions and low fetal birth weight) and can be considered in patients with severe persistent symptoms despite the above interventions. Omeprazole, although designated as class C, has been administered to

women immediately prior to labor and during elective C section without complication, cannot be routinely recommended in pregnancy. The other PPIs—lansoprazole, rabeprazole, pantoprazole, and esomeprazole—have been demonstrated as class B, but have not been tested in clinical trials. Overall, the pharmacologic approach to the pregnant patient with GERD must be individualized and undertaken with care. Fortunately, the condition is temporary and the symptoms often are transient. Major complications are extremely unusual.

REFERENCES

1. Johnson LF, DeMeester TR. Evaluation of the head of the bed, bethanechol, and antacid foam tablets on gastroesophageal reflux. *Dig Dis Sci* 1980;26:673.
2. Stanciu C, Bennett JR. Effects of posture on gastro-oesophageal reflux. *Digestion* 1977;15:104.
3. Khoury RM, Camacho-Lobato LC, Katz PO, et al. Influence of spontaneous sleep positions on nighttime recumbent reflux in patients with gastroesophageal reflux disease. *Am J Gastroenterol* 1999;94:2069–2073.
4. Kapur KC, Trudgill NJ, Riley SA. Mechanism of gastrosophageal reflux in the lateral decubitus position. *Neurogastroenterol Motil* 1998;10:517.
5. Katz LC, Just R, Castell DO. Body position affects recumbent postprandial reflux. *J Clin Gastroenterol* 1994;18:280.
6. VanHerwaarden M, Katzka D, Smout AJPM, et al. Effect of different recumbent positions on postprandial reflux in normal subjects. *Am J Gastroenterol* 2000;95:2731.
7. McArthur K, Hogan D, Isenberg JI. Relative stimulatory effects of commonly ingested beverages on gastric acid secretion in humans. *Gastroenterology* 1982;83:199.
8. Babka JC, Castell DO. On the genesis of heartburn: the effects of specific foods on the lower esophagus sphincter. *Dig Dis* 1973;18:391.
9. Castell DO. Diet and the lower esophageal sphincter. *Am J Clin Nutr* 1975;28:1296.
10. Chernow B, Castell DO. Diet and heartburn. *JAMA* 1979;241:2307.
11. Nebel OT, Castell DO. Lower esophageal sphincter pressure changes after food ingestion. *Gastroenterology* 1972;63:778.
12. Pehl C, Pfeiffer A, Wendl B, et al. The effect of decaffeination of coffee on gastro-esophageal reflux in patients with reflux disease. *Aliment Pharmacol Ther* 1997;11:483.
13. Becker DJ, Sinclair J, Castell DO, et al. A comparison of high and low fat meals on postprandial esophageal acid exposure. *Am J Gastroenterol* 1989;84:782.
14. Nebel OT, Castell DO. Lower esophageal sphincter pressure changes after food ingestion. *Gastroenterology* 1972;63:778.
15. Wright LE, Castell DO. Adverse effect of chocolate on lower esophageal sphincter pressure. *Dig Dis Sci* 1975;20:703.
16. Murphy DW, Castell DO. Chocolate and heartburn: evidence of increased esophageal acid exposure after chocolate ingestion. *Am J Gastroenterol* 1988;83:633.
17. Kjellin A, Ramel S, Rossner S, et al. Gastroesophageal reflux in obese patients is not reduced by weight reduction. *Scand J Gastroenterol* 1996;31:1047.
18. Chow WH, Blot WJ, Vaughan TL, et al. Body mass index and risk of adenocarcinoma of the esophagus and gastric cardia. *J Natl Cancer Inst* 1998;90:150.
19. Perez AR, Moncure AC, Rattner DW. Obesity adversely affects

the outcome of antireflux operations. *Surg Endosc* 2001;15: 986.

20. Vitale GC, Cheadle WG, Patel B, et al. The effect of alcohol on nocturnal gastroesophageal reflux. *JAMA* 1987;258:2077.

21. Pehl C, Pfeiffer A, Wendle B, et al. Different effects of white and red wine on lower esophageal sphincter pressure and gastroesophageal reflux disease. *Scand J Gastroenterol* 1998;33: 118.

22. Meining A, Classen M. The role of diet and lifestyle measures in the pathogenesis and treatment of gastroesophageal reflux disease. *Am J Gastroenterol* 2000;95:2692.

23. Kitchin LI, Castell DO. Rationale and efficacy of conservative therapy for gastroesophageal reflux disease. *Arch Intern Med* 1991;151:448.

24. DeVault KR, Castell DO. Updated guidelines for the diagnosis and treatment of gastroesophageal reflux disease. *Am J Gastroenterol* 1999;94:1434–1442.

25. Tytgat GNJ, Nio CY. The medical therapy of reflux oesophagitis. *Bailleres Clin Gastroenterol* 1987;1:791.

26. Klinkenberg-Knol EC, Festen HPM, et al. Pharmacologic management of gastro-oesophageal reflux disease. *Drugs* 1995;49: 695–710.

27. Furman D, Mensh R, Winan G, et al. A double-blind trial comparing high dose liquid antacid to placebo and cimetidine in improving symptoms and objective parameters in gastroesophageal reflux. *Gastroenterology* 1992;82:A1062.

28. Eslborg L, Beck B, Stubgaard M. Effect of sucralfate on gastroesophageal reflux in esophagitis. *Hepatogastroenterology* 1985;32: 181.

29. Katz PO, Castell DO. Gastroesophageal reflux disease during pregnancy. *Gastroenterol Clin* 1998;27:153.

30. Simon B, Mueller P. Comparison of the effect of sucralfate and ranitidine in reflux esophagitis. *Am J Med* 1987;83:43.

31. Hameeteman W, van de Boomgaard DM, Dekker W, et al. Sucralfate versus cimetidine in reflux esophagitis: single blind multicenter study. *J Clin Gastroenterol* 1987;9:390-394.

32. Barone JA, Jessen LM, Colaizzi JL, et al. Cisapride: a gastrointestinal prokinetic drug. *Ann Pharmacother* 1994;28:488.

33. McCallum RW, Ippoliti AF, Cooner C, et al. A controlled trial of metoclopramide in symptomatic gastroesophageal reflux. *N Engl J Med* 1977;296:354.

34. Bright-Asare P, El-Bassoussi M. Cimetidine, metoclopramide or placebo in the treatment of symptomatic gastroesophageal reflux. *J Clin Gastroenterol* 1980;2:149.

35. Temple JG, Bradby GVH, O'Connor F, et al. Cimetidine and metoclopramide in esophageal reflux disease. *BMJ* 1983;286: 1863.

36. Paull A, Grant AK. A controlled trial of metoclopramide in reflux esophagitis. *Med J Aust* 1974;2:627.

37. Venables CW, Bell D, Eccleston D. A double-blind study of metoclopramide in symptomatic peptic esophagitis. *Postgrad Med J* 1973;49(suppl 4)73.

38. Ramirez B, Richter JE. Review article: promotility drugs in the treatment of gastro-oesophageal reflux disease. *Aliment Pharmacol Ther* 1993;7:5–20.

39. Blackwell JN, Heading RC, Fettes MR. Effects of domperidone on lower oesophageal sphincter pressure and gastro-oesophageal reflux in patients with peptic esophagitis. Progress with domperidone. *International Congress and Symposium Series,* vol. 36. London: Royal Society of Medicine Press, 1981:57.

40. Kahrilas PJ, Quigley EM, Castell DO, et al. The partial 5HT4 agonist HTC 919 reduced acid reflux parameters in patients with GERD. *Gastroenterology* 1999;116:G0881.

41. Richter JE, Sabesin SM, Kogut DG, et al. Omeprazole versus ranitidine or ranitidine/metoclopramide in poorly responsive symptomatic gastroesophageal reflux disease. *Am J Gastroenterol* 1996;91:1766.

42. Vignieri S, Termini R, Leandro G, et al. A comparison of five maintenance therapies for reflux esophagitis. *N Engl J Med* 1995; 333:1106.

43. Bell NJV, Burget DL, Howden CW, et al. Appropriate acid suppression for the management of gastro-esophageal reflux disease. *Digestion* 1992;51(suppl 1):59.

44. Jones DB, Howden CW, Burget DW, et al. Acid suppression in duodenal ulcer: a meta-analysis to define optimal dosing with antisecretory drugs. *Gut* 1987;28:1120.

45. DeVault KR, Castell DO. Guidelines for the diagnosis and treatment of gastroesophageal reflux disease. *Arch Intern Med* 1995;155:2165–2173.

46. Bell NJV, Hunt RH. Role of gastric acid suppression in the treatment of gastro-oesophageal reflux disease. *Gut* 1992;33: 118.

47. Cloud ML, Offen WW. Nizatidine versus placebo in gastroesophageal reflux disease: a six-week, multicenter, randomized, double-blind comparison. *Dig Dis Sci* 1992;37:865.

48. McCarty-Dawson D, Sue So, Morrill B, et al. Ranitidine versus cimetidine in the healing of erosive esophagitis. *Clin Ther* 1996; 18:1150.

49. Roufail W, Belsito A, Robinson M, et al. Ranitidine for erosive esophagitis: a double-blind, placebo controlled study. *Aliment Pharmacol Ther* 1992;6:597.

50. Simon TJ, Roberts WG, Berlin RG, et al. Acid suppression by famotidine 20 mg twice daily or 40 mg twice daily in preventing relapse of endoscopic recurrence of erosive esophagitis. *Clin Ther* 1995;17:1147.

51. Wesdorp ICE, Dekker W, Festen HPM. Efficacy of famotidine 20 mg twice a day versus 40 mg twice a day in the treatment of erosive or ulcerative reflux esophagitis. *Dig Dis Sci* 1993;38: 2287.

52. Euler AR, Murdock RH Jr, Wilson TH, et al. Ranitidine is effective therapy for erosive esophagitis. *Am J Gastroenterol* 1993;88:520.

53. Hallerback B, Glise H, Johansson B, et al. Gastroesophageal reflux symptoms: clinical findings and effect of ranitidine treatment. *Eur J Surg Suppl* 1998;583:6.

54. Vignieri S, Termini R, Leandor G, et al. A comparison of five maintenance therapies for reflux esophagitis. *N Engl J Med* 1995;333:1106–1110.

55. Feldman M, Burton ME. Histamine2-receptor antagonists: standard therapy for acid-peptic diseases. *N Engl J Med* 1990; 323:1672.

56. Lipsy RJ, Fennerty B, Fagan TC. Clinical review of histamine2 receptor antagonists. *Arch Intern Med* 1990;150:745.

57. Robinson M. Review article: current perspectives on hypergastrinemia and enterochromaffin-like-cell hyperplasia. *Aliment Pharmacol Ther* 1999;13(suppl 5):5.

58. Massoomi F, Savage J, Destache CJ. Omeprazole: a comprehensive review. *Pharmacotherapy* 1993;13:46.

59. Lew EA. Review article: pharmacokinetic concerns in the selection of anti-ulcer therapy. *Aliment Pharmacol Ther* 1999:13 (suppl 5):11.

60. Wolfe MM, Sachs G. Acid suppression: optimizing therapy for gastroduodenal ulcer healing, gastroesophageal reflux disease, and stress-related erosive syndrome. *Gastroenterology* 2000;118 (suppl):9.

61. Chiba N, De Gara CJ, Wilkonson JM, et al. Speed of healing and symptom relief in grade II to IV gastroesophageal reflux disease: a meta-analysis. *Gastroenterology* 1997;112:1798.

62. Castell DO, Richter JE, Robinson M, et al. Efficacy and safety of lansoprazole in the treatment of erosive esophagitis. *Am J Gastroenterol* 1996;91:1749–1758.

63. Richter JE, Kahrilas PJ, Johanson J, et al. Efficacy and safety of esomeprazole compared with omeprazole in GERD patients with erosive esophagitis: a randomized controlled study. *Am J Gastroenterol* 2001;96:656.

64. Dekkers CPM, Beker JA, Thjodleifsson B, et al. Double-blind, placebo-controlled comparison of rabeprazole 20 mg vs. omeprazole 20 mg in the treatment of erosive or ulcerative gastro-oesophageal reflux disease. *Aliment Pharmacol Ther* 1999;13:49.

65. Castell DO, Kahrilas PJ, Richter JE, et al. Esomeprazole (40 mg) compared with lansoprazole (30 mg) in the treatment of erosive esophagitis. *Am J Gastroenterol* 2002;97:575.

66. Mossner J, Holscher Ah, Herz R, et al. A double-blind study of pantoprazole and omeprazole in the treatment of reflux oesophagitis: a multicentre trial. *Aliment Pharmacol Ther* 1995; 9:321.

67. Kahrilas PJ, Fennerty MB, Joelsson B. High versus standard dose ranitidine for control of heartburn in poorly responsive acid reflux disease: a prospective, controlled trial. *Am J Gastroenterol* 1999;94:92–97.

68. Harris RA, Kuppermann M, Richter JE. Prevention of recurrences of erosive reflux esophagitis: a cost effectiveness analysis of maintenance proton pump inhibition. *Am J Med* 1997;102: 78–88.

69. Ladas SD, Tassios PS, Raptis SA. Selection of patients for successful maintenance treatment of esophagitis with low dose omeprazole: use of 24-hour gastric pH monitoring. *Am J Gastroenterol* 2000;95:374–380.

70. Lundell LR, Dent J, Bennett JR, et al. Endoscopic assessment of oesophagitis: clinical and functional correlates and further validation of the Los Angeles classification. *Gut* 1999;45:172.

71. Sontag SJ, Hirschowitz BJ, Holt S, et al. Two doses of omeprazole versus placebo in symptomatic erosive esophagitis: the US multicenter study. *Gastroenterology* 1992;102:109.

72. Klinkenberg-Knol EC, Nelis F, Dent J, et al. Long-term omeprazole treatment in resistant gastroesophageal reflux disease: efficacy, safety, and influence on gastric mucosa. *Gastroenterology* 2000;118:661.

73. Hatlebakk JG, Katz PO, Castell DO. Proton pump inhibitors: better acid suppression when taken before a meal than without a meal. *Aliment Pharmacol Ther* 2000;14:1267–1272.

74. Kuo B, Castell DO. Optimal dosing of omeprazole 40 mg daily: Effects on gastric and esophageal pH and serum gastrin in healthy controls. *Am J Gastroenterol* 1996;91:1532–1538.

75. Hatlebakk JG, Katz PO, Kuo B, et al. Nocturnal gastric acidity and acid breakthrough on different regimens of omeprazole 40 mg daily. *Aliment Pharmacol Ther* 1998;12:1235–1240.

76. Katz PO, Hatlebakk JG, Castell DO. Gastric acidity and acid breakthrough with twice daily omeprazole or lansoprazole. *Aliment Pharmacol Ther* 2000;14:709.

77. Howden CW, Henning JM, Huang B, et al. Management of heartburn in a large, randomized, community-based study: Comparison of four therapeutic strategies. *Am J Gastroenterol* 2001;96:1704. Erratum in: *Am J Gastroenterol* 2001 Sep;96: 2809.

78. Inadomi JM, Jamal R, Murata GH, et al. Step-down management of gastroesophageal reflux disease. *Gastroenterology* 2001; 121:1095.

79. Peghini PL, Katz PO, Bracy NA, et al. Nocturnal recovery of gastric acid secretion with twice-daily dosing of proton pump inhibitors. *Am J Gastroenterol* 1998;93:763.

80. Tutuian R, Katz PO, Castell DO. A PPI is a PPI is a PPI: Lessons from prolonged intragastric pH monitoring. *Gastroenterology* 2000;118:A17.

81. Katz PO, Anderson C, Khoury R, et al. Gastro-oesophageal reflux associated with nocturnal gastric acid breakthrough on proton pump inhibitors. *Aliment Pharmacol Ther* 1998;12: 1231–1234.

82. Katz P, Castell DO, Chen Y, et al. Esomeprazole 40 mg twice daily maintains intragastric pH > 4 more than 80% of a 24-hour time period. *Am J Gastroenterol* 2002;97:520.

83. Hatlebakk J, Katz PO, Castell DO. Medical therapy: management of the refractory patient. *Gastroenterol Clin North Am* 1999;28:847.

84. Fass R, Sampliner RE, Malagon IB, et al. Failure of acid control in candidates for Barrett's oesophagus reversal on a very high dose of proton pump inhibitor. *Aliment Pharmacol Ther* 2000; 14:597.

85. Leite LP, Johnston BT, Barrett J, et al. Persistent acid secretion during omeprazole therapy: A study of gastric acid profiles in patients demonstrating failure of omeprazole therapy. *Am J Gastroenterol* 1996;91:1527.

86. Fackler WK, Ours Tm, Vaezi MF, et al. Long-term effect of H2RA therapy on nocturnal gastric acid breakthrough. *Gastroenterology* 2002;122:625.

87. Katz PO, Xue S, Castell DO. Control of intragastric pH with omeprazole 20 mg, omeprazole 40 mg and lansoprazole 30 mg. *Aliment Pharmacol Ther* 2001;15:647–652.

88. Lind T, Havelund T, Carlsson O, et al. Heartburn without oesophagitis: Efficacy of omeprazole therapy and features determining therapeutic response. *Scand J Gastroenterol* 1997;32:974.

89. Bate CM, Griffin SM, Keeling PWN, et al. Reflux symptom relief with omeprazole in patients without unequivocal oesophagitis. *Aliment Pharmacol Ther* 1996;10:547.

90. Carlsson R, Dent J, Watts R, et al. Gastro-oesophageal reflux disease in primary care: An international study of different treatment strategies with omeprazole. *Eur J Gastroenterol Hepatol* 1998;10:119.

91. Achem SR, Kolts BE, MacMath T, et al. Effects of omeprazole versus placebo in treatment of noncardiac chest pain and gastroesophageal reflux. *Am J Gastroenterol* 1997;42:2138.

92. Fass R, Fennerty MB, Ofman JJ, et al. The clinical and economic value of a short course of omeprazole in patients with non-cardiac chest pain. *Gastroenterology* 1998;115:42.

93. Kjellin G, Tibbling L, Wranne B. Effect of conservative treatment of oesophageal dysfunction in bronchial asthma. *Eur J Respir Dis* 1981;62:190.

94. Katz PO. Ambulatory esophageal and hypopharyngeal pH monitoring in patients with hoarseness. *Am J Gastroenterol* 1990;85:38.

95. Larrain A, Carrasco E, Galleguillos F, et al. Medical and surgical treatment of non-allergic asthma associated with gastroesophageal reflux. *Chest* 1991;99:1330.

96. Harper PC, Bergner A, Kaye MD. Antireflux treatment for asthma: improvement in patients with associated gastroesophageal reflux. *Arch Intern Med* 1987;147:56.

97. Ekstrom T, Lindgren BR, Tibbling L. Effects of ranitidine treatment on patients with asthma and a history of gastro-oesophageal reflux: a double blind crossover study. *Thorax* 1989;44:19.

98. Gustafsson PM, Kjellman N-IM, Tibbling L. A trial of ranitidine in asthmatic children and adolescents with or without pathological gastro-oesophageal reflux. *Eur Respir J* 1992;5:201.

99. Irwin RS, Curley FJ, French CL. Chronic cough: the spectrum and frequency of causes, key components of the diagnostic evaluation, and outcome of specific therapy. *Am Rev Respir Dis* 1990;141:640.

100. Irwin RS, Azwacki JK, Curley FJ, et al. Chronic cough as the sole presenting manifestation of gastroesophageal reflux. *Am Rev Respir Dis* 1989;140:1294–1300.

101. Fitzgerald JM, Allen CJ, Craven MA, et al. Chronic cough and gastro-esophageal reflux. *CMAJ* 1989;140:520–524.
102. Waring JP, Lacayo L, Hunter J, et al. Chronic cough and hoarseness in patients with severe gastroesophageal reflux disease. Diagnosis and response to therapy. *Dig Dis Sci* 1995;40:1093–1097.
103. Ekstrom T, Tibbling T. Esophageal acid perfusion, airway function and symptoms in asthmatic patients with marked bronchial hyperactivity. *Chest* 1989;96:995–998.
104. Smyrnios NA, Irwin RS, Curley FJ. Chronic cough with a history of excessive sputum production. *Chest* 1995;108:991–997.
105. Khoury R, Paoletti V, Cohn J, et al. Cisapride improves pulmonary function tests in patients with gastroesophageal (GE) reflux and chronic respiratory symptoms. *Gastroenterology* 1998:114:712.
106. Ford GA, Oliver PS, Prior JS, et al. Omeprazole in the treatment of asthmatics with nocturnal symptoms and gastroesophageal reflux: A placebo-controlled cross-over study. *Postgrad Med J* 1994;70:350–354.
107. Meier JH, McNally PR, Punja M, et al. Does omeprazole (Prilosec) improve respiratory function in asthmatics with gastroesophageal reflux? *Dig Dis Sci* 1994;39:2127–2133.
108. Boree MJ, et al. No effects of high dose omeprazole in patients with severe airway hypersecretion and asymptomatic GER. *Eur Respir J* 1998;11:1070–1074.
109. Harding SM, Richter JE, Guzzo MR, et al. Asthma and gastroesophageal reflux: acid suppression therapy improves asthma outcome. *Am J Med* 1996;100:395–405.
110. Kamal PL, Hanon D, Kahrilas PJ. Omeprazole for the treatment of posterior laryngitis. *Am J Med* 1994;96:321.
111. Hanson DG, Karnel PL, Kahrilas PJ. Outcomes of antireflux therapy for the treatment of chronic laryngitis. *Ann Otol Rhinol Laryngol* 1995;104:550–555.
112. El-Serag HB, Lee P, Buchner A, et al. Lansoprazole treatment of patients with chronic idiopathic laryngitis: a placebo-controlled trial. *Am J Gastroenterol* 2001;96:979.
113. Klinkenberg-Knol E, Meuwissen S. Combined gastric and oesophageal 24 hour monitoring in patients with reflux disease resistant to treatment with omeprazole. *Aliment Pharmacol Ther* 1990;4:485–495.
114. Peghini PL, Katz PO, Castell DO. Ranitidine controls nocturnal gastric acid breakthrough on omeprazole: a controlled study in normal subjects. *Gastroenterology* 1998;115:1335.
115. Katz PO, Castell DO. Gastroesophageal reflux disease during pregnancy. *Gastroenterol Clin North Am* 1998;27:153.

ENDOSCOPIC THERAPIES FOR GASTROESOPHAGEAL REFLUX DISEASE

GEORGE TRIADAFILOPOULOS

Gastroesophageal reflux disease (GERD) is a chronic esophageal condition that affects 7% of the adult population daily and compromises the quality of their life (1,2). Left untreated, GERD not only causes symptoms such as heartburn and acid regurgitation, but also causes complications such as esophagitis, esophageal ulceration, stricture formation, and Barrett's esophagus, a premalignant condition to esophageal adenocarcinoma (3). Medical and surgical therapy may achieve both symptom relief and healing of esophagitis (4,5).

Long-term medical therapy is generally safe and effective for symptom relief, healing of esophagitis, and maintenance of remission. The proton pump inhibitors (PPIs) are the primary agents in the pharmacologic therapy of GERD since their efficacy in healing and symptom control ranges from 80% to 95%, compared to the H_2 receptor antagonists (H_2RAs) that carry a response rate of 50% to 60% (6). However, these drugs need to be taken daily and they may fail to control regurgitation for 10% to 20% of patients. Further, the annual cost of PPI therapy ranges from $1,500 to $2,000.

Laparoscopic antireflux surgery, such as Nissen fundoplication, is an alternative to long-term medical therapy for GERD since it may also effectively lead to healing, symptom control, and maintenance of remission in >90% of cases with reduced perioperative and postoperative morbidity as compared to the open approach with laparotomy or thoracotomy (7). The procedure in experienced hands is safe but requires 1 day of hospitalization and 3 weeks of postoperative recovery with dietary modification and restriction of certain activities. However, the efficacy of Nissen fundoplication may wane over time, with up to 50% of patients requiring medications to control recurrent reflux symptoms 10 years following surgery. After surgery, new symptoms occur in 5% to 8% of patients and may include dysphagia, gas, bloating, increased flatus, and difficulty with belching or vomiting. The cost of surgery ranges from $7,000 to $15,000 (8,9).

The invasiveness and costs and risks of surgery, or, alternatively, the daily dependence on antisecretory drugs, their high cost, the need to escalate dosage over time, and the lack of complete symptom control in some patients, have created an interest in endoscopic therapy for GERD. Over the past 3 years, endoscopically assisted interventional techniques have emerged and have generated considerable interest among physicians and patients. These endoscopic interventions may be viewed as "bridge" therapy for GERD, since patients may still choose to be treated with antisecretory drugs or fundoplication if the endoscopic therapy does not provide symptom relief or if symptoms later recur. These endoscopic therapies include radio-frequency (RF) thermal energy delivery (Stretta), sewing or placation techniques (EndoCinch, Wilson-Cook, NDO plicator), and injection or implantable biopolymer therapies (Enteryx, Gatekeeper, Plexiglas). Since these therapies are under development, most initial studies address symptom relief in short-term follow-up studies performed in GERD patients with minimally compromised esophageal structure and function (Savary stage <III). The true merit of such therapies will be determined in long-term, sham-controlled studies, and with in-depth understanding of their mechanism(s) of action. In addition, cost-effectiveness analyses and postmarketing surveillance of long-term efficacy, tolerability, and complications will be necessary.

In this chapter, I review all endoscopic procedures that have been marketed or are being introduced as novel therapies for GERD. Since all are new, the information pre-

G. Triadafilopoulos: Medical Service, Palo Alto Veterans Affairs Health Care System, Palo Alto, California; and Department of Medicine, Division of Gastroenterology and Hepatology, Stanford University School of Medicine, Stanford, California.

sented may not yet have been published in peer-reviewed journals but it exists in abstract form. Although Stretta, EndoCinch, and the Wilson-Cook plicator are approved by the Food and Drug Administration (FDA), none of these therapies should be considered as routine for the treatment of GERD without careful assessment and consideration of their respective merits for an individual patient (10).

We sequentially review the principles, instrument design, and technical aspects of each procedure, mechanism(s) of action, safety and tolerability, and efficacy in reported preclinical animal and human clinical trials. We conclude by discussing current and future trends in the use of these endoscopic therapies for managing GERD. The various endoscopic techniques reviewed are listed in Table 26.1.

In general, these therapies should be considered for patients who respond well to PPIs but do not wish to take long-term medications, patients who respond partly to PPIs or have regurgitation that is not responsive to PPIs and do not wish to undergo surgery, patients who are afraid of possible long-term sequelae of PPI therapy, patients intolerant to PPIs, and, possibly, patients who have failed fundoplication for GERD. The role of these procedures in the management of extraesophageal manifestations of GERD is currently under evaluation. There is no evidence that these procedures prevent Barrett's esophagus or esophageal adenocarcinoma.

The best candidates for endoscopic therapies are those who have well-established GERD (Savary stages <III and without a hiatal hernia >3cm) documented by endoscopy, pH monitoring, and esophageal motility studies and have, at least in part, responded to PPIs. Other potential candidates, albeit less well studied, are those with PPI-responsive GERD despite normal 24-hour pH study (nonerosive reflux disease, NERD), and possibly patients with PPI-responsive, extraesophageal manifestations of GERD. Until further experience and data become available, the endoscopic procedures currently available are *not* appropriate for the late, complicated disease states of esophageal shortening or stricture; large, fixed hiatal hernia > 3cm in length; poor esophageal function; and persistent dysphagia.

TABLE 26.1. ENDOSCOPIC THERAPIES FOR GERD

- Radiofrequency energy application (Stretta)[a]
- Endoscopic luminal gastroplasty (EndoCinch, Wilson-Cook)[a]
- Biopolymer augmentation therapy (Enteryx)
- Expandable hydrogel prosthesis (Gatekeeper)
- Full thickness plicator (NDO)
- Plexiglass implantation (Plexiglas)
- Per oral Nissen fundoplication

[a]FDA approved.

TABLE 26.2. FEATURES OF AN IDEAL ENDOSCOPIC THERAPY FOR GERD

- Safe and effective
- Easily deliverable
- Durable (>12 months)
- Biologically inert (locally and at distance)
- Non-carcinogenic, non-immunogenic
- Non-biodegradable
- High retention at the site
- Elastic
- Capable of resisting mechanical strain
- Low cost

Adapted from Lehman G. Endoscopic and endoluminal techniques for control of gastro-esophageal reflux: Are they ready for widespread clinical application? *Gastrointest Endosc* 2001;52:808–11.

In the immediate future, many technique modifications will certainly improve the ease, safety, and efficacy profiles of all endoscopic therapies. However, efficacy comparisons and sham trials will be needed in order to show differences among these new endoscopic techniques in GERD management. Comparisons to surgery and long-term drug therapy will probably ensue. Safety and tolerability will continuously be assessed in postmarketing surveillance studies. Longer observations of patients already treated will address the durability of effect over periods >12 months. The general applicability in all GERD groups and their cost-effectiveness will be determined with the wider application and future technological advances. The features of an ideal endoluminal therapy for GERD are outlined in Table 26.2 (11).

At present, many questions about endoscopic therapies for GERD remain unanswered: How exactly do these procedures treat GERD? How well do they work? How safe are they? Who are the best candidates for it? How long do effects last? Can they be repeated? Can they be combined? Are they cost-effective? Answers to all these questions will become available with the increased and widespread utilization of these procedures and the design and execution of well-controlled, randomized clinical trials. Table 26.3 out-

TABLE 26.3. CURRENT AND FUTURE ISSUES IN THE ENDOSCOPIC MANAGEMENT OF GERD

- Emergence of many technologies of variable technical complexity
- Efficacy comparison
- Safety and tolerability issues
- Controlled (sham) trials
- Durability of effect
- Comparisons to surgery and drug therapy
- General applicability in all GERD groups
- Cost-effectiveness

lines current and future issues regarding the endoscopic management of GERD.

RADIOFREQUENCY ENERGY APPLICATION (STRETTA)

Device and Procedure

Radiofrequency (RF) energy has been used since 1921 for general surgical cutting, coagulation, and neural ablation. The most commonly used RF energy waveforms are 400 kHz to 1 MHz. In monopolar RF energy delivery, current flows between the active and return (ground) electrodes, thereby heating tissue due to inductive and frictional heating of water molecules. The Stretta procedure incorporates constant tissue temperature monitoring and automated modulation of RF power output to control tissue heating. A thermocouple (electrical thermometer) resides in the active electrode to provide temperature feedback. A target temperature is preselected (85°C) and power is automatically modulated to achieve, but not exceed, the prescribed temperature. Thermocouple-controlled RF delivery results in the propagation of a circumscribed thermal lesion. Collagen contraction occurs, reaching 65°C, which in turn results in tissue shrinkage. With more prolonged heating, the acute phase of wound healing ensues with influx of macrophages, neutrophils, and myofibroblasts. The wound volume is reduced over time as fibroblasts contract and collagen is deposited. The tensile strength of the wound increases over the first year as remodeling occurs and the collagen matrix aligns according to tissue force vectors.

Temperature-controlled RF energy is currently used for treating benign prostatic hypertrophy, liver tumors, aberrant myocardial conduction pathways, snoring and sleep apnea, and lax joint capsules (12–14). The mechanism of action depends on the specific pathophysiology. In the prostate, for example, both volumetric contraction and alpha-adrenergic fiber ablation occur after RF energy delivery. Conversely, in the treatment of joint capsule laxity, the mechanism of action is purely mechanical shrinkage and remodeling of the ligamentous collagen.

The commercially available Stretta system consists of an RF generator and single-use RF energy catheters (Fig. 26.1). The RF generator (Curon Control Module, Curon Medical, Inc., Sunnyvale, CA) delivers pure sine-wave energy (465 kHz and 2 to 5 watts per channel) (Fig. 26.1, left). There are four RF channels, one powering each needle electrode, a temperature feedback control system, and a peristaltic irrigation pump. The RF energy delivery catheter (Stretta catheter, Curon Medical, Inc., Sunnyvale, CA) is comprised of a soft, 6-mm shaft with a guide wire tip, a balloon-basket assembly that inflates to a maximum 3-cm diameter, and four electrode delivery sheaths positioned radially around the balloon, as well as suction and irrigation (Fig. 26.1, middle). The generator delivers RF in an automated fashion under temperature control using thermocouple monitoring while the power output is regulated by computer algorithm. Target tissue as well as mucosal temperature are achieved and maintained through a special suction and irrigation system. There is a curved, nickel-titanium needle electrode (25 gauge, 5.5-mm length) within each delivery sheath, each with a thermocouple at the tip and base of the needle (Fig. 26.1, right). When the catheter is positioned and the needles deployed into the circular muscle of the distal LES or cardia, RF energy is delivered to each electrode to achieve a temperature of 85°C in the muscle, while irrigation maintains mucosal temperature <50°C. The result is a thermal lesion in the muscle with intact overlying mucosa.

Patients are treated in the endoscopy unit or ambulatory surgery center, most commonly under conscious sedation. In one report, medications used were midazolam (mean 8.5 mg) and fentanyl (mean 157 μg) (15). Endoscopy is first performed, the distance from the incisors to the squamocolumnar junction (z-line) measured, a super-stiff, coated guide wire (0.035 to 0.039 cm thick) is placed in the duodenum and the endoscope removed, leaving the guide wire in place. The Stretta catheter comprised of the bougie tip, balloon-basket assembly, and four electrode delivery sheaths positioned radially around the balloon are then passed transorally over the fixed guide wire into the stomach and then withdrawn to 1 cm proximal to the z-line using the markings on the catheter shaft. The wire is then removed. Endoscopic confirmation of catheter position may be performed. The suction and irrigation lines are connected, the balloon is inflated to 2.5 psi, and the four needle electrodes are deployed into the muscle of the gastroesophageal junction

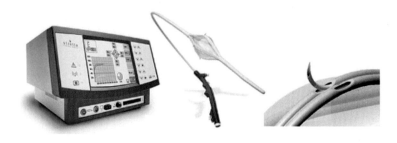

FIGURE 26.1. Technical components of the Stretta system. **Left:** The RF generator. **Middle:** The Stretta disposable catheter carrying the balloon/basket combination. **Right:** Detail of the needle and thermocouple that records the temperature at the mucosa and muscle levels.

(GEJ). There is a reduction in the electrode electrical impedance displayed on the generator screen when the electrodes are delivered into the muscle. RF energy is delivered for 90 seconds to each electrode, while the mucosa is being cooled with irrigation, using the temperature-controlled RF generator system (Color Plate 26.2, left). The needles are then retracted and balloon deflated. The catheter is rotated 45 degrees and a second set of lesions created, establishing the first ring of eight lesions. Three more rings are created in this manner at 0.5 cm above the z-line, the z-line, and 0.5 cm below the z-line. The gastric cardia is treated by positioning the catheter in the stomach, inflating the balloon to 25 cc or 22 cc, respectively, retracting against the hiatus, and deploying the electrodes. The final result is four ante-grade rings in the distal LES and two pull-back rings in the gastric cardia (Color Plate 26.2, middle). Ideally, a total of 14 lesion sets are created, a number determined by previous animal model investigations and individual patient anatomy. Patients then undergo endoscopy immediately after delivery of RF energy to assess the early post-RF appearance of the mucosa. Heat-induced collagen shrinkage will be immediately evident after the Stretta procedure, evidenced by a contraction of the GEJ around the endoscope (Color Plates 26.2 [right] and 26.3A and B).

Mechanism(s) of Action

There are two potential mechanisms of action of Stretta: mechanical alteration of the GEJ and neural modulation of transient lower esophageal sphincter relaxations (tLESRs).

Mechanical

In a porcine model of botulinum-induced LES hypotension, RF energy delivery substantially restored LES pressure by 21% within 8 weeks of treatment. Further, in this porcine model of reflux, RF treatment increased the gastric yield pressure (GYP) by 75% over controls. GYP is the gastric pressure at which the barrier function of the LES is overcome, causing a common cavity event. Augmentation of GYP, similar to that occurring after fundoplication, indicates a more robust antireflux barrier (16). Regarding durability of this response, a separate group of animals in this trial (not treated with botulinum toxin) demonstrated a 68% increase in LES pressure and a 114% increase in GYP at 6 months follow-up. After Stretta, increased muscular wall thickness has been shown histopathologically in a canine model (17) and endosonographically in porcine model (18). A modest increase of the lower esophageal sphincter pressure (LESP) 6 months after Stretta has also been found in a recently reported human trial showing a 60% increase in postprandial LES pressure 12 months after RF treatment (19).

An additional mechanical effect of Stretta in patients with delayed gastric emptying and GERD symptoms was evaluated by Noar et al. (20). After Stretta, gastric emptying normalized in 16 of 17 patients. Augmenting the antireflux barrier with Stretta improves gastric motility efficiency in these patients who demonstrate baseline impairment.

Neurological

Approximately 85% of GERD patients have tLESRs as the primary mechanism of disease. A second, potentially synergistic, mechanism of action for the Stretta procedure is the disruption of the triggering mechanism for tLESRs. Two human Stretta studies incorporating 3-hour postprandial esophageal manometry and pH monitoring after a standard meal (3000kJ, 55% fat) have been reported. DiBaise et al. (21) reported a 75% reduction in stimulated tLESRs in humans after RF delivery, while Tam et al. (22) found a 50% reduction in stimulated reflux events and a 25% reduction in tLESRs. Kim et al. (17) evaluated triggering of tLESRs in awake, upright dogs, finding that RF delivery reduced tLESRs by 54% at 7-month follow-up. Transient LESRs are considered a neurologic event, reduced by vagal blockade and the GABA$_\beta$-receptor agonist baclofen (23); therefore RF energy may disrupt these aberrant intramural vagal afferent nerve pathways within the gastric cardia.

Clinical Experience with Stretta

This procedure is ideally suited for patients with GERD confirmed by pathologic esophageal acid exposure on pH monitoring, gross regurgitation, and esophagitis. It is also indicated for those patients who are considering antireflux surgery, yet are not accepting of general anesthesia and the risk of surgical adverse events. These candidate patients typically present with inadequate GERD symptom control on a properly escalated antisecretory regimen, intolerance to antisecretory therapy, or (less commonly) an unwillingness to continue a long-term high-dose antisecretory regimen. Exclusion criteria for the Stretta procedure include the following: hiatal hernia ≥3 cm, active grade 3 to 4 of esophagitis, long-segment Barrett's metaplasia or dysplasia, or collagen vascular disease. Based on these selection criteria, approximately 40% of all antireflux surgical patients would be candidates for Stretta as a first-line, less-invasive therapy. Importantly, Stretta does not preclude the opportunity to undergo surgery in the future. As of November 2002, more than 3,000 procedures have been performed, many in the context of clinical trials. The safety, effectiveness, and mechanism of action of the Stretta procedure have been evaluated in a number of prospective U.S. and international clinical trials, including a U.S. multicenter, randomized, double-blind, sham-controlled clinical trial (Tables 26.4 to 26.6).

TABLE 26.4. CLINICAL TRIAL DATA SUMMARY WITH STRETTA: GERD SYMPTOM SCORES

| Author | N | Follow-up (months) | GERD Symptom Index | | p value |
			Baseline	After Stretta	
Triadafilopoulos	47	6	26	7	<0.0001
Triadafilopoulos	118	12	27	9	<0.0001
DiBaise	18	12	22	7	<0.001
Tam	20	12	19.5	7	<0.05
Corley	35	12	28	7	<0.003
Mansell	29	11	33	2	<0.001
Meier	25	6	17	6	0.0002
Noar	118	8-12	31.9	9	<0.0001
Wolfsen	558	9 (2-33)	23%[a]	86%[a]	<0.0001
Houston	25	6	3.5[b]	5.5[b]	<0.001
Richards	41	6	3.7[b]	5.1[b]	<0.001

GERD Symptom Index reflects the GERD-HRQL (0-50) with normal<10
[a]indicates % symptom control on-drugs (baseline) vs. off-drugs (after Stretta)
[b]indicates QOLRAD score (0-7, quality of life related to reflux disease, higher numbers=better control)

TABLE 26.5. CLINICAL TRIAL DATA SUMMARY WITH STRETTA: 24-HOUR ESOPHAGEAL ACID EXPOSURE

| Author | N | Follow-up (months) | 24-hr Esophageal Acid Exposure | | p value |
			Baseline	After Stretta	
Triadafilopoulos	47	6	11.7	4.8	<0.0001
Triadafilopoulos	118	12	10.2	6.4	<0.0001
DiBaise	18	12	9.5	6.7	<0.05
Tam	20	12	11.0	6.3	<0.01
Corley	35	12	11.0	5.0	<0.003
Corley	29	6	10.5	4.8	<0.01
Houston	25	6	6.6	0.7	n.a.
Richards	41	6	8.4	4.4	<0.001

TABLE 26.6. CLINICAL TRIAL DATA SUMMARY WITH STRETTA: USE OF PROTON PUMP INHIBITORS

| Author | N | Follow-up (months) | PPI Utilization (% patients) | | p value |
			Baseline	After Stretta	
Triadafilopoulos	47	6	87	13	<0.0001
Triadafilopoulos	118	12	86	30	<0.0001
DiBaise	18	12	90	6	<0.05
Tam	20	12	80	10	<0.01
Reymunde	82	6-11	94	3	<0.05
Mansell	29	11	96	24	<0.001
Meier	25	6	100	38	<0.05
Mavrelis	29	6	100	0	<0.05
Noar	118	8-12	100	<10	<0.0001
Wolfsen	558	8 (2-33)	80	<30	<0.0001
Houston	25	6	100	38	<0.001
Richards	41	6	100	35	<0.001

A U.S. open-label trial assessed, in patients with uncomplicated GERD, the long-term (12 month) effect of Stretta on GERD symptoms and quality of life, medication use, esophageal acid exposure, LESP and esophageal motor function, severity of esophagitis, tolerability, and complications (15). Entry criteria for the trial were age >18, daily heartburn and/or regurgitation requiring daily medication, LESP >5 mm Hg, normal LES relaxation, esophageal body amplitude >30 mm Hg, and a minimum acid exposure time of >4% over 24 hours. Excluded were patients with hiatal hernia of >2 cm long, grade > 3 esophagitis, severe dysphagia, previous esophagogastric surgery, ASA (American Society of Anesthesiologists) class >III, history of collagen vascular disease, or pregnancy.

The study involved objective assessment of symptoms and quality-of-life scores before, and 1, 4, 6, and 12 months after Stretta, as well as endoscopy, esophageal motility, and pH monitoring before and 6 months after the procedure. The study population consisted of 118 patients (72 male and 46 female) and a mean duration of GERD symptoms of 9.5 years. Stretta was performed as an outpatient procedure under conscious sedation and was generally well tolerated with <10% incidence of moderate or severe patient discomfort with either catheter passage or RF delivery. Complications noted with the procedure were superficial mucosal injury (2.5%), fever (1.7%), chest discomfort (1.7%), transient dysphagia (0.8%), sedation-related hypotension (0.8%), and topical anesthesia allergy (0.8%), totaling 8.6%.

Patients had superior satisfaction and GERD scores at 12 months compared to those at baseline while on their original antisecretory medication. A significant improvement in heartburn scores was noted, from a median of 4 (baseline) to 1 (12 months). Median GERD scores improved from 27 to 9. Median patient satisfaction scores improved from 1 to 4. There were also significant improvements at 12 months in mental and physical quality of life, as assessed by the SF-36 questionnaire. There was a significant reduction in distal and proximal esophageal acid exposure. Median distal esophageal acid exposure time improved from 10.6% to 6.4% and proximal esophageal acid exposure improved from 1.9% to 0.9%. At baseline, 90% of these patients used, on average, twice-daily PPI therapy. At 12 months, only 30% of patients used any PPI. Esophagitis, when present, was also improved at 6 months after the procedure. Six patients (5%) who failed opted for laparoscopic fundoplication performed by four different surgeons without additional difficulty or evidence of anatomic abnormality (24).

Corley et al. (25) recently reported the Stretta randomized, double-blind, sham-controlled trial. Sixty-four GERD patients were randomly assigned to RF energy delivery to the gastroesophageal junction (35 patients) or to a sham procedure (29 patients). Principal outcomes were heartburn symptoms and quality of life; secondary outcomes were medication usage and esophageal acid exposure. After 6 months, interested sham patients crossed over to active treatment. At 6 months, active treatment significantly and substantially improved heartburn symptoms, GERD-specific quality of life, and general quality of life. More active versus sham patients were responders (>50% improvement in GERD quality of life; 61% vs. 30%) and more were without daily heartburn symptoms (61% vs. 33%). These improvements persisted at 12 months posttreatment. Esophageal acid exposure was significantly improved in treated patients at 1-year follow-up and in crossover patients 6 months after Stretta treatment. These results confirm that the positive effects of the Stretta procedure are not derived from a placebo effect.

Using a standardized survey instrument, Wolfsen (26) evaluated GERD symptoms, patient satisfaction, and antisecretory drug use in 558 patients treated with the Stretta procedure at 33 U.S. centers from February 1999 to December 2001 (mean follow-up 8 months, range 2 to 33 months). At baseline, 76% patients on antisecretory regimen were dissatisfied with relief of GERD. After Stretta, onset of GERD relief was <2 months (68.7%) or 2 to 6 months (14.6%) after Stretta. Median drug requirement improved from twice-daily PPI to antacids as needed. The percentage of patients with satisfactory GERD control (absent or mild) improved from 26.3% at baseline to 77.0% after Stretta. Median baseline symptom control on-meds was 50%, compared to 90% at follow-up. Baseline patient satisfaction on-drugs was 23.2%, compared to 86.5% at follow-up after Stretta. Subgroup analysis (<1 year vs. >1 year after Stretta) showed a superior effect on symptom control and drug use for those patients beyond 1-year follow-up.

In well-selected patients, Stretta may be an effective alternative to laparoscopic Nissen fundoplication. Patients presenting to Vanderbilt University Medical Center for surgical evaluation of GERD were prospectively offered the Stretta procedure or laparoscopic Nissen fundoplication (27). Patients were studied pre and post-operatively with validated GERD-specific quality-of-life questionnaires (QOLRAD) and short-form health surveys (SF12). Seventy-five patients (age 49±14 years, 56% female) underwent laparoscopic Nissen fundoplication and 65 patients (age 46±12 years, 58% female) underwent the Stretta procedure. At 6 months, the QOLRAD and SF12 scores were significantly improved in both groups. Sixty-two percent of Stretta patients were off PPIs and an additional 30% had reduced their dose significantly while 92% of fundoplication patients were off PPIs. There was a significant reduction in esophageal acid exposure time (8.4±0.9% to 4.4±1.3%) in the Stretta group. Both groups were highly satisfied with their procedure (94% fundoplication vs. 89% Stretta). Adoption of an endoscopic treatment for GERD has allowed the Vanderbilt Surgical Group to stratify the management of their GERD patients according to hiatal hernia size, LES pressure, and disease severity. The decision whether to undergo antireflux surgery or Stretta must be based on the relative risk/benefit of each procedure (27). While antireflux surgery provides better control of esophageal acid exposure than Stretta, the outcomes for GERD symptoms, quality of life, and reduction in PPI use are comparable. Stretta has a low risk of acute adverse events (<0.13%), has no reported cases of long-term dysphagia, and obviates the need for general anesthesia and hospitalization, while antireflux surgery has a reported adverse event rate of approximately 2%, a considerable incidence of dysphagia, and requires general anesthesia and 1 to 2 days in the hospital. Antireflux surgery may always be performed after Stretta in the case of failures.

In an Australian study, Tam et al. (22) reported on 20 patients with chronic GERD who underwent the Stretta procedure. In these patients, esophageal acid exposure was significantly reduced from 10.8% to 6.6% and basal LES pressure was increased by 60%. At 12 months, 75% of patients were able to discontinue all antisecretory medications. There was also significant improvement in esophagitis grade, GERD scores (19 to 6), and quality-of-life scores. DiBaise et al. (21) reported on 18 patients with chronic GERD. A dramatic reduction in symptom scores (113.4 vs. 82.4) and antacid use (14.5/week vs. 2.3/week) was noted with Stretta and was associated with a 75% reduction in tLESRs. Ninety percent of patients discontinued all antisecretory medications.

Since its FDA approval, Stretta has been assessed in several community practice trials. In 82 consecutively treated patients, Reymunde and Santiago (28) reported an overall 70% improvement in GERD quality-of-life scores. A total of 97% of patients were able to discontinued baseline PPI use. Mansell et al. (29) treated 22 women and 7 men with and without hiatal hernia. At follow-up (136±78 days), there were significant improvements in the median heartburn score (4 to 1), GERD score (32 to 9), satisfaction (1 to 5), mental SF-36 (52.5 to 59.4), and physical SF-36 (31.3 to 39.2). Medication use improved from baseline (79% 2×PPI, 17% 1×PPI, and 4% H_2RA) to posttreatment (17% 2×PPI, 7% 1×PPI, 7% H_2RA, and 69% no drug or as needed medication only). There were no adverse effects requiring intervention. One patient had fundoplication for incomplete symptom control. A small study evaluated modified Stretta in ten patients either with >3-cm sliding hiatal hernias or after a failed Nissen fundoplication (30). Ablation was performed in an ante-grade fashion to eliminate the risk of pulling back the balloon into the hiatal hernia. Of the ten patients who were followed for 1 to 8 months, all had no more regurgitation, six discontinued their medication, and four had mild heartburn that was controlled with once-daily PPI. One patient experienced delayed bleeding requiring endoscopic intervention, and another developed chest pain requiring analgesia.

Delayed gastric emptying occurs in a significant number of GERD patients, and Stretta, by improving the barrier function of the GEJ, may benefit gastric emptying. Noar et al. (20) studied patients with severe, drug-refractory GERD and concurrent delayed gastric emptying. Patients were studied at baseline and 8 months after Stretta. In addition to improvements in standardized GERD symptoms scores and reductions in PPI usage, gastric emptying at 90 minutes improved from baseline 34.6±11.8% to follow-up 72.5±21.7%. Overall, 16 patients normalized their gastric emptying studies (94%) and 1 patient improved.

Postmarketing experience with Stretta in the United States has revealed the following complications (31): bleeding, mucosal ulceration, pleural effusion, perforation, and aspiration/death. As has occurred with the introduction of other new techniques, safety and tolerability have improved over time with the natural evolution of the device and technique, physician learning curve, physician training, patient education, and development of posttreatment management guidelines. The initial complication incidence was 2.2%, while in the subsequent 3- and 6-month periods, the incidence of complications decreased significantly to 0.6%, 0.1%, and 0.0%, respectively. In order to prevent complications, patient selection is paramount. Technical considerations such as catheter placement at <1cm above the z-line, balloon distention to >2.5 psi, proper sedation, endoscopy confirmation after the first set or therapy, guide wire catheter placement, and adherence to patient management guidelines have played a role in curtailing the number of complications. There have been no long-term cases of stricture formation, development of achalasia, dysphagia, or bloating, as may be seen after antireflux surgery.

In conclusion, the Stretta procedure offers a minimally invasive, safe, and effective alternative to antireflux surgery for those patients with GERD who are unsatisfactorily controlled on antisecretory medications, who are considering surgery, and who meet the anatomic criteria that make the procedure technically feasible and safe.

ENDOSCOPIC LUMINAL GASTROPLASTY (ELGP, ENDOCINCH)

Device and Procedure

This is an endoscopic suturing method introduced by CR Bard, Inc. (Murray Hill, NJ) under the name EndoCinch, and is FDA approved. The procedure represents the commercial version of miniature endoscopic sewing machines, developed by Paul Swain (32–34). Such sewing machines can be attached to flexible endoscopes and can place single or multiple sutures in the gastrointestinal tract in order to treat perforations, over-sew areas of bleeding, or change anatomy. The Bard EndoCinch is a multicomponent system that is introduced through a 19.7-mm over-tube. The procedure aims at altering the anatomy of the gastroesophageal junction by tightening the cardia within the lesser curve, accentuating the angle of His.

The sewing capsule that is attached to the tip of an endoscope has a hollow chamber into which tissue is suctioned. A handle is attached to the biopsy port on the handle of the endoscope, and drives the needle in order to create a stitch. The handle controls the advance of the hollow-core needle, into which is back-loaded the tilt-tag attached to the end of 3-0 monofilament suture material. The tilt-tag is captured in the tip of the mounted capsule after being driven forward by a stiff wire pushed through the hollow needle and controlled by the handle. In the current model, a small ring and peg-cinching tag eliminate the need for hand tying knots, cutting the suture ends, and cinching together the tag parts at the tissue surface (35).

The procedure is performed in the endoscopy unit but generally takes more time, requires more sedation, two upper endoscopes, and an over-tube. The first endoscope carries the metal sewing capsule on its tip. The second endoscope cinches the sutures through a catheter device that deploys a ceramic plug and ring through which the sutures are threaded. After an initial endoscopy, a guide wire is positioned into the distal stomach. An oroesophageal over-tube is loaded onto a 15-mm Savary esophageal dilator and advanced over the guide wire. The dilator and wire are then removed and the second endoscope with mounted sewing capsule is then passed through the over-tube to the gastroesophageal junction.

Two or three placations are then usually created (Color Plate 26.4, A to C). Each placation is formed by two sutures that are placed into the gastric submucosa, about 1.5 cm apart and then pulled together. Most commonly, circumferential placations are made 1 cm below the gastroesophageal (GE) junction at the three, six, and nine o'clock positions; less frequently placations are made in a linear fashion 1, 2, and 3 cm below the GE junction. A helical configuration is sometimes made, especially if a small hiatal hernia is present. When at the desired location, suction is applied to the capsule, drawing the tissue into the capsule chamber. After 10 seconds of suction, the handle is depressed, forcing the needle through the suctioned tissue; withdrawing the handle leaves the tag captured into the tip of the sewing capsule. Release of suction and forward advancement of the endoscope releases the stitched tissue and the endoscope is withdrawn through the over-tube. The same tilt-tag is reloaded into the hollow-core needle to place a second stitch at a location 1 to 1.5 cm away from the initial stitch. The second stitch is placed in a similar fashion. The two stitches are then pulled together and cinched by the ceramic plug and ring using the second endoscope. Depending on anatomy and technical expertise, the procedure takes 40 to 60 minutes. The majority of the stitches are placed submucosally, not

transmurally, just below the squamocolumnar junction. As the technique is refined, some groups have reported that application of cautery to the lesser curvature before placement of the sutures may reduce the chance of suture pull-through (36).

Mechanism of Action

The precise mechanism by which endoscopic suturing achieves its beneficial effect in GERD is unknown but it may change the anatomy of the cardia and the angle of His. In a study in dogs, a significant increase in LES pressure (form 4.6 to 13.3 mm Hg) and cardiac yield pressure (from 10 to 19 mm Hg) were noted. In a porcine model, the median LES pressure increased from 3 to 6 mm Hg, and the sphincter length from 3 to 3.75 cm. The median time pH was <4 and decreased significantly from 9.3% to 0.2% postprocedure in these pigs (37). Animal studies have shown that most stitches are placed submucosally, not transmurally (mean depth 2.8 mm), regardless of the tissue suction time (10 vs. 30 seconds) (38).

Clinical Experience with EndoCinch

The first multicenter trial that led to approval of the device involved 64 patients from eight U.S. centers (39). For this trial, inclusion criteria were more than three episodes per week of heartburn while off antisecretory drugs (regardless of whether erosive esophagitis was present), partial response to antisecretory therapy, drug dependence for symptom control, and pathologic acid reflux by pH monitoring. Exclusion criteria included dysphagia, esophagitis Savary stage > II while on therapy, body mass index (BMI) >40 kg/m², GERD symptomatically refractory to antisecretory therapy, and a >2-cm long hiatal hernia. Treatment success was defined as a decrease in the heartburn severity score of >50% plus a reduction of antireflux medication use to under four doses per month. Patients were assessed by endoscopy, esophageal manometry, ambulatory pH monitoring, symptom severity scoring, and quality-of-life scoring before and 6 months after therapy, and were randomized to either linear or circumferential placations.

With EndoCinch, the mean heartburn symptom score fell from 62.7 to a mean of 16.7 and 17 at 3 and 6 months, respectively. Regurgitation scores also significantly improved. LES pressure or length did not change. Savary grade II esophagitis was noted at baseline in 25% of cases and in 19% at 6-month follow-up. The percent of total time with pH<4, total number of reflux episodes, and percent of upright time with pH<4 were all significantly improved at 6 months follow-up. Of note, improvement in symptoms did not always correlate to improvement of esophagitis or pH scores. Quality-of-life scores at 6 months postprocedure were significantly improved for social functioning and bodily pain. There was no difference in any outcomes related to linear versus circumferential placement of the stitches. Disrupted placations were associated with poor symptom control. Most importantly, at 6 months follow-up, 62% of patients were taking less than four doses of medications per month and were considered treatment successes. Adverse events included pharyngitis (31%), vomiting (14%), and abdominal and/or chest pain (14% to 16%). Two patients suffered minor mucosal tears probably related to over-tube use. One patient suffered a suture microperforation that was treated conservatively. None of these complications required surgical intervention.

Other centers have presented similar short-term results. In a European study, 102 patients treated with linear placations and followed for a median of 12 weeks had significant improvement in heartburn symptoms, and percent of time with pH<4. In this study, a significant increase in LES length and tone were also noted (40). Eighty-eight patients underwent gastroplication in a U.S. postmarketing multicenter study that included tertiary and community practices (41). ELGP was performed with two placations in 82%, three placations in 18%, 96% circumferentially. Upon short-term follow-up, heartburn resolved completely in 85% of patients and to less than three episodes per week in 6%, while 9% of patients did not improve. Regurgitation resolved in 90%. In this study, 74% of patients discontinued antireflux medications, and an additional 17% used medications occasionally. A small number of patients with Barrett's esophagus and/or hiatal hernia were also treated with favorable results. In another, single-center, community practice study with 55 GERD patients who underwent linear placations and were followed for a mean of 3.7 months (42), a significant reduction in heartburn and regurgitation was noted, and 76% of these patients were completely off PPI.

In a Mayo Clinic study with 23 patients and a mean 6.7-month follow-up, 24% of patients had a second placation, because the first one failed to adequately control GERD. Although most patients had either partial or complete symptom relief, only 20% were off antireflux medications (43).

Long-term studies with EndoCinch have been recently reported. A multicenter U.S. study of 33 patients who were followed for up to 2 years demonstrated persistent improvement in heartburn severity and frequency but failed to show improvement in regurgitation. Twenty-five percent of the patients were completely off antisecretory medications, while 28 percent were on minimal medications to control symptoms. Forty-one percent of patients were on the same doses of antisecretory drugs or had fundoplication (44). In another 2-year follow-up study of 23 patients, 22% were off antisecretory drugs and another 30% required less than half of the

original dose; 6% underwent fundoplication due to treatment failure (45).

ELGP was also evaluated in 20 patients with "refractory" GERD, defined as twice-daily PPI use. Nine patients were treated again at 1 month for continued symptoms. At 3 months, symptoms and esophageal pH exposure improved significantly, and pH studies normalized in seven patients (46). Another study showed similar results (47). EndoCinch has also been compared to laparoscopic fundoplication (48). In this study, 18 patients treated with ELGP were compared with 16 age-matched patients who underwent laparoscopic Nissen fundoplication. As expected, the mean procedure duration (52 vs. 116 minutes) and hospital stay (0.05 vs. 3.3 days) were shorter with gastroplication. Symptoms scores, need for PPIs, and quality of life were significantly improved in both groups, but those undergoing laparoscopic Nissen fundoplication showed greater control of esophageal acid exposure. A preliminary report suggested that EndoCinch may be effective even in patients with hiatal hernias >2 cm, as long as more placations are performed (49).

WILSON-COOK ENDOSCOPIC SUTURING DEVICE

Device and Procedure

This system consists of a flexible Sew-Right device, a flexible Ti-Knot device, an external accessory channel to attach to any flexible upper endoscope, braided 2-0 polyester suture, and titanium knot-clipping devices (Fig. 26.5). There is no need for an over-tube. The Sew-Right and Ti-Knot devices can be reloaded through the accessory channel attached to the endoscope, creating multiple placations with only one intubation. The Sew-Right device contains two needles oriented in tandem and controlled by a toggle switch (Fig. 26.5A). A continuous single suture loop is utilized to stitch two adjacent areas below the squamocolumnar junction. A vacuum cap slides over the distal end of the sewing device once it has been loaded with the suture.

After a standard endoscopy is performed, the endoscope is fitted with the external accessory channel (EAC). The needle selector is toggled to the right side on the handle of the Sew-Right device, and after its tip is lubricated it is inserted and advanced into the EAC until it can be seen endoscopically. After a site in the proximal stomach is selected to be aspirated into the cap of the sewing device, suction is applied through the suction tubing that is attached to the flush/vacuum port on the handle of the device (Fig. 26.5B). While suction is holding the tissue, the handle of the device is squeezed and released, pushing the right needle forward where it picks up the suture end and draws it through the tissue as the needle returns to its initial position. Suction is released, and the left needle is activated by toggling the needle selector to the left

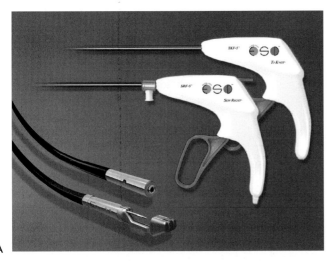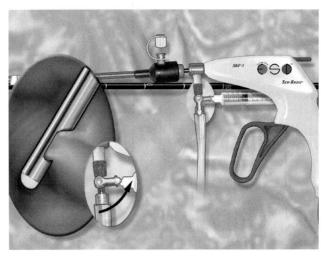

A   B

FIGURE 26.5. Instruments **(A)** and concepts **(B)** for the gastroplasty procedure using the Wilson-Cook endoscopic suturing device.

side of the handle. The sequence is repeated in order to place the second stitch, 1 to 2 cm away from the first. The sewing device is slowly removed from the EAC and the suture ends are kept externally. The two cut ends of the suture are backloaded through the distal end of the Ti-Knot device, and the device is inserted into the EAC and guided over the two suture threads to the tissue surface. The lever of this device is then squeezed and crimps the preloaded titanium knot and simultaneously cuts the excess suture. Two or three additional placations can then be formed by reinserting a reloaded Sew-Right, selecting a new location and repeating the above steps. Animal studies have demonstrated that the sutures are located in the submucosa.

Clinical Experience

The device has been FDA approved for human use but there have been no published studies on its efficacy or safety for the treatment of GERD.

NDO ENDOSCOPIC PLACATION SYSTEM (NDO SURGICAL PLICATOR)

Device and Procedure

Currently in human clinical trials (NDO Surgical Inc., Mansfield, MA) and not yet FDA approved, this device creates a transmural, full-thickness, placation. Such placation is formed with a pretied, suture-based implant that is delivered just below the gastroesophageal junction in a retroflexed manner. The system includes an over-tube through which the plicator device is introduced into the stomach, the plicator, a tissue retracting helical catheter, and pretied suture insert. The plicator has a handle with levers for opening/closing the arms and sliding/locking the pretied suture insert, as well as

a channel for passage of the endoscope and tissue-retracting helical catheter (Color Plate 26.6).

The procedure is performed under direct endoscopic visualization using a 5.9-mm flexible pediatric endoscope that is inserted through the device channel. Because of the need for an over-tube insertion, higher amounts of sedation are required. First, the gastroscope is passed for inspection of the anatomy. A guide wire is then placed into the antrum, the endoscope is withdrawn and a Savary dilator is passed over the guide wire. A 60-F over-tube is inserted into the esophagus; the dilator and guide wire are then removed. The plicator device is loaded with the pretied suture insert, the tissue retracting helical catheter, and the gastroscope, and passed via the over-tube into the proximal stomach, about 12 cm below the gastroesophageal junction. Inflation of the stomach before attempting to retroflex the device is paramount. The distal end of the over-tube is pulled back into the distal esophagus and the plicator device is retroflexed. At the same time the gastroscope is advanced into its retroflexed viewing position facing the anterior site of the cardia (Fig. 26.6). After such positioning, a set of jaws is opened and a catheter with a corkscrew tip is advanced and screwed into the muscularis propria of that area, bringing the gastric wall into the span of the jaws. Upon closure of the jaws, one large placation is accomplished using a double-pronged rivet-like implant opposing two full thickness portions of the cardia wall at a distance about 1.0 to 1.5 cm below the z-line. The instrument arms are then opened to release the device from the tissue. The device is released from its retroflexed position, the arms are closed, and the device is withdrawn from the patient through the over-tube. The total procedure takes 10 to 20 minutes. Over time, the serosal sides of the gastric wall fuse and tighten the cardia and accentuate the angle of His (50). In contrast to other placation devices that are more

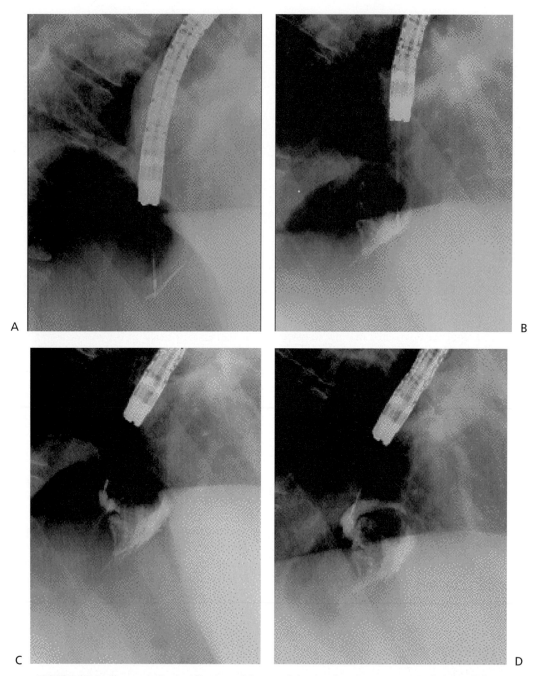

FIGURE 26.8. Fluoroscopic visualization of Enteryx injection for the treatment of GERD, **(A)** to **(F)**. Injection creates a ring of radio-opaque material at the GEJ corresponding to the bulking effect in that region.

superficial in stitch location, the NDO plicator creates a deeper tissue apposition that may increase efficacy durability.

Clinical Experience

In an *ex vivo* porcine stomach model, the full-thickness plicator increased significantly the intragastric pressure required to induce reflux in preventing gastroesophageal reflux with a single placation (50). *In vivo*, 12-week-long

studies in swine demonstrated no complications and confirmed serosal healing (51).

An early human trial with seven GERD patients who were PPI dependent was performed in India (52). Six of the seven were successfully placated without complications, and at 3 months follow-up had a 48% reduction in median heartburn symptom score and a 58% improvement in median regurgitation symptom score. Five of six patients were completely off these antisecretory medications. Upon

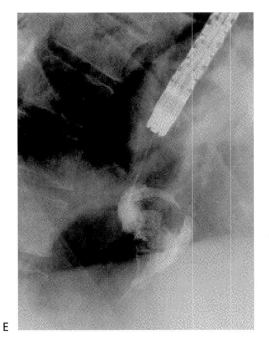

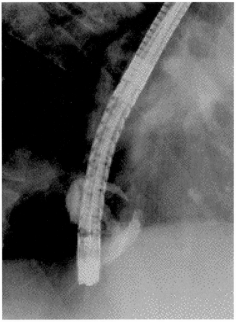

E   F

FIGURE 26.8. *(Continued)*

follow-up 6 months later, the improvements in symptoms, quality of life, and esophageal pH exposure persisted (53).

A North American multicenter trial with 70 patients with mild GERD and no hiatal hernia >2 cm has been just completed. The study involves one placation and comparisons of baseline symptom scores, manometry and pH probe data, endoscopic findings, and quality-of-life scores with follow-up assessments at 12 months.

In summary, several gastroplication approaches have been shown to be feasible and effective in enhancing the antireflux barrier in GERD patients. Further experience with these techniques, refinement of the instrumentation, and efficacy and safety studies will eventually accurately characterize their therapeutic potential.

INJECTION THERAPY WITH ENTERYX

Device and Procedure

The injection of bulking agents that are of low viscosity to traverse a needle and then change to a solid state at the local injection site has been studied for many years. The site of injection is near the squamocolumnar junction in a circumferential fashion (54,55). The injection needle diameter must match implant viscosity. Preferably, 23- to 27-percent gauges are used since they are easier to manipulate and atraumatic enough to minimize back leak of the implantable material from the puncture site. The depth of implant (submucosal or intramuscular) also varies depending on the material that tends to flow 1 to 2 cm up or down from the injection site. If a submucosal injection is made, the endoscopist observes a bulging effect. If not, and a

deeper implantation is desired, fluoroscopy is used. The latter approach is preferred with ethinyl-vinyl alcohol (Enteryx, Enteric Medical Technologies, Palo Alto, CA), an inert, biocompatible polymer, which needs to be placed deeply into the muscle in order to avoid back erosion into the lumen (56).

The Enteryx solution consists of a biocompatible polymer, 8% EVOH dissolved in dimethyl sulfoxide (DMSO) as the solvent (57,58). Since the polymer itself is not radio-opaque, micronized tantalum powder (30%) is added to the polymer/solvent mixture to serve as the contrast for fluoroscopic visualization. Upon injection and contact with aqueous body fluids, the solvent rapidly dissipates causing *in situ* precipitation of the polymer as a spongy mass (Color Plate 26.7). The homopolymers—polyethylene and polyvinyl alcohol (PVA)—from which the copolymer EVOH is derived have a long history as implant materials. Polyethylene is used in numerous implant applications. Similarly, PVA has been used clinically in topical solutions, plasma expanders, and as a particle embolization material (59,60). The EVOH copolymer is used as a hemodialysis and plasmapheresis membrane. DMSO, the carrier solvent, is commercially available for the symptomatic relief of interstitial cystitis an as an antiinflammatory agent for soft tissue injuries, joint pain, and arthritis (61–63). Tantalum powder serves as the radiographic marker because it is insoluble, inert, possesses a high radio density and tissue adherence, and has been used in other long-term implants (64).

The Enteryx injection therapy is performed endoscopically under fluoroscopic control (Fig. 26.8A through F). The injection catheter is introduced through the biopsy channel of the endoscope and its tip is placed at or 1 to 2 mm below the z-line. The 4-mm long, 23-gauge needle is advanced and the mucosa is punctured, in an ante-grade direction, at or below the z-line. Enteryx solution is then injected along the muscle layer or the deep submucosal layer of the cardia. If the material forms an arc or a ring, multiple syringes are then used to add material at the same injection position. Otherwise, multiple discrete injections of 1 to 2 cc each are performed in a circumferential manner until a total of 6 to 8 cc are implanted. If a shallow, submucosal injection that creates a gray color with bulging mass effect into the lumen is observed, the injection is stopped immediately and a new site is chosen. The injection rate should be no faster than 1 cc/minute in order to allow time for polymerization and heat dissipation. The needle remains in place for 1 minute after complete implantation, again to allow complete polymerization and prevent back flow of unpolymerized implant. During the procedure, the use of fluoroscopy allows for optimal visualization of the injection, and confirms that the implant is been placed intramurally by observing the radio-opaque marker in a linear or ring-like distribution. Oral analgesics are typically administered as needed for pain control and PPI therapy is continued for 7 to 10 days following the procedure.

Mechanism of Action

Initial trials with bulking agents were performed using Teflon paste and bovine dermal collagen in a refluxing dog model. These trials showed that there is a transient increase in gastric yield pressure and a decrease in esophagitis. The exact mechanism to account for the clinical efficacy of Enteryx is not known. Although there was no significant change in LES pressure following implantation, the LES length slightly increased. The Enteryx polymer does not appear to cause bulking, but is incorporated into the esophageal wall and encapsulated by fibrosis. This in turn lengthens the LES and possibly alters the compliance in the distal esophagus and/or proximal stomach.

Clinical Experience with Enteryx

Injection of Enteryx through a sclerotherapy needle under fluoroscopy was studied in a multicenter European and North American open-label trial of 81 patients with GERD symptoms partly controlled with PPIs, pathologic acid exposure, and a GERD score of <11 on therapy and >20 off therapy (65). Excluded were patients with hiatal hernia >3cm, grade II to IV esophagitis or Barrett's esophagus, esophageal varices, or obesity (BMI>35). The average procedure time was 30 to 40 minutes with a total fluoroscopy time of 10 to 20 minutes. There were no clinically serious adverse events or infections at the injection site. Ninety-two percent of patients experienced transient retrosternal chest pain that was mild to moderate and resolved within 2 weeks with oral analgesics as needed. Following injection, 17 patients reported mild or moderate dysphagia that typically started 4 days later and fully resolved within 12 weeks. Only one patient required dilation. Ten patients reported transient, low-grade fever. Of note, subjects noted a body odor and taste similar to garlic for several hours after use of DMSO. Seventy-four percent of patients in the trial were able to eliminate and 10% were able to reduce use of PPIs by ≥50% following the Enteryx procedure. At 6 months, 12% of patients reported use of PRN antacids and only three were using H_2 antagonists as needed.

Six months after therapy with Enteryx, patients experienced significant improvements in heartburn compared to baseline off PPIs (median scores 4.0 vs. 24.0) (66). The effect was similar to baseline while taking PPI therapy (median score 4.0 vs. 6.0). Similarly, patients experienced significant improvements in regurgitation compared to baseline off PPIs (1.0 vs. 11.0) and had comparable symptoms to baseline on PPIs (median score 1.0 vs. 2.0). SF-36 mental and physical component summary scores were significantly improved following Enteryx treatment compared to baseline off PPIs (55.9 vs. 52.7, and 50.8 vs. 44.8, respectively) and were comparable to baseline on PPIs (55.9 vs. 54.0, and 50.8 vs. 51.0, respectively).

At 6 months, esophageal acid exposure improved significantly after Enteryx therapy (median time at pH<4 of 9.5% vs. 6.7%) and 26 of 71 (37%) of patients normalized their total time with pH<4. There were no significant changes in LES pressure, peristaltic amplitude, or residual LESP between baseline and 6 months, but the median LES length significantly increased from 2.0 to 3.0 cm. Of interest, 19 patients underwent repeat implantation due to an inadequate initial therapeutic response. Six months after reimplantation, 63% (12 of 19) of these patients had improved symptom scores and were either off PPIs or had reduced PPI use by =50%. FDA approval is pending.

EXPANDABLE HYDROGEN PROSTHESIS (GATEKEEPER)

Device and Procedure

The procedure involves submucosal placement of expandable miniature hydrogel prostheses in the region of the gastroesophageal junction under direct endoscopic visualization (Color Plate 26.9). After placement, the prostheses swell up and bulk the LES region (Gatekeeper, Medtronics, Minneapolis, MN).

The placement of the prostheses in the submucosa of the esophagus can be performed under conscious sedation. After endoscopic inspection of the esophagus, stomach, and duodenum, a guide wire is placed in the duodenum. The Gatekeeper system uses a 16-mm over-tube as a conduit for the endoscope and for the 2.4-mm–diameter hydrogel delivery system. Distally in the over-tube a shelf is present in a rigid segment. Both endoscope (contained within the lumen of the over-tube) and over-tube are passed into the lower esophagus over a guide wire. Once in position, suction is applied via the endoscope, which pulls the esophageal wall into a shelf at the end of the over-tube (Color Plate 26.10).

A conventional injection needle is passed through a second channel in the over-tube and saline is injected into the submucosal tissue, creating a tissue bleb or submucosal pocket. The injection needle is removed and the prosthesis delivery system (1-mm diameter needle, dilator, and 2.4-mm–diameter trocar) is passed through the same channel and advanced into the tissue bleb. The needle assembly and dilator are then removed, leaving the sheath in the submucosal plane. A dry 1.5-mm diameter by 18-mm long hydrogel rod is then loaded into the proximal end of the sheath and advanced with a push rod through the sheath into the submucosa. Once the hydrogel has been delivered the push rod and sheath are removed. Finally the sheath can be pulled out of the submucosa and the fold is removed from the chamber by inflating some air and slight twisting of the over-tube. Axial rotation or further insertion or removal of the over-tube repositions the shelf to place additional prostheses. The complete procedure takes approximately 15 minutes for one hydrogel and 5 minutes for each additional hydrogel. Regardless of the number of deliveries, only one pass of the over-tube and endoscope are required. Within 24 hours, the prostheses expand to their full volume, creating submucosal swellings in the esophageal wall, thus creating a mechanical antireflux barrier (Color Plate 26.11A and B).

Mechanism of Action

In a preliminary study (67), LESP augmentation was noted but the precise mechanism of action is unknown.

Clinical Experience

In preclinical animal studies, the 1-year prosthesis retention rate has varied from 68% to 92% (68). A pilot safety and efficacy study with ten patients has been recently reported (69). After baseline manometry and pH monitoring, patients with GERD and good PPI response were treated under conscious sedation, and oral antibiotics were given around the procedure. Three prostheses (6×15mm) were placed above the z-line. Proper positioning of the prostheses was confirmed by endoscopic ultrasound miniprobe. Placement was successful in 33 of 34 prostheses (97%) and was well tolerated by all patients. However, six prostheses migrated into the lumen of the esophagus within 6 months. The maximum duration of the procedure was 22 minutes. Median symptom scores (GERD-HRQL) improved from 23 at baseline (off PPI) to 9 at 4 weeks (n=9) and 7.5 at 6 months (n=8). The pH-monitoring scores improved at 3 months in five of nine patients and at 6 months in six of

seven patients. Medication use was reduced in seven of nine patients. Four patients were off medications and three reduced their PPI dosage by at least 50%. One patient complained of nausea at 1 week postplacement, which remained unexplained. In this patient, the prostheses were removed 3 weeks after placement. For this, a repeat endoscopy with an endoscopic ultrasound miniprobe was performed for accurate prosthesis localization (70). With a transparent cap on the tip of the endoscope and using a needle-knife sphincterotome, a 2- to 3-mm mucosal incision was made overlying the prosthesis. The cap was then placed over the prosthesis and, with suction, the prosthesis was removed (71). Long-term data are awaited and a multicenter, prospective trial has been initiated (72).

ENDOSCOPIC IMPLANTATION WITH PLEXIGLAS

Device and Procedure

Inert polymer microspheres made of polymethyl acrylate (PMMA, Plexiglas, Rohm and Haas, Philadelphia, PA) have been used in plastic surgery as tissue expanders without causing tissue reaction or migration. This material, dispersed in gelatin solution, has been injected in the mucosa of the lower esophageal sphincter region in ten patients, aiming at persistent bulking of the gastroesophageal junction barrier (73) (Color Plate 26.12, left). The microspheres resist phagocytosis and do not migrate, thereby providing durability of the effect. Endoscopic ultrasound was used to ensure that particles had not migrated at 6 months (Color Plate 26.12, right). The mean follow-up of patients in that study was 7.2 months, and 70% of patients were off medications at last follow-up. GERD symptoms decreased in frequency and severity in nine of ten patients while the mean time with esophageal pH<4 decreased by two thirds. The procedure has not been approved in the United States, and wide-application or long-term data are lacking.

PER-ORAL ENDOSCOPIC FUNDOPLICATION

Device and Procedure

This procedure involves the invagination and fixation of the gastroesophageal junction, creating a functional nipple valve at the lower esophageal sphincter. Using a special device (Boston Scientific/Microvasive, Natick, MA), the distal esophagus and proximal fundus are grasped, folded, and remodeled to create a valvular structure comparable to that of a Nissen fundoplication (74) (Fig. 26.13A and Color Plate 26.13.B). A small-caliber gastroscope is advanced through the lumen of the grasping device so that the procedure can be performed under endoscopic visualization. Bioabsorbable clips are used to fasten the esophageal and gastric tissue together (75).

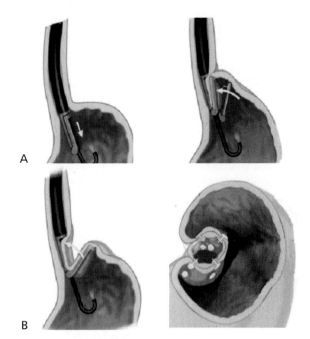

FIGURE 26.13. A: Diagrammatic representation of per oral fun-doplication. (Courtesy of Rodney Mason, M.D.,) **B:** Under direct endoscopic visualization, the gastric mucosa below the GEJ is grasped by the plicator and a full-thickness placation is achieved. (Courtesy of Rodney Mason, M.D., UCLA.)

Clinical Experience

Experience thus far is limited to adult baboons, but the method appears promising.

PRESENT AND FUTURE: A PATIENT-CENTERED APPROACH TO ENDOSCOPIC THERAPIES FOR GERD

In general, the endoscopic therapies should be considered for patients who respond in part to PPIs, but they do not wish to take long-term medication and are considering surgery. In addition, possible candidates are patients who respond partly to PPIs but do not want surgery, patients who are afraid of possible long-term sequelae of PPI therapy, patients with regurgitation not responsive to PPIs who are not yet "ready" for surgery, patients intolerant to PPIs, and possibly patients who have failed fundoplication for GERD.

However, before using them in everyday practice, clinicians need to carefully review the efficacy and safety outcomes of these new therapies. Thus far, studies have been open-label and uncontrolled, with small numbers of subjects studied during the early phases of the learning curve. Almost all studies have been performed in symptomatic patients who are not well controlled on PPIs, but exhibit endoscopically mild, uncomplicated GERD. The feasibility, efficacy, and safety of such therapies in PPI-naïve patients

or patients with complicated GERD, are currently unknown. For example, the use of these techniques in patients with large (>3cm) hiatal hernias or foreshortened esophagus with Barrett's metaplasia may be of limited value or technically impossible. To what degree these therapies will have a role for patients with atypical or extraesophageal manifestations of GERD remains unclear.

Except for the Stretta procedure, no controlled study has yet been performed and future sham-controlled trials will be needed to assess a potential placebo effect. Further, the exact location, configuration, and number of RF treatments, placations, or injections, have not been standardized. Long-term follow-up will be essential to evaluate the cost-effectiveness and durability of these novel approaches compared to medical or surgical therapy. The learning curve for each of these modalities and their respective training requirements need to be defined in order for appropriate credentialing to be established.

Future improvements in device miniaturization and instrumentation will probably eliminate the use of overtubes, minimize endoscope or accessory exchanges, enhance procedure visualization, shorten procedure time, and reduce the need for support personnel. Combination studies may involve augmentation of placations with mucosal cautery, RF with placation, or placation with injection may enhance durability of effect. Repeated "touch-up" procedures and procedures after failed fundoplication may also be considered. Endoscopic therapies have a bright future, as they have opened a new era in the management of GERD and have quickly become a reality.

Disclosure

G. Triadafilopoulos is consultant to almost all major pharmaceutical companies that are active in the area of gastroesophageal reflux. He has received funding for studies, seminars, and travel from such companies and has an equity position in Curon Medical Inc.

REFERENCES

1. Howard PJ, Heading RC. Epidemiology of gastro-esophageal reflux disease. *World J Surg* 1992;16:288–293.
2. Locke GR, Talley NJ, Fett SL, et al. Prevalence and clinical spectrum of gastroesophageal reflux: a population-based study in Olmsted County, Minnesota. *Gastroenterology* 1997;112:1448–1456.
3. Lagergren J, Bergstrom R, Lindgren A, et al. Symptomatic gastro-esophageal reflux as a risk factor for esophageal adenocarcinoma. *N Engl J Med* 1999;340:825–831.
4. Pope CE. Acid reflux disorders. *N Engl J Med* 1995;331:656–660.
5. Richardson WS, Truss TL, Hunter JG. Laparoscopic anti-reflux surgery. *Surg Clin North Am* 1996;76:437–450.
6. Chiba N, DeGara CJ, Wilkinson JM, et al. Speed of healing and symptom relief in grade II–IV gastro-esophageal reflux disease: a meta-analysis. *Gastroenterology* 1997;112:1798–1810.

7. Lundell L, Mietinnen P, Myrvold HE, et al. Continued (5-year) follow-up of a randomized clinical study comparing anti-reflux surgery and omeprazole in gastro-esophageal reflux disease. *J Am Coll Surg* 2001;192:172–179.

8. Peters JH, DeMeester TR, Crookes PA, et al. The treatment of gastro-esophageal reflux with laparoscopic fundoplication: prospective evaluation of 100 consecutive patients with typical symptoms. *Ann Surg* 1998;228:40–50.

9. Spechler SJ, Lee E, Ahnen D, et al. Long-term outcome of medical and surgical therapies for gastro-esophageal reflux disease: follow-up of a randomized controlled trial. *JAMA* 2001;285: 2331–2338.

10. Hogan WJ. Endoscopic treatment modalities for GERD: technologies score or scare? *Gastrointest Endosc* 2001;53:541–545.

11. Lehman G. Endoscopic and endoluminal techniques for control of gastro-esophageal reflux: are they ready for widespread clinical application? *Gastrointest Endosc* 2001;52:808–811.

12. Powell NB, Riley RW, Troell RW, et al. Radiofrequency volumetric tissue reduction of the palate in subjects with sleep-disordered breathing. *Chest* 1998;113:1163–1174.

13. LeVeen H, Wapnick S, Piccone V, et al. Tumor eradication by radiofrequency therapy: response in 21 patients. *JAMA* 1976; 253:2198–2200.

14. Jackman WM, Wang XZ, Friday KJ, et al. Catheter ablation of accessory atrioventricular pathways (Wolff-Parkinson-White syndrome) by radiofrequency current. *N Engl J Med* 1991;324: 1605–1611.

15. Triadafilopoulos G, DiBaise JK, Nostrant TT, et al. Radiofrequency energy delivery to the gastro-esophageal junction for the treatment of GERD. *Gastrointest Endosc* 2001;53:407–415.

16. Utley DS, Kim M, Vierra MA, et al. Augmentation of lower esophageal sphincter pressure and gastric yield pressure after radiofrequency energy delivery to the gastroesophageal junction: a porcine model. *Gastrointest Endosc* 2000;52:81–86.

17. Kim MS, Holloway R, Dent J, et al. Radiofrequency energy (RFe) application to the gastric cardia decreases transient lower esophageal sphincter relaxation (tLESR) frequency in a canine model. *Gastroenterology* 2000;118:A860.

18. Chang KJ, Utley DS. Endoscopic ultrasound (EUS) *in-vivo* assesment of radiofrequency (RF) energy delivery to the gastroesophageal (GE) junction in a porcine model. *Gastrointest Endosc* 2001;53:AB165.

19. Tam WCE, Schoeman MN, Dent J, et al. Control of reflux following radiofrequency energy (RFe) in patients with gastroesophageal reflux disease (GERD): 12 months follow-up. *Gastroenterology* 2002;122:AB387.

20. Noar M, Knight S, Bidlack D. Impaired gastric emptying in GERD patients improved after radiofrequency (RF) energy delivery to the gastroesophageal junction (Stretta procedure). *Gastroenterology* 2002;122:A558.

21. DiBaise JK, Brand RE, Quigley EMM. Endoluminal delivery of radiofrequency energy to the gastro-esophageal junction in uncomplicated GERD: efficacy and potential mechanism of action. *Am J Gastroenterol* 2002;97:833–842.

22. Tam WCE, Schoeman MN, Zhang Q, et al. Delivery of radiofrequency energy (RFe) to the lower esophageal sphincter (LES) and gastric cardia inhibits transient LES relaxations and gastro-esophageal reflux in patients with reflux disease. *Gut* 2003;52 (4):479–485.

23. Martin CJ, Patrikios J, Dent J. Abolition of gas reflux and transient lower esophageal sphincter relaxation by vagal blockade in the dog. *Gastroenterology* 1986;91:890–896.

24. Triadafilopoulos G, DiBaise JK, Nostrant TT, et al. The Stretta procedure for the treatment of GERD: 6 and 12 month follow-up of the U.S. open label trial. *Gastrointest Endosc* 2002;55: 149–156.

25. Corley DA, Katz P, Wo J, et al. Temperature-controlled radiofrequency energy delivery to the gastro-esophageal junction for the treatment of GERD (the Stretta Procedure): a randomized, double-blind, sham-controlled, multi-center clinical trial. *Gastrointest Endosc* 2002;55:AB19.

26. Wolfsen HC. Stretta Procedure Patient Registry: GERD symptom scores, patient satisfaction and medication use in 590 patients. *Gastrointest Endosc* 2002;55:AB113.

27. Houston H, Khaitan L, Scholze S, et al. First year experience of patients undergoing the Stretta procedure: follow-up of 60 patients. *Surg Endosc* 2002;16:S004.

28. Reymunde A, Santiago N. The Stretta procedure is an effective alternative to long-term PPI therapy for patients with GERD: clinical experience after 82 consecutive procedures. *Am J Gastroenterol* 2001;96:S34.

29. Mansell DE. Extended follow-up in patients treated with the Stretta procedure: a report on 29 patients. *Gastrointest Endosc* 2002;55:AB194.

30. Noar MD, Igari Y, Mulock D, et al. The large hiatal hernia and failed Nissen fundoplication: initial report of successful treatment using modified radiofrequency ablation (Stretta) technique. *Am J Gastroenterol* 96:2001;S27.

31. Gersin K, Fanelli R. The Stretta procedure: Review of catheter and technique evolution, efficacy and complications 2 years after introduction. *Surg Endosc* 2002;16(suppl 1):PF199.

32. Swain CP, Brown GJ, Mills TN. An endoscopic stapling device: the development of a new flexible endoscopically controlled device for placing multiple trans-mural staples in gastrointestinal tissue. *Gastrointest Endosc* 1989;35:338.

33. Swain CP, Kadirkamanathan SS, Gong F, et al. Knot tying at flexible endoscopy. *Gastrointest Endosc* 1994;40:722.

34. Kadirkamanathan SS, Evans DF, Gong F, et al. Anti-reflux operations at flexible endoscopy using endo-luminal stitching techniques: an experimental study. *Gastrointest Endosc* 1996;44:133.

35. Swain P, Park PO, Kjellin T, et al. Endoscopic gastroplasty for gastro-esophageal reflux disease. *Gastroint Endosc* 2000;51: AB144.

36. Lehman GA, Dunne DP, Hieston K, et al. Suturing placation of cardia with EndoCinch device: effect of supplemental cautery. A human prospective randomized trial. *Gastrointest Endosc* 2002; 55:AB260(abst).

37. Kadirkamanathan SS, Yazaki E, Evans DF, et al. An ambulant porcine model of acid reflux used to evaluate endoscopic gastroplasty. *Gut* 1999;44:782.

38. Rothstein, RI, Moodie, K. Depth of endoscopically placed sutures. *Gastrointest Endosc* 2000;51:102(abst).

39. Filipi CJ, Lehman GA, Rothstein RI, et al. Trans-oral, flexible endoscopic suturing for treatment of GERD: a multi-center trial. *Gastrointest Endosc* 2001;53:416–422.

40. Swain CP, Park PO, Kjellin T, et al. Endoscopic gastroplasty for the treatment of gastro-esophageal reflux disease. *Gastrointest Endosc* 2001;51:144.

41. Raijman I, Ben-Menachem T, Reddy G, et al. Symptomatic response to endoluminal gastroplication (ELGP) in patients with gastro-esophageal reflux disease (GERD): a multi-center experience. *Gastrointest Endosc* 2001;53:AB74.

42. Patel VM. Clinical utility of endoluminal gastroplication for gastro-esophageal reflux disease in private practice—a prospective study of 55 patients in the Southwest. *Am J Gastroenterol* 2001; 96:S89(abst).

43. Maple JT, Alexander JA, Gostout CJ, et al. Endoscopic gastroplasty for GERD: not as good as billed? A single-center, 6-month report. *Am J Gastroenterol* 2001;96:S22.

44. Rothstein RI, Pohl H, Grove M, et al. Endoscopic gastric placation for the treatment of GERD: two-year follow-up results. *Am J Gastroenterol* 2001;96:S107(abst).

45. Haber GB, Marcon NE, Kortan P, et al. A 2-year follow-up of 25 patients undergoing endoluminal gastric placation (ELGP) for gastro-esophageal reflux disease (GERD). *Gastrointest Endosc* 2000;53:116(abst).

46. Arts J, Slootmaekers S, Sifrim D, et al. Endoluminal gastroplication (EndoCinch) in GERD patients refractory to PPI therapy. *Gastroenterology* 2002;122:A47(abst).

47. Liu JJ, Knapp R, Carr-Lock DL. Treatment of medication refractory gastro-esophageal reflux disease with endoluminal gastroplication. *Gastrointest Endosc* 2002;55:AB257(abst).

48. Mahmood Z, Byrne PJ, McCullough J, et al. A comparison of BARD EndoCinch trans-esophageal endoscopic placation (BETEP) with laparoscopic Nissen fundoplication (LNF) for the treatment of gastro-esophageal reflux disease (GORD). *Gastrointest Endosc* 2002;55:AB90.

49. Raijman I, Ben-Menachem T, Sterol AA, et al. Endo-luminal gastroplication (ELGP) improves GERD symptoms in patients with large hiatal hernias. *Gastrointest Endosc* 2002;55:AB255(abst).

50. Chuttani R, Kozarek R, Polavaram V, et al. A novel endoscopic full thickness plicator for the treatment of GERD: efficacy in an ex-vivo porcine model. *Gastrointest Endosc* 2001;53:132.

51. Chuttani R, Kozarek R, Lo J, et al. A novel endoscopic full thickness plicator for the treatment of GERD: demonstration of safety in pigs. *Gastrointest Endosc* 2001;53:2241.

52. Chuttani R, Kozarek R, Sachdev R, et al. A novel endoscopic full thickness plicator for the treatment of GERD: early clinical results. *Endoscopy* 2001;33S:2200.

53. Chuttani R, Sud R, Sachdev G, et al. Endoscopic full-thickness plication for GERD: Final results of human pilot study. *Gastrointest Endosc* 2002;55:AB258.

54. O'Connor KW, Madison SA, Smith DJ, et al. An experimental endoscopic technique for reversing gastro-esophageal reflux in dogs by injecting inert material in the distal esophagus. *Gastrointest Endosc* 1984;31:275–280.

55. O'Connor KW, Lehman GA. Endoscopic placement of collagen at the lower esophageal sphincter to inhibit gastro-esophageal reflux: a pilot study of 10 medically intractable patients. *Gastrointest Endosc* 1988;34:106–112.

56. Mason RJ, Hughes M, Lehman GA, et al. Endoscopic augmentation of the cardia with a biocompatible injectable polymer (Enteryx) in a porcine model. *Surg Endosc* 2002;16:386–391.

57. Deviere J, Wustenberg W, Hook G, et al. A transgenic mouse model for carcinogenicity testing of Enteryx—an implantable biopolymer for treatment of GERD. Paper presented at 9th United European Gastroenterology Week, October 2001.

58. Deviere J, Pastorelli A, Louis H, et al. Endoscopic implantation of a biopolymer in the lower esophageal sphincter for gastroesophageal reflux: a pilot study. *Gastrointest Endosc* 2002;55:335–341.

59. Elahi MM, Parnes LS, Fox AJ, et al. Therapeutic embolization in the management of neck para-gangliomas. *Laryngoscope* 1997;107:821.

60. Emmett JR. Plasti-pore implants in middle ear surgery. *Otolaryngol Clin North Am* 1995;28:265.

61. Dickman CA, Papadopoulos SM, Crawford NR, et al. Comparative mechanical properties of spinal cable and wire fixation systems. *Spine* 1997;22:596.

62. Swanson BN. Medical use of dimethyl sulfoxide (DMSO). *Rev Clin Basic Pharmacol* 1985;5:1–33.

63. Levi J. Percutaneous recanalization of iliac artery occlusions with the Strecker stent. *Cardiovasc Surg* 1998;39:287.

64. Bobyn JD, Toh KK, Hacking SA, et al. Tissue response to porous tantalum acetabular cups. *J Arthroplasty* 1999;14:347.

65. Lehman GA, Deviere J, Haber G, et al. Lower esophageal sphincter (LES) augmentation therapy for GERD with Enteryx, a biocompatible inert polymer. Initial multi-center human trial results. *Gastrointest Endosc* 2001;53:AB123.

66. Johnson DA, Aisenberg J, Cohen L, et al. Enteryx solution, a minimally invasive injectable treatment for GERD: initial multi-center human trial results. *Am J Gastroenterol* 2001;96:S17.

67. Fockens P, Bruno MJ, et al. Pilot study of the Gatekeeper Reflux Repair System in patients with GERD. *Gastrointest Endosc* 2002;55:AB257.

68. Easter DW, Yurek M, Summers H, et al. Endoscopic prosthesis augmentation of the lower esophageal sphincter in swine. *Am J Surg* 2001;182:697–701.

69. Fockens P, Bruno MJ, Hirsch DP, et al. Endoscopic augmentation of the lower esophageal sphincter. Pilot study of the Gatekeeper system in patients with gastro-esophageal reflux disease. *Am J Gastroenterol* 2001;96S:37.

70. Fockens P, Bruno MJ, Hirsch DP, et al. Endoscopic augmentation of the lower esophageal sphincter. Pilot study of the Gatekeeper Reflux Repair System in patients with GERD. Paper presented at Digestive Disease Week conference, San Francisco, CA, May 19–22, 2002.

71. Fockens P, Bruno MJ, Boeckxstaens GE, et al. Endoscopic removal of the Gatekeeper Reflux Repair System prosthesis. Paper presented at Digestive Disease Week conference, San Francisco, CA, May 19–22, 2002.

72. Lehman G, Watkins JL, Hieston K, et al. Endoscopic gastroesophageal reflux disease (GERD) therapy with Gatekeeper System. Initiation of a multicenter prospective randomized trial. Paper presented at Digestive Disease Week conference, San Francisco, CA, May 19–22, 2002.

73. Feretis C, Benakis P, Dimopoulos C, et al. Endoscopic implantation of Plexiglass (PMMA) micro-spheres for the treatment of GERD. *Gastrointest Endosc* 2001;53:423–426.

74. Mason RJ, Filipi CJ, DeMeester TR, et al. A new intra-luminal anti-reflux procedure. *Gastrointest Endoscopy* 1997;45:283–290.

75. Mason RJ, DeMeester TR, Schurr MO, et al. Per oral endoscopic Nissen fundoplication: The introduction of a new era. *Gastrointest Endosc* 2001;53:AB74.

BARRETT'S ESOPHAGUS

PRATEEK SHARMA
RICHARD E. SAMPLINER

Barrett's esophagus is the premalignant lesion for adenocarcinoma of the esophagus and the esophagogastric junction. The incidence of esophageal adenocarcinoma is rapidly rising and has increased by five- to eight-fold over the last 2 decades (1,2). This has led to an increased awareness of the premalignant lesion with emphasis on screening, surveillance, and treatment, with the ultimate goal of having an impact on mortality from this rapidly rising incidence cancer. Barrett's esophagus occurs in patients with chronic gastroesophageal reflux (GER) symptoms, and the role of acid and bile reflux in the development of Barrett's esophagus has been the subject of many animal and human studies. The traditional definition of Barrett's esophagus or long-segment Barrett's esophagus (LSBE) was arbitrarily an abnormal-appearing columnar mucosa extending for a minimum of 3 cm proximal to the gastroesophageal junction. With the observation that even shorter lengths of intestinal metaplasia could be associated with dysplasia and adenocarcinoma, the term short-segment Barrett's esophagus (SSBE) was developed (3).

DEFINITION AND DIAGNOSIS

The definition and concept of Barrett's esophagus have undergone significant changes from its initial description to the present time where most of the data suggest that it is an acquired disorder caused by reflux of gastroduodenal contents into the distal esophagus. Norman Barrett (4) described autopsy cases of esophageal ulcers surrounded by columnar mucosa and suggested that the ulcers developed in the stomach, which was displaced proximally. Later in 1953, Allison and Johnstone (5) published a paper describing in detail seven cases of a columnar-lined lower esophagus. All these patients had erosive esophagitis and a hiatal

hernia, suggesting that "Barrett's ulcers" might be a consequence of chronic GER.

The presence of a columnar lined distal esophagus of any length, with intestinal metaplasia, characterized by acid mucin-containing goblet cells using combined hematoxylin and eosin-alcian blue pH 2.5 stain is defined as Barrett's esophagus (6). Since the columnar lining should be present in the esophagus, that is, above the gastroesophageal junction (GEJ), it is important to recognize the GEJ. A commonly used landmark for recognizing the GEJ is a pinch at the end of the tubular esophagus that coincides with the proximal margin of the gastric folds (7). Careful identification of the GEJ can potentially prevent inadvertent biopsy of the gastric cardia (i.e., distal to the GEJ), and the incorrect labeling of a patient with Barrett's esophagus who in fact may have cardia intestinal metaplasia (8). Routine histopathologic techniques are unable to distinguish between intestinal metaplasia originating in the stomach, a normal GEJ, or the gastric cardia.

PATHOPHYSIOLOGY

Barrett's esophagus is an acquired condition resulting from severe esophageal mucosal injury. However, it still remains unclear why some patients with gastroesophageal reflux disease (GERD) develop Barrett's esophagus whereas others do not. The current hypothesis is that Barrett's mucosa develops from pleuropotential stem cells, which are present in the basal layer of the esophageal mucosa. Barrett's esophagus seems to be an acquired lesion since the prevalence is very low in childhood and increases with age, confirming that this lesion is acquired and not congenital.

A major advance in the understanding of the pathogenesis of Barrett's esophagus and the importance of GER is from an experiment by Bremner et al. (9) showing that regeneration of esophageal mucosa after severe mucosal injury from chronic GER in dogs occurred with columnar rather than squamous mucosa (9). In humans, clinical stud-

---

P. Sharma: University of Kansas School of Medicine, Kansas City, Missouri; and Veterans Affairs Medical Center, Kansas City, Missouri.

R.E. Sampliner: University of Arizona College of Medicine, Tucson, Arizona; and Southern Arizona VA Health Care System, Tucson, Arizona.

ies have confirmed the presence of severe GER in patients with Barrett's esophagus characterized by decreased lower esophageal sphincter (LES) pressure and delayed esophageal acid clearance, as well as increase in the frequency and duration of esophageal acid exposure. In addition, patients with Barrett's esophagus have frequently associated hiatal hernias and ineffective peristalsis leading to defective clearance of the refluxed gastric contents (10,11). Recent studies have also shown the extent of columnar metaplasia to be related to the severity of GER and inversely to the LES pressure (12). There is no convincing evidence that patients with GERD and Barrett's secrete abnormally high gastric acid or pepsin compared to controls (13). The duration of reflux symptoms appears to be longer in patients with Barrett's than those without Barrett's esophagus. Hirota et al. (14) reported the mean duration of reflux symptoms in patients with SSBE was 3.5 years, compared to 20 years in those with LSBE.

The presence of Barrett's esophagus in patients with achlorhydria and postgastrectomy states has suggested a possible role of duodenal contents in its pathogenesis. Although commonly referred to as bile reflux, reflux of duodenal contents contains more than just bile; therefore, the term "duodenal gastroesophageal reflux" (DGER) has been proposed (15). Reflux of acid parallels DGER and both have been shown to be significantly higher in patients with Barrett's esophagus compared to controls and to GERD patients without Barrett's esophagus (16,17). Thus, both gastric and duodenal contents mix together and reflux into the esophagus in an acid environment. However, the individual contributions and influences of acid, pepsin, bile, and other duodenal contents in patients with Barrett's esophagus remain to be determined.

Studies have shown that relatives of patients with Barrett's esophagus and also relatives of patients with esophageal adenocarcinoma have reflux symptoms two to three times more commonly than controls (18). Also, individuals with Barrett's esophagus and esophageal adenocarcinoma are more likely to have a positive family history of Barrett's esophagus or esophageal adenocarcinoma than individuals without Barrett's esophagus (19). Studies are currently underway to identify a "Barrett's gene."

EPIDEMIOLOGY

The mean age of diagnosis of Barrett's esophagus is approximately 60 years and it is rarely detected in children. From Mayo Clinic data, only one of 679 patients aged 10 to 19 years was diagnosed with Barrett's esophagus and none aged <10 years had Barrett's esophagus (20). Hassal (21) reported the youngest proven case at age 7, and even this childhood condition was acquired and associated with GERD (21). Barrett's esophagus is primarily detected in Caucasians; the

reason for this predominance is not clear. Even in a large black population in South Africa, only 5% of the Barrett's esophagus cohorts were black (22). Barrett's esophagus and adenocarcinoma are rare in the Asian population, and Barrett's esophagus is uncommon outside of North America, Europe, and Australia. It is detected in 0.1% to 0.3% of upper endoscopies in Japan (as opposed to 1% in the United States), and this difference between Eastern and Western populations may be due to differences in the prevalence of GERD (23). For example, in Singapore the prevalence of heartburn in adults is 1.6% (on a monthly basis) compared to 29% to 44% in the Western countries (24).

Both European as well as U.S. studies have reported that the prevalence of Barrett's esophagus is higher in males than in females. The ratio has been documented to vary from 2 to 3 (males) to 1 female (20). The gender ratio for esophageal adenocarcinoma is much higher, at 8:1 (male:female). Thus, Barrett's esophagus appears to be more prevalent in Caucasians, males, and the developed countries.

INCREASING INCIDENCE OF ESOPHAGEAL ADENOCARCINOMA

Patients with Barrett's esophagus have an increased risk of 30 to 125 times of developing esophageal adenocarcinoma compared to the general population. Recent studies from the United States have suggested an incidence of cancer of about 1 in 200 patient years of follow-up (25). Esophageal adenocarcinomas now account for over 50% of esophageal cancers in many reports. Population-based studies from the United States and Western Europe have shown a dramatic increase in the incidence of adenocarcinoma starting in the 1970s to the early 1990s. The exact etiology for this rising incidence is unclear and whether there has been a true increase in the prevalence of Barrett's esophagus is unclear.

GER symptoms have been identified as a risk factor for esophageal adenocarcinoma. Lagergren et al. (26) showed that the more frequent, severe, and long-lasting the symptoms of reflux, the greater the risk for esophageal adenocarcinoma (26). A similar association between adenocarcinoma and GERD symptom duration and frequency has been confirmed in other studies (27). There is increasing evidence of an association between body mass index (BMI) and esophageal adenocarcinoma (28,29). Chow et al. (28) found that BMI was related to an increasing incidence of esophageal adenocarcinoma. The odds ratio for obesity was 2.9 times greater in the heaviest 25% of the population compared to the lightest. Dietary and environmental issues implicated include smoking, and a diet low in fresh fruit (30–32). Gammon et al. (32) reported that the odds ratio for current smoking was 2.2 times greater and for ex-smokers was 2.0 times greater in the cancer cases compared to controls. These authors concluded that smoking could account for 40% of adenocarcinomas and the increased risk persisted up to 30 years after quitting smoking. Drugs that lower LES pressure have also been implicated for such an effect, whereas use of antisecretory medicine does not appear to increase cancer risk (33,34). A protective effect of *Helicobacter pylori* has been suggested as an alternative hypothesis to explain the increasing incidence of this cancer. The incidence of GERD and esophageal adenocarcinoma has increased in recent years, whereas the incidence of *H. pylori*–associated peptic ulcer disease and distal gastric adenocarcinomas has declined. This suggests an inverse relationship between *H. pylori* infection and esophageal disease. Recent studies suggest that infection with *H. pylori*, especially *cagA* strains may protect against the development of Barrett's esophagus dysplasia and adenocarcinoma (35). All the abovementioned factors associated with esophageal adenocarcinoma may also be linked to the development of Barrett's esophagus; but have not yet been well explored.

SCREENING FOR BARRETT'S ESOPHAGUS

Why should we consider screening for Barrett's esophagus? The rationale for diagnosing Barrett's esophagus is driven by population-based studies documenting the association of reflux symptoms with adenocarcinoma of the esophagus and the continuing rising incidence of this cancer (1,2,26). The recognition of Barrett's esophagus and the appropriate treatment for high-grade dysplasia and early cancer may offer the opportunity to improve the survival from a high mortality cancer. Early diagnosis of esophageal adenocarcinoma is critical, given the high likelihood of lymphatic metastasis due to the rich lymphatic supply of the esophagus that extends into the lamina propria. Lymph node metastases may be found in up to 5% of intramucosal carcinoma and up to 24% of submucosal cancers (36). Furthermore, <5% of esophageal adenocarcinomas are diagnosed in patients without a prior diagnosis of Barrett's esophagus (37). The only hope for improved survival of patients with esophageal adenocarcinoma is its detection at an early and potentially curable stage.

Who should we consider screening for Barrett's esophagus? Compared to GERD patients without Barrett's esophagus, Barrett's patients develop reflux symptoms at an earlier age, and have an increased duration of symptoms and increased severity of nocturnal reflux symptoms (38). A community-based study by Lieberman et al. (39) found that compared to patients with reflux symptoms for <1 year, Barrett's esophagus (suspected, that is, not biopsy proven) was five times more common if symptom duration was 5 to 10 years, and 6.4 times more common if symptom duration was >10 years (39). Thus, selectively screening older white

patients with long-standing GERD symptoms is a reasonable approach, but the precise threshold criteria for screening have not been determined. Published guidelines recommend screening for Barrett's esophagus in patients at highest risk for this condition: white men, aged ≥50 years, with long-standing reflux symptoms (40).

Should we even screen for Barrett's esophagus? There are no controlled trials examining the clinical utility or cost-effectiveness of screening for Barrett's esophagus, and screening for Barrett's esophagus has not yet been proven to alter outcomes of this disease. GERD symptoms are highly prevalent in the adult population and using current endoscopic techniques, screening the entire population will probably not be cost-effective. Moreover, the prevalence of Barrett's in patients without GERD may be similar to those as a GERD population (41). Therefore, limiting screening to supposed "high-risk" populations cannot be completely justified based on currently available data and is of unproven value.

What issues need to be addressed in the future? The major issue that should be addressed is whether screening for Barrett's esophagus has an impact on the mortality from esophageal adenocarcinoma. In brief, will screening improve outcomes and is it cost-effective? Endoscopy with biopsy is the only validated technique to diagnose Barrett's esophagus. However, it has clear limitations as a screening tool, considering cost, risk, and complexity. The ideal characteristics of a screening tool include high sensitivity and specificity, low risk to patients, ease of performance, and low cost. Currently, there are no validated alternative techniques to screen for Barrett's esophagus that overcome the cost and risks associated with endoscopy. Future goals are screening a large population for this premalignant lesion at low cost and minimal risk.

Unsedated endoscopy utilizing small-caliber endoscopes is well tolerated, causes minimal discomfort to the patient, can potentially lower costs, and has a high sensitivity and specificity for identifying Barrett's esophagus (42,43). Pilot studies have demonstrated the feasibility of using this technique and if validated further, screening for Barrett's esophagus can potentially be accomplished in an office setting, without the use of sedation, and with acceptable accuracy and safety. Recent data suggest that methylene blue spraying in the distal esophagus can help aid the identification of areas of intestinal metaplasia, which can then be targeted for biopsy (44,45). Use of techniques that combine spraying of vital stains in the distal esophagus, along with a zoom endoscope to demonstrate specific mucosal patterns, may also be of value (46). A variety of endoscopic optical techniques, including spectroscopy, optical coherence tomography, and light-induced fluorescence endoscopy have the potential to obtain "real-time" biopsies of Barrett's esophagus (47–49). Mass screening with balloon cytology is well described in China for the detection of esophageal squamous cell carcinoma/dysplasia; preliminary results using this technique in patients with Barrett's esophagus have been promising for the detection of high-grade dysplasia, but the yield for intestinal metaplasia was lower (50). Another new nonendoscopic technique can optically recognize the proximally displaced squamocolumnar junction, but needs further validation before it can be used in the clinical setting (51). Finally, advances in family and genetic studies could also lead to a simple blood test for the detection of Barrett's esophagus.

SURVEILLANCE OF BARRETT'S ESOPHAGUS

The concept of surveillance endoscopy in Barrett's esophagus is driven by a number of assumptions.

- Barrett's esophagus is a premalignant disease for adenocarcinoma of the esophagus.
- The incidence of adenocarcinoma of the esophagus is increasing.
- Dysplasia precedes the development of adenocarcinoma of the esophagus.
- Intervention for dysplasia or early adenocarcinoma will impact the survival of patients with Barrett's esophagus.

Not all patients with adenocarcinoma have Barrett's esophagus documented before or after the development of cancer. In fact, <5% of patients presenting with adenocarcinoma have a prior diagnosis of Barrett's esophagus (52,53). In one population-based study with histology available in 97% of cases, 38% of adenocarcinoma cases had no detectable Barrett's esophagus (26). Yet, adenocarcinoma may overgrow a preexisting Barrett's esophagus. This possibility is supported by the finding of Barrett's esophagus more commonly in shorter adenocarcinoma of the esophagogastric junction than in more extensive cancer (54). The sequence of progression from intestinal metaplasia, to low-grade dysplasia, to high-grade dysplasia, and subsequently adenocarcinoma of the esophagus is well recognized. Yet, a significant subgroup of patients progress to adenocarcinoma without high-grade dysplasia having been documented (55,56).

INCIDENCE OF ADENOCARCINOMA

A more accurate estimate of the incidence of adenocarcinoma in patients with Barrett's esophagus is emerging. A large prospective cohort and a registry of Barrett's esophagus each demonstrated a lower incidence than previously observed—0.5% and 0.4% per year, respectively (57,58). A funnel diagram analysis of reports of cancer risk suggested a publication bias—selective reporting of higher cancer risks (59). The point of the funnel was a 0.5% incidence per patient year, which supported the referenced series.

RATIONALE FOR SURVEILLANCE

It is a matter of faith that early intervention for cancer will result in better survival. However, only a small percent of patients with Barrett's esophagus die of adenocarcinoma—2.5% in one series of 155 patients followed a mean of 9.3 years without surveillance endoscopy (60). In a smaller retrospective study, only 9% and 1% of patients with Barrett's esophagus developed adenocarcinoma in those with and without surveillance, respectively (61). In contrast, retrospective surgical series suggest that patients with Barrett's esophagus undergoing surveillance endoscopy have early-stage cancer with better survival than patients presenting with both adenocarcinoma and Barrett's esophagus (62–66). Additionally, two cohort studies with 23 patients and 49 patients with prior Barrett's esophagus documented earlier-stage disease and improved survival in patients with a prior endoscopic diagnosis of Barrett's esophagus (67,68), suggesting that endoscopy offered the opportunity for intervening in earlier-stage disease.

Given the above controversy and the lack of prospective data, it may seem surprising that two surveys of gastroenterologists showed that 96% perform endoscopic surveillance (69,70). However, agreement on the frequency of endoscopy, the technique of biopsy, and the histologic threshold for clinical intervention is far from complete. Even 18 months after the publication of practice guidelines for the management of Barrett's esophagus, only 55% of gastroenterologists were aware of them, and practice in accordance with the guidelines rose from only 27% to 38% (71).

SURVEILLANCE INTERVALS

The endoscopy and biopsy surveillance intervals are driven by the grade of dysplasia. Dysplasia is a microscopic change in cell cytology and glandular architecture that is the first step in the neoplastic process. The time interval of progression from one grade of dysplasia to another is difficult to determine. The interval in only 31 patients can be gleaned from six prospective trials (ten patients are included twice in the low-grade dysplasia [LGD] to cancer and the high-grade dysplasia [HGD] to cancer) (55,72–75). These are from a total of 1613 patients followed for a mean of 2.9 to 7.3 years. Table 27.1 shows that the mean interval for Barrett's progression is years; however, the range is broad and the lower limit of the time frame is from 0.2 to 2.5 years. In the older series, the definition of Barrett's esophagus was 3 cm to 5 cm of columnar epithelium, and intestinal metaplasia was not present in all patients (72,74). Four-quadrant biopsies were not necessarily performed (72,73).

The surveillance intervals for different grades of dysplasia should be determined by the time and risk of progression. There are inadequate data on the time and risk of progression for patients with dysplasia. There is information

TABLE 27.1. TIME COURSE OF PROGRESSION OF DYSPLASIA (YEARS)

	n	Range	Mean
IM → HGD	4	2.5–4.5	3.3
IM → Ca	6	1–8.5	5.7
LGD → Ca	15	1–9.6	4.3
HGD → Ca	16	0.2–10	3.0

Ca, cancer; HGD, high-grade dysplasia; IM, intestinal metaplasia; LGD, low-grade dysplasia.
Sources: Schnell TG, Sontag SJ, Chejfec G, et al. Long-term nonsurgical management of Barrett's esophagus with high-grade dysplasia. *Gastroenterology* 2001;120:1607–1619; Robertson CS, Mayberry JF, Nicholson DA, et al. Value of endoscopic surveillance in the detection of neoplastic change in Barrett's oesophagus. *Br J Surg* 1988;75:760–763; Hammeetman W, Tytgat JN, Houthoff HJ, et al. Barrett's esophagus: development of dysplasia and adenocarcinoma. *Gastroenterology* 1989;69:1249–1256; Miros M, Kerlin MM, Walker N. Only patients with dysplasia progress to adenocarcinoma in Barrett's oesophagus. *Gut* 1991;32:1441–1446; Reid B, Levine D, Longton G, et al. Predictors of progression to cancer in Barrett's esophagus: baseline histology and flow cytometry identify low- and high-risk patient subsets. *Am J Gastroenterol* 2000;95:1669–1676.

from larger numbers of patients that HGD has a risk of progressing to cancer that is a multiple of the progression of no dysplasia or LGD (40). The suggested intervals represent an empiric working approach that will need to be altered based on emerging data. The recommended intervals of surveillance are lengthening, although practice fails to keep up with even the conservative recommendations (71).

The sampling of the surface of Barrett's esophagus remains a major challenge. Only 15% to 17% of gastroenterologists use large-capacity biopsy forceps (70,71). The majority do perform four-quadrant biopsies. The median surface area of 30 patients undergoing esophagectomy without visible cancer is informative: Barrett's esophagus, 32 sq cm; LGD, 13 sq cm; HGD, 1.3 sq cm; and adenocarcinoma, 1.1 sq cm (76). This decreasing area of distribution of higher-risk lesions contributes to the sampling problem.

Because HGD and cancer are often focal, two endoscopies are recommended to classify the patient's highest grade of dysplasia. The updated American College of Gastroenterology guidelines recommend a 3-year interval between surveillance endoscopies in patients with no dysplasia after two endoscopic evaluations (40). If LGD is the highest grade after two evaluations, then annual endoscopy until no dysplasia is found is recommended. If HGD is present, assuming no mucosal irregularities, then a repeat endoscopy within 3 months is necessary to rule out cancer. If mucosal irregularities are present, an endoscopic mucosal resection is appropriate to ensure the absence of cancer, or if cancer is present in the specimen, to more accurately stage it (77,78). In the absence of cancer, HGD can be assessed as focal versus diffuse (79). Diffuse HGD has 3.7 times the risk of cancer as focal. The treatment options for HGD are discussed below.

The cost-effectiveness of surveillance is sensitive to the incidence of esophageal adenocarcinoma in patients with Barrett's esophagus, the health-related quality of life following intervention, and the accuracy of the diagnosis (HGD and/or cancer) (80). Accurate risk stratification of patients, that is, identifying those at highest risk of developing cancer, would reduce the number of patients requiring surveillance. Both risk stratification and accuracy of diagnosis could be enhanced by the use of validated biomarkers.

BIOMARKERS FOR RISK STRATIFICATION

Many biomarkers—proliferation indices, growth factors, flow cytometry abnormalities, and genetic mutations—have been assessed in relation to progression to cancer. Most studies evaluate the marker in a series of patients or biopsies with the spectrum of dysplasia: none, LGD, HGD, and adenocarcinoma. One center has studied markers in a large prospective cohort of patients with Barrett's esophagus in relation to the clinically important outcome of cancer. In 322 Barrett's esophagus patients, the relative risk of cancer with increased 4N by-flow cytometry (7.5×) or aneuploidy (abnormal cell DNA content, 5×) was significantly greater than in patients without flow abnormalities (81). The cumulative cancer incidence at 5 years was 0 in patients with negative, indefinite, or LGD, lacking flow cytometric abnormalities. Confirming this predictive value would enable the extension of surveillance in patients with LGD and no-flow cytometric abnormalities to 5 years. In 269 patients from the same cohort, 17p (*p53*) loss of heterozygosity identified patients with a 3-year cumulative incidence of cancer of 38% versus 3.3% in patients with two 17p alleles (82). This genetic mutation offers another possible stratification factor.

THERAPY FOR BARRETT'S ESOPHAGUS

The goals of therapy for patients with Barrett's esophagus include the control of reflux symptoms and the healing of erosive esophagitis. The prevention of adenocarcinoma is the ultimate goal of Barrett's esophagus therapy. To date the only intervention with evidence documenting decreased development of cancer is photodynamic therapy.

Medical Therapy

On average, patients with Barrett's esophagus have greater esophageal acid exposure than other reflux patients (10). Proton pump inhibitors (PPIs) are the mainstay treatment for Barrett's esophagus. Although successful in controlling heartburn, regurgitation may remain a problem (83). Dose escalation may be necessary to control symptoms (84). Even bid dosing in patients with Barrett's esophagus does not reduce esophageal acid exposure to normal in 25% of patients (85,86).

With the introduction of PPI there was an expectation that acid reduction might lead to regression of Barrett's esophagus. However, in 100 patients with Barrett's esophagus treated for 12 to 68 months with 20 mg to 80 mg of omeprazole per day or 60 mg of lansoprazole, only three patients reportedly had complete reversal of Barrett's esophagus (87–91). Squamous islands are commonly seen in the Barrett's esophagus, but intestinal metaplasia may underlie these (92), leading to questions about whether islands represent true regression.

The abovementioned studies used fixed doses of PPIs and a minority of patients had esophageal pH exposure assessed. In the PPI arm of one trial, 26 patients were treated with omeprazole 40 mg bid for 2 years (91). The percent pH<4 during 24 hours was 0.1. There was an observed 6% decrease from baseline in length and 8% in estimated area of Barrett's. Squamous islands were not measured as part of the area of Barrett's mucosa, potentially exaggerating the impact of therapy. These statistically significant but minor changes were accomplished in patients whose reflux symptoms could be controlled with ranitidine 150 mg bid alone or in combination with cisipride 10 mg qid.

If long-term PPI therapy does not lead to clinically important regression, perhaps it can prevent neoplastic progression. Barrett's patients with symptom relief and normal esophageal pH on PPI have a significant decrease in proliferation as measured by proliferating cell nuclear antigen and increased villin expression in contrast to unchanged proliferation and villin expression in a group with symptom control but abnormal esophageal pH (93). Although this may infer a reduction in dysplasia, it has not been documented. In a retrospective study, PPI therapy was associated with significantly lower expression levels of key cell-cycle proteins—cyclin D1 and E (94). In contrast, another report suggested that acid suppression therapy only reduced oxidative DNA damage in patients lacking the *p53* mutation (95). The ultimate impact of acid reduction on the molecular biology of Barrett's esophagus awaits the clarification of future studies.

Surgical Therapy

The surgical therapy of Barrett's esophagus includes antireflux surgery for symptom control and resectional surgery for HGD and/or adenocarcinoma. Laparoscopic antireflux surgery is an option for patients with Barrett's esophagus. It can provide excellent symptom relief equivalent to results in patients without Barrett's esophagus (96). There may be a higher failure rate requiring a redo procedure (97). Even in the hands of experts, recurrent symptoms developed in 20% of patients at a median follow-up of 5 years (98). Postoperative esophageal pH monitoring was abnormal in a similar percentage of patients.

In spite of excellent short-term symptomatic results, antireflux surgery does not prevent the progression to neoplasia. Continuation of surveillance endoscopy remains necessary (99,100). The lack of impact on progression of neoplasia is most dramatically indicated in a retrospective Swedish population-based study. The incidence of esophageal adenocarcinoma in male patients treated medically for GERD was sixfold that of the general population. In male patients undergoing antireflux surgery the rate was 14-fold (101). These risk estimates were based on more than 196,000 and 49,000 person-years of follow-up, respectively, for the medical and surgical groups. Unfortunately, endoscopic data were not available, so the contribution of Barrett's esophagus is unknown. However, a literature meta-analysis shows that patients with documented Barrett's esophagus with antireflux surgery had the same incidence of adenocarcinoma as in medically treated patients with Barrett's esophagus (102).

Although the threshold for undergoing esophagectomy in patients with Barrett's esophagus remains controversial, the majority of gastroenterologists recommend this procedure for patients with HGD (70,71). The relationship of hospital volume to operative mortality for esophagectomy is so dramatic that it cannot be overlooked (103). In high-volume hospitals (more than six esophagectomies per year) the mortality was 3.4% versus 17.3% in low-volume hospitals. In a recent confirmatory study, "very high" volume hospitals had an operative mortality for esophagectomy of 8% versus 23% for "very low" volume hospitals (104).

Endoscopic Therapy

Innovations over the past decade have demonstrated that Barrett's esophagus can be reversed by a combination of endoscopic therapy aimed at injuring the Barrett's and acid reduction therapy using PPI or antireflux surgery (105,106). Such a reversal had not been systematically accomplished by medical or surgical therapy. Specifically, when using photodynamic therapy (PDT) with porfimer sodium as the photosensitizer, there is preliminary evidence documenting reduction in the development of adenocarcinoma in patients with HGD (107). This reduction of cancer in a randomized trial of PDT versus no endoscopic therapy would represent a dramatic breakthrough—a nonsurgical approach that could prolong the life of individual patients at high risk of developing esophageal adenocarcinoma.

Many forms of mucosal injury have been documented to remove cancer, HGD, LGD, or nondysplastic Barrett's esophagus. Ranging from deep to superficial are PDT with porfimer sodium (108), endoscopic mucosal resection (77), argon plasma coagulation (APC) (109), multipolar electrocoagulation (MPEC) (110), PDT with 5-aminolevulinic acid (111), and argon laser (106). The only randomized trials using an endoscopic ablation technique compared to no endoscopic therapy used PDT. The largest trial included 138 patients with HGD treated with porfimer sodium (107). Another trial included 18 patients with LGD treated with 5-aminolevulinic acid (112). The other trials have not been randomized, and are based on smaller numbers of patients and patients with varying grades of dysplasia. The side effects of these procedures correlate with depth of injury. Stricture requiring dilation is common with PDT with porfimer sodium (108). Perforation (113) and a mediastinis syndrome (114) have occurred with APC.

Endoscopic ablative therapy has raised many questions. What amount of esophageal acid reduction is necessary for successful reversal (115)? How durable is the new squamous epithelium? It can be long lasting, but what conditions are necessary (116)? What technique is most effective with the fewest side effects? What are the appropriate indications for endoscopic therapy? Finally, the most important unanswered question is whether endoscopic therapy reduces the risk of developing cancer. A minimum of 5 years of follow-up data will be necessary to answer this question.

Therapy of High-Grade Dysplasia

HGD therapy highlights many of the complex issues of decision making in Barrett's esophagus in the race between cancer and comorbidity—endoscopic techniques, pathologic interpretation, the threshold for surgical intervention, and weighing the odds. The problem of sampling is greater for HGD than LGD (76). Most endoscopists do not use large-capacity biopsy forceps and do not follow the suggested University of Washington protocol of four-quadrant biopsies every 1 cm (117). The optical recognition of dysplasia is being assessed by techniques ranging from the simple, but not necessarily reproducible, such as methylene blue chromoendoscopy (118), to the technically complex, such as spectroscopy (119). Pathologists' interobserver variability of reading dysplasia in Barrett's esophagus is a problem for surveillance and for therapeutic decisions. Interobserver agreement is near perfect (mean kappa 0.8) when separating Barrett's esophagus indefinite and LGD from HGD and cancer (120). However, separating HGD from intramucosal cancer can be a major problem even for experts. When using four categories rather than two, the agreement was only moderate (kappa 0.43 to 0.46).

One option is frequent surveillance endoscopy—every 3 months—with an intensive biopsy protocol, large-capacity biopsy forceps, four quadrant every 1 cm (Table 27.2). The threshold for intervention with surgical resection has been rising with the recognized increasing variability of the natural history of HGD, sensitivity of operative mortality to volume, and more effective staging with endoscopic mucosal resection (EMR). In the short run, focal HGD has a lesser risk of progressing to cancer than multifocal. HGD with mucosal nodularity has a greater risk of having associated cancer (79,121) than with a regular Barrett's mucosa.

TABLE 27.2. HIGH-GRADE DYSPLASIA TREATMENT OPTIONS

Frequent surveillance without intensive biopsy protocol
Endoscopic therapy: Photodynamic
                              Thermal
Esophagectomy

Mucosal irregularities are now amenable to EMR, providing the depth of tissue that allows the clear distinction between intramucosal cancer—a lesion potentially curable by EMR—and cancer invading below the muscularis mucosa—a lesion associated with regional lymph node metastasis 25% of the time (122). The former lesion can be treated endoscopically; the latter requires surgical resection. The option of esophagectomy is attractive in the younger surgically fit candidate with multifocal HGD that is persistently present and confirmed by an expert gastroenterologic pathologist. This surgery needs to be performed at a high-volume institution.

The first clinically accepted role of endoscopic ablative therapy is likely to be PDT in patients with HGD. This offers retention of swallowing function, no immediate procedure-related mortality, and a reduction in cancer development. In the future, less deep thermal techniques may accomplish the same outcomes.

Weighing the odds involves deciding whether a given patient is a fit candidate for esophagectomy, and whether a patient's major comorbidity will result in death prior to his developing cancer, among other issues. Making these difficult decisions requires individualization and precision judgments involved in the art of medicine.

REFERENCES

1. Devesa SS, Blot WJ, Fraumeni JF. Changing patterns in the incidence of esophageal and gastric carcinoma in the United States. *Cancer* 1998;83:2049–2053.
2. Blot WJ, Devesa SS, Fraumeni JF Jr. Continuing climb in rates of esophageal adenocarcinoma: an update [Letter]. *JAMA* 1993; 270:1320.
3. Sharma P, Morales TG, Sampliner RE. Short segment Barrett's esophagus—the need for standardization of the definition and of endoscopic criteria. *Am J Gastroenterol* 1998;93:1033–1066.
4. Barrett NR. Chronic peptic ulcer of the oesophagus and "esophagitis." *Br J Surg* 1950;38:175–182.
5. Allison PR, Johnstone AS. Oesophagus lined with gastric mucous membrane. *Thorax* 1953;8:87–93.
6. Weinstein WM, Ippoliti AF. The diagnosis of Barrett's esophagus: goblets, goblets, goblets. *Gastrointest Endosc* 1996;44: 91–95.
7. McClave SA, Boyce HW, Gottfried MR. Early diagnosis of columnar-lined esophagus: a new endoscopic criterion. *Gastrointest Endosc* 1987;33:413–416.
8. Sharma P, Weston AP, Morales T, et al. Relative risk of dysplasia for patients with intestinal metaplasia in the distal esophagus and in the gastric cardia. *Gut* 2000;46:9–13.

9. Bremner CG, Lynch VP, Ellis FH. Barrett's esophagus: congenital or acquired? An experimental study of esophageal mucosal regeneration in the dog. *Surgery* 1970;68:209–216.

10. Iascone C, DeMeester TR, Little AG, et al. Functional assessment, proposed pathogenesis and surgical therapy. *Arch Surg* 1983;118:543–549.

11. Parrilla P, Ortiz A, Martinez DE, et al. Evaluation of the magnitude of gastro-oesophageal reflux in Barrett's esophagus. *Gut* 1990;31:964–967.

12. Oberg S, DeMeester TR, Peters JH, et al. The extent of Barrett's esophagus depends on the status of the lower esophageal sphincter and the degree of esophageal acid exposure. *J Thorac Cardiovasc Surg* 1999;117:572–580.

13. Hirschowitz BI. Gastric acid and pepsin secretion in patients with Barrett's esophagus and appropriate controls. *Dig Dis Sci* 1996;41:1384–1391.

14. Hirota WK, Loughney TM, Lazas DJ, et al. Specialized intestinal metaplasia dysplasia and cancer of the esophagus and esophagogastric junction: prevalence and clinical data. *Gastroenterology* 1999;116:277–285.

15. Singh S, Bradley LA, Richter JE. Determinants of oesophageal "alkaline" pH environment in controls and patients with gastro-oesophageal reflux disease. *Gut* 1993;34:309–316.

16. Vaezi MF, Richter JE. Role of acid and duodenogastroesophageal reflux in gastroesophageal reflux disease. *Gastroenterology* 1996;111:1192–1199.

17. Marshall REK, Anggiansah A, Owen WA, et al. The relationship between acid and bile reflux and symptoms of gastro-oesophageal reflux disease. *Gut* 1997;40:182–187.

18. Romero Y, Cameron AJ, Locke GR III, et al. Familial aggregation of gastroesophageal reflux in patients with Barrett's esophagus and esophageal adenocarcinoma. *Gastroenterology* 1997;113:1449–1456.

19. Chak A, Lee T, Kinnard MF, et al. Familial aggregation of Barrett's oesophagus, oesophageal adenocarcinoma and oesophagogastric junctional adenocarcinoma in Caucasian adults. *Gut* 2002;51:323–328.

20. Cameron AJ, Lomboy CT. Barrett's esophagus; age, prevalence and the extent of columnar epithelium. *Gastroenterology* 1992;103:1241–1245.

21. Hassell E. Barrett's esophagus: congenital or acquired? *Am J Gastroenterol* 1993;88:819–824.

22. Mason RJ, Bremner CG. The columnar-lined (Barrett's) oesophagus in black patients. *S Afr J Surg* 1998;36:61–62.

23. Shoji T, Hongo M, Fukudo S, et al. Increasing incidence of Barrett's esophagus and Barrett's carcinoma in Japan. *Gastroenterology* 1999;116:A312.

24. Ho KY, Kang JY, Seow A. Prevalence of gastrointestinal symptoms in a multiracial Asian population, with particular reference to reflux-type symptoms. *Am J Gastroenterol* 1998;93:1816–1822.

25. Sharma P. Risk of cancer in Barrett's esophagus. *Clin Perspect Gastroenterol* 2002;5:248–250.

26. Lagergren J, Bergstrom R, Lindgren A, et al. Symptomatic gastroesophageal reflux as a factor for esophageal adenocarcinoma. *N Engl J Med* 1999;340:825–831.

27. Farrow DC, Vaughan TL, Sweeney C, et al. Gastroesophageal reflux disease, use of H2 receptor antagonists and risk of esophageal gastric cancer. *Cancer Causes Control* 2000;11:231–238.

28. Chow WH, Blot WJ, Vaughan TL, et al. Body mass index and risk of adenocarcinoma of the esophagus and gastric cardia. *J Natl Cancer Inst* 1998;90:150–155.

29. Lagergren J, Bergstrom R, Lindgren A, et al. Association between body mass and adenocarcinoma of the esophagus. *Ann Intern Med* 1999;130:883–890.

30. Brown LM, Swanson CA, Gridley G, et al. Adenocarcinoma of the esophagus: role of obesity and diet. *J Natl Cancer Inst* 1995;87:104–109.

31. Kuczmarski RJ, Flegal KM, Campbell SM, et al. Increasing incidence of overweight among US adults. The National Health and Nutrition Examination Surveys, 1960 to 1991. *JAMA* 1994;272:205–211.

32. Gammon MD, Schoenberg JB, Ahsan H, et al. Tobacco, alcohol and socioeconomic status and adenocarcinomas of the esophagus and gastric cardia. *J Natl Cancer Inst* 1997;89:1277–1284.

33. Lagergren J, Bergstrom R, Adami HO, et al. Association between medications that relax the lower esophageal sphincter and esophageal adenocarcinoma. *Ann Intern Med* 2000;133:165–175.

34. Chow WH, Finkle WD, McLaughlin JK, et al. The relation of gastroesophageal reflux disease and its treatment to adenocarcinomas of the esophagus and gastric cardia. *JAMA* 1996;274:474–477.

35. Vicari JJ, Peek RM, Falk GW, et al. The seroprevalence of cagA positive Helicobacter pylori strains in the spectrum of gastroesophageal reflux disease. *Gastroenterology* 1998;115:50–57.

36. Sabik JF, Rice TW, Goldblum JR, et al. Superficial esophageal carcinoma. *Ann Thorac Surg* 1995;60:896–902.

37. Dulai GS, Guha S, Kahn KL, et al. Preoperative prevalence of Barrett's esophagus in esophageal adenocarcinoma: a systematic review. *Gastroenterology* 2002;122:26–33.

38. Eisen GM, Sandler RS, Murray S, et al. The relationship between gastroesophageal reflux disease and its complications with Barrett's esophagus. *Am J Gastroenterol* 1997;92:27–31.

39. Lieberman DA, Oehlke M, Helfand M, et al. Risk factors for Barrett's esophagus in community-based practice. *Am J Gastroenterol* 1997;92:1293–1297.

40. Sampliner RE, Practice Parameters Committee of the American College of Gastroenterology. Updated guidelines for the diagnosis, surveillance, and therapy of Barrett's esophagus. *Am J Gastroenterol* 2002;97:1888–1895.

41. Gerson LB, Shetler K, Triadafilopoulos G. Prevalence of Barrett's esophagus in asymptomatic individuals. *Gastroenterology* 2002;123:461–467.

42. Dean R, Dua K, Massey B, et al. A comparative study of unsedated transnasal esophagogastroduodenoscopy and conventional EGD. *Gastrointest Endosc* 1996;44:422–424.

43. Saeian K, Staff DM, Vasilopoulos S, et al. Unsedated transnasal endoscopy accurately detects Barrett's metaplasia and dysplasia. *Gastrointest Endosc* 2002;56:472–478.

44. Sharma P, Mayo M, Topalovski M, et al. Methylene blue chromoendoscopy for the detection of patients with short segment Barrett's esophagus. *Gastrointest Endosc* 2001;54:289–293.

45. Canto MI, Setrakian S, Willis J, et al. Methylene-blue directed biopsies improve detection of intestinal metaplasia and dysplasia in Barrett's esophagus. *Gastrointest Endosc* 2000;51:560–568.

46. Sharma P, Weston AP, Sampliner RE. Magnification chromoendoscopy for the detection of intestinal metaplasia and dysplasia in Barrett's esophagus—preliminary results. *Gut* 2003 (in press).

47. Poneros JM, Brand S, Bouma BE, et al. Diagnosis of specialized intestinal metaplasia by optical coherence tomography. *Gastroenterology* 2001;120:7–12.

48. Wallace MB, Perelman LT, Backman V, et al. Endoscopic detection of dysplasia in patients with Barrett's esophagus using light-scattering spectroscopy. *Gastroenterology* 2000;119:677–682.

49. Panjehpour M, Overholt BF, Vo-Dinh T, et al. Endoscopic fluorescence detection of high-grade dysplasia in Barrett's esophagus. *Gastroenterology* 1996;111:93–101.

50. Falk GW, Chittajallu R, Goldblum JR, et al. Surveillance of

patients with Barrett's esophagus for dysplasia and cancer with balloon cytology. *Gastroenterology* 1997;112:1787–1797.

51. Dattamajumdar AK, Blout PL, Myer JA, et al. A low-cost fiberoptic instrument to colorimetrically detect patients with Barrett's esophagus for early detection of esophageal adenocarcinoma. *IEEE Trans Biomed Eng* 2001;48:695–705.

52. Bytzer P, Christensen PB, Damkier P, et al. Adenocarcinoma of the esophagus and Barrett's esophagus: a population based study. *Am J Gastroenterol* 1999;94:86–91.

53. Conio M, Cameron AJ, Romero Y, et al. Secular trends in the epidemiology and outcome of Barrett's oesophagus in Olmsted County, Minnesota. *Gut* 2001:304–309.

54. Cameron AJ, Lomboy CT, Pera M, et al. Adenocarcinoma of the esophagastric junction in Barrett's esophagus. *Gastroenterology* 1995;109:1541–1546.

55. Schnell TG, Sontag SJ, Chejfec G, et al. Long-term nonsurgical management of Barrett's esophagus with high-grade dysplasia. *Gastroenterology* 2001;120:1607–1619.

56. Sharma P, Weston A, Falk GA, et al. Can two upper endoscopies negative for dysplasia eliminate the need for future surveillance in patients with Barrett's esophagus? *Am J Gastroenterol* 2001; 96:536.

57. Drewitz DJ, Sampliner RE, Garewal HS. The incidence of adenocarcinoma in Barrett's esophagus—a prospective study of 170 patients followed 4.8 years. *Am J Gastroenterol* 1997;92:212–215.

58. O'Connor JB, Falk GW, Richter JE. The incidence of adenocarcinoma and dysplasia in Barrett's esophagus. *Am J Gastroenterol* 1999;94:2037–2042.

59. Shaheen NJ, Crosby MA, Bozymski EM. Is there publication bias in the reporting of cancer risk of Barrett's esophagus? *Gastroenterology* 2000;119:333–338.

60. VanDerBurgh A, Doos J, Hop WJC, et al. Oesophageal cancer is an uncommon cause of death in patients with Barrett's oesophagus. *Gut* 1996;39:5–8.

61. MacDonald CE, Wicks AC, Playford RJ. Final results from 10 year cohort of patients undergoing surveillance for Barrett's oesophagus: observational study. *BMJ* 2000;321:1252–1255.

62. Streitz JM, Andrews CW, Ellis FH. Endoscopic surveillance of Barrett's esophagus: does it help? *J Thorac Cardiovasc Surg* 1993; 105:383–388.

63. Peters JH, Clark GWB, Ireland AP, et al. Outcome of adenocarcinoma arising in Barrett's esophagus in endoscopically surveyed and nonsurveyed patients. *J Thorac Cardiovasc Surg* 1994;108:813–822.

64. Lerut T, Coosemans W, VanRaemdonck D, et al. Surgical treatment of Barrett's carcinoma. *J Thorac Cardiovasc Surg* 1994;107: 1059–1066.

65. vanSandick JW, vanLanschot JJB, Kuiken BW, et al. Impact of endoscopic biopsy surveillance of Barrett's oesophagus on pathological stage and clinical outcome of Barrett's carcinoma. *Gut* 1998;43:216–222.

66. Fitzgerald RC, Saeed IB, Khoo D, et al. Rigorous surveillance protocol increases detection of curable cancers associated with Barrett's esophagus. *Dig Dis Sci* 2001;46:1892–1898.

67. Corley DA, Levin TR, Habel LA, et al. Surveillance and survival in Barrett's adenocarcinomas: a population-based study. *Gastroenterology* 2002;122:633–640.

68. Cooper GS, Yuan Z, Chak A, et al. Association of prediagnosis endoscopy with stage and survival in adenocarcinoma of the esophagus and gastric cardia. *Cancer* 2002;95:32–38.

69. Gross GP, Canto MI, Hixson J, et al. Management of Barrett's esophagus: a national study of practice patterns and their cost implications. *Am J Gastroenterol* 1999;94:3440–3447.

70. Falk GW, Ours TM, Richter J. Practice patterns for surveillance of Barrett's esophagus in the United States. *Gastrointest Endosc* 2000;52:197–203.

71. Correa-Cruz M, Gross GP, Canto MI, et al. The impact of practice guidelines in the management of Barrett esophagus. *Arch Intern Med* 2001;161:2588–2595.

72. Robertson CS, Mayberry JF, Nicholson DA, et al. Value of endoscopic surveillance in the detection of neoplastic change in Barrett's oesophagus. *Br J Surg* 1988;75:760–763.

73. Hammeetman W, Tytgat JN, Houthoff HJ, et al. Barrett's esophagus: development of dysplasia and adenocarcinoma. *Gastroenterology* 1989;69:1249–1256.

74. Miros M, Kerlin MM, Walker N. Only patients with dysplasia progress to adenocarcinoma in Barrett's oesophagus. *Gut* 1991; 32:1441–1446.

75. Reid B, Levine D, Longton G, et al. Predictors of progression to cancer in Barrett's esophagus: baseline histology and flow cytometry identify low- and high-risk patient subsets. *Am J Gastroenterol* 2000;95:1669–1676.

76. Cameron AJ, Carpenter HA. Barrett's esophagus, high-grade dyspalsia, and early adenocarcinoma: a pathological study. *Am J Gastroenterol* 1997;92:586.

77. Ell C, May A, Gossner L, et al. Endoscopic mucosal resection of early cancer and high grade dysplasia in Barrett's esophagus. *Gastroenterology* 2000;118:670–677.

78. Nijhawan PK, Wang KK. Endoscopic mucosal resection for lesions with endoscopic features suggestive of malignancy and high-grade dysplasia within Barrett's esophagus. *Gastroenterology* 2000;52:328–332.

79. Buttar NS, Wang KK, Sebo TJ, et al. Extent of high-grade dysplasia in Barrett's esophagus correlates with risk of adenocarcinoma. *Gastroenterology* 2001;120:1630–1639.

80. Sonnenberg A, Soni A, Sampliner RE. Medical decision analysis of endoscopic surveillance of Barrett's oesophagus to prevent oesophageal adenocarcinoma. *Aliment Pharmacol Ther* 2002;16: 41–50.

81. Reid BJ, Blount PL, Rubin CE, et al. Flow-cytometric and histological progression to malignancy in Barrett's esophagus: prospective endoscopic surveillance of a cohort. *Gastroenterology* 1992;102:1212–1219.

82. Reid B, Prevo L, Galipeau P, et al. Predictors of progression in Barrett's esophagus II: Baseline 17p (p53) loss of heterozygosity identifies a patient subset at increased risk for neoplastic progression. *Am J Gastroenterol* 2001;96:2839–2848.

83. Sampliner RE. Effect of up to three years of high dose lansoprazole on Barrett's. *Am J Gastroenterol* 1994;89:1844–1848.

84. Katzka DA, Paoletti V, Leite L, et al. Prolonged ambulatory pH monitoring in patients with persistent gastroesophageal reflux disease symptoms: testing while on therapy identifies the need for more aggressive anti-reflux therapy. *Am J Gastroenterol* 1996; 91:2110–2113.

85. Fass R, Sampliner RE, Malagon IB, et al. Failure of oesophageal acid control in candidates for Barrett's oesophagus reversal on a very high dose of proton pump inhibitor. *Aliment Pharmacol Ther* 2000;14:597–602.

86. Sharma P, Weston A, Keeton S, et al. Control of esophageal acid exposure in patients with Barrett's esophagus on rabeprazole. *Am J Gastroenterol* 2001;96:S36(110).

87. Neumann CS, Iqbal TH, Cooper BT. Long term continuous omeprazole treatment of patients with Barrett's esophagus. *Aliment Pharmacol Ther* 1995;9:451–454.

88. Sharma P, Sampliner RE, Camargo E. Normalization of esophageal pH with high dose proton pump inhibitor therapy does not result in regression of Barrett's esophagus. *Am J Gastroenterol* 1997;92:582–585.

89. Malesci A, Savarino V, Ventilin P, et al. Partial regression of Barrett's esophagus by long-term therapy with high dose omeprazole. *Gastrointest Endosc* 1996;44:700–705.

90. Wilkinson SP, Biddlestone L, Gore S, et al. Regression of

columnar lined (Barrett's) oesophagus with omeprazole 40mg daily: results of 5 years of continuous therapy. *Aliment Pharmacol Ther* 1999;13:1205–1209.

91. Peters FTM, Ganesh S, Kuipers EJ, et al. Endoscopic regression of Barrett's oesophagus during omeprazole treatment: a randomised double blind study. *Gut* 1999;45:489–494.

92. Sharma P, Morales TG, Bhattacharyya A, et al. Squamous islands in Barrett's esophagus: what lies underneath? *Am J Gastroenterol* 1998;93:332–335.

93. Ouatu-Lascar R, Fitzgerald RC, Triadafilopoulos G. Differentiation and proliferation in Barrett's esophagus and the effects of acid suppression. *Gastroenterology* 1999;117:327–335.

94. Umansky M, Yasui W, Hallak A, et al. Proton pump inhibitors reduce cell cycle abnormalities in Barrett's esophagus. *Oncogene* 2001;20:7987–7991.

95. Carlson N, Lechago J, Richter J, et al. Acid suppression therapy may not alter malignant progression in Barrett's metaplasia showing p53 protein accumulation. *Am J Gastroenterol* 2002;97:1340–1345.

96. Yau P, Watson D, Devitt PG, et al. Laparoscopic antireflux surgery in the treatment of gastroesophageal reflux in patients with Barrett's esophagus. *Arch Surg* 2000;135:801–805.

97. Farrell TM, Smith CD, Metreveli RE, et al. Fundoplication provides effective and durable symptom relief in patients with Barrett's esophagus. *Am J Surg* 1999;178:18–21.

98. Hofstetter WL, Peters JH, DeMeester T, et al. Long-term outcome of antireflux surgery in patients with Barrett's esophagus. *Ann Surg* 2001;234:532–538; discussion 538–539.

99. Wiliamson WA, Ellis FH, Gibb SP, et al. Effect of antireflux operation on Barrett's mucosa. *Ann Thorac Surg* 1990;49:537–542.

100. McDonald ML, Trastek VF, Allen MS, et al. Barrett's esophagus: Does an antireflux procedure reduce the need for endoscopic surveillance? *J Thorac Cardiovasc Surg* 1996;111:1135–40.

101. Ye W, Chow WH, Lagergren J, et al. Risk of adenocarcinomas of the esophagus and gastric cardia in patients with gastroesophageal reflux disease and after antireflux surgery. *Gastroenterology* 2001;121:1286–1293.

102. Corey KE, Schmitz SM, Shaheen NJ. Does a surgical antireflux procedure decrease the incidence of esophageal adenocarcinoma in Barrett's esophagus? A meta-analysis. *Gastroenterology* 2002;122:A292(abst).

103. Begg CB, Cramer LD, Hoskins WJ, et al. Impact of hospital volume on operative mortality for major cancer surgery. *JAMA* 1998;280:1747–1751.

104. Birkmeyer JD, Siewers AE, Finlayson EVA, et al. Hospital volume and surgical mortality in the United States. *N Engl J Med* 2002;346:1128–1137.

105. Sampliner RE, Hixson LJ, Fennerty MB, et al. Regression of Barrett's esophagus by laser ablation in an antacid environment. *Dig Dis Sci* 1993;38:365–368.

106. Berenson MM, Johnson TD, Markowitz NR, et al. Restoration of squamous mucosa after ablation of Barrett's esophagus epithelium. *Gastroenterology* 1993;104:1686–1691.

107. Overholt B. A multicenter, partially blinded, randomized study of the efficacy of photodynamic therapy using porfimer sodium for the ablation of high grade dysplasia in Barrett's esophagus: results of 6-month follow-up. *Gastroenterology* 2001;120:A79.

108. Overholt BF, Panjehpour M, Haydek JM. Photodynamic therapy for Barrett's esophagus: follow-up in 100 patients. *Gastrointest Endosc* 1999;49:1–7.

109. Schulz H, Miehlke S, Antos D, et al. Ablation of Barrett's epithelium by endoscopic argon plasma coagulation in combination with high-dose omeprazole. *Gastrointest Endosc* 2000;51:659–663.

110. Sampliner RE, Faigel D, Fennerty MB, et al. Effective and safe endoscopic reversal of nondysplastic Barrett's esophagus with thermal electrocoagulation combined with high-dose acid inhibition: a multicenter study. *Gastrointest Endosc* 2001;53:554–558.

111. Gossner L, Stolte M, Sroka R, et al. Photodynamic ablation of high-grade dysplasia and early cancer in Barrett's esophagus by means of 5-aminolevulinic acid. *Gastroenterology* 1998;114:448–455.

112. Ackroyd R, Brown NJ, Davis MF, et al. Photodynamic therapy for dysplastic Barrett's oesophagus: a prospective, double blind, randomised, placebo controlled trial. *Gut* 2000;47:612–617.

113. Byrne JP, Armstrong GR, Attwood SEA. Restoration of the normal squamous lining in Barrett's esophagus by argon beam plasma coagulation. *Am J Gastroenterol* 1998;93:1810–1815.

114. Pereiera-Lima J, Busnello JV, Saul C, et al. High power setting argon plasma coagulation for the eradication of Barrett's esophagus. *Am J Gastroenterol* 2000;95:1661–1668.

115. Sampliner RE, Camargo L, Fass R, et al. Impact of esophageal acid exposure on the endoscopic reversal of Barrett's esophagus. *Am J Gastroenterol* 2002;97:270–272.

116. Sharma P, Bhattacharyya A, Garewal HS, et al. Durability of new squamous epithelium following endoscopic reversal of Barrett's esophagus. *Gastrointest Endosc* 1999;50:159–164.

117. Levine DS, Haggitt RC, Blount PL, et al. An endoscopic biopsy protocol can differentiate high grade dysplasia from early adenocarcinoma in Barrett's esophagus. *Gastroenterology* 1993;105:40–50.

118. Canto M, Setrakian S, Willis J, et al. Methylene blue staining of dysplastic and nondysplastic Barrett's esophagus: an in vivo and ex vivo study. *Endoscopy* 2001;33:391–400.

119. Georgakoudi I, Jacobson BC, VanDam J, et al. Fluorescence, reflectance, and light–scattering spectroscopy for evaluating dysplasia in patients with Barrett's esophagus. *Gastroenterology* 2001;120:1620–1629.

120. Montgomery E, Bronner MP, Goldblum JR, et al. Reproducibility of the diagnosis of dysplasia in Barrett's esophagus: a reaffirmation. *Hum Pathol* 2001;32:368–378.

121. Nigro JJ, Hagen JA, DeMeester TR, et al. Occult esophageal adenocarcinoma. Extent of disease and implications for effective therapy. *Ann Surg* 1999;230:433–440.

122. Holscher AH, Bollschweiler E, Schneider PM, et al. Early adenocarcinoma in Barrett's oesophagus. *Br J Surg* 1997;84:1470–1473.

ESOPHAGEAL STRICTURES

MARK H. JOHNSTON
ROY WONG

Approximately 60% to 70% of all esophageal strictures are peptic in origin and are located at the squamocolumnar junction (Color Plate 28.1 and Fig. 28.2). These strictures develop secondary to gastroesophageal reflux disease (GERD) and by definition are a fibrotic narrowing caused by "digestive juices." The remaining strictures are postsurgical, related to corrosive injury, radiation, sclerotherapy, or photodynamic therapy (1) (Table 28.1).

Peptic strictures occur two to three times more frequently in men than woman (2), are tenfold more common in whites than African Americans or Asians (3), and complicate the course of GERD in 10% to 15% of patients (4). Most patients with peptic strictures are older, have had a longer duration of GERD symptoms, and have abnormal esophageal motility when compared to GERD patients without peptic strictures (1).

PATHOPHYSIOLOGY

Strictures related to GERD can be attributed to the breakdown of the three primary areas of defense: antireflux barriers, luminal clearance, and epithelial resistance. The reflux barriers can be weakened by any of the following: inappropriate transient lower esophageal sphincter (LES) relaxations, a hypotensive resting LES, or a hiatal hernia. Although transient LES relaxations are found in normal individuals, they occur more often and represent the majority of reflux episodes in GERD patients (5). A hypotensive LES is found in 4% to 25% of GERD patients (6). When LES pressure is compared in GERD patients with and without stricture, stricture patients have significantly lower LES pressure. In one study none exceeded 8 mmHg with a mean of 4.9, whereas in the controls, the mean was 20 mmHg (7). Hiatal hernias are more common in peptic stricture patients and are found in as many as 85%. The prevalence in controls is estimated to be 10% to 15% (8). Hiatal hernias contribute to GERD and stricture formation through several mechanisms: increasing acid contact time via trapping of the refluxate in the hiatal hernia sac, reducing the basal LES pressure, and shortening the length of the high pressure zone of the LES (9). GERD patients with peptic strictures, relative to controls, have particularly poor esophageal acid clearance as measured by 24-hour esophageal pH and manometric studies (10). In addition to the low LES pressure mentioned above, the most common manometric finding associated with peptic strictures is abnormal peristalsis. Abnormal peristalsis includes simultaneous and repetitive contractions, which are the most common finding and more rarely aperistalsis (11). Factors contributing to the compromise of epithelial resistance are many and include the medications listed in Table 28.1, alkaline reflux, and lack of salivary bicarbonate, such as in the scleroderma patient. Alkaline reflux of trypsin, bile, and pancreatic enzymes has been implicated as a contributing factor to both GERD and esophageal strictures. Attwood et al. (12) found through prolonged ambulatory pH monitoring that Barrett's patients with complications, including 92% with peptic strictures, had significant alkaline reflux defined as pH>7.

The pathophysiology of photodynamic therapy and radiation-induced strictures is different and follows the sequence of vascular damage, consequent ischemia, apoptosis, and development of fibrosis (13).

In a study correlating esophageal stricture diameter that was measured radiographically, grade of esophagitis as determined endoscopically, and severity of dysphagia estimated using a numerical scoring system, Dakkak et al. (14) found that stricture diameter alone could not explain the variation in dysphagia score, whereas the combination of stricture diameter and severity of esophagitis could account for 66% of that variation. The authors concluded that the degree of esophagitis is as important as stricture diameter in causing dysphagia.

M. H. Johnston: National Naval Medical Center, Division of Gastroenterology, Bethesda, Maryland.

R. Wong: Uniformed Services University of the Health Sciences, Walter Reed Army Medical Center, Washington, DC.

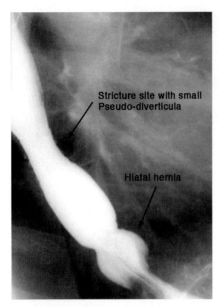

FIGURE 28.2. Peptic stricture with hiatal hernia and pseudo-diverticula at the stricture site (Case courtesy of Perry J. Pickhardt, M.D.,.)

TABLE 28.1. DIFFERENTIAL DIAGNOSES OF ESOPHAGEAL STRICTURES

Gastroesophageal reflux
Corrosive injury: lye, batteries, HCL, sulfuric acid
Postsurgical
  Anastomotic
  Heller myotomy for achalasia
Radiation
Band ligation of esophageal varicies
Photodynamic therapy
Crohn's disease
Eosinophilic esophagitis
Epidermolysis bullosa
Esophageal atresia
Gastric inlet patch
Nasogastric tube
Sclerotherapy
Steven–Johnson syndrome
Infections
  Candida
  Tuberculosis
  Typhoid
Medications
  Alendronate
  Ferrous sulfate
  NSAIDs
  Phenytoin
  Potassium chloride
  Quinidine
  Tetracycline
Ascorbic acid

NSAID, nonsteroidal antiinflammatory drugs.

GERD initially produces an inflammatory reaction and edema in the lamina propria. In some patients, chronic GERD progresses to destruction of the muscularis mucosae, with the formation of fibrosis down to and including the circular muscle layer. Eventually, transmural inflammation results in the scarring of the outer longitudinal muscle layer, causing shortening and narrowing of the distal esophagus (15).

PREDISPOSING MEDICAL CONDITIONS

There are numerous conditions associated with esophageal strictures. They include but are not limited to Barrett's esophagus, scleroderma, Zollinger-Ellison syndrome, Schatzki's rings, gastric inlet patches, postachalasia treatment, and although not a medical condition, the presence of a nasogastric tube. All of these are associated with acid-peptic damage.

In Barrett's esophagus, retrospective studies have suggested an association with peptic strictures, while a more recent prospective study suggests no such association, as the prevalence of intestinal metaplasia was 23.9% in patients without strictures and 25% in patients with peptic strictures (*p*=NS) (16).

Scleroderma (Color Plate 28.3 and Fig. 28.4) is associated with esophageal symptoms in >70% of patients and peptic strictures in almost 50% (17). These strictures are particularly problematic in that the underlying esophageal

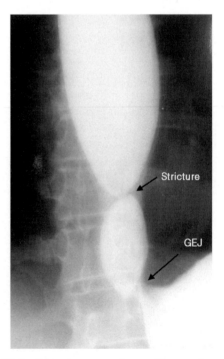

FIGURE 28.4. Scleroderma patient with patulous gastroesophageal junction with "tight" peptic stricture above (Case courtesy of Perry J. Pickhardt, M.D.,.)

defect, aperistalsis, and low LES pressure are predisposing to prolonged acid exposure in the esophagus.

Zollinger-Ellison (ZE) syndrome has been associated with a prevalence of esophageal stricture in 8% to 13% of cases in older literature (18). More recent studies, and specifically a report of 235 patients that included a review of 984 patients from the literature, report a stricture prevalence of only 3%. In this same study, esophageal stricture was associated with an even higher basal acid output (BAO) than ZE patients without stricture. None of the patients who had gastric acid–reducing surgery developed peptic strictures (19).

Aspirin (ASA) and nonsteroidal antiinflammatory drug (NSAID) use, even low-dose ASA and over-the-counter use of NSAIDs, are independently associated with esophageal strictures (20). Heller et al. demonstrated a 31% prevalence of esophageal strictures in NSAID and ASA users compared to14% in controls (21). Wilkens et al. found that approximately 50% of patients with benign esophageal strictures had ingested NSAIDs within the previous 12 months compared to only 12% of controls (21a). However, no studies to evaluate esophageal acid exposure were performed in these cases.

A Schatzki's ring (also known as B-ring) is almost always associated with a hiatal hernia and not uncommonly progresses to a peptic stricture. Marshall et al. (22) reported that 65% of patients with Schatzki's rings had ambulatory pH confirmation of significant GERD. Chen et al. (23) reported that 40% of patients with barium esophagram documented lower esophageal rings progressed to strictures over 1 to 5 years.

Gastric inlet patches located in the mid or proximal esophagus have been associated with increased acid secretion and the development of esophageal strictures (24–26). Treatment with dilation followed by acid suppression with lansoprazole, ranitidine, or sucralfate slurry has been associated with healing and resolution of symptoms.

Although discussed in chapter 11, achalasia postpneumatic dilation may be complicated by the development of a peptic stricture due to the disruption of the LES and consequent development of GERD (27). These should be treated as peptic strictures as detailed below.

Prolonged use of nasogastric tubes (NGT) may be associated with the development of long esophageal strictures due to NGT-impaired LES function and prolonged acid exposure to the esophageal mucosa (28). These can be particularly difficult to dilate and may require multiple, sequential dilations.

Clinical Presentation

Careful history alone can accurately diagnose the cause of dysphagia in 80% of cases (29). The typical presentation of an esophageal stricture includes the insidious onset of dysphagia to solid foods with antecedent pyrosis. However, in up to 25% of cases there is no prior history of pyrosis (30). In some patients, pyrosis may resolve over time secondary to progression of fibrosis and esophageal narrowing only to return after therapeutic dilation. Additionally, not all pyrosis is secondary to GERD; patients with achalasia frequently complain of pyrosis that may be caused by abnormal motor activity as well as by esophageal acid exposure (31). Over time both solid and liquid dysphagia may develop due to progressive narrowing of the stricture and the associated inflammation affecting esophageal motility. The perception that a bolus of food is sticking at the suprasternal notch does not help in localizing the point of obstruction in the esophagus, as the bolus may be located at any point distal to the suprasternal notch. However, the perception that the bolus is below the suprasternal notch correlates well with location of the esophageal abnormality (32). Intermittent dysphagia, separated by long periods of no dysphagia is most characteristic of a Schatzki's ring (Fig. 28.5). Ingestion of doxycycline, potassium chloride preparations, NSAIDs, or quinidine is more frequently associated with esophageal strictures (33). Other symptoms and conditions associated with peptic stricture of the esophagus are regurgitation, hiccups, water brash, chest pain, chronic cough, recurrent aspiration pneumonia, interstitial lung disease, and asthma. Weight loss is an ominous sign and mandates exclusion of a neoplasm.

Physical exam uncommonly delineates the cause of dysphagia. However, signs of joint abnormalities, calcinosis, sclerodactyly, or telangiectasias are supportive of an esophageal abnormality secondary to scleroderma or other collagen vascular disease. A Virchow's node (palpable left supraclavicular lymph node) suggests an intraabdominal neoplasm, such as adenocarcinoma of the gastroesophageal junction. Severe dental erosions suggest GERD and consequent peptic stricture.

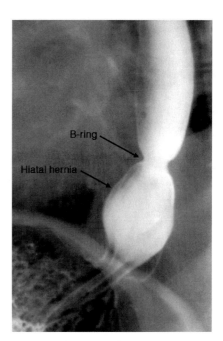

FIGURE 28.5. Hiatal hernia with prominent Schatzki's ring.

DIAGNOSIS

Barium Swallow

On barium swallow, esophageal strictures of peptic origin are usually smooth, tapered, concentric narrowings confined to the distal esophagus. Barium reliably identifies location, diameter, and length of lesion in peptic strictures. Yet, the debate continues regarding the role of barium swallow relative to endoscopy in the evaluation of solid food dysphagia. Should all patients with dysphagia undergo barium swallow prior to endoscopy, or should endoscopy alone be performed since only endoscopy can reliably diagnose other lesions associated with GERD such as Barrett's esophagus? There are proponents for both approaches. Regardless, it should be kept in mind that a barium swallow is more sensitive than endoscopy for the detection of relatively "open" strictures >10 mm in diameter (34), and is generally regarded as the initial procedure of choice, when achalasia, a proximal esophageal lesion, or a motility disorder is suspected (Fig. 28.6). In one study, barium swallow accurately diagnosed achalasia in 18 of 19 cases (95%) and diffuse esophageal spasm in five of seven cases (71%) (35). Barium swallow may also more accurately identify Zenker's or epiphrenic diverticula and paraesophageal hernias. Yet, no study to date has demonstrated that the barium swallow performed prior to endoscopy improves outcome or decreases complications.

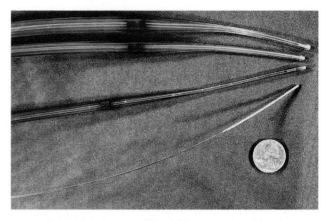

FIGURE 28.7. Savary-Gilliard dilators with guide wire.

Endoscopy

Nearly all patients with dysphagia should undergo upper endoscopy unless contraindicated. It is more sensitive than barium swallow for detection of subtle mucosal lesions (36) such as esophagitis, and enables the use of various therapeutic devices requiring passage of a guide wire or "through-the-scope balloon" (Figs. 28.7 and 28.8). The appearance of a peptic stricture is characterized by a smooth narrowing in the distal esophagus with decreased mucosal vascular pattern that

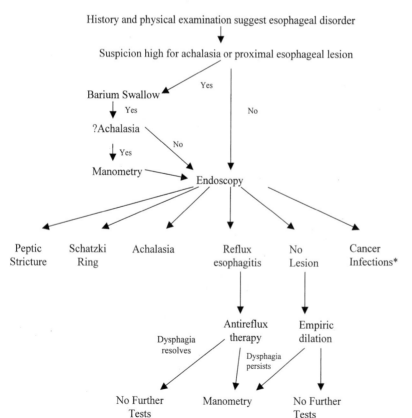

FIGURE 28.6. American Gastroenterological Association medical position statement on treatment of patients with dysphagia caused by benign disorders of the distal esophagus. (From Spechler SJ. American gastroenterological association medical position statement on treatment of patients with dysphagia caused by benign disorders of the distal esophagus. *Gastroenterology* 1999;117:229–233, with permission.)

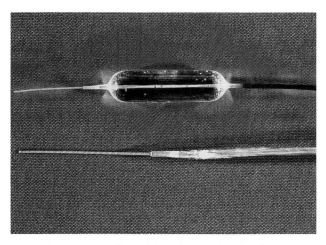

FIGURE 28.8. Balloon dilator pre- and post-inflation.

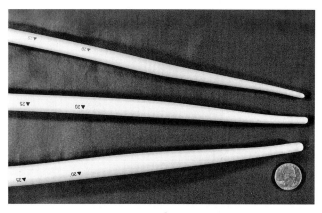

FIGURE 28.9. American dilators.

is difficult to distend with air insufflation. Proximal esophagitis may be associated with peptic strictures in 50% of fibrous band and pseudo-diverticula cases (37). Some investigators have noted an association between peptic strictures and Barrett's esophagus, while others have not (17,38). Peptic strictures are always located at the squamocolumnar junction. Location elsewhere calls into question its peptic etiology. Biopsy of strictures is important to rule out an associated neoplasm, although rare in benign-appearing strictures. Biopsy does not preclude subsequent dilation and has not been associated with an increased perforation risk.

MEDICAL Rx

Dysphagia in patients with peptic stricture is due to both decreased luminal diameter and often coexistent esophagitis resulting in dysmotility. This is supported by multiple studies in which use of proton pump inhibitors (PPIs), which are superior to H_2 blockers, have resulted in healed esophagitis, improved dysphagia, decreased need for esophageal dilation, and prolonged interval between esophageal dilations (39–41). Prior to PPIs, 60% of patients dilated required repeat dilations to maintain alleviation of dysphagia (30,42–44). PPIs have reduced the need for repeat dilation to approximately 30% (40). Patients dilated for peptic strictures should be maintained on long-term PPIs to maintain healing of esophagitis and reduce the need for future esophageal dilation.

BOUGIENAGE

Esophageal dilation has been practiced since at least the 16th century for the treatment of esophageal strictures. The use of tapered wax wands and whalebones to dislodge material stuck in the esophagus is well documented (45). Whalebones and wax wands have been replaced with Maloney dilators, Hurst dilators, wire-guided Savary-Gilliard dila-

tors, American dilators, and balloon dilators passed through the scope or over a guide wire (Figs. 28.8 and 28.9) (46).

Dilation can be performed in either the sitting position or in the left lateral decubitus position following the "rule of threes." A typical algorithm for treatment is depicted in Fig. 28.10. The initial dilator should approximate the estimated diameter of the stricture. Sequential dilation should then be performed with moderate resistance marking the first dilation followed by two additional dilators of increasing size (2F increments). Although the "rule of threes" for sequential dilation is standard dogma, studies achieving the targeted diameter at the first session with low complication rates have been reported. In one series using polyvinyl (American) dilators, 606 wire-guided dilations, on 354 adult patients were performed. Peptic strictures were dilated sequentially to their maximum target size, 45 to 51 Fr (determined by the individual endoscopist) in one session in 195 of 253 instances (77.1%). The remainder of cases were dilated over more than one session and were strictures that did not permit passage of the endoscope on first session. No perforations or other serious complications occurred in this series. Flouroscopy was used in only 5.3% of cases and only when the endoscope could not be passed through the stricture (47).

Small diameter (<10 mm) and complicated esophageal strictures are best treated with either balloon or wire-guided polyvinyl bougies, as Maloney dilators of ≤10 mm diameter are usually too floppy and often curl up in the esophagus. In one study comparing perforation rates of Maloney, balloon, or Savary dilators, all perforations that occurred were with Maloney dilators passed blindly into complex strictures, leading the authors to conclude that they should not be used in such cases (48). Yet, for uncomplicated esophageal strictures with diameters >10 to 12 mm, evidence supports the use of mercury-filled or tungsten bougies as the dilators of choice as they are equally safe, effective, and less costly (18,49,50).

The best dilation technique for peptic strictures remains controversial. However, regardless of technique, dysphagia relief can generally be achieved in nearly 95% of cases. Strictures that are peptic in origin not uncommonly require repeat dilations up to a median of three sessions to achieve

Management of Peptic Esophageal Strictures

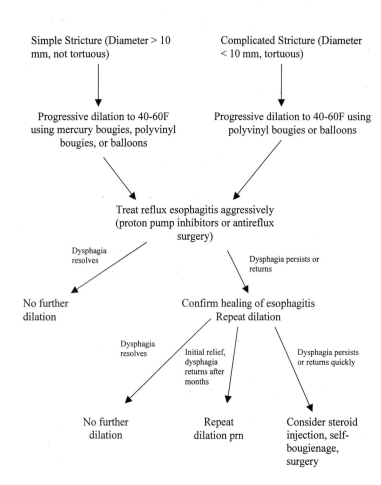

Simple Stricture (Diameter > 10 mm, not tortuous)

Complicated Stricture (Diameter < 10 mm, tortuous)

Progressive dilation to 40-60F using mercury bougies, polyvinyl bougies, or balloons

Progressive dilation to 40-60F using polyvinyl bougies or balloons

Treat reflux esophagitis aggressively (proton pump inhibitors or antireflux surgery)

Dysphagia resolves

Dysphagia persists or returns

No further dilation

Confirm healing of esophagitis Repeat dilation

Dysphagia resolves

Initial relief, dysphagia returns after months

Dysphagia persists or returns quickly

No further dilation

Repeat dilation prn

Consider steroid injection, self-bougienage, surgery

FIGURE 28.10. American Gastroenterological Association medical position statement on treatment of patients with dysphagia caused by benign disorders of the distal esophagus. (From Spechler SJ. American Gastroenterological Association medical position statement on treatment of patients with dysphagia caused by benign disorders of the distal esophagus. *Gastroenterology* 1999;117:229–233, with permission.)

adequate dilation; whereas strictures that are postsurgical or caustic in nature require a median of five sessions for adequate treatment (51).

In some studies, fluoroscopy has been advocated for Maloney dilation of esophageal strictures. Tucker (52) evaluated 145 patients for the importance of fluoroscopic monitoring during Maloney dilation. In 35 patients (24%), fluoroscopy altered the dilation technique. In 26 of 35 cases, successful redirection of the dilator and passage under fluoroscopy was accomplished. In nine patients, Maloney dilation was impossible, and use of Savary wire-guided dilators was needed. For 36% of peptic stricture dilations, fluoroscopy resulted in a change of dilation technique versus 11% of Schatzki's ring dilations ($p<0.05$). Patients with larger hiatal hernias (6.5 vs. 4.3 cm, $p<0.05$) also benefited from fluoroscopy. There was no reported morbidity or mortality in this study. The authors advised the use of fluoroscopy for Maloney dilation of peptic strictures and large hiatal hernias.

The usual endpoint for defining success of dilation is subjective relief of dysphagia. Yet, strictures commonly recur using this criterion. Additionally, there are few postdilation studies that help predict the durability of dilation. Consequently, investigators have evaluated predetermined

endpoints in an attempt to improve outcome and tried to identify predictors for restricturing. At best, the results are mixed and no clear conclusion can be made. Saeed et al. (53) demonstrated improved outcomes utilizing the passage of a 12-mm barium pill test as an objective endpoint. They noted reduced stricture recurrence and need for subsequent dilation utilizing this criterion. Marks and Shukla (1) evaluated whether the maximum diameter achieved at initial stricture dilation affected either stricture recurrence or the requirement for subsequent dilation and found no significant influence. Predictors of restricturing after dilation have been tight stricture at the initial dilation, a long history of reflux symptoms, and a short history of dysphagia (54). Other studies have not found reflux symptoms predictive of restricturing but report that a lack of heartburn or a history of weight loss at the time of initial presentation as predictive for need of repeat dilation (55). To date, no clear-cut criteria exist to identify those who will require repeat dilations.

There is no significant difference in efficacy or complication rate between balloon dilators and rigid dilators in the treatment of benign esophageal strictures and Schatzki's rings (56) (Table 28.2).

TABLE 28.2. COMPARISON OF VARIOUS DILATORS

Author	N	Stricture Description	Dilators Compared	Investigators' Conclusion	Complications
Kelly (45)	71	Benign esophageal strictures	Through the scope balloons (TTS) vs. Celestin and Eder Puestow	Bougie better than balloon for reduction of dysphagia and maintenance of stricture patency	None
Tytgat (46)	60	Benign esophageal strictures	Savary vs. TTS	Bougie modestly better than balloon for reduction of dysphagia	None
McBride and Ergun (63)	71	Benign esophageal strictures	Eder-Puestow vs. TTS	No significant difference	None
Tulman and Boyce (49)	93	Benign esophageal strictures	TTS vs. Celestin and Eder Puestow	Bougie modestly better than ballon for reduction of dysphagia and maintenance of stricture patency	Perforation: 1 in the TTS and 1 bougie
Saedd et al. (81)	34	All peptic	Savary vs. TTS	Both devices effective in relieving dysphagia, but balloons may have a long-term advantage due to reduced need for repeat dilation and improved patient comfort	None
Cox et al. (82)	71	Benign esophageal strictures	Maloney vs. TTS	Maloney dilatation is more effective in reducing dysphagia and maintaining stricture patency	No difference
Cox et al. (83)	93	Benign esophageal strictures	Maloney vs. TTS	There is no significant difference in safety or patient acceptability. Balloons are probably more costly to use than bougies. Bougie dilatation is to be preferred to balloon dilatation in adults except in special circumstances	No difference
Scolapio et al. (56)	251	Benign esophageal strictures	Savary (n=88), Microvasive (n=81), or Bard (n=82) TTS dilator	Both rigid and balloon dilators are equally effective and safe in the treatment of benign lower esophageal strictures caused by acid reflux and Schatzki rings	No difference
Shemesh and Czerniak (84)	60	Benign esophageal strictures	Savary vs. through-the-scope balloons (TTS)	Both methods were highly effective and well tolerated, yet Savary-Gilliard dilators were slightly more effective and simpler to use than balloons	None
Yamamoto et al. (85)	31	All peptic	Eder-Puestow or Medi-Tech balloon dilation	Eder-Puestow and balloon dilations of benign esophageal strictures are associated with similar outcomes, but repeated dilations and the Eder-Puestow technique may be associated with an increased risk of complications	Higher complication with Eder-Puestow

Management of Lower Esophageal Mucosal Ring

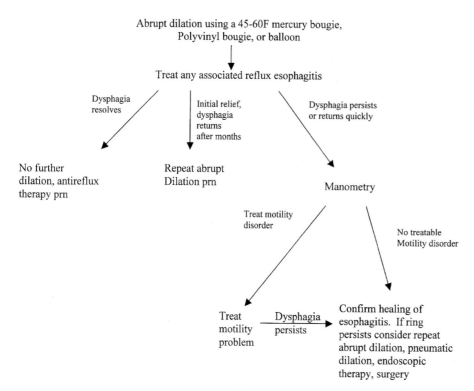

Abrupt dilation using a 45-60F mercury bougie, Polyvinyl bougie, or balloon

Treat any associated reflux esophagitis

Dysphagia resolves

Initial relief, dysphagia returns after months

Dysphagia persists or returns quickly

No further dilation, antireflux therapy prn

Repeat abrupt Dilation prn

Manometry

Treat motility disorder

No treatable Motility disorder

Treat motility problem

Dysphagia persists

Confirm healing of esophagitis. If ring persists consider repeat abrupt dilation, pneumatic dilation, endoscopic therapy, surgery

FIGURE 28.11. American Gastroenterological Association medical position statement on treatment of patients with dysphagia caused by benign disorders of the distal esophagus. (From Spechler SJ. American Gastroenterological Association medical position statement on treatment of patients with dysphagia caused by benign disorders of the distal esophagus. *Gastroenterology* 1999;117:229–233, with permission.)

Metallic stents can be considered as a therapeutic alternative in selected patients with severe benign esophageal strictures that are refractory to conventional treatment. Unfortunately, once a metallic stent has been in the esophagus for an extended period of time it becomes nearly impossible to retrieve. In a small series of ten patients who received metallic stents for benign disease, all achieved marked improvement in their dysphagia. Chest pain was reported as an early complication and proximal or distal stent migration as a late complication. The best results were achieved in postradiation strictures (57).

The standard therapy for Schatzki's rings is depicted in Fig. 28.11. In the rare case of a Schatzki's ring refractory to conventional dilation, electrosurgical endoscopic incision via a sphincterotome has been advocated by some investigators with excellent results. In one series of 17 patients, 14 were asymptomatic at nearly 4 years after a single treatment. The only complication reported was mild bleeding in one patient (58). In a smaller series of seven patients, all of whom were refractory to standard dilation, 100% achieved resolution of symptoms with electrosurgical endoscopic incision with only one recurrence at 6 months. Transient chest pain was the only reported complication (59).

STEROIDS

Theoretically, steroids injected into an esophageal stricture may reduce inflammation with delay or prevention of fibrosis, thus decreasing the re-stenosis rate after esophageal dilation. Unfortunately, there are no randomized controlled trials of adequate size that have assessed the role of intralesional steroids for the treatment of difficult esophageal strictures. Their efficacy is supported only by anecdotal reports using the patient as a historical control. Kochhar et al. (60) demonstrated that in 17 patients intralesional triamcinolone injections augmented the effects of endoscopic dilation in patients with corrosive esophageal strictures. Zein et al. (61) described dramatic improvement in five of seven pediatric patients with peptic stricture after injection with intralesional steroids. Lee et al. (62) demonstrated significant improvement in 31 esophageal stricture patients treated with intralesional steroids, 12 of which were peptic in origin. A typical regimen utilized was triamcinolone (10 mg per mL in 0.5-mL aliquots) injected in four quadrants in the narrowest area of the stricture.

SBE PROPHYLAXIS

Of all procedures performed by gastroenterologists, esophageal dilation of peptic strictures is associated with the

TABLE 28.3. ANTIBIOTIC PROPHYLAXIS IN ENDOSCOPY: AMERICAN SOCIETY FOR GASTROINTESTINAL ENDOSCOPY GUIDELINES

Patient Condition	Procedure Contemplated	Antibiotic Prophylaxis	Comments
Prosthetic valve Hx endocarditis Syst-pulm shunt Syn vasc grant (>1 yr old)	Stricture dilation, Varix sclerosis ERCP/obstructed biliary tree	Recommended	High-risk conditions for development of infectious complication; procedures are associated with relatively high bacteremia rates
Rheumatic valvular dysfunction Mitral valve prolapse with insufficiency Hypertrophic cardiomyopathy Most congenital cardiac malformations	Stricture dilation, Varix sclerosis ERCP/obstructed biliary tree	Insufficient data to make firm recommendation; endoscopists may choose on case-by-case basis	Conditions pose lesser risk for infectious complications than prosthetic valve, etc.
Cirrhosis and ascites Immunocompromised patient	Stricture dilation, Varix sclerosis ERCP/obstructed biliary tree	Insufficient data to make firm recommendation; endoscopists may choose on case-by-case basis	Risk for infectious complications related to endoscopic procedures unestablished

highest degree of bacteremia, reported to be between 11% and 45% (63–66). Consequently, antibiotic prophylaxis should be used as outlined by the American Society for Gastrointestinal Endoscopy (ASGE) in its recommendations for antibiotic prophylaxis for endoscopic procedures (Table 28.2) (67).

COMPLICATIONS OF DILATION

One of the most serious complications after esophageal dilation for peptic stricture of the esophagus is perforation. In some studies, perforation is reported to be as high as 1%. Consequently, some experts recommend routine CXR after all dilations (68). In the 1974 survey of members of the ASGE, the complication rate for dilation of the esophagus with mercury-filled dilators was 0.4%. The most common complication in the group using mercury-filled dilators was bleeding. In the same survey, the perforation rate was 0.03% with a mortality rate of 0.001%. In the 1984 ASGE survey of balloon dilation in 456 patients, there were two perforations and ten hemorrhages reported by those responding to the survey. This represented an overall complication rate of 2.5% (69). However, based on the overall data reviewed to date, the serious complication rate for esophageal dilation is estimated to be 0.5% (70). Predisposing factors for perforation include the presence of anterior cervical osteophytes, Zenker's diverticulum, esophageal strictures, and malignancies (71). Subsequent prospective studies comparing rigid to balloon dilators have not demonstrated a significant difference in complication rates (72) (Table 28.3).

SURGICAL TREATMENT OF GERD AND RECURRENCE OF PEPTIC STRICTURES

A small surgical series published in 1975 (73) demonstrated a significant improvement in dysphagia and a substantial increase in stricture diameter for patients treated with antireflux surgery alone (without stricture dilation). This report received relatively little attention from gastroenterologists at that time.

Laparoscopic fundoplication is effective in GERD patients for treatment of moderate to severe dysphagia secondary to peptic esophageal stricture. This treatment has shown a reduced requirement for repeat dilation—10% at 1.5 years with significantly improved dysphagia and heartburn scores relative to controls (74). Yet, in other studies the requirement for repeat dilation varies considerably, at 1% to 31% (75–80). In spite of these favorable results, there has been no significant study comparing PPIs and surgical treatment for esophageal peptic strictures.

REFERENCES

1. Marks RD, Shukla M. Diagnosis and management of peptic esophageal strictures. *Gastroenterologist* 1996;4:223.
2. Vasudeva R, Deal DR. Esophageal stricture. *Med* 2002;3.
3. El-Serag HB, Sonnenberg A. Associations between different forms of gastro-oesophageal reflux disease. *Gut* 1997;41:594–599.
4. Barkun AN, Mayrand S. The treatment of peptic esophageal strictures. *Can J Gastroenterol* 1997;11(suppl):94–97.
5. Grossi L. Transient lower esophageal sphincter relaxations and gastroesophageal reflux episodes in healthy subjects and GERD patients during 24 hours. *Dig Dis Sci* 2001;46:815–821.
6. Kahrilas PJ, Dodds WJ, Hogan WJ, et al. Esophageal peristaltic dysfunction in peptic esophagitis. *Gastroenterology* 1986;91:897–804.
7. Ahtaridis G, Snape WJ, Cohen S. Clinical and manometric findings in benign peptic strictures of the esophagus. *Dig Dis Sci* 1997;24:858–861.
8. Bergstad A, Weberg R, Froyshov I, et al. Relationship of hiatus hernia to reflux esophagitis: a prospective study of incidence using endoscopy. *Scand J Gastroenterol* 1986;21:55–60.
9. Mittal RK, McCallum RW. Identification and mechanism of

delayed esophageal clearance in subjects with hiatal hernia. *Gastroenterology* 1987;92:130–135.

10. Barham CP, Gotley DC, Mills A, et al. Oesophageal acid clearance in patients with severe reflux oesophagitis. *Br J Surg* 1995; 82:333–337.

11. Zaninotto G, DeMeester TR, Bremner CG, et al. Esophageal function in patients with reflux-induced strictures and its relevance to surgical treatment. *Ann Thorac Surg* 1989;47:362–370.

12. Attwood SEA, DeMeester TR, Bremner CG, et al. Alkaline gastroesophageal reflux: Implications in the development of complications in Barrett's columnar lined lower esophagus. *Surgery* 1989;106:764–770.

13. Wang KK. Current status of photodynamic therapy of Barrett's esophagus. *Gastrointest Endosc* 1999;49:S20–S23.

14. Dakkak M, Hoare RC, Maslin SC, et al.Oesophagitis is as important as oesophageal stricture diameter in determining dysphagia. *Gut* 1993;34:152–155.

15. Awad ZT, Filipi CJ. The short esophagus: pathogenesis, diagnosis, and current surgical options. *Arch Surg* 2001;136:113–114.

16. Kim SL, Wo JM, Hunter JG, et al. The prevalence of intestinal metaplasia in patients with and without peptic strictures. *Am J Gastroenterol* 1998;93:53–55.

17. Treacy WL, Baggenstass AM, Slocumb CM, et al. *Ann Intern Med* 1963;59:351–356.

18. Marks RD, Richter JE. Peptic strictures of the esophagus. *Am J Gastroenterol* 1993;88:1160–1173.

19. Roy PK, Venzon DJ, Feigenbaum KM, et al. Gastric secretion in Zollinger-Ellison syndrome. Correlation with clinical expression, tumor extent and role in diagnosis—a prospective NIH study of 235 patients and a review of 984 cases in the literature. *Medicine (Baltimore)* 2001;80:189–222.

20. Kim SL, Hunter JG, Wo JM, et al. NSAIDs, aspirin, and esophageal strictures: are over-the-counter medications harmful to the esophagus? *J Clin Gastroenterol* 1999;29:32–34.

21. Heller SR, Fellows IW, Ogilvie AL, et al. Non-steroidal anti-inflammatory drugs and benign oesophageal stricture. *Br Med J* 1982;285:167–168.

21a. Wilkins WE, Ridley MG, Pozniak Al. Benign stricture of the oesophagus: role of non-steroidal anti-inflammatory drugs. *Gut* 1984;25:478–480.

22. Marshall JB, Kretschmar JM, Kiaz-Arias AA. Gastroesophageal reflux as a pathogenic factor in the development of symptomatic lower esophageal rings. *Arch Intern Med* 1990;150:1669.

23. Chen YM, Gelfand DW, Ott DJ. Natural progression of the lower esophageal mucosal ring. *Gastrointest Radiol* 1987;12:93–98.

24. Galan AR, Katzka DA, Castell DO. Acid secretion from an esophageal inlet patch demonstrated by ambulatory pH monitoring. *Gastroenterology* 1998;115:1574–1576.

25. Yarborough CS, McLane RC. Stricture related to an inlet patch of the esophagus. *Am J Gastroenterol* 1993;88:275–276.

26. Steadman C, Kerlin P, Teague C, et al. High esophageal stricture: a complication of "inlet patch" mucosa. *Gastroenterology* 1988; 94:521–524.

27. Meijssen MA, Tilanus HW, van Blankenstein M, et al. Achalasia complicated by oesophageal squamous cell carcinoma: a prospective study in 195 patients. *Gut* 1992;33:155–158.

28. Beg MH. Distal esophageal stricture due to indwelling nasogastric tube. *Indian J Chest Dis Allied Sci* 1988;30:64–66.

29. Castell DO, Donner MW. Evaluation of dysphagia: a careful history is crucial. *Dysphagia* 1987;2:65–71.

30. Patterson DJ, Graham DY, Lacy-Smith J, et al. Natural history of benign esophageal stricture treated by dilatation. *Gastroenterology* 1983;85:346–350.

31. Spechler SJ, Souza RF, Rosenberg SJ, et al. Heartburn in patients with achalasia. *Gut* 1995;37:305–308.

32. Wilcox CM, Alexander LN, Clark WS. Localization of an obstructing esophageal lesion. Is the patient accurate? *Dig Dis Sci* 1995;40:2192–2196.

33. Kikendall JW, Johnson LF. The esophagus. 2nd ed. Boston: Little Brown, 1995:619–633.

34. Ott DJ, Chen YM, Wu WC, et al. Endoscopic sensitivity in the detection of esophageal strictures. *J Clin Gastroenterol* 1985;7: 121–125.

35. Ott DJ, Richter JE, Chen YM, et al. Esophageal radiography and manometry: correlation in 172 patients with dysphagia. *AJR Am J Roentgenol* 1987;149:307–311.

36. Ott DJ. Radiographic techniques and efficacy in evaluating esophageal dysphagia. *Dysphagia* 1990;5:192–203.

37. Richter JE. Peptic strictures of the esophagus. *Gastroenterol Clin North Am* 1999;28:875–891.

38. Spechler SJ, Sperber H, Doos WG, et al. The prevalence of Barrett's esophagus in patients with chronic peptic esophageal strictures. *Dig Dis Sci* 1983;28:769–774.

39. Marks RD, Richter JE, Rizzo J, et al. Omeprazole versus H-2 receptor antagonists in treating patients with peptic stricture and esophagitis. *Gastroenterology* 1994;106:907–915.

40. Smith PM, Kerr GD, Cockel R, et al. A comparison of omeprazole and ranitidine in the prevention of recurrence of benign esophageal stricture. *Gastroenterology* 1994;107:1312–1318.

41. Barbezat GO, Schlup M, Lubcke R. Omeprazole therapy decreases the need for dilatation of peptic oesophageal strictures. *Aliment Pharmacol Ther* 1999;13:1041–1045.

42. Ogilvie AL, Ferguson R, Atkinson M. Outlook with conservative treatment of peptic oesophageal stricture. *Gut* 1980;21:23–25.

43. Benedict EB. Peptic stenosis of the esophagus. A study of 233 patients treated with bougienage, surgery, or both. *Am J Dig Dis* 1966;11:761–770.

44. Hands LJ, Dennison AR, Papavramidis S, et al. The natural hisory of peptic oesophageal stricture treated by dilation and antireflux therapy alone. *Ann R Coll Surg Engl* 1989;71:306–309.

45. Kelly HD. Origins of oesophagology. *Proc R Soc Med* 1969;62: 781–786.

46. Tytgat GN. Dilation therapy of benign esophageal stenoses. *World J Surg* 1989;13:142–148.

47. Marshall JB, Afridi SA, King PD, et al. Esophageal dilation with polyvinyl (American) dilators over a marked guidewire: practice and safety at one center over a 5-yr period. *Am J Gastroenterol* 1996;91:1503–1506.

48. Hernandez LJ. Comparison among the perforation rates of Maloney, balloon, and savary dilation of esophageal strictures. *Gastrointest Endosc* 2000;51:460–462.

49. Tulman AB, Boyce HW Jr. Complications of esophageal dilation and guidelines for their prevention. *Gastrointest Endosc* 1981;27: 229–234.

50. Nostrant TT. Esophageal dilatation. *Dig Dis* 1995;13:337–355.

51. Pereira-Lima JC, Ramires RP, Zamin I, et al. Endoscopic dilation of benign esophageal strictures: report on 1043 procedures. *Am J Gastroenterol* 1999;94:1497–1501.

52. Tucker LE. The importance of fluoroscopic guidance for Maloney dilation. *Am J Gastroenterol* 1992;87:1709–1711.

53. Saeed ZA, Ramirez FC, Hepps KS, et al. An objective end point for dilation improves outcome of peptic esophageal strictures: a prospective randomized trial. *Gastrointest Endosc* 1997;45: 354–359.

54. Farup PG, Modalsli B, Tholfsen J. The natural restricturing process after dilatation of peptic esophageal strictures. *Dis Esophagus* 1998;11:116–119.

55. Agnew SR, Pandya SP, Reynolds RP, et al. Predictors for frequent esophageal dilations of benign peptic strictures. *Dig Dis Sci* 1996; 41:931–936.

56. Scolapio JS, Pasha TM, Gostout CJ, et al. A randomized prospec-

tive study comparing rigid to balloon dilators for benign esophageal strictures and rings. *Gastrointest Endosc* 1999;50:13–17.

57. Fiorini A, Fleischer D, Valero J, et al. Self-expandable metal coil stents in the treatment of benign esophageal strictures refractory to conventional therapy: a case series. *Gastrointest Endosc* 2000; 52:259–262.

58. Guelrud M, Villasmil L, Mendez R. Late results in patients with Schatzki ring treated by endoscopic electrosurgical incision of the ring. *Gastrointest Endosc* 1987;33:96–98.

59. Burdick JS, Venu RP, Hogan WJ. Cutting the defiant lower esophageal ring. *Gastrointest Endosc* 1993;39:616–619.

60. Kochhar R, Ray DM, Parupudi DM, et. al. Intralesional steroids augment the effects of endoscopic dilation in corrosive esophageal strictures. *Gastrointest Endosc* 1999;49:509–513.

61. Zein NN, Greseth JM, Perrault J. Endoscopic intralesional steroid injections in the management of refractory esophageal strictures. *Gastrointest Endosc* 1995;41:596–598.

62. Lee M, Kubik CM, Polhamus CD, et al. Preliminary experience with endoscopic intralesional steroid injection therapy for refractory upper gastrointestinal strictures. *Gastrointest Endosc* 1995; 41:598–601.

63. McBride MA, Ergun GA. The endoscopic management of esophageal strictures. *Gastrointest Endosc Clin North Am* 1994;4: 595–621.

64. Zuccaro G Jr. Viridans streptococcal bacteremia after esophageal stricture dilation. *Gastrointest Endosc* 1998;48:568–573.

65. Nelson DB, Sanderson SJ, Azar MM. Bacteremia with esophageal dilation. *Gastrointest Endosc* 1998;48:563–567.

66. Botoman VA, Surawicz CM. Bacteremia with gastrointestinal endoscopic procedures. *Gastrointest Endosc* 1986;32:342–346.

67. American Society for Gastrointestinal Endoscopy. Infection control during gastrointestinal endoscopy: guidelines for clinical application. *Gastrointest Endosc* 1999;49:836–841.

68. Foster DR. Routine chest radiography following endoscopic oesophageal dilatation for benign peptic oesophageal strictures. *Aust Radiol* 1998;42:33.

69. Kozarek RA. Hydrostatic balloon dilation of gastrointestinal stenoses: a national survey. *Gastrointest Endosc* 1986;32:15–19.

70. American Gastroenterological Association. AGA technical review on treatment of patients with dysphagia caused by benign disorders of the distal esophagus. *Gastroenterology* 1999;117:233–254.

71. Silvis SE, Nebel O, Rogers G, et al. Endoscopic complications. Results of the 1974 American Society for Gastrointestinal Endoscopy Survey. *JAMA* 1976;235:928.

72. Scolapio JS. A randomized prospective study comparing rigid to balloon dilators for benign esophageal strictures and rings. *Gastrointest Endosc*.1999;50:13–17.

73. Larrain A, Csendes A, Pope CE 2d. Surgical correction of reflux: an effective therapy for esophageal strictures. *Gastroenterology* 1975;69:578–583.

74. Spivak H, Farrell TM, Trus TL, et al. Laparoscopic fundoplication for dysphagia and peptic esophageal stricture. *J Gastrointest Surg* 1998;2:555–560.

75. Little AG, Naunheim KS, Ferguson MK, et al. Surgical management of esophageal strictures. *Ann Thorac Surg* 1988;45: 144–147.

76. Mercer CD, Hill LD. Surgical management of peptic esophageal stricture. Twenty-year experience. *J Thorac Cardiovasc Surg* 1986; 91:371–378.

77. Payne WS. Surgical management of reflux-induced oesophageal stenoses: results in 101 patients. *Br J Surg* 1984;71:971–973.

78. Orringer MB, Orringer JS. The combined Collis-Nissen operation: early assessment of reflux control. *Ann Thorac Surg* 1982; 33:534–539.

79. Hollenbeck JI, Woodward ER. Treatment of peptic esophageal stricture with combined fundic patch–fundoplication. *Ann Surg* 1975;182:472–477.

80. Maher JW, Hocking MP, Woodward ER. Long-term follow-up of the combined fundic patch fundoplication for treatment of longitudinal peptic strictures of the esophagus. *Ann Surg* 1981;194:64–69.

81. Saedd ZA, Winchester CB, Ferro PS, et al. Prospective randomized comparison of polyvinyl bougies and through the scope balloons for dilatation of peptic strictures of the esophagus. *Gastrointest Endosc* 1995;41:189–195.

82. Cox JGC, Winter RK, Maslin SC, et al. Balloon or bougie for dilatation of benign esophageal stricture? An interim report of a randomized controlled trial. *Gut* 1988;29:1741–1747.

83. Cox JG, Winter RK, Maslin SC, et al. Balloon or bougie for dilatation of benign esophageal stricture? *Dig Dis* 1994;39: 776–781.

84. Shemesh E, Czerniak A. Comparison between Savary-Gilliard and balloon dilatation of benign esophageal strictures. *World J Surg* 1990;14:518–522.

85. Yamamoto H, Hughes RW, Schroeder KW, et al. Treatment of benign esophageal strictures by Eder-Peustow or balloon dilators: a comparison between randomized and prospective nonrandomized trials. *Mayo Clin Proc* 1992;67:228–236.

GASTROESOPHAGEAL REFLUX LARYNGITIS

HARJOT SIDHU
REZA SHAKER
WALTER J. HOGAN

Esophagopharyngeal reflux of gastric acid has been implicated in the pathogenesis of a variety of otolaryngologic and respiratory disorders. "Reflux laryngitis" is the most commonly diagnosed of these disorders. The relationship between gastroesophageal reflux (GER) and laryngitis is still a matter of controversy because of lack of reliable, accepted criteria defining reflux-induced laryngitis and unavailability of a validated technique for documenting contact of acid refluxate with laryngeal structures. The suspicion of a linkage between acid reflux and vocal cord inflammation is not new.

In 1903, L.A. Coffin (1) was one of the first to associate GER with laryngeal disorders. He speculated that the "eructation of gases" from the stomach and hyperacidity were responsible for the symptoms of "post-nasal catarrh." He stated that the problem was overlooked, as most patients did not have gastrointestinal symptoms.

Jackson and Margulies (2) first described the "contact ulcer" in 1928. At that time the etiology of this disorder was thought to be vocal abuse. Cherry and Margulies (3) in 1937 reported three patients with persistent contact ulcer of the larynx who were refractory to accepted treatment of vocal rehabilitation. "Pharyngolaryngeal reflux" of gastric contents into the larynx was determined to be the etiology based on barium esophagram. These patients responded to treatment with antacids, dietary modification, and elevation of head of bed. Delahunty and Cherry (4) in 1943 reported reproducing vocal cord granulomas by application of gastric acid to the vocal cords of dogs.

Over the last 2 decades, the role of acid reflux has gained further status as a cause of chronic laryngitis with the increased recognition of gastroesophageal reflux disease (GERD) and its complications. How significant this relationship is remains to be proven.

H. Sidhu, R. Shaker, W. J. Hogan: Medical College of Wisconsin, Division of Gastroenterology & Hepatology, Milwaukee, Wisconsin.

PREVALENCE

GERD is the most common malady of the esophagus. Frequently cited figures for prevalence of heartburn are obtained from survey of 335 hospital employees in Philadelphia, Pennsylvania (5). Heartburn was experienced monthly by 15%, weekly by 14%, and daily by 7%. These data have been since corroborated by several recent population-based studies of reflux disease. A Gallup poll (6) in 1988 of U.S. adults reported monthly heartburn in 44% of respondents. A recent Gallup poll (7) 1000 adults exeriencing heartburn at least once a week conducted for the American Gastroenterology Association showed that 79% of all respondents with regular heartburn reported experiencing heartburn at night, 65% both day and night, 15% night only, and 20% day only. 45% of all respondents reported sleep difficulties due to heartburn during the prior 30 nights. These sleeping difficulties were present every night in 29%, three to six times per week in 30%, and one to two times per week in 23% of this group. Forty percent reported that sleeping difficulty had some effect on their ability to function well the next day. Thirty-four percent reported sleeping in a chair or sitting up during the night. Daily heartburn was reported by 24% of the respondents. Supraesophageal symptoms were reported by 20% three to six times per week, and 43% reported symptoms once or twice per week. This survey provides an overview of the extent of the problem and impairment of quality of life.

A population-based study by Locke et al. (8) from Olmstead County, Minnesota, determined a prevalence of occasional heartburn episodes in 59% and weekly heartburn in 20% of the respondents. Only 5% of the people who experienced symptoms within the previous year had visited the physician because of the symptoms. On the basis of recent information about the incidence of esophagitis in a large group of patients and extrapolation of these findings to the prevalence of GER observed in database studies, Johanson (9)

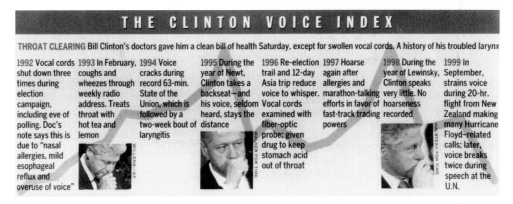

FIGURE. 29.1. Clinton voice index. (From *Time* 1999;154:42, with permission, Time Life Syndication.)

estimated that if " every patient with daily reflux symptoms" was examined with endoscopy, the prevalence of esophagitis in the general population would be approximately 1.4% (3.4 million people). Case control study of a large veteran population by El-Serag and Sonnenberg (10) showed that laryngeal disorders were twice as likely in patients with esophagitis compared to those without esophagitis.

In an uncontrolled study by Koufman (11) using 24-hour pH monitoring in a large group of patients with laryngopharyngeal disorders and suspected acid reflux, the incidence of GERD ranged from 78% in patients with laryngeal stenosis to 52% in patients with chronic cough. In a study in which GER was demonstrated with barium esophagram, esophagogastroduodenoscopy, or 24-hour pH monitoring, 80% of patients had refractory hoarseness and 50% had globus sensation; cancer of the larynx was found in a smaller percentage (12).

Supraesophageal complications of GERD are more common than we suspect. Perhaps the most noteworthy case was first reported in the June 9, 1993, edition of the *Milwaukee Journal Sentinel* (13). During the end of Bill Clinton's first presidential campaign, a severe bout of laryngitis had impeded his ability to speak. Reporters uncovered the information that president took "'antacids' and occasionally prescription medication to reduce the condition's [acid reflux] effects." Furthermore, Clinton was reported to sleep with the head of the bed elevated 30 degrees to reduce nighttime reflux, which typified the chronicity of this problem. Additional bouts of "presidential laryngitis" were chronicled in *Time* (14) (Fig. 29.1).

MECHANISM OF GASTROESOPHAGEAL REFLUX LARYNGITIS

Two major mechanisms of GER–associated laryngeal disorders have been proposed: (a) direct laryngeal contact with acid, pepsin, or nonacid injurious substance present in the gastroesophageal refluxate; and (b) acid stimulation of vagal afferents nerves in the distal and, or proximal esophagus producing a transient decrease in upper esophageal sphincter pressure (UESP).

Direct contact of acid refluxate on the pharyngeal surfaces of oral cavity could conceivably be the mechanism of injury for structures located there. However, there is little direct evidence to support this theory and the literature relative to this theory is confusing.

As early as the 1940s, Delahunty and Cherry (4) had made the observation that application of gastric juice to vocal cords of two dogs caused granulomas to develop. In one report, a group of 117 patients with GER were screened for concurrent oral lesions. Endoscopic examination and 24-hour pH monitoring showed oral lesions in 28 patients with the most severe reflux episodes (15).

In another study, however, Gudmundsson et al. (16) recorded 24-hour pH from both the esophageal body and the oral cavity of 14 patients with teeth erosion from suspected GER. No alterations in oral pH were detected, despite the occurrence of 339 acid reflux events recorded within the esophagus.

Investigations with the use of radio isotopic–labeled meals and lung scans the day after ingestion to document microaspiration have also yielded divergent results. In one study of a group of patients with nocturnal asthma, there was no radioactivity on the lung scans for the majority of the patients the morning after ingestion of the tracer meal (17). In another recent study in which scintigraphic techniques were used, lung contamination with gastric radio-labeled contents was detected with scanning in 75% of a group of 32 patients with chronic bronchial problems ranging from recurrent unexplained cough to pulmonary infections (18).

Pharyngeal reflux of gastric acid and the ratio of proximal to distal esophageal acid reflux episodes were shown to be significantly increased in patients with posterior laryngitis compared to controls in a study using a triple pH probe system with the proximal probe situated in the pharynx (19).

Adhami et al. (20) evaluated the role of gastric and duodenal ingredients on laryngeal tissue injury in dogs. They concluded that pepsin at pH 1 to 2 caused more severe histologic damage and visual changes than at pH 4 to 7. Duodenal ingredients caused no or a minimal degree of histologic damage at all pH values. However, conjugated bile acids and unconjugated bile acids showed significant visual changes but no histologic inflammation. Trypsin caused neither histologic inflammation nor visual changes. Of the three laryngeal tissue sites—right vocal cord, medial arytenoids wall, and posterior cricoid wall—the vocal cords were most sensitive to acid-related injury. Microaspiration of gastric contents into supraesophageal structures can occur during reflux episodes (21). Laboratory investigations with animal models have substantiated the deleterious effects of acid on the bronchopulmonary system by both mechanisms (22,23).

A vagal reflex arc that extends from the esophageal body to the bronchopulmonary system can be stimulated by GER events that trigger cough or bronchial constriction (24). The role of the vagus afferent nerve sensitization by acid reflux and its effect on upper esophageal sphincter pressure (UESP) remains controversial. The UESP has been reported to be unchanged (25) with spontaneous and experimental acid exposure. UESP decreased in response to distention with air boluses and increased in response to fluid boluses. Mucosal anesthesia did not alter the upper esophageal (UES) response to esophageal distention with gas or liquid, making it unlikely that these substances are differentiated by mucosal receptors. Rapid distention of the proximal esophagus with a cylindrical balloon (15 cm long) elicited UES relaxation. These findings suggest that the rapidity and spatial pattern of esophageal distention, rather than discrimination of the type of material causing the distention, determines whether UES relaxation occurs (26). Torrico et al. (27) showed that in GERD patients and control subjects all intraesophageal pressure increase events irrespective of pH drop were associated with abrupt increase in UES pressure. Although both acidic and nonacidic reflux events induce UES contraction, intraluminal pH<4 seemed to augment the contractile response (27).

Recently, preliminary observations were reported on the manometric correlates of spontaneous gastroesophago-pharyngeal acid regurgitation in patients in whom pharyngeal acid regurgitation has been previously demonstrated using dual (pharyngo-esophageal) pH monitoring (more than two episodes of acid regurgitation per 24 hours). Using a sophisticated 13-channel manometric assembly and dual pH catheter with the proximal sensor placed 2 cm above the UES midpoint and Dent sleeve sensors in both sphincters, a total of eight episodes of spontaneous esophagopharyngeal acid reflux were recorded in two of seven subjects. All eight episodes occurred abruptly. The mean time between esophageal reflux and onset of pharyngeal acidification was 8 seconds (range 0.5 to 30 seconds). In all episodes of regurgitation, retrograde transsphincteric flow was associated with a nonswallow-related UES relaxation. This UES relaxation occurred at a mean duration of 7 seconds of the initiation of esophageal reflux and in all instances pharyngeal acidification was observed to occur following the onset of UES relaxation. No episodes of abdominal straining were recorded with these regurgitation episodes, but an intraesophageal pressure increase (common cavity) was recorded with four of the eight regurgitation episodes. These results suggest that the dominant mechanism underlying esophagopharyngeal acid regurgitation is the nonswallow-related transient UES relaxation. Obviously, additional sophisticated studies of this nature may reveal more information about the mechanism of these transient UES relaxations and their relationship to supraesophageal complications of GERD (28).

Thus, at best the role of UESP, UES reflexes, or pharyngeal protective reflexes in patients with GERD and laryngitis remains incompletely defined.

SUPRAESOPHAGEAL DEFENSES

A number of reflex mechanisms within the supraesophageal area have been discovered and appear to be a part of an integrated network that prevents aspiration of gastric refluxate. For example, during belching and regurgitation of gastric fluid, the airway is protected by two reflex actions that occur at the tracheal introitus: (a) complete adduction of the true vocal cords and arytenoids, and (b) approximation of the adducted arytenoids at the base of the epiglottis, which occludes entry to the closed vocal cords (29). Abrupt distention of the esophagus (either regional or generalized) has been shown to cause brief closure of the glottis (30). This esophagoglottal closure reflex may prevent the aspiration of a larger volume of refluxate that escapes the esophagus. Finally, stimulation of the pharynx by fluid triggers a swallowing response (pharyngeal swallow) that clears the pharyngeal space while it induces complete closure of the glottis (31). Stimulation of the pharynx itself results in closure of the vocal cords, that is, the pharyngo-glottal reflex. In addition to these potential defense mechanisms in the pharyngoglottal axis, there are intrinsic laryngeal reflex mechanisms, including the cough reflex, laryngeal adduction reflex, and mucociliary action of the bronchotracheal surface. These responses obviously are important in limiting spread of the aspirate and in the enhancement of subsequent clearance.

CLINICAL SYMPTOMS

Reflux laryngitis can be associated with multiple symptoms including morning hoarseness, prolonged voice warm-up time (>20 to 30 minutes), halitosis, excessive phlegm, frequent throat clearing, dry mouth, coated tongue, sensation of a lump in the throat (globus sensation), throat tickle, dysphagia, regurgitation of food, chronic sore throat, nocturnal cough, chronic or recurrent cough, difficulty breathing especially at night, aspiration, closing off of the airway (laryngospasm), poorly controlled asthma, pneumonia, recurrent airway problems in infants, and occasionally dyspepsia (epigastric discomfort) or pyrosis (heartburn) (32, 72,73).

PHYSICAL EXAMINATION

General

Physical examination of patients with throat and voice complaints must be comprehensive. A thorough head and neck examination is always included, with attention to ears and hearing, nasal patency, oral cavity, temporomandibular joints, larynx, and neck. A limited general physical examination should include observation for signs of systemic or neurologic dysfunction that may present as throat or voice complaints.

LARYNGEAL EVALUATION

Functional

When the patient has complaints of vocal difficulties, laryngeal examination may also include formal assessment of the speaking and singing voice and strobovideolaryngoscopy for slow-motion evaluation of the vibratory margin of the vocal folds. Objective voice analysis quantifies voice quality, pulmonary function, valvular efficiency of the vocal folds, harmonic spectral characteristics, and neuromuscular function on electromyography (33).

Structural

It is estimated that 4% to 10% of patients presenting to otolaryngologists have symptoms or problems related in part to GERD. Hoarseness caused by GERD is suspected in 10% of all cases seen by them. Laryngoscopic examination typically reveals erythema and edema of mucosa overlying the arytenoid cartilages, the posterior aspect of the larynx, and often the posterior portion of the true vocal folds.

In severe cases, the erythema and edema may be more extensive. Mild, diffuse, nonspecific laryngitis and halitosis are also commonly present (Color Plate 29.2). In some patients with laryngopharyngeal reflux severe enough to involve the oral cavity, there is also loss of dental enamel. This transparency of the lower portion of the central incisors may be seen occasionally in supraesophageal reflux patients, although it may be more common in patients with bulimia and those who habitually eat lemons.

A number of relatively recent developments, such as direct per oral intubation techniques, introduction of narrow-caliber high-resolution video instruments, and the increasing number of otolaryngologists who perform transnasal fiberoptic laryngoscopy, afford new opportunities to recognize oropharyngeal pathology (34). It has also sparked increasing interest in the pharyngolaryngeal zone among gastroenterologists.

The ability of gastroenterologists to recognize laryngeal abnormalities has been sharply criticized (35,36). Interpretation of endoscopic photographs of the larynx can vary greatly between gastroenterologists and otolaryngologists. Otolaryngologists are more critical in assessing the adequacy of laryngeal views for interpretation. This is predictable given gastroenterologists' lack of experience with laryngeal pathology and examination techniques. Efforts to educate gastroenterologists regarding normal laryngeal anatomy and abnormalities associated with laryngeal anatomy and abnormalities associated with GER should improve detection of GER-related laryngeal disorders during endoscopy (Color Plate 29.3).

The pharyngolaryngeal area is best visualized during insertion of an endoscope through the pharynx. The endoscopic procedure may induce significant edema and erythema due to trauma from manipulation of instrument during diagnostic study. This is particularly important when considering the endoscopic criteria for "posterior laryngitis," which can be reproduced by the posterior laryngeal trauma created during routine upper endoscopic examination.

The spectrum of laryngeal findings attributed to reflux include:

- Vocal fold edema/polypoid degeneration
- Posterior commisure hypertrophy
- Diffuse laryngeal edema
- Laryngeal erythema/hyperemia
- Pseudo sulcus vocalis
- Excessive mucous
- Granuloma/granulation formation (37)

Laryngopharyngeal reflux (LPR) is the nomenclature adopted by the American Academy of Otolaryngology/Head and Neck Surgery for reflux induced laryngeal disorders. Investigations in this discipline have attempted to quantify laryngeal physical findings detected during fiberoptic laryngoscopy and to attribute them to reflux injury. A reflux finding score (RFS) has been developed (Table 29.1) This eight-item RFS has been validated based on a clinical severity scale of laryngeal inflammation

TABLE 29.1. REFLUX FINDING SCORE

Pseudosulcus vocalis	0 = absent
	2 = present
Ventricular obliteration	0 = none
	2 = partial
	4 = complete
Erythema/hyperemia	0 = none
	2 = arytenoids only
	4 = diffuse
Vocal fold edema	0 = none
	1 = mild
	2 = moderate
	3 = severe
	4 = polypoid
Diffuse laryngeal edema	0 = none
	1 = mild
	2 = moderate
	3 = severe
	4 = obstructing
Posterior commisure	0 = none
Hypertrophy	1 = mild
	2 = moderate
	3 = severe
	4 = obstructing
Granuloma/granulation	0 = absent
	2 = present
Thick endolaryngeal mucus fold lesion	0 = absent
	2 = present
	Total

Source: Belafsky PC, Postma GN, Koufman JA. The validity and reliability of the reflux finding score (RFS). *Laryngoscope* 2001;111: 1313, with permission.

(38). Independent items of the RFS are nonspecific because they can be caused by a number of other sources of laryngeal inflammation, such as infection, allergy, and environmental toxins. An RFS>5 is considered abnormal. This rating scale is considered to be reproducible and reliably documents treatment efficacy among laryngopharyngeal reflux. Although the RFS scale provides a useful framework for describing reflux-induced laryngeal tissue injury, nevertheless it has not been shown to be a sensitive/specific diagnostic tool for confirming this association.

Edema of the ventral surface of the vocal fold extending from the anterior commisure to the posterior larynx is termed "pseudo sulcus vocalis." A recent investigation reported that the presence of pseudo sulcus alone has a positive predictive value for LPR of 90% (39).

Although the current practice of ENT physicians in diagnosing and managing patients suspected of GERD-related ENT disorders is based on laryngoscopic findings, up to 50% of patients with laryngoscopic "signs" suggesting GERD does not respond to aggressive acid suppression nor do they have abnormal acid reflux on 24-hour esophageal pH monitoring. This results in frustration on the part of subspecialists (ENT/GI) and confusion for the patient. Although some investigators and clinicians believe that laryngeal signs are specific for GERD-related problems, there is paucity of information relating to the inter- and intra-variability of laryngoscopists in accurately identifying these "signs."

Vaezi et al. (40) recently investigated the baseline prevalence of laryngeal signs in a prospective study of 50 healthy subjects without acid reflux or laryngeal complaints. The majority of subjects did not have normal laryngeal findings; 43 of 50 (86%) had one or more findings often considered pathognomic of GERD-related laryngeal complaints, suggesting the overdiagnosis of GERD due to the poor specificity of these laryngeal "signs." In a more recent comparison of the laryngoscopic findings associated with GERD with normal controls, posterior cricoid wall erythema, true/false vocal cord erythema, and edema and arytenoid medial wall erythema/edema were significantly more often detected in patients suspected of reflux injury versus control subjects (41). Importantly, these signs improved or resolved on acid suppressive therapy. These observations highlight the existing confusion on the role of the laryngeal findings in the diagnosis of supraesophageal reflux.

Endoscopic detection of inflammation of the esophageal lining does not indicate that GER, per se, is responsible for the suspected supraesophageal disorder. However, documentation of acid reflux injury does help build a plausible scenario for the association of supraesophageal reflux and alerts the physician to a possible explanation for the problem and a potential target for treatment.

Finding esophagitis during an esophagogastroduodenoscopy examination is an inconsistent finding in patients with suspected supraesophageal complications of GERD. Only 40% incidence of esophageal mucosa damage was reported in patients with asthma in a comprehensive literature review (42). Although a recent study of U.S. military veterans showed a significant association between esophagitis and various pulmonary and laryngeal problems (10), the absence of physical damage to the esophagus has been noted in the majority of patients with suspected supraesophageal complications of GERD. At first glance, this is an apparent paradox. Nonetheless, most clinicians have come to accept that there is a disparity of esophageal symptoms and signs in many patients in whom acid reflux does cause supraesophageal problems. Certain factors may explain the absence of macroscopic inflammation of the esophagus. Patients may have been treated previously for reflux with potent acid-suppressing medication at doses that heal inflammation but were inadequate to effectively treat the reflux laryngitis. Often, the presence of discrete esophageal surface scarring or pitting in the area immediately above the gastroesophageal junction is a hallmark of chronic GER injury (Color Plates 29.4 and 29.5).

The posterior surface of the arytenoids and the posterior commissure are most likely to come in contact with acid reflux. The lining of the larynx is believed to be stratified squamous epithelium in the area of true vocal cords and pseudo stratified columnar (respiratory type) in the remainder of the larynx. Laryngeal tissue is not adapted to an acid milieu. It has been suggested that frequent or long exposure to gastroesophageal refluxate may result in both benign and malignant changes at the sites. The exact time required for acid exposure to damage structures above the esophagus is unknown (43).

Although reflux laryngitis is believed to be a consequence of supraesophageal reflux, a direct cause-and-effect relationship is difficult to document. Nonetheless, clinical suspicion of a connection continues to grow despite this lack of validation.

DIAGNOSTIC STUDIES/AMBULATORY pH STUDIES

Ambulatory 24-hour pH monitoring is considered the current "gold standard" for reflux testing. There is agreement that a single distal probe is not adequate for evaluation of supraesophageal disorders. The use of a distal and pharyngeal pH probe appears critical to making a diagnosis of pharyngeal acid reflux. The feasibility and efficacy of combined dual, hypopharyngeal and esophageal pH monitoring in documenting hypopharyngeal acid exposure was demonstrated in patients with chronic hoarseness (44). Seven of ten patients monitored with the dual system demonstrated at least one episode of hypopharyngeal reflux preceded by an episode of esophageal reflux. Three of these seven patients had "normal" esophageal reflux frequency, but hypopharyngeal reflux was associated with the few esophageal episodes that did occur (44).

A study of normal subjects with five pH probes placed at 3-cm increments above the lower esophageal sphincter demonstrated a linear decrease in the percentage of the time that pH was <4 from the 3-cm level to the 15-cm level. The number of reflux episodes likewise decreased with more proximal positioning (45). Generally the proximal pH is positioned by mapping UES at manometry, but it may be reasonable to position the proximal probe with endoscopic visualization without the use of manometry. This technique may help standardize the recording site and the data derived from proximal location (46).

The currently accepted criteria for defining pharyngeal reflux events were recently defined as follows:

- pH reduction to <4.0 in the pharynx
- Pharyngeal pH drop during or immediately after distal esophageal acid exposure
- pH drop does not occur during an episode of eating or swallowing
- Proximal sensor pH drop is rapid and sharp, not gradual
- Hypo pharyngeal pH drop should be greater than 2 pH units (47)

Williams et al. (47) determined that 92% of pharyngeal pH decreases of 1 to 2 pH units and 66% of pH decreases

of this magnitude reaching a nadir pH<4.0 were artifactual. The study also demonstrated that most esopharyngeal regurgitation events occur in an upright position and the most prevalent pattern of acid regurgitation is an abrupt continuous transfer of acid refluxate from stomach to pharynx. The study also found a poor correlation between what is perceived by the patient as pharyngeal regurgitation and demonstrable acid regurgitation into the pharynx. The patients reported only 44% of pharyngeal acid regurgitation events detected by pharyngeal sensor. Conversely, of 27 reports of regurgitation, only 4 (15%) were actually associated with pharyngeal acidification and just over half were associated with esophageal acidification.

Validation of pharyngeal pH criteria is more difficult than validation of esophageal pH criteria in diagnosis of GERD, a disease in which endoscopic esophagitis correlates well with acid exposure and symptoms are highly specific and reasonably sensitive for the disease (48–50). In contrast, throat symptoms believed to be attributable to acid regurgitation are protean and these symptoms and laryngitis have multiple causes. Pharyngeal symptoms, particularly during sleep are unreliable. Also, laryngoscopically demonstrable laryngitis is not appropriate for validation of pH criteria because posterior laryngitis is nonspecific for acid-related injury. The true prevalence of esopharyngeal acid regurgitation in patients with laryngitis remains unknown.

PH MEAUREMENT VARIABILITY

Extraesophageal reflux is often intermittent. A negative pH study does not rule out extraesophageal reflux (11,51). The difficulty in confirming the diagnosis of extraesophageal reflux is well demonstrated in the study by Vaezi et al. (52), which showed that there was a significant day-to-day variability of pH in the proximal esophagus. Healthy volunteers had good intrasubject reproducibility (91% to 100%). Those with distal reflux and proximal reflux had poor reproducibility (distal 70% to 90%; proximal 55%). The outcome demonstrated good specificity (91%), but poor sensitivity and reproducibility (55%) for proximal pH probe for identifying an abnormal amount of proximal esophageal acid reflux. Therefore, a negative test result does not exclude proximal reflux.

ROLE OF THREE-SITE AMBULATORY PHARYNGO-ESOPHAGEAL pH MONITORING

Several studies to determine the role of gastroesophageal reflux in reflux laryngitis have been performed at our center.

A study using simultaneous three-site pharyngo-esophageal pH monitoring demonstrated that, pharyngeal reflux of gastric acid is significantly more prevalent and

TABLE 29.2. PHARYNGEAL pH MONITORING IN PATIENTS WITH POSTERIOR LARYNGITIS

Patient No.	Videostroboscopy	Diagnostic Workup Results		
		Barium Esophagram	T-EGD Esophageal Findings	Pharyngeal Acid Exposure
1	PL, VCN	GER (−)	No abnormality	Positive
2	PL	GER (−)	No abnormality	Positive
3	PL, LTS	GER (−)	No abnormality	Positive
4	PL, VCN	GER (−)	No abnormality	Negative
5	PL, LTS	GER (−)	No abnormality	Positive
6	PL, LTS	GER (−)	No abnormality	Negative
7	PL	GER (−)	No abnormality	Negative
8	PL	GER (+), HH	HH	Positive
9	PL	AM	No abnormality	Negative
10	PL	GER (−)	No abnormality	Negative
11	PL	AM	No abnormality	Negative
12	PL, LTS	GER (−)	—	Positive
13	PL, VCN	GER (+), HH	HH, Esophagitis	Positive
14	PL	GER (+), AM, HH	HH	Positive
15	PL, LTS	GER (+)	No abnormality	Positive
16	PL	AM	Esophagitis	Positive
17	PL	GER (+), HH	—	Positive
18	PL, VFP	GER (−)	—	Positive
19	PL, VCN	GER (−)	—	Positive
20	PL	GER (−)	—	Positive

AM, abnormal motility; GER, gastroesophageal reflux; HH, hiatal hernia; LTS, laryngotracheal stenosis; PL, posterior laryngitis; T-EGD, transnasal esophago-gastro-duodeno-endoscopy, or transnasal endoscopy; VCN, vocal cord nodules; VFP, vocal fold polyp.
Adapted from Ulualp SO, Toohill RJ, Hoffman R, et al. Pharyngeal pH monitoring in patients with posterior laryngitis. *Otolaryngol Head Neck Surg* 1999;120:672–677, with permission.

the ratio of proximal to distal esophageal acid reflux episodes is significantly increased in patients with posterior laryngitis compared to normal controls and patients with GERD (19). A subsequent study (53) showed pharyngeal acid reflux to be more prevalent in patients with posterior laryngitis than in healthy controls (Table 29.2). The authors noted that patients with posterior laryngitis infrequently have esophageal inflammatory sequelae of reflux disease, which was determined using unsedated transnasal pharyngoesophagoduodenoscopy. Another study (54) determined the prevalence of pharyngeal acid reflux events to be significantly higher in patients with vocal cord nodules compared with normal controls. This study used barium esophagram and ambulatory 24-hour, three-site pharyngoesophageal pH monitoring in patients and controls (Table 29.3). This confirms a contributory

TABLE 29.3. PHARYNGEAL ACID REFLUX EVENTS IN PATIENTS WITH VOCAL CORD NODULES

Patient No.	Age (Years)	Sex	Results of Diagnostic Evaluation		
			Endoscopy	Barium Esophagram	Pharyngeal Acid Reflux
1	51	M	VCN, PL	GER, HH	Positive
2	17	F	VCN, PL	GER	Positive
3	22	F	VCN, PL	Normal	Negative
4	39	F	VCN, PL	Normal	Positive
5	78	F	VCN, PL	Normal	Positive
6	32	F	VCN, PL	Normal	Positive
7	73	M	VCN, PL	GER, HH	Positive
8	30	F	VCN	Normal	Negative
9	41	F	VCN, PL	GER	Positive
10	34	F	VCN	Abnormal motility	Negative
11	51	F	VCN, PL	GER	Negative

GER, gastroesophageal reflux; HH, hiatal hernia; PL, posterior laryngitis; VCN, vocal cord nodules.
Source: Kuhn J, Toohill RJ, Ulualp SO, et al. Pharyngeal acid reflux events in patients with vocal cord nodules. *Laryngoscope* 1998;108:1146–1149, with permission.

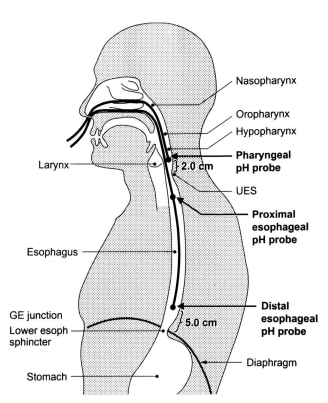

FIGURE. 29.6. Schema of ambulatory three-site pH probe technique. The standard dual pH probe is placed so that the distal probe is 5.0 cm above the lower esophageal sphincter; the proximal esophageal probe is situated beneath the upper esophageal sphincter (UES) zone. The pharyngeal pH probe (which frequently requires a separate tube) is placed in the hypopharynx approximately 2.0 cm above the UES.

A recent study (55) evaluated the diagnostic role of simultaneous pharyngeal pH monitoring and laryngoscopy in gastrolaryngeal reflux as a cause of respiratory symptoms. A total of 76 patients with respiratory symptoms and 10 control patients were evaluated with a symptomatology questionnaire, direct laryngoscopy using the RFS to grade laryngeal injury, esophageal manometry, and 24-hour esophagopharyngeal pH monitoring. Control subjects had significantly lower RFS (2.1 vs. 9.6, $p<0.01$) and fewer episodes of pharyngeal reflux episodes (0.2 vs. 3.4, $p<0.01$) than patients. Patients were divided into three groups: group I=RFS–/PR–, group II=RFS–/PR+, and group III=RFS+/PR+. Patients in group III had significantly higher heartburn scores and distal esophageal acid exposure. Eighty-three percent of patients in group III but only 44% in group I had improvement in their respiratory symptoms as a result of antireflux therapy. The study suggests that agreement between PR and RFS helps establish or refute the GER diagnosis as cause of laryngeal symptoms. Patients who are RFS+ and PR– may have laryngeal injury from another source, whereas patients who are RFS–/PR+ may not have acid entering the larynx despite the presence of pharyngeal reflux. Patients who are RFS+ and PR+ have reflux causing laryngeal damage. Thus, laryngoscopy and pharyngeal pH monitoring should be considered complimentary studies in establishing the diagnosis of laryngeal injury induced by GER (55).

MANAGING LARYNGEAL COMPLICATIONS OF REFLUX DISEASE

Medical Management

Laryngeal complications of reflux disease are most effectively treated with a proton pump inhibitor (PPI). PPIs are the most effective drugs in treating GERD involving the esophagus. Acid reflux events are decreased by greater than 80% and healing of esophagitis is reported in 80% to 90% of patients. Their efficacy in patients with suspected laryngeal complications of GERD is significantly lower than that noted in esophageal complications of GERD. It is a general clinical observation that PPIs appear to be most effective at

role for supraesophageal acid reflux in the pathogenesis of vocal cord nodules (54).

We routinely use simultaneous three-site ambulatory pH monitoring at our center to determine the possibility of pharyngeal reflux (Fig. 29.6). Over the last year and half, three-site ambulatory pH studies have been performed in 108 patients; 76 studies were done to exclude supraesophageal reflux. There were 16 positive studies; all except one patient was off all acid-suppressive treatment (Fig. 29.7).

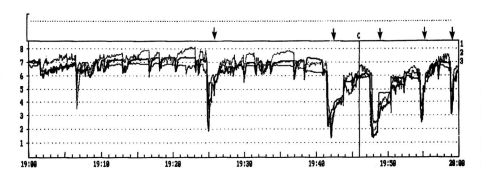

FIGURE. 29.7. Trace segment of three-site ambulatory pH study noting five episodes of retrograde pharyngeal reflux during 1-hour period. One episode was followed by a cough *(c)* . (Time in minutes on horizontal scale, and pH units on vertical scale.)

higher doses for laryngeal complications, and a longer duration of therapy is necessary compared to that required for esophageal GERD.

Based on these clinical experiences, a similar approach for the treatment of suspected supraesophageal complications of GERD was recommended by Hogan et al. (56) for the working group at the first multidisciplinary symposium on supraesophageal complications of reflux disease. The recommendations call for a double dose of PPI therapy, initially for patients with suspected supraesophageal complications of GERD, and a duration of therapy for at least 3 and possibly 6 months. At the completion of this initial therapeutic trial, assessment of the patient's symptoms and response to therapy should be critically evaluated. This is considered both a diagnostic and therapeutic trial.

An uncontrolled study reported the results of PPI therapy in 16 patients with persistent posterior laryngitis who had previously failed H2 receptor antagonist (H2RA) therapy. Omeprazole treatment ranged from 6 to 24 weeks with dosage of 40 mg of omeprazole at nighttime. This was increased to 40 mg bid for 6 weeks in four patients with continuing symptoms. At the conclusion of the study, both laryngoscopy scores and esophageal symptom indices improved significantly. Symptoms recurred, however, after the discontinuation of acid-suppressant therapy, suggesting that acid reflux was indeed the underlying etiology (57).

The importance of long-term treatment for laryngeal complications of reflux disease is stressed because injury to the epithelium is a chemical burn that can take weeks to months to resolve. For most patients, an 8-week course of antisecretory treatment, used for esophageal reflux injury, is inadequate. Recurrence of symptoms is common in patients who require PPI therapy for initial treatment (58).

Currently, it is difficult to interpret the evidence from trials using PPIs for treatment of patients with suspected laryngeal complications of GERD. This is because studies contain small groups of patients, treatment durations are very short, and no control groups have been included. Furthermore, studies using PPIs in patients with suspected supraesophageal complications of GERD require properly designed, controlled protocols to fully evaluate treatment efficacy.

H2RAs and prokinetic medications have not, for the most part, found an effective role in treating patients with suspected laryngeal GERD complications. Because sensitivity/accuracy of diagnostic testing is not uniformly successful in substantiating the role of acid reflux in laryngeal disorders, a therapeutic trial may be the only recourse.

Table 29.4 shows key features of the nine studies that evaluated the efficacy of antireflux medical treatment on reflux laryngitis. Only one of these studies was a randomized placebo-controlled study.

Before medical therapy can be considered a "failure," adequate esophageal and gastric acid suppression should be documented. We recommend a three-site, simultaneous pharyngoesophageal pH monitoring with patient on acid-suppressive therapy to document whether the current dose of medical therapy is adequate (Fig. 29.8).

Surgical Therapy

The apparent advantage of operative therapy is that it corrects the antireflux barrier at the gastroesophageal junction, it repairs the hiatal hernia, and prevents the reflux of most stomach contents, thus preventing acid and nonacidic material from coming in contact with the pharyngolaryngeal mucosa.

TABLE 29.4. OUTCOMES REPORTED BY TRIALS OF ANTIREFLUX TREATMENT OF REFLUX LARYNGITIS, 1991–2001

Author	N	Pharmacologic Intervention	Treatment Duration	Symptom Improvement Laryngeal	Symptom Improvement Esophageal	Laryngoscopic Improvement	Follow-up
Koufman (11)	33	Ranitidine 300–600 mg/d or famotidine 80 mg/d	24 wk	85%	—	85%	44 wk
Kamel et al. (57)	16	Omeprazole 40 mg/d	6–24 wk	79%	96%	56%	6 wk
Hanson et al. (59)	182	Stepwise treatment: Famotidine 20 mg/d and omeprazole 20–40 mg/d	6–12 wk	96%	—	96%	>6–12 wk
Shaw et al. (60)	68	Omeprazole 20 mg bid	12 wk	Significant improvement	40%	Significant improvement	None
Wo et al. (61)	21	Omeprazole 40 mg/d	8 wk	40%	48%	50%	8 wk
Metz et al. (62)	10	Omeprazole 20 mg bid	4 wk	60%	100%	—	—
Hanson et al. (63)	16	Omeprazole 20 mg/d	6–9 wk	Significant improvement, acoustic parameters	—	—	
Jaspersen et al. (64)	21	Omeprazole 40 mg/d, maintenance 20 mg bid	4 wk	100%	100%	100%	1 yr
El-Serag et al. (65)	20	Omeprazole 30 mg bid	3 mo	50%	—	58%	3 mo

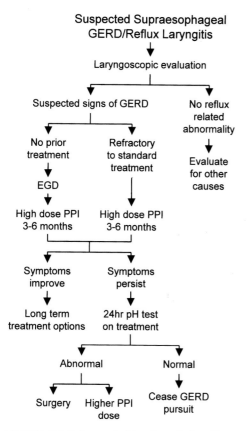

FIGURE. 29.8. Suggested treatment algorithm.

with H₂RA, and included those with previous laryngeal carcinoma (38%) and leukoplakia (46%). Symptoms resolved and laryngoscopic abnormalities disappeared in 73% of patients when followed for 11 months. So et al. (68) evaluated improvement in symptom scores over an average of 22 months in 35 patients with cervical or thoracic symptoms, the majority of whom had pharyngeal acid reflux, by a 24-hour pH study. Heartburn requiring antacids was reported by 86% of patients and 36% had evidence of esophagitis. Although 93% of patients were relieved of heartburn, only 58% of them showed an improved supraesophageal symptom score. A symptom response to preoperative acid-suppressive treatment was a significant predictor of postoperative improvement.

The recent introduction of "minimally invasive" laparoscopic fundoplication has, for the most part, replaced conventional open fundoplication operation. Because many surgeons with little experience in esophageal physiology have begun to perform this procedure, not unexpectedly, the number and severity of complications resulting from laproscopic fundoplication have increased. For this reason, this operation should not be the "first-line" therapy for patients with "suspected" supraesophageal complications of GERD. Exceptions to this approach would be dramatic situations such as obvious regurgitation and aspiration or laryngospasm. In fact, demonstration of the effectiveness of acid-suppression therapy should be the major criteria for predicting successful outcome to fundoplication. The morbidity associated with fundoplication varies but may be significant. In large reported series, the frequency of postoperative dysphagia ranges from 0% (69) to 17% (70).

Finally, fundoplication surgery is championed as the treatment of choice particularly for the young patient with significant GERD who faces a "lifetime" of medical treatment with a potentially negative impact on lifestyle. Although this notion seems reasonable, few have questioned the long-term integrity of the fundoplication wrap structure. Reports vary concerning the long-standing durability of the fundoplication wrap, but at least one long-term study showed a significant "breakdown" of the fundoplication wrap 20 years after the open fundoplication operation (71).

SUMMARY

The prevalence of supraesophageal GERD and reflux laryngitis is unknown. While there is a clear association between acid reflux and structural injury to laryngeal tissues, there is no specific or sensitive test to serve as a totally reliable marker. The standard two-site, 24-hour ambulatory pH study has served as the "gold standard" in the past to help identify patients with potential reflux laryngitis. The three-site pH probe test to detect pharyngeal acid events is an improvement, but it also has limitations. Despite the lack of

Candidates for antireflux surgery are often patients who require continuous or increasing doses of medication to maintain their response to acid-suppressive therapy. The case has been made for young patients, noncompliant patients, and those who choose to have this type of therapy. Oftentimes, financial concerns of the patient have been a reason for fundoplication. Except for two studies reporting the result of Nissen fundoplication in patients with laryngopharyngeal complications of reflux disease, the published reports generally deal with efficacy and long-term outcomes of operations in patients with esophageal complications of reflux. Although the long-term efficacy of laparoscopic fundoplication is not available, 80% to 90% of patients are reported to be asymptomatic or have minimal symptoms following a conventional open fundoplication. In a 10-year follow-up after open fundoplication surgery, 91% of patients continued to have control of their symptoms. Short-term outcome results following laproscopic fundoplication indicate symptom control in 85% to 90% of patients with acceptable low morbidity rates (66).

Two prospective uncontrolled clinical trials evaluated the efficacy of Nissen fundoplication for patients with GERD-related laryngeal disorders. Deveney et al. (67) studied 13 consecutive patients with symptomatic laryngitis and objective evidence of GERD who were refractory to treatment

objective parameters, many otolaryngologists have now equated subtle laryngeal changes at laryngoscopy (e.g., erythematous arytenoids) as being caused solely by acid reflux. Attempts are being made to score a variety of laryngeal changes to provide a more objective parameter of GERD-related injury, but a head-to-head comparison with concurrent acid reflux measurement studies remains to be done to confirm these ENT findings.

Presently, in the context of a negative history, endoscopic and radiologic exam and three-site ambulatory pH study, the only alternative for the physician in charge is empiric treatment of presumed reflux laryngitis with high-dose PPI therapy for a prolonged period. Lacking a successful outcome (see algorithm), the physician(s) involved in patient care should cease the further pursuit of GER as the potential etiology (74,75). When disagreement between physician specialists continues concerning the cause of the patient's symptoms of laryngitis, the patient becomes both confused and frustrated.

GER can be a cause for chronic laryngeal injury and laryngitis. Unfortunately, the diagnostic tools available are imperfect and often unreliable. Until this situation is remedied, we must attempt to avoid overdiagnosing this entity and thus to use appropriate restraint.

REFERENCES

1. Coffin LA. The relationship of upper airway passages to diseases of gastrointestinal tract. *Ann Otol Rhinol Laryngol* 1903;12: 521–526.
2. Jackson C, Margulies SI. Contact ulcer of larynx. *Ann Otol Rhinol Laryngol* 1928;37:227–230.
3. Cherry J, Margulies SI. Contact ulcer of the larynx. *Laryngoscope* 1968;78:1937–1940.
4. Delahunty JE, Cherry J. Experimentally produced vocal cord granulomas. *Laryngoscope* 1968;78:1941–1947.
5. Nebel OT, Fornes MF, Castell DO. Symptomatic gastroesophageal reflux: incidence and precipitating factors. *Am J Dig Dis* 1976;21:953–956.
6. Gallup Organization. *A Gallup survey on heartburn across America.* Princeton, NJ: Gallup Organization, Inc., 1988.
7. Shaker R, Castell D, Schoenfeld PS, et al. Nighttime heartburn is an underappreciated clinical problem that impacts sleep and daytime function. *Gastroenterology* 2001;120(suppl 1):A420.
8. Locke GR III, Talley NJ, Fett SL, et al. Prevalence and clinical spectrum of gastroesophageal reflux: a population-based study in Olmsted County, Minnesota. *Gastroenterology* 1997;112: 1448–1456.
9. Johanson JF. Epidemiological review of esophageal and supraesophageal reflux injuries. *Am J Med* 2000;108(suppl 4a): 99s–103s.
10. El-Serag HB, Sonnenberg A. Comorbid occurrence of laryngeal or pulmonary disease with esophagitis in United States military veterans. *Gastroenterology* 1997;113:755–760.
11. Koufman JA. The otolaryngolic manifestation of gastroesophageal reflux (GERD): a clinical investigation of 225 patients using ambulatory 24-hour pH monitoring and an experimental investigation of the role of acid and pepsin in the development of laryngeal injury. *Laryngoscope* 1991;101(suppl 53):1–78.
12. Gaynor EB. Otolaryngologic manifestations of gastroesophageal reflux. *Am J Gastroenterol* 1991 Jul;86(7):801–8.
13. Resler J. Clinton's hoarse voice. *Milwaukee Journal-Sentinel*, June 9, 1993.
14. The Clinton voice index. *Time* 1999;154(14):42.
15. Meurman JH, Toskala J, Nuutinen P, et al. Oral and dental manifestations in gastroesophageal reflux disease. *Oral Surg Oral Med Oral Pathol* 1994;78:583–589.
16. Gudmundsson K, Kristleifsson G, Theodor A, et al. Tooth erosion, gastroesophageal reflux and salivary buffer capacity. *Oral Surg Oral Med Oral Pathol Oral Radiol Endod* 1995;79:185–189.
17. Greyson ND, Reid RH, Lui YC, et al. Radionucleide assessment in nocturnal asthma. *Clin Nucl Med* 1982;7:318–319.
18. Crausaz FM, Favez G. Aspiration of solid food particles into lungs of patients wit gastroesophageal reflux and chronic bronchial disease. *Chest* 1988;93:376–378.
19. Shaker R, Milbrath M, Ren J, et al. Esophagopharyngeal distribution of refluxed gastric acid in patients with reflux laryngitis. *Gastroenterology* 1995;109:1575–1582.
20. Adhami T, Goldblum J, Richter J, et al. Role of gastric and duodenal ingredients in laryngeal tissue injury: an experimental study in dogs. *Gastroenterology* 2002;122:A-50.
21. Belsey R. The pulmonary complications of oesophageal disease. *Br J Dis* Chest 1960;54:342–348.
22. Tuchman DN, Boyle JT, Pack AI, et al. Comparisons of airway responses following tracheal or esophageal acidification in the cat. *Gastroenterology* 1984;87:872–881.
23. Mansfield LE, Hameister HH, Spaulding NS, et al. The role of the vagus nerve in airway narrowing caused by intraesophageal hydrochloric acid provocation and esophageal distention. *Ann Allergy* 1981;47:431–434.
24. Mansfield LE, Stein MR. Gastroesophageal reflux and asthma: a possible reflex mechanism. *Ann Allergy* 1978;41:224–226.
25. Vakil NB, Kahrilas PJ, Dodds WJ, et al. Absence of an upper esophageal sphincter response to acid reflux. *Am J Gastroenterol* 1989;84:606–610.
26. Kahrilas PJ, Dodds WJ, Dent J, et al. Upper esophageal sphincter function during belching. *Gastroenterology* 1986;91:133–140.
27. Torrico S, Kern M, Aslam M, et al. Upper esophageal sphincter function during gastroesophageal reflux events revisited. *Am J Physiol Gastrointest Liver Physiol* 2000;279(2):G262–7.
28. Rohan W, Cook IJ. Preliminary observations on the mechanisms of esophago-pharyngeal acid regurgitation in humans subjects. *Gastroenterology* 2002;122:A-190(abst).
29. Shaker R, Ren J, Kern M, et al. Mechanisms of airway protection and upper esophageal sphincter opening during belching. *Am J Physiol* 1992;262:G621–G628.
30. Shaker R, Dodds WJ, Ren J, et al. Esophagoglottal closure reflex: a mechanism of airway protection. *Gastroenterology* 1992;102: 857–886.
31. Kelly JH. Management of upper esophageal sphincter disorders: indications and complications of myotomy. *Am J Med* 2000; 108(suppl 4a):43s–46s.
32. Castell DO, Richter JE. *The esophagus.* 3rd ed. Philadelphia, PA: Lippincott–Raven Publishers, 1999.
33. Sataloff RT. *Professional voice: the science and art of clinical care.* 2nd ed. San Diego, CA: Singular Publishing Group, 1997.
34. Johnson DA, Schecter GL, Katz PO, et al. ENT and GI specialists' interpretation of possible reflux laryngitis—coalition or confusion? *Gastroenterology* 1992;102(suppl):A91(abst).
35. Johnson DA, Katz PO, Castell DO. Interobserver variability among GI specialists in evaluation of the larynx. *Am J Gastroenterol* 1991;86,1296(abst).
36. Young JL, Shaw GY, Searl JP, et al. Laryngeal manifestations of gastroesophageal reflux disease:endoscopic appearance and management. *Gastrointest Endosc* 1995;43:225–230.

Color Plates

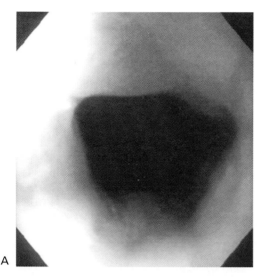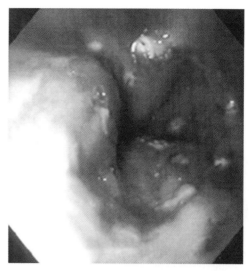

COLOR PLATE 26.3. Endoscopic appearance of the gastroesophageal junction (GEJ) before and immediately after Stretta. **A:** Patulous GEJ. **B:** Mucosal burn marks straddling the GEJ. These marks disappear within 10 days after Stretta.

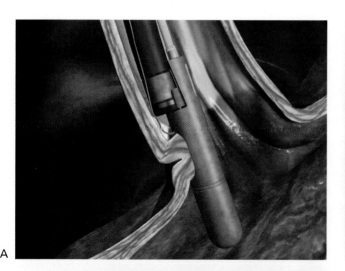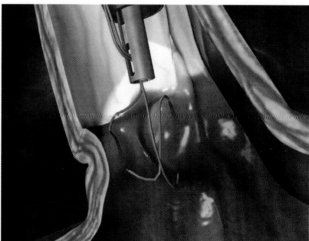

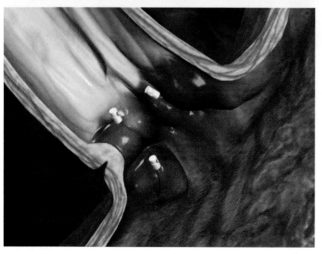

COLOR PLATE 26.4. Sequential steps **(A)** to **(C)** in the gastroplasty procedure using EndoCinch.

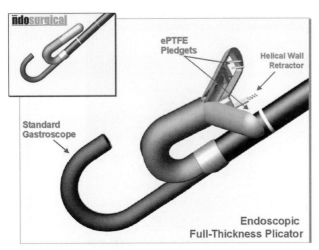

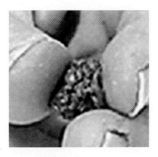

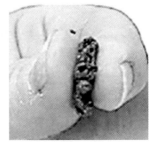

COLOR PLATE 26.6. Diagrammatic representation of the NDO placation system. Under direct endoscopic visualization, the gastric mucosa below the GEJ is retracted within the jaws of the plicator and a full-thickness placation is achieved. (Courtesy of NDO Surgical, Mansfield, MA.)

COLOR PLATE 26.7. A: Features of Enteryx. **B:** Upon contact with water, the material precipitates into a spongy mass.

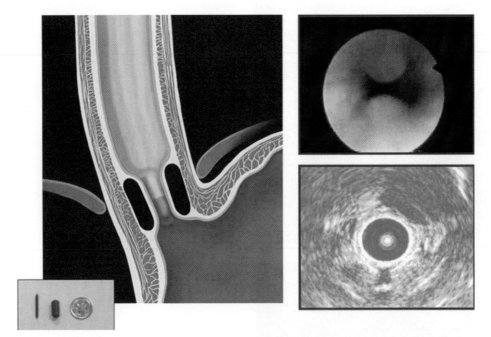

COLOR PLATE 26.9. The Gatekeeper reflux repair system. **Left:** Placement of the prosthesis in the submucosa of the gastroesophageal junction (GEJ) creates a bulking effect. **Top right:** Endoscopic image after placement. **Bottom right:** Endoscopic ultrasonographic image of the prosthesis after placement in the submucosa of the GEJ.

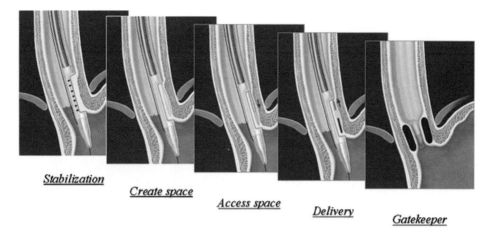

Stabilization

Create space

Access space

Delivery

Gatekeeper

COLOR PLATE 26.10. Steps in the placement of hydrogel prosthesis. (Courtesy of Paul Fauckens, AMC, Amsterdam, Netherlands.)

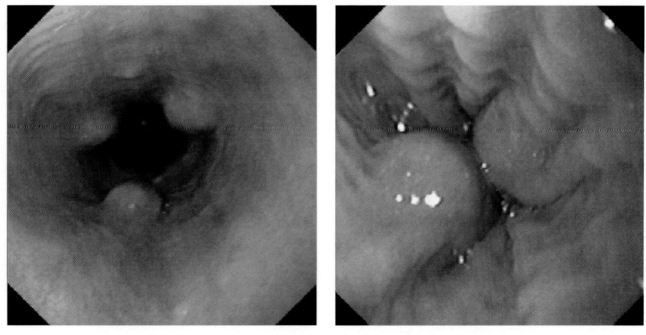

A

B

COLOR PLATE 26.11. Endoscopic appearance of the hydrogel prostheses in place at the gastroesophageal junction, **(A)** and **(B)**. (Courtesy of Paul Fauckens, AMC, Amsterdam, Netherlands.)

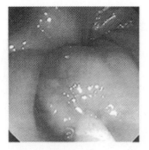

U/S at 6 months

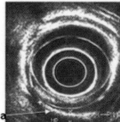

Plexiglas injection

Plexiglas in submucosa

COLOR PLATE 26.12. **Left:** Endoscopic visualization of Plexiglas injection at the level of the gastroesophageal junction. **Right:** Endoscopic ultrasonographic image of Plexiglas in the submucosa 6 months after implantation. (From Feretis C, Benakis P, Dimopoulos C, et al. Endoscopic implantation of Plexiglass (PMMA) micro-spheres for the treatment of GERD. *Gastrointest Endosc* 2001;53:423–426.)

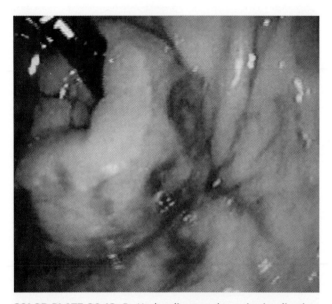

COLOR PLATE 26.13. B: Under direct endoscopic visualization, the gastric mucosa below the GEJ is grasped by the plicator and a full-thickness placation is achieved. (Courtesy of Rodney Mason, M.D., .)

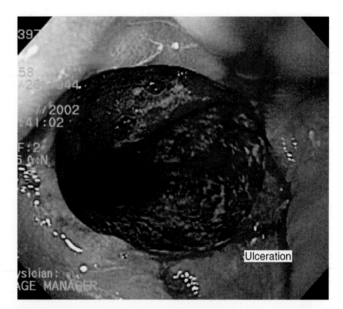

Ulceration

COLOR PLATE 28.1. Peptic stricture and ulceration in patient with long-standing GERD and dysphagia.

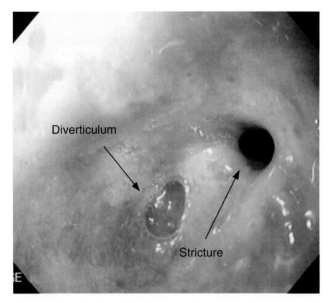

COLOR PLATE 28.3 Peptic stricture in patient with long-standing scleroderma.

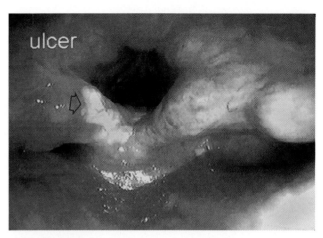

COLOR PLATE 29.2. Ulcers on epiglottal folds (*arrow*).

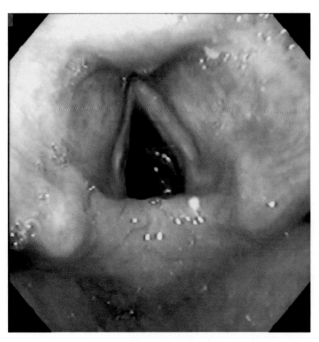

COLOR PLATE 29.3. Endoscopic view of normal vocal cords.

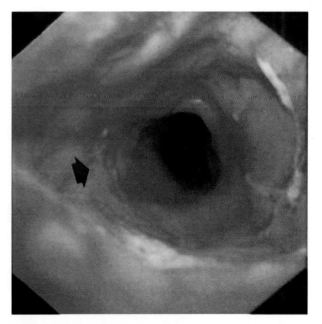

COLOR PLATE 29.4. Endoscopic detection of esophageal mucosal changes indicative of chronic esophagitis. The distal esophagus shows several pit-like depressions (*arrow*) caused by chronic inflammation.

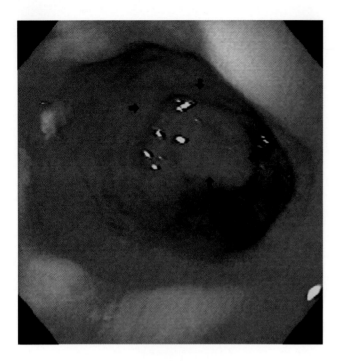

COLOR PLATE 29.5. The prolapse of fundic mucosa into the distal esophagus during endoscopic inspection is heavily weighted for acid reflux disease despite the absence of active inflammatory changes. The finding of patulous esophageal junction or hiatal hernia does not necessarily indicate GERD.

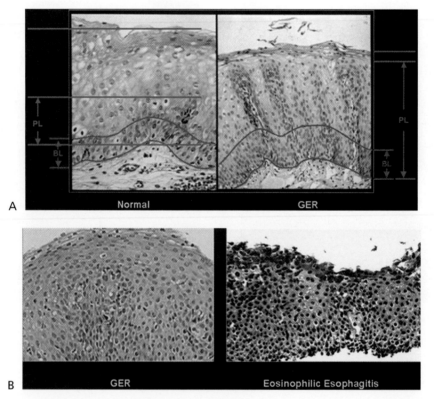

COLOR PLATE 31.2. Morphometric histologic parameters of reflux esophagitis compared to normal esophagus **(A)**[B, basal layer thickness; P, Papillary height. Normal: P > 40% of epithelial height, B > 15%. GER: P > 90% of epithelial height, B > 30%.] and eosinophilic esophagitis **(B)**.

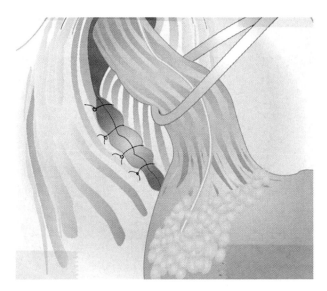

COLOR PLATE 33.3. Reconstruction of the hiatus by crural repair. In this situation the nonabsorbable sutures are applied posterior to the entrance of the esophagus.

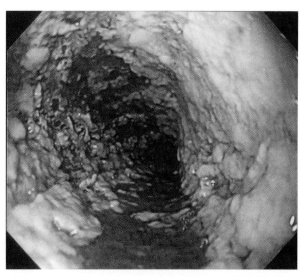

COLOR PLATE 35.1. Candida esophagitis. Endoscopic photograph demonstrating a large amount of yellowish material circumferentially coating the esophagus. One portion of the material has been removed with the endoscope documenting normal underlying mucosa.

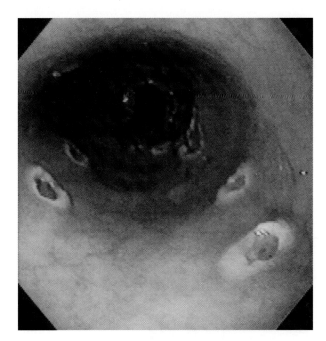

COLOR PLATE 35.2. Herpes esophagitis. Multiple small, raised lesions with central ulceration typical for herpes simples esophagitis. Note that the intervening mucosa is normal.

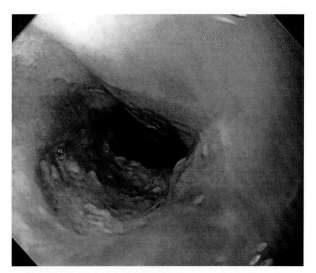

COLOR PLATE 35.3. Cytomegalovirus esophagitis. Large ulceration in the proximal esophagus typical for cytomegalovirus. Idiopathic esophageal ulcer may have a similar endoscopic appearance.

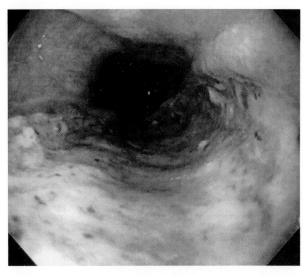

COLOR PLATE 35.4 Idiopathic esophageal ulcer. Large deep ulcer with heaped-up margins in the mid-esophagus. The surrounding mucosa is normal. This lesion is typical for either an idiopathic ulcer or cytomegalovirus.

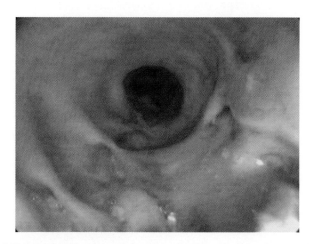

COLOR PLATE 37.4. Endoscopic finding in a patient with Crohn's disease complaining of dysphagia. Irregular mucosal ridges and prominent scarring were noted in the mid-esophagus. (Courtesy Gerald Dryden, University of Louisville, Louisville, KY.)

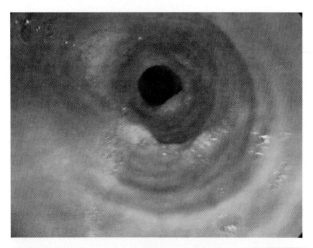

COLOR PLATE 37.5. Endoscopic finding in a patient with eosinophilic esophagitis complaining of solid food dysphagia. The esophageal lumen has a corrugated appearance with circumferential mucosal ridges throughout the entire esophagus.

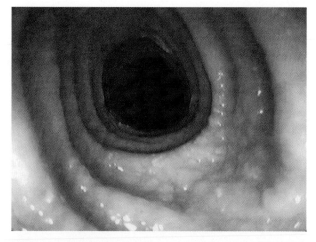

COLOR PLATE 37.6. Another patient with eosinophilic esophagitis with food impaction. The mucosa surface was irregular, and biopsy revealed extensive intraepithelial eosinophilic inflammation.

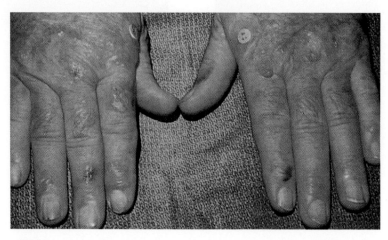

COLOR PLATE 40.1. Epidermolysis bullosa acquisita. Bullous lesions and scarring resemble those seen in porphyria cutanea tarda.

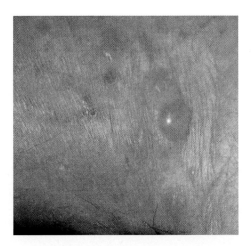

COLOR PLATE 40.2. Bullous pemphigoid. Tense bullae on the wrist.

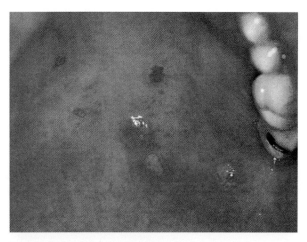

COLOR PLATE 40.3. Bullous pemphigoid. Bullous lesions on the palate.

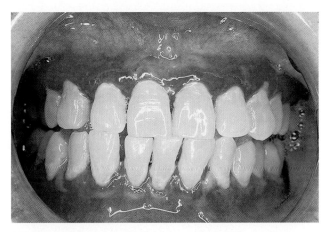

COLOR PLATE 40.4. Cicatricial pemphigoid, presenting as severe inflammatory desquamative gingivitis.

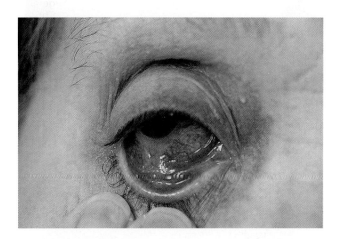

COLOR PLATE 40.5. Ocular cicatricial pemphigoid with conjunctivitis and early formation of scar between bulbar and palpebral conjunctivae (symblepharon).

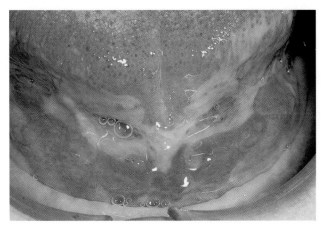

COLOR PLATE 40.6. Pemphigus vulgaris. Typical locations of superficial erosions with fibropurulent membrane in floor of mouth and ventral tongue.

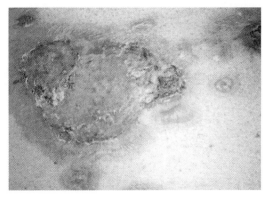

COLOR PLATE 40.7. Pemphigus vulgaris. Erosions and crusting are often more evident than intact blisters.

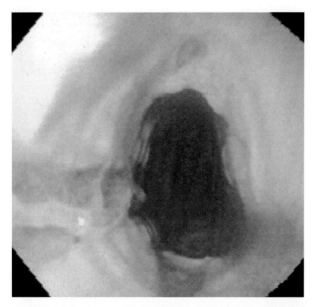

COLOR PLATE 40.8. Endoscopic view of pemphigus vulgaris of esophagus shows raised white blistered areas; the epithelium peels away easily with pressure.

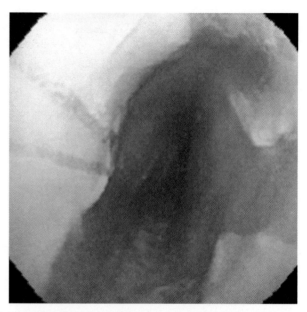

COLOR PLATE 40.9. Endoscopic view of pemphigus vulgaris of esophagus demonstrates longitudinal red streaks.

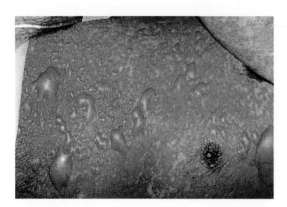

COLOR PLATE 40.10. Toxic epidermal necrolysis. Widespread bullae and erythema, in this case secondary to trimethoprim-sulfamethoxazole.

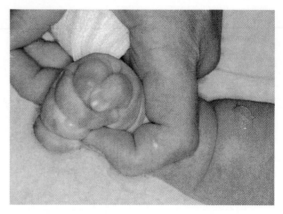

COLOR PLATE 40.11. Epidermolysis bullosa dystrophica. Blisters and erosions on fingers and arms of newborn infant.

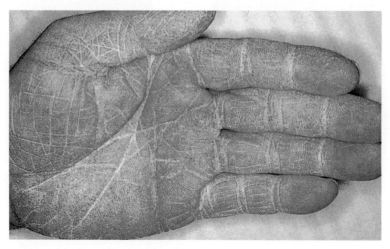

COLOR PLATE 40.12. Tylosis, or acquired palmar keratoderma, in patient with esophageal carcinoma.

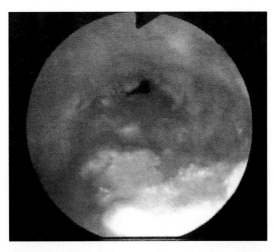

COLOR PLATE 40.13. Endoscopy demonstrating typical endoscopic features of esophageal cancer. The lumen is narrowed and irregular.

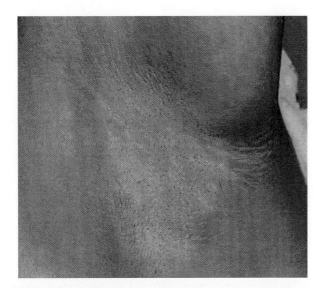

COLOR PLATE 40.14. Acanthosis nigricans. Note brown hyperpigmentation of the axilla.

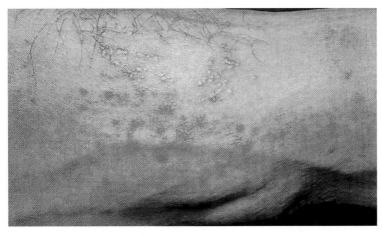

COLOR PLATE 40.15. Lichen planus. Small violaceous papules on the ankle.

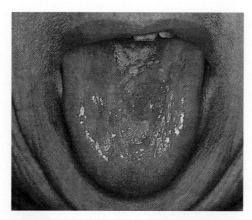

COLOR PLATE 40.16. Lichen planus. Hyperkeratosis and erosion on the tongue. There is also Candida infection present.

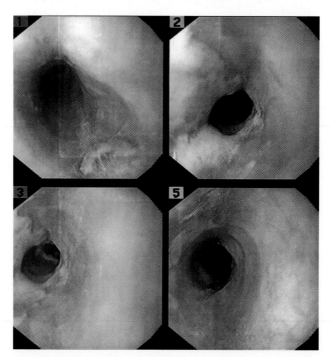

COLOR PLATE 40.17. Endoscopic views of lichen planus of the esophagus show white striae and erosion (top left) and white papules and plaques in a stricture (top right).

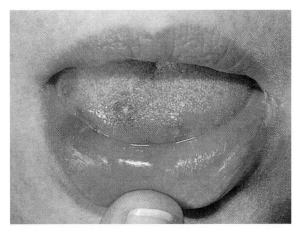

COLOR PLATE 40.18. Aphthous stomatitis. Punctate aphthae of the tongue and lip mucosae.

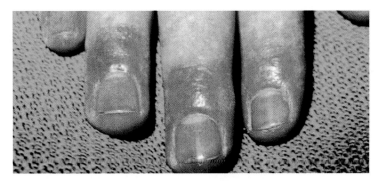

COLOR PLATE 40.19. Dermatomyositis. Note periungual atrophy and telangiectasia.

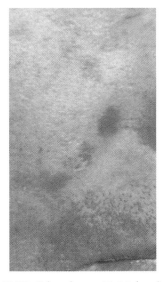

COLOR PLATE 40.20. Scleroderma. Mat telangiectasia and taut skin of the face in patient with progressive systemic sclerosis.

37. Jaffe PE. Abnormal endoscopic findings in pharynx and larynx. ASGE clinical symposium. *Gastroenterology* 2002;122(suppl):48.

38. Belafsky PC, Postma GN, Koufman JA. The validity and reliability of the reflux finding score (RFS). *Laryngoscope* 2001;111: 1313–1317.

39. Hickson C, Simpson CB, Falcon R. Laryngeal pseudo sulcus as a predictor of gastroesophageal reflux. *Laryngoscope* 2001;111: 1742–1745.

40. Vaezi MF, Ours TM, Hicks DM, et al. Laryngoscopic signs of gastroesophageal reflux disease: science or fiction? *Am J Gastroenterol* 1999;94:2601.

41. Vaezi MF, Hicks DM, Ours TM, et al. Are there specific laryngeal signs for gastroesophageal reflux disease. *Gastroenterology* 2000;118(suppl 2):A490.

42. Sontag SJ. Why do the published data fail to clarify the relationship between GER and asthma? *Am J Med* 2000;108(suppl 4a): 159s–169s.

43. Ward PH, Hanson DG. Reflux as an etiologic factor of carcinoma of the laryngopharynx. *Laryngoscope* 1988;98:1195–1199.

44. Katz PO. Ambulatory esophageal and hypopharyngeal pH monitoring in patients with hoarseness. *Am J Gastroenterol* 1990; 85:38–40.

45. Weusten BL, Akkermans LM, VanBerge-Henegouwen GP, et al. Spatiotemporal characteristics of physiological gastroesophageal reflux. *Am J Physiol* 1994;266:G357–G362.

46. Smit CF, Tan J, Devriese PP, et al. Ambulatory pH measurements at the upper esophageal sphincter. *Laryngoscope* 1998;108:299–302.

47. Williams RB, Ali GN, Wallace KL, et al. Esophagopharyngeal acid regurgitation: dual pH monitoring criteria for its detection and insight into mechanisms. *Gastroenterology* 1999;117: 1051–1061.

48. Anderson LI, Madsen PV, Dalgaard P, et al. Validity of clinical symptoms in benign esophageal disease, assessed by questionnaire. *Acta Med Scand* 1987;221:171–177.

49. Johanssen T, Petersen H, Kleveland PM, et al. The predictive value of history in dyspepsia. *Scand J Gastroenterol* 1990;25: 689–697.

50. Klauser AG, Schindlebeck NE, Muller-Lissner SA. Symptoms in gastro-oesophageal reflux disease. *Lancet* 1990;335:205–208.

51. Richter JE. Ambulatory esophageal pH monitoring. *Am J Med* 1997;103:130S–134S.

52. Vaezi MF, Schroeder PL, Richter JE. Reproducibility of proximal probe pH parameters in 24-Hour Ambulatory esophageal pH monitoring. *Am J Gastroenterol* 1997;92:825–829.

53. Ulualp SO, Toohill RJ, Hoffman R, et al. Pharyngeal pH monitoring in patients with posterior laryngitis. *Otolaryngol Head Neck Surg* 1999;120:672–677.

54. Kuhn J, Toohill RJ, Ulualp SO, et al. Pharyngeal acid reflux events in patients with vocal cord nodules. *Laryngoscope* 1998; 108:1146–1149.

55. Oelschlager BK, Thomas RE, Maronian N, et al. Laryngoscopy and pharyngeal pH are complementary in the diagnosis of gastroesophageal-laryngeal reflux. *J Gastrointest Surg* 2002;6: 189–194.

56. Hogan WJ, Hinder R, Dent JD, et al. First multidisciplinary international symposium on supraesophageal complications of gastroesophageal reflux disease: workshop consensus reports. *Am J Med* 1997;103:149s–150s.

57. Kamel PL, Hanson D, Kahrilas PJ. Omeprazole for treatment of posterior laryngitis. *Am J Med* 1994;96:321–326.

58. Hanson DG, Jiang JJ. Diagnosis and management of chronic laryngitis associated with reflux. *Am J Med* 2000;108(suppl 4a): 112S–119S.

59. Hanson DG, Kamel PL, Kahrilas PJ. Outcome of antireflux therapy for the treatment of chronic laryngitis. *Ann Otol Rhinol Laryngol* 1995;104:550–555.

60. Shaw GY, Searl JP, Young JL, et al. Subjective, laryngoscopic and acoustic measurements of laryngeal reflux before and after treatment with omeprazole. *J Voice* 1996;10:410–418.

61. Wo JM, Grist WJ, Gussack G, et al. Empiric trial of high-dose omeprazole in patients with posterior laryngitis: a prospective study. *Am J Gastroenterol* 1997;92:2160–2165.

62. Metz DC, Childs ML, Ruiz C, et al. Pilot study of the oral omeprazole test for reflux laryngitis. *Otolaryngol Head Neck Surg* 1997;116:41–46.

63. Hanson DG, Jiang JJ, Chen J, et al. Acoustic measurement of change in voice quality with treatment for chronic posterior laryngitis. *Ann Otol Rhinol Laryngol* 1997;106:279–285.

64. Jaspersen D, Weber R, Hammar CH, et al. Effects of omeprazole on the course of associated esophagitis and laryngitis. *J Gastroenterol* 1996;31:765–767.

65. El-Serag HB, Lee P, Buchner A, et al. Lansoprazole treatment of patients with chronic idiopathic laryngitis: a placebo controlled trial. *Am J Gastroenterol* 2001;96:979–983.

66. Peters JH, Heimbucher J, Incarbone R, et al. Clinical and physiological comparison of laprascopic and open nissen fundoplication. *J Am Coll Surg* 1995;180:385–393.

67. Deveney CW, Benner K, Cohen J. Gastroesophageal reflux and laryngeal disease. *Arch Surg* 1993;128:1021–1025.

68. So JB, Zeitels SM, Rattner DW. Outcomes of atypical symptoms attributed to gastroesophageal reflux treated by laprascopic fundoplication. *Surgery* 1998;124:28–32.

69. Cadiere GB, Houben JJ, Bruyns J, et al. Laparoscopic Nissen fundoplication: technique and preliminary results. *Br J Surg* 1994;81:400–403.

70. Jamieson CG, Watson DI, Brittin-Jones R, et al. Laparoscopic Nissen fundoplication. *Ann Surg* 1994;220:137–145.

71. Luostarinen M, Isolauri J, Laitinen J, et al. Fate of Nissen fundoplication after 20 years: a clinical, endoscopical and functional analysis. *Gut* 1993;34:1015–1020.

72. Walter HJ, Shaker R. Supraesophageal complications of gastroesophageal reflux. *Dis Mon* 2000;46:193–232.

73. Jailwala JA, Shaker R. Reflux laryngitis. *Prac Gastroenterol* 2000; 24:15–41.

PULMONARY COMPLICATIONS
OF GASTROESOPHAGEAL REFLUX

SUSAN M. HARDING

Gastroesophageal reflux disease (GERD) may trigger, cause, or be a co-morbid factor in many pulmonary diseases (1). The tracheobronchial tree and the esophagus have common embryonic foregut origins and share autonomic innervation through the vagus nerve (2). Both GERD and pulmonary disease are prevalent in the human population and can coexist without direct interaction.

To solidify the association between GERD and pulmonary disease, three criteria should be considered. First, patients with GERD should have a higher prevalence of pulmonary disease than patients without GERD. Second, pathophysiologic mechanisms between GERD and pulmonary disease should explain how the disease processes interact. Esophageal acid should exacerbate the pulmonary process. Third, if GERD is a contributor to the pulmonary process, then antireflux therapy should improve or even resolve the pulmonary process in many patients. Since the cause and exacerbating factors of many pulmonary diseases may be multifactorial, predictive variables should identify subsets of patients who respond dramatically to antireflux therapy.

Pulmonary disease and GERD do coexist. For example, El-Serag and Sonnenberg (3) performed a case-control study involving inpatients treated in 172 Veterans Administration hospitals in the United States comparing the frequency of asthma, chronic bronchitis, chronic obstructive pulmonary disease (COPD), pulmonary fibrosis, bronchiectasis, pulmonary collapse, and pneumonia in 101,366 patients having erosive esophagitis or esophageal stricture, to a control population of 101,366 random subjects without GERD who were admitted during the same time period (3) (Table 30.1). Veterans with erosive esophagitis or stricture had a higher risk of having pulmonary disease. Similarly, in children without neurologic

defects, a case-control study of 1980 GERD subjects and 7920 controls without GERD, showed that children with GERD were more likely to have asthma (13.2% vs. 6.8%, $p<0.0001$), pneumonia (6.3% vs. 2.3%, $p<0.0001$), and bronchiectasis (1.0% vs. 0.1%, $p<0.0001$) (4). This chapter reviews the prevalence, pathogenesis, diagnosis, and management of GERD-related chronic cough and asthma. Finally, pertinent data in other pulmonary disorders where GERD may be a co-morbid disorder will also be discussed.

GERD-RELATED CHRONIC COUGH
Prevalence

Using a systematic protocol evaluating the anatomy of the cough reflex prospectively, Irwin et al. (5) found the cause of cough in all patients, and specific therapy directed toward the cause resulted in cough resolution in 98% of patients. Further developing this protocol, they found that postnasal drip, asthma, and GERD caused cough in 99.4% of patients if they were not receiving angiotensin-converting enzyme inhibitors, were nonsmokers, and had a normal chest radiograph (6). Irwin et al. (5) also found that cough was due to a single condition in 73%, to multiple disorders in 26%, and to unknown causes in 1% of patients. The prevalence of GERD in patients with chronic cough is 10% if the diagnosis was made by history, endoscopy, or barium esophagogram. Adding 24-hour esophageal pH testing to the diagnostic protocol, GERD was the cause of cough in 40% of patients (7). Cough may be the sole manifestation of GERD, so that GERD is "clinically silent." Utilizing 24-hour esophageal pH testing, Irwin et al. (6) found that 43% of patients with GERD-related cough denied heartburn or a sour taste in their mouth. Kiljander et al. (8) noted that 28% of patients did not have typical reflux symptoms. In yet another study population, Irwin et al. (9) confirmed that

S. M. Harding: Division of Pulmonary, Allergy & Critical Care Medicine, University of Alabama at Birmingham, Birmingham, Alabama.

TABLE 30.1. PULMONARY DISORDERS ASSOCIATED WITH ESOPHAGITIS OR STRICTURE[a]

Pulmonary Variable	Odds Ratio	Cases (N=101,366)	Controls (N=101,366)
Asthma	1.51	4,314	2,602
Pulmonary fibrosis	1.36	1,511	952
Pulmonary collapse	1.31	2,463	1,595
Chronic bronchitis	1.28	8,659	4,931
Bronchiectasis	1.26	522	280
COPD	1.22	8,557	4,920
Pneumonia	1.15	17,283	12,794

[a]All *p* values <0.002.
COPD, chronic obstructive pulmonary disease.
Source: El-Serag HB, Sonnenberg A. Comorbid occurrence of laryngeal or pulmonary disease with esophagitis in United States military veterans. *Gastroenterology* 1997;113:755–760, with permission.

chronic cough may be the only manifestation of GERD, finding that GERD was clinically silent in 75% of patients. Clinically silent GERD is also prevalent in elderly subjects with cough (10).

Pathogenesis

Two pathophysiologic mechanisms play a role in GERD-related cough: esophagotracheobronchial cough reflex and microaspiration. Irwin et al. (11), using dual-probe esophageal pH monitoring, noted that cough occurred simultaneously with acid in the distal esophagus 28% of the time versus 6% of the time in the proximal esophagus. Also, endoscopy showed distal, but not proximal esophagitis. Bronchoscopy failed to reveal evidence of microaspiration (9). They hypothesized that acid stimulated distal esophageal mucosal receptors. Ing et al. (12) also noted that distal reflux occurred simultaneously with coughing in 78% of cough episodes. No evidence of aspiration was noted on chest radiographs and laryngeal examinations. Ing et al. (13) noted that cough patients had more reflux episodes and prolonged esophageal acid clearance times compared to control subjects. Fouad et al. (14) examined 43 chronic cough patients and 66 GERD patients without cough, finding that ineffective esophageal motility was present in 49% of cough patients compared to 20% of GERD patients without cough. Prolonged esophageal acid contact times were also present in the cough patients (14).

Ing et al. (15) examined the afferent pathway of the cough reflex in 22 patients with GERD-related cough. There was a significant increase in cough frequency with esophageal acid (n=36) versus saline (n=8) infusions. Blocking the afferent pathway of the cough reflex with esophageal lidocaine inhibited acid-induced coughs. Blocking the efferent cough reflex with inhaled ipratropium (an anticholinergic agent) also inhibited cough, but esophageal

ipratropium did not, further supporting the presence of a vagally mediated cough reflex (15).

Microaspiration may also play a role, especially since Paterson and Murat (16) observed that gastrohypopharyngeal reflux occurred in 9 of 15 cough patients. GERD-associated chronic cough is also linked to laryngeal injury, as based on higher laryngitis scores and lower/upper esophageal sphincter pressure in patients with GERD-associated cough compared to GERD subjects without chronic cough (17). When aspiration does occur, cough can be initiated by irritating the cough receptors present in the lower airway or by triggering, through a vagally mediated reflex, lower airway secretions that can irritate cough receptors (18).

Multiple investigators have proposed a self-perpetuating positive feedback cycle between cough and GERD, where cough precipitates reflux (15).

Treatment Outcome

If reflux plays a key role in cough, then aggressive reflux treatment should result in cough resolution. Table 30.2 (5,6,8,11,19–23) outlines medical trials evaluating the outcome of antireflux therapy on GERD-related cough. Only two trials were placebo-controlled and many trials did not utilize proton pump inhibitors (PPIs), so that the time between initiating antireflux therapy and cough resolution was prolonged, up to 50 days. When using omeprazole 40 mg in the morning and at bedtime in subjects with a positive esophageal pH test, 2 weeks was an adequate time to access a treatment response. Combining the reported medical treatment trials in adults, 112 of 135 (approximately 83%) subjects had cough resolution. It is hard to compare the reported trials as a meta-analysis because of differences in subject selection criteria, treatment regimens, and outcome measurement. One common pitfall of chronic cough management is failure of the clinician to recognize that

TABLE 30.2. OUTCOME OF MEDICAL ANTIREFLUX THERAPY FOR GASTROESOPHAGEAL REFLUX DISEASE–RELATED COUGH IN ADULTS[a]

Study	Study Design	Patient Number	Intervention	Response Rate (%)	Time to Cough Resolution (Days)
Irwin et al. (5)	Prospective	5	Conservative, AA or H_2	100	—
Irwin et al. (11)	Prospective	9	Conservative, H_2 and/or PK	100	161
Fitzgerald et al. (19)	Prospective	20	Conservative, AA, H_2 and PK	70	90
Irwin et al. (6)	Prospective	28	Conservative, H_2 and/or PK	100	179
Waring et al. (20)	Prospective	25	Conservative, H_2, PPI	80	—
Smyrnios et al. (21)	Prospective	20	Conservative, H_2 with/without PK	97	—
Vaezi and Richter (22)	Retrospective	11	H_2 or PPI	100	53
Ours et al. (23)	Prospective	17	PPI	35	14
Kiljander et al. (8)	Prospective	21	PPI	Unclear	Improved at 56

[a]All studies were unblinded and lacked controls.
AA, antacid; H_2, H_2 antagonist; PK, prokinetic agent; PPI, proton pump inhibitor.

multiple conditions may simultaneously contribute to cough (24).

Fundoplication outcomes for GERD-related chronic cough have also been reported. Table 30.3 reviews all trials reported. All trials were uncontrolled, without a placebo arm (25–33). Overall, antireflux surgery improves or resolves cough associated with GERD in 51% to 100% of adult patients. Combined results of nine trials examining 199 patients resulted in a response rate of 77%, with 153 subjects showing improvement (Table 30.3). The surgically treated patients were from highly selected patient populations. Some investigators noted that there was a better cough response in subjects who preoperatively had normal esophageal motility and/or response with medical antireflux therapy.

Two reports indicate that nonacidic reflux may play a role in GERD-associated cough. Fitzgerald et al. (19) reported four medical therapy nonresponders (H_2 antagonist and prokinetic agents) who underwent fundoplication, and all four had cough resolution 3 months postoperatively. Furthermore, Irwin et al. (32) reported eight subjects whose chronic cough did not respond to medical therapy despite

esophageal pH testing showing minimal esophageal acid and no acid reflux events lasting >4 minutes. Fundoplication resulted in cough resolution in six subjects, and marked cough improvement in two subjects. Their findings suggest that mediators other than acid may play a role. Simultaneous esophageal pH and impedance testing could determine whether this hypothesis is true. Data are inadequate at present to recommend fundoplication in subjects who are cough nonresponders, despite adequate control of esophageal acid.

CLINICAL PRESENTATION, DIAGNOSTIC EVALUATION, AND MANAGEMENT

All patients with chronic cough should have a history and physical examination targeted toward the most common causes of cough, including postnasal drip, cough-variant asthma, and GERD. A chest radiograph and other tests as outlined by the American College of Chest Physicians' Consensus Statement on Chronic Cough should be performed (34). Patients should be questioned for symptoms

TABLE 30.3. EFFICACY OF FUNDOPLICATION IN GASTROESOPHAGEAL REFLUX DISEASE–RELATED COUGH IN ADULTS

Study	Study Design[a]	Patient Number	Response Rate (%)
Pellegrini et al. (25)	Prospective	5	100
DeMeester et al. (26)	Prospective	17	100
Guidicelli et al. (27)	Prospective	13	85
Johnson et al. (28)	Prospective	40	76
Allen and Anvari (29)	Prospective	42	51
So et al. (30)	Prospective	16	56
Novitsky et al. (31)	Prospective	21	86
Irwin et al. (32)	Prospective	8	100
Thoman et al. (33)	Retrospective	37	91

[a]Studies were unblinded and lacked controls.

of GERD, including heartburn, regurgitation, and worsening cough with foods that decrease lower esophageal sphincter (LES) pressure. Mello et al. (7), using a prospective design, found that detailed questions about cough characteristics and timing were not useful in determining the cause of cough. Many patients with GERD-related cough do not have esophageal reflux symptoms. Irwin and Madison (24) described the clinical profile of patients with cough due to silent GERD as someone who is not immunocompromised, has a normal or near-normal chest radiograph, is a nonsmoker, is not taking an angiotensin-converting enzyme inhibitor, and is not exposed to environmental irritants. Additionally, asthma (negative methacholine challenge test or cough not improved with asthma therapy), rhinosinus diseases (cough not improved with therapy utilizing a first generation H_1 antagonist, and silent sinusitis has been ruled out), and eosinophilic bronchitis (negative sputum studies for eosinophilia or cough not improved with inhaled or systemic corticosteroids) have been ruled out or treated (24).

In subjects with GERD symptoms and in those who fit the clinical profile as outlined for silent GERD, an aggressive empiric trial of antireflux therapy should be initiated. This trial should include diet and lifestyle changes, as well as high-dose PPI therapy. Esophageal pH testing should be performed while on therapy in the cough nonresponders after a 3-month therapeutic trial. Esophageal pH testing in GERD-associated cough patients has positive and negative predictive values of 83% and 90%, respectively (34). Ambulatory 24-hour esophageal pH testing also allows correlation of coughs with reflux events. Irwin et al. (9) found that correlation of cough episodes with simultaneous reflux events is more helpful than total esophageal acid contact times, which may be normal in some patients.

Ours et al. (23) concluded that 2 weeks of omeprazole, 40 mg twice daily, was three- to five-fold less costly than esophageal pH testing at onset. Treatment failures may be due to nonacid reflux, inadequate acid suppression, and/or failure to recognize and treat other conditions that cause chronic cough. Therapy should continue an additional 3 months after cough resolution, and then gradually tapered and discontinued. Since GERD is a chronic disease, cough may return when medication is stopped, so episodic and prolonged therapy may be required (34). Surgery may be considered in selected patients.

ASTHMA AND GERD

Gastroesophageal reflux also plays a role in asthma (1,35,36). In a prospective cohort of 6590 adult asthmatics, heartburn was associated with a higher rate of future asthma hospitalizations (odds ratio [OR]=1.10; 95% confidence interval, 0.87–1.39) (37). In a population-based study of 2661 adults participating in the European Community Respiratory Health Survey, nocturnal GERD symptoms were linked with wheezing (adjusted OR=2.5) and asthma (adjusted OR=2.2), so that GERD appears to influence asthma (38).

Prevalence

The prevalence of GERD in asthmatics is estimated to be between 34% and 89% (39–48). Many asthmatics complain of GERD symptoms. Field et al. (40) examined GERD symptom prevalence in 109 asthmatics and two control groups (68 patients visiting their family physicians and 67 patients with other medical disorders). Among the asthmatics, 77% experienced heartburn, 55% complained of regurgitation, and 24% had swallowing difficulties; these percentages were higher than in the two control groups. In the week prior to completing the questionnaire, 41% of asthmatics noted reflux-associated respiratory symptoms and 28% used inhalers while experiencing GERD symptoms. Respiratory symptoms also correlate with esophageal acid events. Our laboratory noted that of 151 respiratory symptoms, 119 (79%) were associated with esophageal acid (49). Furthermore, Avidan et al. (50) noted in 128 asthmatics that cough was associated with esophageal acid 46% of the time and wheezing 48% of the time. As in the chronic cough population, asthmatics may have significant GERD without classic esophageal reflux symptoms. Irwin et al. (41) reported that GERD was clinically silent in 24% of difficult-to-control asthmatics. Furthermore, our laboratory reported that 62% of consecutive asthmatics without GERD symptoms had abnormal esophageal acid contact times (51).

There is also a high prevalence of esophagitis and abnormal esophageal acid contact times in asthmatics. Sontag et al. (48) examined 186 consecutive adult asthmatics with endoscopy and esophageal biopsy and found that 79 (43%) had esophagitis or Barrett's esophagus. The same group evaluated 104 consecutive asthmatics and 44 control subjects with esophageal manometry and 24-hour esophageal pH tests and found that 82% of asthmatics had abnormal amounts of acid reflux (47). The asthmatics compared to normal controls had significantly lower LES pressure (p=0.0001), more frequent reflux episodes (p=0.0001), and higher esophageal contact times (p=0.0001). Proximal esophageal acid exposure is also common in asthmatics. Tomonaga et al. (52) noted that 27 (48%) of 56 asthmatics had abnormal esophageal acid contact times at both the distal and proximal pH probes.

In conclusion, reflux symptoms, LES hypotension, and abnormal esophageal acid contact times are more prevalent in asthmatics compared to normal control groups. Furthermore, that esophageal acid events are temporally correlated with respiratory symptoms helps to substantiate the association between GERD and asthma.

PATHOGENESIS OF ESOPHAGEAL ACID–INDUCED BRONCHOCONSTRICTION

There are three proposed mechanisms whereby esophageal acid produces bronchoconstriction, including an esophago-bronchial vagal reflex, heightened bronchial reactivity, and microaspiration. These three mechanisms may interact and further augment airway responses. Interestingly, the vagus nerve is involved in all three mechanisms, including microaspiration. Esophageal acid may also induce neuroinflammatory mediators, including substance P, which lead to airway inflammation.

Vagal Reflex

Airway reflexes may be protective in order to avoid exposure to noxious agents (53). In a dog model, Mansfield and Stein (54) noted that esophageal acid increased respiratory resistance, which was ablated with bilateral vagotomy. They also examined 15 asthmatics with GERD. When reflux symptoms appeared with esophageal acid, there was an increase in total respiratory resistance and a decrease in airflow at 25% of vital capacity, which returned to baseline after reflux symptoms were relieved with antacids (55). The same group performed a double-blinded, acid infusion study in four subject groups: normal controls, asthmatics with GERD, asthmatics without GERD, and subjects with GERD alone (56). The asthmatics with a positive Bernstein test group had a 10% increase in total respiratory resistance. The changes in total respiratory resistance were even more pronounced (72% over baseline) in asthmatics with GERD, in whom asthma attacks were associated with reflux symptoms ($p < 0.0001$) (56). Kjellen et al. (57) found that esophageal acid caused a 0.2-liter decrease in vital capacity and an increase in alveolar plateau by 0.9% in asthmatics with GERD. Likewise, Wright et al. (58) studied 136 individuals, measuring airflow and arterial oxygen saturation both before and after esophageal acid infusions, and found significant reductions in airflow and arterial oxygen saturation. Atropine pretreatment abolished these findings, providing more evidence for an acid-induced, vagally mediated esophagobronchial reflex (58).

Because previous studies failed to control for microaspiration, we performed a series of studies utilizing dual-probe esophageal pH testing (59–61). Peak expiratory flow (PEF) rates decreased with esophageal acid infusion in normal control subjects, asthmatics with GERD, asthmatics without GERD, and subjects with GERD alone (61). Esophageal acid clearance improved PEF in all groups except for the asthma with GERD group, which had further deterioration. These effects were not dependent on a positive Bernstein test or evidence of proximal esophageal acid exposure, a prerequisite for microaspiration. The asthma with GERD group also had an increase in specific airway resistance with esophageal acid infusion, which continued to increase despite acid clearance. Subsequently, we infused esophageal acid into subjects in the supine position, and again, esophageal acid decreased PEF and increased specific airway resistance in asthmatics with GERD, which did not improve despite esophageal acid clearance (59). In a third study, vagolytic doses of intravenous atropine partially ablated the bronchoconstrictive response to esophageal acid, implying the importance of a vagally mediated reflex (60).

To further evaluate the role of the autonomic nervous system in esophageal acid–induced bronchoconstriction, we performed autonomic function testing in 15 asthmatics with GERD, hypothesizing that asthmatics with GERD have exaggerated vagal responsiveness compared to 23 age-matched controls (62). All asthmatics with GERD had at least one autonomic function test display a hypervagal response. Seventy-three percent of asthmatics with GERD had a hypervagal response during the deep-breathing maneuver, 31% had a hypervagal response during the Valsalva maneuver, and 6% had a hypervagal response during the tilt test (62). The overall response scores showed that no asthmatic with GERD had a normal or hyperadrenergic score. These data suggest that asthmatics with GERD have heightened vagal responsiveness, which may be partially responsible for the airway responses to esophageal acid.

However, other reports show conflicting data. Tan et al. (63) studied 15 nocturnal asthmatics with esophageal acid infusions, measuring respiratory flow, tidal volume, and airflow resistance during sleep, and found no significant changes in airflow resistance when esophageal acid was present.

Heightened Bronchial Reactivity

Herve et al. (64) examined the effect of esophageal acid on expiratory flow with methacholine challenge testing in asthmatics with and without GERD. The total dose of methacholine required to reduce the forced expiratory volume in 1 second (FEV_1) by 20% (PD_{20}) was significantly lower when esophageal acid was infused versus normal saline. Furthermore, the response to esophageal acid was abolished with atropine pretreatment. They proposed that stimulated esophageal acid–sensitive receptors interact with cholinergic bronchial tone by a vagally mediated reflex, suggesting that GERD aggravates asthma by increasing bronchomotor responsiveness to other stimuli (64). Vincent et al. (65) noted in 105 consecutive asthmatics that the PD_{20} correlated with the number of reflux episodes during esophageal pH testing. Even in mild asthmatics, esophageal acid alters airway reactivity. Wu et al. (66) examined seven mild asthmatics without GERD symptoms or esophagitis and performed methacholine challenge tests while infusing esophageal acid or saline. Airway responsiveness as measured by the cumulative dose of methacholine at the inflection point where respiratory conductance decreases linearly (D_{min}) and the dose of methacholine required for a 35% fall in respiratory conductance were both decreased significantly with esophageal acid. Increased airway reactivity with esophageal acid was also noted during the sleep period. Cuttitta et al. (67) monitored esophageal pH and respiratory resistance in seven asthmatics with GERD. Esophageal acid was associated with an increase in lower respiratory resistance. There was also a correlation between the length of the reflux episode and the increase in lower airway resistance. The sleep-wake state had no impact on this reflux-induced bronchoconstriction.

Microaspiration

It is well established that mechanical stimulation of the upper airway or instillation of saline into the trachea increases airway resistance (68,69). Chernow et al. (70) instilled technetium-99 sulfur colloid into the stomachs of six patients while monitoring overnight esophageal pH, finding that patients with abnormal lung scans had prolonged episodes of acid reflux. One of the most convincing studies examining the role of microaspiration was performed in a cat model by Tuchman et al. (71). Instilling 10 mL of acid into the esophagus resulted in a 1.5-fold increase in total lung resistance compared to a nearly a fivefold increase if 0.5 mL of tracheal acid was instilled (71). Furthermore, the esophageal acid response occurred in only 60% of animals versus 100% of animals given tracheal acid (71). Interestingly, the effect of tracheal acidification on total lung resistance was abolished with bilateral cervical vagotomy, so even in the microaspiration model, the vagus nerve plays a role (71). In a human study, Varkey et al. (72) examined 19 consecutive asthmatics and seven normal controls with dual esophageal pH monitoring and a probe in the pharynx 2 cm above the upper esophageal sphincter. In asthmatics, 31% of reflux episodes were associated with a fall in pH at the proximal esophagus. and 5% of these episodes were associated with a fall in pH at the pharyngeal probe, documenting that microaspiration occurs more frequently in asthmatics than in normal controls (72).

Even more convincing evidence of microaspiration was provided by Jack et al. (73), who monitored simultaneous tracheal and esophageal pH in four patients with severe asthma. Thirty-seven episodes of esophageal reflux lasting >5 minutes were observed, and five of these episodes were associated with a fall in tracheal pH. Peak respiratory flow rate decreased to 84 liters a minute when esophageal acid and tracheal acid were present versus 8 liters a minute with esophageal acid alone. Episodes of tracheal microaspiration were associated with significant deterioration in pulmonary function (73).

Conclusion

Data suggest that all three mechanisms play a role in esophageal acid–induced bronchoconstriction. Both human and animal data show evidence of bronchoconstriction with esophageal acid in the distal esophagus. This bronchoconstriction is modest but when present, the PEF decreases approximately 10 liters per minute. Numerous studies show that airway resistance also increases with esophageal acid. Atropine inhibits these responses to esophageal acid. There is also evidence of heightened bronchial reactivity, with atropine inhibiting this response. Microaspiration causes significant alterations in pulmonary mechanics in human and animal studies. The magnitude of the airway responses to tracheal acidification is fivefold over baseline in an animal model, and in a human study, tracheal acidification caused a tenfold worsening in airflow, with PEF decreasing to 84 liters a minute. The vagus nerve has also been implicated in the microaspiration model. Fig. 30.1 shows how all three

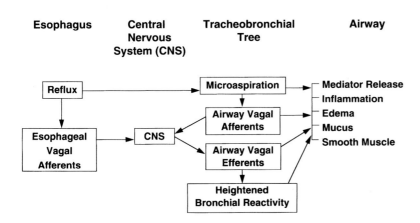

FIGURE. 30.1. Pathophysiologic mechanisms of esophageal acid-induced bronchoconstriction. The three mechanisms include a vagally mediated reflex, heightened bronchial reactivity, and microaspiration, resulting in bronchoconstriction and airway inflammation. The vagus nerve plays a role in all three mechanisms. (From Harding SM. Pulmonary abnormalities in gastroesophageal reflux disease. In: Richter JE, ed. *Ambulatory esophageal pH monitoring: practical approach and clinical applications.* Baltimore: Williams & Wilkins, 1997: 149–164, with permission.)

mechanisms interact through the vagus nerve, leading to airway inflammation.

POSSIBLE FACTORS PROMOTING GERD IN ASTHMATICS

There are a number of physiologic factors that contribute to GERD development in asthmatics, including autonomic dysfunction, an increased pressure gradient between the thorax (esophagus) and abdominal cavity (stomach), alterations in crural diaphragm function, and asthma medications.

Asthmatics show evidence of autonomic dysfunction. Our laboratory showed that asthmatics with GERD have hypervagal responses (62). Autonomic dysregulation could result in decreased LES pressure and transient relaxations of the LES, major mechanisms of GERD (74).

As noted, an increased pressure gradient between the thorax and the abdomen may play a role in GERD development. At the end of expiration, the pressure gradient between the stomach (abdominal cavity) and esophagus (thorax) is 4 to 5 mm Hg (74). Therefore, a normal LES pressure of 10 to 35 mm Hg is sufficient to counteract this pressure gradient (74). However, during an acute asthma exacerbation, wide pressure swings are generated, where there is a more negative intrathoracic pressure during inspiration, which could potentially overcome the LES pressure (75).

Another factor that may be altered is crural diaphragmatic function. Multiple investigators have shown that transient relaxations of the LES and the crural diaphragm are responsible for GERD (76,77). There is relaxation of the LES associated with an inhibition of the diaphragmatic electromyogram and an increase in esophageal pressure, resulting in a reflux episode (77). Hyperinflation associated with bronchospasm places the diaphragm at a functional disadvantage because of geometric flattening (78). Flattening and stretching of the diaphragmatic crura may also occur with chronic hyperinflation and air trapping.

Medications used to treat asthma may also promote GERD. Theophylline increases gastric acid secretion and decreases LES pressure (79–81); however, there is debate about its clinical importance. In a randomized, double-blind, crossover study, Hubert et al. (82) administered oral theophylline or placebo in asthmatics, finding no difference in the number of reflux episodes or total acid exposure time, while pulmonary function improved while on theophylline. However, Ekström et al. (83) examined 25 asthmatics with GERD using 24-hour esophageal pH testing and found that asthmatics with therapeutic theophylline levels had a 24% increase in total esophageal acid exposure and a 170% increase in reflux symptoms.

Oral beta$_2$-adrenergic agents may also decrease LES pressure (84). Schindlbeck et al. (85) found no significant difference in GERD parameters or esophageal motility in normal controls taking inhaled albuterol. Likewise, Michoud et al. (86) found that inhaled albuterol had no effect on LES pressure or esophageal function in both normal controls and asthmatics. However, repeated doses of nebulized albuterol, similar to what is utilized during an acute asthma exacerbation, alters esophageal manometric parameters. Crowell et al. (87) performed a prospective, randomized, double-blind, placebo-controlled crossover trial evaluating the effects of sequential doses of nebulized albuterol (2.5 mg to 10 mg) on esophageal manometry in nine healthy volunteers. Nebulized albuterol produced a dose-dependent reduction in LES pressure from 17.0 mm Hg at baseline to 8.9 mm Hg at the maximum cumulative dose (10 mg). Similarly, the amplitude of esophageal contractions at 5 cm and 10 cm above the LES also decreased. There was no significant difference in the number of transient LES relaxations.

Oral corticosteroids may also affect GERD. Lazenby et al. (88) performed a prospective, placebo-controlled crossover trial in 20 stable moderate persistent asthmatics and noted that prednisone, 60 mg a day for 7 days resulted in significant increases in esophageal acid contact times at both the proximal and distal esophageal pH probes as shown in Fig. 30.2. Despite evaluation of multiple variables, including esophageal manometry and basal and stimulated gastric acid secretion, the mechanism of this finding remains unclear.

There are three studies evaluating GERD in asthmatics while taking multiple asthma medications. Sontag et al. (48) examined the frequency of esophagitis in 186 consecutive asthmatics using bronchodilators versus not on bronchodilators, finding that 38% of asthmatics had esophagitis on bronchodilators compared to 39% of asthmatics not on bronchodilators. The same group also evaluated 104 consecutive asthmatics with esophageal manometry and 24-hour esophageal pH testing, finding no significant difference in LES pressure, esophageal acid contact times, or number of reflux episodes in asthmatics on versus not on chronic bronchodilator therapy (47). Finally, Field et al. (40) examined GERD symptoms in 109 consecutive asthmatics, and no asthma medication was associated with an increased likelihood of having heartburn or regurgitation.

In conclusion, there are physiologic alterations associated with asthma that may promote GERD, which may partially explain the increased prevalence of GERD in asthmatics.

TREATMENT OUTCOME

If GERD triggers asthma, then adequate control of reflux should improve asthma outcome in selected patients. There

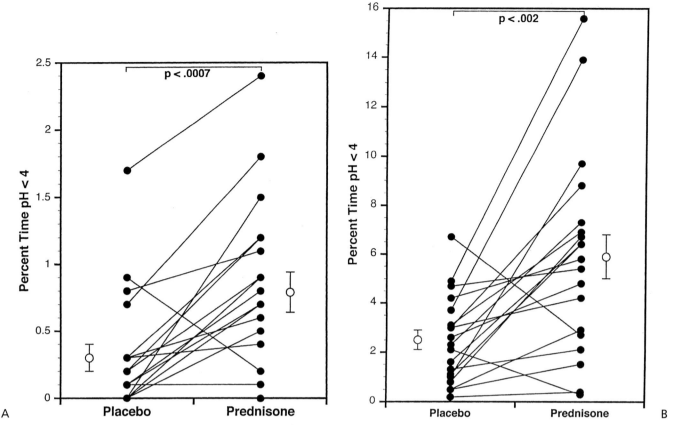

FIGURE. 30.2. Individual esophageal acid contact times at the proximal **(A)** and distal **(B)** probe during the placebo phase and the prednisone phase. Mean ± standard errors and *p* values are also displayed. (From Lazenby JP, Guzzo MR, Harding SM, et al. Oral corticosteroids increase esophageal acid contact times in patients with stable asthma. *Chest* 2002;121:625–634, with permission.)

have been numerous medical and surgical trials evaluating asthma outcome.

Medical Therapy

Table 30.4 (89–101) reviews medical therapy trials in asthmatics with GERD. Many studies have design limitations, including the absence of a control group, use of a crossover design, small or selected patient populations, inconsistent outcome parameters, and lack of objective evidence of acid suppression. More importantly, many trial durations are too short to assess asthma outcome. Despite these limitations, many studies show modest improvement in asthma symptoms and some show objective improvement in pulmonary function.

All placebo-controlled trials using PPIs reported to date have utilized a crossover design allowing for carryover effect. Field and Sutherland (102) reviewed all English-language studies from the Medline database from 1966 to 1996, evaluating asthma outcome with medical GERD therapy. Their search resulted in 12 studies evaluating 326

treated subjects. Antireflux therapy resulted in asthma symptom improvement in 67%, asthma medication reduction in 62%, and evening PEF improvement in 26% of subjects. Furthermore, Coughlan et al. (103) examined randomized, placebo-controlled trials in the Cochrane Airways Groups Clinical Trials Register and confirmed that most studies had significant design flaws; however, they also noted that selected asthmatics may benefit from antireflux therapy. Their power analysis revealed that a sample size of 506 subjects would be necessary to detect a 20-liter-per-minute improvement in PEF.

Our laboratory performed a prospective, pretest/posttest evaluation of 30 asthmatics with GERD with 3 months of acid-suppressive therapy (omeprazole 20 to 60 mg per day). Seventy-three percent of asthmatics with GERD had a 20% increase in PEF and/or a 20% decrease in asthma symptoms (96). The asthma responders had improvement in pulmonary function studies, including FEV_1 and midexpiratory flow rates. Asthma symptoms required time to improve. After 1 month of acid-suppressive therapy, there was a 30% reduction in asthma symptoms compared to

TABLE 30.4. MEDICAL THERAPY TRIALS FOR GASTROESOPHAGEAL REFLUX DISEASE–RELATED ASTHMA IN ADULTS

Study	Study Design	Number	Patient Intervention	Document Acid Suppression	Therapy Duration	Asthma Outcome
Kjellen et al. (89)	Randomized, placebo controlled	65	Antacids, postural therapy	No	—	54% improved symptoms, no change in PFTs
Goodall et al. (90)	Double blind, placebo controlled, crossover	18	Cimetidine 200 mg qid	No	6 weeks	78% responded, decreased symptom score
Harper et al. (91)	Open label, prepost comparison	15	Ranitidine 150 mg bid	Endoscopy	8 weeks	Increase in FEV_1, decreased symptoms
Nagel et al. (92)	Double blind, placebo controlled, crossover	15	Ranitidine 450 mg qd	No	1 week	No change
Ekström et al. (93)	Placebo controlled, crossover	5	Ranitidine 150 mg bid	No	4 weeks	Improvement in night asthma score, no change in PFTs, mild decrease in β_2 agonist rescue
Meier et al. (94)	Placebo controlled, crossover	5	Omeprazole 20 mg bid	Endoscopy	6 weeks	29% increased FEV_1 by 20%, only if esophagitis healed
Ford et al. (95)	Placebo controlled, crossover	11	Omeprazole 20 mg bid	No	4 weeks	No improvement
Harding et al. (96)	Prospective, pretest, posttest	30	Omeprazole 20–60 mg qd for acid suppression	pH testing	3 months	73% increased PEF or decreased symptoms by 20%
Teichtahl et al. (97)	Placebo controlled, crossover	20	Omeprazole 40 mg qd	pH testing but still had acid	4 weeks	Mild improvement in evening PEF
Boeree et al. (98)	Double blind, placebo controlled, parallel	36 includes COPD	Omeprazole 40 mg bid	Yes	3 months	Improvement in nocturnal cough, 31% took <75% of study drug, no change in PFTs
Kiljander et al. (99)	Double blind, placebo controlled, crossover	52	Omeprazole 40 mg qd	No	8 weeks	Reduction in nighttime asthma symptoms, 35% responded
Harmanci et al. (100)	Prospective placebo controlled, single blinded crossover	5	Omeprazole 40 mg qd	No	4 weeks	No improvement in PFTs
Levin et al. (101)	Randomized placebo controlled, crossover study	9	Omeprazole 20 mg qd	No	8 weeks	Improved morning and evening PEF and improved quality of life

FEV_1, forced expiratory volume at 1 second; PEF, peak expiratory flow rate; PFT, pulmonary function test.

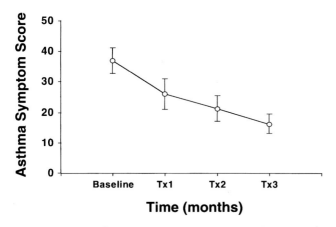

FIGURE. 30.3. Asthma symptom score response to omeprazole over time. Asthma symptom score at baseline, at omeprazole treatment month 1 *(Tx 1)*, treatment month 2 *(Tx 2)*, and treatment month 3 *(Tx 3)* in 22 asthma responders to antireflux therapy. Mean ± standard error shown. Asthma responders had a 30% reduction in asthma symptoms at month 1, a 43% reduction at month 2, and a 57% reduction after 3 months of therapy. (From Harding SM, Richter JE, Guzzo MR, et al. Asthma and gastroesophageal reflux: acid suppressive therapy improves asthma outcome. *Am J Med* 1996;100:395–405, with permission.)

baseline; at 2 months, a 43% reduction; and by 3 months, a 57% reduction (Fig. 30.3). Although not a placebo-controlled trial, acid-suppressive therapy can improve asthma symptoms in nearly 75% of asthmatics with GERD, similar to the reported success rates with antireflux surgery (96).

Surgical Therapy

Table 30.5 reviews studies examining outcomes of surgical therapy. Most studies have design flaws, including lack of a control group, poor documentation of airflow obstruction both preoperatively and postoperatively, poor documentation of asthma severity, and no proof that reflux was adequately controlled in the postoperative state. Despite these flaws, combining the results of 12 trials (26,42,46, 104–112), which include 297 asthmatics with GERD, 235 (70%) had asthma improvement. Field et al. (113) also examined asthma outcome with antireflux surgery. In 24 trials identifying 417 asthmatics, antireflux surgery resulted in improvement in GERD variables in 90%, improvement in asthma symptoms in 79%, asthma medication reduction in 80%, and improvement in pulmonary function in 27%.

Combined Medical and Surgical Trials

Two studies examined medical and surgical therapy response in GERD–related asthma using a placebo-controlled design (114,115). Unfortunately, PPIs were not available when these studies were performed. Larrain et al. (114) examined the effect of cimetidine 300 mg four times a day versus surgery in a placebo-controlled trial in nonallergic asthmatics. After 6 months, there was improvement in FEV$_1$ and PEF in the cimetidine and surgically treated groups but not in the placebo group. Medication scores also dropped significantly in both treatment groups compared to the placebo group. Asthma was considered improved in 36% of the control subjects versus 74% in the medically treated subjects and 77% in the surgically treated subjects (114). Likewise, Sontag et al. (115) performed a placebo-controlled, randomized study comparing ranitidine 150 mg three times a day to surgery (Nissen fundoplication) in 73 asthmatics with GERD. In

TABLE 30.5. SURGICAL THERAPY TRIALS FOR GASTROESOPHAGEAL REFLUX DISEASE–RELATED ASTHMA IN ADULTS

Study	Study Design	Patient Number	Surgical Intervention	Monitoring Time	Asthma Outcome
Kennedy (42)	Case series	15	Unknown	—	15 (100%) improved
Overholt and Ashraf (46)	Case series	28	Transthoracic repair	>6 months	23 (82%) improved or cured
Urschel and Paulson (104)	Case series	27	Unknown	—	24 (89%) improved
Lomasney (105)	Case series	129	Unknown	—	97 (75%) improved
Sontag et al. (106)	Case series	13	Nissen fundoplication	1 to 5 years	6/11 (55%) improved
Tardif et al. (107)	Case series	10	Unknown	21 months	5 (50%) improved
Perrin-Fayolle et al. (108)	Case series	44	Unknown	>5 years	37 (84%) improved
DeMeester et al. (26)	Case series of subjects who failed medical therapy	17	14 Nissen fundoplication, Belsen Mark IV	36 to 103 months	14 (82%) improved
Johnson et al. (109)	Case series	14	Nissen or Belsey fundoplication	3 years	Group had improvement
So et al. (110)	Case series	16	Laparoscopic fundoplication	12-month minimum	48% improved
Patti et al. (111)	Case series	39	Laparoscopic fundoplication	28 months median follow-up	64% had resolution of wheezing
Spivak et al. (112)	Case series	39	Fundoplication	2.7 years median follow-up	Decrease in asthma symptom score; use of oral corticosteroids decreased in 78% of subjects taking daily steroids

the surgically treated group, 75% had resolution or improvement in asthma symptoms versus 9% of the ranitidine group and 4% of the control group at 5-year follow-up. They concluded that surgical treatment of GERD in asthmatics improved pulmonary function and decreased medication usage more often than medical therapy or placebo.

Conclusion

Aggressive antireflux therapy results in asthma improvement in approximately 70% of asthmatics with GERD. Since there are design flaws in many of the outcome studies performed to date, future studies should be multicentered and placebo controlled, using acid-suppressive therapy for at least 3 months with documentation of asthma outcome, cost analysis, and quality-of-life assessment.

PREDICTORS OF ASTHMA RESPONSE

Many studies report predictors of asthma response. Some studies examined subgroups that had excellent asthma response, while others examined predictors using sophisticated statistical analysis techniques. All of these potential predictors need to be verified in independent study populations. Table 30.6 reviews these potential predictors. Meier et al. (94) found that only patients with complete endoscopic healing of esophagitis had asthma improvement (*p*<0.01). Larrain et al. (114) performed a trial in a subset of nonallergic asthmatics with <grade 1 esophagitis who had asthma improvement. Another asthma subset with improvement included the difficult-to-control asthmatics (who require prednisone 10 mg every other day for at least 3 consecutive months per year) (41). Ekström et al. (93) found that a history of reflux-associated respiratory symptoms predicted asthma improvement in 48 moderate to severe asthmatics.

TABLE 30.6. PREDICTORS OF ASTHMA RESPONSE

Healing of esophagitis with antireflux therapy
Asthmatics with <grade 1 esophagitis at study entry
Nonallergic asthma/intrinsic asthma
Difficult-to-control asthma
Reflux-associated respiratory symptoms
Nocturnal asthma
Pulmonary symptoms occur during or within 3 min of reflux event
Presence of proximal reflux on pH testing
Presence of regurgitation >once a week
Obesity/high body mass index
More severe distal esophageal reflux (total time or upright)

Perrin-Fayolle et al. (108) reported predictors of asthma response in 44 asthmatics with GERD more than 5 years after fundoplication. They found that younger asthmatics who had nocturnal and/or intrinsic asthma had improved outcomes. GERD symptom onset before respiratory symptoms, severe GERD, and medical therapy response also predicted asthma improvement (104). DeMeester et al. (26) performed fundoplication in patients who were unresponsive to medical antireflux therapy. Patients with normal esophageal motility and who had pulmonary symptoms during or within 3 minutes of reflux events or patients who had pulmonary symptoms unrelated to reflux events had a higher success rate than patients who had pulmonary symptoms 3 minutes before reflux events. This study showed that 24-hour esophageal pH testing predicted which patients improve with aggressive antireflux therapy (26).

Schnatz et al. (116) also found that esophageal pH testing was able to predict asthma improvement with antireflux therapy. Nine out of 11 (82%) asthmatics with distal only reflux and four out of four (100%) with proximal-only reflux events had a favorable response. None of the five patients with normal esophageal acid contact times had asthma improvement.

We examined predictors of asthma response and found that higher amounts of total proximal reflux, higher baseline asthma symptom score, higher baseline reflux symptom score, the presence of regurgitation, asthma exacerbated by upper respiratory tract infection, and asthma exacerbated by allergies showed a trend toward asthma improvement (96). Forward linear regression analysis found that the presence of regurgitation more than once a week and/or excessive amounts of proximal reflux (i.e., esophageal proximal pH<4 over 1.1% of the time) predicted >20% improvement in asthma symptoms. These two variables had 100% sensitivity, 100% negative predictive value, specificity of 44%, and positive predictive value of 79% (96).

Kiljander et al. (117) reported that a higher BMI (≥29.7 kg/m^2) and higher esophageal acid contact times at the distal probe (total and upright only) predicted asthma improvement. In their multivariate analysis, adding more than one predictor did not improve their prediction model.

In conclusion, there are many possible predictors. These predictors need to be reexamined in an independent study population. This would allow further characterization of which patients to target for antireflux therapy.

DIAGNOSTIC AND THERAPEUTIC APPROACH

All asthmatics should be treated in accordance with the *Guidelines for the Diagnosis and Management of Asthma,*

Expert Panel Report 2, and the *Update on Selected Topics 2002* supported by the National Institutes of Health (35,118). These include aggressive therapy with bronchodilators and antiinflammatory agents. All asthmatics should be asked about the presence of reflux symptoms. A recent American Thoracic Society Workshop on Refractory Asthma recommended that GERD be investigated in selected refractory asthmatics (119).

Since antireflux therapy has the potential to improve asthma symptoms in up to 70% of asthmatics, individual asthmatics should be considered for an empiric medical trial that should include conservative lifestyle therapy and a PPI for at least 3 months. During this time, patients should monitor asthma and GERD symptoms, daily PEF, and asthma medication usage.

If after the therapeutic trial both GERD and asthma are improved, then GERD is an important asthma trigger. If GERD is improved but asthma is not, then GERD is most likely not a trigger of asthma. In the asthma nonresponders, 24-hour esophageal pH testing should be considered to see if there is adequate acid suppression while on antireflux therapy. This paradigm is reasonable since O'Connor et al. (120) performed a cost-effectiveness analysis comparing 11 diagnostic strategies and found that the most cost-effective approach was to start an empiric trial of omeprazole 20 mg daily for 3 months with esophageal pH testing reserved for the asthma nonresponders while on reflux therapy to see if there is adequate acid suppression (120).

If there is a therapeutic response with aggressive antireflux therapy, then the patient should be placed on chronic maintenance therapy, which may include PPIs, a prokinetic agent, or H_2 antagonists with or without a prokinetic agent. Surgical therapy should be reserved for patients who are good surgical risks, whose asthma responds to medical antireflux therapy, who do not have a long esophageal stricture, and who have normal esophageal motility with a hypotonic LES pressure. Chronic treatment should be individualized for each patient. There are no data examining chronic maintenance therapy for GERD-related asthma.

ROLE OF GERD IN OTHER PULMONARY DISEASES

Gastroesophageal reflux may also have an impact or be a comorbid condition in other pulmonary diseases, including aspiration pneumonia, ventilator-associated pneumonia, bronchiectasis, bronchitis, COPD, cystic fibrosis, and interstitial lung diseases, including idiopathic pulmonary fibrosis and scleroderma.

Aspiration of esophageal contents has long been recognized as a cause of lung abscess and pneumonia (121).

Diagnosis is usually straightforward because patients often describe regurgitation. Risk factors for aspiration pneumonia include disruption of normal deglutition and airway protective mechanisms (122). Pellegrini et al. (123) examined GERD in 48 patients suspected of being aspirators. Eight patients had documented episodes of aspiration during the monitoring period and 75% had esophageal dysmotility. Antireflux surgery improved both aspiration and reflux. Recurrent lung injury from GERD may result from direct contact with caustic reflux gastric contents (acid and pepsin) and possibly aspirated gastric, esophageal, or pharyngeal bacteria (124–126). This may be especially true in ventilator-associated pneumonia (126–128). Recurrent episodes of aspiration and pneumonitis may lead to bronchiectasis. Although prokinetic agents and acid-secretion inhibitors may decrease regurgitant volume and acid content, selected patients are encouraged to undergo surgical fundoplication for chronic recurring aspiration pneumonia if they are surgical candidates (124). Raiha et al. (129) examined chest radiographs in 95 adults aged >60 years undergoing 24-hour esophageal pH testing. Subjects with total reflux times of >10% compared with those with a total reflux times of <10% had more frequent respiratory symptoms (OR=8.7), more pleural thickening (OR=3.1), and more pulmonary scars (OR=5.8) (129).

There is a small body of evidence suggesting a possible relationship between GERD and chronic bronchitis. Crausaz and Favez (130) performed scintiscans showing reflux in 27 patients (84%) versus five control subjects (38%). Lung contamination was seen in 24 patients (75%) and two control subjects (15%) ($p<0.001$) 15 hours after eating a labeled solid meal. Although the two associated phenomena may not be causally related, pulmonary aspiration did correlate with GERD, suggesting that GERD may contribute to chronic bronchial disease (130). Tibbling (131) also further examined the association between GERD with aspiration and bronchitis. She examined 119 patients who underwent fundoplication and 90 patients treated with omeprazole, examining bronchial symptoms. Patients treated with omeprazole did not have significant relief of bronchial symptoms, whereas patients who underwent fundoplication with crural repair, showed a marked reduction in bronchitis. She concluded that the main reason for chronic bronchitis in patients with GERD was intermittent aspiration due to partial mis-swallowing (131). Further research is needed in this area.

Gastroesophageal reflux may also be a co-morbid factor in COPD. Utilizing a validated GERD questionnaire, Mokhlesi et al. (132) reported that COPD patients have an increased prevalence of heartburn and/or regurgitation (19%), dysphagia (17%), and used antireflux medication (50%) more frequently than the control group. A higher number of altered swallowing maneuvers compared to historical controls was also noted (133).

Cystic fibrosis patients also have a high prevalence of GERD with estimates ranging between 24% and 50%. Studies show that cystic fibrosis patients with GERD have more severe pulmonary dysfunction than those without GERD. Further investigation is needed, however; antireflux therapy should be considered since therapy has the potential to slow the rate of decline in pulmonary function in these individuals (134).

Gastroesophageal reflux has also been implicated in the pathogenesis of interstitial pulmonary fibrosis. Mays et al. (135) examined 48 patients with idiopathic pulmonary fibrosis (IPF) and showed that 54% had reflux on barium esophagogram versus 8.5% in a normal control group. Patients with IPF also have a high prevalence of GERD. Tobin et al. (136) performed dual-probe esophageal pH testing in 17 consecutive biopsy-proven IPF patients and 8 control patients with interstitial lung disease from other etiologies. Sixteen of 17 IPF patients compared to four of eight control subjects had abnormal esophageal acid contact times. Twenty-five percent of GERD subjects with IPF had "clinically" silent GERD. Episodes of reflux in IPF patients tended to occur at night and into the proximal esophagus (136). Animal models showed that aspiration of acid and/or gastric contents induces epithelial injury and intraalveolar and interstitial fibrosis (137,138). Although there are no prospective trials reported examining antireflux therapy in IPF patients, therapy should be considered in selected patients since there is no known effective therapy for IPF.

Esophageal dysfunction and pulmonary interstitial disease are common manifestations of systemic sclerosis (scleroderma). Johnson et al. (139) studied 13 patients with scleroderma and interstitial lung disease (ILD) with esophageal pH testing and found that 11 had evidence of proximal esophageal reflux. They also found a correlation between proximal acid reflux and a decrease in lung diffusion capacity. Marie et al. (140) examined high-resolution CT scans of the lung, and pulmonary function tests in systemic sclerosis (SSc) patients with severe esophageal motor abnormalities and in SSc patients with normal esophageal motor function. At baseline, 57% of SSc patients with severe esophageal motor abnormalities had evidence of ILD compared to 18% of those with normal esophageal motor function. In follow-up 2 years later, 70% of SSc patients with severe esophageal motor abnormalities had ILD compared to 25% of SSc patients with normal esophageal motility. Pulmonary function also deteriorated in the individuals with esophageal motor abnormalities. Troshinsky et al. (141) examined 39 patients with systemic sclerosis with 24-hour esophageal pH and pulmonary function tests, finding no difference in total lung capacity or diffusion capacity between patients with versus without GERD. Further research is needed in this area.

CONCLUSION

In conclusion, GERD should be aggressively examined as a cause of chronic persistent cough and as a trigger of asthma. In these two diseases, there is evidence showing that GERD therapy may improve outcome in selected patients. In other respiratory diseases, GERD may be an important co-factor or co-morbid condition; however, more research is needed to clarify GERD's role.

REFERENCES

1. Harding SM. Gastroesophageal reflux and asthma: insight into the association. *J Allergy Clin Immunol* 1999;105:251–259.
2. Cunningham ET Jr, Ravich WJ, Jones B, et al. Vagal reflexes referred from the upper aerodigestive tract: an infrequently recognized cause of common cardiorespiratory responses. *Ann Intern Med* 1992;116:575–582.
3. El-Serag HB, Sonnenberg A. Comorbid occurrence of laryngeal or pulmonary disease with esophagitis in United States military veterans. *Gastroenterology* 1997;113:755–760.
4. El-Serag HB, Gilgen M, Kuebeler K, et al. Extraesophageal association of gastroesophageal reflux disease in children without neurologic defects. *Gastroenterology* 2001;121;1294–1299.
5. Irwin RS, Corrao WM, Pratter MR. Chronic persistent cough in the adult: the spectrum and frequency of causes and successful outcome of specific therapy. *Am Rev Respir Dis* 1981;123: 413–417.
6. Irwin RS, Curley FJ, French CL. Chronic cough: the spectrum and frequency of causes, key components of the diagnostic evaluation, and outcome of specific therapy. *Am Rev Respir Dis* 1990;141:640–647.
7. Mello CJ, Irwin RS, Curley FJ. Predictive values of the character, timing and complications of chronic cough in diagnosing its cause. *Arch Intern Med* 1996;156:997–1003.
8. Kiljander TO, Salomaa ERM, Hietanen EK, et al. Chronic cough and gastro-oesophageal reflux: a double-blind placebo-controlled study with omeprazole. *Eur Respir J* 2000;16:633–638.
9. Irwin RS, French CL, Curley FJ, et al. Chronic cough due to gastroesophageal reflux disease: clinical, diagnostic, and pathogenetic aspects. *Chest* 1993;104:1511–1517.
10. Raiha IJ, Impivaara O, Seppala M, et al. Prevalence and characteristics of symptomatic gastroesophageal reflux disease in the elderly. *J Am Geriatr Soc* 1992;40:1209–1211.
11. Irwin RS, Zawacki JK, Curley FJ, et al. Chronic cough as the sole presenting manifestation of gastroesophageal reflux. *Am Rev Respir Dis* 1989;140:1294–1300.
12. Ing AJ, Ngu MC, Breslin ABX. Chronic persistent cough and gastroesophageal reflux. *Thorax* 1991;46:479–483.
13. Ing AJ, Ngu MC, Breslin ABX. Chronic persistent cough and clearance of esophageal acid. *Chest* 1992;102:1668–1671.
14. Fouad YM, Katz PO, Hatlebakk JF, et al. Ineffective esophageal motility: the most common motility abnormality in patients with GERD-associated respiratory symptoms. *Am J Gastroenterol* 1999;94:1466–1467.
15. Ing AJ, Ngu MC, Breslin ABX. Pathogenesis of chronic persistent cough associated with gastroesophageal reflux. *Am J Respir Crit Care Med* 1994;149:160–167.
16. Paterson WG, Murat BW. Combined ambulatory esophageal manometry and dual-probe pH-metry in evaluation of patients with chronic unexplained cough. *Dig Dis Sci* 1994;39: 1117–1125.

17. Rolla G, Colagrande P, Magnano M, et al. Extrathoracic dysfunction in cough associated with gastroesophageal reflux. *J Allergy Clin Immunol* 1998;102:204–208.

18. Irwin RS, Madison JM, Fraire AE. The cough reflex and its relationship to GE reflux. *Am J Med* 2000;108(suppl4a):73S–78S.

19. Fitzgerald JM, Allen CJ, Craven MA, et al. Chronic cough and gastroesophageal reflux. *CAMJ* 1989;140:520–524.

20. Waring JP, Lacayo L, Hunter J, et al. Chronic cough and hoarseness in patients with severe gastroesophageal reflux disease. Diagnosis and response to therapy. *Dig Dis Sci* 1995;40:1093–1097.

21. Smyrnios NA, Irwin RS, Curley, FJ. Chronic cough with a history of excessive sputum production: the spectrum and frequency of causes, key components of the diagnostic evaluation, and outcome of specific therapy. *Chest* 1995;108:991–997.

22. Vaezi MF, Richter JE. Twenty-four hour ambulatory esophageal pH monitoring in the diagnosis of acid reflux-related chronic cough. *South Med J* 1997;90:305–311.

23. Ours TM, Kavaru MS, Schilz RJ, et al. A prospective evaluation of esophageal testing and a double-blind, randomized study of omeprazole in a diagnostic and therapeutic algorithm for chronic cough. *Am J Gastroenterol* 1999;94:3131–3138.

24. Irwin RS, Madison JM. Clinical commentary: the persistently troublesome cough. *Am J Respir Crit Care Med* 2002;165:1468–1147.

25. Pellegrini CA, DeMeester TR, Johnson LF, et al. Gastroesophageal reflux and pulmonary aspiration: incidence, functional abnormality, and results of surgical therapy. *Surgery* 1979;86:110–119.

26. DeMeester TR, Bonavina L, Iascone C, et al. Chronic respiratory symptoms and occult gastroesophageal reflux: a prospective clinical study and results of surgical therapy. *Ann Surg* 1990;211:337–345.

27. Guidicelli R, Dupin B, Surpas P, et al. Gastroesophageal reflux and respiratory manifestations;diagnostic approach, therapeutic indications and results. *Ann Chir* 1990;42:552–554.

28. Johnson WE, Hagen JA, DeMeester TR, et al. Outcome of respiratory symptoms after anti-reflux surgery on patients with gastroesophageal reflux disease. *Arch Surg* 1996;131:489–492.

29. Allen CJ, Anvari M. Gastro-oesophageal reflux related cough and its response to laparoscopic fundoplication. *Thorax* 1998;53:963–968.

30. So JBY, Zeitel SM, Rattner DW. Outcome of atypical symptoms attributed to gastroesophageal reflux treated by laparoscopic fundoplication. *Surgery* 1998;124:28–32.

31. Novitsky YW, Zawacki JK, Irwin RS, et al. Chronic cough due to gastroesophageal reflux disease: efficacy of antireflux surgery. *Surg Endosc* 2002;16:567–571.

32. Irwin RS, Zawacki JK, Wilson MM, et al. Chronic cough due to gastroesophageal reflux disease: failure to resolve despite total/near-total elimination of esophageal acid. *Chest* 2002;121:1132–1140.

33. Thomam DS, Hui TT, Spyrou M, et al. Laparoscopic antireflux surgery and its effect on cough in patients with gastroesophageal reflux disease. *J Gastrointest Surg* 2002;6:17–21.

34. Irwin RS, Boulet LP, Cloutier MM, et al. Managing cough as defense mechanism and as a symptom: a consensus panel report of the American College of Chest Physicians. *Chest* 1998;114:133S-181S.

35. National Asthma Education and Prevention Program. Guidelines for the diagnosis and management of asthma: expert panel report 2. Bethesda MD: National Institutes of Health, 1997 (publication 97-4051).

36. Harding SM, Richter JE. The role of gastroesophageal reflux in chronic cough and asthma. *Chest* 1997;111:1389–1402.

37. Diette GB, Krishnan JA, Dominici F, et al. Asthma in older patients: factors associated with hospitalization. *Arch Intern Med* 2002;121:8–10.

38. Gislason T, Janson C, Vermeire P, et al. Respiratory symptoms and nocturnal gastroesophageal reflux: a population-based study of young adults in three European countries. *Chest* 2002;121:158–163.

39. Davis MV. Relationship between pulmonary disease, hiatal hernia and gastroesophageal reflux. *N Y State J Med* 1972;72:935–938.

40. Field SK, Underwood M, Brant R, et al. Prevalence of gastroesophageal reflux symptoms in asthma. *Chest* 1996;109:316–322.

41. Irwin RS, Curley FJ, French CL. Difficult-to-control asthma: contributing factors and outcome of a systematic management protocol. *Chest* 1993;103:1662–1669.

42. Kennedy JH. "Silent" gastroesophageal reflux. *Dis Chest* 1962;42:42–45.

43. Kjellen G, Brundin A, Tibbling L, et al. Oesophageal function in asthmatics. *Eur J Respir Dis* 1981;62:87–94.

44. Mansfield LE. Gastroesophageal reflux and asthma. *Postgrad Med* 1989;86:265–269.

45. Mays EE. Intrinsic asthma in adults: association with gastroesophageal reflux. *JAMA* 1976;236:2626–2628.

46. Overholt RH, Ashraf MM. Esophageal reflux as a trigger in asthma. *N Y State J Med* 1966;66:3030–3032.

47. Sontag SJ, O'Connell S, Khandelwal S, et al. Most asthmatics have gastroesophageal reflux with or without bronchodilator therapy. *Gastroenterology* 1990;99:613–620.

48. Sontag SJ, Schnell TG, Miller TO, et al. Prevalence of oesophagitis in asthmatics. *Gut* 1992;33:872–876.

49. Harding SM, Guzzo MR, Richter JE. 24-hour pH testing in asthmatics: respiratory symptoms correlate with esophageal acid events. *Chest* 1999;115:654–659.

50. Avidan B, Sonnenberg A, Schnell TG, et al. Temporal associations between coughing or wheezing and acid reflux in asthmatics. *Gut* 2001;49:767–772.

51. Harding SM, Guzzo MR, Richter JE. The prevalence of gastroesophageal reflux in asthma patients without reflux symptoms. *Am J Respir Crit Care Med* 2000;162:34–35.

52. Tomonaga T, Awad ZT, Filipi CJ, et al. Symptom predictability of reflux-induced respiratory disease. *Dig Dis Sci* 2002;47:9–14.

53. Karlsson JA, Sant' Ambrogio G, Widdicombe J. Afferent neural pathways in cough and reflex bronchoconstriction. *J App Physiol* 1998;65:1007–1023.

54. Mansfield LE, Stein MR. Gastroesophageal reflux and asthma: a possible reflex mechanism. *Ann Allergy* 1978;41:224–226.

55. Mansfield LE, Hameister HH, Spaulding HS, et al. The role of the vagus nerve in airway narrowing caused by intraesophageal hydrochloric acid provocation and esophageal distention. *Ann Allergy* 1981;47:431–434.

56. Spaulding MS Jr, Mansfield LE, Stein MR, et al. Further investigation of the association between gastroesophageal reflux and bronchoconstriction. *J Allergy Clin Immunol* 1982;69:516–521.

57. Kjellen G, Tibbling L, Wranne B. Bronchial obstruction after esophageal acid perfusion in asthmatics. *Clin Physiol* 1981;1:285–292.

58. Wright RA, Miller SA, Corsello BF. Acid-induced esophagobronchial cardiac reflexes in humans. *Gastroenterology* 1990;99:71–73.

59. Harding SM, Schan CA, Guzzo MR, et al. Gastroesophageal reflux-induced bronchoconstriction: is microaspiration a factor? *Chest* 1995;108:1220–1227.

60. Harding SM, Guzzo MR, Maples RV, et al. Gastroesophageal reflux induced bronchoconstriction: vagolytic doses of atropine diminish airway responses to esophageal acid infusion. *Am J Respir Crit Care Med* 1995;151:A589(abst).

61. Schan CA, Harding SM, Haile JM, et al. Gastroesophageal reflux-induced bronchoconstriction: an intraesophageal acid infusion study using state-of-the-art technology. *Chest* 1994;106:731–737.

62. Lodi U, Harding SM, Coghlan HC, et al. Autonomic regulation in asthmatics with gastroesophageal reflux. *Chest* 1997;111:65–70.

63. Tan WC, Martin RJ, Pandey R, et al. Effects of spontaneous and stimulated gastroesophageal reflux on sleeping asthmatics. *Am Rev Respir Dis* 1990;141:1394–1399.

64. Herve P, Denjean A, Jian R, et al. Intraesophageal perfusion of acid increases the bronchomotor response to methacholine and to isocapnic hyperventilation in asthmatic subjects. *Am Rev Respir Dis* 1986;134:986–989.

65. Vincent D, Cohen-Jonathan AM, Leport J, et al. Gastro-oesophageal reflux prevalence and relationship with bronchial reactivity in asthma. *Eur Respir J* 1997;10:2255–2259.

66. Wu D-N, Tamifugi Y, Kobayashi H, et al. Effects of esophageal acid perfusion on airway hyperresponsiveness in patients with bronchial asthma. *Chest* 2000;118:1553–1556.

67. Cuttitta G, Cibella F, Visconti A, et al. Spontaneous gastroesophageal reflux and airway patency during the night in adult asthmatics. *Am J Respir Crit Care Med* 2000;161:177–181.

68. Colebatch HJH, Halmagyi DFJ. Reflex airway reaction to fluid aspiration. *J Appl Physiol* 1962;17:787–787.

69. Tomori Z, Widdicombe JG. Muscular, bronchomotor and cardiovascular reflexes elicited by mechanical stimulation of the respiratory tract. *J Physiol (Lond)* 1969;200:25–49.

70. Chernow B, Johnson LF, Janowitz WR, et al. Pulmonary aspiration as a consequence of gastroesophageal reflux: a diagnostic approach. *Dig Dis Sci* 1979;24:839–844.

71. Tuchman DN, Boyle JT, Pack AI, et al. Comparison of airway responses following tracheal or esophageal acidification in the cat. *Gastroenterology* 1984;87:872–881.

72. Varkey B, Pathial K, Shaker R, et al. Pharyngoesophageal reflux index in asthmatics. *Chest* 1992;102:152S(abst).

73. Jack CI, Calverley PM, Donnelly RJ, et al. Simultaneous tracheal and oesophageal pH measurements in asthmatic patients with gastro-esophageal reflux. *Thorax* 1995;50:201–204.

74. Mittal RK, Balaban DH. The esophagogastric junction. *N Engl J Med* 1997;336:924–932.

75. Holmes PW, Campbell AM, Barter CE. Acute changes of lung volumes and lung mechanics in asthma and normal subjects. *Thorax* 1978;33:394–400.

76. Mittal RK, Holloway RH, Penagiri R, et al. Transient lower esophageal sphincter relaxation. *Gastroenterology* 1995;109:601–610.

77. Mittal RK, Rochester DF, McCallum RW. Electrical and mechanical activity in the human lower esophageal sphincter during diaphragmatic contraction. *J Clin Invest* 1988;81:1182–1189.

78. Roussos C, Macklem PT. The respiratory muscles. *N Engl J Med* 1982;307:786–789.

79. Ekström T, Tibbling L. Can mild bronchospasm reduce gastroesophageal reflux? *Am Rev Respir Dis* 1989;139:52–55.

80. Johannesson N, Andersson KE, Joelsson B, et al. Relaxation of lower esophageal sphincter and stimulation of gastric secretion and diuresis by antiasthmatic xanthines: role of adenosine antagonism. *Am Rev Respir Dis* 1985;131:26–30.

81. Stein MR, Towner TG, Weber RW, et al. The effect of theophylline on the lower esophageal sphincter pressure. *Ann Allergy* 1980;45:238–241.

82. Hubert D, Gaudric M, Guerre J, et al. Effect of theophylline on gastroesophageal reflux in patients with asthma. *J Allergy Clin Immunol* 1988;81:1168–1174.

83. Ekström T, Tibbling L. Influence of theophylline on gastroesophageal reflux and asthma. *Eur J Clin Pharmacol* 1988;35:353–356.

84. DiMarino AJ Jr, Cohen S. Effect of an oral beta-2 adrenergic agonist on lower esophageal sphincter pressure in normals and in patients with achalasia. *Dig Dis Sci* 1982;27:1063–1066.

85. Schindlbeck NE, Heinrich C, Huber RM, et al. Effects of albuterol (salbutamol) on esophageal motility and gastroesophageal reflux in healthy volunteers. *JAMA* 1988;260:3156–3158.

86. Michoud MC, Leduc T, Proulx F, et al. Effect of salbutamol on gastroesophageal reflux in healthy volunteers and patients with asthma. *J Allergy Clin Immunol* 1991;87:762–767.

87. Crowell MD, Zayat EN, Lacy BE, et al. The effects of an inhaled beta(2)-adrenergic agonist on lower esophageal function: a dose–response study. *Chest* 2001;120:1184–1189.

88. Lazenby JP, Guzzo MR, Harding SM, et al. Oral corticosteroids increase esophageal acid contact times in patients with stable asthma. *Chest* 2002;121:625–634.

89. Kjellen G, Tibbling L, Wranne B. Effect of conservative treatment of oesophageal dysfunction on bronchial dysfunction on bronchial asthma. *Eur J Respir Dis* 1981;62:190–197.

90. Goodall RJ, Earis JE, Cooper DN, et al. Relationship between asthma and gastroesophageal reflux. *Thorax* 1981;36:116–121.

91. Harper PC, Bergren A, Kaye MD. Anti-reflux treatment in asthma: improvement in patients with associated gastroesophageal reflux. *Arch Intern Med* 1987;147:56–60.

92. Nagel RA, Brown P, Perks WH, et al. Ambulatory pH monitoring of gastro-esophageal reflux in "morning dipper" asthmatics. *BMJ* 1988;297:1371–1373.

93. Ekström T, Lindgren BR, Tibbling L. Effects on ranitidine treatment on patients with asthma and a history of gastroesophageal reflux: a double blind crossover study. *Thorax* 1989;44:19–23.

94. Meier JH, McNally PR, Punja M, et al. Does omeprazole (Prilosec) improve respiratory function in asthmatics with gastroesophageal reflux? A double-blind, placebo-controlled crossover study. *Dig Dis Sci* 1994;39:2127–2133.

95. Ford GA, Oliver PS, Prior JS, et al. Omeprazole in the treatment of asthmatics with nocturnal symptoms and gastroesophageal reflux: a placebo-controlled cross-over study. *Postgrad Med J* 1994: 70;350–354.

96. Harding SM, Richter JE, Guzzo MR, et al. Asthma and gastroesophageal reflux: acid suppressive therapy improves asthma outcome. *Am J Med* 1996;100:395–405.

97. Teichtahl H, Kronbert IJ, Yeomans ND, et al. Adult asthma and gastroesophageal reflux: the effects of omeprazole therapy on asthma. *Aust N Z J Med* 1996;26:671–676.

98. Boeree MJ, Peters FTM, Postma DS, et al. No effects of high-dose omeprazole in patients with severe airway hyperresponsiveness and (a) symptomatic gastro-oesophageal reflux. *Eur Resp J* 1998;11:1070–1074.

99. Kiljander T, Salomaa E-R, Hietanen E, et al. Gastroesophageal reflux in asthmatics: a double-blind, placebo-controlled crossover study with omeprazole. *Chest* 1999: 116:1257–1264.

100. Harmanci E, Entok E, Metintas M, et al. Gastroesophageal reflux in patients with asthma. *Allergol Immunopathol (Madr)* 2001;29:123–128.

101. Levin TR, Sperling RM, McQuaid KR. Omeprazole improves peak expiratory flow rate and quality of life in asthmatics with gastroesophageal reflux. *Am J Gastroenterol* 1998;93:1060–1063.

102. Field SK, Sutherland LR. Does medical anti-reflux therapy improve asthma in asthmatics with gastro esophageal reflux: a critical review of the literature. *Chest* 1998;114:275–285.

103. Coughlan JL, Gibson PG, Henry RL. Medical treatment for reflux oesophagitis does not consistently improve asthma control: a systematic review. *Thorax* 2001;56:198–204.

104. Urschel HC, Paulson DL. Gastroesophageal reflux and hiatal hernia: complications and therapy. *J Thorac Cardiovasc Surg* 1967;53:21–32.

105. Lomasney TL. Hiatus hernia and the respiratory tract. *Ann Thorac Surg* 1977;24:448–450.

106. Sontag S, O'Connell S, Greenlee H, et al. Is gastroesophageal reflux a factor in some asthmatics? *Am J Gastroenterol* 1987;82: 119–126.

107. Tardif C, Nouvet G, Denis P, et al. Surgical treatment of gastroesophageal reflux in 10 patients with severe asthma. *Respiration* 1989;56:110–115.

108. Perrin-Fayolle M, Gormand F, Braillon G, et al. Long-term results of surgical treatment for gastroesophageal reflux in asthmatic patients. *Chest* 1989;96:40–45.

109. Johnson WE, Hagan JA, DeMeester TR, et al. Outcome of respiratory symptoms after antireflux surgery on patients with gastroesophageal reflux disease. *Arch Surg* 1996;131:489–492.

110. So JBY, Zeitel SM, Rattner DW. Outcome of atypical symptoms attributed to gastroesophageal reflux treated by laparoscopic fundoplication. *Surgery* 1998;124:28–32.

111. Patti MG, Arcerito M, Tamburini A, et al. Effect of laparoscopic fundoplication on gastroesophageal reflux disease-induced respiratory symptoms. *J Gastrointestinal Surg* 2000;4:143–149.

112. Spivak H, Smith CD, Phichith A, et al. Asthma and gastroesophageal reflux: fundoplication decreases need for systemic corticosteroids. *Gastrointest Surg* 1999;3:477–482.

113. Field SK, Gelfand GAJ, McFadden SD. The effects of antireflux surgery on asthmatics with gastroesophageal reflux. *Chest* 1999;116:766–774.

114. Larrain A, Carrasco E, Galleguillos F, et al. Medical and surgical treatment of nonallergic asthma associated with gastroesophageal reflux. *Chest* 1991;99:1330–1335.

115. Sontag S, O'Connell S, Khandelwal S, et al. Anti-reflux surgery in asthmatics with reflux (GER) improves pulmonary symptoms and function. *Gastroenterology* 1990;98:A128(abst).

116. Schnatz PF, Castell JA, Castell DO. Pulmonary symptoms associated with gastroesophageal reflux: use of ambulatory pH monitoring to diagnose and to direct therapy. *Am J Gastroenterol* 1996;91:1715–1718.

117. Kiljander TO, Salomaa ER, Hietanen EK. Asthma and gastroesophageal reflux: can the response to anti-reflux therapy be predicted? *Respir Med* 2001;95:387–392.

118. National Asthma Education and Prevention Program. Executive summary of the NAEPP expert panel report, guidelines for the diagnosis and management of asthma: update on selected topics 2002. Bethesda, MD: National Institutes of Health, June 2002 (NIH publication no. 02-5075).

119. American Thoracic Society. Proceedings of the ATS workshop on refractory asthma. Current understanding, recommendations, and unanswered questions. *Am J Respir Crit Care Med* 2000;162:2341–2351.

120. O'Connor JRF, Singer ME, Richter JE. The cost-effectiveness of strategies to assess gastroesophageal reflux as an exacerbating factor in asthma. *Am J Gastroenterol* 1999;94:1472–1480.

121. Allen CJ, Newhouse MT. Gastroesophageal reflux and chronic respiratory disease: clinical commentary. *Am Rev Respir Dis* 1984;129:645–647.

122. Martin BJW, Robbins JA. Physiology of swallowing: protection of the airway. *Semin Respir Crit Care Med* 1995;16:448–458.

123. Pellegrini CA, DeMeester TR, Johnson LF, et al. Gastroesophageal reflux and pulmonary aspiration: incidence, functional abnormality, and results of surgical therapy. *Surgery* 1979;86:110–119.

124. Finegold SM. Aspiration pneumonia. *Semin Respir Crit Care Med* 1995;16:475–483.

125. Patti MG, Debas HT, Pellegrini CA. Esophageal manometry and 24-hour pH monitoring in the diagnosis of pulmonary aspiration secondary to gastroesophageal reflux. *Am J Surg* 1992;163:401–406.

126. Torres A, Serra-Battles J, Ros E, et al. Pulmonary aspiration of gastric contents in patients receiving mechanical ventilation: the effect of body position. *Ann Intern Med* 1992;116:540–543.

127. Garrouste-Orgeas M, Chevret S, Arlet G, et al. Oropharyngeal or gastric colonization and nosocomial pneumonia in adult intensive care unit patients: a prospective study based on genomic DNA analysis. *Am J Respir Crit Care Med* 1997;156: 1647–1655.

128. Valles J, Artigas A, Rello J. Continuous aspiration of subglottic secretions in preventing ventilation-associated pneumonia. *Ann Intern Med* 1995;122:179–186.

129. Raiha IJ, Ivaska K, Sourander LB. Pulmonary function in gastro-oesophageal reflux disease of elderly people. *Age Ageing* 1992;21:368–373.

130. Crausaz FM, Favez G. Aspiration of solid food particles into the lungs of patients with gastroesophageal reflux and chronic bronchial disease. *Chest* 1988;93:376–378.

131. Tibbling L. Wrong-way swallowing as a possible cause of bronchitis in patients with gastroesophageal reflux disease. *Acta Otolaryngol* 1993;113:405–408.

132. Mokhlesi B, Morris AC, Huang C-F, et al. Increased prevalence of gastroesophageal reflux symptoms in patients with COPD. *Chest* 2001;119:1043–1048.

133. Mokhlesi B, Logemann JA, Rademaker AW, et al. Oropharyngeal deglutition in stable COPD. *Chest* 2002;121:361–369.

134. Brodzicki J, Trawinska M, Korzon M. Frequency, consequences and pharmacological treatment of gastroesophageal reflux in children with cystic fibrosis. *Med Sci Monit* 2002;8: CR529–CR537. (Available at *www.MedSciMonit.com*.)

135. Mays EE, Dubois JJ, Hamilton GB. Pulmonary fibrosis associated with tracheobronchial aspiration: a study of the frequency of hiatal hernia and gastroesophageal reflux in interstitial pulmonary fibrosis of obscure etiology. *Chest* 1976;69:512–515.

136. Tobin RW, Pope II CE, Pellegrini CA, et al. Increased prevalence of gastroesophageal reflux in patients with idiopathic pulmonary fibrosis. *Am J Respir Crit Care Med* 1998;158: 1804–1808.

137. Popper H, Juettner F, Pinter J, et al. The gastric juice aspiration syndrome (Mendelson syndrome): aspects of pathogenesis and treatment in the pig. *Virchows Arch* 1986;409:105–117.

138. Mitsuhashi T, Shimazaki M, Chanoki Y, et al. Experimental pulmonary fibrosis induced by trisodium citrate and acid-citrate-dextrose. *Exptl Mol Path* 1985;42:261–271.

139. Johnson DA, Drane WE, Curran J, et al. Pulmonary disease in progressive systemic sclerosis: a complication of gastroesophageal reflux and occult aspiration. *Arch Intern Med* 1989; 149:589–593.

140. Marie I, Dominique S, Levesque H, et al. Esophageal involvement and pulmonary manifestations in systemic sclerosis. *Arthritis Rheum* 2001;45:346–354.

141. Troshinsky MB, Kane GC, Varga J, et al. Pulmonary function and gastroesophageal reflux in systemic sclerosis. *Ann Intern Med* 1994;121:6–10.

142. Harding SM. Pulmonary abnormalities in gastroesophageal reflux disease. In: Richter JE, ed. *Ambulatory esophageal pH monitoring. Practical approach and clinical applications*. Baltimore: Williams & Wilkins, 1997:149–164.

GASTROESOPHAGEAL REFLUX DISEASE IN INFANTS AND OLDER CHILDREN

SEEMA KHAN
SUSAN R. ORENSTEIN

Gastroesophageal reflux disease (GERD) is the most common esophageal disorder in children of all ages, and is one of the most common pediatric disorders of any kind. It has a broad spectrum of clinical presentations: occasional episodes of physiologic gastroesophageal reflux (GER) occur in normal infants, and GERD develops in those with more frequent or persistent episodes producing esophageal complications, and mishandled episodes producing extraesophageal complications. The evaluation of most infants and children with GER is based on a thorough history; those requiring investigative tests are usually patients with factors exacerbating reflux and its complications.

In this chapter we review the expanding concept of pediatric GERD, the advances made in the diagnostic armamentarium, and optimal strategies of reflux treatment in children. Optimal management strategies in pediatric GERD are as yet unclear, due largely to the dearth of randomized and controlled clinical therapeutic trials in children, prompting extrapolation from knowledge regarding GERD management in adults, but with recognition of important distinctions between adult and pediatric, especially infantile, GERD.

EPIDEMIOLOGY AND NATURAL HISTORY

The prevalence of GERD depends on the gold standard for its identification. Pediatric GERD has been variously defined as an abnormal quantity of acid reflux as measured by distal esophageal pH monitoring, by abnormal frequency of regurgitation, by presence of esophagitis, or by occurrence of other complications of reflux. These definitions are complicated by the quantitative variation in these

S. Khan, S. R. Orenstein: Division of Pediatric Gastroenterology, University of Pittsburgh School of Medicine, Children's Hospital of Pittsburgh, Pittsburgh, Pennsylvania.

parameters during maturation. Esophageal pH probe monitoring of healthy infants during a screening program related to sudden infant death syndrome (SIDS) in Belgium disclosed the range of normal values for distal esophageal acid exposure during infancy; these values can be compared to those from studies of healthy adults (1–3) (Figure 31.1). Regurgitation peaks at 4 to 6 months of age. It may occur two or more times daily in approximately 50% of normal 2-month-old infants, and 67% of infants until 4 months, but persists in only 1% to 5% of normal 10- to 12-month-olds, resolving spontaneously in almost all infants by 12 months (4,5). About 90% of older children who have GERD are reported to have had emesis as a prominent symptom before 6 weeks of age. Symptoms persisting beyond infancy tend to be chronic and resemble adult patterns of GERD, with persistent or recurrent symptoms in half (6). A recent 28-month follow-up of 67 children aged 2 to 17 years with GERD showed no worsening of mild histologic esophagitis during that time, although symptoms persisted in 75% of the children (7).

PATHOPHYSIOLOGY

Pathophysiologic differences between infants and adults will be highlighted here, with the understanding that older children likely manifest intermediate pathophysiology, with more similarities to adult than to infantile GERD.

The gastroesophageal refluxate in children contains hydrochloric acid, pepsin, trypsin, and bile in quantities comparable to adults. However, infants' gastric acid is buffered by the neutral pH of infant formulas and breast milk, in contrast to the acidity of most beverages consumed by adults. The pathologic significance of nonacid reflux in infants is controversial, particularly with respect to the airway complications of reflux.

The lower esophageal sphincter (LES), a functional antireflux barrier, measures only a few millimeters in length

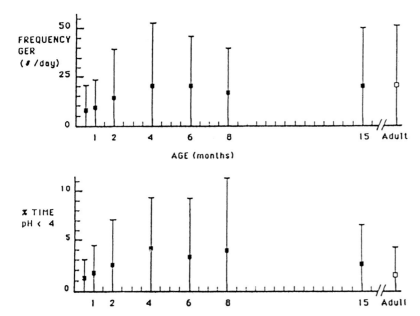

FIGURE. 31.1. Physiologic reflux: range of normal values (mean ±2 standard deviations) in children of various ages (n=285) and adults (n=15). **Top:** Frequency of reflux episodes. **Bottom:** Total duration of esophageal acidification throughout the day, during normal activities and diet. (From Orenstein SR. Gastroesophageal reflux. In: Stockman J, Winter R, eds. *Current problems in pediatrics.* Chicago: Mosby Year Book, 1991:193–241, with permission. Data from Vandenplas Y, Sacre-Smits L. Continuous 24-hour esophageal pH monitoring in 285 asymptomatic infants 0–15 months old. *J Pediatr Gastroenterol Nutr* 1987;6:220–224, and Johnson LF, DeMeester TR. Twenty-four-hour pH monitoring of the distal esophagus: a quantitative measure of gastroesophageal reflux. *Am J Gastroenterol* 1974; 62:325–332.)

in infants, compared to 3 to 4 cm in adults. As in adults, it relaxes in response to initiation of a swallow, maintaining nadir pressure of <2 mm Hg above intragastric pressure for <10 seconds. The LES is reinforced by the diaphragmatic crura and the acute angle of His in healthy children and adults; this angle is less acute in infants.

The transient lower esophageal sphincter relaxation (TLESR), as in adults, is the major mechanism underlying reflux episodes in children, including healthy premature infants. A TLESR can be conceptualized as a mechanism for dispelling gastric pressure, much as occurs with a belch. A TLESR occurs independently of swallowing, with LES pressure <2 mm Hg above intragastric pressure, and usually lasts >10 seconds. It remains unclear if a higher frequency of TLESRs, or a greater incidence of reflux during TLESRs, determines who develops GERD pathophysiology. The reported frequency with which acid reflux episodes are associated with a TLESR in various pediatric studies is 62% to 94% (8–11). Recent investigations have also confirmed their presence in premature babies near the very onset of viability, at 26 weeks gestational age (12,13). The frequency of TLESRs, and thus the frequency of reflux episodes, is increased by the seated position in children, and also by gastric distention from large and hyperosmolar meals (14).

Delayed gastric emptying has been reported in approximately half of children with GERD. It may engender GERD by increasing gastric residual volume and distension and thus triggering TLESRs, or it may increase intraluminal pressure, which then overrides LES pressure, particularly in children with moderate to severe GERD, whose tonic LES pressure is more likely to be abnormally

low. Children with delayed gastric emptying, compared to those with normal gastric emptying, manifest a greater frequency of prolonged reflux episodes postprandially (15).

The ratio of meal volume to gastric capacity is huge in infants compared to adults, due to the infants' need to consume adequate calories to triple their weight in 12 months. This large meal volume combines with a decreased gastric compliance and the frequently slowed gastric emptying to provide a powerful stimulus for TLESRs in young children. The exacerbation of reflux, however, is somewhat ameliorated by the buffering of the refluxate provided by the infant's meals.

Increased abdominal pressure is pronounced in children during random squirming movements or crying in infants, and during coughing or wheezing in children with chronic respiratory disease. When such straining occurs during a TLESR, it is more likely to produce acid reflux than when straining occurs independently of a TLESR (probably because of inhibition of the crural diaphragm by the TLESR) (16). Similarly, when a reflux episode (and thus probably a TLESR) occurs during straining, the refluxate is more likely to be ejected from the mouth as regurgitation than if the reflux episode occurs in the absence of straining (probably because of the propulsive force transmitted to the refluxate by the straining) (17). These phenomena help to explain some of the characteristics of regurgitant reflux in infants and young children.

Hiatal hernia occurs in children with GERD in an estimated prevalence of 6% to 41% in pediatric studies (18–20), but in practice the identification of a fixed and significant hernia is uncommon in children in the absence of complications of GERD. Hiatal hernia removes the crural support of the LES (by raising the LES cephalad to the diaphragmatic crura), impairs the flap valve mechanism, and delays esophageal clearance once reflux has occurred. Delayed esophageal clearance of acid reflux has been demonstrated in children with reflux and hiatal hernia compared to those without hiatal hernia (20). In adults, hiatal hernia is associated with more severe reflux esophagitis, especially Barrett's esophagus and stricture (21), so the presence of hiatal hernia may indicate the need for more intense antireflux management, repeated clinical evaluation, and long-term follow-up. It has been further proposed that hiatal herniation may also be a result, rather than simply a cause, of severe reflux esophagitis, and thus might be more likely to develop in adults after protracted reflux than to occur *de novo* in young children.

Clearance of refluxed material is accomplished by gravity, esophageal peristalsis, and salivary "washdown"; saliva also aids in neutralization of acidic reflux. The large proportion of time that infants spend recumbent, and the semisupine character of even the seated position because of infants' developmental deficits in torso tone, impair the ability of gravity to assist clearance in this age group (22,23). In older children with GERD, nonspecific esophageal motility defects have been reported; these motility defects become more pronounced with increasing GERD severity. These defects include both reduction in pressure wave amplitude and disturbances in pressure wave propagation, although a lack of pediatric normative data makes interpretation of these reports difficult (24). Salivary neutralization of acidic refluxate is impaired during sleep because of the reduction of salivation and swallowing; the greater sleep time of young children compared to adults may diminish these clearance functions (24).

GENETICS OF GERD

The possibility of a genetic basis for GERD and its complications in children, as well as in adults, has received attention recently (25). One such study mapped a severe pediatric GERD phenotype as an autosomal dominant condition linked to chromosome 13q14 in several families (26), but a follow-up study excluded a proposed candidate gene (27). In addition, another study used linkage analysis of probands with infantile reflux esophagitis and a history of similarly affected family members to exclude association with 13q14 locus (28), but identified an area on chromosome 9q22-q31 as a locus for this pediatric phenotype (29). Further research into the genetic loci underlying familial pediatric GERD, and thus into the responsible molecular mechanisms, should markedly improve our understanding, and thus our management, of this common and costly disorder.

CLINICAL PRESENTATIONS

The clinical spectrum of GERD in infants and children continues to evolve, with a growing recognition of the extraesophageal (generally airway) presentations.

Esophageal and Other Nonairway Presentations

Infants

Regurgitation, often termed vomiting, though distinct from vomiting in its physiology, is the most easily recognizable presentation of GER in nonverbal infants. This regurgitation usually appears in the postprandial period, although some episodes may occur several hours after meals. Although two-thirds of normal 4-month-old infants regurgitate daily, less than 15% continue this symptom by 7 months of age (30). The character of regurgitation varies from drooling to effortless regurgitation, and in some cases to apparently projectile expulsion of gastric contents (31). If the refluxate is expelled from the mouth, it may produce loss of calories, malnutrition, and failure to thrive. On the other hand, refluxate that remains in the esophagus produces esophagitis, while refluxate that escapes the esophagus but is not regurgitated may reach the upper and lower airways to produce airway manifestations of GERD.

Esophagitis typically presents in infants with irritability, arching, hiccups, and feeding aversion (32,33). Hematemesis is uncommon, but is the most striking presentation of erosive esophagitis in infants. An infant with reflux esophagitis is at high risk for malnutrition and failure to thrive due to the combination of regurgitant loss of calories, inadequate intake associated with odynophagia, and, in some cases, to the parents' hesitancy to feed in anticipation of repeated regurgitation and irritability.

Children Beyond Infancy

Regurgitation may still be an occasional manifestation of reflux in preschool children, but abdominal pain and chest pain supervene during later childhood and adolescence (7,34). In an epidemiologic survey of reflux symptoms in unselected healthy children, abdominal pain was a common complaint, reported by 24% of parents of 3- to 9-year-olds, 15% of parents of 10- to 17-year-olds, and 28% of the older children themselves (34). Other common complaints in 3- to 9-year-olds were epigastric pain (7.2 %), regurgitation (2.3 %), and heartburn (1.8%).

Sandifer's syndrome is a relatively rare manifestation of acid reflux in childhood. The esophageal pain causes stereotypical repetitive posturing, particularly of the neck, which may resemble seizure activity (35).

Airway GERD

Much of our understanding of the complex relationship between reflux and airway disorders is based on epidemiologic studies, pH monitoring to assess temporal relationships, and response to trials of therapy for GERD. Most epidemiologic studies are retrospective, inadequately powered, and biased by examination of referred patient populations. Twenty-four-hour esophageal pH monitoring may miss events that occur even as frequently as every few days. Trials of therapy have often been hampered by limitations in the efficacy of current therapeutic modalities. Consideration of GERD as the cause of respiratory, otolaryngologic, and dental presentations may also be challenging because typical GERD symptoms may be absent in these patients, while benign reflux symptoms are quite common in healthy children. Therefore, one must have a high index of suspicion for GERD, while maintaining appropriate skepticism regarding GERD as the cause, in evaluating children with unexplained or refractory airway complaints.

Apnea and Laryngospasm

Apparent life-threatening events (ALTEs), sudden infant death syndrome (SIDS), and regurgitation all occur largely during the first 6 months of life, making it tempting to suspect a relation between these phenomena. While SIDS generally occurs in sleeping babies and most commonly in the prone position, thus making it unlikely to be caused by reflux, ALTEs often occur awake, in the postprandial interval, and in the supine or semisupine seated position, making them more likely to be causally linked to reflux. It has been estimated that one baby in 30 experiences an ALTE, which has been defined as an episode occurring in an infant that is frightening to the observer and characterized by a combination of apnea, change in color, change in muscle tone, or choking and gagging and requires intervention by the caretaker (36). In a large study of 3,799 infants carefully studied following an ALTE, reflux was determined to be the triggering factor in 20% of these episodes (37).

ALTEs are probably manifestations of apneic events. Reflux-induced apneas are obstructive in nature, usually involving episodes of laryngospasm. Conceptually, this is a protective response but clearly an exaggerated one when it engenders hypoxemia and cyanosis. Mixed apnea, in which obstructive apnea is superceded by central apnea, might also occur in some cases. The classic history is that of an infant whose apnea transpires in a supine or semisupine seated position in the postprandial period, and is manifested as cyanosis, despite continued efforts to breathe. The pathophysiology of the induction of such laryngospasm and subsequent apnea by reflux episodes probably involves the refluxate stimulating esophageal, pharyngeal, or laryngeal receptors mediating laryngospasm via a vagal reflex (38,39).

It appears that acidity of the refluxate is not required for such events.

Intraluminal esophageal pH monitoring in combination with pneumocardiography (polysomnography) has been used to attempt to demonstrate a temporal relationship between reflux episodes and such events, but their episodic nature challenges detection during a 24-hour study. Moreover, the detection of reflux episodes is flawed by the insensitivity of pH-metry for nonacid reflux, which is the most common type of reflux in infants, particularly in the postprandial period while the gastric contents are neutralized for up to 2 hours by the liquid meals of breast milk or infant formula. Thus, to date there are conflicting data regarding the association between reflux episodes and these apneic episodes in babies.

Intraluminal esophageal impedance, used in combination with pH-metry and pneumocardiography, has the potential for obviating this flaw, by identifying volumetric movement of refluxate within the esophagus, without requiring an acid pH (40).

Reflux Laryngitis and Other Otolaryngologic Manifestations

The prevalence of reflux laryngitis and its associated complaints such as hoarseness is 4% to 10% in adult otolaryngology practice (41), but information is not available concerning the extent of these laryngeal complications of GERD in children. Children are referred for GERD evaluation with complaints of sinusitis, recurrent otitis media, chronic cough, hoarseness, stridor, and globus (42). In a huge case-controlled study of 1,980 neurologically normal children with GERD aged 2 to 18 years, the frequency of sinusitis, laryngitis, and lower respiratory diseases (asthma, bronchiectasis, pneumonia), but not otitis media, were significantly increased in children with GERD (43). Despite the negative results regarding otitis in that epidemiologic study, other authors have reported an abnormal quantity of esophageal acid reflux measured by 24-hour pH monitoring in nearly half of 27 children with chronic tubotympanic disorders (44). An association has also been reported between GERD and both laryngomalacia and tracheomalacia (45). A possible mechanism is via airflow obstruction generating negative intrathoracic pressure, in turn causing reflux across a hypotensive LES (46). Studies employing the response of various laryngeal symptoms to antireflux therapy have also suggested a likely role for reflux, but were limited by small numbers of patients, retrospective designs, and selection bias (47). Some laryngeal sequellae of reflux are believed caused by direct acid-peptic injury to the supraglottic structures; others by vagally mediated reflexes in response to acid contacting the esophagus or upper airway. The mechanisms of symptoms involving the sinuses and middle ears are controversial, but also may involve direct acid-mediated injury and swelling of the orifices to these structures.

Dental Erosions

The reported prevalence of dental erosions attributed to GERD in children varies between 2% and 57% (48). Gastroesophageal reflux constitutes an important source of acid that may contact the teeth; other sources of oral acid are extrinsic—acidic foods and beverages. Nearly all beverages other than milk or water have a pH of <4 (49). Oral hygiene practices, salivary secretions, and presence or absence of fluoride also influence the process of dental erosions (48). In 53 children with pH-metry–proven acid reflux, typical dental erosions were present in 17%. Others have reported dental erosions in 20 of 24 (83%) children with biopsy-proven reflux esophagitis (50). The typical lesion is on the lingual surface, thus distinguishing it from other causes of dental erosion. With increasing exposure to gastric acid refluxate, the dental lesions progress from superficial erosions to dissolution and enamel loss (51).

Asthma

Whereas apnea as a response to GERD predominates in infancy, asthma occurs more often as a response to GERD in older children. Asthma is attributed to GERD in approximately half of asthmatic children (38,47,52), similar to the prevalence in adults. The most powerful evidence for asthma being caused or exacerbated by reflux in particular individuals is the improvement in asthma symptoms and pulmonary function in response to antireflux pharmacotherapy and surgery (53–55). A substantial number of patients with reflux-induced asthma have predominantly respiratory symptoms, lacking symptoms suggesting esophagitis. In children, more reflux disease has been detected in those with nocturnal exacerbations of asthma, and in those with worse asthma (56,57). The mechanisms by which reflux provoke asthma include vagally mediated bronchoconstriction in response to distal esophageal acid and actual aspiration of refluxed gastric material. Despite our sizeable diagnostic armamentarium, the clear definition of reflux causing asthma in individual children often proves difficult.

DIFFERENTIAL DIAGNOSIS

A broader differential diagnosis must be entertained in evaluating infants and children with GERD than in adults, but it can be narrowed according to the child's age at presentation and the predominant clinical presentation (Tables 31.1 and 31.2).

TABLE 31.1. DIFFERENTIAL DIAGNOSIS OF PEDIATRIC GASTROESOPHAGEAL REFLUX DISEASE ORGANIZED ACCORDING TO ESOPHAGEAL SYMPTOMATIC PRESENTATIONS

Vomiting, regurgitation	Dietary protein allergy
	Gastroenteritis
	Gastritis/peptic ulcer disease
	Achalasia
	Hepatobiliary disorders
	Pancreatitis
	Pyloric stenosis
	Malrotation
	Metabolic disorders
	Ureteropelvic junction obstruction
	Increased intracranial pressure
	Toxins
	Extraintestinal infections
	Rumination
	Functional vomiting
	Cyclic vomiting syndrome
Esophagitis (pain and irritability)	"Colic"
	Food intolerance
	Gastritis/peptic ulcer disease
	Infections
	Diffuse esophageal spasm
	Hepatobiliary disorders
	Pancreatitis
	Cardiac pain
	Costochondritis
	Functional abdominal pain
Failure to thrive	Feeding disorder
	Malabsorption
	Metabolic disorder
	Chromosomal anomaly/genetic syndrome

DIAGNOSTIC EVALUATION

History and Physical Examination

In most typical pediatric GERD presentations, a thorough history and physical examination by a practitioner knowledgeable in the manifestations and differential diagnosis of pediatric GERD suffice to reach the right diagnosis. The aspects of this evaluation are aimed at identifying the pertinent positives in support of GERD and its complications, negatives that make other diagnoses unlikely, and in arriving at a specific management plan. Questionnaires have been developed to facilitate comprehensive and consistent history, and have enabled normative values to be established regarding symptoms of infant regurgitation (30,31,32).

Radiographic Tests

Upper gastrointestinal series are performed in children with vomiting or dysphagia, to evaluate for achalasia, esophageal strictures or stenosis, hiatal hernia, and gastric outlet, or intestinal obstruction. These series are also useful in assessing gastric motility.

TABLE 31.2. DIFFERENTIAL DIAGNOSIS OF PEDIATRIC GASTROESOPHAGEAL REFLUX DISEASE ORGANIZED ACCORDING TO EXTRAESOPHAGEAL SYMPTOMATIC PRESENTATIONS

Apnea/ALTE	Prematurity
	Bronchopulmonary disease
	RSV, pertussis
	Sepsis
	Cardiac disease
	Laryngomalacia
	Tracheomalacia
	Choanal atresia
	Micrognathia
	Macroglossia
	Foreign body aspiration
	Adenoidal and tonsillar hypertrophy
Otitis	Infections
Sinusitis	Infections
	Allergies
	Cystic fibrosis
	Immotile cilia syndrome
	Immune deficiency
Chronic cough	Allergies
	Asthma
	Postnasal drip
	Pneumonia
	Bronchitis, bronchiectasis
Stridor	Viral croup
	Subglottic stenosis
	Laryngomalacia
	Tracheomalacia
	Laryngeal cyst
	Vascular ring
Wheezing	Bronchial asthma
	Cystic fibrosis
	Foreign body aspiration
	Immotile cilia syndrome
Dental erosions	Acidic foods and drinks
	Acidic medications (chewable vitamin C tablets, aspirin)
	Bulimia
	Rumination

ALTE, apparent life-threatening event.

Milk scan is performed by using a technetium-labeled age-appropriate solid or liquid meal and evaluates episodes of acid and nonacid reflux, aspiration, and quantitative gastric emptying time. It may be more sensitive for detection of aspiration if performed over a prolonged period of time, especially overnight. It differs from pH-metry both in its sensitivity for nonacid events and its insensitivity for fasting reflux.

Intraesophageal pH Probe

A prolonged pH probe study identifies the occurrence, duration, and degree of acid reflux episodes, thus providing extremely useful information. However, pH studies have lim-

ited reproducibility and predictive value; therefore, now they are not considered the gold standard for diagnosis they once were (58). Other challenges for pH studies in children also include partial obstruction of the nostrils of small infants, the duration (18 to 24 hour) of the study, and the failure to detect acid reflux in the postprandial period in infants receiving neutral formula. To counter the latter problem, some experts recommend enhancing the sensitivity of pH probe studies by using apple juice meals, (pH <4) alternating with formula feedings, a technique that itself may produce exaggerated results. Currently, the most important indications for performing a pH study are to assess the efficacy of acid suppression, to identify reflux-associated apneic episodes (in conjunction with a pneumocardiogram), and to assess the role of gastroesophageal reflux in atypical GERD presentations (such as chronic cough, stridor, and asthma).

In children, the pH probe is placed in the distal esophagus at a level corresponding to several centimeters above the gastroesophageal junction used in adults by localizing it at 87% of the nares–LES distance. In practice, this is usually done by use of one of several regression equations using the patient's height (59–61), but the placement may also be verified fluoroscopically, using anatomic markers such as the right atrium or vertebral bodies, or manometrically. Dual pH probes involve placement of a proximal probe at a distance of 5 to 15 cm above the distal one, depending on the child's size. The use of dual pH probes may improve the diagnostic accuracy for reflux-associated otolaryngologic and respiratory diseases, but more normative data are needed (62).

Endoscopy and Esophageal Biopsy

Endoscopy allows detection of erosive esophagitis and its complications, as well as other inflammatory conditions of the upper gastrointestinal tract. In children, endoscopy is always accompanied by histologic evaluation, to identify the degrees of nonerosive esophagitis (more common in children) and to differentiate reflux esophagitis from disorders such as eosinophilic esophagitis. Some studies in infants have even utilized blind esophageal suction biopsies, because of the infrequency of endoscopic, compared with histologic, findings at this age. Morphometric histologic parameters for reflux esophagitis in children are basal layer thickening (normal <53% of the epithelial thickness), papillary lengthening (normal <25% of the epithelial thickness), and the presence of "squiggle" lymphocytes and eosinophils (63). An eosinophil density of >15 eosinophils per high power field indicates a different entity, eosinophilic esophagitis (64) (Color Plate 31.2A and B).

Multiple Intraluminal Electrical Impedance

The multiple intraluminal esophageal impedance technique (IMP) is a new method that uses closely arranged electrodes to detect bolus flow during antegrade or retrograde passage of intraluminal material. Combined with a pH probe, it adds several advantages for detecting pediatric reflux, including detection of nonacid as well as acid episodes, identification of the direction of the bolus flow and the height reached as well as the degree of acidity, distinction between reflux and swallowing of a bolus, and simultaneous evaluation of esophageal clearance of volume and acid. In infant studies, IMP demonstrated many postprandial reflux episodes undetected by pH monitoring because of neutral pH (65), a phenomenon predicted by scintigraphy (66) and by pH probe studies using apple juice. This technique, used in combination with polysomnography and pH probe, also has great potential to clarify the temporal relationship between apnea episodes and reflux in infants (40,67,68). At present, IMP use is limited in the routine clinical setting by the lack of widespread availability of the technique, the cumbersome visual analysis of tracings, and the limited normative data available. With its increasing use in clinical trials, these drawbacks are likely to be overcome.

Miscellaneous

Laryngobronchoscopy is useful in the evaluation of airway disease. Postglottic and arytenoid edema and erythema are laryngeal findings regarded as suggestive of GERD (25,69), although the subtle subjectivity of these findings prompts some skepticism. More severe damage is represented by vocal cord nodules and subglottic stenosis. Abnormal quantities of lipid-laden macrophages, containing dietary lipid, may be found in bronchoalveolar lavage fluid obtained during bronchoscopy or by deep suctioning via a tracheostomy of children with silent aspiration presenting as chronic pulmonary infections or difficult-to-control asthma (70,71).

Esophageal manometry is useful in evaluating esophageal dysmotility, particularly in preparation for antireflux surgery.

Empiric Antireflux Therapy

Recent data in adults support a trial of high-dose proton pump inhibitor (PPI) as a cost-effective strategy for diagnosis (72). A failure to respond to such empiric treatment mandates formal diagnostic tests.

MANAGEMENT

Conservative Therapy and Lifestyle Modifications

Lifestyle modifications are the cornerstone of antireflux therapy in all ages, but among infants these nonpharmacologic measures have shown some of the strongest evidence for efficacy, and are used for GER as well as GERD.

Dietary measures include normalization of feeding volumes and frequencies for infants being fed unnecessarily large meals, and thickening of infant formula. Thickening of formula with a tablespoon of rice cereal per ounce of formula results in fewer reflux episodes, greater caloric density (30 kcal/oz compared to 20 for the unthickened formula), and reduced crying time (73). Prethickened infant formulas are now available for this use (74). A short trial of a hypoallergenic diet is a means of differentiating milk allergy from GERD, as both may cause regurgitation and irritability (75). In older children, as in adults, dietary recommendations include avoidance of acidic foods (tomatoes, citrus, chocolate, mint) and beverages (juices, carbonated and caffeinated drinks, alcohol). Other crucial measures include weight reduction for obese patients and elimination of smoke exposure.

Positioning for management of reflux is complicated. Esophageal pH monitoring has shown more reflux episodes in infants in the supine or side positions compared to the prone position (76). However, as the supine position reduces the risk of SIDS, the American Academy of Pediatrics recommends nonprone positioning during sleep, reserving prone position for observed periods (77). The efficacy of positioning for older children is unclear but there may be some benefit to left side positioning and head elevation during sleep, similar to adults.

Pharmacotherapy

Infants and children with GERD are candidates for antireflux pharmacotherapy in addition to conservative therapy. The important classes of pharmacotherapy and their recommended pediatric doses and important side effects are shown in Table 31.3. Until very recently, the lack of pediatric studies and Food and Drug Administration (FDA) evaluation meant that all such pediatric antireflux pharmacotherapies were "off label," and dosing was relatively empiric. With the institution of the FDA Modernization Act of 1997, this barrier to optimal pediatric therapy is beginning to be removed, as pharmaceutical companies begin to study antireflux drugs in children.

Antacids are readily available as over-the-counter antireflux therapies. They provide rapid but transient relief of symptoms by their acid-neutralization properties. However, side effects of diarrhea (magnesium-based), constipation (aluminum), rickets, and aluminum toxicity, and the availability of better treatment alternatives mitigate against their long-term use in children (78,79).

Histamine-2 receptor antagonists (H-2RAs), cimetidine, famotidine, ranitidine, and nizatidine are the most widely used antisecretory agents in infants and children, being considered the first line of pharmacotherapy. They act by selective inhibition of H-2 receptors on gastric parietal cells. Several placebo-controlled studies have shown a benefit for H-2RAs in the treatment of mild to moderate

TABLE 31.3. PHARMACOTHERAPY FOR PEDIATRIC GASTROESOPHAGEAL REFLUX DISEASE

Medications	Doses	Side Effects
Prokinetics		
Metoclopramide	0.1 mg/kg/dose qid: AC, HS	Drowsiness, restlessness, dystonia, gynecomastia, galactorrhea
Cisapride	0.2 mg/kg/dose qid: AC, HS	Diarrhea, cramps, cardiac arrhythmias
Erythromycin	3–5 mg/kg/dose tid qid: AC, HS	Diarrhea, vomiting, cramps, antibiotic effect, pyloric stenosis
Domperidone	Pediatric doses not defined	Hyperprolactinemia, dry mouth, rash, headache, diarrhea, nervousness
Bethanechol	0.1–0.3 mg/kg/dose tid qid: AC, HS	Hypotension, bronchospasm, salivation, cramps, blurred vision, bradycardia
Acid neutralization		
Antacids	1 ml/kg/dose, 3–8 ×/day	Constipation, diarrhea
H₂ receptor antagonists		
Cimetidine	10–15 mg/kg/dose qid: AC, HS	Headache, confusion, pancytopenia, gynecomastia
Ranitidine	3–5 mg/kg/dose bid tid: AC, HS	Headache, rash, constipation, diarrhea, malaise, elevated transaminases, dizziness, thrombocytopenia
Famotidine	Pediatric doses not defined	Headache, dizziness, constipation, diarrhea, nausea
Nizatidine	Pediatric doses not defined	Headache, dizziness, constipation, diarrhea, nausea, anemia, urticaria
Proton pump inhibitors		
Omeprazole	0.7–3.5 mg/kg/day, 1–2 divided doses: AC	Headache, rash, diarrhea, nausea, abdominal pain, vitamin B12 deficiency
Lansoprazole	1.4 mg/kg/day, 1–2 divided doses: AC	Headache, diarrhea, abdominal pain, nausea
Pantoprazole	Pediatric doses not defined	Headache, diarrhea, abdominal pain, nausea, flatulence
Rabeprazole	Pediatric doses not defined	Headache, diarrhea, abdominal pain, nausea
Esomeprazole	Pediatric doses not defined	Headache, diarrhea, nausea, abdominal pain, flatulence, dry mouth, constipation

reflux in children (80,81). Because of the predominance of nonacid reflux and regurgitation, infants are often treated with a four-times-daily dose of a prokinetic; in this case, administration of cimetidine at a similar frequency simplifies the regimen. As the pharmacodynamics and pharmacokinetics for these widely used drugs are explored in children, it is becoming clear that children will likely benefit from more frequent and higher doses than used in adults or in children previously, as has been shown for ranitidine (82,83). Similar studies are needed for other H-2RAs.

PPIs currently provide the most potent anti-GER effect by blocking the H^+, K^+-ATPase channels in the final common pathway in H^+ secretion. Although there are extensive data on the use of PPIs in adults, showing them to be superior to H-2RAs in treating erosive esophagitis (84), the scant data on the use of PPIs in children have been largely devoid of pharmacokinetic or pharmacodynamic explorations of optimal dosing, and efficacy studies have been generally retrospective, uncontrolled, and lacking in endoscopic proof of healing. In an open multicenter study in children aged 1 to 16 years with erosive reflux esophagitis, omeprazole doses required for healing were between 0.7 to 3.5 mg/kg/day, higher than those used in adults on a milligram per kilogram basis (85). The healing dose correlated with the grade of esophagitis but not with age or underlying disease. Omeprazole is well tolerated in addition to

being highly effective for the treatment of GERD refractory to other medical and surgical treatments (54,86). The ideal time to administer omeprazole is with the first meal of the day after an overnight fast, when the H^+, K^+-ATPase pumps are maximally active. In children with neurologic disorders and inability to swallow intact capsules, the granules are suspended in an acidic medium (such as yogurt, apple sauce, or apple, cranberry, or orange juices) at the time of administration and swallowed without chewing to prevent dissolution of the protective enteric coating. For patients with jejunal tubes, the granules are dissolved in an alkaline medium to provide rapid absorption and effective pH control (87). Lansoprazole will soon be available as a liquid formulation, facilitating dosage and administration in children; the recommended starting dose is 1.4 mg/kg (30 mg/m²) (88). Pantoprazole is the only PPI available for intravenous administration, and hence is indicated for efficient acid suppression in critically ill patients, especially those not receiving enteral nutrition, but has not yet been studied in children (84). Other drugs in this class—rabeprazole and esomeprazole—appear to have similar efficacy but there are no studies in children.

Prokinetic drugs would seem ideally suited for pediatric GERD because of the pathophysiologic importance of large meal size, delayed gastric emptying, and volumetric regurgitation. Initially used for increasing LES pressure when a hypotonic LES was believed responsible for most GERD, the ability of prokinetics to decrease reflux episodes has been ambiguous. Other actions of prokinetic drugs potentially ameliorating reflux in children are improved esophageal peristalsis and gastric emptying (89). Prokinetic drugs used in children include metoclopramide (dopamine-2 and 5HT-3 antagonist), cisapride (5HT-4 agonist), domperidone (peripheral dopamine-2 antagonist), bethanecol (cholinergic agonist), and erythromycin (motilin receptor agonist). None have been definitively shown to be effective in GERD, and safety issues exist for each. Cisapride and domperidone are not available in the United States. Baclofen, a gamma-amino-butyric acid β receptor (GABAβ) agonist significantly reduces TLESRs and the frequency of both acid and nonacid reflux (90), raising hope for the first effective therapy directed against the basic pathophysiologic mechanism in GER. The efficacy and safety of this drug have yet to be explored in studies involving children with GERD.

Surgery

The potential risks, benefits, and costs of surgery versus medical therapy have not been well studied in children. It appears from some case series that children with refractory esophagitis and those at risk for significant morbidity from chronic pulmonary diseases benefit from either a partial or complete Nissen fundoplication (54). Neurologic disorders, respiratory disease, delayed gastric emptying, retching, and esophageal dysmotility may predispose the patient to postfundoplication complications (91). In one pediatric study the antireflux effects of a Nissen fundoplication were observed to be due to incomplete LES relaxations and a reduction in the frequency of TLESRs (92). Infants may require a venting gastrostomy, due to their lower gastric compliance and to provide supplemental nutrition. Children with delayed gastric emptying may benefit from a pyloroplasty or other gastric drainage procedure, although the act of performing a fundoplication itself seems to speed gastric emptying by decreasing compliance. Laparoscopic fundoplication is comparable to open fundoplication in terms of efficacy against GERD, and is associated with less operating time and earlier initiation of postoperative feeding, even in infants (93). There are limited but positive reports of the feasibility of robotic surgery for performing laparoscopic fundoplication in children with GERD (94).

COMPLICATIONS

The incidence of GERD complications in children is low compared to adults because of the shorter acid exposure times. Esophageal complications, strictures, Barrett's esophagus, and adenocarcinoma, arise due to severe or protracted esophagitis.

Strictures

Prolonged and severe esophagitis leads to formation of strictures, which are generally located in the distal esophagus, and produce obstructive symptoms. Diagnosis of stricture may be delayed in infants, due to their liquid and soft diet. The incidence of pediatric esophageal strictures may have decreased in recent years due to improved diagnosis and treatment of GERD (95).

Barrett's Esophagus and Adenocarcinoma

Long-standing esophagitis predisposes to Barrett's esophagus, an intestinal metaplastic transformation of the esophageal squamous epithelium that is a precursor of esophageal adenocarcinoma. Although Barrett's esophagus and adenocarcinoma occur largely in older white male adults, and are associated with increased duration, frequency and severity of reflux symptoms, they do occur in children. In one study, the prevalence of pediatric cases of Barrett's esophagus was 0.02% compared to 12% of all adults who had biopsies at the time of endoscopies (96). The prevalence and density of the goblet cells in the metaplastic tissue increases with age until about 40 years, and then remains stable. Pediatric populations at particular risk are those with neurologic disability and chronic respiratory diseases. Surveillance protocols following identification of Barrett's esophagus in children should probably mirror those in adults, with endoscopy and multiple biopsies every few years in Barrett's cases without dysplasia and much more frequently in the presence of dysplasia (97).

Adenocarcinoma of the esophagus as a complication of Barrett's esophagus has rarely been reported in children (98). It may present as an esophageal mass or stricture, but may not come to attention until metastatic disease supervenes.

Better understanding and management of pediatric GERD has the potential to reduce the impact of this disease, not only in childhood itself, but also in adulthood, by impacting the incidence of complications of long-standing disease.

REFERENCES

1. Orenstein SR. Gastroesophageal reflux. In: Stockman J, Winter R, eds. *Current problems in pediatrics.* Chicago: Mosby Year Book, 1991:193–241.
2. Vandenplas Y, Sacre-Smits L. Continuous 24-hour esophageal pH monitoring in 285 asymptomatic infants 0–15 months old. *J Pediatr Gastroenterol Nutr* 1987;6:220–224.
3. Johnson LF, DeMeester TR. Twenty-four-hour pH monitoring of the distal esophagus: a quantitative measure of gastroesophageal relfux. *Am J Gastroenterol* 1974;62:325–332.
4. Jadcherla SR. Gastroesohageal reflux in the neonate. Recent advances in neonatal gastroenterology. *Clin Perinatol* 2002;29: 135–158.

5. Orenstein SR. Infantile reflux: different from adult reflux. *Am J Med* 103;1997:114S–119S.

6. Treem WR, Davis PM, Hyams JS. Gastroesophageal reflux in the older child: presentation, response to treatment and long-term follow-up. *Clin Pediatr* 1991;30:435–440.

7. Ashorn M, Ruuska T, Karikoski R, et al. The natural course of gastroesophageal reflux disease in children. *Scand J Gastroenterol* 2002;37:638–641.

8. Cucchiara S, Staiano A, Di Lorenzo C, et al. Pathophysiology of gastroesophageal reflux and distal esophageal motility in children with gastroesophageal reflux disease. *J Pediatr Gastroenterol Nutr* 1988;7:830–836.

9. Cucchiara S, Bortolotti M, Minella R, et al. Fasting and post-prandial mechanisms of gastroesophageal reflux in children with gastroesophageal reflux. *Dig Dis Sci* 1993;38:86–92.

10. Kawahara H, Dent J, Davidson G. Mechanisms responsible for gastroesophageal reflux in children. *Gastroenterology* 1997;113: 399–408.

11. Davidson G, Omari TI. Pathophysiological mechanisms of gas-troesophageal reflux disease in children. *Curr Gastroenterol Rep* 2001;3:257–262.

12. Omari T, Benninga M, Barnett C, et al. Characterization of esophageal body and lower esophageal sphincter motor function in the very premature neonate. *J Pediatr* 1999;135:517–521.

13. Omari T, Benninga M, Barnett C, et al. Acid associated transient lower esophageal sphincter relaxations (TLESRs) are the cause of GERD in premature infants. *Gastroenterology* 2000;118: A2626(abst).

14. Salvia G, De Vizia B, Manguso F, et al. Effect of intragastric vol-ume and osmolality on mechanisms of gastroesophageal reflux in children with gastroesophageal reflux disease. *Am J Gastroenterol* 2001;96:1725–1732.

15. Estevao-Costa J, Campos M, Dias JA, et al. Delayed gastric emp-tying and gastroesophageal reflux: a pathophysiologic relation-ship. *J Pediatr Gastroenterol Nutr* 2001;32:471–474.

16. Kawahara H, Dent J, Davidson G, et al. Relationship between straining, transient lower esophageal sphincter relaxation, and gastroesophageal reflux in children. *Am J Gastroenterol* 2001;96: 2019–2025.

17. Orenstein SR, Dent J, Deneault LG, et al. Regurgitant reflux, vs. non-regurgitant reflux, is preceded by rectus abdominis contrac-tion in infants. *Neurogastroenterol Motil* 1994;6:271–277.

18. Stewart RJ, Johnston BT, Boston VE, et al. Role of hiatal hernia in delaying acid clearance. *Arch Dis Child* 1993;68:662–664.

19. Thomas PS, Carre IJ. Findings on barium swallow in younger siblings of children with hiatal hernia (partial thoracic stomach). *J Pediatr Gastroenterol Nutr* 1991;12:174–177.

20. Gorenstein A, Cohen AJ, Witzling M, et al. Hiatal hernia in pediatric gastroesophageal reflux. *J Pediatr Gastroenterol Nutr* 2001;33:554–557.

21. Ben Rejeb M, Bouche O, Zeiton P. Study of 47 consecutive patients with peptic esophageal stricture compared with 3880 cases of reflux esophagitis. *Dig Dis Sci* 1992;37:733–736.

22. Orenstein SR. Effects on behaviour state of prone versus seated positioning for infants with gastroesophageal reflux. *Pediatrics* 1990;85:765–767.

23. Orenstein SR, Whitington PF, Orenstein DM. The infant seat as treatment for gastroesophageal reflux. *N Engl J Med* 1983; 309:760–763.

24. Vandenplas Y, Hassall E. Mechanisms of gastroesophageal reflux and gastroesophageal reflux disease. *J Pediatr Gastroenterol Nutr* 2002;35:119–136.

25. Orenstein SR, Shalaby TM, Barmada MM, et al. Genetics of gas-troesophageal reflux disease: a review. *J Pediatr Gastroenterol Nutr* 2002;34:506–510.

26. Hu FZ, Preston RA, Post JC, et al. Mapping of a gene for severe pediatric gastroesophageal reflux to chromosome 13q14. *JAMA* 2000;284:325–334.

27. Hu FZ, Post CJ, Johnson S, et al. Refined localization of a gene for pediatric gastroesophageal reflux makes HTR2A an unlikely candidate gene. *Hum Genet* 2000;107:519–525.

28. Orenstein SR, Shalaby TM, Finch R, et al. Autosomal dominant infantile gastroesophageal reflux disease: Exclusion of a 13q14 locus in 5 well-characterized families. *Am J Gastroenterol* 2002; 97:2725–2732.

29. Orenstein SR, Suman A, Shalaby TM, et al. Infantile GERD maps to chromosome 9. *J Pediatr Gastroenterol Nutr* 2002;35: 440–441.

30. Nelson SP, Chen EH, Syniar GM, et al. Prevalence of symptoms of gastroesophageal reflux in infancy: a pediatric practice based survey. *Arch Pediatr Adolesc Med* 1997;151:569–572.

31. Orenstein SR, Cohn JF, Shalaby TM, et al. Reliability and valid-ity of an infant gastroesophageal reflux questionnaire. *Clin Pedi-atr* 1993;32:472–484.

32. Orenstein SR, Shalaby T, Cohn J. Reflux symptoms in 100 nor-mal infants: diagnostic value of the Infant Gastroesophageal Reflux Questionnaire. *Clin Pediatr* 1996;35:607–614.

33. Hyman PE. GER: one reason why baby won't eat. *J Pediatr* 1994;125:S103–S109.

34. Nelson SP, Chen EH, Syniar GM, et al. Prevalence of symptoms of gastroesophageal reflux during childhood: a pediatric prac-tice–based survey. Pediatric Research Group. *Arch Pediatr Adolesc Med* 2000;154:150–154.

35. Olguner M, Akgur FM, Hakguder G, et al. Gastroesophageal reflux associated with dystonic movements: Sandifer's syndrome. *Pediatr Int* 1999;41:321–322.

36. Spitzer AR, Boyle JT, Tuchman DN, et al. Awake apnea associ-ated with gastroesophageal reflux: a specific clinical syndrome. *J Pediatr* 1984;104:200–205.

37. Kahn A, Rebuffat E, Franco P, et al. Apparent life threatening events and apnea of infancy. In: Beckerman R, Brouilette R, Hunt C, eds. *Respiratory control disorders in infants and children.* Baltimore: Williams & Wilkins, 1992:178–189.

38. Orenstein SR. Update on gastroesophageal efflux and respiratory disease in children. *Can J Gastroenterol* 2000;14:131–135.

39. Orenstein SR. An overview of reflux-associated disorders in infants: apnea, laryngospasm, and aspiration. *Am J Med* 2001; 111:60S–63S.

40. Peter CS, Sprodowski N, Bohnhorst B, et al. Gastroesophageal reflux and apnea of prematurity: no temporal relationship. *Pedi-atrics* 2002;109:8–11.

41. Wong RKH, Hanson DG, Patrick JW, et al. ENT manifestations of gastroesophageal reflux. *Am J Gastroenterol* 2000;95 (suppl):S15–S22.

42. Zalesska-Krecicka M, Krecicki T, Iwanczak B, et al. Laryngeal manifestations of gastroesophageal reflux disease in children. *Acta Otolaryngol* 2002;122:306–310.

43. El-Serag HB, Gilger M, Kuebler M, et al. Extraesophageal asso-ciations of gastroesophageal reflux disease in children without neurologic defects. *Gastroenterology* 2001;121:1294–1299.

44. Rozmanic V, Velepic M, Ahel V, et al. Prolonged esophageal pH monitoring in the evaluation of gastroesophageal reflux in chil-dren with chronic tubotympanal disorders. *J Pediatr Gastroen-terol Nutr* 2002;34:278–280.

45. Bibi H, Khvolis E, Shoseyov D, et al. The prevalence of gastroe-sophageal reflux in children with tracheomalacia and laryngoma-lacia. *Chest* 2002;119:409–413.

46. Wang W, Tovar JA, Eizaguirre I, et al. Airway obstruction and gastroesophageal reflux: an experimental study on the pathogen-esis of the association. *J Pediatr Surg* 1993;28:995–998.

47. Sontag SJ. Gastroesophageal reflux disease and asthma. *J Clin Gastroenterol* 2000;30:S9–S30.

48. Linnett V, Seow WK. Dental erosion in children: a literature review. *Pediatr Dent* 2001;23:37–43.

49. Feldman M, Barnett C. Relationships between the acidity and osmolality of popular beverages and reported postprandial heartburn. *Gastroenterology* 1995;108:125–131.

50. Dahshan A, Patel H, Delaney J, et al. Gastroesophageal reflux and dental erosions in children. *J Pediatr* 2002;140:474–478.

51. Lazarchik DA, Filler SJ. Dental erosion: predominant oral lesion in gastroesophageal reflux disease. *Am J Gastroenterol* 2000;95: S33–S38.

52. Suskind DL, Zeringue GP III, Kluka EA, et al. Gastroesophageal reflux and pediatric otolaryngologic disease. The role of antireflux surgery. *Arch Otolaryngol Head Neck Surg* 2001;127: 511–514.

53. Tucci F, Resti M, Fontana R, et al. Gastroesophageal reflux and bronchial asthma: prevalence and effect of cisapride therapy. *J Pediatr Gastroenterol Nutr* 1993;17:265–270.

54. Bowrey DJ, Peters JH, DeMeester TR. Gastroesophageal reflux disease in asthma: effects of medical and surgical antireflux therapy on asthma control. *Ann Surg* 2000;21:161–172.

55. Andze GO, Brandt ML, St. Vil D, et al. Diagnosis and treatment of gastroesophageal reflux in 500 children with respiratory symptoms: the value of pH monitoring. *J Pediatr Surg* 1991;26: 295–300.

56. Martin ME, Grunstein MM, Larsen GL. The relationship of gastroesophageal reflux to nocturnal wheezing in children with asthma. *Ann Allergy* 1982;49:318–322.

57. Harding SM. Nocturnal asthma: role of nocturnal gastroesophageal reflux. *Chronobiol Int* 1999;16:641–662.

58. Bauman NM, Bishop WP, Sandler AD, et al. Value of pH probe testing in pediatric patients with extraesophageal manifestations of gastroesophageal reflux disease: a retrospective review. *Ann Otol Rhinol Laryngol* 2000;109:18–24.

59. Putnam PE, Orenstein SR. Crown-rump length and pH probe length [Letter]. *J Pediatr Gastroenterol Nutr* 1992;15:222–223.

60. Strobel CT, Byrne JT, Tuchman DN, et al. Correlation of esophageal lengths in children with height: application to the Tuttle test without prior esophageal manometry. *J Pediatr* 1979; 94:81–84.

61. Jolley SG, Tunnell WP, Carson JA, et al. The accuracy of abbreviated esophageal pH monitoring in children. *J Pediatr Surg* 1984;19:848–854.

62. Arana A, Bagucka B, Hauser B, et al. pH monitoring in the distal and proximal esophagus in symptomatic infants. *J Pediatr Gastroenterol Nutr* 2001;32:259–264.

63. Black DD, Haggitt RC, Orenstein SR. Esophagitis in infants. Morphometric histological diagnosis and correlation with measures of gastroesophageal reflux. *Gastroenterology* 1990; 98:1408–1414.

64. Orenstein SR, Shalaby TM, Di Lorenzo C, et al. The spectrum of pediatric eosinophilic esophagitis beyond infancy: a clinical series of 30 children. *Am J Gastroenterol* 2000;95:1422–1430.

65. Skopnik H, Silny J, Heiber O, et al. Gastroesophageal reflux in infants: evaluation of a new intraluminal impedance technique. *J Pediatr Gastroenterol Nutr* 1996;23:591–598.

66. Orenstein SR, Klein HA, Rosenthal MS. Scintigraphy vs. pH probe for quantification of pediatric gastroesophageal reflux: a study using concurrent multiplexed data and acid feedings. *J Nucl Med* 1993;3:1228–1234.

67. Wenzl TG. Investigating esophageal reflux with the intraluminal impedance technique. *J Pediatr Gastroenterol Nutr* 2002;34: 261–268.

68. Wenzl TG, Moroder C, Trachterna M, et al. Esophageal pH monitoring and impedance measurement: a comparison of two diagnostic tests for gastroesophageal reflux. *J Pediatr Gastroenterol Nutr* 2002;34:519–523.

69. Carr MM, Nagy ML, Pizzuto MP, et al. Correlation of findings at direct laryngoscopy and bronchoscopy with gastroesophageal reflux disease in children. A prospective study. *Arch Otolaryngol Head Neck Surg* 2001;127:369–374.

70. Sacco O, Fregonese B, Silvestri M, et al. Bronchoalveolar lavage and esophageal pH monitoring data in children with "difficult to treat" respiratory symptoms. *Pediatr Pulmonol* 2000;30: 313–319.

71. Ahrens P, Noll C, Kitz R, et al. Lipid-laden alveolar macrophages (LLAM): a useful marker of silent aspiration in children. *Pediatr Pulmonol* 1999;28:79–82.

72. Gerson LB, Robbins AS, Garber A, et al. A cost-effectiveness analysis of prescribing strategies in the management of gastroesophageal relfux disease. *Am J Gastroenterol* 2000;95:395–407.

73. Orenstein SR, Magill HL, Brooks P. Thickening of infant feedings for therapy of gastroesophageal reflux. *J Pediatr* 1987;110: 181–186.

74. Vanderhoof JA, Moran JR, Harris CL, et al. Efficacy of prethickened infant formula: a multi-center, double-blind, randomized, placebo-conrolled parallel group trial in 104 infants with symptomatic gastroesphoageal reflux. *Clin Pediatr (Phila)* 2003; 42:483–495.

75. Hill DJ, Heine RG, Cameron DJ, et al. Role of food protein intolerance in infants with persistent distress attributed to reflux esophagitis. *J Pediatr* 2000;136:641–647.

76. Vandenplas Y, Sacre SL. Seventeen-hour continuous esophageal pH monitoring in the newborn: evaluation of the influence of position in asymptomatic and symptomatic babies. *J Pediatr Gastroenterol Nutr* 1985;4:356–361.

77. Rudolph CD, Mazur LJ, Liptak GS, et al. Pediatric gastroesophageal reflux clinical practice guidelines. *J Pediatr Gastroenterol Nutr* 2001;32:S1–S31.

78. Pivnick E, Kerr N, Kaufman R, et al. Rickets secondary to phosphate depletion: a sequela of antacid use in infancy. *Clin Pediatr* 1995;34:73–78.

79. Tsou V, Young R, Hart M, et al. Elevated plasma aluminum levels in normal infants receiving antacids containing aluminum. *Pediatrics* 1991;87:148–151.

80. Chiba N, De Gara CJ, Wilkinson JM, et al. Speed of healing and symptom relief in grade II to IV gastroesophageal reflux disease: a meta analysis. *Gastroenterology* 1997;112:1798–1810.

81. Orenstein SR, Shalaby TM, DeVandry SN, et al. Famotidine for infant gastrooesopheal reflux: a multi-centre, randomized, placebo-controlled, withdrawal trial. *Aliment Pharmacol Ther* 2003;17:1–11.

82. Orenstein SR, Blumer JL, Fassel HM, et al. Rantidine, 75mg, over-the-counter does: pharmacokinetic and pharmacodynamic effects in children with symptoms of gastrooesophageal reflux. *Aliment Pharmacol Ther* 2002;16:899–907.

83. Khan S. Orenstein SR, Shalaby TM. the effects of increasing doses of rantidine on gastric pH in children. *Gastroenterology* 2001;120:1212.

84. Vanderhoff BT, Tahboub RM. Proton pump inhibitors: an update. *Am Fam Physician* 2002;66:273–280.

85. Hassall E, Israel D, Shepherd R, et al. Omeprazole for treatment of chronic erosive esophagitis in children: a multicentre study of efficacy, safety, tolerability and dose requirements. International Pediatric Omeprazole Study Group. *J Pediatr* 2000;137: 800–807.

86. Scaillon M, Cadranel S. Safety data required for proton pump inhibitor use in children. *J Pediatr Gastroenterol Nutr* 2002;35:113–118.

87. Israel D, Hassall E. Omeprazole and other proton pump inhibitors: pharmacology, efficacy, and safety, with special reference to use in children. *J Pediatr Gastroenterol Nutr* 1998;27: 568–579.

88. Faure C, Michaud L, Khan Shaghaghi E, et al. Lansoprazole in children: pharmacokinetics and efficacy in reflux esophagitis. *Aliment Pharmacol Ther* 2001;15:1397–1402.

89. Cucchiara S, Staiano A, Boccieri A, et al. Effects of cisapride on parameters of esophageal motility and on the prolonged intraesophageal pH test in infants with gastroesophageal reflux disease. *Gut* 1990;31:21–25.

90. Lidums I, Lehmann A, Checklin H, et al. Control of transient lower esophageal sphincter relaxations and gastroesophageal reflux by the GABA(β) agonist baclofen in normal human subjects. *Gastroenterology* 2000;118:1–8.

91. Orenstein SR, Di Lorenzo C. Postfundoplication complications in children. *Curr Treatment Options Gastroenterol* 2001;4:441–449.

92. Kawahara H, Imura K, Yagi M, et al. Mechanisms underlying the antireflux effect of Nissen fundoplication in children. *J Pediatr Surg* 1998;33:618–622.

93. Somme S, Rodriguez JA, Kirsch DG, et al. Laparoscopic versus open fundoplication in infants. *Surg Endosc* 2002;16:54–56.

94. Gut CN, Markus B, Kim ZG, et al. Early experiences of robotic surgery in children. *Surg Endosc* 2002;16:1083–1086.

95. Rode H, Millar AJW, Brown RA, et al. Reflux strictures of the esophagus in children *J Pediatr Surg* 1992;27:462–465.

96. Qualman S, Murray R, McClung J, et al. Intestinal metaplasia is age related in Barrett's esophagus. *Arch Pathol Lab Med* 1990;114:1236–1240.

97. Montgomery E, Goldblum JR, Greenson JK, et al. Dysplasia as a predictive marker for invasive carcinoma in Barrett esophagus: a follow-up study based on 138 cases from a diagnostic variability study. *Hum Pathol* 2001;32:379–388.

98. Hassall E, Dimmick JE, Magee JF. Adenocarcinoma in childhood Barrett's: case documentation and the need for surveillance in children. *Am J Gastroenterol* 1993;88:282–288.

32

REGURGITATION AND RUMINATION

HEATHER J. CHIAL
MICHAEL CAMILLERI
JOSEPH A. MURRAY

Physicians frequently evaluate patients with persistent regurgitation and/or vomiting. In this chapter, we discuss the diagnosis of the frequently encountered symptom of chronic regurgitation and the often overlooked rumination syndrome.

CHRONIC REGURGITATION

Regurgitation refers to the action of bringing up previously ingested food from the esophagus and/or stomach into the pharynx. Regurgitation may be distinguished from vomiting by a lesser volume of regurgitant and the absence of forceful contractions of abdominal and thoracic musculature. Regurgitation is also a quiet process. The absence of autonomic symptoms of diaphoresis, tachycardia, and pallor is also more suggestive of regurgitation than vomiting. However, it is sometimes difficult to distinguish regurgitation from vomiting in the clinical setting; a thorough history will clarify most situations. Rumination is a very characteristic form of repetitive regurgitation that occurs during and immediately after meals and may be followed by reswallowing.

Chronic regurgitation may be due to a variety of underlying conditions including primary abnormalities of the esophagus and gastroesophageal reflux disease (GERD). Esophageal etiologies include structural abnormalities, such as diverticula (e.g., epiphrenic), or motility disorders, such as achalasia, a hypertensive lower esophageal sphincter (LES), and diffuse esophageal spasm. Esophageal regurgitation as in achalasia is usually nonacid, in contrast to GERD. Complications of chronic regurgitation include aspiration, nocturnal coughing, secondary pneumonia, interstitial lung disease, and dental problems.

H.J. Chial, M. Camilleri, J. Murray: Clinical Enteric Neuroscience Translational and Epidemiological Research Program, Mayo Clinic Rochester, Rochester, Minnesota.

Solids or liquid may accumulate in the pharynx and present a picture that mimics regurgitation. This is called pseudoregurgitation, and it may occur in the setting of structural lesions of the pharynx such as Zenker's diverticula and inflammation of the nasal passages.

A detailed clinical history may help to identify the underlying etiology. Many patients with an underlying abnormality of the esophagus will describe symptoms of dysphagia or odynophagia. A complaint of chest pain may point to an esophageal motility disorder or underlying GERD. Regurgitation of food ingested several hours earlier suggests gastric retention, but may also be associated with a pharyngeal or epiphrenic diverticulum or achalasia. History of a restrictive bariatric surgical procedure would suggest a very specific syndrome of acute food impaction at the level of the proximal gastric pouch. This results in the somewhat abrupt regurgitation of an intact food bolus (often described by patients as "upchucking"), and is often associated with acute high epigastric or low retrosternal chest pain.

Diagnosis may require a structural assessment of the upper gastrointestinal tract such as a barium study (with or without food), endoscopy, or physiologic testing using esophageal manometry, 24-hour esophageal pH testing, or assessment of gastric emptying.

Treatment of chronic regurgitation is based on the underlying etiology as described in other chapters of this textbook.

RUMINATION SYNDROME
Definition

Rumination is a well-known phenomenon that occurs in animals such as sheep, cattle, and goats with compartmentalized stomachs consisting of multiple chambers (1,2). In these animals, food residue in the proximal two chambers of the stomach moves by retrograde peristalsis into the mouth in a coordinated manner associated with relaxation of the LES. The animals then rechew and reswallow the

TABLE 32.1. ROME II DIAGNOSTIC CRITERIA FOR RUMINATION SYNDROME IN INFANTS

Infant rumination syndrome is defined by at least 3 months of stereotypical behavior beginning with repetitive contractions of the abdominal muscles, diaphragm, and tongue, and culminating in regurgitation of gastric contents into the mouth which is either expectorated or rechewed and reswallowed, and three or more of the following:
1. Onset between 3 and 8 months of age
2. Does not respond to management for gastroesophageal reflux disease, anticholinergic drugs, hand restraints, formula changes, and gavage or gastrostomy feedings
3. Unaccompanied by signs of nausea or distress
4. Does not occur during sleep and when the infant is interacting with individuals in the environment

regurgitated food. This process aids in the digestion and absorption of food by reducing particle size and enhancing acid exposure (3).

In humans, rumination syndrome is a condition characterized by the effortless regurgitation of recently ingested food into the mouth followed by rechewing and reswallowing or expulsion (4). Although initially described in infants (5–8) and the developmentally disabled (9–11), it is now widely recognized that rumination syndrome occurs in males and females of all ages and cognitive abilities (1,12–17). In general, rumination is more common in females than males (13–15).

Diagnostic Criteria

The diagnosis of rumination syndrome is based on signs and symptoms. The Rome II diagnostic criteria for rumination syndrome in infants and adults are shown in Tables 32.1 and 32.2, respectively. Diagnostic criteria for rumination syndrome in children and adolescents are lacking. However, with the availability of large data sets describing the manifestations of rumination in these age groups (13–15), we anticipate that such criteria will be developed in the future.

Associated Symptoms

The primary symptom in rumination syndrome is regurgitation of recently ingested food. The frequency of regurgitation can be quite variable; some patients will regurgitate following nearly every meal, while others may have intermittent episodes of regurgitation. Many individuals with rumination have additional symptoms including nausea, heartburn, abdominal discomfort, diarrhea, and/or constipation (13–15,18). Patients with additional symptoms may require further medical evaluation before rumination syndrome can be confidently confirmed as a singular diagnosis.

Weight loss can also be a prominent feature of rumination syndrome, particularly in the adolescent population (13–15,18). Considering the female predominance of the condition and the frequent occurrence of weight loss, patients are often misdiagnosed as having bulimia and/or anorexia nervosa (19,20). Although weight loss is a concerning symptom, particularly in children and adolescents, we do not believe that weight loss alone is an indication for more exhaustive diagnostic testing in the presence of classical clinical features of rumination syndrome. Fig. 32.1 summarizes the typical clinical approach to a patient with suspected rumination.

Pathophysiology

Normally, there is active contraction at the esophagogastric junction and increased LES pressure during periods of increased intraabdominal pressure. Tonic contraction of the crural diaphragm is the proposed mechanism for this response (21). In patients with rumination syndrome,

TABLE 32.2. ROME II DIAGNOSTIC CRITERIA FOR RUMINATION SYNDROME IN ADULTS

At least 12 weeks, which need not be consecutive, in the preceding 12 months of:
1. Persistent of recurrent regurgitation of recently ingested food into the mouth with subsequent remastication and swallowing
2. Absence of nausea and vomiting
3. Cessation of process when regurgitated material becomes acidic
4. Absence of pathologic gastroesophageal reflux, achalasia, or other motility disorder with a recognized pathologic basis as the primary disorder

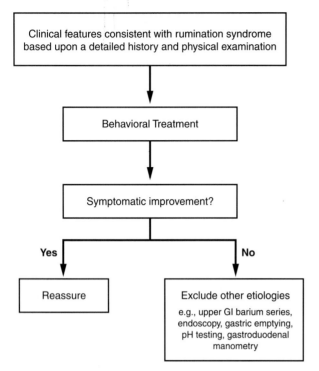

FIGURE. 32.1. Clinical approach to the patient with suspected rumination syndrome.

shown in Fig. 32.2. Thus, one hypothesis proposes simultaneous relaxation of the LES during episodes of increased intraabdominal pressure (16). A second hypothesis is a learned, voluntary relaxation of the diaphragmatic crura that allows the normal postprandial increase in intragastric pressure to overcome the resistance to retrograde flow provided by the LES.

Thumshirn et al. (23) demonstrated that patients of normal intelligence with rumination syndrome required significantly lower fundic pressures to induce LES relaxation and had increased gastric sensitivity to balloon distention compared to healthy controls. The data suggest that the pressure of food within the fundus may result in reflex inhibition of lower esophageal pressure leading to the induction of a modified belch reflex.

In some cases, stressful life events can be identified around the time of symptom onset (15). However, in most cases, rumination occurs in the absence of such identifiable predisposing factors.

In individuals with developmental disabilities, the etiology of rumination is often multifactorial. It is not uncommon for these individuals to have concomitant structural abnormalities of the upper gastrointestinal tract in addition to oropharyngeal dysfunction (11).

Smout and Breumelhof (22) demonstrated transient LES relaxations following abdominal straining events, suggesting that the usual mechanisms that prevent reflux of gastric content are altered.

Although several theories have been proposed, the pathophysiologic mechanisms involved in rumination syndrome remain somewhat unclear, although all observations suggest that there is an adaptation of the belch reflex (14) as

Diagnosis

Rumination syndrome is a clinical diagnosis. No specific tests can be performed to definitively diagnose rumination syndrome. Perhaps the most convincing diagnosis is based on identifying the syndrome and successful treatment or cure obtained exclusively with behavioral modification (discussed below). Although many patients undergo extensive and sometimes invasive testing prior to diagnosis, such tests

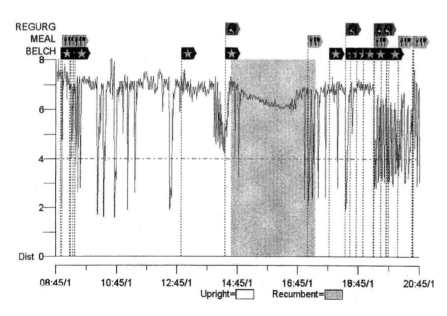

FIGURE. 32.2. Esophageal pH tracing from a patient with rumination syndrome. Note the frequent episodes of postprandial regurgitation.

can only rule out other causes of regurgitation. Blood tests in patients with rumination are nearly always normal with the exception of mild abnormalities in electrolytes such as sodium and potassium with prolonged and severe rumination. Commonly performed clinical tests include barium studies of the upper gastrointestinal tract, abdominal x-rays, esophagogastroduoenoscopy (EGD), scintigraphic assessment of gastric emptying, prolonged esophageal pH monitoring, and other specialized testing. In patients with rumination syndrome, these studies are nearly always normal (1,15,17,18). However, there are many important pitfalls to consider when these tests are requested.

When gastric emptying is performed in patients with rumination syndrome, several caveats exist. For example, some patients will have mildly delayed gastric emptying due to the to-and-fro motion of food that occurs during rumination, which slows the transfer of stomach contents into the distal stomach for trituration before emptying into the small bowel. These patients may be misdiagnosed as having gastroparesis. Another caveat is the potential for expulsion of the radio-labeled meal; when the majority of the meal is expelled, the study cannot be interpreted. Therefore, results of scintigraphic gastric emptying studies should be interpreted cautiously in patients with rumination syndrome.

In general, esophageal pH testing is not advocated in patients with rumination as changes in esophageal pH are a consequence of rumination, rather than a cause for symptoms. As shown in Fig. 32.2, when such testing is performed for suspected GERD, rumination syndrome is characterized by numerous episodes of postprandial acid regurgitation and drops in esophageal pH that occur in the upright position only, rather than recumbent or nocturnal reflux that indicates GERD. In our experience, nocturnal regurgitation is extremely rare in patients with rumination syndrome (15). The other clue is that despite repetitive changes in pH, the total time that the esophageal pH is <4 may be paradoxically low, since food buffers the gastric acid and the pH of gastric contents may be >4 during the postprandial period when repetitive regurgitation occurs.

Gastroduodenal manometry with simultaneous esophageal pH testing has been advocated as a diagnostic test in patients with rumination syndrome (4). In approximately 40% to 60% of patients with rumination syndrome, characteristic rumination or "R-waves" are evident on manometry as shown in Fig. 32.3. (14,15,18). The term R-wave refers to pressure spikes recorded simultaneously at all levels in the stomach and small intestine, presumed to represent a generalized increase in intraabdominal pressure that occurs at the time of rumination. R-waves are typically associated with a sudden decrease in the esophageal pH due to regurgitation of stomach content into the esophagus and pharynx. Although the presence of R-waves is highly suggestive of rumination syndrome, up to 50% of patients will not show these waves during the test, suggesting that the diagnostic utility of this invasive test is low. The informa-

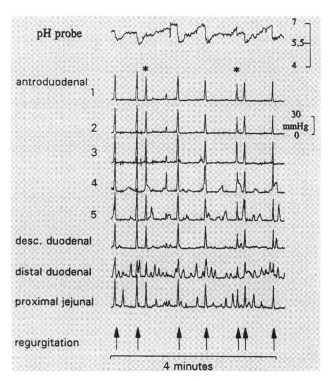

FIGURE. 32.3. Gastroduodenal manometry tracing from a patient with rumination syndrome. Note the characteristic R-waves (indicated by *). (From Malcolm A, Thumshirn MB, Camilleri M, et al. Rumination syndrome. *Mayo Clin Proc* 1997;72: 646–652, with permission.)

tion obtained by taking a sufficient clinical history is often adequate to make the diagnosis of rumination syndrome (14). In addition, gastroduodenal manometry is an invasive test requiring significant technical and interpretive expertise, and is only available in tertiary care centers. Therefore, we believe that gastroduodenal manometry should be limited to cases of suspected intestinal pseudo-obstruction, a very rare cause of chronic regurgitation.

Alternative Diagnoses

The differential diagnosis for persistent regurgitation, rumination, and vomiting is broad and includes gastroparesis, GERD, disorders of the central nervous system, mechanical obstruction, intestinal pseudo-obstruction, eating disorders such as anorexia and bulimia nervosa, cyclic vomiting syndrome, and medication side effects. However, the typical pattern and timing of symptoms allow the differentiation of rumination syndrome from other conditions.

Complications of Rumination Syndrome

The common medical complications of rumination syndrome are relatively mild and variable and include weight loss, vitamin and mineral deficiencies, and dental problems including cavities and erosion of enamel by stomach acid

(24). Fortunately, with appropriate treatment, many of the complications associated with rumination syndrome are reversible.

Significant medical complications resulting from rumination syndrome itself are unusual. However, complications may result from extensive and sometimes invasive testing or treatment before the diagnosis is made. Patients frequently miss school/work due to symptoms, and may even require hospitalization for evaluation and/or management of symptoms prior to diagnosis (4,13,15). We have noted significant functional disability related to weight loss, school and work absenteeism, social consequences and embarrassment related to rumination behavior at mealtime, hospitalization, and extensive diagnostic testing in pediatric and adolescent patients with rumination syndrome (15). Early recognition of the clinical features of rumination is key to avoiding adverse consequences.

Treatment and Prognosis

The mainstay of treatment for rumination syndrome involves behavioral modification. The preferred behavioral treatment for rumination syndrome consists of habit reversal using special diaphragmatic breathing techniques to compete with the urge to regurgitate (25,26). Habit reversal techniques are used in such a way that the target behavior (rumination) is eliminated by the consistent use of an incompatible or competing behavior. The rumination behavior is eliminated because rumination and the competing response cannot be performed at the same time. After proper training, consistent practice of diaphragmatic breathing during rumination effectively eliminates rumination activity in both habit reversal and diaphragmatic breathing. Rumination complicated by co-morbid medical, psychological, or psychiatric conditions may require additional medical and/or psychotherapeutic interventions.

Treatment of rumination syndrome in infants and the developmentally disabled also involves behavioral modification. In infants, increasing social interaction between the infant and caregiver(s) and increased holding during and following meals have been shown to be beneficial (5,27). Aversive therapies incorporating unpleasant stimuli when regurgitation occurs have also been tried when other treatments fail (28). In individuals who are developmentally disabled, dietary modification (29) to adjust food consistency and behavioral intervention (30) are often combined. When these techniques are unsuccessful, food satiation approaches to increase the caloric content of meals in underweight individuals and aversive therapies can be implemented (31–33).

In general, medications including acid-blocking agents (antacids, H_2-receptor blockers, and proton pump inhibitors) and prokinetic medications (cisapride and metoclopramide) are not helpful at improving symptoms in patients with rumination syndrome. Operations such as fundoplication to inhibit regurgitation of stomach contents have not proven to be effective either, and adult patients who have received the operation have considerable upper abdominal discomfort after meals, although the regurgitation may stop.

In general, early intervention with behavioral treatment is recommended in order to reduce adverse consequences related to school/work absenteeism, weight loss, extensive diagnostic testing, social embarrassment, and hospitalization (18).

Although controlled treatment trials are lacking, the outcome for patients with rumination syndrome who undergo behavioral treatment appears to be quite good (14–18,25, 34). The vast majority of patients will have significant improvement of their symptoms, and many report complete resolution of symptoms following treatment.

Nutritional Issues

The severity of regurgitation in patients with rumination syndrome is quite variable. For some, regurgitation occurs at nearly every meal and the amount of weight loss can be significant. On the other hand, many patients with rumination syndrome are able to maintain and even gain weight despite frequent regurgitation. In rare situations, patients with severe symptoms and associated weight loss require supplemental enteral or parenteral nutrition. However, after rumination syndrome is diagnosed and behavioral treatment is initiated, such measures are almost never required (13). In general, it is recommended that patients with rumination syndrome eat a balanced diet. Dietary restrictions are rarely needed. After behavioral treatment is initiated, gradual reintroduction of foods under supervision by the behavioral therapist or a dietitian would be advantageous.

CONCLUSIONS

Rumination syndrome is an underrecognized condition in otherwise healthy pediatric, adolescent, and adult patients. Insufficient awareness of the clinical features of rumination syndrome contributes to the underdiagnosis of this important medical condition. The diagnosis of rumination syndrome is based on clinical features, and extensive diagnostic testing is unnecessary. Early behavioral therapy is advocated, and patient outcomes are generally favorable (Tables 32.1 and 32.2).

REFERENCES

1. Levine DF, Wingate DL, Pfeffer JM, et al. Habitual rumination: a benign disorder. *BMJ* 1983;287:255–256.
2. Winship DH, Shoralski FF, Weber WN, et al. Esophagus in rumination. *Am J Physiol* 1964;207:1189–1194.

3. Dougherty RW. Eructation in ruminants. *Ann N Y Acad Sci* 1968;150:22–26.
4. Malcolm A, Thumshirn MB, Camilleri M, et al. Rumination syndrome. *Mayo Clin Proc* 1997;72:646–652.
5. Whitehead WE, Drescher VM, Morrill-Corbin E, et al. Rumination syndrome in children treated by increased holding. *J Pediatr Gastroenterol Nutr* 1985;4:550–556.
6. Sheagren TG, Mangurten HH, Brea F, et al. Rumination—a new complication of neonatal intensive care. *Pediatrics* 1980;66:551–555.
7. Fleisher DR. Infant rumination syndrome: report of a case and review of the literature. *Am J Dis Child* 1979;133:266–269.
8. Fleisher DR. Functional vomiting disorders in infancy: innocent vomiting, nervous vomiting, and infant rumination syndrome. *J Pediatr* 1994;125:S84–S94.
9. Fredericks DW, Carr JE, Williams WL. Overview of the treatment of rumination disorder for adults in a residential setting. *J Behav Ther Exp Psychiatry* 1998;29:31–40.
10. Ball TS, Hendricksen H, Clayton J. A special feeding technique for chronic regurgitation. *Am J Ment Defic* 1974;78:486–493.
11. Rogers B, Stratton P, Victor J, et al. Chronic regurgitation among persons with mental retardation: a need for combined medical and interdisciplinary strategies. *Am J Ment Retard* 1992;96:522–527.
12. Brown WR. Rumination in the adult. A study of two cases. *Gastroenterology* 1968;54:933–939.
13. Khan S, Hyman PE, Cocjin J, et al. Rumination syndrome in adolescents. *J Pediatr* 2000;136:528–531.
14. O'Brien MD, Bruce BK, Camilleri M. The rumination syndrome: clinical features rather than manometric diagnosis. *Gastroenterology* 1995;108:1024–1029.
15. Chial HJ, Camilleri M, Williams DE, et al. Rumination syndrome in children and adolescents: diagnosis, treatment, and prognosis. *Pediatrics* 2003;111:158–162.
16. Shay SS, Johnson LF, Wong RK, et al. Rumination, heartburn, and daytime gastroesophageal reflux. A case study with mechanisms defined and successfully treated with biofeedback therapy. *J Clin Gastroenterol* 1986;8:115–126.
17. Soykan I, Chen J, Kendall BJ, et al. The rumination syndrome: clinical and manometric profile, therapy, and long-term outcome. *Dig Dis Sci* 1997;42:1866–1872.
18. Amarnath RP, Abell TL, Malagelada JR. The rumination syndrome in adults. A characteristic manometric pattern. *Ann Intern Med* 1986;105:513–518.
19. Larocca FE, Della-Fera MA. Rumination: its significance in adults with bulimia nervosa. *Psychosomatics* 1986;27:209–212.
20. Eckern M, Stevens W, Mitchell J. The relationship between rumination and eating disorders. *Int J Eat Disord* 1999;26:414–9.
21. Mittal RK, Fisher M, McCallum RW, et al. Human lower esophageal sphincter pressure response to increased intra-abdominal pressure. *Am J Physiol* 1990;258:G624–G630.
22. Smout AJ, Breumelhof R. Voluntary induction of transient lower esophageal sphincter relaxations in an adult patient with the rumination syndrome. *Am J Gastroenterol* 1990;85:1621–1625.
23. Thumshirn M, Camilleri M, Hanson RB, et al. Gastric mechanosensory and lower esophageal sphincter function in rumination syndrome. *Am J Physiol* 1998;275:G314–G321.
24. White DK, Hayes RC, Benjamin RN. Loss of tooth structure associated with chronic regurgitation and vomiting. *J Am Dent Assoc* 1978;97:833–835.
25. Wagaman JR, Williams DE, Camilleri M. Behavioral intervention for the treatment of rumination. *J Pediatr Gastroenterol Nutr* 1998;27:596–598.
26. Johnson WG, Corrigan SA, Crusco AH, et al. Behavioral assessment and treatment of postprandial regurgitation. *J Clin Gastroenterol* 1987;9:679–684.
27. Murray ME, Keele DK, McCarver JW. Behavioral treatment of ruminations. A case study. *Clin Pediatr* 1976;15:591–593, 595.
28. Sajwaj T, Libet J, Agras S. Lemon-juice therapy: the control of life-threatening rumination in a six-month-old infant. *J Appl Behav Anal* 1974;7:557–563.
29. Greene KS, Johnson JM, Rossi M, et al. Effects of peanut butter on ruminating. *Am J Ment Retard* 1991;95:631–645.
30. Luiselli JK, Haley S, Smith A. Evaluation of a behavioral medicine consultative treatment for chronic, ruminative vomiting. *J Behav Ther Exp Psychiatry* 1993;24:27–35.
31. Foxx RM, Snyder MS, Schroeder F. A food satiation and oral hygiene punishment program to suppress chronic rumination by retarded persons. *J Autism Dev Disord* 1979;9:399–412.
32. White JC Jr, Taylor DJ. Noxious conditioning as a treatment for rumination. *Ment Retard* 1967;5:30–33.
33. Bright PJ, George GC, Smart DE. Suppression of regurgitation and rumination with aversive events. *Mich Ment Health Res Bull* 1968;11:17.
34. Prather CM, Litzinger KL, Camilleri M, et al. An open trial of cognitive behavioral intervention in the treatment of rumination syndrome. *Gastroenterology* 1997;112:A808(abst).

33

SURGICAL TREATMENT OF GASTROESOPHAGEAL REFLUX DISEASE

LARS R. LUNDELL

Surgical treatment of gastroesophageal reflux disease (GERD) has previously been limited to patients with chronic complicated reflux in patients with very long-standing severe symptoms. There is now an increasing tendency in many countries to utilize surgery in early stages of the disease (1–3). This changing clinical practice may be due to a variety of factors but partly due to changes in surgical technique (the laparoscopic approach) but may also paradoxically be due to the improvement in medical therapy. With the efficacy and availability of modern medical therapy, the focus and opportunity of therapy in GERD, have changed, as well as recognition of the magnitude of the impairment of quality of life in these patients when not on adequate therapy (4–6). This increased awareness might well be the most important cause behind the suggested increase in prevalence of the disease among the Western adult population.

An important background factor for the strategic decisions to be taken in the long-term management of GERD patients is the fact that there are shortcomings and drawbacks with pharmacologic maintenance therapy. Medical therapies at present and into the foreseeable future are entirely targeted on control of acid reflux, rather than correcting the underlying motor abnormalities of the upper alimentary canal. An additional issue of potential concern is the prevailing controversy on the significance of nonacid reflux components (biliary-pancreatic juice constituents) and their probable effects on the occurrence of columnar metaplasia and the impact on the perpetuation of meta-plastic-dysplastic processes leading to the rapidly increasing incidence of adenocarcinoma of the esophagus (7–10). These concerns have already convinced some that complete control of reflux is necessary and will definitely convince others in the future. Together all these factors seem to indicate that there is a growing demand for the complete and durable control of reflux based on the principle of reconstructing the physiology of the gastroesophageal junction, which seems to be a reachable goal when carrying out a proper antireflux operation.

SELECTION OF PATIENTS FOR ANTIREFLUX SURGERY

Potential candidates for surgery may, for the sake of simplicity, be categorized into three general groups.

1. Patients whose symptoms are fully controlled by medications but who do not wish to continue life-long medication.
2. Patients who have failed to respond (or have responded only partially) to medical therapy.
3. Patients who present with a significant complication of GERD.

The first group of patients are those who have had an excellent response to therapy but who do not wish to rely on drugs to be free of symptoms. These patients are often relatively young and face the prospect of taking acid suppression therapy for the rest of their lives. This also raises cost implications. Although costs vary, there is no doubt that decades of reflux medication are more costly than a laparoscopic antireflux operation (11,12).

The second group refers to those who can be classified as partial or complete failures of medical treatment, which can be defined as continuing symptoms (purely from each individual's perspective) of reflux while on an adequate dose of acid suppression. Typically, this means at least standard doses of a proton pump inhibitor (PPI) for a minimum of 3 months. In some countries, governments limit the availability of PPIs. Consequently, some patients selected for surgery have been treated only with H_2-receptor antagonists. Furthermore, despite the fact that PPIs are very effective in controlling symptoms, volume regurgitation problems may remain and this symptom is often the dominant

L. R. Lundell: Department of Surgery, Sahlgren's University Hospital, Gothenburg, Sweden.

problem in patients who fail on medical therapy (13). If patients do not respond at all to PPIs, one has to carefully consider the possibility that the patient should by all means avoid an anti-reflux operation.

The third group of patients present with the complication of gastroesophageal reflux. Some patients present with difficulties in swallowing due to stricture formation. The treatment of peptic esophageal strictures has been greatly altered since PPIs became available (14). In the past, surgery was the only effective treatment for strictures. If a stricture was densely fibrotic and undilatable, this usually meant resection of the esophagus. Fortunately, these patients are presently very rare. For young and fit patients, many would argue that optimal treatment is antireflux surgery and dilatation. However, many patients presenting with strictures are elderly and fragile and have concomitant complicated diseases, and the use of PPIs with dilatation is usually very effective. Gastroesophageal regurgitation spilling over into the respiratory area can cause chronic respiratory illness such as recurrent pneumonia and asthma, which may constitute an important indication for antireflux surgery (15–17). Problems such as chronic cough, chronic laryngitis, chronic pharyngitis, chronic sinusitis and loss of dental enamel can sometimes be attributed to gastroesophageal reflux.

Presently whether Barrett's esophagus alone is an indication for antireflux surgery remains an open question. There is little argument that patients with Barrett's esophagus who have reflux symptoms can be good candidates for surgery, largely as outlined previously, on the basis of their symptoms and their response to medication, but not simply because they have a columnar-lined esophagus. Experimental evidence suggests that continuing reflux may be deleterious regarding malignant change in the metaplastic epithelium of the esophagus, and trials have suggested that antireflux surgery is somewhat superior to medial treatment in these groups of patients as well. There is, however, no evidence to support the contention that neither surgical nor medical treatment of reflux in patients with Barrett's esophagus consistently leads to regression of the columnar lining and to a significant decrease in the risk for development of dysplasia and neoplasia (18).

PREOPERATIVE INVESTIGATIONS

Fundoplication operations are designed to correct anatomical deficiencies and defects in the pathophysiology of the gastroesophageal junction, with permanent control of GERD and minimal postfundoplication complaints. Therefore, the precision by which the diagnosis of chronic GERD is established is vital for the subsequent success rate of therapy. In recent years, the response to medical therapy has achieved greater importance, and in the future it will occupy an even more significant clinical role as a selection tool.

ENDOSCOPY

Endoscopy is the most readily available diagnostic tool for GERD but its strengths and limitations should be appreciated (19,20). The advantage of endoscopy includes the ability to directly assess esophageal mucosal damage complications and structural abnormalities resulting from and/or associated with GERD (ulcer, stricture, columnar-lined esophagus). In these contexts it is important to emphasize that there is no relationship between the postoperative success rate after antireflux surgery and the preoperative grading of esophagitis (21). There is consensus among surgeons that endoscopy should be done before referral for antireflux surgery. In the case of Barrett's esophagus, the histopathologic characteristics of the columnar-lined esophagus will have an impact on the subsequent follow-up strategy (22,23).

MANOMETRY

Manometry should be used to exclude primary motility disorders such as achalasia. It is also possible to document the adequacy of esophageal peristalsis and clearance function with the use of manometry (24–26). The presence of weak peristaltic amplitudes or poor propagation of peristalsis is not a contraindication to antireflux surgery. Although many surgeons have recommended a tailored approach to patient selection by choosing a partial fundoplication in patients with poor peristalsis, there is no strong scientific evidence to support this approach (27–31). Nevertheless, common sense suggests that a partial fundoplication procedure is likely to be safer in patients with a true adynamic esophagus. Manometry also assists in the precise placement of a pH probe at the time of ambulatory 24-hour pH monitoring.

ESOPHAGEAL pH MONITORING

Twenty-four-hour pH monitoring has been considered important for establishing the diagnosis of GERD in patients with or without normal or equivocal endoscopic findings (32). This test is particularly helpful in patients who have reflux symptoms or supposed reflux symptoms that are relieved insufficiently by acid suppression therapy. The monitoring needs to be carried out before surgery in endoscopy-negative reflux disease and in patients with atypical symptoms such as noncardiac chest pain and supposed respiratory complications of GERD where dual probe positioning may be useful (33). The role of bile reflux monitoring has yet to be defined in GERD, although in the future bile reflux measurements may be helpful in patients who fail to respond to acid suppression therapy (34,35).

OTHER FUNCTION TESTS

For routine clinical practice, the assessment of gastric emptying cannot be recommended in the preoperative evaluation of patients before antireflux surgery. Even in patients with delayed gastric emptying, significant improvement in gastric motor function will ensue after the fundoplication procedure (36,37). Moreover, until now no clear-cut picture has emerged that relates the preoperative motor characteristics of the stomach to the long-term outcome after antireflux surgery.

ANTIREFLUX OPERATIONS

The fundoplication procedure that is most commonly used at present was introduced by Rudolf Nissen in 1956 (38). Total fundoplications such as the Nissen and partial anterior or posterior fundoplications work in similar fashions and these may be as much mechanical as physiological (39). The basic technical aspects of fundoplication operations comprise mobilization of the lower esophagus and then wrapping the fundus of the stomach either partially or totally around the esophagus (Fig. 33.1). An enlarged esophageal hiatus is narrowed by sutures to pre-

vent paraesophageal herniation postoperatively and also to prevent the wrap from being pulled up into the chest. However, a fundoplication will work even when located in the chest, but other complications may develop in these instances, such as gastric ulcerations and severe gastric obstruction (40).

Fibrotic stricturing with or without shortening of the esophagus is seen much less frequently today than in the past. In this circumstance, in order to ensure that the esophagus reaches the abdomen, an esophageal lengthening (Collies) procedure may be undertaken (41). The upper less curvature of the stomach is used to produce the length of the new esophagus, and the stomach is then wrapped around this neoesophagus (Fig. 33.2).

Total, partial, or posterior fundoplications are effective not only when placed in the chest but also when tested in animal viscera. Antireflux procedures focus on three main components. First, we have the anatomic repositioning of the LES into the abdominal positive pressure environment with the reduction of the hiatal hernia sack by dissection, mobilization, and positioning of the crural sutures (Color Plate 33.3). This anatomical restoration per se might also have the potential to prevent reflux by reducing the hiatal hernia (42) and by improving the esophageal clearance and crural function. Whether this repair always should be done posterior or anterior to the esophageal entrance into the abdominal cavity has yet to be clarified (43).

Second, it has been suggested that peristaltic amplitude and other esophageal mechanical functions may improve after antireflux operations (44,45). It is doubtful, however, that these observations are entirely

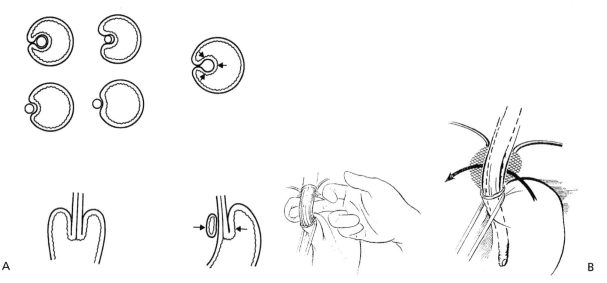

FIGURE 33.1. Principles behind construction of fundoplication with mobilization of the abdominal portion of the esophagus and subsequently wrapping the fundus around the distal esophagus to various extent.

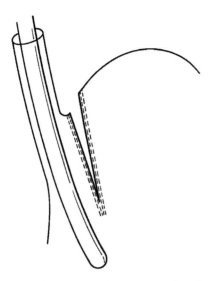

FIGURE 33.2. Esophageal lengthening procedure by tubulizing the upper portion of the minor curvature of the stomach.

explained by secondary compensatory mechanisms resulting from subclinical outflow obstruction in the gastroesophageal junction caused by, for instance, total fundoplication (46). Third, the resting pressure of the LES and the lengthening of the abdominal portion of the high-pressure zone are important consequences of these operations (47). Rydberg et al. (48) assessed LES tone over a long period of time, and showed that pressure was considerably higher after total fundoplication than after a partial, posterior fundoplication. In this study, the pressure level of the LES region was very close to what is seen in healthy individuals. Total fundoplication might overcorrect the mechanical deficiencies in the gastroesophageal junction, thereby creating a supercompetent cardia. After a successful antireflux operation, LES pressure never reaches a level at which free reflux is considered to occur. Furthermore, the number of transient LES relaxations and also the proportion of those associated with reflux are substantially reduced by an antireflux operation (49). After these operations, gas insufflation into the stomach or meal ingestion seldom elicit transient LES relaxations; in unoperated GERD patients, these stimuli may trigger repeated relaxation of the LES accompanied by reflux (50–52). Air venting from the stomach may be a problem after some antireflux operations. This problem is reduced after a partial fundoplication compared to a total fundic wrap, as indicated by the common occurrence of cavities during manometry after gas insufflation into the stomach.

Delayed gastric emptying may be a contributing pathogenetic factor in up to 40% of GERD cases (53,54). Postfundoplication studies have consistently demonstrated an accelerated gastric emptying after these operations. This is probably caused by a high gastric tone postprandially that accelerates the transfer of chyme to the distal part of the stomach, thus facilitating emptying (55).

PROCEDURE SELECTION

Fundoplications usually produce maintained control of reflux, and the efficacy of these operations has been established by clinical and endoscopic follow-up as well as 24-hour pH monitoring, irrespective of whether these are performed by open conventional techniques or by use of modern laparoscopic technology. Based on data from controlled clinical trials, there are no major and obvious clinical differences in the efficacy between different antireflux procedures when the outcome of interest is the accumulated relapse rate (56). Excellent control of the gastroesophageal reflux can be obtained with the total fundic wrap, 270° fundoplication, or 180° fundoplication, provided that each operation involves the reduction of the hiatal hernia coupled with reconstruction of the reflux-preventing mechanisms to reestablish gastroesophageal competence. However, one remaining issue is that published outcomes usually present the best results in the field of antireflux surgery, whereas local expertise can vary considerably (57,58).

CONVERSION RATES AND LEARNING CURVES

The laparoscopic antireflux surgery technique requires that surgeons learn a new range of operating skills. During the learning curve period, operation times are longer and there is increased risk of complications. A learning curve of 50 procedures and individual learning curves of 20 operations have been identified (59). Importantly, similar studies have clearly suggested that the adverse effect of the learning curve could be prevented if new surgeons commence laparoscopic antireflux surgery under the direct supervision of an experienced surgeon.

In a comprehensive review of laparoscopic Nissen fundoplications, a conversion rate of 5.8% to open surgery has been reported. Conversion to the open operation was necessary because of difficulty with the exposure or dissection in almost 4%, and in a few cases equipment failure was reported as the reason for conversion. Direct injuries to the intraabdominal viscera that necessitated conversion were rare, but sometimes CO_2 retention might require an open operation (0.2%) (60).

POSTOPERATIVE ASSESSMENTS

Few controlled studies have been performed that provide sound guidance for the design of a follow-up program after antireflux surgery. In general terms, there is a good correlation between symptom relief and objective assessment of the outcomes in the form of endoscopy and/or 24-hour pH monitoring. Follow-ups of these patients are warranted as part of each institution's quality control program, particularly when alternative therapeutic strategies may be indicated and highly relevant. In patients with Barrett's esophagus, it can be argued that 24-hour pH monitoring is of particular importance for several reasons. For instance, some investigators have reported quite inferior results in patients with Barrett's esophagus compared to those without columnar-lined esophagus (61,62). In cases of suggested failure, endoscopy and barium swallow are mandatory in order to fully explore the anatomical deficiencies occurring in the postsurgical situation. Furthermore, eventual reflux relapse should also be documented by the use of 24-hour pH monitoring. Issues such as tight fundoplication or slipped fundoplication can be addressed more comprehensively by manometry using a sleeve sensor to monitor pressure at the gastroesophageal junction (63). A sustained and high basal pressure with an increased nadir pressure or incomplete relaxation, frequently combined with a compensatory increase in peristaltic amplitudes, suggest that the wrap may be too tight. Scintigraphic investigations of the esophageal function that are also directed toward gastric motor function may sometimes be indicated. Some investigators have reported a significant incidence of severe vagal damage in patients with failed antireflux procedures, which leads to delayed gastric emptying (64).

BENEFITS OF LAPAROSCOPY

The laparoscopic approach to antireflux surgery has gained more or less instant acceptance as the preferred surgical treatment (65). Few direct comparisons of clinical outcome, surgical morbidity, and cost-effectiveness have been attempted between laparoscopic and open surgical procedures (66–69). Nonrandomized comparisons have shown that laparoscopic antireflux surgery reduces hospital treatment costs and early surgical morbidity. Similar results have been obtained from other surgical areas such as inguinal hernia repair, appendectomy, and cholecystectomy. However, these advantages seen in uncontrolled trials have not been firmly supported by data from prospective, randomized clinical trials. Although laparoscopic antireflux surgery generally requires more operating time than open surgical procedures, this difference diminishes with increasing experience. The incidence of postoperative complications has been reduced by at least 50% and length of the postoperative hospital stay has usually been reported to be shortened. It can also be concluded from a recent comprehensive review that the two surgical approaches are very similar with regard to effective reflux control in the short, medium, and long term (70,71). However, a current nationwide survey

indicated a somewhat inferior result after the laparoscopic approach to antireflux surgery (58).

Hiatal repair (crural repair) was not a major issue during the era of open fundoplication, but it seems as though this maneuver has become more important when the operations are done laparoscopically. The incidence of up to 10% of early paraesophageal hiatal herniation in patients undergoing laparoscopic operations seems to be higher than previously recognized (65). Circumstantial evidence, however, exists from the earlier open surgical literature to suggest that hiatal repair should always be added to the operation. In light of these experiences it seems therefore advisable to perform some form of hiatal repair during all antireflux procedures (56).

REDUCING RISK OF ADVERSE CONSEQUENCES OF ANTIREFLUX PROCEDURE

The most frequent postfundoplication symptoms are dysphagia, inability to belch (72–74), postprandial fullness, bloating and pain, and socially embarrassing rectal flatus (67–69). The frequency by which these postfundoplication symptoms have been reported varies considerably between series (Table 33.1). Dysphagia is frequently reported during the early postoperative period but seems to diminish with the passage of the time as do many other postfundoplication symptoms (75). A recent randomized clinical trial suggested that laparoscopic total fundoplications were associated with more obstructive complaints in the early postoperative period than open procedures (66). Other similar trials have not been able to confirm these potential hazards of laparoscopic operations (67–69). At any rate, since we lack effective treatment of established, severe postfundoplication symptoms, prevention is of great importance. There is widespread consensus among experienced surgeons that if a complete wrap is done, it must be both floppy and short. Large randomized trials had reported that posterior partial fundoplications are associated with less troublesome complaints of gas/bloating and rectal flatus (76,77). Furthermore, the laparoscopic anterior partial fun-

TABLE 33.1. SYMPTOM CONTROL AND ADVERSE SIDE EFFECTS OF NISSEN FUNDOPLICATION— SUMMARY OF LITERATURE REVIEW (N=2,230)

	% Mean (Range)
Control of heartburn	89.5 (63–100)
Control of regurgitation	92.5 (81–100)
Dysphagia	24.5 (0–71)
Flatulence	44.9 (9–88)
Inability to belch	25.9 (3–50)
Inability to vomit	36.8 (8–90)

doplication has recently also been reported to have similar advantages (78). However, recent trial data strongly indicates potential weaknesses with the anterior approach to a partial fundoplication (79).

Failure of fundoplication to control reflux occurs in a minority of patients (≤15%) (80). There are reports with a considerably higher failure rate and it is important to emphasize that essentially all failures occur early in the postoperative period, indicating the importance of adhering to technical details and expertise (64). There are no data available to suggest that the failure rate is higher after laparoscopic fundoplication than after open operations. The success rates after redo surgery for failed primary operations are generally lower than after the index operations (64,81–84). This should seriously be taken into consideration along with the fact that postoperative morbidity and mortality are many times higher than after the index operation. These facts should form a strong justification for referring patients who need reoperations to specialized, tertiary referral centers for assessment and careful investigation, as well as adequate surgical expertise to minimize the risk and to optimize the subsequent functional outcome.

SURGICAL VERSUS MEDICAL THERAPY

Unfortunately, very few randomized controlled clinical trials have been carried out comparing antireflux surgery with modern medical therapy. Thus far, only one study has performed a head-to-head comparison between a modern PPI-based therapy (omeprazole) and antireflux surgery in 310 esophagitis patients, in which a slight advantage for operative treatment was observed after a minimal follow-up of 5 years (85). In the United States, a similar trial was initiated many years ago in severe reflux patients recruited from Veterans Administration hospitals at a time when medical therapy was quite different from the present level of efficacy (86). The 2-year follow-up data showed that surgical therapy was more effective. A fairly high proportion of patients randomized to antireflux surgery who could be located for the 10-year follow-up took antisecretory drugs, which suggested suboptimal control of reflux disease (87). Recently, however, we have learned that recording only whether patients take antisecretory drugs after surgery is insufficient, since the reasons for drug use may vary considerably (88). Furthermore, it was reported that patients allocated to antireflux surgery had a survival curve that was significantly inferior to that of medically treated patients (87). The enhanced mortality of patients who had the surgery was mainly due to cardiovascular events. The much larger Nordic GERD trial showed that there is no survival difference whatsoever between operated and nonoperated patients after 7 years of follow-up (85).

In order to obtain a comprehensive and adequate picture of the merits of antireflux surgery in general, and also of the relative merits of various long-term therapeutic alternatives, cost aspects have to be brought into focus. There are inherent methodologic problems in assessing the true costs of a certain therapeutic strategy (12). For instance, the societal perspective is rarely applied, including assessment of both direct and indirect costs. It is obvious that all costs for medical as well as surgical treatment of GERD vary among countries, and likely from one time to another (12). In a prospective, randomized controlled clinical trial, it was observed that in one country, where the relative cost of an open operation was lowest, the subsequent 5-year direct cost of the surgical strategy was significantly lower than the corresponding cost of medical therapy, where the reverse was true in the other participating countries. It is clear that the surgical treatment is associated with a huge initial investment followed by low annual costs; thus, with the passage of time, it becomes relatively less expensive when compared with medical therapy (89–93). Regardless of the methodology used, time spans to be applied when comparing different therapeutic alternatives and treatment options are debatable. With the introduction of the laparoscopic approach to antireflux surgery, it is obvious that cost estimates must be changed (91). Many studies have suggested that the laparoscopic antireflux surgery is less costly than open surgery, based on the fact that days in hospital and missed work/school days are reduced (89,90). In a recent prospective controlled clinical trial, total costs of open laparoscopic surgery were assessed. It was found that by applying the laparoscopic operative technique, total societal cost was reduced during the first postoperative year by 40% (91). Based on similar calculations, it can be concluded that laparoscopic antireflux operations seem to be more cost-effective than available medical therapy after 3 to 5 years, depending on which country the relative estimates are derived from. Furthermore, it must be emphasized that these calculations are based on operative procedures carried out with an acceptable level of experience and expertise.

REFERENCES

1. Shirvani VN, Ouatu-Lascar R, Kaur BS, et al. Cyclooxygenase 2 expression in Barrett's esophagus and adenocarcinoma: ex vivo induction by bile salts and acid exposure. *Gastroenterology* 2000;118:487–496.
2. Viljakka M, Luostarinen M, Isolauri J. Incidence of antireflux surgery in Finland 1988–1993. *Scand J Gastroenterol* 1997;32:415–418.
3. Sandbu R, Haglund U, Arvidsson D, et al. Antireflux surgery in Sweden 1987–1997: decade of change. *Scand J Gastroenterol* 2002;35:345–348.
4. Klinkenberg-Knol E, Festen H, Jansen J, et al. Long-term treatment with omeprazole for refractory reflux esophagitis: efficacy and safety. *Ann Intern Med* 1994;121:161–233.
5. Bardhan KD. The role of the proton pump inhibitors in the treatment of gastroesophageal reflux disease. *Aliment Pharmacol Ther* 1995;9(suppl 1):15–25.

6. Lundell L. Acid suppression in the long term treatment of peptic strictures in Barrett's oesophagus. *Digestion* 1992;51(suppl 1): 49–58.

7. Attwood SE, Smyrk TC, DeMeester TR, et al. Duodenoesophageal reflux and the development of adenocarcinoma in rats. *Surgery* 1992;111:503–510.

8. Lagergren J, Bergström R, Lindgren A, et al. Symptomatic gastroesophageal reflux as a risk factor for esophageal adenocarcinoma. *N Engl J Med* 1999;18:340:825–831.

9. Pera AM, Cameron AJ, Trastec VF. Increasing incidence in adenocarcinoma of the esophagus and esophago-gastric junction. *Gastroenterology* 1993;104:510–513.

10. Rantanen TK, Halme TV, Luostarinen ME, et al. The long-term results of open antireflux surgery in a community-based health care centre. *Am J Gastroenterol* 1999;94:1777–1781.

11. Viljakka M, Nevalainen J, Isolauri J. Lifetime costs of surgical versus medical treatment of severe gastrooesophageal reflux disease in Finland. *Scand J Gastroenterol* 1999;32:776–772.

12. Myrvold HE, Lundell L, Liedman B, et al. The cost of omeprazole versus open antireflux surgery in the long-term management of reflux esophagitis. *Gut* 2001;49:488–494.

13. Lundell L, Dalenbäck J, Hattlebakk J, et al. Nordic GORD-study Group. Outcome of open antireflux surgery as assessment in a Nordic multicenter, prospective clinical trial. *Eur J Surg* 1998;164:751–757.

14. Marks RD, Richter JE, Rizzo J, et al. Omeprazole versus H$_2$-receptor antagonists in treating patents with peptic stricture and oesophagitis. *Gastroenterology* 1994;106:907–915.

15. DeMeester TR, Bonavina L, Lascone C, et al. Chronic respiratory symptoms and occult gastroesophageal reflux: a prospective clinical trial and results of surgical therapy. *Ann Surg* 1990;211: 337–345.

16. Ruth M, Bake B, Sandberg N, et al. Pulmonary function in gastroesophageal reflux disease. Effects of reflux controlled by fundoplication disease of the esophagus. *Dis Esophagus* 1994;7: 268–275.

17. Jamieson GG, Duranceau AC, Dechamps C. Surgical treatment of gastroesophageal reflux disease. In: Jamieson GG, Duranceau AC, eds. *Gastroesophageal reflux*. Philadelphia: WB Saunders, 1988:10–35.

18. Lundell L. Prevention of cancer by control of reflux. In: *Barrett's oesophagus*. Kluwer Academic Publishers, 2000:231–238.

19. Armstrong D, Bennett JR, Blum AL, et al. The endoscopic assessment of esophagitis: a progress report on observer agreement. *Gastroenterology* 1996;111:85–92.

20. Lundell LR, Dent J, Bennett JR, et al. Endoscopic assessment of oesophagitis: clinical and functional correlates and further validation of the Los Angeles classification. *Gut* 1999;45:2:172–180.

21. Watson DI, Foreman D, Devitt PG, et al. Preoperative endoscopic grading of oesophagitis vs. outcome after laparoscopic Nissen fundoplication. *Am J Gastroenterology* 1997;92:222–225.

22. Öberg S, Peters JH, DeMeester TR, et al. Determinants of intestinal metaplasia within the columnar lined esophagus. *Arch Surgery* 2000;135:651–655.

23. Öberg S, Johansson J, Wenner J, et al. Endoscopic surveillance of columnar-lined esophagus: frequency of intestinal metaplasia detection and impact of antireflux surgery. *Ann Surg* 2001; 234:619–626.

24. Kahrilas PJ, Dodds WJ, Hogan WJ. Effect of peristaltic dysfunction on esophageal volume clearance. *Gastroenterology* 1988;94: 73–80.

25. Jacob P, Kahrilas PJ, Vanagunas A. Peristaltic dysfunction associated with non-obstructive dysphagia in reflux disease. *Dig Dis Sci* 1990;35:939–942.

26. Olsen AM, Schlegel JF. Motility disturbances caused by oesophagitis. *J Thorac Cardiovasc Surg* 1965;150:706–712.

27. Fuchs KH, Heimbucher J, Freys SN, et al. Management of gastro-oesophageal reflux disease 1995. Tailored concept of antireflux operations. *Dis Esophagus* 1994;7:250–254.

28. Kauer WKH, Peters JH, DeMeester TR, et al. A tailored approach to antireflux surgery. *J Thorac Cardiovasc Surg* 1995: 110:141–146;discussion 146–147.

29. Mughal MM, Bancewicz J, Marpies M. Oesophageal manometry and pH recording does not predict the bad results of Nissen fundoplication. *Br J Surg* 1990;77:43–45.

30. Baigrie RJ, Watson DI, Meyers JC, et al. Outcome of laparoscopic Nissen fundoplication in patients with disordered preoperative peristalsis. *Gut* 1997;40:381–385.

31. Rydberg L, Ruth M, Abrahamsson H, et al. Tailoring of antireflux surgery. A concept subjective to a randomised clinical trial. *World J Surg* 1999;23:612–618.

32. Armstrong D, Emde C, Inauen W, et al. Diagnostic assessment of gastrooesophageal reflux disease: what is possible vs. what is practical? *Hepatogastroenterology* 1992;39:3–13.

33. Dobhan R, Castell DO. Normal and abnormal proximal esophageal acid exposure: results of ambulatory dual-probe pH monitoring. *Am J Gastroenterology* 1993;88:25–29.

35. Shaker R, Milbrath M, Ren J, et al. Esophagopharyngeal distribution of refluxed gastric acid in patients with reflux laryngitis. *Gastroenterology* 1995;19:1575–1582.

36. Maddern GJ, Jaimeson GG. Fundoplication enhances gastric emptying. *Ann Surg* 1985:301:296–299.

37. Jaimeson GG, Maddern GJ, Meyers JC. Gastric emptying after fundoplication with and without proximal gastric vagotomy. *Arch Surg* 1991;126:1414–1417.

38. Nissen R. Eine einfasche operation zur B-einsflussung der reflux-esophagitis. *Schweiz Med Wochen* 1956;86:590–592.

39. Watson DI, Mathew G, Pike GK, et al. Comparison of anterior, posterior and total fundoplication using a viscera model. *Dis Esophagus* 1997;10:110–114.

40. Herrington JL Jr, Meacham PW, Hunter RM. Gastric ulceration after fundic wrapping. Vagal nerve entrapment, a possible causative factor. *Ann Surg* 1982;195:574–581.

41. Hendersson H, Track NS, Marryatt G. Gastro plastic tube and its rolling reflux control experimentally and clinical study. *Can J Surg* 1980;23:63–66.

42. Kahrilas PJ, Lin S, Chen J. The effect of hiatus hernia on gastroesophageal junction pressure. *Gut* 1999;4:476–482.

43. Watson DI, Jamieson GG, Devitt PG, et al. A prospective randomized trial of laparoscopic Nissen fundoplication with anterior vs posterior hiatal repair. *Arch Surg* 2001;136:745–751.

44. Stein HJ, Bremner RM, Jameson J, et al. Effect of Nissen fundoplication on esophageal motorfunction. *Ann Surgery* 1992;127: 788–791.

45. Escandell AO, deHaro LFM, Paricio PP, et al. Surgery improves the effective oesophageal peristalsis in patient with gastric oesophageal reflux. *Br J Surg* 1991;78:1095–1097.

46. Rydberg L, Ruth M, Lundell L. Does oesophageal motor function improve with time after successful antireflux surgery? Results of a prospective, randomised clinical study. *Gut* 1997;41:82–86.

47. DeMeester TR, Wernly JA, Brian GH, et al. Clinical and in vitro analysis of determinants of gastroesophageal competence: a study of principles of antireflux surgery. *Am J Surg* 1979;137:39.

48. Rydberg L, Ruth M, Lundell L. Mechanism of action of antireflux procedures. *Br J Surg* 1999;86:405–410.

49. Johnsson F, Holloway RH, Ireland AC, et al. Effect of fundoplication on transient lower oesophageal sphincter relaxation and gas reflux. *Br J Surg* 1997;84:686–689.

50. Mittal RK, Holloway RH, Penagini R, et al. Transient lower esophageal sphincter relaxation. *Gastroenterology* 1995;109: 601–610.

51. Schoeman MN, Tippett MD, Akkermans LM, et al. Mechanisms

of gastroesophageal reflux in ambulant healthy human subjects. *Gastroenterology* 1995;108:83–91.

52. Holloway RH, Kocyan P, Dent J. Provocation of transient lower esophageal reflux by meals in patients with symptomatic gastro-sophageal reflux. *Dig Dis Sci* 1991;36:1034–1039.

53. Mc Callum RW, Berkowitz DM, Lerner E. Gastric emptying in patients with gastrooesophageal reflux. *Gastroenterology* 1981;80: 285–291.

54. Velasco N, Hill LD, Ganna RM, et al. Gastric emptying and gas-troesophageal reflux. *Am Surg* 1982;144:58–62.

55. Pu MK, Straathof JWA, Schaar PJ, et al. Motor and sensory func-tion of the approximal stomach in reflux disease and after laparo-scopic Nissen fundoplication. *Am J Gastroenterology* 1999;94: 1481–1489.

56. Lundell LR. Surgical treatment of gastroesophageal reflux dis-ease. In: Orlando RC, ed. *Gastroesophageal reflux disease*. New York: Marcel Dekker Inc., 2000:311–329.

57. Loustarinen MES, Isolauri JO. Surgical experience improve the long-term results of Nissen fundoplication. *Scand J Gastroenterol* 1999;34:117–120.

58. Sandbu R, Khamis HJ, Gustavsson S, et al. Long-term results of antireflux surgery. The benefits of laparoscopic technique under question. *Br J Surg* 2002;89:225–230.

59. Watson DI, Baigrie RJ, Jaimeson GG. A learning curve for laparoscopic fundoplication. Definable, avoidable, or a waste of time? *Ann Surg* 1996;224:198–203.

60. Viljakka M. *Studies on surgical treatment of gastroesophageal reflux disease*. Acta Universitatis Tamperensis 606. Tampere, Finland: University of Tampere, 1998.

61. Franzen J, Bostrom J, Tibbling Grahn L, et al. Prospective study of symptoms and gastroesophageal reflux 10 years after posterior partial fundoplikation. *Br J Surg* 1999;86:956–960.

62. Csendes A, Braghetto I, Burdiles P, et al. Long-term results of clas-sic antireflux surgery in 152 patients with Barrett's esophagus: clin-ical, radiologic, endoscopic, manometric and acid reflux test analy-sis before and late after operation. *Surgery* 1998;123:645–657.

63. Dent J. New technique for continues sphincter pressure mea-surement. *Gastroenterology* 1976;71:263–267.

64. Rieger NA, Jamieson GG, Britten-Jones R. Re-operation after failed antireflux surgery. *Br J Surg* 1994;81:1159–1161.

65. Watson DI, Jamieson GG. Antireflux surgery in the laparoscopic area. *Br J Surg* 1998;85:1173–1184.

66. Bais JE, Bartelsman JFWM, Bonjer HJ, et al. Laparoscopic or conventional Nissen fundoplication for gastroesophageal reflux disease: randomised clinical trial. *Lancet* 2000;355: 170–174.

67. Laine S, Rantala A, Gullichsen R, et al. Laparoscopic vs conven-tional Nissen fundoplication. A prospective randomized study. *Surg Endosc* 1997;11:441–444.

68. Watson DI, Gourlay R, Globe J, et al. Prospective randomised trial of laparoscopic (LNF) versus open (ONF) Nissen fundopli-cation. *Gut* 1994;35(suppl 2):S15(abst).

69. Nilsson G, Larsson S, Johnsson F. Randomised clinical trial of laparoscopic versus open fundoplication: blind evaluation of recovery and discharge period. *Br J Surg* 2000.

70. Lundell L. Laparoscopic fundoplication is the treatment of choise for GORD, the view of a protagonist. *Gut* 2002;51:468–471.

71. Bammer T, Hinder RA, Klaus A, et al. Five- to eight-year out-come at the first laparoscopic Nissen fundoplication. *J Gastroin-test Surg* 2001;5:42–48.

72. DeMeester TR, Stein HJ. Minimizing the side effects of anti-reflux surgery. *World J Surg* 1992;16:335–336.

73. Garstin WI, Hohnston GW, Kennedy TL, et al. Nissen fundo-plication: the unhappy 15%. *J R Coll Surg Edinb* 1986;31:207.

74. Negre JB. Post fundoplication symptoms. Do they restrict the success of Nissen fundoplication? *Ann Surg* 1983;198:698.

75. Bessell JR, Gotley DC, Smithers BM, et al. Chronic dysphagia following laparoscopic fundoplication. *Br J Surg* 2000;87: 1341–1345.

76. Lundell L, Abrahamsson H, Ruth M, et al. Long-term results of a prospective randomised comparison of total fundic wrap (Nis-sen-Rossetti) or semi-fundoplication (Toupet) for gastro-oesophageal reflux. *Br J Surg* 1996;83:830–835.

77. Hagedorn C, Lönroth H, Rydberg L, et al. Long-term efficacy of a total (Nissen-Rossetti) and a posterior partial fundoplication (Toupét). Results of a randomised clinical trial. *J Gastrointest Surg* 2002;6:540–545.

78. Watson DI, Jamieson GG, Pike GK, et al. Prospective randomized double-blind trial between laparoscopic Nissen fundoplication and anterior partial fundoplication. *Br J Surg* 1999;86:123–130.

79. Hagedorn C, Jönson C, Lönroth H, et al. The efficacy of an ante-rior as compared as compared to a posterior laparoscopic partial fundoplication. Results of a randomised, controlled clinical trial. *Ann Surgery* 2003 *(in press)*.

80. Peridikis G, Hinder RA, Lund RJ, et al. Laparoscopic Nissen fundoplication: where do we stand? *Surg Laparosc Endosc* 1997; 7:17–21.

81. Deschamps C, Trastec VF, Allen MS, et al. Long-term results after re-operation for failed antireflux procedures. *J Thorac Car-diovasc Surg* 1997;113:545–551.

82. Stein HJ, Feussner H, Siewert JR. Failure of antireflux surgery: causes and management strategies. *Am J Surg* 1996;171:36–40.

83. Luostarinen ME, Isolauri JO, Koskinen MO, et al. Re-fundopli-cation for recurrent gastroesophageal reflux. *World J Surg* 1993; 17:587–594.

84. Watson DI, Jamieson PA, Game PA, et al. Laparoscopic reoper-ation following failed antireflux surgery. *Br J Surg* 1999;86: 98–101.

85. Lundell L, Miettinen P, Myrvold HE, et al. Continued (5-year) follow-up of a randomised clinical study comparing antireflux surgery and omeprazole in gastroesophageal reflux disease. *J Am Coll Surg* 2001;192:172–179.

86. Spechler SJ. Comparison of medical and surgical therapy for complicated gastroesophageal reflux disease in veterans. *N Engl J Med* 1992;326:786–792.

87. Spechler SJ, Lee E, Ahnen D, et al. Long-term outcome of med-ical and surgical therapies for gastroesophageal reflux disease. *JAMA* 2001;285:2331–2338.

88. Lord RV, Kaminski A, Bowrey DJ, et al. Absence of gastroe-sophageal reflux disease in a majority of patients taking acid sup-pression medications after Nissen fundoplication. *Gastroenterol-ogy* 2001;120(suppl 1):A44.

89. van der Boom G, Go PM, Hameeteman W, et al. Cost effective-ness of medical versus surgical treatment in patients with severe or refractory gastroesophageal reflux disease in the Netherlands. *Scand J Gastroenterol* 1996;31:1–9.

90. Heudebert G, Marks R, Wilcox C, et al. Choice of long-term strategy in the management of patients with severe esophagitis: a cost utility analysis. *Gastroenterology* 1996;112:1078–1086.

91. Blomqvist AMK, Lönroth H, Dalenbäck J, et al. Laparoscopic or open fundoplication? A complete cost analysis. *Surg Endosc* 1998;12:1209–1212.

92. Incarbone R, Peters JH, Heimbucher J, et al. A contemporane-ous comparison of hospital charges for laparoscopic and open Nissen fundoplication. *Surg Endosc* 1995;9:151–155.

93. Laycock WS, Oddsdottir M, Franco A, et al. Laparoscopic Nis-sen fundoplication is less expensive than open Belsey Mark IV. *Surg Endosc* 1995;9:426–429.

PILL-INDUCED ESOPHAGEAL INJURY

JAMES WALTER KIKENDALL

Most oral medications are administered as nonchewable tablets or capsules because these solid, compact pills are easily stored, transported, and consumed, and may be modified to regulate absorption. The tablets and capsules are designed to pass rapidly through the mouth and esophagus and to release their contents in the stomach or more distal regions of the gastrointestinal tract. On occasion, tablets and capsules may lodge in the esophagus and dissolve therein, releasing their undiluted contents directly onto the esophageal mucosa. If the concentrated medication thus released is sufficiently caustic, the esophageal wall may be injured, either directly or through interaction with refluxed gastric contents. This process is known as pill-induced esophageal injury (1). In this chapter, I review evidence from 1,088 reported cases of pill-induced esophageal injury caused by more than 100 different medications.

CLINICAL PRESENTATION AND DIFFERENTIAL DIAGNOSIS

The abrupt onset of odynophagia in a patient taking potentially injurious pills is highly suggestive of pill-induced esophageal injury, the principal differential being infectious esophagitis (1). The typical injured patient has no prior esophageal symptoms but experiences the sudden onset and progression over 1 to 4 days of retrosternal pain. The pain is almost always exacerbated by swallowing and may be perceived only with swallowing. The pain may remain mild or become so severe as to make swallowing impossible, compromising hydration and alimentation (3–6). Symptoms typically resolve in a few days to a few weeks.

Many patients relate that the tablet or capsule seemed to stick in the esophagus prior to the onset of symptoms. Others admit that they have taken their pills with little or no water. Those patients who have been awakened from sleep by pain may relate that they took their pills immediately

prior to going to bed. Many injured patients, however, have taken their pills entirely properly, and the absence of these predisposing features does not constitute evidence against the diagnosis of pill-induced esophageal injury.

Less typical symptoms may lead to diagnostic confusion. A burning quality to the pain may result in confusion with gastroesophageal reflux disease (GERD). Constant pain may suggest myocardial infarction (7–9). Slowly progressive painless dysphagia is uncommon but has been observed, particularly with injury due to alendronate, quinidine, or potassium chloride pills, and this history may suggest neoplasia. Hemorrhage occurs in less than 5% of reported cases, but pill-induced ulcers have indeed penetrated the left atrium and major vessels (10–13). Mediastinitis and free esophageal perforation have complicated injuries due to alendronate (14), an aspirin–caffeine compound pill (15), sustained-release ferrous sulfate (16), and sustained-release sodium valproate (17).

DIAGNOSIS, PATHOLOGY, AND COMPLICATIONS

When a patient states that a swallowed pill had become lodged in the chest prior to the onset of rapidly progressive retrosternal pain clearly exacerbated by swallowing, the diagnosis of pill-induced esophagitis is apparent. The evaluation of such a patient will be directed toward discovery of possible predisposing factors or complications and toward the planning of appropriate alternatives to the implicated oral medication.

While endoscopy may not be necessary for the patient with a typical, uncomplicated presentation and rapid recovery, endoscopy is indicated when symptoms are gradual rather than acute in onset, atypical, or inordinately persistent, or when the relationship of symptoms to a previously reported potentially injurious pill is unclear. Endoscopy is also indicated in immunocompromised patients or in patients with hemorrhage.

Endoscopy is more sensitive than barium esophagography for subtle pill-induced esophageal lesions. With its

J. W. Kikendall: Gastroenterology Service, Walter Reed Army Medical Center, Washington, DC.

biopsy capability, endoscopy is also more likely to provide a definitive alternative diagnosis such as infectious esophagitis, cancer, or GERD. The only apparent advantages of esophagography over endoscopy are its lower initial cost and its higher sensitivity for extrinsic compression, which might lead to a recurrence of injury if undetected. The higher diagnostic yield of endoscopy will make it the most cost-effective procedure if diagnostic testing is reserved for difficult cases as suggested above.

Endoscopy typically reveals one or more discrete ulcers with normal surrounding mucosa (1). Discrete ulcers range from pinpoint to several centimeters in size. At times, diffuse inflammation is observed either without ulceration or surrounding the ulcer(s). Remnants of the offending pill may occasionally be identified (15,18–23). Biopsies reveal acute inflammation without evidence for infection or neoplasia.

In contrast to this typical pattern of injury, exudates, edema, and nodularity may be so profuse that neoplasia is suggested, either at endoscopy or on barium swallow (1,16,24–27). Such inflammatory pseudotumors have been observed in patients injured by quinidine, especially the sustained-release form of quinidine (1,24,27,28); sustained-release ferrous sulfate (16); and sustained-release naproxen (25). Even such flamboyant inflammatory stenoses tend to resolve spontaneously if the offending pill is withdrawn. More ominously, large circumferential ulcers or repetitive injuries may lead to fibrotic strictures requiring dilatation or surgery.

Several cases of alendronate-induced esophageal injuries have demonstrated an unusual, thick, white pseudomembranous exudate (7,29). Biopsies in some of these cases have shown granulation tissue and birefringent, polarizable, crystalline material similar to a component of the alendronate tablet (7,29).

Any area of the esophagus may be injured (1). The most common site of injury is the junction of the proximal and middle thirds of the esophagus where peristaltic amplitude is relatively low and where the esophagus may be compressed anteriorly by the aortic arch. Patients with left atrial enlargement are susceptible to injury at the site where the esophagus is compressed by the left atrium (30–32). The most distal esophagus has uncommonly been reported as the site of injury, perhaps because of the difficulty in differentiating pill-induced injury from GERD in this location.

THERAPY AND CLINICAL COURSE

The obvious first step in the treatment of pill-induced esophageal injury is withdrawal of the offending pill. Empiric antireflux therapy may be administered to prevent exacerbation of injury by refluxing acid. Swallowing a topical anesthetic will temporarily relieve severe pain. Most patients will become asymptomatic within a few days to a few weeks if the injury is not repeated (1). Rarely, patients require parenteral hydration or parenteral alimentation. Complications of esophageal perforation, mediastinitis, hemorrhage, or fibrotic stricture require specific treatment.

EPIDEMIOLOGY AND PATHOGENESIS

Pill-induced esophageal injury was first reported in 1970 (22,33,34). To date, 1,088 cases have been reported or summarized in the medical literature. These cases represent only the tip of the iceberg. Cases are reported selectively, usually because of an unusual quality such as a clustering of cases, a newly implicated pill, or a complication. The best estimate of the incidence of pill-induced esophageal injury is derived from 109 cases diagnosed in a region of Sweden during a 4-year period in the 1970s (35), an incidence of 4 cases per 100,000 population per year. The incidence of injury today is probably higher because of more frequent administration of medications. Still, pill-induced esophageal injury is an uncommon event considering the number of pills consumed each year.

Patients of all ages (3 to 98 years) have been injured (Tables 34.1 to 34.4). Women have been injured in 71% of cases for which gender has been reported. More women than men have been injured by antibiotics, nonsteroidal antiinflammatory drugs (NSAIDs), alendronate (indicated for osteoporosis), and emepronium bromide (indicated for urinary frequency due to bladder irritability).

Most injured patients have normal esophageal structure and function. This is possible because pill transit through the esophagus is commonly interrupted even in normal subjects. When swallowed with water by upright subjects, gelatin capsules were retained in the esophagus longer than 5 minutes by 11 of 18 subjects (36). Chasing pills with more water makes them more likely to pass rapidly to the stomach but does not guarantee transit (36). Pills are even more likely to stick in the esophagus if taken without water or while supine, and these predisposing factors are frequently documented in literature case reports. Other factors favoring esophageal retention of pills include advanced patient age, decreased esophageal peristalsis, and extrinsic esophageal compression. Gelatin capsules are more likely to stick in the esophagus than tablets, and large pills are more likely to stick than small ones (37).

When a pill is retained in the esophagus, it may dissolve there and release its contents. If the contents are sufficiently caustic, injury will occur. The pathogenic mechanism for some pills including the tetracyclines, ascorbic acid, and ferrous sulfate may be production of an acid burn. Any of these pills dissolved in 10 ml of water produces a solution with a pH of ≤3.0 (36,38). Phenytoin sodium, 100 mg, dissolved in 10 ml of water produced a solution with a pH of 10.4, suggesting that it might pro-

TABLE 34.1. ESOPHAGEAL INJURY DUE TO ANTIBIOTIC AND ANTIVIRAL PILLS

Pill Type	Cases	Gender M	Gender F	# for whom Reported	Age (Yr) Range	Age (Yr) Mean	Hemorrhage	Stricture	Death	References
Doxycycline	302	51	104	142	10–98	30	1	2	1	[a]
Tetracycline HCl	44	11	25	25	18–72	35	5	1	—	[b]
Unspecified tetracyclines	72	—	—	—	—	—	—	—	—	58,59
Oxytetracycline	10	3	2	5	25–32	30	—	—	—	59,60–64
Demethylchlortetracycline	1	1	—	1	—	24	—	—	—	65
Minocycline	8	1	—	2	16–21	18	—	—	—	66–69
Florocycline	1	1	—	1	—	19	—	—	—	70
Metacycline	1	0	1	1	—	49	—	—	—	71
Methylenecycline	1	0	1	1	—	30	—	—	—	72
Pivmecillinam	32	2	30	32	—	35	—	—	—	73,74
Penicillin	5	—	2	4	18–31	23	—	1	—	35,75–78
Ampicillin	2	1	1	2	20–28	24	—	—	—	79,80
Pivampicillin	2	1	—	1	—	35	—	—	—	80,81
Amoxicillin	3	2	—	2	39–70	51	—	—	—	82–84
Apocillin	2	—	—	—	—	—	—	—	—	62
Cloxacillin	1	—	—	—	—	—	—	—	—	68
Ampicillin/cloxacillin	2	2	0	2	21–24	22	—	—	—	85
Dicloxacillin + danzen	1	—	—	—	—	—	—	—	—	68
Trimethoprim-sulfamethoxazole	2	1	1	2	14–63	38	—	—	—	86,87
Clindamycin	5	4	1	4	22–35	29	—	—	—	8,61,88–90
Lincomycin	1	—	1	1	—	28	—	—	—	91
Spiramycine	1	1	0	1	—	70	—	—	—	92
Erythromycin	1	—	—	—	—	—	—	—	—	35
Rifampicin	2	1	1	2	23–70	46	—	1	—	61,93
Sulfamethoxypyridazine	1	—	—	1	—	24	—	1	—	94
Tinidazole	1	—	—	—	—	—	—	—	—	35
Metronidazole	1	0	1	1	—	25	—	—	—	95
Cephalexin	1	0	1	1	—	15	—	—	—	96
Grouped antibiotics[c]	4	3	1	2	33–77	55	1	—	—	97
Unidentified antibiotic	1	—	—	—	—	—	—	—	—	98
Nelfinavir	1	1	0	1	—	25	—	—	—	99
Zalcitibine	2	2	0	2	20–32	26	—	—	—	100,101
Zidovudine	3	3	0	3	33–38	35	—	—	—	102
Totals	516	92	173	242	10–98	31	7	6	1	

[a]References for doxycycline: 1,4,6,7,28,35,40,58,61,64,67,68,71,75,85,88,89,97,98,103–166.
[b]References for tetracycline: 1,10,36,62,65,67,75,85,105,110,112,118,119,139,167–176.
[c]Erythromycin (two cases), josamycine (one case), and clindamycine (one case).

duce an alkaline burn (36). Other dissolved pills produce neutral solutions, so other mechanisms must be invoked. Postulated mechanisms include induction of GERD by anticholinergics and theophylline, production of local hyperosmolarity by potassium chloride (39), and intracellular poisoning after uptake of doxycycline (40), NSAIDs (41), and alprenolol (42,43) directly from the esophageal lumen into the mucosa.

Several observations suggest that sustained-release medications may be more injurious to the esophagus than standard-release pills of the same medications. First, sustained-release preparations of potassium chloride, quinidine, ferrous sulfate, and alprenolol have caused most of the reported esophageal injuries and most of the reported complicated injuries due to these medications despite the widespread availability and use of standard-release preparations of the latter three medications. Isolated cases of complicated esophageal injury due to other sustained-release pills have also been reported: esophageal hemorrhage and pseudotumor due to slow-release naproxen (25), esophageal perforation due to sustained-release sodium valproate (17), and deep, circumferential esophageal ulceration and hemorrhage due to sustained-release morphine sulfate (44). Finally, two small prospective clinical trials suggest that sustained-release pamidronate may be more injurious to the esophagus than the standard preparation of this drug (45).

TABLE 34.2. ESOPHAGEAL INJURY DUE TO ASPIRIN AND OTHER NONSTEROIDAL ANTIINFLAMMATORY DRUG PILLS

Pill Type	Cases	Gender M	Gender F	Age (Yr) # for whom Reported	Age (Yr) Range	Age (Yr) Mean	Number of Complications Hemorrhage	Number of Complications Stricture	Number of Complications Death	References
Aspirin	19	12	4	10	16–89	40	8	2	—	1,23,34,35, 36,75, 101,177, 178
Aspirin, caffeine	1	1	—	1	—	26	—	—	—	15
Aspirin, phenacetin, caffeine	1	1	—	1	—	54	1	—	—	179
Aspirin, Anacin	1	0	1	1	—	41	1	—	—	180
Aspirin, ibuprofen	1	1	0	1	—	20	1	—	—	180
Doleron[a]	7	—	—	—	—	—	—	1	—	35
Decagesic[b]	1	1	—	1	Adolescent	—	—	—	—	181
Paraflex compound[c]	1	—	—	—	—	—	—	—	—	35
Naproxen										
Literature case reports	3	1	2	3	29–87	62	2	—	—	25,182, 183
FDA reporting program	81	16	65	—	—	36	—	—	—	48
Indomethacin	15	4	1	5	28–82	62	2	—	1	46,106, 170,181,18 4,185
Ibuprofen	6	3	2	5	18–63	33	1	1	—	98,105, 116,180, 186
Piroxicam	5	4	1	5	20–79	33	—	1	—	187,188
Meclofenamate sodium	2	0	2	2	36–47	41	—	—	—	189,190
Mefenamic acid	2	2	0	2	35–63	49	1	1	—	191,192
Tolmetin	2	2	0	2	11–27	19	—	—	—	193,194
Diclofenac	2	0	2	2	20–23	22	—	—	—	195,196
Sulindac	1	1	0	1	—	36	—	—	—	197
Flurbiprofen	1	1	0	1	—	26	—	—	—	198
Phenylbutazone + prednisone	1	0	1	1	—	75	1	—	—	33
Grouped nonsteroidal agents[d]	6	3	3	2	21–75	48	4	—	—	97
Unspecified nonsteroidals	8	—	—	—	—	—	—	—	—	59
Mesalamine	1	0	1	1	—	32	—	—	—	199
Acetaminophen	2	—	1	1	—	55	—	—	—	62,85
Acemetacin[e]	1	0	1	1	—	77	—	—	1	47
Percogesic[f]	1	0	1	1	—	31	—	—	—	200
Totals	172	53	88	50	11–89	43	22	6	2	

[a]Components of Doleron: aspirin, dextropropoxyphene, phenothiazine carboxyl-10-hydrochloride, antipyrene, and vinbarbital.
[b]Components of Decagesic: aspirin, dexamethasone, and aluminum hydroxide gel.
[c]Components of Paraflex compound: aspirin, dextropropoxyphene, and chlorzoxazone.
[d]Oxyphenbutazone (three cases), indomethacin (two cases), and diclofenac (one case).
[e]Patient also took verapamil, ferrous sulfate, and prednisone, but acemetacin was most closely related and likely causative.
[f]Components of Percogesic: acetaminophen, and phenyltoloxamine citrate.

TABLE 34.3. ESOPHAGEAL INJURY DUE TO OTHER PILLS AVAILABLE IN UNITED STATES

Pill Type	Cases	Gender M	Gender F	# for whom Reported	Age (Yr) Range	Age (Yr) Mean	Hemorrhage	Stricture	Death	References
Potassium chloride (KCl)	33	9	16	23	14–77	55	4	17	6	a
Alendronate	127	7	117	112	23–90	68	3	26	1	b
Pamidronate	5	0	5	5	64–74	69	—	—	—	45
Etidronate	3	1	1	3	66–81	72	—	1	—	54–56
Ferrous sulfate or succinate	24	4	10	14	62–89	79	4	6	1	16,18,35, 142
Quinidine	13	6	5	11	12–76	60	—	7	—	1,19,26,27, 36,118, 201–203
Quinidine + KCl	2	—	2	2	49–73	61	—	2	—	204,205
Quinidine + other pills	3	—	3	3	69–77	73	—	2	—	24,170
Mexiletine	4	1	2	3	72–77	74	—	—	—	97,206–208
Captopril	1	0	1	1	—	84	1	—	—	209
Nifedipine	2	1	—	1	—	69	—	1	—	97,210
Verapamil (+ zolpidem)	1	0	1	1	—	50	—	—	—	211
Bepridil	1	—	—	—	—	—	—	—	—	97
Unidentified antihypertensive	1	—	—	—	—	—	—	—	—	98
Theophylline/ aminophylline	7	2	1	3	28–31	30	—	—	—	5,59,212, 213
Corticosteroids	6	4	2	3	42–81	66	—	—	—	97,214
Multivitamin + iron or minerals	3	2	—	3	3–62	29	—	—	—	75,215, 216
Ascorbic acid	3	0	3	3	24–61	47	—	2	—	36,217,218
13-cis-Retinoate	3	3	0	3	17–74	46	—	1	—	219,220
Tryptophan	1	0	1	1	—	81	1	—	—	221
Valproic acid	1	1	0	1	—	49	—	—	—	17
Phenytoin sodium	1	1	0	1	—	36	—	1	—	36
Phenytoin + phenobarbital	1	0	1	1	—	41	1	—	—	222
Warfarin	1	1	0	1	—	58	1	—	—	223
Lansoprazole	1	0	1	1	—	21	—	—	—	224
Thioridazine, slow release	1	1	0	1	—	22	—	—	—	80
Clorazepate	1	0	1	1	—	25	—	—	—	225
Diazepam	1	0	1	1	—	45	—	—	—	226
Morphine sulfate, slow release	1	—	—	—	—	—	1	—	—	44
Glyburide (glibenclamide)	2	—	1	1	—	82	—	—	—	80,81
Estramustine phosphate	2	—	—	—	—	—	—	—	—	35
Eucalyptus-menthol	2	1	1	2	9–33	21	—	—	—	227,228
Oral contraceptives	4	—	3	3	19–24	21	—	—	—	82,229,230
Sildenafil	1	1	0	1	—	61	—	—	—	231
"Fat burner"	1	0	1	1	—	34	—	—	—	85
Totals	264	46	180	211	3–90	63	16	66	8	

[a]References for potassium chloride: 11–13,20,22,30,31,35,36,57,59,97,98,162,201,232–238.
[b]References for alendronate: 2,3,14,29,49–52,54,139,239–254.

TABLE 34.4. ESOPHAGEAL INJURY DUE TO PILLS NOT AVAILABLE IN UNITED STATES

| Pill Type | Cases | Gender | | Age (Yr) | | | Number of Complications | | | References |
		M	F	# for whom Reported	Range	Mean	Hemorrhage	Stricture	Death	
Emepronium bromide	90	11	52	67	5–89	34	2	2	—	[a]
Alprenolol	12	—	3	3	32–73	59	—	7	—	35,59,255
Pinaverium bromide	14	4	7	11	17–48	33	—	—	—	97,163, 256–259
Thiazinium	5	1	3	4	21–53	30	—	—	—	97,260
Naftidrofuryl	3	1	2	2	17–21	19	—	—	—	9,28,261
Pantogan[b]	1	0	1	1	—	21	—	—	—	141
Rhinasal[c]	3	2	—	1	—	27	—	—	—	262–264
Clomethiazol	1	1	0	1	—	55	—	—	—	80
Diltenate-tetra[d]	1	—	—	1	—	75	—	—	—	265
Traumanase-cyklin[e]	1	—	—	1	—	45	—	—	—	265
Acenocoumarol	1	—	—	—	—	—	—	—	—	97
Calcium dobesilate	1	—	—	1	—	45	—	—	—	266
Pantozyme	1	—	—	—	—	—	—	—	—	68
Minidril	1	—	—	—	—	—	—	—	—	82
Chlormadinone	1	0	1	1	—	50	—	—	—	267
Totals	136	20	69	94	5–89	35	2	9	—	

[a]References for emepronium bromide: 35,64,67,71,80,81,137,141,268–293.
[b]Components of Pantogar: thiamine HCl, calcium pantothenate, paraaminobenzoic acid, cystin, faex, and keratin.
[c]Components of Rhinasal: thiazinium methylsulfate, acetaminophen, and norephedrine chlorhydrate.
[d]Components of Diltenate-tetra: tetracycline, theophylline, etafedrine, doxylamine succinate, phenylephrine, and guaifenesin.
[e]Components of Traumanase-cyklin: tetracycline and bromelaine.

Taken together, these observations demonstrate enhanced causticity for some sustained-release preparations.

INJURIES DUE TO SPECIFIC PILLS

Antibiotics and Antiviral Pills

Antibiotics and antivirals have caused 516 of the 1,088 reported cases of pill-induced esophageal injury (Table 34.1), nearly 50% of the esophageal injuries due to all medicinal pills combined. Doxycycline (most frequently the large-capsule form of this drug) and other tetracyclines have caused over 400 of these cases, but 20 nontetracycline antibiotics and antivirals have also been implicated. Injured patients tend to be younger (mean age 31 years) than those injured by other pills. Predisposing factors other than improper pill-taking behavior have been rare. Almost all injured patients have presented with acute, severe retrosternal pain and/or odynophagia. Mucosal injury is usually superficial, and symptoms almost always resolve in a few days to a few weeks. Only 2.5% of reported cases have been complicated, seven by hemorrhage and six by stricture.

Aspirin and Other Nonsteroidal Antiinflammatory Drugs

Table 34.2 documents 91 literature case reports of NSAID pill-induced esophageal injury and 81 cases compiled by the U.S. Food and Drug Administration. Considering only the case reports, aspirin and other NSAIDs have caused less than 10% of the literature reports of pill-induced esophageal injury, but 22 of these NSAID-induced injuries have been complicated by hemorrhage. In contrast, only 25 esophageal injuries due to all other medications combined have been complicated by hemorrhage. NSAIDs are thus strikingly more likely than other pill classes to cause hemorrhage when they injure the esophagus.

Several of the NSAID-induced injuries have been devastating. A patient taking indomethacin suffered a fatal esophageal hemorrhage (46), and a patient whose injury was most likely due to acemetacin, a derivative of indomethacin, died of recurrent pulmonary infections due to a pill-induced bronchoesophageal fistula (47). A patient taking aspirin required surgery for a bleeding pill-induced esophageal ulcer (23), and a patient taking pills containing aspirin and caffeine suffered an esophageal perforation (15). Six other patients injured by NSAIDs developed esophageal strictures.

Nearly half of the cases of NSAID-related esophageal injury documented in Table 34.2 are due to over-the-counter naproxen sodium. These were not reported as literature case reports but were detected by the U.S. Food and Drug Administration's Spontaneous Reporting System (48). This system is a more sensitive surveillance system than review of literature case reports, especially for less serious injuries. Consequently, these 81 cases do not necessarily imply that naproxen is more likely than other NSAIDs to injure the esophagus. None of these 81 patients is known to have suffered a hemorrhage or stricture.

Bisphosphonates

Alendronate, pamidronate, etidronate, and risedronate are bisphosphonate inhibitors of bone resorption, and all but risedronate have been reported to cause pill-induced esophageal injury (Table 34.3). Since the initial marketing of alendronate in late 1995, 76 esophageal injuries due to this medication have been reported as case reports or case series in the medical literature, making alendronate the most commonly reported cause of pill-induced esophageal injury in the past decade. Twenty-four of the injured patients developed esophageal strictures. In one patient, an extensive stricture failed to respond to repetitive attempts at dilatation (49). Another patient taking alendronate suffered fatal esophageal perforation (14). Postmarketing surveillance reports compiled by the manufacturer of alendronate document 51 additional patients with "serious" or "severe" adverse esophageal effects (50). Two of these patients developed strictures, and two suffered hemorrhage. Most patients injured by alendronate appear to have taken their pills improperly, either failing to remain upright after swallowing the pills or taking the pills with less than the 6 ounces of water recommended by the manufacturer. Nonetheless, some patients appear to have been injured despite taking their pills entirely appropriately (3,14,49–52).

Even though alendronate is a frequent offender compared to other medications, an individual patient taking alendronate properly is at only remote risk for serious esophageal injury. In 1998, only 65 patients were known to have been injured out of more than 500,000 patients for whom prescriptions had been written (53).

Two controlled clinical trials provide the only documentation of esophageal injury due to oral pamidronate (45). In these trials, 4 of 33 subjects taking timed-release pamidronate and 1 of 33 subjects taking standard pamidronate developed severe chest pain, dysphagia, and vomiting. Endoscopy revealed erosive and exudative distal esophagitis in each. No complications occurred.

Etidronate has been reported as causative in three cases of pill-induced esophageal injury (54–56), including one complicated by an esophageal stricture.

Potassium Chloride, Quinidine, Ferrous Sulfate or Succinate, and Alprenolol

Many of the 87 patients injured by potassium chloride, quinidine, ferrous sulfate or succinate, and alprenolol (a beta blocker) (Tables 34.3 and 34.4) have presented with progressive dysphagia, often with little or no pain. Esophageal strictures have occurred in 41 (47%) of the patients injured by

these four medications. This is nearly equal to the 46 strictures caused by all other medications combined.

At least 26 of the 33 patients injured by potassium chloride tablets (Table 34.3) have been predisposed to esophageal retention of pills by virtue of extrinsic esophageal compression or esophageal motor dysfunction. At least 21 had previously undergone cardiac surgery, which can result in entrapment of the esophagus between the aorta and vertebral column (31). When the esophagus is fixed in position by adhesions and neighboring structures, it is especially susceptible to compression by an enlarged left atrium, predisposing these patients to pill retention and injury (31).

Potassium chloride–induced esophageal injuries have often been devastating. Seventeen patients have developed esophageal strictures, four have presented with hemorrhage, and six have died as a result of their injuries. Four patients suffered fatal esophageal hemorrhage, including one patient each with penetration of the aorta (12), the left atrium (13), and a bronchial collateral artery (11). Another death was due to penetration of the mediastinum (57), and a patient with a potassium chloride–induced esophageal stricture died 1 week after surgical placement of a feeding jejunostomy (31). All six deaths occurred in patients with cardiomegaly, and four of the six patients had previously undergone cardiac surgery.

Thirteen cases of pill-induced esophageal injury in patients taking no caustic pill other than quinidine have been reported, and 7 of the 13 injured patients developed esophageal strictures. In contrast to the injuries due to potassium chloride, predisposing factors were identified in only two of these subjects.

An unusual feature of quinidine-induced esophageal injury is the occasional presentation with flamboyant exudate that is so thick and tenacious as to suggest neoplasia on barium swallow (1,24,26,27). This exudate may break up at endoscopy and reveal edematous, ulcerated underlying mucosa. Similar presentations have been documented in injuries due to sustained-release ferrous sulfate (16) and sustained-release naproxen (25). Although these patients sometimes present with painless dysphagia suggesting a stricture or carcinoma, the lesions and symptoms may resolve without dilatation.

PREVENTION OF PILL-INDUCED ESOPHAGEAL INJURY

Pills will not injure the esophagus directly unless they dissolve in the esophagus, so physicians, nurses, and pharmacists should instruct patients in a few simple and prudent steps to enhance esophageal transit of prescribed pills:

1. Patients should drink at least 4 ounces of fluid with any pill, and twice this amount with pills that are especially likely to cause injury.

2. Patients should remain upright for at least 10 minutes after taking most pills and for 30 minutes after taking pills likely to cause injury.
3. Pills implicated as causing frequent or severe esophageal injury should be avoided in bedridden patients or patients with esophageal compression, stricture, or dysmotility.

These steps will greatly reduce the frequency of pill-induced esophageal injury but will not completely eliminate injury. A high index of suspicion is required to recognize pill-induced esophageal injury when it occurs, so that repetitive injury may be avoided by prompt withdrawal of the offending pill.

Disclaimer: The opinions and assertions contained herein are the personal views of the author and are not to be construed as reflecting the views of the U.S. Department of the Army or Department of Defense. This work was written by a government employee using government resources and is therefore not subject to copyright restrictions. All previous writings by this author on this subject have similarly been written by a government employee using government resources.

REFERENCES

1. Kikendall JW, Friedman AC, Oyewole MA, et al. Pill-induced esophageal injury: case reports and review of the medical literature. *Dig Dis Sci* 1983;28:174–182.
2. Yue Q-Y, Mortimer O. Alendronate—risk for esophageal stricture. *J Am Geriatr Soc* 1998;46:1581–1582.
3. Abdelmalek MF, Douglas DD. Alendronate-induced ulcerative esophagitis. *Am J Gastroenterol* 1996;91:1282–1283.
4. Jost PM. Drug-induced esophagitis. *JAMA* 1985;254:508.
5. Stoller JL. Oesophageal ulceration and theophylline. *Lancet* 1985;2:328–329.
6. Tankurt IE, Akbaylar H, Yenicerioglu Y, et al. Severe, long-lasting symptoms from doxycycline-induced esophageal injury. *Endoscopy* 1995;27:626.
7. Amendola MA, Spera TD. Doxycycline-induced esophagitis. *JAMA* 1985;253:1009–1011.
8. Froese EH. Oesophagitis with clindamycin. *S Afr Med J* 1979;56:826.
9. McLean D. Drug-induced oesophageal ulceration. *BMJ* 1981;282:1975–1976.
10. Cummin ARC, Hangartner JRW. Oesophago-atrial fistula: a side effect of tetracycline? *J R Soc Med* 1990;83:745–746.
11. Henry JG, Shinner JJ, Martino JH, et al. Fatal esophageal and bronchial artery ulceration caused by solid potassium chloride. *Pediatr Cardiol* 1983;4:251–252.
12. McCall AJ. Slow-K ulceration of oesophagus with aneurysmal left atrium. *BMJ* 1975;3:230.
13. Sumithran E, Lim KH, Chiam HL. Atrio-oesophageal fistula complicating mitral valve disease. *BMJ* 1979;2:1552–1553.
14. Famularo G, De Simone C. Fatal esophageal perforation with alendronate. *Am J Gastroenterol* 2001;96:3212–3213.
15. Corsi PR, de Aguiar JR, de S Kronfly F, et al. Lesao esofagica provocada por ingestao de pilula. *Rev Assoc Med Bras* 1995;41:360–364.
16. Serck-Hanssen A, Stray N. Jerntablettinduserte oesophaguslesjoner. *Tidsskr Nor Laegeforen* 1994;114:2129–2131.
17. Yamaoka K, Takenawa H, Tajiri K, et al. A case of esophageal perforation due to a pill-induced ulcer successfully treated with conservative measures. *Am J Gastroenterol* 1996;91:1044–1045.
18. Abbarah TR, Fredell JE, Ellenz GB. Ulceration by oral ferrous sulfate. *JAMA* 1976;236:2320.
19. Bohane TD, Perrault J, Fowler RS. Oesophagitis and oesophageal obstruction from quinidine tablets in association with left atrial enlargement. *Aust Paediatr J* 1978;14:191–192.
20. Howie AD, Strachan RW. Slow release potassium chloride treatment. *BMJ* 1975;2:176.
21. Lubbe WF, Cadogan ES, Kannemeyer AHR. Oesophageal ulceration due to slow-release potassium in the presence of left atrial enlargement. *N Z Med J* 1979;90:377–379.
22. Pemberton J. Oesophageal obstruction and ulceration caused by oral potassium therapy. *Br Heart J* 1970;32:267–268.
23. Schreiber JB, Covington JA. Aspirin-induced esophageal hemorrhage. *JAMA* 1988;259:1647.
24. Ravich WJ, Kashima H, Donner MW. Drug-induced esophagitis simulating esophageal carcinoma. *Dysphagia* 1986;1:13–18.
25. Sacca N, Rodino S, De Medici A, et al. NSAIDS-induced digestive hemorrhage and esophageal pseudotumor: a case report. *Endoscopy* 1995;27:632.
26. Teplick JG, Teplick SK, Ominsky SH, et al. Esophagitis caused by oral medication. *Radiology* 1980;134:23–25.
27. Wong RKH, Kikendall JW, Dachman AH. Quinaglute-induced esophagitis mimicking an esophageal mass. *Ann Intern Med* 1986;105:62–63.
28. Rodrigo Moreno M, Pleguezuelo Diaz J, et al. Ulceraciones esofagicas de origen medicamentoso. Aportacion de dos casos y descripcion de un nuevo agente etiologico. *Gastroenterol Hepatol* 1985;8:311–315.
29. Ribeiro A, DeVault KR, Wolfe JT III, et al. Alendronate-associated esophagitis: endoscopic and pathologic features. *Gastrointest Endosc* 1998;47:525–528.
30. Chesshyre MH, Braimbridge MV. Dysphagia due to left atrial enlargement after mitral Starr valve replacement. *Br Heart J* 1971;33:799–802.
31. Whitney B, Croxon R. Dysphagia caused by cardiac enlargement. *Clin Radiol* 1972;23:147–152.
32. Channer KS, Bell J, Virjee JP. Effect of left atrial size on the oesophageal transit of capsules. *Br Heart J* 1984;52:223–227.
33. Juncosa L. Ulcus peptico yatrogeno del esofago. *Rev Esp Enferm Apar Dig* 1970;30:457–458.
34. Knauer CM, McLaughlin WT, Mark JBD. Esophago-esophageal fistula in a patient with achalasia. *Gastroenterology* 1970;58:223–228.
35. Carlborg B, Kumlien A, Olsson H. Medikamentella esofagusstrikturer. *Lakartidningen* 1978;75:4609–4611.
36. Bonavina L, DeMeester TR, McChesney L, et al. Drug-induced esophageal strictures. *Ann Surg* 1987;206:173–183.
37. Hey H, Jorgensen F, Sorensen K, et al. Oesophageal transit of six commonly used tablets and capsules. *BMJ* 1982;285:1717–1719.
38. Carlborg B. Biverkningar vid accidentell losning av lakemedel i esofagus och bronker. *Lakartidningen* 1976;73:4201–4204.
39. Boley SJ, Allen AC, Schultz L, et al. Potassium-induced lesions of the small bowel. *JAMA* 1965;193:997–1000.
40. Giger M, Sonnenberg A, Brandli H, et al. Das tetracyclin-ulkus der speiserohre. *Dtsch Med Wochenschr* 1978;103:1038.
41. Semble EL, Wu WC, Castell DO. Nonsteroidal antiinflammatory drugs and esophageal injury. *Semin Arthritis Rheum* 1989;19:99.
42. Olovson SG, Bjorkman JA, Ek L, et al. The ulcerogenic effect on the esophagus of three B-adrenoceptor antagonists, investigated in a new porcine oesophagus test model. *Acta Pharmacol Toxicol (Copenh)* 1983;53:385–391.

43. Olovson SG, Havu N, Regardh CG, et al. Oesophageal ulcerations and plasma levels of different alprenolol salts: potential implications for the clinic. *Acta Pharmacol Toxicol (Copenh)* 1986;58:55–60.

44. Hiraoka T, Okita M, Koganemaru S, et al. Hemorrhagic esophageal ulceration associated with slow-release morphine sulfate tablets. *Nippon Shokakibyo Gakkai Zasshi* 1991;88:1231.

45. Lufkin EG, et al. Pamidronate: an unrecognized problem in gastrointestinal tolerability. *Osteoporosis Int* 1994;4:320–322.

46. Agdal N. Mediciniducerede esophagusskader. *Ugeskr Laeger* 1979;141:3019–3021.

47. McAndrew NA, Greenway MW. Medication-induced oesophagial injury leading to broncho-oephageal fistula. *Postgrad Med J* 1999;75:379–381.

48. Kahn LH, Chen M, Eaton R. Over-the-counter naproxen sodium and esophageal injury. *Ann Intern Med* 1997;126:1006.

49. Ryan JM, Kelsey P, Ryan BM, et al. Alendronate-induced esophagitis: case report of a recently recognized form of severe esophagitis with esophageal stricture—radiographic features. *Radiology* 1998;206:389–391.

50. de Groen PC, Lubbe DF, Hirsch LJ, et al. Esophagitis associated with the use of alendronate. *N Engl J Med* 1996;335:1016–1021.

51. Colina RA, Smith M, Kikendall JW, et al. A new, probably increasing cause of esophageal ulceration: alendronate. *Am J Gastroenterol* 1997;92:704–706.

52. Levine J, Nelson D. Esophageal stricture associated with alendronate therapy. *Am J Med* 1997;102:489–491.

53. Kikendall JW. Pill-induced esophageal injury. In: Castell DO, Richter JE, eds. *The esophagus.* 3rd ed. Philadelphia: Lippincott Williams & Wilkins, 1999:527–537.

54. Larsen K-O, Stray N, Engh V, et al. Oesophagus lesions associated with bisphosphonates. *Tidsskr Nor Laegeforen* 2000;120:2397–2399.

55. Macedo G, Azevedo F, Ribeiro T. Ulcerative esophagitis caused by etidronate. *Gastrointest Endosc* 2001;53:250–251.

56. Maroy B. Ulcere geant de l'oesophage probablement du a la prise d'etidronate. *Gastroenterol Clin Biol* 2001;25:917–918.

57. Rosenthal T, Adar R, Militianu J, et al. Esophageal ulceration and oral potassium chloride ingestion. *Chest* 1974;65:463–465.

58. Carlborg B, Densert O, Lindqvist C. Tetracycline induced esophageal ulcers. A clinical and experimental study. *Laryngoscope* 1983;93:184–187.

59. Ollyo J-B, Fontolliet C, Monnier P, et al. L'oesophagite medicamenteuse et ses complications. *Schweiz Rundsch Med Prax* 1990;79:394–397.

60. Bretzke G. Tetrazyklin-ulkus der speiserohre. *Z Gesamte Inn Med* 1982;37:574–575.

61. Chen CY, Wang LY, Liu HW, et al. Esophageal ulcers caused by antibiotics. *J Formos Med Assoc* 1982;81:618–625.

62. Djupesland G, Rolstad EA. Etsskader i oesophagus forarsaket av medikamenter. *Tidsskr Nor Laegeforen* 1978;98:696–697.

63. Haefeli W. Der fall aus der praxis. *Praxis* 1982;71:1396–1397.

64. Kato S, Komatsu K, Harada Y. Medication-induced esophagitis in children. *Gastroenterol Jpn* 1990;25:485–488.

65. Berli DE, Salis GB, Chiocca JC. Lesion esofagica por drogas. *Acta Gastroenterol Latinoam* 1986;16:109–114.

66. Algayres JP, Valmary J, Chabierski M, et al. Ulcère oesophagien après prise de minocycline. *Presse Med* 1989;18:541.

67. Jeffery PC, Cullis SNR. Drug-induced oesophagitis. *S Afr Med J* 1983;64:1081.

68. Ovartlarnporn B, Kulwichit W, Hiranniramol S. Medication-induced esophageal injury: report of 17 cases with endoscopic documentation. *Am J Gastroenterol* 1991;86:748–750.

69. Stillman AE, Martin RJ. Tetracycline-induced esophageal ulcerations. *Arch Dermatol* 1979;115:1005.

70. Maroy B. Ulcère oesophagien après prise de florocycline. *Gastroenterol Clin Biol* 1983;7:324.

71. Hugel HE, Schinko H, Bischof HP. Das medikamentos bedingte osophagusulkus. *Z Gastroenterol* 1982;20:599–603.

72. Papazian A, Descombes P, Capron JP. Oesophagite ulcérée et mycotique après prise de Physiomycine[R]. *Gastroenterol Clin Biol* 1984;8:389.

73. Matteo A, Eyssautier B, Rodor F, et al. Oesophagite ulcérée après prise de Selexid[R]. *Gastroenterol Clin Biol* 1988;12:670–671.

74. Mortimer O, Wiholm BE. Oesophageal injury associated with pivmecillinam tablets. *Eur J Clin Pharmacol* 1989;37:605–607.

75. Bova JG, Dutton NE, Goldstein HM, et al. Medication-induced esophagitis: diagnosis by double-contrast esophagography. *Am J Roentgenol* 1987;148:731–732.

76. Brochet E, Croisier G, Grimaldi A, et al. Stenose oesophagienne liée à la prise de phenoxylmethylpenicilline chez une diabetique insulino-dependante. *Presse Med* 1984;13:2392.

77. Gould PC, Bartolomeo RS, Sklarek HM. Esophageal ulceration associated with oral penicillin in Marfan's syndrome. *N Y State J Med* 1985;85:199–200.

78. Suissa A, Parason M, Lachter J, et al. Penicillin VK-induced esophageal ulcerations. *Am J Gastroenterol* 1987;82:482–483.

79. Rambaud S, Elkharrat D, Gajdos P. Ulcération oesophagienne après prise d'ampicilline. *Ann Med Interne (Paris)* 1990;141:275.

80. Rohner HG, Berges W, Wienbeck M. Clomethiazol tablets induce ulcers in the esophagus. *Z Gastroenterol* 1982;20:469–473.

81. Hunert H, Ottenjann R. Drug-induced esophageal ulcers. *Gastrointest Endosc* 1979;25:41.

82. Cocheton J-J, Bigot J-M, Penalba C. Les avatars du transit oesophagien des medicaments solides. *Le Concours Médical* 1984;106:3895–3901.

83. Palop V, Mir IM, Morales-Olivas FJ, et al. Esofagitis relacionada con tabletas de amoxicilina de 750 mg. *Med Clin (Barc)* 1998;110:118–119.

84. Treille C. Ulcéres de l'oesophage secondaires à la prise d'amoxycilline (1 cas) et de mequitazine (1 cas). *Acta Endosc* 1985;15:41–49.

85. Yap I, Guan R, Kang JY, et al. Pill-induced esophageal injury. *Singapore Med J* 1993;34:257–258.

86. Bjarnason I, Bjornsson S. Oesophageal ulcers. *Acta Med Scand* 1981;209:431–432.

87. Seibert D, Al-Kawas F. Trimethoprim-sulfamethoxazole, hiccups, and esophageal ulcers. *Ann Intern Med* 1986;105:976.

88. Kimura K, Sakai H, Ido K, et al. Drug-induced esophageal ulcer. *Nippon Shokakibyo Gakkai Zasshi* 1978;75:64–70.

89. Sakai H, Seki H, Yoshida T, et al. [Radiological study of drug-induced esophageal ulcer. (author's translation)] *Rinsho Hoshasen* 1980;25:27–34.

90. Sutton DR, Gosnold JK. Oesophageal ulceration due to clindamycin. *BMJ* 1977;1:1598.

91. Seaman WB. The case of the antibiotic dysphagia. *Hosp Pract* 1979;14:206, 208.

92. Perreard M, Klotz F. Oesophagite ulcérée après prise de spiramycine. *Ann Gastroenterol Hepatol (Paris)* 1989;25:313–314.

93. Smith SJ, Lee AJ, Maddix DS, et al. Pill-induced esophagitis caused by oral rifampin. *Ann Pharmacother* 1999;33:27–31.

94. Voilque G. Oesophagite stenosante apparue au cours d'accidents digestifs graves par intolerance à la sulfamethoxypyridazine. *J Fr Otorhinolaryngol* 1973;22:923–925.

95. Marin Pineda R, Vila G. Ulcera esofagica inducida por metronidazol. Informe de un caso. *Rev Gastroenterol Mex* 1998;63:106–107.

96. Engmann C, Kadish M, Truding RM. Picture of the month. *Arch Pediatr Adolesc Med* 2001;155:729–730.

97. Netter P, Paille F, Trechot P, et al. Les complications oesophagiennes d'origine medicamenteuse. *Therapie* 1988;43: 475–479.

98. Mohandas KM, Swaroop VS, et al. Medication-induced esophageal injury. *Indian J Gastroenterol* 1991;10:20–22.

99. Hutter D, Akgun S, Ramamoorthy R, et al. Medication bezoar and esophagitis in a patient with HIV infection receiving combination antiretroviral therapy. *Am J Med* 2000;108:684–685.

100. Blanco JR, Ibarra V, Oteo JA. Ulcera esofagica en paciente con SIDA. *Enferm Infec Microbiol Clin* 1997;15:269–270.

101. Indorf A, Pegram PS. Esophageal ulceration related to Zalcitabine (ddC). *Ann Intern Med* 1992;117:133–134.

102. Edwards P, Turner J, Gold J, et al. Esophageal ulceration induced by zidovudine. *Ann Intern Med* 1990;112:65–66.

103. Aarons B, Bruns BJ. Oesophageal ulceration associated with ingestion of doxycycline. *N Z Med J* 1980;91:27.

104. Adverse Drug Reactions Advisory Committee. Doxycycline-induced oesophageal ulceration. *Med J Aust* 1994;161:490.

105. Agha FP, Wilson JAP, Nostrand TT. Medication-induced esophagitis. *Gastrointest Radiol* 1986;11:7–11.

106. Alvares JF, Kulkarni SG, Bhatia SJ, et al. Prospective evaluation of medication-induced esophageal injury and its relation to esophageal function. *Indian J Gastroenterol* 1999;18:115–117.

107. Anonymous. Esophageal injury in treatment with Doryx. *Lakartidningen* 1997;94:2665.

108. Barbier P, Dumont A, Dony A, et al. Ulcérations oesophagiennes induites par la doxycycline. *Acta Gastroenterol Belg* 1981;44: 424–429.

109. Baumer VF, Kellner R, Neumaier U. Doxycyclin-induzierte ulzerose Osophagitis. *Fortschr Med* 1997;115:26–30.

110. Bell RL. Tetracycline induced esophagitis. *Alabama Med* 1986;55:47–50.

111. Bezuidenhout DJJ. Iatrogene esofagitis. *S Afr Med J* 1980;57: 1023.

112. Biller JA, Flores A, Buie T, et al. Tetracycline-induced esophagitis in adolescent patients. *J Pediatr* 1992;120:144–145.

113. Bissonnette B, Biron P. Ulcère oesophagien causé par la doxycycline. *CMAJ* 1984;131:1186–1188.

114. Bokey L, Hugh TB. Oesophageal ulceration associated with doxycycline therapy. *Med J Aust* 1975;1:236–237.

115. Cleau D. Ulcère oesophagien après prise de doxycycline. *Gastroenterol Clin Biol* 1982;6:510–511.

116. Coates AG, Nostrant TT, Wilson JAP, et al. Esophagitis caused by nonsteroidal antiinflammatory medication: case reports and review of the literature on pill-induced esophageal injury. *South Med J* 1986;79:1094–1097.

117. Craig JM, Giaffer MH, Talbot MD. Drug-induced oesophageal ulceration in a patient with acquired immunodeficiency syndrome. *Int J STD AIDS* 1996;7:370–371.

118. Creteur V, Laufer I, Kressel HY, et al. Drug-induced esophagitis detected by double-contrast radiography. *Radiology* 1983;147:365–368.

119. Crowson TD, Head LH, Ferrante WA. Esophageal ulcers associated with tetracycline therapy. *JAMA* 1976;235:2747–2748.

120. Daunt N, Brodribb TR, Dickey JD. Oesophageal ulceration due to doxycycline. *Br J Radiol* 1985;58:1209–1211.

121. de Celis G, Sanchez J, Roig J, et al. Ulceracion esofagica unica por doxiciclina. *Med Clin (Barc)* 1998;110:118.

122. Delpre G. Esophageal ulcers due to tetracycline. *Harefuah* 1981;101:281–282.

123. Delpre G, Kadish U. Esophageal ulceration due to enterocoated doxycycline therapy—further considerations. *Gastrointest Endosc* 1984;30:44.

124. Evenepoel C. Slokdarmzweren door gebruik van doxycycline. *Tijdschr Gastroenterol* 1977;20:293–296.

125. Florent C, Chagnon JP, Vivet P, et al. Accidents oesophagiens

126. Foucaud P, Vincent MH, Scart G, et al. Premier cas chez l'enfant d'ulcère aigu oesophagien après pris de doxycycline. *Med Infantile* 1980;87:233–238.

127. Fraser GM, Odes HS, Krugliak P. Severe localised esophagitis due to doxycycline. *Endoscopy* 1987;19:86.

128. Garcia Molinero MJ, Vidal Ruiz JV, Garcia Cabezudo J. Ulcera esofagica por doxiciclina. *Gastroenterol Hepatol* 1981;4:383.

129. Geschwind A. Oesophagitis and oesophageal ulceration following ingestion of doxycycline tablets. *Med J Aust* 1984;1:223.

130. Golindano C, Villalobos MM. Doxycycline esophageal ulcers: are they due to an irritant effect? *Gastrointest Endosc* 1985;31: 408.

131. Hatheway GJ. Doxycycline-induced esophagitis. *Drug Intell Clin Pharmacy* 1982;16:879–880.

132. Herrerias JM, Bonet M, Jimenez M, et al. Oesophagite ulcérative et doxycycline. *Acta Endosc* 1984;14:141–143.

133. Huizar JF, Podolsky I, Goldberg J. Ulceras esofagicas inducidas por doxiciclina. *Rev Gastroenterol Mex* 1998;63:101–105.

134. Isler M. Doxycycline-induced esophageal ulceration. *Mil Med* 2001;166:203, 222.

135. Kalar JG, Redwine JN, Persaud MV. Iatrogenic esophagitis. *Iowa Med* 1988;78:323–326.

136. Kato S, Kobayashi M, Sato H, et al. Doxycycline-induced hemorrhagic esophagitis: a pediatric case. *J Pediatr Gastroenterol Nutr* 1988;7:762–765.

137. Kavin H. Oesophageal ulceration due to emepronium bromide. *Lancet* 1977;1:424–425.

138. Keegan AD. Drug-induced oesophageal ulceration. *Med J Aust* 1990;152:383.

139. Kikendall JW. Pill esophagitis. In: Brandt LJ, ed. *Clinical practice of gastroenterology*. Philadelphia: Current Medicine, 1999: 91–96.

140. Klegar KL, Young TL. Pill-Induced esophageal injury. *J Tenn Med Assoc* 1992;85:417–418.

141. Kobler E, Buhler H, Nuesch HJ, et al. Medikamentos induzierte osophagusulzera. *Dtsch Med Wochenschr* 1978;103: 1035–1037.

142. Kobler E, Nuesch HJ, Buhler H, et al. Medikamentos bedingte osophagusulzera. *Schweiz Med Wochenschr* 1979;109:1180–1182.

143. Llanos O, Guzman S, Duarte I. Doxycycline esophageal ulcer. *Gastrointest Endosc* 1985;31:407–408.

144. Macdonald L. Bulletin canadien sur les effets indesirables des medicaments. *CMAJ* 1998;158:945–946.

145. Maffioli C, Segal S, Diot J, et al. Oesophagite ulcéreuse a la doxycycline. *Acta Endosc* 1980;10:285–288.

146. Maffioli C, Segal S, Renard A, et al. Ulcères oesophagiens à la doxycycline. *Nouv Presse Med* 1979;8:1264.

147. Markin RS, al-Turk M, Zetterman RK. Esophageal ulceration following doxycycline ingestion. *Postgrad Med* 1992;91:179–180.

148. Merino Angulo J, Perez de Diego I, Varas R, et al. Dolor retrosternal y esofagitis inducida por doxiciclina. A proposito de dos observaciones. *Rev Clin Esp* 1986;179:431.

149. Meyboom RHB. Slokdarmbeschadiging door doxycycline en tetracycline. *Ned Tijdschr Geneeskd* 1977;121:1770.

150. Morris TJ, Davis TP. Doxycycline-induced esophageal ulceration in the U.S. military service. *Mil Med* 2000;165:316–319.

151. Muller KD. Ulzerose osophagitis durch doxycyclin. *Z Arztl Fortbild Qualitatssich* 1990;84:659–660.

152. Mur Villacampa M, Guerrero Navarro L, Cabeza Lamban F. Ulcera esofagica por doxiciclina. *Rev Esp Enferm Apar Dig* 1989;76:67–69.

153. O'Meara TF. A new endoscopic finding of tetracycline-induced esophageal ulcers. *Gastrointest Endosc* 1980;26:106–107.

154. Palmer KM, Selbst SM, Shaffer S, et al. Pediatric chest pain

induced by tetracycline ingestion. *Pediatr Emerg Care* 1999;15: 200–201.

155. Papazian A, Capron JP, Dupas JL. Doxycycline-induced esophageal ulcer. *Gastrointest Endosc* 1981;27:201.

156. Petigny A, Moulinier B. Ulcères oesophagiens après prise de doxycycline. *Nouv Presse Med* 1979;8:439.

157. Pinos T, Figueras C, Mas R. Doxycycline-induced esophagitis: treatment with liquid sucralphate. *Am J Gastroenterol* 1990;85: 902.

158. Schneider R. Doxycycline esophageal ulcers. *Am J Dig Dis* 1977;22:805–807.

159. Shiff AD. Doxycycline-induced esophageal ulcers in physicians. *JAMA* 1986;256:1893.

160. Stricker BHC, van Overmeeren AB, Vegter AW. Doxycycline, tabletten of capsules? *Ned Tidschr Geneeskd* 1982;126:2200–2201.

161. Tan HJ. Drug-induced oesophageal injury. *Hosp Med* 1998;59:938–939.

162. Tanaka S, Yamada A, Yoshida M, et al. Drug-induced esophageal ulcer—clinical report of 3 cases. *I To Cho* 1980;15:255–260.

163. Tournier C, Lapuelle J, Gerardin A, et al. Ulcères oesophagiens medicamenteux. *Rev Med Limoges* 1981;12:160.

164. Tzianetas I, Habal F, Keystone JS. Short report: severe hiccups secondary to doxycycline-induced esophagitis during treatment of malaria. *Am J Trop Med Hyg* 1996;54:203–204.

165. Ullah R, Golchin K, Hampton S, et al. Oesophageal ulceration caused by doxycycline: an unusual complication. *J Laryngol Otol* 2000;114:467–468.

166. Viver JM, Bory F, Forne M, et al. Ulceraciones esofagicas medicamentosas a proposito de tres casos secundarios a ingestion de doxiciclina. *An Med Intern (Madrid)* 1986;3:600–602.

167. Bliss MR. Tablets and capsules that stick in the oesophagus. *J R Coll Gen Pract* 1984;34:301.

168. Burke EL. Acute oesophageal damage from one brand of tetracycline tablets. *Gastroenterology* 1975;68:1022.

169. Channer KS, Hollanders D. Tetracycline-induced oesophageal ulceration. *BMJ* 1981;282:1359–1360.

170. Doman DB, Ginsberg AL. The hazard of drug-induced esophagitis. *Hosp Pract* 1981;16:17–25.

171. Ginaldi S. Drug-induced esophagitis. *Am Fam Physician* 1984; 30:169–170.

172. Khan SA. Esophageal ulceration related to oral ingestion of tetracycline capsules. *Gastrointest Endosc* 1983;29:163.

173. Khera DC, Herschman BR, Sosa F. Tetracycline-induced esophageal ulcers. *Postgrad Med* 1980;68:113, 115.

174. Lee MG, Hanchard B. Tetracycline-induced proximal oesophagitis. *West Indian Med J* 1990;39:124–127.

175. Scapa E, Shemesh E, Batt L. Fsophageal ulceration caused by tetracycline. *Harefuah* 1980;99:373–374.

176. Schmidt-Wilcke HA. Tetracyclin-ulkus der speiserohre. *Dtsch Med Wochenschr* 1978;103:2053.

177. Rodino S, Sacca N, De Medici A, et al. Multiple esophageal ulcerations caused by a granular formulation of aspirin. *Endoscopy* 1994;26:509–510.

178. Wilcox CM, Schwartz DA, Clark WS. Esophageal ulceration in human immunodeficiency virus infection. *Ann Intern Med* 1995;122:143–149.

179. Williams JG. Drug-induced oesophageal injury. *BMJ* 1979;2:273.

180. Sugawa C, Takekuma Y, Lucas CE, et al. Bleeding esophageal ulcers caused by NSAIDs. *Surg Endosc* 1997;11:143–146.

181. Division of Drug Experience. *Drug experience report. Spontaneous reporting program (1969–1980)*. Rockville, MD: Division of Drug Experience, Food and Drug Administration.

182. Ecker GA, Karsh J. Naproxen induced ulcerative esophagitis. *J Rheumatol* 1992;19:646–647.

183. Vazquez Valdes E, Baptista MA, Barradas Guevara MC. Ulceras

esofagicas producidas por medicamentos. Informe de un paciente. *Rev Gastroenterol Mex* 1987;52:119–121.

184. Bataille C, Soumagne D, Loly J, et al. Esophageal ulceration due to indomethacin. *Digestion* 1982;24:66–68.

185. Gardies A, Gevaudan J, Le Roux C, et al. Ulcére iatrogene de l'oesophage. *Nouv Presse Med* 1978;7:1032.

186. Levine MS, Borislow SM, Rebesin SE, et al. Esophageal stricture caused by a Motrin tablet (Ibuporfen). *Abdom Imaging* 1994;19:6–7.

187. Dertinger SH, Glossmann H, Reichsollner F, et al. Ulcerative esophagitis and stricture due to long-term piroxicam therapy. *Gastroenterology* 1998;114:A101.

188. Santucci L, Patoia L, Fiorucci S, et al. Oesophageal lesions during treatment with piroxicam. *BMJ* 1990;300:1018.

189. Minocha A, Greenbaum DS. Pill-esophagitis caused by nonsteroidal antiinflammatory drugs. *Am J Gastroenterol* 1991;86: 1086–1089.

190. Santalla Pecina F, Gomez Huelgas R, Sanchez Robles C. Sodium meclofenamate-induced esophageal ulcerations. *Am J Gastroenterol* 1991;86:786.

191. de Caestecker JS, Heading RC. Iatrogenic oesophageal ulceration with massive haemorrhage and stricture formation. *Br J Clin Pract* 1988;42:212–214.

192. Katsinelos P, Dimiropoulos S, Vasiliadis T, et al. *Eur J Gastroenterol Hepatol* 1999;11:1431–1432.

193. Cunningham JT. Induced esophageal ulceration. *Gastrointest Endosc* 1982;28:49–50.

194. Palop V, Juan-Martinez J, Andreu-Alapont E, et al. Tolmetin-induced esophageal ulceration. *Ann Pharmacother* 1997;31:929.

195. Imada T, Aoyama N, Amano T, et al. Esophageal ulceration associated with Voltaren therapy. *I To Cho* 1983;18:227–230.

196. Isler M, Bahceci M. Cataflam-induced esophageal ulceration. *Am J Gastroenterol* 2001;96:1300–1301.

197. Levine MS, Rothstein RD, Laufer I. Giant esophageal ulcer due to Clinoril. *Am J Roentgenol* 1991;156:955–956.

198. Takehana T, Imada T, Kubo A, et al. A case of drug-induced esophageal ulcer developed at the esophageal constriction due to the right aortic arch. *Nippon Kyobu Geka Gakkai Zasshi* 1992;40:1131–1134.

199. Lopez-Cepero Andrada JM, Lopez Silva M, Salado Fuentes M, et al. Ulcera esofagica por mesalazine. *Gastroenterol Hepatol* 2000;23:362.

200. Nwakama PE, Jenkins HJ Jr, Bailey RT Jr, et al. Drug-induced esophageal injury: a case report of Percogesic. *Drug Intell Clin Pharmacy* 1989;23:227–229.

201. Boyce HW Jr. Dysphagia after open heart surgery. *Hosp Pract* 1985;20:40–50.

202. Mason SJ, O'Meara TF. Drug-induced esophagitis. *J Clin Gastroenterol* 1981;3:115.

203. Stanely AJ, Eade OE, Hardwick D. Oesophageal ulceration secondary to potassium tablets. *Scott Med J* 1994;39:118–119.

204. Lambert JR, Newman A. Ulceration and stricture of the esophagus due to oral potassium chloride (slow release tablet) therapy. *Am J Gastroenterol* 1980;73:508–511.

205. Riker J, Swanson M, Schweigert B. Esophageal ulceration caused by wax-matrix potassium chloride. *West J Med* 1978; 128:542–543.

206. Adler JB, Goldberg RI. Mexiletine-induced pill esophagitis. *Am J Gastroenterol* 1990;85:629–630.

207. Penalba C. Ulcérations oesophagiennes induites par le chlorhydrate de mexiletine. *Ann Gastroenterol Hepatol (Paris)* 1986;22: 267–268.

208. Rudolph R, Seggewiss H, Seckfort H. Oesophagus-ulcus durch Mexiletin. *Dtsch Med Wochenschr* 1983;108:1018–1020.

209. Al Mahdy H, Boswell GV. Captopril-induced oesophagitis. *Eur J Clin Pharmacol* 1988;34:95.

210. Simko V, Joseph D, Michael S. Increased risk in esophageal obstruction with slow-release medications. *J Assoc Acad Minority Physicians* 1997;8:38–42.

211. Jacques JP, Llau ME, Mercier JF, et al. Ulcération oesophagienne d'origine medicamenteuse. *Therapie* 1993;48:513.

212. Enzenauer RW, Bass JW, McDonnell JT. Esophageal ulceration associated with oral theophylline. *N Engl J Med* 1984;310:261.

213. Shaikh YM, Khan AH, Rao N, et al. Phyllocontin (theophylline) induced esophagitis. *J Pakistan Med Assoc* 1993;43:183.

214. de Witte C, Dony A, Serste JP. Ulcere oesophagien iatrogene. *J Belge Radiol* 1972;55:655–656.

215. Ewert B, Ewert G, Glas JE, et al. Medikamentell hypofarynxskada. *Lakartidningen* 1979;76:739–740.

216. Perry PA, Dean BS, Krenelok EP. Drug induced esophageal injury. *Clin Toxicol* 1989;27:281–286.

217. Kikendall JW, Schmidt M, Graeber GM, et al. Pill-induced esophageal ulceration and stricture following cardiac surgery. *Mil Med* 1986;151:539–542.

218. Walta DC, Giddens JD, Johnson LF, et al. Localized proximal esophagitis secondary to ascorbic acid ingestion and esophageal motor disorder. *Gastroenterology* 1976;70:766–769.

219. Amichai B, Grunwald MH, Odes SH, et al. Acute esophagitis caused by isotretinoin. *Int J Dermatol* 1996;35,528–529.

220. Fennerty B, Sampliner R, Garewal H. Esophageal ulceration associated with 13-cis-retinoic acid therapy in patients with Barrett's esophagus. *Gastrointest Endosc* 1989;35:442–443.

221. Piccione PR, Winkler WP, Baer J, et al. Pill-induced intramural esophageal hematoma. *JAMA* 1987;257:929.

222. Walsh J, Kneafsey DV. Phenobarbitone induced oesophagitis. *Ir Med J* 1980;73:399.

223. Loft DE, Stubington S, Clark C, et al. Oesophageal ulcer caused by warfarin. *Postgrad Med J* 1989;65:258–259.

224. Maekawa T, Ohji G, Inoue R, et al. Pill-induced esophagitis caused by lansoprazole. *J Gastroenterol* 2001;36:790–791.

225. Maroy B, Moullot P. Esophageal burn due to chlorazepate dipotassium (Tranxene). *Gastrointest Endosc* 1986;32:240.

226. Herrerias JM, Bonet M. Esofagitis por diacepam. *Med Clin (Barc)* 1984;83:690.

227. Fiedorek SC, Casteel HB. Pediatric medication-induced focal esophagitis. *Clin Pediatr* 1988;27:455–456..

228. Sharara AI. Lozenge-induced esophagitis. *Gastrointest Endosc* 2000;51:622–623.

229. Allmendinger G. Esophageal ulcer caused by the "pill." *Z Gastroenterol* 1985;23:531–533.

230. Oren R, Fich A. Oral contraceptive-induced esophageal ulcer. Two cases and literature review. *Dig Dis Sci* 1991;36:1489–1490.

231. Higuchi K, Ando K, Kim SR, et al. Sildenafil-induced esophageal ulcers. *Am J Gastroenterol* 2001;96:2516–2518.

232. Ashour M, Salama FD, Morris A, et al. Acute dysphagia induced by bendrofluazide-K. *Practitioner* 1984;228:524.

233. Barbier P, Pringot J, Heimann R, et al. Ulcérations digestives induites par le chlorure de potassium. *Acta Gastroenterol Belg* 1976;39:261–274.

234. Eng J, Sabanathan S. Drug-induced esophagitis. *Am J Gastroenterol* 1991;86:1127–1133.

235. Learmonth I, Weaver PC. Potassium stricture of the upper alimentary tract. *Lancet* 1976;1:251–252.

236. Lowry N, Delaney P, O'Malley E. Oesophageal ulceration occurring secondary to slow release potassium tablets. *Ir J Med Sci* 1975;144:366.

237. Peters JL. Benign oesophageal stricture following oral potassium chloride therapy. *Br J Surg* 1976;63:698–699.

238. Ryan JR, McMahon FG, Akdamar K, et al. Mucosal irritant potential of a potassium-sparing diuretic and of wax-matrix potassium chloride. *Clin Pharmacol Ther* 1984;35:90–93.

239. Abraham SC, Cruz-Correa M, Lee LA, et al. Alendronate-associated esophageal injury: pathologic and endoscopic features. *Mod Pathol* 1999;12:1152–1157.

240. Cameron RB. Esophagitis dissecans superficialis and alendronate: case report. *Gastrointest Endosc* 1997;46:562–563.

241. Duques P, Araujo RSA, de Amorim WPD. Ulceracao de anastomose esofago-enterica causada por alendronato. *Arq Gastroenterol* 2001;38:129–131.

242. Ferrari Junior AP, Domingues SH. Esophageal ulcer and alendronate. *Rev Paul Med* 1998;116:1882–1884.

243. Girelli C, Reguzzoni G, Rocca F. Esofagite da alendronato. *Recenti Prog Med* 1997;88:223–225.

244. Kessenich CR. Differential diagnosis of chest pain: a case report. *Gastroenterol Nurs* 1999;22:10–12.

245. Larzilliere I, Gargot D, Zleik T, et al. Oesophagite medicamenteuse: responsabilite de l'alendronate. *Gastroenterol Clin Biol* 1999;23:1098–1099.

246. Lilley LL, Guanci R. Avoiding alendronate-related esophageal irritation. *Am J Nurs* 1997;97:12, 14.

247. Luciani J, Pigatto V, Naves A, et al. [Esophagitis associated with use of alendronate in 5 postmenopausic patients.] *Acta Gastroenterol Latinoam* 2001;31:59–63.

248. Maconi G, Bianchi Porro G. Multiple ulcerative esophagitis caused by alendronate. *Am J Gastroenterol* 1995;90:1889–1890.

249. Naylor G, Davies MH. Oesophageal stricture associated with alendronic acid. *Lancet* 1996;348:1030–1031.

250. Pizzani E, Valenzuela G. Esophagitis associated with alendronate sodium. *Va Med Q* 1997;124:181–182.

251. Rimmer DE, Rawls DE. Improper alendronate administration and a case of pill esophagitis. *Am J Gastroenterol* 1996;91:2648–2649.

252. Sorrentino D, Trevisi A, Bernardis V, et al. Esophageal ulceration due to alendronate. *Endoscopy* 1996;28:529.

253. Toth E, Fork F-T, Lindelow K, et al. Alendronate-induced oesophagitis; a rare, serious, but reversible side-effect. *Lakartidningen* 1998;95:3676–3680.

254. Tursi A, Cuoco L, Cammarota G, et al. Ulcerative oesophagitis due to alendronate. *Ital J Gastroenterol Hepatol* 1997;29:477–478.

255. Stiris MG, Oyen D. Oesophagitis caused by oral ingestion of Aptin (alprenolol chloride) Durettes. *Eur J Radiol* 1982;2:38–40.

256. Andre JM, Voiment YM, Marti RG. Ulcéres oesophagiens après prise de bromure de pinaverium. *Acta Endosc* 1980;10:289–291.

257. Lamouliatte H, Plane D, Quinton A. Ulcére oesophagien après pris orale de bromure de pinaverium. *Gastroenterol Clin Biol* 1981;5:812–813.

258. Rodriguez Agullo JL, Vidal Ruiz JV, Benita Leon V. Ulceras esofagicas causadas por una capsula de bromuro de pinaverium. *Gastroenterol Hepatol* 1983;6:362–365.

259. Stricker BHC. Slokdarmbeschadiging door pinaveriumbromide. *Ned Tijdschr Geneeskd* 1983;127:603–604.

260. Pen J, Van Meerbeeck J, Pelckmans P, et al. Thiazinium-induced oesophageal ulcerations. *Acta Clin Belg* 1986;41:278–283.

261. McCloy EC, Kane S. Drug-induced oesophageal ulceration. *BMJ* 1981;282:1703.

262. Allard C. Ulcére iatrogene de l'oesophage. *Gastroenterol Clin Biol* 1982;6:712.

263. Penalba C, Eugene C. Oesophagite medicamenteuse due au Rhinasal. *Presse Med* 1983;12:1725–1726.

264. Rives JJ, Olives JP, Ghisolfi J. Oesophagite aigue medicamenteuse. *Arch Fr Pediatr* 1985;42:33–34.

265. Winckler K. Tetracycline ulcers of the oesophagus. Endoscopy, histology and roentgenology in two cases, and review of the literature. *Endoscopy* 1981;13:225–228.

266. Fernandez Rodriguez C, Moreira V, Boixeda D, et al. Ulcera esofagica por dobexilato calcico. *Gastroenterol Hepatol* 1986;9:102.

267. Daghfous R, Hedi Loueslati M, El Aidli S, et al. Atteinte inflammatoire du tractus digestif superieur probablement due à un progestatif de synthese. *Gastroenterol Clin Biol* 1995;19:853–854.

268. Barrison IG, Trewby PN, Kane SP. Oesophageal ulceration due to emepronium bromide. *Endoscopy* 1980;12:197–199.

269. Bennett JR. Oesophageal ulceration due to emepronium bromide. *Lancet* 1977;1:810.

270. Chapman K. Emepronium bromide and the treatment of urge incontinence. *Med J Aust* 1978;1:103.

271. Collins FJ, Matthews HR, Baker SE, et al. Drug-induced oesophageal injury. *BMJ* 1979;1:1673–1676.

272. Cowan RE, Wright JT, Marsh F. Drug-induced oesophageal injury. *BMJ* 1979;2:132–133.

273. Eichenberger P, Blum AL. Drug-induced esophageal lesions. *Acta Endosc* 1980;10:273–283.

274. Fellows IW, Ogilvie AL, Atkinson M. Oesophageal stricture associated with emepronium bromide therapy. *Postgrad Med J* 1982;58:43–44.

275. Freysteinsson H, Thorsson AV. Oesophageal ulcerations in two children taking emepronium bromide. *Acta Paediatr Scand* 1982;70:513–514.

276. Guignard A, Savary M. L'oesophagite d'origine medicamenteuse. *Acta Endosc* 1980;10:263–272.

277. Habeshaw T, Bennett JR. Ulceration of mouth due to emepronium bromide. *Lancet* 1972;2:1422.

278. Hale JE, Barnardo DE. Ulceration of mouth due to emepronium bromide. *Lancet* 1973;1:493.

279. Halter F, Scheurer U. Veratzung des distalen osophagus durch ein anticholinergikum. *Z Gastroenterol* 1978;16:699.

280. Higson RH. Oesophagitis as a side effect of emepronium. *BMJ* 1978;2:201.

281. Hillman LC, Scobie BA, Pomare EW, et al. Acute oesophagitis due to emepronium bromide. *N Z Med J* 1981;94:4–6.

282. Hughes R. Drug-induced oesophageal injury. *BMJ* 1979;2:132.

283. Johnsen S, Koefoed-Nielsen B, Tos M. Emepron (Cetiprin) og aetsskader i mund og spiseror. *Ugeskr Laeger* 1982;144:1477–1479.

284. Kenwright S, Norris ADC. Oesophageal ulceration due to emepronium bromide. *Lancet* 1977;1:548.

285. Kunert H. Medikamentos induzierte osophagusulzera. *Dtsch Med Wochenschr* 1978;103:1278.

286. Leonard RCF, Adams PC, Parker S, et al. Oesophageal injury associated with emepronium bromide (Ceteprin). *Br J Clin Pract* 1984;38:429–430.

287. Lind O. Medikamentindusert osofagitt. *Tidsskr Nor Laegeforen* 1978;98:742.

288. Morck HI, Nielsen VM, Kirkegaard P. Ulcus esophagei forarsaget af emeproniumbromid (Cetiprin). *Ugeskr Laeger* 1981;143:623.

289. Murray K. Severe dysphagia from emepronium bromide associated with oesophageal diverticulum. *Br J Surg* 1982;69:439.

290. Puhakka HJ. Drug-induced corrosive injury of the oesophagus. *J Laryngol Otol* 1978;92:927–931.

291. Rose JDR, Tobin GB. Drug-induced oesophageal injury. *BMJ* 1980;1:110.

292. Shepperd HWH. Iatrogenic reflux oesophagitis. *J Laryngol Otol* 1977;91:171–172.

293. Tobias R, Cullis S, Kottler RE, et al. Emepronium bromide-induced oesophagitis. *S Afr Med J* 1982;61:368–370.

35

ESOPHAGITIS IN THE IMMUNOCOMPROMISED HOST

C. MEL WILCOX

Despite the great strides in immunosuppressive therapy that now can more selectively target selective components of the immune system, use of antimicrobial prophylaxis for high-risk transplant patients, and the development of highly active antiretroviral therapy (HAART) for human immunodeficiency virus (HIV)–infected patients, esophageal infections remain important for the clinician. Infections of the esophagus are a relatively new problem. Before the 1960s, esophageal infections were uncommon and most often identified at autopsy (1). The prevalence of these infections increased markedly from the 1970s through 1990s as organ transplantation grew and acquired immunodeficiency syndrome (AIDS) exploded. Fortunately, the concurrent development and widespread adoption of endoscopy with biopsy defined the spectrum of causes, helped characterize these infections endoscopically and histologically, and became the gold standard for diagnosis.

More recently, there has been a reversal in the prevalence of esophageal infections. The incidence of esophagitis has been evolving in patients undergoing transplantation due to the widespread administration of antimicrobial prophylaxis, particularly the use of strategies to prevent cytomegalovirus (CMV) disease (2,3). In the first 2 decades of the AIDS epidemic in the United States, esophageal infections were one of the primary manifestations of the disease. However, since the availability of protease inhibitors in 1996, there has been a striking reduction overall in the incidence of opportunistic infections including those involving the esophagus (4,5).

Given the efficacy of therapies for virtually all esophageal infections, timely and accurate diagnosis is essential. This chapter focuses on esophagitis in the immunocompromised host, and reviews epidemiology, pathology, presentation, diagnosis, and therapy for specific infections. Esophageal infections occurring in the normal host are briefly discussed. Selected esophageal disorders associated with HIV and AIDS are also reviewed.

EPIDEMIOLOGY

The epidemiology of esophageal infections is rapidly changing. Much of the early data on the etiology and prevalence of esophageal infections were acquired from retrospective autopsy and radiographic series. Studies performed in the 1970s and 1980s that documented the incidence of esophageal infections following transplantation are now largely outdated because of refinements in immunosuppressive therapy and overall management of the transplant patient. Similarly, the high incidence of esophageal infections, especially *Candida*, previously documented in patients with AIDS, is not accurate today since the era of HAART (5).

Esophageal infection is rare in an otherwise healthy person in whom no permissive factor is present. In this setting, the most common pathogen is herpes simplex virus (HSV) (6). Although candidiasis may be observed in elderly patients without any predisposing factors, almost uniformly, immunocompetent patients who develop esophageal infection have conditions that either weaken esophageal defense mechanisms and/or alter esophageal flora such as disorders of esophageal emptying (achalasia, diverticula) or treatment with broad-spectrum antimicrobial agents.

Esophageal infection following solid organ transplantation is usually due to *Candida* or herpes viruses (CMV, HSV) (7,8); coinfections have been described. The causes of esophageal infection following bone marrow transplantation are generally similar to other transplant patients (9). As immunosuppressive therapy becomes even more targeted, it is likely that the prevalence of esophageal infection in all transplant patients will continue to decline (10).

Candida is the most common cause of esophageal infection associated with malnutrition, broad-spectrum antibiotics, and corticosteroids, both inhaled and ingested. Patients with cancer as well as lymphoproliferative diseases are well recognized to develop esophageal infections following chemotherapy, but *Candida* and viral esophagitis may also occur prior to such treatment.

C. M. Wilcox: Department of Medicine, University of Alabama at Birmingham; and Division of Gastroenterology, University Hospital, Birmingham, Alabama.

Esophageal infections were common gastrointestinal complications of HIV infection, but as mentioned above, the efficacy of HAART has resulted in a striking reduction in the incidence of all opportunistic infections (4). Before the development of these antiretroviral regimens and the widespread use of antifungal agents, prospective series of symptomatic patients found that *Candida* esophagitis was the most frequent cause of disease, seen in approximately 50% of patients (11–13). Coinfections of *Candida* and viruses are common (14). In contrast to other immunocompromised hosts, HSV esophagitis is less common than CMV esophagitis (15). Patients with AIDS are also susceptible to a number of other unusual pathogens that cause esophagitis, and these patients are commonly affected by idiopathic esophageal ulcer (see below).

PREDISPOSING FACTORS

Esophageal infections are generally the result of humoral or cellular immune dysfunction, or less commonly, arise from alterations in the normal esophageal flora. Numerous conditions are associated with immune dysfunction predisposing to infections, including diabetes mellitus, alcoholism, malnutrition, malignancies, and advanced age. In diabetes mellitus, hyperglycemia and ketoacidosis impair granulocyte function. Corticosteroids have many deleterious effects on the immune system that result in both lymphocyte and granulocyte dysfunction. Mucosal disruption of the oropharynx and esophagus commonly follows chemotherapy or radiation therapy, providing a portal of entry for pathogens. Depending on the specific type, transplantation predisposes to infection through both qualitative and quantitative effects on B and T cells due to immunosuppressive agents, chemotherapy, and neutropenia. Major risk factors for infection are episodes of rejection in recipients of solid organ transplant and graft versus host disease following allogeneic bone marrow transplantation, because these patients require additional potent immune suppression. Broad-spectrum antibiotics and antiacid therapy, as well as surgical trauma, further predispose to esophageal infections in the immunocompromised host.

Infection following solid organ transplantation has a relatively predictable time course (16). Bacterial and fungal infections are most common during the initial months after transplantation, because it is during this period that granulocyte numbers and/or function are most compromised. HSV infection also tends to occur early after transplantation due to reactivation of disease, whereas CMV typically presents 2 to 6 months following transplantation at a time when neutropenia is common and T-cell function is most impaired. For HIV-infected patients, opportunistic infections reflect severe immunodeficiency (i.e., AIDS); esophageal infections typically become clinically manifest when the CD4 lymphocyte count falls below 200/mm³, with most occurring below 100/mm³ (15,17,18).

GENERAL CONSIDERATIONS

A number of factors guide the approach to the immunosuppressed patient with suspected esophageal infection. Given the breadth of potential causes of infection (Table 35.1), the differential diagnosis should be based on the cause, severity, and timing of immunodeficiency, character of esophageal complaints, and findings on physical examination, particularly of the oropharynx. For HIV-infected patients, the absolute value of the CD4 lymphocyte count stratifies the risk for esophageal infection or other HIV-related process. Odynophagia is the most common presenting symptom of esophageal infection, and disorders resulting in esophageal ulceration almost uniformly cause odynophagia. Dysphagia may be observed with esophageal infections, especially *Candida* esophagitis, or may represent esophageal obstruction or dysmotility from some other cause. Bleeding may be the initial manifestation of esophageal ulceration especially when there is an associated coagulopathy. Inspection of the oropharynx is essential when esophageal infection is suspected. Oropharyngeal candidiasis is commonly associated with esophageal candidiasis (19,20). However, the presence of oropharyngeal candidiasis does not prove that *Candida* is the only cause of symptoms, nor does the absence of oropharyngeal candidiasis exclude *Candida* esophagitis. Coexistent oropharyngeal ulceration is common in patients with HSV esophagitis but is rarely observed in patients with CMV esophagitis (20,21). Patients with AIDS often have multiple coexisting

TABLE 35.1. REPORTED ETIOLOGIES OF ESOPHAGEAL INFECTIONS

Fungal	Viral	Bacterial	Mycobacterial	Parasitic
Candida sp.	CMV	Oral flora	TB	*Cryptosporidia*
Histoplasma	HSV	*Nocardia*	MAC	*Pneumocystis*
Blastomycosis	EBV	*Actinomyces*		*Leishmania*
Mucormycosis	HPV	*Bartonella*		*Trympanosoma*
Aspergillus	Varicella			

CMV, cytomegalovirus; HSV, herpes simplex virus; EBV, Epstein-Barr virus; HPV, human papilloma virus; TB, tuberculosis; MAC, *Mycobacterium avium* complex.

esophageal disorders, which further complicates management (11,14).

Documentation of an infectious agent in tissue biopsies is the most specific means of diagnosis. Although barium radiography may suggest infectious esophagitis, rarely will these studies be definitive. Likewise, the clinical presentation may favor an infectious esophagitis, but the specific etiology can rarely be determined by history and physical examination alone.

At the time of endoscopy, the characteristics of the esophageal lesion(s) will provide diagnostic clues. The location, size, and appearance of all endoscopic abnormalities should be documented, because these features form the basis of the differential diagnosis and are useful for comparison on follow-up endoscopic examinations. The differential diagnosis of the lesion will dictate how the lesion(s) is sampled and what recommendations for diagnostic testing on the biopsy and/or cytologic specimens should be made. Based on the suspected cause clinically, endoscopically, and pathologically, additional stains for pathogens may be required, thereby necessitating close collaboration with the pathologist to accurately diagnose these infections (22). Since most esophageal infections can be diagnosed on tissue biopsy alone, multiple biopsies should be performed of endoscopic abnormalities to increase diagnostic yield. Esophageal brushings with cytologic evaluation may be diagnostically helpful in certain diseases such as those due to *Candida* and HSV. Viral culture of biopsy specimens may increase the diagnostic yield, although both false positives and false negatives occur. Serologic testing plays no significant role in the diagnosis of acute infectious esophagitis.

FUNGAL INFECTIONS

Candida Species

Epidemiology

Candida species are the most frequent esophageal pathogens. While *C. albicans* is most common, other reported species include *C. dublenis, C. tropicalis, C. parapsilosis,* and *C. glabrata.* Conditions predisposing to *Candida* esophagitis in

the normal host include antibiotics; inhaled or ingested corticosteroids; antiacid therapy or hypochlorhydric states; diabetes mellitus; alcoholism; malnutrition; old age; radiation therapy to the head, neck, and chest; and esophageal motility disturbances. Alterations in cellular immunity lead to candidal colonization and superficial infection, whereas humoral immunity (granulocytes) prevents invasive disease and dissemination. Chronic mucocutaneous candidiasis, a congenital immunodeficiency, is typically complicated by *Candida* esophagitis. As stated above, the use of immunosuppressive regimens (i.e., cyclosporine), which better target the immune system, combined with prophylactic antifungal therapy have reduced the incidence of candidal infections following solid organ and bone marrow transplantation (3,23). The incidence of *Candida* esophagitis in transplant patients administered prophylactic oral nystatin or azole therapy is <5% (24). For HIV-infected patients, the primary risk factor for esophageal candidiasis is the level of immunodeficiency (25).

Pathology

The gross pathologic appearance of esophageal candidiasis ranges from a few white or yellow plaques on the mucosal surface to a dense, thick plaque coating the mucosa and encroaching on the esophageal lumen. Although occasionally misinterpreted as "ulcer," this plaque material is composed of desquamated squamous epithelial cells, admixed with fungal organisms, inflammatory cells, and bacteria (26). True ulceration (granulation tissue) is rarely caused by *Candida* alone, and has been documented most commonly in immunosuppressed patients with profound granulocytopenia or when *Candida* is a coinfection with another cause of ulceration (27).

Clinical Manifestations

Although esophageal candidiasis may be an incidental finding in an asymptomatic patient, the usual clinical presentation is odynophagia with dysphagia (13,19,21) (Table 35.2). Symptoms vary in severity, ranging from mild difficulty with swallowing to severe pain resulting in an inability to eat and secondary dehydration. When odynophagia is very severe,

TABLE 35.2. PRESENTATIONS AND COMPLICATIONS OF ESOPHAGEAL INFECTIONS

	Common	Uncommon
Candida sp.	Dysphagia, odynophagia	Bleeding, chest pain
Other fungi	Dysphagia, odynophagia	Fistula
Viral	Odynophagia, chest pain	Fever, bleeding
Mycobacterial	Odynophagia, dysphagia, fever	Fistula
Bacterial	Odynophagia, fever	Dissemination
Parasitic	Odynophagia	—

however, one must always consider causes other than *Candida* or coinfections, particularly in patients with AIDS.

Physical examination may be helpful in suggesting the diagnosis. Approximately two-thirds of patients with AIDS and esophageal candidiasis have oral candidiasis (thrush) (19,20). In other immunocompromised patients, oropharyngeal candidiasis is also commonly associated with esophageal candidiasis (21). It should be recognized, however, that thrush may be absent if antifungal therapy, such as nystatin, is currently administered. Patients with chronic mucocutaneous candidiasis may have fungal involvement of various mucous membranes, hair, nails, and skin, and have a history of adrenal or parathyroid dysfunction.

Complications

Complications from esophageal candidiasis are rare. Hemorrhage may occur when the disease is severe (erosion/ulcer) and there is an associated coagulopathy. Lumenal obstruction secondary to a mycetoma has also been described (28). Fibrosis and stricture formation, and fistulization into the bronchial tree have also been reported (29–31), but these lesions probably represent *Candida* colonization of anatomic abnormalities caused by other underlying disorders or unrecognized coinfections.

Diagnosis

Esophageal candidiasis should be suspected in any patient at risk for esophageal infection, especially the immunocompromised patient who complains of dysphagia or odynophagia. The presence of thrush further supports this diagnosis, but the absence of thrush does not exclude esophageal disease. Before endoscopy was developed, radiographic examination (barium esophagram) was the only diagnostic modality. The most characteristic radiographic feature of *Candida* esophagitis is the appearance of diffuse plaque-like lesions usually in a linear configuration. With disease progression, these plaques become confluent causing a "shaggy" appearance of the esophagus often described as ulcerations (31–34) (Color Plate 35.1). Additional radiographic findings that have been reported include pseudomembranes, cobblestoning, polypoid nodules, fungus balls, strictures, esophagopulmonary fistulas, mucosal bridges, or large neoplastic-appearing esophageal ulcers and masses (27,29,30–33). A large, well-circumscribed ulceration should not be attributed to *Candida*. Importantly, a normal barium esophagram does not exclude esophageal candidiasis. In any patient, the presence of severe odynophagia limits the ability to drink barium, thereby hampering the utility of barium studies.

Cytology brush and balloon devices that can be placed through the nose to sample the esophagus, and thus do not require endoscopy, have been developed for the rapid diagnosis of esophageal infections. Although appealing, these devices have not been widely adopted. When compared to endoscopy, they have been found to be sensitive for the diagnosis of *Candida*, less sensitive for the detection of HSV, and unreliable for CMV (35). The frequency of esophageal coinfections and the idiopathic esophageal ulcer (see below) are likely one explanation for the limited acceptance of these techniques.

Endoscopic examination of the esophagus is the most sensitive and specific method of diagnosing esophageal candidiasis (Table 35.3). The gross endoscopic appearance of *Candida* esophagitis is pathognomonic and may be graded according to recently published criteria (26). During endoscopy, mucosal lesions can be brushed and submitted for cytologic evaluation or biopsied for histologic diagnosis (36). When ulceration is identified endoscopically, multiple biopsies should be performed of the ulcer to exclude coexisting disorders. The use of periodic acid-Schiff or Gomori methenamine silver stains helps highlight the organisms. Cytologic examination of esophageal brushings is more sensitive than histologic examination of biopsy specimens in mild superficial candidiasis (i.e., grades 1 and 2) because organisms may be washed off tissue surfaces during processing of biopsy specimens (37). A positive cytology but negative endoscopy and histology indicate colonization rather than infection. Skin testing and serologic tests for candidiasis are not useful for the diagnosis of *Candida* esophagitis.

In patients with AIDS and thrush, the presence of dysphagia and/or odynophagia usually indicates *Candida* esophagitis (13,38). Therefore, in the symptomatic patient with associated thrush, an empirical trial of antifungal therapy should be instituted, reserving endoscopy for those patients who fail to respond. Further evaluation should be delayed no longer than 1 week for patients with severe persistent symptoms since the response to antifungal therapy is rapid, with clinical improvement occurring in the majority of patients within days (13,39). If patients fail to improve with empirical antifungal therapy, endoscopy should be performed since disorders other than *Candida* are identified

TABLE 35.3. PATHOLOGIC FINDINGS OF ESOPHAGEAL INFECTIONS

	Common	Uncommon
Candida	Plaques	Ulcer (rare)
Other fungi	Plaques, ulcer	Fistula
Viral	Ulcer	Mass lesions; nodules[a]
Mycobacteria	Ulcer	Fistula
TB	Ulcer, fistula	Mass lesions
MAC	Ulcer	—
Bacteria	Ulcer, plaques	—
Parasites	Plaques, ulcer	—

TB, *Mycobacterium tuberculosis*; MAC, *Mycobacterium avium* complex.
[a]Human papilloma virus.

in most patients (13,40). This empirical strategy has not been critically studied in the transplant setting, yet clinical experience suggests that it is effective.

Treatment

A number of highly efficacious oral and intravenous medications are available for the treatment of *Candida* esophagitis (Table 35.4). In general, oral therapies should be initiated first, reserving intravenous treatment for refractory disease or when there are contraindications to orally administered medication. Although candidal species other than *C. albicans* cause esophagitis, speciation is neither widely employed nor necessary, as reliable culturing and sensitivity testing are lacking at most centers and treatment is generally similar. For patients with mild disease, minimal immunocompromise, and/or readily reversible immunodeficiency, an abbreviated course of therapy with an oral azole should be given. Immunocompromised transplant patients and AIDS patients with *Candida* esophagitis are best treated with systemically active agents (azoles). In addition, patients with granulocytopenia are at significant risk for disseminated candidal infection, warranting the use of systemically acting agents. Drug interactions must always be kept in mind, particularly in transplant patients.

Orally administered systemically active agents, all of which have efficacy for the treatment of *Candida* esophagitis, include ketoconazole (Nizoral), fluconazole (Diflucan), and itraconazole (Sporanox). These agents, like other azoles, alter fungal cell membrane permeability by cytochrome P-450–dependent interference with ergosterol biosynthesis, resulting in fungal cell injury and death. The newer triazoles

(itraconazole and fluconazole) have greater affinity than the imidazoles (miconazole and ketoconazole) for fungal P-450 enzymes (41). Although other agents such as clotrimazole and nystatin are effective for oral candidiasis and provide prophylaxis against esophageal involvement (42), they are significantly less effective than azoles as primary therapy for esophageal candidiasis. Ketoconazole therapy (200 to 400 mg per day) requires an acid milieu for optimal absorption, which limits its use in many patients (43). Itraconazole absorption is also reduced by an increasing gastric pH (44).

Large randomized studies of patients with AIDS suggest that fluconazole (100 mg per day) has significantly greater efficacy than both ketoconazole (200 mg per day) and itraconazole for the treatment of *Candida* esophagitis (45,46). Unlike ketoconazole and itraconazole, fluconazole is highly water soluble, is minimally protein bound or metabolized, and is excreted unchanged in the urine. The half-life of fluconazole is approximately 30 hours if renal function is normal, and the presence of food or hypochlorhydria does not alter absorption. Fluconazole is available in oral and intravenous preparations, and both fluconazole and itraconazole are also available in equally effective oral solutions (47).

Adverse effects of ketoconazole, fluconazole, and itraconazole are primarily dose dependent and include nausea, hepatotoxicity, and inhibition of steroid production and cyclosporine metabolism (41). Due to the effects on hepatic microsomal enzymes, all three azoles inhibit the metabolism of cyclosporine, potentially resulting in an increase in cyclosporine blood levels; this effect is most pronounced with ketoconazole (41). In standard doses, however, fluconazole has no significant effect on cyclosporine metabolism. A number of other important drug interactions have

TABLE 35.4. RECOMMENDED TREATMENT REGIMENS FOR ESOPHAGEAL INFECTIONS

Pathogen	Drug	Dosage	Route	Duration	Efficacy (%)
Candida	Ketoconazole	200–400 mg/d	PO	7–14 d	<80
	Fluconazole	100 mg/d	PO/IV	7–14 d	~80
	Itraconazole	200 mg/d	PO	7–14 d	~80
	Amphotericin B	0.5 mg/kg/d	PO/IV	7 d	>95
Histoplasma	Amphotericin B	—	IV	—	>90
	Ketoconazole	—	—	—	>90
Other fungi	Amphotericin B	—	IV	—	>90
CMV	Ganciclovir	5 mg/kg b.i.d.	IV	2–4 wk	~75
	Foscarnet	90 mg/kg b.i.d.	IV	2–4 wk	~75
	Valganciclovir	900 mg b.i.d.	PO	14 d	>90
HSV	Acyclovir	400 mg 5× daily	PO/IV	14 d	>90
	Valacyclovir	1 gm t.i.d.	PO	14 d	>90
	Famciclovir	500 mg t.i.d.	PO	14 d	>90
	Foscarnet	90 mg/kg b.i.d.	IV	14 d	>95
	Ganciclovir	5 mg/kg b.i.d.	IV	14 d	>95
Mycobacteria	Same as for pulmonary disease				
Bacteria	Based on infecting species				
Idiopathic ulcer	Prednisone	40 mg/d taper	PO	4 wk	>90
	Thalidomide	200–300 mg/d	PO	4 wk	>90

CMV, cytomegalovirus; HSV, herpes simplex virus; b.i.d., twice a day; t.i.d., three times a day.

been noted with these agents, although these tend to be more common with ketoconazole.

The other major family of antifungal agents is made up of the polyene antibiotics, represented by amphotericin and nystatin. These agents bind irreversibly to sterols in fungal cell membranes, thereby altering the permeability characteristics of the membrane and causing cell death. Nystatin is effective for treating thrush, but less so for esophageal disease. The efficacy, safety, and ease of administration of azoles have made nystatin a second-line agent. Although amphotericin B (Fungizone) is the most effective agent for systemic mycoses, its severe side effects in conjunction with the availability of azoles have limited its use for the treatment of esophageal candidiasis. When there is resistance to treatment with fluconazole or other azoles, low doses of intravenous amphotericin B (10 to 20 mg daily) are effective. Renal toxicity, which is usually reversible, is the most serious adverse effect of continued use of amphotericin B and can be troublesome in patients receiving cyclosporine. The liposomal form of amphotericin B is less toxic, but the high cost has limited its use to patients with contraindications to amphotericin B (48). The total dose of amphotericin B for the treatment of esophageal candidiasis is approximately 100 to 200 mg. An oral suspension of amphotericin B is no longer available.

Flucytosine (Ancobon) is a fluorinated pyrimidine with a narrow spectrum of antifungal activity that acts by interfering with fungal translation of RNA. This oral agent, which is rarely used today, can be combined with amphotericin B or itraconazole (49), but it should not be used alone because fungi rapidly become resistant. Caspofungin, a new broad-spectrum antifungal agent, has been found to be as effective as amphotericin B for candidal esophagitis (50).

Prophylaxis

The prophylactic use of ketoconazole or nystatin for esophageal candidiasis in cancer and transplant patients has yielded mixed results (51). While the frequency of candidal infections is generally reduced, other mycoses still occur, and reductions in mortality have been difficult to establish. The use of azole prophylaxis in transplant patients may also be problematic in those receiving cyclosporine. Low doses of intravenous amphotericin B have been used successfully for prophylaxis in high-risk patients. While effective (52), primary prophylaxis against oropharyngeal and esophageal candidiasis is not currently recommended for patients with AIDS.

Drug Resistance

Because of widespread use, azole resistance has become an important clinical problem especially in AIDS patients. Both the cumulative dose of azole and severe immunode- ficiency have been shown to be highly associated with the development of resistance and cross-resistance (53,54), and clinical resistance correlates with *in vitro* resistance. Prophylactic fluconazole has similarly been associated with resistance in transplant patients. When resistance occurs, increasing the dose of azole is often helpful. If higher doses fail, switching to another azole or use of an oral solution such as itraconazole (55) may be tried, but higher doses are often necessary because of cross-resistance. Intravenous amphotericin B is usually required to achieve a satisfactory response rate when high-dose (>400 mg per day fluconazole) therapy fails. Resistance to amphotericin is rare. With the availability of effective therapy for HIV infection, the current focus in these patients is on improving immune function with HAART as "therapy" for resistant candidal infections as well as prophylaxis for esophageal candidiasis (56).

Other Fungi

Epidemiology

Esophageal involvement with other fungi is rare (57–66), and results from contiguously infected mediastinal lymph nodes, pulmonary parenchymal infection, primary esophageal disease, or widespread dissemination. Most instances of histoplasmosis and blastomycosis esophagitis represent secondary esophageal involvement from mediastinal lymph nodes rather than primary esophageal infection (57). Although no particular geographic distribution within the United States has been reported for aspergillosis, blastomycosis, or mucormycosis, histoplasmosis is endemic in the midwestern states and the Mississippi Valley. *Aspergillus*, principally a lung pathogen, has been reported to involve the esophagus in patients with leukemia and profound neutropenia (58) after bone marrow transplantation (59) and in AIDS (66); contiguous pulmonary disease is usually present. Mucormycosis has been reported to involve the esophagus in a patient with AIDS (61), and only a few cases have been described in other immunocompromised patients (60).

Pathology, Clinical Manifestations, and Complications

Other than the development of fistula, there are no unique pathologic features for these fungi (Table 35.3). The principal clinical manifestation is usually odynophagia and/or dysphagia, and as such is nonspecific. Pulmonary symptoms may predominate when there is fistula formation to the tracheobronchial tree or coexistent pulmonary involvement. With large lesions or fistulization, bleeding or perforation may occur (58,62). Histoplasmosis and blastomycosis are more likely to cause focal lesions as a consequence of extension from mediastinal lymph nodes, but multiple lesions can occur during the course of dissemination (63). Other sites of gastrointestinal involvement are common with disseminated histoplasmosis in immunocompromised patients (57).

Diagnosis

Histoplasmosis should be considered in the endemic areas or in patients who have previously resided in these regions especially if extraesophageal manifestations such as hilar adenopathy, calcified mediastinal lymph nodes, atelectasis of adjacent pulmonary tissue, or splenic calcification are present. Esophageal blastomycosis should be considered in patients with skin involvement and dysphagia; pulmonary disease may be present.

Recognition of these fungi depends on appropriate staining of endoscopic biopsy specimens with the identification of the characteristic fungal elements. Barium esophagram or endoscopy may show changes suggestive of *Candida* (64), malignancy (65), extrinsic compression due to lymph nodes usually in the region of the carina, or ulcer with or without fistula. Ulcerative lesions, which may be extensive, are common with all these fungi. Chest radiography may demonstrate acute or chronic pulmonary parenchymal changes, which frequently coexist in patients with esophageal histoplasmosis and aspergillosis. Endoscopy with biopsies and histologic examination (with cytologic brushings) may establish the diagnosis if the pathologist is able to differentiate the septate hyphae of *Aspergillus* species from the pseudohyphae of *Candida* species. Other fungi can be suggested by their appearance on staining of esophageal biopsies. Culture of biopsy material using fungal media can be diagnostic. Because *Histoplasma capsulatum* does not generally invade the esophageal mucosa and fibrosis is often marked, endoscopic brushings or biopsies are often nondiagnostic, thereby requiring thoractomy or thorascopy (57). Serologic tests are not useful because of the high prevalence of positive results in endemic areas. A urine antigen test has been developed that is sensitive and highly specific for disseminated histoplasmosis in patients with AIDS.

Treatment

Although in the normal host pulmonary histoplasmosis may spontaneously resolve, therapy is required in those who are immunocompromised or when there is extrapulmonary disease. Ketoconazole, itraconazole, and amphotericin B are effective against both histoplasmosis and blastomycosis (41). Systemic aspergillosis should be treated with high-dose amphotericin B, although itraconazole has significant *in vitro* activity. Surgery may be required for drainage of abscesses or excision of fistulas. Amphotericin should be administered with mucormycosis, and surgical debridement may be necessary.

VIRAL INFECTIONS

With the implementation of *Candida* prophylaxis in selected patients undergoing transplantation and the widespread use of oral antifungal therapies in AIDS, viral esophagitis has assumed more etiologic importance in these immunosuppressed patients. Nevertheless, in the transplant setting, the incidence of clinically apparent viral esophageal disease, both HSV and CMV, has also been falling. One explanation for the decrease in herpetic esophagitis in the transplant patient is the frequent use of HSV prophylaxis. The reduced incidence of CMV disease is likely the result of using CMV-seronegative organs and blood products for seronegative recipients, use of leukocyte-depleted platelets for patients following bone marrow transplantation, and the administration of preemptive ganciclovir or more recently, valganciclovir for high-risk transplant patients (2,3). Without antiviral prophylaxis, viral esophagitis is more common in bone marrow than solid organ transplant recipients because of the greater degree of immunosuppression required for these patients.

Herpes Simplex Virus

Epidemiology

HSV type 1 is one of three herpes viruses that affect the esophagus, the others being CMV and varicella-zoster virus. HSV type 2 rarely involves the esophagus. After *Candida* species, HSV is the next most frequent infectious agent that causes esophagitis. Although well recognized as an esophageal pathogen in otherwise healthy people (6), HSV esophagitis occurs most often in patients with some predisposing factor(s). After transplant, HSV and CMV occur with equal frequency as causes of esophagitis (7,67), whereas in patients with AIDS, HSV esophagitis is relatively uncommon and far less frequent than CMV. In a study of 100 HIV-infected patients with esophageal ulcer, HSV was only found in nine, and in four of the latter it was a copathogen with CMV (15).

Pathology

HSV infection is generally limited to squamous mucosa, where the earliest manifestation is a vesicle. As these vesicles enlarge and ulcerate, they coalesce to form larger superficial lesions that are typically focal, which often leave the intervening mucosa normal (68). Microscopic examination of the squamous epithelial cells at the ulcer edge reveals multinucleation, ground-glass nuclei, and eosinophilic Cowdry's type A inclusion bodies that may take up half of the nuclear volume. Over time, these inclusion bodies may be surrounded by halos and become more basophilic, filling, enlarging, and deforming the nucleus (68).

Clinical Manifestations and Complications

HSV esophageal infection commonly presents with the sudden onset of severe odynophagia, heartburn, or chest pain. Autopsy studies, however, suggest that esophageal symptoms may be absent (69). Herpes labialis (i.e., cold sores) and oropharyngeal ulcers may coexist, antedate, or develop during the esophageal infection, whereas skin infection is rare (20,21). A number of systemic manifestations including low-grade fever or symptoms of an upper respiratory infection may precede the onset of esophageal symptoms. In untreated immunocompetent persons, spontaneous resolution of HSV esophageal infection occurs within 2 weeks of the onset of symptoms (6,21,70). Complications are rare and include bleeding (6,71), perforation (6,72), tracheoesophageal fistula in association with other pathogens (73), or dissemination (69).

Diagnosis

Esophageal disease caused by HSV appears in barium radiographic studies as focal small ulceration(s) on a background of normal mucosa; vesicles are infrequently observed. These ulcers have been described as stellate or volcano-like in appearance, often with a thin halo of edema at the margin (70,74). There is less propensity to form the longitudinal or linear lesions that are typical for CMV infection (74). Severe, diffuse herpetic esophagitis may result in a cobblestone or "shaggy" mucosal appearance resembling *Candida* esophagitis (75) (Color Plate 35.2). Although the radiographic appearance may be suggestive, definitive diagnosis of herpetic esophagitis requires endoscopic mucosal biopsies. The endoscopic characteristics of herpetic esophagitis reflect the pathologic changes (Table 35.3), appearing as discrete, usually small (<1 cm), well-circumscribed shallow ulcers (76,77), a diffuse erosive esophagitis, or rarely vesicles. Small-scattered lesions covered with exudate mimic esophageal candidiasis. Deep ulcers, as seen with CMV, are very rare. Cytologic brushings (22) and endoscopic mucosal biopsies should be taken from the ulcer edge, as the viral cytopathic effect is best identified in epithelial cells rather than granulation tissue in the ulcer bed. Immunohistochemical staining on biopsy samples using specific monoclonal antibodies to HSV will help confirm the diagnosis when the viral cytopathic effect is difficult to appreciate. Viral culture of biopsy specimens helps establish a definitive diagnosis but takes several days for the results. As with other etiologies of infectious esophagitis, serologic tests play no role in establishing the diagnosis.

Treatment

Numerous uncontrolled trials and vast clinical experience in both immunocompetent and immunodeficient patients suggest the efficacy of acyclovir (Zovirax), a nucleoside analog, for the therapy of esophageal disease. In the largest study, which evaluated 34 patients with AIDS and HSV esophagitis, a clinical response was seen in essentially all treated patients (78). More recently, valacyclovir, a prodrug of acyclovir, and famciclovir have been released. The advantage of these agents over acyclovir is that they can be administered three times per day at an equivalent cost. While large studies evaluating the use of these agents for esophagitis are lacking, trials for genital disease suggest equivalence to acyclovir (79). Although spontaneous resolution of HSV esophagitis is common in the normal host, therapy is usually instituted regardless of immune status. When oral intake is hampered by severe odynophagia or when there is a question of drug absorption, intravenous administration is required. Side effects of these agents are few. Although rare, resistance should be suspected when there is clinical failure; in this setting, foscarnet (Table 35.4) is the drug of choice and will lead to clinical cure in most patients (80). These agents are effective prophylaxis for HSV-antibody–positive patients undergoing transplantation (3). Long-term secondary prophylaxis should be considered when immunodeficiency persists, because the relapse rate is high.

Cytomegalovirus

Epidemiology

Until the advent of transplantation, CMV disease was uncommon and is extremely rare in normal individuals (81,82). Currently, CMV is regarded as one of the most common opportunistic infections. Studies from developed countries have shown seropositivity rates of ≥50%, and up to 90% seropositivity has been found in homosexual men, reflecting sexual transmission of the virus (83). In transplant patients who receive no antiviral prophylaxis, CMV and HSV are equally common esophageal pathogens (2,7, 67). As already noted, CMV is the most frequent cause of esophageal ulcer in patients with AIDS, comprising >50% of esophageal ulcers in these patients (15).

Pathology

The histologic hallmark of CMV esophagitis is mucosal ulceration (Table 35.3). Although variable, deep ulcers are very characteristic for disease in AIDS, whereas in other immunocompromised patients, lesions tend to remain more superficial. In contrast to HSV, the viral cytopathic effect of CMV is located in endothelial and mesenchymal cells in the granulation tissue of the ulcer base rather than squamous cells. Inclusions are large (cytomegalo) and often have an eosinophilic appearance that may be located either in the nucleus or cytoplasm (22). Because these inclusions can appear atypical, especially in patients with AIDS (84,85), immunohistochemical stains play a valuable role in selected patients for confirming the presence of CMV and often highlight more infected cells than are appreciated by routine hematoxylin and eosin staining. As with other esophageal infections, CMV may coexist with HSV or *Candida*, especially in patients with AIDS (14,15). The pathogenesis of CMV disease is not well understood. Mucosal ischemia has been hypothesized as an etiologic mechanism given the involvement of endothelial cells (86). The high mucosal concentration of tumor necrosis factor-α found in association with CMV esophagitis, which falls after ganciclovir treatment and ulcer healing, suggests an etiologic role for this proinflammatory cytokine (87).

Clinical Manifestations and Complications

Odynophagia is almost uniformly present and is characteristically severe (Table 35.2). Chest pain, weight loss, and fever may be reported. The onset of symptoms is often more subacute than the acute presentation of HSV. A prior or coexistent diagnosis of CMV infection in another organ (e.g., retinitis or colitis) is not infrequent. Although rare in transplant patients, retinitis may be observed in approximately 15% of AIDS patients at the time of diagnosis of gastrointestinal disease (88). Complications include gastrointestinal bleeding (5% of patients) and rarely strictures, or fistulas to the tracheobronchial tree (89,90).

Diagnosis

Like HSV, the radiological appearance of CMV esophagitis is that of either focal or extensive ulceration, and will depend in large part on the epidemiologic setting. Barium esophagography of CMV esophagitis may reveal only thickening of mucosal folds, but more typically, well-circumscribed ulcers are present that may be vertical, linear with central umbilication, solitary, and deep, or occasionally diffuse and superficial (75,91,92). In patients with AIDS, these ulcers are often large and deep, exceeding 2 cm in size (Color Plate 35.3). Rarely, the exuberant inflammatory response results in a lesion suggestive of a malignancy (93). The endoscopic appearance of CMV esophagitis is similarly variable, ranging from multiple shallow ulcers, to solitary giant ulcers, to a diffuse superficial esophagitis (94). Given the high rate of prior exposure to CMV, serologic testing is not helpful. In addition, some immunosuppressed transplant patients fail to develop a brisk antibody response with acute infection. The absence of CMV DNA or antigenemia in the blood would, however, suggest an alternative diagnosis.

Identification of viral cytopathic effect in mucosal biopsies is the best diagnostic method. Multiple biopsies (up to ten) may be required to establish the diagnosis in patients with AIDS and should be taken from the base of the ulcer (22,95). Viral culture of mucosal biopsies is less sensitive and specific than histology (96). Use of shell vial techniques improves the turnaround time for the viral culture to 48 hours. In contrast to *Candida* and HSV, cytologic specimens from esophageal lesion have very poor sensitivity for the diagnosis of CMV. Since retinitis may coexist with gastrointestinal disease, a diagnosis of CMV gastrointestinal disease in any patient with AIDS warrants ophthalmologic examination.

Therapy

The therapies available for the treatment of CMV disease are generally efficacious but require intravenous administration and include ganciclovir, foscarnet, and cidofovir. A prospective open-label trial of ganciclovir therapy for CMV esophagitis in 35 AIDS patients documented clinical and endoscopic improvement in 77% of patients (88). The time course of the clinical response to ganciclovir is variable; 1 week of therapy may be required before there is symptom improvement. The total treatment duration should be based on the clinical and endoscopic response, and a 2- to 4-week treatment course is usually adequate. If retinitis is absent and there has been a complete response, the patient may be followed closely without maintenance therapy. Because of low bioavailability (<10%), oral ganciclovir is not effective for the treatment of active infections, including those of the gastrointestinal tract (97). Following acute CMV disease in transplantation patients, treatment should be given for 1 to 2 months until the immunosuppressive regimen is significantly reduced. Ganciclovir is well tolerated, with its major side effect being myelosuppression, which may be severe when other bone marrow–suppressive drugs, such as azidothymidine, are coadministered. Clinical as well as virologic resistance has been recognized, usually in patients receiving prolonged therapy (98). Combination therapy with foscarnet has been used to treat refractory disease or when side effects are limiting, as lower doses of each agent may be utilized (99).

Foscarnet inhibits viral DNA polymerase and reverse transcriptase. A randomized trial comparing ganciclovir to foscarnet for AIDS patients with gastrointestinal CMV disease found clinical improvement in over 80% of patients, and there were no significant differences in efficacy between the two agents (100). There is less information on the use of foscarnet in non-AIDS immunosuppressed patients. Foscarnet has been most frequently utilized when there is clinical resistance to ganciclovir or a major contradiction to ganciclovir use. The major side effect of foscarnet is reversible renal insufficiency (101). This may be prevented by vigorous saline hydration prior to and during drug administration in combination with dose adjustments based on creatinine clearance. Electrolyte disturbances, which include hypocalcemia and hypophosphatemia, are also common during or shortly after infusion. Because of these side effects as well as higher cost, foscarnet remains second-line therapy.

Cidofovir is the newest systemic agent available for the therapy of CMV but has only undergone evaluation for the treatment of retinitis in AIDS (102,103). Because of its long half-life, once-weekly administration is adequate, which makes it an ideal agent for selected patients. Like foscarnet, this drug is associated with renal insufficiency.

Valganciclovir is a recently released oral agent for the treatment and prophylaxis of CMV infections. In contrast to oral ganciclovir, this agent has excellent oral absorption achieving therapeutic concentrations (104,105). While effective for retintitis, large studies for active gastrointestinal disease are lacking. Because of its low toxicity and oral bioavailability, it has become the agent of choice for prophylaxis in the transplant patient.

All drugs for herpes viruses only inhibit viral replication; thus, relapse is frequent when therapy is discontinued. The relapse rate for transplant patients also remains high until immunosuppressive therapy is reduced. In patients with AIDS, the relapse rate of CMV esophagitis is approximately 50%, similar to HSV (78,88,100). With the advent of HAART, successful treatment of HIV-associated immunosuppresion will serve to prevent relapse, thus negating the need for long-term antiviral therapy for CMV (106).

Prophylaxis

High-dose acyclovir has been used with some success for the prophylaxis of CMV infection in transplant patients, although intravenous ganciclovir has been shown to be superior (107). Because of its cost, potential side effects, and intravenous route of administration, at most transplant centers intravenous prophylaxis is limited to high-risk patients including CMV-seropositive patients, CMV seronegative-recipients who receive CMV-seropositive organs and/or blood products, and patients receiving potent immunosuppression for episodes of rejection (2). With the availability of valganciclovir, most of these patients now receive this agent negating the need for intravenous therapy. While oral ganciclovir prophylaxis has been shown to decrease CMV disease in high-risk patients after liver transplantation (108), valganciclovir is now the drug of choice for such patients. Oral ganciclovir is effective prophylaxis for CMV retinitis in AIDS patients with a CD4 lymphocyte count of <200/mm^3, but is untested for either primary or secondary prophylaxis of gastrointestinal CMV disease (97). Fortunately, despite long-term administration, resistance of CMV to ganciclovir and foscarnet is uncommon.

Other Viruses

The frequency of esophageal involvement caused by varicella-zoster virus during the course of chicken pox or herpes zoster infections is unknown but clinically uncommon (109,110). The esophagitis usually occurs when skin lesions are present rather than antedating the cutaneous disease.

Culture of mucosal biopsies is required to differentiate HSV from varicella-zoster virus. The disease is self-limited in the immunocompetent patient. Papilloma virus may infect the esophagus in both normal and immunocompromised patients and characteristically causes small polypoid lesions (111), usually asymptomatic or symptomatic ulcers (112). Esophageal ulcers have been reported due to Epstein-Barr virus in patients with AIDS (113).

MYCOBACTERIAL INFECTIONS

Epidemiology

Mycobacterial involvement of the esophagus is rare in both immunocompromised and immunocompetent patients with advanced pulmonary tuberculosis, even in countries with high prevalence rates. Previously, *Mycobacterium tuberculosis* (TB) involvement of the esophagus was considered a rare autopsy finding, found in <0.15% of necropsies (114). In developing countries, the rate of TB is much higher, and extrapulmonary manifestations, including esophageal disease, are more common. The upsurge in reported cases of TB linked to the AIDS epidemic has increased the incidence of esophageal infection worldwide. *Mycobacterium avium* complex (MAC), a pathogen principally restricted to patients with AIDS, is primarily a small bowel pathogen with few reported cases of esophageal involvement (115–118).

Pathology

Most commonly, TB involves the mid-esophagus at the level of the carina. Esophageal disease is caused by spread of infection from contiguous TB-infected mediastinal lymph nodes by way of a draining fistula or obstructed lymphatics, resulting in tracheoesophageal fistula. Rarely, TB involves the upper third of the esophagus by direct extension from tuberculous pharyngitis or laryngitis. Primary esophageal TB in the absence of extraesophageal disease is exceedingly rare (119,120). Granulomas are often present in ulcer tissue, with bacilli identifiable by mycobacterial staining. Unless multiple biopsies are taken, the diagnosis can be easily missed, especially if there is a significant fibrotic response.

Clinical Manifestations and Complications

The symptoms of esophageal TB depend on the degree and type of involvement. Systemic symptoms of fever and weight loss are common. Pulmonary complaints often predominate due to a fistula to the trachea, bronchus, or pleural space. Dysphagia may be prominent with the formation of long strictures or traction diverticula resulting from the fibrotic response or mediastinitis may be the cause of dysphagia (121). Upper gastrointestinal hemorrhage from tuberculous esophageal ulcers (122) and tuberculous arterioesophageal fistulas (123) has been reported. Bleeding caused by extensive mucosal disease has been described in an AIDS patient with esophageal MAC (124).

Diagnosis

Esophageal TB should be suspected in patients with pulmonary or systemic TB who develop esophageal symptoms. Barium esophagram findings of ulceration and stricture are nonspecific. A sinus tract or fistulous connection to the bronchial tree or mediastinum at the level of the hilum is highly suggestive of TB but may be attributed to malignancy, which appears similarly, potentially delaying the diagnosis. An ulcerated tuberculous granulomatous mass may also mimic an esophageal neoplasm at endoscopy (120). When a fistula is present, sputum staining and culture can make the diagnosis of TB. Chest radiography is often abnormal and may suggest the diagnosis. Computed tomography of the chest usually demonstrates mediastinal lymphadenopathy, but again, the appearance of carcinoma is similar. Ulceration is usually present at the site of fistula. Endoscopic biopsies from the edge of the lesions may reveal granulomas and/or acid-fast bacilli, and biopsy material should be cultured for further confirmation of the diagnosis and determination of sensitivities to antimycobacterial agents. Cytologic specimens may also be helpful.

Treatment

Even in the presence of immunodeficiency, a 9-month course of multidrug therapy (in the absence of drug resistance) will often cure esophageal TB and close fistulas. If fistulas do not close with medical therapy alone, surgical intervention will be required. Multidrug-resistant TB is becoming an increasingly complex problem; thus, knowing drug sensitivities to antituberculous therapy is essential to guide therapy.

The most effective agents for the treatment of MAC are clarithromycin and ethambutol (125). Although a clinical and bacteriologic response is common, long-term therapy for MAC is required if immune function cannot be improved with highly active antiretroviral therapy.

BACTERIAL INFECTIONS

Epidemiology

Bacterial esophagitis is a very rare cause of esophageal disease (126–129). For the most part, this is a polymicrobial infection consisting of oral flora, particularly gram-positive organisms, including *Streptococcus viridans*, staphylococci, and other bacilli. Bacterial esophagitis with these organisms occurs almost exclusively in patients with hematologic malignancies complicated by severe granulocytopenia (126), but occasionally occurs following bone marrow transplantation (67), diabetic ketoacidosis (127), or steroid therapy. It is likely that these bacteria colonize and then invade mucosa damaged either from reflux disease, radiation therapy, or following chemotherapy, which leads to local infection; dissemination may occur when granulocyte function is poor and/or there is absolute granulocytopenia.

Other bacteria have been reported to involve the esophagus. *Brucella* presenting as a distal submucosal esophageal mass with dysphagia and fever has been noted in a normal host (130). In patients with AIDS, *Bartonella hensellae* (the cause of cat scratch disease [131]), actinomycoses (66,132,133), and *Nocardia* (134) have been described.

Pathology

The gross pathologic appearance of the esophagus in bacterial infection depends on the specific pathogen and ranges from diffuse, shallow ulcerations to ulcers associated with erythema, plaques, pseudomembranes, nodules, or hemorrhage (129). Microscopic examination reveals pseudomembranes and bacterial invasion that may be superficial and limited to squamous epithelium or may be invasive and transmural with infiltration of blood vessels (i.e., phlegmonous esophagitis). Esophageal actinomycosis is characterized by ulceration and sinuses leading from abscess cavities with sulfur granules and filamentous gram-positive branching bacteria seen on tissue biopsies (66). In the one reported case, *B. hensellae* esophagitis resulted in multiple nodules resulting from a lobulated proliferation of capillary vessels lined by plump endothelial cells (131).

Clinical Manifestations and Complications

Bacterial esophagitis presents with odynophagia and dysphagia typical for any infectious esophagitis. Esophageal infection may serve as a focus for bacteremia and seeding of other organs (129). Perforation has not been reported.

Diagnosis

The diagnosis of bacterial esophagitis should be considered in the clinical settings described above. Radiographic findings are nonspecific, and endoscopic biopsy is required to establish this diagnosis. Additional stains including Gram's stain will be necessary to identify the etiologic bacteria. When suspected, bacterial cultures of biopsy material should be submitted. Positive blood cultures will also pinpoint the bacterial pathogen(s) and direct antimicrobial therapy.

Treatment

Since the infection may be polymicrobial, broad-spectrum antibiotics, which effectively treat both gram-positive and gram-negative oropharyngeal flora, are required. Treatment of other bacteria found in these patients is similar to infection in other locations.

Treponema pallidum

Although esophageal involvement by *Treponema pallidum* was well recognized many years ago, this disease is unheard of today in developed countries and is primarily of historical interest. The rarity of this esophageal infection has also not been altered by the AIDS epidemic. Tertiary syphilis of the esophagus may present as a submucosal gumma or diffuse inflammatory reaction with fibrosis, which often affects the upper third of the esophagus, and may be associated with mucosal ulcers and strictures (135,136). Given the rarity of esophageal syphilis, most patients with infectious esophagitis and positive serologic tests for syphilis will have another cause of esophagitis.

PROTOZOAL INFECTIONS

In developed countries, protozoal infections of the esophagus are very rare, having been reported almost exclusively in AIDS patients. In these patients, reported pathogens include *Pneumocystis carinii* (137), *Cryptosporidium parvum* (138), and *Leishmania donovani* (139); coinfections were present in two of these cases (137,138). The clinical presentation is similar to other causes of infectious esophagitis. Ulceration(s) is the most common endoscopic finding, and the diagnosis is established by appropriate histologic staining of mucosal biopsies. In normal hosts from endemic areas in South America, *Trypanosoma cruzi* may involve the myenteric plexus of the esophagus resulting in Chagas' disease. This disease is indistinguishable clinically, radiographically, manometrically, and endoscopically from idiopathic achalasia. This diagnosis may be established by antibody testing.

SELECTED HIV-RELATED ESOPHAGEAL DISORDERS

In addition to the infections described above, there are other unique disorders causing esophageal disease in these patients.

Disorders Associated with Primary HIV Infection

Although primary HIV infection is largely asymptomatic, in some patients, a mononucleosis-like illness occurs around the time of infection consisting of fever, sore throat, and myalgias associated with a maculopapular rash (140). Spontaneously resolving oropharyngeal and esophageal aphthous ulceration, candidal infection, or CMV esophagitis may also be observed with this seroconversion illness (141–143). During this primary infection, a brief period of immunodeficiency occurs and is likely the explanation for the development of opportunistic infections. Endoscopically, these aphthous esophageal ulcerations are multiple, small, and shallow (141,143). In some of these patients, electron microscopic examination of biopsy specimens revealed enveloped virus like particles with morphologic features compatible with retroviruses (143). The diagnosis can be established at the time of presentation by the detection of HIV RNA in serum (140). Serologic testing is unhelpful, as antibody positive to HIV is delayed 3 to 18 months after the illness.

Idiopathic Esophageal Ulcer

Epidemiology

Large, usually isolated esophageal ulcerations in which no specific etiology could be identified were recognized early in the AIDS epidemic. These ulcers, termed idiopathic esophageal ulcers (IEU) or aphthous ulcers, are very common, comprising approximately 40% of esophageal ulcers in HIV-infected patients (15). Like other esophageal infections in AIDS, IEU are observed in patients with AIDS, when the CD4 lymphocyte count is <100/mm^3 (15). These lesions appear to be unique to AIDS.

Pathology

IEU are variable in size, may be quite large, and are uniformly well circumscribed (144,145). Ulcer tissue resembles that in cases of CMV and HSV esophagitis, except that viral cytopathic effect is absent. *Candida* coinfection is common (14). The presence of a superficial candidal infection overlying a large, well-circumscribed lesion with histopathologic findings of granulation tissue but without viral cytopathic effect should still strongly suggest the diagnosis of IEU rather than *Candida* esophagitis. Since HIV has been observed in ulcer tissue by immunohistochemical staining, it has been suggested that HIV is the direct cause of these lesions (141). However, studies have found HIV histopathologically in esophageal biopsies from patients with *Candida*, CMV, and HSV esophagitis (146,147). HIV has been uniformly identified in inflammatory cells rather than in squamous epithelial cells, and the infected cells are few in number (146,147). In aggregate, these studies suggest that HIV does not cause IEU, at least based on a direct cytopathic mechanism.

Clinical Manifestations and Complications

The presentation of IEU is indistinguishable from other causes of esophageal ulcer. Coexistent oropharyngeal aphthous ulcers are infrequent (20), whereas thrush is common, especially if the patient has not received empirical antifungal therapy. Complications of IEU include bleeding and fistula to the stomach, but not to the tracheobronchial tree (144,148), and esophageal strictures (90).

Diagnosis

The findings of IEU on barium esophagram are characteristically large, well circumscribed, and often deep ulcers (149,150) (Color Plate 35.4). Because of the similarity to CMV esophagitis, a definitive diagnosis cannot be made on the radiographic appearance alone. As IEU is a diagnosis of exclusion, endoscopy with biopsy is required. Endoscopically, these ulcers are variable in size and appearance, and larger ulcers are indistinguishable from CMV esophagitis (94,145). Pill-induced esophagitis must be excluded by history since the pathologic findings of esophageal biopsies are similar. Likewise, distal esophageal ulcer may suggest gastroesophageal reflux disease, and the histopathologic features cannot distinguish IEU from gastroesophageal reflux disease. However, the clinical history is different, and the endoscopic appearance helps suggest reflux disease.

Treatment

These ulcers respond rapidly to either prednisone or thalidomide, with clinical and endoscopic cure seen in >90% of cases (151,152). The prednisone regimen consists of 40 mg per day tapering to 10 mg per week for a 1-month treatment course. Intermittent azole therapy should be coadministered to reduce the likelihood of *Candida*, complicating the use of high-dose corticosteroids. Steroid injection into the ulcers is effective, but requires repetitive endoscopy (144). Thalidomide is given in a dose of 200 mg/day for 4 weeks. The main side effects are drowsiness, skin rash, and neurotoxicity. The horrific teratogenic effects are well recognized and limit its cautious use to male patients. The relapse rate for IEU is approximately 50%, and retreatment is usually successful. Long-term daily maintenance therapy may be required for the patient with frequent relapses. Like other opportunistic diseases in AIDS, improvement in immune function with HAART should prevent relapse (56).

REFERENCES

1. Wong TW, Warner NE. Cytomegalic disease in adults. *Arch Pathol* 1962;74:403.
2. Hibberd PL, Tolkett-Rubin NE, Centi D, et al. Preemptive ganciclovir therapy to prevent cytomegalovirus disease in cytomegalovirus-positive renal transplant recipients. *Ann Intern Med* 1995;123:18–26.
3. Momin F, Chandrasekaar PH. Antimicrobial prophylaxis in bone marrow transplantation. *Ann Intern Med* 1995;123:205–215.
4. Brodt HR, Kamps BS, Gute P, et al. Changing incidence of AIDS-defining illness in the era of antiretroviral combination therapy. *AIDS* 1997;11:1731–1738.
5. Monkemuller KE, Call SA, Lazenby AJ, et al. Declining prevalence of opportunistic gastrointestinal disease in the era of combination antiretroviral therapy. *Am J Gastroenterol* 2000;95:457–462.
6. Ramanathan J, Rammouni M, Baran J Jr, et al. Herpes simplex virus esophagitis in the immunocompetent host: an overview. *Am J Gastroenterol* 2000;95:2171–2176.
7. Alexander JA, Brouillette DE, Chien MC, et al. Infectious esophagitis following liver and renal transplantation. *Dig Dis Sci* 1988;33:1121–1126.
8. Bernabeu-Wittel M, Naranjo M, Cisneros JM, et al. Infections in renal transplant recipients receiving mycophenolate versus azathioprine-based immunosuppression. *Eur J Clin Microbiol Infect Dis* 2002;21:173–180.
9. Vishny ML, Blades EW, Creger RJ, et al. Role of upper endoscopy in evaluation of upper gastrointestinal symptoms in patients undergoing bone marrow transplantation. *Cancer Invest* 1994;12:384–389.
10. Hofflin JM, Potasman, I, Baldwin, et al. Infectious complications in heart transplant recipients receiving cyclosporine and corticosteroids. *Ann Intern Med* 1987;106:209–216.
11. Bonacini M, Young T, Laine L. The causes of esophageal symptoms in human immunodeficiency virus infection. *Arch Intern Med* 1991;151:1567–1572.
12. Connolly GM, Hawkins D, Harcourt-Webster JN, et al. Oesophageal symptoms, their causes, treatment, and prognosis in patients with the acquired immunodeficiency syndrome. *Gut* 1989;30:1033–1039.
13. Wilcox CM, Alexander LN, Clark WS, et al. Fluconazole compared with endoscopy for human immunodeficiency virus-infected patients with esophageal symptoms. *Gastroenterology* 1996;110:1803–1809.
14. Wilcox CM. Evaluation of a technique to evaluate the underlying mucosa in patients with AIDS and severe Candida esophagitis. *Gastrointest Endosc* 1995;42:360–363.
15. Wilcox CM, Schwartz DA, Clark WS. Esophageal ulceration in human immunodeficiency virus infection: causes, diagnosis, and management. *Ann Intern Med* 1995;123:143–149.
16. Rubin RR. Infections in the liver and renal transplant patient. In: Rubin RH, Young LS, eds. *Clinical approach to infection in the compromised host.* 2nd ed. New York: Plenum Publishing, 1988:561.
17. Bacellar H, Munoz A, Hoover DR, et al., for Multicenter AIDS Cohort Study. Incidence of clinical AIDS conditions in a cohort of homosexual men with CD4+ cell counts <100/mm³. *J Infect Dis* 1994;170:1284–1287.
18. Bashir RM, Wilcox CM. Symptom-specific use of upper gastrointestinal endoscopy in human immunodeficiency virus-infected patients yields high dividends. *J Clin Gastroenterol* 1996;23:292–298.
19. Lopez-Dulpa M, et al. Clinical, endoscopic, immunologic, and therapeutic aspects of oropharyngeal and esophageal candidiasis in HIV-infected patients: a survey of 114 cases. *Am J Gastroenterol* 1992;87:1771–1774.
20. Wilcox CM, Straub RF, Clark WS. Prospective evaluation of oropharyngeal findings in human immunodeficiency virus-infected patients with esophageal ulceration. *Am J Gastroenterol* 1995;90:1938–1941.
21. Baehr PH, McDonald GB. Esophageal infections: risk factors, presentation, diagnosis, and treatment. *Gastroenterology* 1994;106:509–532.
22. Lazenby AJ. Gastroenterologist/pathologist partnership. *Tech Gastrointest Endosc* 2002;4:95–100.

23. Slavin MA, Osborne B, Adams R, et al. Efficacy and safety of fluconazole prophylaxis for fungal infections after marrow transplantation—a prospective, randomized, double-blind study. *J Infect Dis* 1995;171:1545–1552.

24. Frick T, Fryd DS, Goodale RL, et al. Incidence and treatment of Candida esophagitis in patients undergoing renal transplantation. Data from the Minnesota prospective randomized trial of cyclosporine versus antilymphocyte globulin-azathioprine. *Am J Surg* 1988;155:311–313.

25. Abgrall S, Charreau I, Joly V, et al. Risk factors for esophageal candidiasis in a large cohort of HIV-infected patients treated with nucleoside analogues. *Eur J Clin Microbiol Infect Dis* 2001; 20:346–349.

26. Wilcox CM, Schwartz DA. Endoscopic–pathologic correlates of Candida esophagitis in acquired immunodeficiency syndrome. *Dig Dis Sci* 1996;41:1337–1345.

27. Eras P, Goldstein MJ, Sherlock P. Candida infection of the gastro-intestinal tract. *Medicine (Baltimore)* 1972;51:367–379.

28. Bhalodia MV, Vega KJ, DaCosta J, et al. Esophageal candidoma in a patient with acquired immunodeficiency syndrome. *J Assoc Acad Minor Phys* 1998;9:69–71.

29. Lewicki AM, Moore JP. Esophageal moniliasis: a review of common and less frequent characteristics. *Am J Roentgenol* 1975; 125:218–225.

30. Ott DJ, Gelfand DW. Esophageal stricture secondary to candidiasis. *Gastrointest Radiol* 1978;2:323–325.

31. Sheft DJ, Shrago G. Esophageal moniliasis: the spectrum of the disease. *JAMA* 1970;231:1859–1862.

32. Levine MS, Macones AJ Jr, Laufer I. Candida esophagitis: accuracy of radiographic diagnosis. *Radiology* 1985;154:581–587.

33. Roberts L Jr, Gibbons R, Gibbons G, et al. Adult esophageal candidiasis: a radiographic spectrum. *Radiographics* 1987;7:289–307.

34. Glick SN. Barium studies in patients with Candida esophagitis: pseudoulcerations simulating viral esophagitis. *Am J Roentgenol* 1994;163:349–352.

35. Brandt LJ, Coman E, Schwartz E, et al. Use of a new cytology balloon for diagnosis of esophageal disease in acquired immunodeficiency syndrome. *Gastrointest Endosc* 1993;4:559–561.

36. Geisinger KR. Endoscopic biopsies and cytologic brushings of the esophagus are diagnostically complementary. *Am J Clin Pathol* 1995;103:295–299.

37. Kodsi BE, Wickremesinghe C, Kozinn PJ, et al. Candida esophagitis: a prospective study of 27 cases. *Gastroenterology* 1976;71:715–719.

38. Lai YP, Wu MS, Chen MY, et al. Timing and necessity of endoscopy in AIDS patients with dysphagia or odynophagia. *Hepatogastroenterology* 1998;45:186.

39. Wilcox CM. Time course of clinical response to fluconazole for Candida oesophagitis in AIDS. *Aliment Pharmacol Ther* 1994;8:347–350.

40. Wilcox CM, Straub RF, Alexander LN, et al. Etiology of esophageal disease in human immunodeficiency virus-infected patients who fail antifungal therapy. *Am J Med* 1996;101:599–604.

41. Como JA, Dismukes WE. Oral azole drugs as systemic antifungal therapy. *N Engl J Med* 1994;330:263–272.

42. Shepp DH, Klosterman A, Siegel MS. Comparative trial of ketoconazole and nystatin for prevention of fungal infection in neutropenic patients treated in a protective environment. *J Infect Dis* 1985;152:1257–1263.

43. Tavitian A, Raufman JP, Rosenthal LE. Ketaconazole-resistant Candida esophagitis in patients with acquired immunodeficiency syndrome. *Gastroenterology* 1986;90:443–445.

44. Lim SG, Sawyer AM, Hudson M, et al. The absorption of fluconazole and itraconazole under conditions of low intragastric acidity. *Aliment Pharmacol Ther* 1993;7:317–321.

45. Laine L, Dretler RH, Contea CN, et al. Fluconazole compared to ketoconazole for the treatment of Candida esophagitis in AIDS. *Ann Intern Med* 1992;117:655–660.

46. Barbaro G, Barbarini G, Calderon W, et al. Fluconazole versus itraconazole for Candida esophagitis in acquired immunodeficiency syndrome. *Gastroenterology* 1996;111:1169–1177.

47. Wilcox CM, Darouiche RO, Laine L, et al. A randomized, double-blind comparison of itraconazole oral solution and fluconazole tablets in the treatment of esophageal candidiasis. *J Infect Dis* 1997;176:227–232.

48. Johnson PC, Wheat LJ, Cloud GA, et al. Safety and efficacy of liposomal amphotericin B compared with conventional amphotericin B for induction therapy of histoplasmosis in patients with AIDS. *Ann Intern Med* 2002;137:105–9.

49. Barbaro G, Barbarini G, Di Lorenzo G. Fluconazole vs. itraconazole-flucytosine association in the treatment of esophageal candidiasis in AIDS patients. A double-blind, multicenter placebo-controlled study. The Candida Esophagitis Italian Study (CEMIS) Group. *Chest* 1996;110:1507–1514.

50. Dinubile MJ, Lupinacci RJ, Berman RS, et al. Response and relapse rates of candidal esophagitis in HIV-infected patients treated with caspofungin. *AIDS Res Hum Retroviruses* 2002;18: 903–908.

51. Lumbreras C, Cuervas-Mons V, Jara P, et al. Randomized trial of fluconazole versus nystatin for the prophylaxis of Candida infection following liver transplantation. *J Infect Dis* 1996;174: 583–588.

51. Biancofiore G, Bindi ML, Baldassarri R, et al. Antifungal prophylaxis in liver transplant recipients: a randomized placebo-controlled study. *Transpl Int* 2002;7:341–347.

52. Powderly WG, Finkelstein D, Feinberg J, et al. A randomized trial comparing fluconazole with clotrimazole troches for the prevention of fungal infections in patients with advanced human immunodeficiency virus infection. *N Engl J Med* 1995; 332:700–705.

53. Fichtenbaum CJ, Koletar S, Yiannoutsos C, et al. Refractory mucosal candidiasis in advanced human immunodefiency virus infection. *Clin Infect Dis* 2000;30:749–756.

54. Goldman M, Cloud GA, Smedema M, et al. Does long-term intraconazole prophylaxis result in in vitro azole resistance in mucosal Candida albicans isolates from persons with advanced human immunodeficiency virus infection? The National Institute of Allergy and Infectious Diseases Mycoses study group. *Antimicrob Agents Chemother* 2000;44:1585–1587.

55. Cartledge JD, Midgley J, Gazzard BG. Itraconazole cyclodextrin solution: the role of in vitro susceptibility testing in predicting successful treatment of HIV-related fluconazole-resistant fluconazole-susceptible oral candidosis. *AIDS* 1997;11:163–168.

56. Bini EJ, Micale PL, Weinshel EH. Natural history of HIV-associated esophageal disease in the era of protease inhibitor therapy. *Dig Dis Sci* 2000;45:1301–1307.

57. Marshall JB, Singh R, Demmy TL, et al. Mediastinal histoplasmosis presenting with esophageal involvement and dysphagia: case study. *Dysphagia* 1995;10:53–58.

58. Young RC, Bennett JE, Vogel CL, et al. Aspergillosis. The spectrum of the disease in 98 patients. *Medicine (Baltimore)* 1970; 49:147–173.

59. Choi JH, Yoo JH, Chung IJ, et al. Esophageal aspergillosis after bone marrow transplant. *Bone Marrow Transplant* 1997;19: 293–294.

60. Neame P, Rayner D. Mucormycosis. *Arch Pathol* 1960;70:143.

61. Margolis PS, Epstein A. Mucormycosis esophagitis in a patient with the acquired immunodeficiency syndrome. *Am J Gastroenterol* 1994;89:1900–1902.

62. Washington K, Gottfried MR, Wilson MI. Gastrointestinal cyptococcosis. *Mod Pathol* 1991;4:707–711.

63. Forsmark CE, Wilcox CM, Darragh TM, et al. Disseminated histoplasmosis in AIDS: an unusual case of esophageal involvement and gastrointestinal bleeding. *Gastrointest Endosc* 1990; 36:604–605.

64. Murata K, Sekigawa T, Sakamoto T, et al. Opportunistic esophagitis caused by Aspergillus fumigatus. *Radiat Med* 1984; 2:24–26.

65. Khandekar A, Moser D, Fidler WJ. Blastomycosis of the esophagus. *Ann Thorac Surg* 1980;30:76–79.

66. Spencer GM, Roach D, Skucas J. Actinomycosis of the esophagus in a patient with AIDS: findings on barium esophagograms. *Am J Roentgenol* 1993;161:795–796.

67. McDonald GB, Sharma P, Hackman RC, et al. Esophageal infections in immunosuppressed patients after marrow transplantation. *Gastroenterology* 1985;88:1111–1117.

68. Nash G, Ross JS. Herpetic esophagitis: a common cause of esophageal ulceration. *Hum Pathol* 1974;5:339–345.

69. Buss DH, Scharyj M. Herpes virus infection of the esophagus and other visceral organs in adults: incidence and clinical significance. *Am J Med* 1979;66:457–462.

70. Shortsleeve MJ, Levine MS. Herpes esophagitis in otherwise healthy patients: clinical and radiologic findings. *Radiology* 1992;182:859–861.

71. Byard RW, Champion MC, Orizaga M. Variability in the clinical presentation and endoscopic findings of herpetic esophagitis. *Endoscopy* 1987;19:153–155.

72. Cronstedt JL, Bouchama A, Hainau et al. Spontaneous esophageal perforation in herpes simplex esophagitis. *Am J Gastroenterol* 1992;87:124–127.

73. Obrecht WF, Richter JE, Olympio GA, et al. Tracheoesophageal fistula: a serious complication of infectious esophagitis. *Gastroenterology* 1984;83:1174–1179.

74. Levine MS, Loevner LA, Saul SH, et al. Herpes esophagitis: sensitivity of double–contrast esophagography. *Am J Roentgenol* 1988;151:57–62.

75. Levine MS. Radiology of esophagitis: a pattern approach. *Radiology* 1991;179:1–7.

76. Agha FP, Horchang HL, Nostrant TT. Herpetic esophagitis: a diagnostic challenge in immunocompromised patients. *Am J Gastroenterol* 1986;81:246–253.

77. McBane RD, Gross JR Jr. Herpes esophagitis: clinical syndrome, endoscopic appearance, and diagnosis in 23 patients. *Gastrointest Endosc* 1991;37:600–603.

78. Genereau T, Lortholary O, Bouchaud O, et al. Herpes simplex esophagitis in patients with AIDS: report of 34 cases. *Clin Infect Dis* 1996;22:926–931.

79. Spruance SL, Tyring SK, DeGregorio B, et al. A large-scale, placebo-controlled, dose-ranging trial of peroral valaciclovir for episodic treatment of recurrent herpes genitalis. *Arch Intern Med* 1996;156:1729–1735.

80. Chatis PA, Miller CH, Schrager LE, et al. Successful treatment with foscarnet of an acyclovir-resistant mucocutaneous infection with herpes simplex virus in a patient with acquired immuno-deficiency syndrome. *N Engl J Med* 1989;320:297–300.

81. Altman C, Bedossa P, Dussaix E, et al. Cytomegalovirus infection of esophagus in immunocompetent adults. *Dig Dis Sci* 1995;40:606–608.

82. Venkataramani A, Schlueter AJ, Spech TJ, et al. Cytomegalovirus esophagitis in an immunocompetent host. *Gastrointest Endosc* 1994;40:392–393.

83. Shepp DH, Moses JE, Kaplan MH. Seroepidemiology of cytomegalovirus in patients with advanced HIV disease: influence on disease expression and survival. *J AIDS Hum Retroviruses* 1996;11:460–468.

84. Schwartz DA, Wilcox CM. Atypical cytomegalovirus inclusions in gastrointestinal biopsy specimens from patients with the acquired immunodeficiency syndrome: diagnostic role of in situ nucleic acid hybridization. *Hum Pathol* 1992;23:1019–1026.

85. Monkemuller KE, Bussian AH, Lazenby AJ, et al. Special histologic stains are rarely beneficial for the evaluation of HIV-related gastrointestinal infections. *Am J Clin Pathol* 2000;114:387–94.

86. Henson D. Cytomegalovirus inclusion bodies in the gastrointestinal tract. *Arch Pathol* 1972;93:477–482.

87. Wilcox CM, Harris PR, Redman TK, et al. High mucosal levels of tumor necrosis factor alpha messenger RNA in AIDS-associated cytomegalovirus-induced esophagitis. *Gastroenterology* 1998;114:77–82.

88. Wilcox CM, Straub RF, Schwartz DA. Cytomegalovirus esophagitis in AIDS: a prospective study of clinical response to ganciclovir therapy, relapse rate, and long-term outcome. *Am J Med* 1995;98:169–176.

89. Chalasani N, Parker KM, Wilcox CM. Bronchoesophageal fistula as a complication of cytomegalovirus esophagitis in AIDS. *Endoscopy* 1997;29:S28–S29.

90. Wilcox CM. Esophageal strictures complicating ulcerative esophagitis in patients with AIDS. *Am J Gastroenterol* 1999;94: 339–343.

91. Balthazar EJ, Megibow AJ, Hulnick D, et al. Cytomegalovirus esophagitis in AIDS: radiographic features in 16 patients. *Am J Roentgenol* 1987;149:919–923.

92. Teixidor HS, Honig CL, Norsoph E, et al. Cytomegalovirus infection of the alimentary canal: radiologic findings with pathologic correlation. *Radiology* 1987;163:317–323.

93. Laguna F, Garcia-Samaniego J, Alonso MJ, et al. Pseudotumoral appearance of cytomegalovirus esophagitis and gastritis in AIDS patients. *Am J Gastroenterol* 1993;88:1108–1111.

94. Wilcox CM, Straub RA, Schwartz DA. Prospective endoscopic characterization of cytomegalovirus esophagitis in patients with AIDS. *Gastrointest Endosc* 1994;40:481–484.

95. Wilcox CM, Straub RF, Schwartz DA. A prospective evaluation of biopsy number for the diagnosis of viral esophagitis in patients with HIV infection and esophageal ulcer. *Gastrointest Endosc* 1996;44:587–593.

96. Goodgame RW, Genta RM, Estrada R, et al. Frequency of positive tests for cytomegalovirus in AIDS patients: endoscopic lesions compared with normal mucosa. *Am J Gastroenterol* 1993;88:338–343.

97. Crumpacker CS. Ganciclovir. *N Engl J Med* 1996;335: 721–729.

98. Erice A, Chous S, Biron KK, et al. Progressive disease due to ganciclovir-resistant cytomegalovirus in immunocompromised patients. *N Engl J Med* 1989;320:289–293.

99. Dieterich DT, Poles MA, Lew EA, et al. Concurrent use of ganciclovir and foscarnet to treat cytomegalovirus infection in AIDS patients. *J Infect Dis* 1993;167:1184–1188.

100. Blanshard C, Benhamou Y, Dohin E, et al. Treatment of AIDS-associated gastrointestinal cytomegalovirus infection with foscarnet and ganciclovir: a randomized comparison. *J Infect Dis* 1995;172:622–628.

101. Jacobson MA. Review of the toxicities of foscarnet. *J Acquir Immune Defic Syndr* 1992;5:S11–S17.

102. Lalezari JP, Stagg RJ, Kuppermann BD, et al. Intravenous cidofovir for peripheral cytomegalovirus retinitis in patients with AIDS. *Ann Intern Med* 1997;126:257–263.

103. Studies of Ocular Complications of AIDS Research Group. Parenteral cidofovir for cytomegalovirus retinitis in patients with AIDS: the HPMPC peripheral cytomegalovirus retinitis trial. *Ann Intern Med* 1997;126:264–269.

104. Martin DF, Sierra-Madero J, Walmsley S, et al. A controlled trial of valganciclovir as induction therapy for cytomegalovirus retinitis. *N Engl J Med* 2002;11:1119–1126.

105. Czock D, Scholle C, Rasche FM, et al. Pharmacokinetics of valganciclovir and ganciclovir in renal impairment. *Clin Pharmacol Ther* 2002;72:142–150.

106. Kirk O, Reiss P, Uberti-Foppa U, et al. Safe interruption of maintenance therapy against previous infection with four common HIV-associated opportunistic pathogens during potent antiretroviral therapy. *Ann Intern Med* 2002;137:239–250.

107. Winston DJ, Wirin D, Shaked A, et al. Randomised comparison of ganciclovir and high-dose acyclovir for long-term cytomegalovirus prophylaxis in liver-transplant recipients. *Lancet* 1995;346:69–74.

108. Gane E, Saliba F, Valdecasas GJC, et al. Randomised trial of efficacy and safety of oral ganciclovir in the prevention of cytomegalovirus disease in liver transplant recipients. *Lancet* 1997; 350:1729–1733.

109. Kroneke MK, Cuadrado MR. Esophageal stricture following esophagitis in a patient with herpes zoster: case report. *Mil Med* 1984;149:479–481.

109. Obrecht WF Jr, Richter JE, Olympio GA, et al. Tracheoesophageal fistula: a serious complication of infectious esophagitis. *Gastroenterology* 1984;83:1174–1179.

110. Gill RA, Gebhard RL, Dozenman RL, et al. Shingles esophagitis: endoscopic diagnosis in two patients. *Gastrointest Endosc* 1984;30:26–27.

111. Orlowska J, Jarosz D, Gugulski A, et al. Squamous cell papillomas of the esophagus: report of 20 cases and literature review. *Am J Gastroenterol* 1994;89:434–437.

112. Schechter M, Pannain VLN, de Oliveira AV. Papovavirus-associated esophageal ulceration in a patient with AIDS. *AIDS* 1991;5:238.

113. Kitchen VS, et al. Epstein-Barr virus associated oesophageal ulcers in AIDS. *Gut* 1990;31:1223–1225.

114. Lockard LB. Oesophageal tuberculosis: a critical review. *Laryngoscope* 1913;23:561.

115. de Silva R, Stoopack PM, Raufman JP. Esophageal fistulas associated with mycobacterial infection in patients at risk for AIDS. *Radiology* 1990;175:449–453.

116. El-Serag HB, Johnston DE. Mycobacterium avium complex esophagitis. *Am J Gastroenterol* 1997;92:1561–1563.

117. Gray JR, Rabeneck L. Atypical mycobacterial infection of the gastrointestinal tract in AIDS patients. *Am J Gastroenterol* 1989; 89:1521–1524.

118. Stoopack PM, de Silva R, Raufman JP. Inflammatory double-barrelled esophagus in two patients with AIDS. *Gastrointest Endosc* 1990;36:394–397.

119. Seivewright N, Feehally J, Wicks ACB. Primary tuberculosis of the esophagus. *Am J Gastroenterol* 1984;79:842–843.

120. Laajam MA. Primary tuberculosis of the esophagus: pseudotumoral presentation. *Am J Gastroenterol* 1984;79:839–841.

121. Ramakantan R, Shah R. Dysphagia due to mediastinal fibrosis in advanced pulmonary tuberculosis. *Am J Roentgenol* 1990; 154:61–63.

122. Porter JC, Friedland JS, Freedman AR. Tuberculosis bronchoesophageal fistulae in patients infected with the human immunodeficiency virus: three case reports and review. *Clin Infect Dis* 1994;19:954–957.

123. Catinella FP, Kittle F. Tuberculous esophagitis with aortic aneurysm fistula. *Ann Thorac Surg* 1988;45:87–88.

123. Rattner HM, Cooper DJ, Zaman MB. Severe bleeding from herpes esophagitis. *Am J Gastroenterol* 1985;80:523–525.

124. Cappell MS, Gupta A. Gastrointestinal hemorrhage due to gastrointestinal Mycobacterium avium intracellulare of esophageal candidiasis in patients with the acquired immunodeficiency syndrome. *Am J Gastroenterol* 1992;87:224.

125. Shafran SD, Singer J, Zarowny DP, et al. A comparison of two regimens for the treatment of Mycobacterium avium complex bacteremia in AIDS: rifabutin, ethambutol, and clarithromycin versus rifampin, ethambutol, clofazimine, and ciprofloxacin. *N Engl J Med* 1996;335:377–383.

126. Gilver RL. Esophageal lesions in leukemia and lymphoma. *Dig Dis Sci* 1970;15:31.

127. Ezzell JH, Bremer J, Adamec TA. Bacterial esophagitis: an often forgotten cause of odynophagia. *Am J Gastroenterol* 1990;85: 296.

128. Howlett SA. Acute streptococcal esophagitis. *Gastrointest Endosc* 1979;25:150–151.

129. Walsh TJ, Belitsos NJ, Hamilton SR. Bacterial esophagitis in immunocompromised patients. *Arch Intern Med* 1986;146: 1345–1348.

130. Laso FJ, Cordero M, Giarcia-Sanchez. Esophageal brucelosis: a new location of Brucella infection. *Clin Invest* 1994;72: 393–395.

131. Chang AD, Drachenberg CI, James SP. Bacillary angiomatosis associated with extensive esophageal polyposis: a new mucocutaneous manifestation of acquired immunodeficiency disease (AIDS). *Am J Gastroenterol* 1996;91:2220–2223.

132. Poles MA, McMeeking AA, Scholes JV, et al. Actinomyces infection of a cytomegalovirus esophageal ulcer in two patients with acquired immunodeficiency syndrome. *Am J Gastroenterol* 1994;89:1569–1572.

133. Ng FH, Wong SY, Chang CM, et al. Esophageal actinomycosis: a case report. *Endoscopy* 1997;29:133.

134. Kim J, Minamoto GY, Grieco MH. Nocardial infection as a complication of AIDS: report of six cases and review. *Rev Infect Dis* 1991;13:624–629.

135. Hudson TR, Head JR. Syphilis of the esophagus. *J Thoracic Surg* 1950;20:216.

136. Stone J, Friedberg SA. Obstructive syphilitic esophagitis. *JAMA* 1961;177:7116.

137. Grimes MM, LaPook JD, Bar MH, et al. Disseminated Pneumocystis carinii infection in a patient with acquired immunodeficiency syndrome. *Hum Pathol* 1987;18:307–308.

138. Kazlow PG, Shah K, Benkov KJ, et al. Esophageal cryptosporidiosis in a child with acquired immune deficiency syndrome. *Gastroenterology* 1986;91:1301–1303.

139. Villanueva JL, TorreCisnero J, Jurado R, et al. Leishmania esophagitis in an AIDS patient: An unusual form of visceral leishmaniasis. *Am J Gastroenterol* 1994;89:273–275.

140. Schacker T, Collier AC, Hughes J, et al. Clinical and epidemiologic features of primary HIV infection. *Ann Intern Med* 1996; 125:257–264.

141. Fusade T, Liony C, Joly P, et al. Ulcerative esophagitis during primary HIV infection. *Am J Gastroenterol* 1992;87: 1523–1524.

142. Kinloch-de-Los S, de Saussure P, Saurat JH, et al. Symptomatic primary infection due to human immunodeficiency virus type 1: review of 31 cases. *Clin Infect Dis* 1993;17:59–65.

143. Rabeneck L, Popovic M, Gartner S, et al. Acute HIV infection presenting with painful swallowing and esophageal ulcers. *JAMA* 1990;263:2318–2322.

144. Kotler DP, Reka S, Orenstein JM, et al. Chronic idiopathic esophageal ulceration in the acquired immunodeficiency syndrome: characterization and treatment with steroids. *J Clin Gastroenterol* 1992;15:284–290.

145. Wilcox CM, Schwartz DA. Endoscopic characterization of idiopathic esophageal ulceration associated with human immunodeficiency virus infection. *J Clin Gastroenterol* 1993;16:251–256.

146. Smith PD, Eisner MS, Manischewitz JG, et al. Esophageal disease in AIDS is associated with pathologic processes rather than mucosal human immunodeficiency virus type 1. *J Infect Dis* 1993;167:547–552.

147. Wilcox CM, Zaki SR, Coffield LM, et al. Evaluation of idio-

pathic esophageal ulcer for human immunodeficiency virus. *Mod Pathol* 1995;8:568–572.

148. Kimmel ME, Boylan JJ. Fistulous degeneration of a giant esophageal ulcer in a patient with acquired immunodeficiency syndrome. *Am J Gastroenterol* 1991;86:898–900.

149. Frager D, Kotler DP, Baer J. Idiopathic esophageal ulceration in the acquired immunodeficiency syndrome: radiologic reappraisal in 10 patients. *Abdom Imaging* 1994;19:2–5.

150. Levine MS, Loercher G, Katzka DA, et al. Giant, human immunodeficiency virus-related ulcers in the esophagus. *Radiology* 1991;180:323–326.

151 Wilcox CM, Schwartz DA. Comparison of two corticosteroid regimens for the treatment of idiopathic esophageal ulcerations associated with HIV infection. *Am J Gastroenterol* 1994;89:2163–2167.

152. Alexander LN, Wilcox CM. A prospective trial of thalidomide for the treatment of HIV-associated idiopathic esophageal ulcers. *AIDS Res Hum Retroviruses* 1997;13:301–304.

36

CAUSTIC INJURIES OF THE ESOPHAGUS

JOSEPH R. SPIEGEL
ROBERT THAYER SATALOFF

The Caustic Substances Labeling Act, passed in 1927, was perhaps the first consumer protection legislation. This law was enacted in large part due to the efforts of Chevalier Jackson, who recognized the hazards of caustic ingestion with the increasing prevalence of caustic substances (1). Lye, used in soap making, was the original offending agent. In 1967, the introduction of liquid drain cleaners with their much higher alkaline concentrations greatly increased the risk of severe injuries secondary to ingestion. Some control of the problem was achieved as manufacturers reduced the concentration of caustic substances in their products in response to reports of injuries, and with the Poison Prevention Packaging Act and the Hazardous Substances Act of 1970. In some countries, lye has been outlawed, and the number of caustic ingestions has been reduced greatly, resulting in a trend toward a predominance of acid-induced injuries (2). However, caustic substances remain ubiquitous and available in the United States and throughout most of the world.

Caustic ingestion can result in a range of injuries from a mild oral burn or sore throat to rapidly progressive life-threatening complications. After recovery from the initial injury, esophageal stricture may develop. Reducing the morbidity of these serious injuries depends on accurate early diagnosis, aggressive treatment of life-threatening complications, and attentive, long-term follow-up (Fig. 36.1).

INCIDENCE

Most caustic ingestions occur in children. The average age of an injured child is <3 years, and this problem has been reported in neonates (3–5). It is estimated that there are over 5,000 accidental caustic ingestions each year in the United States (6). In Denmark, the incidence of pediatric caustic ingestion has been measured at 34.6/100,000, with

esophageal burns in 15.8/100,000 (7). Children are almost always the innocent victims of experimentation with substances found around the home. Even though traditional caustics, such as lye and drain cleaners, are now sold in child-protective containers, they are often transferred to cups or bottles. Other potential caustics, such as dishwasher detergent, denture cleanser, and small batteries, can be found easily by an adventurous toddler. In some cases, toxic ingestions can be part of a pattern of child abuse or neglect.

Caustic ingestions in adults are less common and almost always associated with suicide attempts. In one study, 92% of 484 adults with caustic swallowing injuries treated in France were found to be suicide attempts (8). In Denmark, incidence of caustic ingestion in adults has been measured at 1/100,000 with 61% representing suicide attempts. The remaining cases were mostly accidental ingestion by alcoholics (9). In India, corrosive ingestion is a common mode of poisoning (10).

PATHOPHYSIOLOGY

Alkali Ingestion

The sequence of injury in lye burns of the esophagus was first described by Bosher et al. (11): edema and congestion, principally of the submucosa; inflammation of the submucosa with thrombosis of its vessels; sloughing of the superficial layers; necrosis of the muscularis in varying degrees; organization and fibrosis of the deep layers; and delayed reepithelialization. Superficial mucosal burns often heal without sequelae. Deeper burns into the muscularis can result in delayed healing with fibrosis. Usually only circumferential burns result in strictures. For as long as 2 weeks, inflammation persists, necrotic tissue sloughs, granulation tissue forms, and new collagen is laid down. Between 3 and 4 weeks after the initial injury, the collagen begins to contract, and thus, the process of cicatrization begins (12). When the liquefaction necrosis is transmural, esophageal perforation can result with its attendant high morbidity and mortality rates.

J.R. Spiegel, R.T. Sataloff: Department of Otolaryngology, Head and Neck Surgery, Thomas Jefferson University, Philadelphia, Pennsylvania.

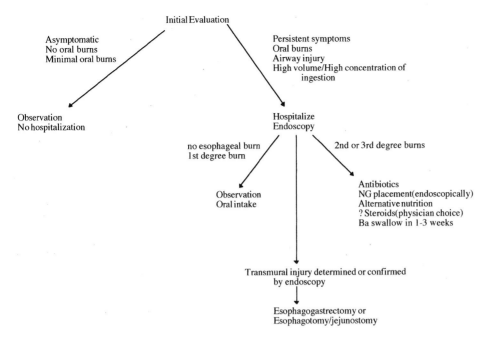

FIGURE 36.1. Algorithm for care of caustic ingestion.

A clinical grading system for esophageal burns has been borrowed from the descriptions of thermal injuries of the skin. First-degree esophageal burns have superficial erythema and edema with only minimal tissue sloughing. Second-degree burns involve the muscularis with ulceration, necrosis, and usually some full-thickness mucosal slough. Third-degree burns are transmural with possible extension to extraesophageal structures (13).

The extent of injury is dependent on two factors: the concentration of the corrosive and the duration of expo-sure. Esophageal stricture has been induced experimentally with as little as a 0.5% NaOH solution (pH 13) and with an 8.8% ammonia solution (pH 12.5) (14). However, most serious esophageal injuries result from ingestion of substances with a pH of 14, and the closer the pH to 14, the more likely the patient is to have an injury requiring treatment (15).

A list of common household products with their corrosive components and concentrations can be found in Table 36.1. Even after safety improvements made in the 1970s, all

TABLE 36.1. COMMON ALKALINE HOUSEHOLD CORROSIVES

Type of Corrosive	Product	Caustic Ingredient
Bleaches	Chlorox	Sodium hypochlorite (5.25%)
	Peroxide	Hydrogen peroxide (3%)
	Minute mildew remover	Calcium hypochlorite (48%)
	Tilex Instant mildew remover	Sodium hypochlorite (5%), sodium hydroxide (1%)
Detergents	Oxydol laundry detergent	Sodium tripolyphosphates (25%–49%)
	Electrasol dishwasher detergent	Sodium tripolyphosphates (20%–40%)
	Calgonite dishwasher detergent	Sodium phosphates (<50%)
	Cascade dishwasher detergent	Phosphates (25%–50%)
	Comet cleanser	Trisodium phosphate (14.5%)
	Polident powder	Sodium tripolyphosphate (<15%)
Alkalis	Drano (liquid)	Sodium hydroxide (9.5%)
	Drano Professional (liquid)	Sodium hydroxide (32.0%)
	Liquid Plummer	Sodium hydroxide (0.5%–2%), sodium hypochlorite (5%–10%)
	Dow oven cleaner (liquid)	Sodium hydroxide (4.0%)
	Crystal Drano (granular)	Sodium hydroxide (54.0%)
Thermal alkalis	Clinitest tablets	Sodium hydroxide (223 mg)
	Efferdent extra-strength tablets	Sodium hydroxide (0.5%–1%)

Source: Moore WR. Caustic ingestions. *Clin Pediatr* 1986;25:192, with permission.

TABLE 36.2. COMMON ACIDIC HOUSEHOLD CORROSIVES

Type of Corrosive	Products	Caustic Ingredient
Acidic cleaners	Mister Plumber (liquid)	Sulfuric acid (99.5%)
	SnoBol toilet cleaner (liquid)	Hydrochloric acid (15%)
	Lysol toilet cleaner (liquid)	Hydrochloric acid (8.5%)
	Cost Cutter toilet cleaner (liquid)	Hydrochloric acid (9.55%)
	Saniflush toilet cleaner (granular)	Sodium bisulfate (75%)
	Vanish toilet cleaner (granular)	Sodium bisulfate (75%)

Source: Moore WR. Caustic ingestions. *Clin Pediatr* 1986;25:192, with permission.

drain cleaners, oven cleaners, and detergents remain sufficiently concentrated to exert their toxic effects at a pH of 14 if swallowed in granular or solid form (16,17). Products with less concentrated alkali, such as Clinitests and denture cleaning tablets, can cause severe esophageal injury because their solid form allows them to lodge in the digestive tract and prolong the duration of action (18). The most common sites of these injuries are at the three natural points of anatomic narrowing in the esophagus: cricopharyngeus, aortic arch, and cardia. Because foreign bodies can lodge at these sites, substances other than traditional caustics can also lead to corrosive injury. A recent report reviewed nearly 100 pill-induced esophageal injuries (19). Antibiotics were the most common offenders, but antiinflammatories, potassium chloride, and quinidine led to a high incidence of secondary complications. There is an increased risk of pill-induced injuries in patients with left atrial enlargement, especially after cardiac surgery (19). Similarly, there have now been many reports of esophageal injury secondary to ingestion of small disk batteries (20). These batteries are a problem in the pediatric population because they are small, shiny, and nonthreatening in appearance. Over one-third of pediatric disk-battery ingestions have been found in children who wear hearing aids (21). The injury in disk battery ingestion is secondary to both a caustic burn from leakage of alkali from inside the battery and a thermal burn from electrical discharge of the battery before it dissolves (22). Because the battery lodges in the esophagus as a foreign body, its effects are concentrated and may lead to esophageal perforation or tracheoesophageal fistula (23,24).

The liquid bleaches are much less concentrated, but they have also been shown to have the potential to cause esophageal injury in both experimental (25) and clinical settings (26). It has long been thought that more viscous liquids, such as the liquid drain cleaners, are more dangerous because of their ability to coat the mucosal surface and thus have an increased duration of effect. However, this concept has recently been questioned in a study that found that relative viscosity of offending agents made no difference when their pH was also considered (14). In recent years, hair relaxants have been involved commonly in caustic ingestions. Hair relaxants are mild alkalis, and although they can cause severe oral burns, they have never been

implicated as a source of esophageal or more distal injury (27).

Acid Ingestion

Esophageal injuries secondary to acid ingestion have been reported far less commonly than injuries due to alkaline products. The mechanism of injury differs, with a predominance of coagulation necrosis and the rapid formation of a protective eschar in tissues exposed to acid. This delays the progression of necrosis into the deeper tissues (28). Additionally, most ingested acids have a rapid transit time in the esophagus, further limiting the opportunity for injury.

Table 36.2 lists the household products involved most often in acid ingestions. Sulfuric acid and hydrochloric acid are the most common offenders by far, but gastric injuries secondary to nitric and trichloroacetic acid, potassium and sodium hydroxide, sodium hypochloride, phenol, zinc chloride, mercurial salts, and formaldehyde have all been reported (29). Even household vinegar has caused injury in young children (2).

Acid injuries have long been thought to relatively spare the esophagus, although they can cause severe gastric injury (30,31). However, a study done in India, where acid ingestion is more common, revealed significant esophageal injury in as many as 85% of patients with gastric or duodenal injuries, and almost one-third of these patients went on to develop esophageal stricture (32). Thus, patients with acid ingestion require the same rigorous assessment and follow-up as patients with caustic alkaline injuries.

EVALUATION

History

Establishing an accurate history of the time of ingestion and the nature of the caustic substance is critical. Since these injuries are common in young children, this often involves sending a parent or guardian back to the home to retrieve a sample of the offending agent, ideally including the labeled bottle. An infant may demonstrate the same level of general distress initially whether a mild or severe corrosive was swallowed, so identifying the substance that was swallowed is often the single most important factor in determining the risk of severe injury. Victims of attempted suicide are often uncooperative historians, and family members or authorities who can investigate the scene of the incident must be interviewed.

Signs and Symptoms

A wide variety of signs and symptoms are associated with caustic ingestion. Since the earliest investigations, there has been little correlation between the severity of presenting symptoms and the extent of the esophageal injury. As many as 10% of patients with significant esophageal injuries may have no early signs or symptoms (33,34), while up to 70% of patients with oral and oropharyngeal burns will not have any significant distal lesion (35). However, recent reviews of pediatric patients alone have shown that there is little risk of subsequent problems in children without symptoms appearing within hours following the ingestion (2,36).

Table 36.3 shows the mild to moderate signs and symptoms of caustic injuries categorized by the anatomic site affected. Oral and pharyngeal findings are established easily by observation and the use of a tongue depressor. Fiberoptic laryngoscopy provides a safe, easy method to complete the laryngeal and pharyngeal examination in almost any setting. Esophageal and gastric examinations must often be repeated to assess findings for signs of complications or long-term sequelae.

Life-threatening complications of airway obstruction, aspiration, or esophagogastric perforation can occur within seconds of the ingestion, or on a delayed basis as inflammation and necrosis progress. Table 36.4 lists the signs and symptoms of the most severe sequelae of caustic ingestions. Death is related to the amount and concentration of caustic substance ingested and has been noted uniformly in patients swallowing >6 ml of a concentrated substance, usually alkaline (37).

Endoscopy

Endoscopy is the single most valuable tool in the assessment of caustic trauma of the esophagus. The key is avoiding iatrogenic perforation of the weakened esophageal wall. Fear of endoscopic injury prompted some authors to suggest that endoscopy on patients suspected of having severe burns is contraindicated (32) or that, in children, it be restricted to patients with significant injuries 2 weeks after the ingestion (38). A review of 115 children evaluated for caustic ingestion in Denmark has suggested that endoscopy is unnecessary in asymptomatic patients (39). However, even earlier studies showed large numbers of patients who safely underwent diagnostic esophagoscopy for caustic injuries. Daly (40) reported 105 consecutive patients and Yarrington (41) reported 70 consecutive patients all having rigid esophagoscopy. More recently, Di Costanzo et al. (42) reported 81 consecutive patients and Rappert et al. (43) reported 102 consecutive patients who underwent evaluation for caustic injuries by flexible esophagoscopy, all without complication.

There are two important factors in performing safe esophagoscopy. First, use the procedure for diagnosis only. The procedure should be terminated before passing the scope beyond any area of severe or circumferential burn. Second, perform the endoscopy within 48 hours of the ingestion, while the lumen wall retains its greatest strength. Some authors suggest a more aggressive approach with full esophagogastroscopy in all patients with severe injuries due to the risk of progressively more severe distal lesions that would otherwise be missed (44,45). The decision to proceed with endoscopy after encountering a severe circumferential burn must be made by an experienced endoscopist with full regard for the possible risks. With these caveats in mind, esophagoscopy is indicated if the history or any of the signs or symptoms raises the index of suspicion for a distal esophageal injury (46).

Either flexible or rigid instrumentation can be used. The flexible esophagoscope is easier to pass and is better tolerated in an awake patient in most cases. A flexible, fiberoptic system is required to assess fully the cardia and stomach due to the anatomic narrowing and the need to "turn" the scope. However, it can be difficult to maintain visualization with the flexible scope in the presence of bleeding and necrotic tissue, so rigid instrumentation is sometimes necessary. An experienced endoscopist can often perform full rigid esophagoscopy with sedation alone, but general anesthesia with muscle relaxation is usually required. Endoscopic findings in the evaluation of acute caustic injuries are shown in Table 36.5.

TABLE 36.3. MILD TO MODERATE SIGNS AND SYMPTOMS OF CAUSTIC INGESTION

Oral/Pharyngeal	Laryngeal	Esophageal	Gastric
Pain	Hoarseness	Dysphagia	Abdominal pain
Odynophagia	Aphonia	Odynophagia	Vomiting
Mucosal ulceration	Stridor	Chest pain	Hematemesis
Drooling		Back pain	
Tongue edema			

TABLE 36.4. SEVERE SIGNS AND SYMPTOMS OF CAUSTIC INGESTION

Airway Obstruction	Aspiration	Perforation
Stridor	Cough	Pain
Agitation	Hypoxia	Tachycardia
Cyanosis	Fever	Fever
Hypoxia	Leukocytosis	Leukocytosis
		Shock

Radiology

A chest x-ray is probably the single most important radiographic study in the earliest stages of severe caustic injuries. Chest x-ray can reveal pulmonary infiltrates secondary to aspiration and signs of esophageal perforation (pneumothorax, pneumomediastinum, subcutaneous emphysema).

Contrast swallowing studies appear to be of little use in the early evaluation of caustic esophageal injuries. Findings of atonic dilatation, intramural contrast dissection, and aperistalsis have been reported in severe injuries and have occasionally been precursors of perforation (47,48). However, even though the correlation of positive radiologic findings to endoscopic findings is reasonably high in some studies (49), other authors have found very high false-negative rates (50). In the evaluation of acute injuries, contrast esophagograms are most useful to rule out and localize perforations. Initial examinations are performed with water-soluble contrast medium due to the risk of extravasation (51). Once perforation is ruled out, studies with barium can proceed.

Contrast swallowing studies are much more important in the evaluation and treatment planning in the later stages of caustic esophageal injury. As patients with moderate to severe injuries are followed, smooth strictures can be noted radiologically as soon as 10 days to 2 weeks after ingestion. Other findings such as diverticulae and aperistaltic segments are not uncommon (46,49). Contrast studies can demonstrate functional deficits such as loss of muscle func-

TABLE 36.5. ENDOSCOPIC FINDINGS IN ESOPHAGEAL BURNS

First degree (superficial)	Nonulcerative esophagitis
	Mild mucosal erythema and edema
Second degree (transmucosal)	Shallow to deep ulceration with possible extension to muscularis
	White exudate
	Severe erythema
Third degree (transmural)	Deep ulceration with possible perforation
	Dusky or blackened transmural tissue
	Little remaining mucosa
	Possible obliteration of lumen

tion or coordination, as well as demonstrate all areas of stricture without the risk of endoscopy (52).

New modalities are being studied to provide additional information about the depth of injury in the early stages. Technetium 99m–labeled sucralfate was used as an indicator of esophageal injury and was found to correlate with endoscopic findings in all cases (53). Endosonography has also been used to assess depth of injury in the esophageal wall (54).

TREATMENT

Initial Management

All patients who are thought to have suffered a serious caustic ingestion are hospitalized. Intravenous fluids are started, and if hypovolemia is present, central venous access is obtained. Intravenous antibiotics should be given prophylactically in any patient being treated for a presumed caustic ingestion.

Airway injury is not very common in adult caustic ingestions, but it is much more frequent in the pediatric population. Moulin et al. (55) found significant laryngeal lesions in 14 of 33 children assessed after caustic ingestions, and 7 children required intubation. Obstruction may not be present initially but may develop over 24 hours with progressive edema of the tongue and supraglottic larynx. If administered early, intravenous steroids can reduce upper airway swelling. If airway support is necessary, intubation is preferred when adequate visualization is possible. However, "blind" nasotracheal intubation should not be attempted because of the potential presence of necrotic tissue in the upper airway. Emergency tracheotomy is indicated in cases of rapidly progressive upper airway obstruction and when there has been a severe laryngeal burn.

After the patient has been stabilized, esophagoscopy should optimally take place within 24 hours. Treatment is then determined based on the patient's general condition and the endoscopic findings. No treatment is necessary in patients with first-degree injuries. As soon as they are tolerating oral fluids, patients can be discharged from the hospital. A follow-up barium swallow study is performed approximately 3 weeks after the injury. Further study is necessary only if symptoms develop or if the barium study identifies an abnormality. Strictures will rarely, if ever, occur in this group (31,56).

In more extensive esophageal burns, the risk of severe complications and stricture is higher. Once the patient has been stabilized, there are many therapeutic options that can be considered.

Nutrition

Most clinicians agree that patients who can swallow should be allowed to take oral nutrition after they are stabilized.

Patients unable to swallow should receive total parenteral nutrition (TPN) or have a nasogastric (NG) tube placed under endoscopic guidance, or undergo gastrostomy. If an NG tube is utilized, it should never be placed blindly due to the risk of perforation. It has been suggested that adequate nutrition alone is the most important factor in promoting healing of an esophageal burn (41).

Steroids

Steroids were originally advocated after they were found to be effective in preventing esophageal stricture in animal models with caustic injury (57–59). Infectious complications of perforation and pneumonia were encountered, but were overcome by the addition of antibiotics (60,61). Subsequently, many clinical reports have supported the use of steroids to prevent the development of secondary esophageal stricture (33,35,52,62,63). A recent review analyzing 13 prior studies (10 retrospective, 3 prospective) found evidence that steroids can prevent strictures in second- and third-degree burns (64). Summarizing the findings of the studies that support steroid use, the following clinical suggestions are noted: steroids are unnecessary in first-degree superficial burns, steroids are not beneficial and potentially dangerous in third-degree severe burns involving perforation or transmural necrosis, steroids should be given early and in high doses (e.g., prednisone 2 mg per kg per day or its equivalent), and steroids should always be given concomitantly with antibiotics. Finally, at least one study suggests that there may be increased effectiveness when steroids are used in conjunction with sucralfate and H_2 blockers (65).

Despite both the scientific logic and the clinical support for steroid use, other reports have questioned the effectiveness of this treatment. Ferguson et al. (66) and Kirsh et al. (67) found no difference in complication rates. Di Costanzo et al. (42) avoided steroid use, advocating "therapeutic nihilism." In this study, 94 patients were treated with supportive care alone, TPN in patients unable to swallow, and oral nutrition in the remaining patients. There were four deaths and five cases of stenosis, four of which required surgery. More recently, Anderson et al. (68) reported a prospective study in which steroids were found to have no effect on stricture rates in patients with moderate and severe circumferential burns.

Thus, there is contradictory evidence regarding the efficacy of steroid use in caustic ingestions. However, if their use is limited to patients with endoscopically confirmed partial thickness injuries, they can be used safely in most cases and may help prevent late sequelae of the injury.

Stenting

The easiest and simplest stent is an NG tube. The endoscopically placed tube can be used to prevent stricture formation as well as provide nutrition (69,70). In patients with deep partial thickness or transmural burns without perforation, a wider intraluminal stent can be considered. This practice was first described in animal models (71,72) and has subsequently been used successfully in both children and adults (73–75). Silicone-rubber or silastic is used. The stent can be placed endoscopically, but some surgeons routinely position the tube through a gastrostomy. Steroids and antibiotics have been utilized routinely, but a recent report by Berkovits et al. (76) described excellent results using a custom-made, twin-tube silicone-rubber stent without steroids.

Dilation

At one time, dilation was considered part of the early therapeutic regimen in caustic ingestions. This practice was abandoned due to the risk of perforation. Dilation is now utilized as the initial treatment for secondary esophageal strictures. The stenotic segments can often be managed with antegrade dilation. A rigid or mercury-weighted bougie system can be used. When stenotic segments are multiple, extensive, or involve the esophagogastric junction, retrograde dilation should be considered. The procedure was first popularized by Tucker (77) in the 1920s and involves having the patient swallow a string that is retrieved through a gastrostomy. Serial dilators are then passed over the string and pulled retrograde into the mouth.

All dilations should be gentle with a goal of slow, progressive improvement. Perforation is a hazard with all manipulations of the stenotic lumen. Steroid and antibiotic treatment is not usually necessary in the secondary treatment of strictures. However, one report did describe an advantage with intralesional steroid injections in conjunction with dilations (78).

The development of dysphagia after the initial injury may be multifactorial, rather than due to stricture alone. Dantas and Mamede (79) reported disordered esophageal motility in almost all patients studied 1 to 53 years after their injury. Other investigative studies such as esophageal manometry, gastric emptying studies, and pH monitoring should be considered in these patients.

Surgery

Surgical treatment is divided into emergency procedures to treat esophagogastric necrosis and perforation, and delayed reconstruction. Widespread necrosis with paraesophageal contamination secondary to a third-degree injury is life-threatening due to the rapid onset of mediastinitis, sepsis, tracheobronchial involvement, and shock. Patients with such severe injuries have routinely responded very poorly to conservative therapy, and thus an aggressive surgical philosophy has been adopted in many institutions (80–83). Gastric necrosis with or without esophageal injury is seen in a high percentage of acid ingestions (84). Often a laparotomy is indicated to diagnose the extent of the intraabdominal complications. These patients undergo emergency esophagogastrectomy and have reconstruction usually with a colon interposition graft on a delayed basis (at least 4 to 6 weeks later). Esophagectomy can be accomplished "bluntly," sparing the patient a thoracotomy (83,85), but the esophagus can be left *in situ* if it is minimally burned (86), and it should not be resected when the trachea is involved. This aggressive approach has greatly reduced mortality and morbidity, and has also yielded acceptable swallowing rehabilitation (10,65,77). A review of patients severely injured by caustic ingestion has shown excellent results utilizing early cervical esophagostomy and feeding jejunostomy, avoiding esophagectomy in most cases (87).

Reconstruction of the esophagus and pharynx is performed either as a planned second stage after an emergency resection or as an alternative to failed conservative treatment of a secondary stricture. If any swallowing can be preserved with periodic dilation, surgery should be avoided (88). If esophageal replacement is necessary, the best results are obtained with vascularized grafts from the stomach or bowel. Colon interposition utilizes the right or transverse colon, on a mesenteric pedicle. The bowel is passed through a retrosternal tunnel into the neck for esophagocolonic or pharyngocolonic anastomosis (89). When the stomach has not been damaged, it can be elongated, passed through the posterior mediastinum, and sutured to the pharynx for total esophageal replacement (a gastric "pull-up" procedure) (90). This has been a useful reconstructive procedure in children as well as adults (91).

Over the past decade, the use of microvascular, free jejunal grafts for reconstruction of the pharynx and cervical esophagus has become popular (92,93). Although this method is used predominantly after cancer resections, it has also been utilized successfully in patients with caustic strictures (82,94). Recent refinements in the procedure may allow free jejunal grafts to be used for total esophageal reconstruction as well (95).

CONCLUSIONS

Caustic ingestion continues to be a complex clinical challenge. Even though most severe injuries are caused by lye or other solid alkalis, all caustic products have the potential to do harm. Acid ingestion must be evaluated with the same concern for serious complications.

Early diagnostic esophagoscopy is the crucial component of the initial evaluation. Contrast radiography is the mainstay of diagnosis in secondary strictures.

Superficial burns require no treatment and limited follow-up. Partial thickness injuries are treated with nutritional support and close follow-up. Most clinicians also utilize steroids and antibiotics during the initial treatment interval. Long segments with circumferential burns can be successfully treated with intraluminal stents. Life-threatening perforations and severe, widespread necrosis are best treated by radical surgical resection and delayed reconstruction. Secondary strictures are treated with dilation or esophageal reconstruction.

Although there have been important advances in the diagnosis and treatment of caustic injuries, much remains unknown. Even the use of steroids and antibiotics remains controversial. Studies of optimal management of caustic injuries are needed, and further refinements in clinical management should be anticipated.

REFERENCES

1. Jackson C. Esophageal stenosis following the swallowing of caustic alkalis. *JAMA* 1921;77:22.
2. Nuutinen M, Uhari M, Karvali T, et al. Consequences of caustic ingestions in children. *Acta Paediatr* 1997;83:1200.
3. Casasnovas BA, Martinez E, Cives V. A retrospective analysis of ingestion of caustic substances by children. *Eur J Pediatr* 1997;156:410.
4. Kushimo T, Ekanem MM. Acid ingestion in a 2-day old baby. *W Afr J Med* 1997;16:121.
5. Turan C, Ozkan U, Ozokutan BH, et al. Corrosive injuries of the esophagus in newborns. *Pediatr Surg Int* 2000;16:483–484.
6. Moore WR. Caustic ingestions. *Clin Pediatr* 1986;25:192.
7. Christesen HB. Epidemiology and prevention of caustic ingestion in children. *Acta Paediatr* 1994;83:212.
8. Sarfati E, Gossot D, Assens P, et al. Management of caustic injuries in adults. *Br J Surg* 1987;74:146.
9. Christesen HB. Caustic ingestion in adults—epidemiology and prevention. *J Toxicol* 1994;32:557.
10. Zargar SA, Kochhar R, Nagi B, et al. Ingestion of strong corrosive alkalis: spectrum of injury to upper gastrointestinal tract and natural history. *Am J Gastroenterol* 1992;87:337.
11. Bosher LH, Burford TH, Ackerman L. The pathology of experimentally produced lye burns and strictures of the esophagus. *J Thorac Surg* 1951;21:483.
12. Waggoner LG. Diagnosis and management of chemical burns of the esophagus. *Laryngoscope* 1958;68:1790.
13. Holinger PH, Management of esophageal lesions caused by chemical burns. *Ann Otol Rhinol Laryngol* 1968;77:819.
14. Krey H. On treatment of corrosive lesions in the esophagus: experimental study. *Acta Otolaryngol Suppl* 1952;102:1.
15. Vancura EM, Clinton JE, Ruiz E, et al. Toxicity of alkaline solutions. *Ann Emerg Med* 1980;9:118.
16. Kynaston JA, Patrick MK, Shepherd RW, et al. The hazards of automatic-dishwasher detergent. *Med J Aust* 1989;151:5.
17. Vadarikan BA. Ingestion of dishwasher detergent by children. *Br J Clin Pediatr* 1996;44:35.
18. Burrington JD. Clinitest burns of the esophagus. *Ann Thorac Surg* 1975;20:400.
19. Kikendall JW. Pill esophagitis. *J Clin Gastroenterol*, 1999;28:298–305.
20. Litovitz TL. Button battery ingestions: a review of 56 cases. *JAMA* 1983;249:2495.
21. Litovitz TL. Battery ingestions: product accessability and clinical course. *Pediatrics* 1985;75:469.
22. Yasui T. Hazardous effects due to alkaline button battery ingestion: an experimental study. *Ann Emerg Med* 1986;15:901.
23. Maves MD, Carithers JS, Brick HG. Esophageal burns secondary to disc battery ingestion. *Ann Otol Rhinol Laryngol* 1984;93:364.

24. Sigalet D, Lees G. Tracheoesophageal injury secondary to disc battery ingestion. *J Pediatr Surg* 1988;23:996.

25. Weeks RS, Ravitch MM. The pathology of experimental injury to the cat esophagus by liquid chlorine bleach. *Laryngoscope* 1971;81:1532.

26. Klein JD. Caustic injury from household bleach too [letter]. *J Pediatr* 1986;108:328.

27. Cox AJ 3rd, Eisenbeis JF. Ingestion of caustic hair relaxer: is endoscopy necessary? *Laryngoscope* 1997;107:897.

28. Ashcraft KW, Padula RT. The effect of dilute corrosives on the stomach. *Pediatrics* 1974;53:226.

29. Gray HK, Holmes CL. Pyloric stenosis caused by ingestion of corrosive substances: report of a case. *Surg Clin North Am* 1948; 28:1041.

30. Chodak GW, Passaro E. Acid ingestion: need for gastric resection. *JAMA* 1978;239:225.

31. Penner GE. Acid ingestion: toxicology and treatment. *Ann Emerg Med* 1980;9:374.

32. Zargar SA, Kochhar R, Nagi B, et al. Ingestion of corrosive acids. *Gastroenterology* 1989;97:702.

33. Crain EF, Gershel JC, Mezey AP. Caustic ingestions: symptoms as predictors of esophageal injury. *Am J Dis Child* 1984;138:863.

34. Ferguson MK, Megliore M, Staszak VM, et al. Early evaluation and therapy for caustic esophageal injury. *Am J Surg* 1989;157: 116.

35. Haller JA, Andrews G, White JJ, et al. Pathophysiology and management of acute corrosive burns of the esophagus: results of treatment in 285 children. *J Pediatr Surg* 1971;6:578.

36. Clausen JO, Nielsen TL, Fogh A. Admission of Danish hospitals after suspected ingestion of corrosives: a nationwide survey (1984–1988) comprising children aged 0–14 years. *Dan Med Bull* 1994;41:234.

37. Berthet B, Castellani P, Brioche MI, et al. Early operation for severe corrosive injury of the upper gastrointestinal tract. *Eur J Surg* 1996;162:951.

38. Borja AR, Ransdell HT, Thomas TV, et al. Lye injuries of the esophagus. *J Thorac Cardiovasc Surg* 1969;57:533.

39. Christesen HB. Prediction of complications following unintentional caustic ingestion in children. Is endoscopy always necessary? *Acta Paediatr* 1995;84:1177.

40. Daly JF. Corrosive esophagitis. *Otolaryngol Clin North Am* 1968; 1:119.

41. Yarrington C. Steroids, antibiotics and early esophagoscopy in caustic esophageal trauma. *NY State J Med* 1963;2960.

42. Di Costanzo J, Noirclerc M, Jouglard J, et al. New therapeutic approach to corrosive burns of the upper gastrointestinal tract. *Gut* 1980;21:370.

43. Rappert P, Preier L, Korab W, et al. Diagnostic and therapeutic management of esophageal and gastric caustic burns in childhood. *Eur J Pediatr Surg* 1993;3:202.

44. Sellars SL, Spence RAJ. Chemical burns of the oesophagus. *J Laryngol Otol* 1987;101:1211.

45. Thompson J. Corrosive eophageal injuries I. A study of nine cases of concurrent accidental caustic ingestion. *Laryngoscope* 1987;97:1060.

46. Friedman EM, Lovejoy FH. The emergency management of caustic ingestions. *Emerg Med Clin North Am* 1984;2:77.

47. Chen YM, Ott DJ, Thompson JN, et al. Progressive roentgenographic appearance of caustic esophagitis. *South Med J* 1988;81: 724.

48. Franken EA. Caustic damage of the gastrointestinal tract: roentgen features. *Am J Radiol* 1973;118:77.

49. Stannard MW. Corrosive esophagitis in children. *Am J Dis Child* 1978;132:596.

50. Mansson I. Diagnosis of acute corrosive lesions of the oesophagus. *J Laryngol Otol* 1978;92:499.

51. Martel WM. Radiologic features of esophagogastritis secondary to extremely caustic agents. *Radiology* 1972;103:31.

52. Ott DJ, Gelfand DW, Wu WC, et al. Radiologic evaluation of dysphagia. *JAMA* 1986;256:2718.

53. Millar AJ, Numanoglu A, Mann M, et al. Detection of caustic oesophageal injury with technetium 99m-labelled sucralfate. *J Pediatr Surg* 2001:36:262–5.

54. Bernhardt J, Ptok H, Wilhelm L, et al. Caustic acid burn of the upper gastrointestinal tract: first use of endosonography to evaluate the severity of the injury. *Surg Endosc* 2002;16:1004.

55. Moulin D, Bertrand JM, Buts JP, et al. Upper airway lesions in children after accidental ingestion of caustic substances. *Pediatrics* 1985;106:408.

56. Hawkins DB, Demeter MJ, Barnett TE. Caustic ingestion: controversies in management: a review of 214 cases. *Laryngoscope* 1980;90:98.

57. Floberg LE, Koch H. The effect of cortisone on the scarification in corrosive lesions of the esophagus. *Acta Otolaryngol Suppl* 1953;109:33.

58. Rosenberg N, Kunderman PJ, Vroman L, et al. Prevention of experimental lye strictures of the esophagus by cortisone. *Arch Surg* 1951;63:147.

59. Weisskopf A. Effects of cortisone on experimental lye burn of the esophagus. *Ann Otol Rhinol Laryngol* 1952;61:681.

60. Haller JA, Bachman K. The comparative effect of current therapy on experimental caustic burns of the esophagus. *Pediatrics* 1964; 34:236.

61. Rosenberg N, Kunderman PJ, Vroman L, et al. Prevention of experimental lye strictures of the esophagus by cortisone II. Control of suppurative complications by penicillin. *Arch Surg* 1953; 66:593.

62. Campbell GS, Burnett HF, Ransom JM, et al. Treatment of corrosive burns of the esophagus. *Arch Surg* 1977;112:495.

63. Cleveland WW, Chandler JR, Lawson RB. Treatment of caustic burns of the esophagus. *JAMA* 1963;186:182.

64. Howell JM, Dalsey WC, Hartsell FW, et al. Steroids for the treatment of corrosive esophageal injury. *Am J Emerg Med* 1992;10: 421.

65. Reddy AN, Budhraja M. Sucralfate therapy for lye-induced esophagitis. *Am J Gastroenterol* 1988;83:71.

66. Ferguson MK, Migliore M, Staszak VM, et al. Early evaluation and therapy for caustic esophageal injury. *Am J Surg* 1989;157: 116.

67. Kirsh MM, Peterson A, Brown JW, et al. Treatment of caustic injuries of the esophagus: a ten-year experience. *Ann Surg* 1978; 188:675.

68. Anderson KD, Rouse TM, Randolph JG. A controlled trial of corticosteroids in children with corrosive injury of the esophagus. *N Engl J Med* 1990;323:637.

69. Wijburg FA, Beukers MM, Heymans HS, et al. Nasogastric intubation as sole treatment of caustic esophageal lesions. *Ann Otol Rhinol Laryngol* 1985;94:337.

70. Wijburg FA, Heymans HS, Urbanus NA. Caustic esophageal lesions in childhood: prevention of stricture formation. *J Pediatr Surg* 1989;24:171.

71. Fell SC, Denize A, Becker NH, et al. The effect of intraluminal splinting in the prevention of caustic stricture of the esophagus. *J Thorac Cardiovasc Surg* 1966;52:675.

72. Reyes HM, Lin CY, Schlunk FF, et al. Experimental treatment of corrosive esophageal burns. *J Pediatr Surg* 1974;9:317.

73. Coln D, Chang, JHT. Experience with esoophageal stenting for caustic burns in children. *J Pediatr Surg* 1986;21:588.

74. Hill JL, Norberg HP, Smith MD, et al. Clinical technique and success of the esophageal stent to prevent corrosive stenosis. *J Pediatr Surg* 1976;11:443.

75. Mills LJ, Estrera AS, Platt MR. Avoidance of esophageal stricture

following severe caustic burns by the use of an intraluminal stent. *Ann Thorac Surg* 1979;28:60.

76. Berkovits RN, Bos CE, Wijburn FA, et al. Caustic injury of the oesophagus. Sixteen years experience, and introduction of a new model oesophageal stent. *J Laryngol Otol* 1996;110:1041.

77. Tucker G. Cicatricial stenosis of the esophagus. *Ann Otol Rhinol Laryngol* 1924;33:1180.

78. Holder TM, Ashcraft KW, Leape L. The treatment of patients with esophageal strictures by local steroid injections. *J Pediatr Surg* 1969;4:646.

79. Dantas RO, Mamede RC. Esophageal motility in patients with esophageal caustic injury. *Am J Gastroenterol* 1996;91:2450.

80. Andreoni B, Farina ML, Biffi R, et al. Esophageal perforation and caustic injury: emergency management of caustic ingestion. *Dis Esophagus* 1997;10:95.

81. Estrera A, Taylor W, Mills LJ, et al. Corrosive burns of the esophagus and stomach: a recommendation for an aggressive surgical approach. *Ann Thorac Surg* 1986;41:276.

82. Gossot D, Sarfati E, Celerier M. Early blunt esophagectomy in severe caustic burns of the upper digestive tract. *J Thorac Cardiovasc Surg* 1987;94:188.

83. Ray JF, Myers WO, Lawton BR, et al. The natural history of liquid lye ingestion: rationale for an agressive surgical approach. *Arch Surg* 1974;109:436.

84. Horvath OP, Olah T, Zentai G. Emergency esophagogastrectomy for treatment of hydrochloric acid injury. *Ann Thorac Surg* 1991;52:98.

85. Hwang TL, Shen-Chen SM, Chen MF. Nonthoracotomy esophagectomy for corrosive esophagitis with gastric perforation. *Surg Gynecol Obstet* 1987;164:537.

86. Ribet ME. Esophagogastrectomy for acid injury [letter]. *Ann Thorac Surg* 1992;53:738.

87. Ribet M, Chambon JP, Pruvot FR. Oesophagectomy for severe corrosive injuries: is it always legitimate? *Eur J Cardiothorac Surg* 1990;4:347.

88. Braghetto ACI. Surgical management of esophageal strictures. *Hepatogastroenterology* 1992;39:502.

89. Postlethwait RW, Sealy WC, Dillon ML, et al. Colon interposition for esophageal substitution. *Ann Thorac Surg* 1971;12:89.

90. Heimlich HJ. Esophagoplasty with reversed gastric tube. *Am J Surg* 1972;123:80.

91. Ein SH. Gastric tubes in children with caustic esophageal injury: a 32-year review. *J Pediatr Surg* 1998:33:1363–1365.

92. Fisher, SR, Cameron R, Hoyt DJ, et al. Free jejunal interposition graft for reconstruction of the esophagus. *Head Neck Surg* 1990;12:126.

93. Gluckman JL, McDonough J, Donegan JO. The role of the free jejunal graft in reconstruction of the pharynx and cervical esophagus. *Head Neck Surg* 1982;4:360.

94. Wang TD, Sun YE, Chen Y. Free jejunal grafts for reconstruction of the pharynx and cervical esophagus. *Ann Otol Rhinol Laryngol* 1986;95:348.

95. Gorbunov GN, Marinichev VL, Volkov ON, et al. Microvascular reconstruction of the esophagus with pedicled small intestine. *Ann Plast Surg* 1993;31:439.

ESOPHAGEAL INVOLVEMENT IN SYSTEMIC DISEASES

JOHN M. WO

Esophageal abnormalities occur in many systemic diseases. However, the clinical presentation of the esophageal involvement varies a great deal. Some patients may have debilitating esophageal symptoms, while others may be asymptomatic despite having impaired esophageal function. In this chapter, I review the esophageal manifestations of the connective tissue diseases, endocrine and metabolic diseases, inflammatory diseases, and neuromuscular diseases.

CONNECTIVE TISSUE DISEASES

Systemic Sclerosis

Systemic sclerosis (SSc) is a generalized disorder of the small arteries with the proliferation of fibrosis affecting the skin and multiple organs. Systemic sclerosis is classified into two subsets, diffuse and limited cutaneous SSc (1). Diffuse cutaneous SSc is characterized by rapidly advancing disease with truncal and acral skin manifestation. The onset of Raynaud's phenomenon, cold-induced peripheral vasospasm with pallor and cyanosis of the digits, occurs within 1 year of the skin changes, as does the presence of antitopoisomerase (Scl-70) antibodies and early visceral involvement (1,2). Limited cutaneous SSc is a stable disease characterized by skin involvement limited to the hands, face, feet and forearms. Raynaud's is usually present for many years, along with the presence of anticentromere antibodies, and a late onset of visceral involvement (1,2). The limited cutaneous SSc includes the CREST variant (calcinosis, Raynaud's, esophageal dysmotility, sclerodactyly, and telangiectasias). Morphea and linear sclerodermas are localized cutaneous forms of scleroderma without esophageal or visceral involvement (3).

The gastrointestinal tract is the third most common organ affected in SSc after the thickening of the skin and Raynaud's phenomenon (4,5). In approximately 8% of cases, gastrointestinal symptoms precede the skin changes (6). Esophageal symptoms are very common, occurring in 50% to 80% of the patients (5,7–9). Other gastrointestinal manifestations include gastroparesis, chronic intestinal pseudo-obstruction, bacteria overgrowth, constipation, and fecal incontinence (2). In a multicenter study of 264 patients with SSc by Altman et al. (10), advanced age, decreased renal function, anemia, pulmonary disease, and hypoalbuminemia were found to be predictors of decreased survival rate. The prognosis in patients with gastrointestinal manifestations of scleroderma is only slightly reduced (10).

Pathology and Pathophysiology

Histologic findings in the esophagus are dependent on the severity of SSc. In the early stages, there are arteriolar changes consisting of a disruption of the internal elastic lamina, a thickened capillary basement membrane, platelet aggregates, swollen endothelial cells, and arteriole sclerosis (11,12). The myenteric plexus is usually unaffected (4,13), but cases of inflammatory infiltration have been reported (11,12). Initially, muscle atrophy and fibrosis are scattered and patchy. In the later stages, extensive collagen infiltration and fibrosis of the smooth muscle occurs. The striated muscle remains unaffected in the proximal esophagus (11,13).

Physiologic and anatomic studies suggest that neural dysfunction precedes the smooth muscle fibrosis in the esophagus. As a result, impaired esophageal peristalsis is present despite normal smooth muscle histology (11). In a study by Cohen et al. (14), the response of the lower esophageal sphincter (LES) was determined by various stimuli. The stimuli used were methacholine to directly stimulate the smooth muscle; edrophonium, a cholinesterase inhibitor, to enhance the effect of acetylcholine; and gastrin I, a hormone that requires endogenous acetylcholine and an intact neural pathway to take effect. In the early stage of SSc, the response of the LES was diminished with gastrin I, but was normal with methacholine and

---

J.M. Wo: Swallowing and Motility Center, Division of Gastroenterology/Hepatology, University of Louisville School of Medicine, Louisville, Kentucky.

edrophonium, suggesting that neural dysfunction occurs before smooth muscle fibrosis (14). In a study by Bortolotti et al. (15), the myoelectric activity was disorganized and hyperactive in early SSc, but the amplitude of the activity was preserved. Parasympathetic impairment and sympathetic hyperactivity can be present, even in early SSc (16). However, the pathologic evidence of neural damage is scarce (12). The vascular changes appear to precede the muscle atrophy and fibrosis (12). One hypothesis is that vascular insufficiency may be the underlying cause of the neural dysfunction (15).

In the late stages of SSc, both neural and muscle dysfunction are present. The response of the LES to edrophonium and gastrin I is more impaired than in early SSc (14). In patients with severe fibrosis and aperistalsis, the direct smooth muscle response to methacholine is also impaired (14). There is a marked decrease in the myoelectric activity in the late stage of SSc, especially in the patients with a dilated esophagus (15). In a study by Miller et al. (17), the degree of esophageal peristaltic dysfunction was correlated with the extent of fibrosis in the muscularis propria by using high-resolution endoluminal ultrasound.

The severity of gastroesophageal reflux disease (GERD) in SSc seems to be associated with the degree of impairment in esophageal peristalsis. In a study of 36 patients by Yarze et al. (18), the severity and proximal extent of reflux were closely associated with the integrity of the distal esophageal peristalsis rather than the diminished LES pressure. While the LES pressures were similar between patients with absent and retained peristalsis, those with aperistalsis had significantly greater proximal and distal esophageal acid exposure (Fig. 37.1A and B). Patients with an aperistaltic esophagus have poor acid clearance and a significant amount of recumbent acid exposure (19). Esophageal sensation appears to be preserved in patients with SSc, even in patients with impaired peristalsis (20).

Clinical Manifestations

Heartburn is reported in 50% to 79% and dysphagia in 25% to 53% of scleroderma patients selected from large series (5,7,21,22). Esophageal involvement does not correlate with the age at diagnosis, gender, duration of disease, or the presence of Raynaud's phenomenon (23). The extent of skin involvement, either diffuse or limited, does not appear to correlate with the prevalence of esophageal manifestations (7,18,22). However, the degree of esophageal dysfunction and erosive esophagitis are generally more severe in patients with diffuse cutaneous SSc (7,22). The clinical progression of esophageal disease in SSc is unclear. In most patients, esophageal dysmotility does not progress in longitudinal studies (24); however, other investigators have reported deterioration over time (25). Patients with diffuse cutaneous SSc may be more likely to progress to severe esophageal dysfunction and aperistalsis. An end-stage dilated esophagus is uncommon in SSc, occurring in about 6% of the patients (5).

The contribution of acid reflux to pulmonary disease in SSc is unclear. Johnson et al. (26) reported an association between the severity of acid reflux and severity of pulmonary disease. However, Troshinsky et al. (27) reported no significant correlation. Complications of GERD are common. The prevalence of erosive esophagitis varies in the literature from 36% to 63% of patients with SSc (5,22,28). In a study of 53 patients by Zamost et al. (28), patients with erosive esophagitis have significantly reduced LES pressure

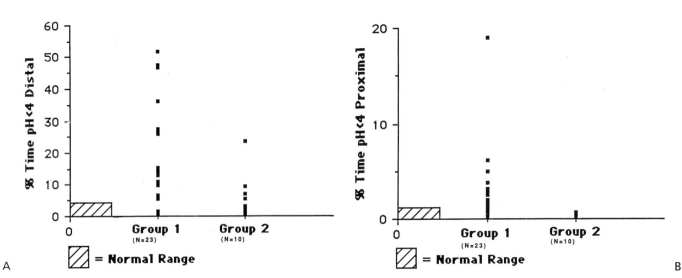

FIGURE 37.1. A: Twenty-four-hour distal esophageal acid exposure in patients with systemic sclerosis (SSc) having absent (*group 1*) and retained (*group 2*) distal esophageal peristalsis. **B:** Twenty-four-hour proximal esophageal acid exposure in patients with SSc having absent (*group 1*) and retained (*group 2*) distal esophageal peristalsis.

and greater acid exposure. The patients with normal peristalsis exhibited no signs of erosive esophagitis (28). The presence of erosive esophagitis may indicate impaired esophageal peristalsis (28). Esophageal peptic stricture has been reported in 3% to 30% of the patients studied (5,9,28).

The risk for Barrett's esophagus and adenocarcinoma in SSc is controversial. The prevalence of Barrett's esophagus varies greatly from 6% to 37% in patients with SSc (5,29); however, esophageal adenocarcinoma is rare. In a review of 2,141 patients, Duncan and Winklemann (30) reported that only one patient had esophageal adenocarcinoma. In a review of 680 patients, Segel et al. (31) also reported only one patient with undifferentiated esophageal carcinoma. In two other series, in a total of 770 patients with SSc, no adenocarcinoma was found (5,32).

Diagnostic Features

Esophageal symptoms are unreliable in judging the presence or extent of esophageal dysfunction (22,33). Occasionally, an air-filled esophagus may be noted on a chest radiograph, but this finding is not sensitive or specific for SSc (34). In the late stages of SSc, a dilated atonic esophagus and the absence of longitudinal mucosal folds may be present. However, the radiographic findings are less sensitive than esophageal scintigraphy and manometry (35). More importantly, barium radiography can detect structural defects, such as an esophageal stricture, hiatal hernia, or small bowel diverticulosis.

Esophageal scintigraphy is a noninvasive test to quantify esophageal emptying. An abnormal esophageal scintigraphy has been reported in approximately 85% of the patients (7,33). The scintigraphy technique varies from liquid (36) to semisolid boluses (33,37). In a study by Kaye et al. (33), 301 patients were evaluated with scintigraphy using a semisolid ingested bolus to quantify the severity of esophageal dysfunction and to detect early dysfunction in asymptomatic patients. Esophageal scintigraphy is reported to be comparable to manometry in SSc (38,39). Scintigraphy can also provide information on gastric emptying and whole gut transit simultaneously (36,37).

Esophageal manometric disturbances of SSc are characterized by hypomotility of the smooth muscle (Figs. 37.2 and 37.3). A diminished LES pressure is very common, occurring in approximately 80% of patients (5,22), and the distal esophageal peristaltic amplitude is reduced in 60% to 86% of the patients with SSc (5,6,35). On the other hand, a normal esophageal manometry is uncommon in SSc, occurring in only 14% to 20% of the patients (5,22). Diffuse esophageal spasms and nontransmitted contractions have been reported but are uncommon (15). The presence of aperistalsis is more common in patients with diffuse cutaneous SSc compared to those with the limited variant (22). Aperistalsis with very low LES pressure distinguishes SSc from primary achalasia. Peristalsis in the striated proximal esophagus and upper esophageal sphincter pressure are preserved (18). The manometric findings in SSc are not specific, occurring also in mixed connective tissue disorder, Sjögren's syndrome, and rheumatoid arthritis (40).

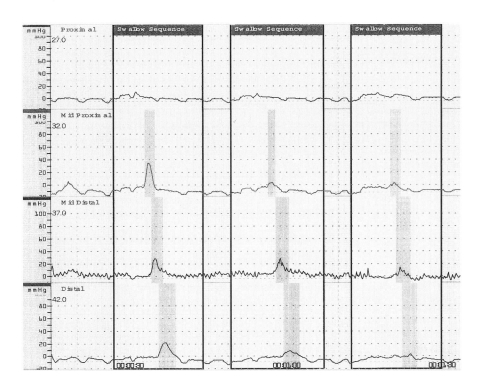

FIGURE 37.2. Esophageal manometric tracing in a patient with limited cutaneous systemic sclerosis. Peristalsis is present, but the distal esophageal peristaltic pressures are diminished.

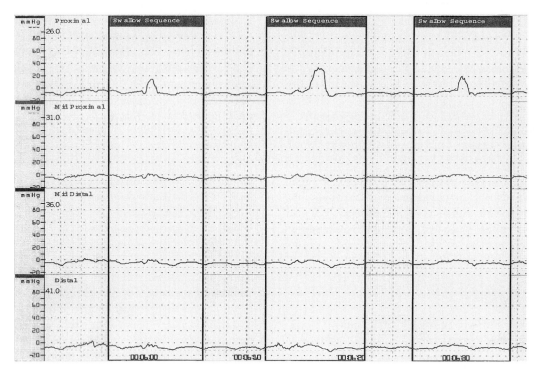

FIGURE 37.3. Esophageal manometric tracing in a patient with diffuse cutaneous systemic sclerosis. The contractions of the striated muscle in the proximal esophagus are preserved but esophageal peristalsis in the distal smooth muscle is absent.

Ambulatory pH monitoring is the most sensitive and specific test for detecting acid reflux. In a study of 55 SSc patients by Stentoft et al. (41), a positive pH test was reported in 67% of the patients with heartburn and in 25% of those without heartburn. The severity of heartburn and regurgitation, however, does not correlate with the severity of GERD by pH monitoring (18). Endoscopy should be performed on patients with dysphagia and odynophagia to detect erosive esophagitis, peptic stricture, and Barrett's esophagus. Impaired esophageal function may be appreciated during endoscopy. The LES tends not to close completely, and lumen-occluding contractions are mostly absent in the distal esophagus (42).

Treatment

The medical treatment of acid reflux in SSc is similar to that of patients with typical GERD without SSc. In uncontrolled studies (5), symptoms improved in 59% of patients with SSc by using histamine-2 receptor antagonists (H2RAs) and 94% improvement with proton pump inhibitors (PPIs). Patients treated with PPIs may be at a higher risk of developing esophageal candidiasis, but the clinical significance of this is uncertain (43). Oral doses of metoclopramide can increase the LES pressure, but have a minimal effect on esophageal function (44). If gastroparesis is present, prokinetic medications such as metoclopramide

and erthyromycin are appropriate. The treatment of skin manifestations in SSc with penicillamine does not improve esophageal manifestations (45).

The role of antireflux surgery in SSc is very controversial. Most reported surgical series consist of open antireflux procedures with few patients, all being performed before the availability of PPIs (46–49). These surgical series have reported improvement of symptoms and acid exposure (46–48). However, LES pressure was mostly unchanged or just minimally improved (47,48). Esophageal body function has shown no significant deterioration after antireflux surgery (48), but recurrence of reflux symptoms and esophagitis is common (49). With the effectiveness and proven safety of PPI therapy, antireflux surgery is best avoided in patients with SSc.

Mixed Connective Tissue Disease

Mixed connective tissue disease (MCTD) is a syndrome characterized by overlapping clinical features of systemic sclerosis (SSc), systemic lupus erythematosus (SLE), idiopathic inflammatory myopathy, and rheumatoid arthritis with the presence of antibodies against the U1-small nuclear ribonucleoprotein (snRNP) complex (50). The clinical features of MCTD are Raynaud's phenomenon, polyarthritis, swelling of the hands, myalgia, and esophageal dysfunction. Unlike those with SSc, patients with MCTD may respond to corticosteroids. Gastrointestinal symptoms such as heartburn, regurgitation, dysphagia, dyspepsia, vomiting, diarrhea, and constipation are common in patients with MCTD (51).

Pathology and Pathophysiology

Similar to the overlapping clinical features of MCTD, histologic changes seem to overlap as well. Histologic findings of the skin consist of vascular alterations and luminal thrombosis similar to SSc (52). Biopsies of the skeletal muscle reveal inflammatory infiltration and focal interstitial myositis that are similar to polymyositis (53). Abnormal autonomic testing suggesting parasympathetic dysfunction is frequently seen in MCTD (54). One hypothesis suggests that the cause of esophageal manifestations is an overlap of the neural dysfunction and smooth muscle atrophy as seen in SSc and striated muscle weakness as seen in idiopathic inflammatory myopathy (51).

Clinical Manifestations

Heartburn and regurgitation are common, occurring in 24% to 48% of the patients with MCTD (51,55). Dysphagia may be present (51,55). In a study by Doria et al. (55), symptoms of oropharyngeal and esophageal dysphagia were both present. In a study of 61 patients with MCTD by Marshall et al. (51), one patient (2%) developed recurrent aspiration, and three (5%) developed esophageal stricture during a mean follow-up of 6.3 years.

Diagnostic Findings

The barium esophagram findings in MCTD are similar to SSc with diminished esophageal peristalsis and a dilated esophagus (51,56). Esophageal strictures can be accurately identified. Dilated small bowel and gastric bezoar have been reported, indicating a more diffuse gastrointestinal dysmotility (51). Videofluoroscopic pharyngeal studies may detect oropharyngeal dysfunction similar to that of patients with polymyositis. The esophageal motility pattern in patients with MCTD is similar to patients with SSc. The LES pressure is diminished but not as severe when compared to patients with SSc (55). Distal esophageal peristaltic pressure is also reduced (55). Aperistalsis has been reported in 17% to 29% of patients (51,57). Water-perfused manometry findings are inconsistent in the striated upper esophagus. The upper esophageal sphincter pressure was reduced in some studies but elevated in others (51,55,57).

Treatment

Corticosteroids and alkylating agents have been used with some success for the skin and systemic manifestations of MCTD (52). In a study of ten patients by Marshall et al.

(51), the effect of corticosteroids on the esophagus was minimal, with the LES pressure improving but the esophageal peristaltic pressures not changing. Pharmacologic acid suppression can be used when heartburn or complications of acid reflux are identified.

Idiopathic Inflammatory Myopathies

Idiopathic inflammatory myopathies consist of a heterogeneous group of acquired disorders including dermatomyositis (DM), polymyositis (PM), and inclusion-body myositis (IBM). Dermatomyositis and PM are more prevalent in women, whereas IBM is more prevalent in men (58,59). Polymyositis and DM are characterized by proximal muscle weakness with difficulty lifting the arms, climbing steps, and arising from chairs. Polymyositis affects mainly adults aged >20 years, whereas DM may affect both children and adults (58,59). Dermatomyositis can be recognized by the characteristic heliotrope rash, periorbital edema, and papular scaly lesions over the knuckles (Gottren's signs). Inclusion body myositis causes a slowly progressive weakness of proximal and distal muscles in patients aged >50 years (58,59).

The diagnosis of inflammatory myopathy is based on elevated muscle enzymes, electromyography, and muscle biopsy. Dermatomyositis and PM can present as an isolated entity or may be associated with an overlapping connective tissue disorder (58). Adult patients with DM and to a lesser extent with PM are associated with the paraneoplastic syndrome (58,59). It may be difficult to differentiate the histologic and clinical manifestations of various inflammatory myopathies because of their heterogeneous nature. Oropharyngeal dysphagia is the most prominent gastrointestinal complaint in inflammatory myopathies (60), with other intestinal manifestations including vasculitis, ulcerations, perforation, and intestinal bleeding (59).

Pathology and Pathophysiology

The histologic changes of the striated cricopharyngeus and the upper esophagus in PM and DM consist of mononuclear inflammatory infiltration, patchy area of necrosis, fiber degeneration, and prominent fibrosis (61,62). The inflammatory invasion of the muscle fibers is more characteristic of PM (59). Involvement of the upper aerodigestive tract may cause weak pharyngeal muscles and uncoordinated oropharyngeal swallowing. Rare cases of smooth muscle fibrosis have been reported, but some patients may have an overlapping connective tissue disorder or a paraneoplastic syndrome (63). Functional disturbances of the distal esophagus have also been reported (64,65). In an autopsy and chart review of 18 patients, de Merieux et al. (64) found that smooth muscle fibrosis was mostly absent despite the presence of radiographic dysfunction of the distal esophagus.

Clinical Manifestations

Dysphagia has been reported in approximately one-third of the patients with DM and PM (66–70) and in 40% of patients with IBM (71,72). In some cases, dysphagia can be the presenting complaint rather than the proximal weakness of skeletal muscles (70,73). Dysphagia is mostly oropharyngeal with choking, nasal regurgitation, dysphonia, and aspiration. Heartburn and regurgitation are uncommon (66). In rare cases, an inflammatory pseudotumor can cause neck swelling and anatomical obstruction (74).

Diagnostic Features

A videofluoroscopic swallowing study is important to detect oropharyngeal dysfunction, such as nasal regurgitation, laryngeal penetration, and residual barium in the piriform sinuses. Assessment of the cricopharyngeus is particularly important to identify poor relaxation during swallowing, prominent cricopharyngeal bar, and Zenker's diverticulum (61,62). Barium esophagram findings may be normal, but impaired peristalsis and aperistalsis have been reported (63,64,67). Manometric abnormalities consist of weak pharyngeal pressures and poor relaxation of the cricopharyngeal muscle with swallowing (61,65,67). The proximal and distal esophageal peristaltic pressures may both be reduced (67). The LES pressure is usually normal (67). Esophageal scintigraphy transit may be delayed (65). The serum creatinine kinase is a sensitive test to detect elevated muscle enzymes in DM and PM (58,72).

Treatment

Corticosteroid therapy is the first line of treatment for patients with PM and DM (58–60). Patients with IBM are usually refractory to corticosteroid therapy (59). Oropharyngeal dysphagia in DM and PM may respond well with corticosteroid treatment (75). Cricopharyngeal myotomy has been successful in selected patients with evidence of poor cricopharyngeal relaxation (61,62).

Sjögren's Syndrome

Sjögren's syndrome is a chronic autoimmune inflammatory disorder associated with the destruction of salivary and lacrimal glands, causing xerostomia and keratoconjunctivitis sicca. Other systemic manifestations include dysphagia, arthralgia, and pulmonary involvement. Sjögren's syndrome can present as a primary disorder or as a secondary disorder associated with other autoimmune diseases. Autoantibody anti-Ro and anti-La are frequently present in Sjögren's syndrome.

The histologic findings of the salivary and lacrimal glands in Sjögren's syndrome consist of lymphocytic infiltration, acinar atrophy, and hypertrophy of the ductal epithelial cells (76). The precise mechanism causing dysphagia is unclear. Many hypotheses have been proposed, such as a lack of saliva, esophageal dysmotility, and a proximal esophageal web. It is believed that the absence of saliva, acting as a lubricant, may lead to impaired solid bolus transit through the esophagus (76). Some investigators have found a significant correlation between esophageal and salivary gland dysfunction (77), but many others have not (78,79). Dysphagia cannot be explained by esophageal dysmotility in most patients. Many case-controlled studies have failed to detect any differences in esophageal peristalsis when compared to normal volunteers (78,79). A cervical esophageal web has been reported in approximately 10% of patients with Sjögren's syndrome (80).

The precise prevalence of dysphagia in Sjögren's syndrome is unclear. In the literature, dysphagia has been reported in 32% to 92% of the patients (76–81). Dysphagia with solids is much more common than liquids (77–80). Most patients localize the dysphagia sensation to the pharyngeal and upper esophageal region (77,79,80). Barium esophagrams are normal in most patients. Close attention to the upper esophagus is needed to detect the subtle proximal esophageal web. Esophageal manometry, with dry and wet swallows, is usually normal in Sjögren's syndrome (78,79,81,82). Lower esophageal sphincter pressure varies, from being low (77) to normal (80,82) to elevated (78), while esophageal peristaltic pressures are usually normal, even when dysphagia is present (77,78). Rosztóczy et al. (77) reported in a study of 25 patients with primary Sjögren's syndrome that propagation velocity was slower than in normal controls. Simultaneous esophageal contractions (79,80,82) and aperistalsis (81,82) have been reported, but these occurrences are rare.

The treatment of Sjögren's syndrome is directed at correcting the lack of saliva. Patients are advised to increase intake of fluids with swallowing (76). Other strategies include a change in diet, chewing sugarless gum, mucous-containing lozenges, and pharmacologic agents such as muscarinic cholinergic agonists (83).

Systemic Lupus Erythematosus

Anorexia, nausea, vomiting, and abdominal pain are common gastrointestinal symptoms associated with systemic lupus erythematosus (SLE). Esophageal involvement is less frequent. Approximately 16% of the patients studied with SLE have an overlapping diagnosis of SSc, rheumatoid arthritis, polymyositis, or MCTD, which are all syndromes that can affect the esophagus (84).

Histologic findings of the esophagus are infrequent in patients with SLE. Harvey et al. (85) reported that only 4 of 105 (4%) patients had arteritis in the esophagus. Salivary gland dysfunction has been identified in SLE, which may contribute to symptoms of dysphagia or acid clearance (86). Esophageal spasms have been suggested to be the cause of unexplained chest pain (87). Reduced LES pressure and impaired peristalsis may contribute to heartburn and dysphagia. However, the correlation between esophageal symptoms and dysfunction has been poor with esophageal scintigraphy (84) and manometry (86,88).

Dysphagia is uncommon, occurring in 1.5% to 8% of patients with SLE (84,89). The prevalence of heartburn and chest pain is unclear. Physiologic esophageal dysfunction appears more common than the presence of esophageal symptoms. Esophageal scintigraphy may detect impaired esophageal transit in about 30% of the patients, including those with no esophageal complaints (84). An abnormal esophageal manometry can be found in 32% to 72% of patients with SLE (57,84,88). Some patients have a manometric pattern similar to SSc with reduced LES and esophageal peristaltic pressures (57,84). However, manometric abnormalities are less frequent in SLE than in SSc (90) and MCTD (57). The prevalence of esophageal aperistalsis is rare, only 4% to 7% (57,88). Symptomatic patients should be evaluated for treatment. Therapy for acid suppression is reasonable when acid reflux is present.

Rheumatoid Arthritis

Gastrointestinal manifestations of rheumatoid arthritis (RA) are rare, if complications of aspirin and nonsteroidal antiinflammatory drugs are excluded. Dysphagia has been reported in 10% to 38% of RA patients in a few small series studies, but usually does not require medical attention (91,92). There are many potential causes of dysphagia in RA. The prevalence of cricoarytenoid arthritis is estimated to be 26% (93). The immobility of the cricoarytenoid joint can affect the coordination of oropharyngeal swallowing. Rheumatoid arthritis may cause an inflammatory mass from chronic synovial inflammation that invades the adjacent laryngeal structures (94,95). This inflammatory mass consists of palisading histocytes, necrosis, confluent rheumatoid nodules, and destroyed cartilage (94,95). The anterior cervical spine spur may cause extrinsic compression on the upper esophagus, but in most cases it is an incidental finding rather than the cause of dysphagia. Geterud et al. (91) reported that RA patients have reduced stimulated saliva production compared to normal controls, but this abnormality was not associated with dysphagia. Bassotti et al. (92) reported that esophageal motility disorders were common in RA, but the clinical significance was uncertain because the symptom correlation was poor.

The presence of dysphagia associated with hoarseness, nasal regurgitation, or stridor should alert clinicians to the possibility that oropharyngeal dysfunction may be present. Radiating pain to the ears and pain with speech may indicate cricoarytenoid arthritis (93). A videofluoroscopic study is helpful to identify functional abnormality. A laryngoscopic and physical exam may identify acute cricoarytenoid arthritis with erythema and edema over the arytenoids,

immobile vocal processes, and tenderness on compressing the thyroid cartilage (93). However, the exam in patients with chronic cricoarytenoid arthritis may be normal with minimal thickening over the arytenoids (93,94). An inflammatory rheumatoid mass may not be apparent on exam and usually requires a computed tomography of the neck (94). Esophageal manometry is likely to be normal in RA (96). Some patients have nonspecific triple peaked waves, spasms, and spontaneous contractions (92), but distal peristaltic pressures are normal in most patients (91,92). The treatment of dysphagia in RA depends on the identifiable underlying etiology. Medical therapy of an inflammatory rheumatoid mass is usually ineffective, and surgical debridement is required in most patients (95).

ENDOCRINE AND METABOLIC DISEASES

Diabetes Mellitus

Nausea, vomiting, diarrhea, and fecal incontinence are well-recognized gastrointestinal manifestations of diabetes mellitus, but the association with esophageal symptoms is not as clear. Bytzer et al. (97) reported that esophageal symptoms were more prevalent in the diabetic patients than nondiabetic controls in a population-based study in Australia. However, a U.S. population-based study by Maleki et al. (98) failed to find such an association.

Pathology and Pathophysiology

The myelinated and unmyelinated nerve fibers, endoneural vessels, and perineurium are all affected in diabetic neuropathy (99). Morphologically, there is progressive axonal atrophy and segmental demyelination of the parasympathetic fibers in the esophagus, similar to that found in somatic diabetic peripheral neuropathy (99,100). The esophageal myenteric plexus is preserved (100). Autonomic neuropathy is very common in diabetes. Some investigators report a significant correlation between autonomic neuropathy and esophageal dysfunction (101,102). However, many other investigators were unable to find any significant correlation (103–106).

The most common esophageal motility abnormality in diabetic patients is ineffective peristalsis (107). The underlying cause remains unclear, but it is believed that diabetic polyneuropathy causes impairment of the autonomic pathways of the esophagus (108). Hyperglycemia also has a significant effect on esophageal motor function (109,110). In normal volunteers, the induction of acute hyperglycemia reduces LES pressure and prolongs peristaltic velocity (110). Furthermore, the response to edrophonium is suppressed, suggesting that impaired vagal cholinergic activity occurs with acute hyperglycemia (110).

The sensory function of the esophagus is impaired in diabetes. Electrical stimulation of the esophagus in diabetic patients with autonomic neuropathy produces erratic or absent cortical evoked potentials, indicative of vagal afferent sensory neuropathy (111,112). Diabetics also have a higher perception threshold for the electrical stimuli (111). The cardiac response to esophageal electrical stimulation appears to be normal, suggesting that the subcortical reflex circuit is intact (112). Acute hyperglycemia may also alter the esophageal visceral sensation. In experimental studies with normal subjects, acute hyperglycemia can enhance the cortical evoked potential response to esophageal balloon distension (113).

The pathophysiology of GERD in diabetes appears to be different than that of typical GERD (114). Silent acid reflux is common in diabetes. In a study of diabetics without heartburn, Lluch et al. (115) reported that 39% of the patients with autonomic neuropathy had pH tests that were abnormal, compared to only 11% of the patients without autonomic neuropathy. The difference was not related to the pressure or the length of the LES (115).

Clinical Manifestations

Heartburn, dysphagia, and chest pain are infrequent symptoms among diabetic patients. The prevalence of heartburn is approximately 14% (116) and dysphagia is 8% to 27% in diabetic outpatients (117,118). Despite having no symptoms, many patients have esophageal motility abnormalities (119). The clinical significance of this silent esophageal dysmotility is still unclear. The presence or absence of reflux symptoms is also an unreliable indicator for acid reflux (120).

Diagnostic Features

The barium esophagram is usually normal in diabetics. Esophageal transit by scintigraphy may be delayed in 30% to 63% of patients with diabetes (101,105,106,117). Approximately one-third of diabetic patients have esophageal manometric abnormalities (121). The predominant finding is diminished muscular tone, indicated by a diminished LES pressure (106,122), and distal peristaltic amplitude (103). There seems to be a close relationship between the level of peristaltic failure and the degree of bolus transit failure, as shown by esophageal scintigraphy (107). Other manometry abnormalities include simultaneous contractions (119,122) and multipeaked contractions (103,119). Esophageal aperistalsis is rarely reported in diabetes (119).

Treatment

Treatment of esophageal dysmotility is usually not required since most patients are asymptomatic. Patients with reflux symptoms should be treated with acid suppression. Prokinetic medications can be used if esophageal symptoms coexist with diabetic gastroparesis. Intensive therapy to control hyperglycemia can effectively delay the onset and slow the progression of diabetic autonomic neuropathy (123). However, the effectiveness of glycemic control for preventing the esophageal manifestations of diabetes is not yet known.

Hypothyroidism

Hypothyroidism is a known cause of hypomotility of the gastrointestinal tract. Constipation, small bowel ileus, and megacolon have also been reported in patients with hypothyroidism (124,125). Reports of esophageal manifestations of hypothyroidism are rare and consist of dysphagia (126–128) and secondary achalasia (129). The underlying histology in myxedema small bowel ileus is the infiltration of the stroma, muscle fibers, and myenteric plexus by mucinous protein complexes (125,130). The precise mechanisms for the esophageal symptoms are unclear. Myxedematous infiltration of the cricopharyngeus has been postulated (127). Myxedema of the vocal cords has been documented in a case report (131).

Oropharyngeal dysphagia has been reported in patients with myxedma who also exhibit characteristic features such as edematous facies and periorbital edema (127,128). Barium videofluoroscopy may identify a delay of pharyngeal swallowing and aspiration (128). The cricopharyngeal muscle may not relax adequately with swallowing during barium esophagram or solid-state esophageal manometry (127). Other reported manometric abnormalities include diminished LES pressure (124,129) and low peristaltic amplitude (124). Esophageal aperistalsis has been reported (129). Dysphagia responds well with thyroid replacement therapy (127,128), and the manometric abnormalities are reversible (127,129).

Hyperthyroidism

Hyperthyroidism can cause a variety of neurologic manifestations, such as thyrotoxic myopathy and periodic paralysis (132). Proximal muscle weakness and wasting of the striated muscles are common. Histologic changes consist of focal myofibril degeneration and mitochondria hypertrophy (132). Thyrotoxic myopathy involving the bulbar muscles can cause progressive oropharyngeal dysphagia (133–136). Solid food dysphagia with esophageal dysfunction is rare (137). The precise cause of dysphagia may be difficult to determine because myasthenia gravis, hypercalcemia, and hypokalemia periodic paralysis may coexist in thyrotoxicosis (132).

Dysphagia is usually progressive and associated with dysphonia, nasal regurgitation, and choking while swallowing (138). The degree of hyperthyroidism in patients with dysphagia is usually severe with marked weight loss and muscle wasting. Videofluoroscopic studies can identify reduced pharyngeal movement, pooling of barium, and laryngeal penetration (135,136). Impaired esophageal peristalsis has been described with barium esophagram (137,139). Meshkinpour et al. (140) reported that the velocity of the propagation contraction by manometry was prolonged in the patients with hyperthyroidism compared to normal controls, but the proximal and distal esophageal peristaltic amplitudes were similar. However, most of the patients did not complain of dysphagia (140). The details of the esophageal manometry in symptomatic patients are scarce (133,134). Dysphagia usually resolves completely after the patient is treated for hyperthyroidism, but improvement may take several months (138). Radiographic abnormalities return to normal when the patient becomes euthyroid (135–137,139).

Hypercalcemia

Hypercalcemia is a common manifestation of many disorders, such as hyperparathyroidism, paraneoplastic syndrome, and increased bone turnover. Gastrointestinal symptoms of hypercalcemia include constipation, anorexia, nausea, and vomiting. Esophageal manifestations are rare. Chronic hypercalcemia results in the depression of the nervous system because the neuronal membrane becomes impermeable to sodium ions; thus it is unable to generate action potentials (141). Therefore, striated and smooth muscle contractility is reduced. Dysphagia to solids has been reported in patients with hypercalcemia associated with a paraneoplastic syndrome (141,142). Heartburn was reported to be common by some investigators (143). Esophageal manometry may reveal a low LES pressure (143); however, manometry of the esophageal body is grossly normal (142). The treatment of hypercalcemia depends on the underlying cause. Dysphagia readily improves after the correction of hypercalcemia (141,142). Serial esophageal manometries have documented the improvement of the LES pressure during the treatment of hypercalcemia (143).

Hypomagnesemia

Magnesium deficiency is a complication of nutritional deficiency states, such as alcoholism, starvation, short-bowel syndrome, and diseases of malabsorption. Hypomagnesemia causes irritability, myoclonic spasm, convulsions, ataxia, and dysphagia (144). Magnesium inhibits the liberation of acetylcholine at the neuromuscular junction and sympathetic ganglia (145), thereby relaxing smooth muscles in the uterus, blood vessels, and bronchial airways (146). Magnesium deficiencies result in enhanced neuronal excitability. Dysphagia to solids and chest pain has been reported in patients with hypomagnesemia (145,147,148). Pharyngeal and hypopharyngeal dyskinetic movements can be seen with videofluoroscopy (147). Barium esophagrams have demonstrated rare cases of diffuse esophageal spasms (145) and aperistalsis (147). Dysphagia and esophageal spasms are reversible after replenishing the body's supply of magnesium (145,147).

Alcoholism

Excessive alcohol ingestion is associated with multiple abnormalities in the gastrointestinal tract. The most recognized complications in the esophagus are the development of esophageal varices from liver damage and Mallory-Weiss tears from vomiting; both are indirect effects of alcohol (149). Direct effects of acute and chronic alcohol ingestion include esophageal motor abnormalities (150–153) and gastroesophageal reflux (GER) (154,155).

The pathophysiology of the effects of alcohol on the esophagus is complex. Alcohol causes direct damage of the mucosa by impairing the epithelial active ion transport and barrier function, leading to the breakdown of mucosal resistance (156). In a rabbit model by Bor et al. (156), the detrimental mucosa effect is dependent on the concentration of alcohol and exposure time. Multiple animal studies have demonstrated that acute alcohol exposure predisposes the esophagus to acid and bile mucosal injury (157–159).

Acute alcohol ingestion causes transient esophageal dysmotility. In a study of normal volunteers by Hogan et al. (150), acute intoxication with oral and intravenous ethanol caused impairment of the primary esophageal peristalsis and reduction of LES pressure (150). In a study by Mayer et al. (152), esophageal motor abnormalities were dependent on the serum alcohol concentration, and the LES pressure was reduced in response to a protein meal. Acute alcohol ingestion appears to exert a direct effect on esophageal motility, rather than a neurally mediated process (160,161). In a cat model by Keshavarzian et al. (161), acute alcohol exposure suppressed the contractility of esophageal smooth muscle, which was not abolished by bilateral vagal vagotomy or intravenous tetrodotoxin (161).

In chronic alcohol abuse, esophageal peristaltic amplitude and LES pressures tend to be elevated, rather than diminished, during intoxication and alcohol withdrawal (162–164). Interestingly, the esophageal dysmotility persisted in individuals with ongoing alcoholism, while it normalized in those who abstain from alcohol (163,164). Winship et al. (151) reported that alcoholic neuropathy was associated with impaired distal esophageal peristalsis, but other investigators found no correlation (163,164).

Nocturnal (155) and postprandial (154) GER are increased with acute alcohol ingestion in normal volunteers. However, the associations between alcohol consumption complications of acid reflux, such as erosive esophagitis (165,166) and Barrett's esophagus (165,167–169), are lacking in case-controlled studies. The prevalence of heartburn is common in actively drinking alcoholics presenting to treatment centers, occurring in 33% to 52% of the patients (164,170). Esophageal symptoms decrease significantly with alcohol abstinence (170). Patients with reflux symptoms should be treated with acid suppression. Treatment of esophageal dysmotility is usually not required since most patients are asymptomatic (163).

INFLAMMATORY DISEASES

Crohn's Disease

Crohn's disease is a systemic inflammatory disorder affecting the entire gastrointestinal tract. The prevalence of esophageal involvement is only 0.2% to 1.8% from two large retrospective series of patients with Crohn's disease (171,172). However, the true prevalence of esophageal involvement is unclear, since most cases were discovered during the evaluation of esophageal symptoms (172). In a study of 41 unselected patients with Crohn's disease regardless of the presence or absence of esophageal symptoms, 2 patients (5%) had esophageal involvement by upper endoscopy (173).

Pathology and Pathophysiology

The histologic findings in the esophagus consist of polymorphic inflammatory cells in the squamous epithelium and lamina propria (174). The infiltrate consists of lymphocytes, eosinophils, mast cells, and neutrophils (171). A proliferation of histocytes and noncaseating granulomas may be present. Epithelial basal zone hyperplasia is usually absent (171,174). The inflammation can be transmural causing extensive fibrosis with anatomical obstruction of the esophageal lumen (175). Fissures may penetrate deep into the muscularis forming fistulas to adjacent organs.

Clinical Manifestations

Dysphagia, odynophagia, retrosternal pain, and epigastric discomfort are symptomatic complaints associated with esophageal Crohn's disease (172). Dysphagia can be severe with marked weight loss in patients with a long narrowed stricture (176,177). Esophageal erosions and ulcerations are the most common lesions found at endoscopy (171,172). The ulcers are usually superficial aphthous ulcers, but deep penetrating ulcers may occur (178). Crohn's fistulas to the bronchopulmonary tree (178), mediastinum (179), pleura (180), and gastric cardia (181) have been reported. Ileitis or colitis is present in 95% to 100% of the patients with esophageal involvement (171,172,174). Isolated esophageal Crohn's disease is very rare (175,182).

Diagnostic Features

A double-contrast barium esophagram is needed to adequately visualize the mucosa, but it can be normal in up to 50% of the patients with documented esophageal involvement (172). Aphthous ulcers appear as punctate, slit-like, or ring-like collections of barium (183). Occasionally, thickened, irregular, and nodular mucosa folds may be seen. Strictures and fistulas can be identified with a barium esophagram. Endoscopy is very helpful to identify and biopsy the mucosa lesions. Endoscopic findings vary, consisting of multiple, shallow, irregular erosions and ulcers. Ulcerations with polypoid cobblestone features can be present. Other findings include irregular longitudinal mucosal ridges and prominent scarring of the esophagus (Color Plate 37.4). Endoscopic biopsy findings are not specific. Some investigators have found noncaseating granuloma in more than 50% of the cases (171,174) while others found none (172).

Treatment

There is no prospective study on the treatment of esophageal Crohn's disease. Some patients with esophageal ulcers have responded well to 5-aminosalicylates or corticosteroids (171,172). In a study of 14 patients by D'Haens et al. (174), esophageal ulcers were healed in 64% treated with corticosteroids. During follow-up endoscopies, 57% of their patients remained in remission, 21% had a relapse, and 21% had refractory ulcers (174). Immune-modifying agents have been successful in a few cases (172). Esophageal dilation can improve dysphagia in patients with strictures (172,179). Long stenotic strictures and fistulas may require surgical intervention.

Behçet's Disease

Behçet's disease is a systemic vasculitis with chronic relapsing symptoms. Patients with Behçet's disease cluster along the ancient Silk Road from eastern Asia to the Mediterranean basin. The prevalence of Behçet's disease is highest in Turkey at 80 to 370 cases per 100,000 (184). The prevalence in Japan, Korea, China, Iran, and Saudi Arabia is approximately 13.5 to 20 cases per 100,000 (184). Major clinical features of Behçet's disease are recurrent oral ulcers, genital ulcers, uveitis, erythema nodosum, and papulopustular skin lesions. Other features include thrombophlebitis and arthritis. The prevalence of gastrointestinal involvement varies, from a low frequency in Turkey (3% to 5%) to a high frequency in Japan (50% to 60%) (184). Ileocecal ulcerations are the most common lesions. Esophageal involvement is uncommon, reported to be 2% to 11% of the patients with Behçet's disease (185).

Pathology and Pathophysiology

The etiology of Behçet's disease is unknown but most likely involves immune mechanisms, infectious agents, and genetic factors (186). Systemic vasculitis, hyperfunction of neutrophils, and autoimmune inflammatory response are the predominant features (184). Histologic findings in the esophagus consist of nonspecific ulcerations in the squamous mucosa with a neutrophilic inflammatory infiltrate (187). Proliferative arteriolitis has been identified (187). The inflammatory process can be transmural with significant fibrosis resulting in esophageal stenosis (187).

Clinical Manifestations

Esophageal symptoms of Behçet's disease consist of dysphagia, chest pain, and odynophagia (185,187). The most common lesions are recurrent esophageal erosions and ulcers (188,189). Deep penetrating ulcers can develop and dissect into the deep layers (190) and form a fistula to the adjacent organs (187). In rare cases, hematemesis and esophageal perforation may occur (187). Luminal esophageal strictures can develop causing persistent dysphagia (187,189). Esophageal lesions usually parallel oral ulcerations in Behçet's disease (185). A rare complication of Behçet's disease is the formation of esophageal varices from thrombosis of the superior vena cava or portal vein (185,190).

Diagnostic Features

Diagnostic features in the esophagus are similar to esophageal Crohn's disease. Barium esophagram findings include mucosal ulcerations, irregular strictures, and fistula to the adjacent organs (187). Endoscopic screening in patients without esophageal symptoms is usually normal and not clinically helpful (189). Endoscopic findings consist of multiple discrete ulcers, which can be anywhere along the esophagus (190). Esophageal strictures may be present along with mucosal bridges and prominent scarring. Endoscopic biopsies are not specific for Behçet's disease (187). There are no signs, symptoms, or laboratory tests specific to Behçet's disease.

Treatment

The treatment of esophageal symptoms is to treat the underlying Behçet's disease. Resolution of esophageal ulcers has been reported with corticosteroid therapy (188). Spontaneous remission of esophageal ulcers can occur. Long stenotic strictures and fistulas may require surgical intervention.

Sarcoidosis

Sarcoidosis is a systemic disorder of unknown etiology. It affects nearly all ages, ethnicities, and geographical regions (191). In the United States, patients are predominately African American. Sarcoidosis is characterized by accumulation of T-lymphocytes, macrophages, and noncaseating epithelial granuloma. It affects the lungs in 90% of patients,

and less frequently affects the lymph nodes, skin, eyes, nasopharynx, and liver (191). In a review of 1,254 cases of sarcoidosis, Mayock et al. (192) did not identify a single case of esophageal involvement. However, sporadic cases of esophageal sarcoidosis have been reported (193–202).

Pathology and Pathophysiology

Sarcoidosis can affect the esophagus in many different ways. The mid-esophagus may be compressed extrinsically by mediastinal lymphadenopathy (194,195). Direct granulomatous infiltration of the esophagus can result in a markedly thickened esophagus (199,201). Development of strictures may occur. The histologic findings consist of mononuclear inflammatory cells and noncaseating granuloma (199,201). Direct involvement of the myenteric plexus has been reported (193,197), producing an achalasia-like picture. The number of neurons appears to be normal, but there may be extensive demyelinization and axonal loss of the myenteric nerve fibers (197). Sarcoid myopathy of the striated upper esophagus has been reported, but the diagnosis was made indirectly by biopsying muscles from the quadriceps (203). Direct granulomatous infiltration of the larynx may cause oropharyngeal dysphagia (204,205). Sarcoidosis can present as an inflammatory mass affecting the brainstem and cranial nerves that are critical for oropharyngeal swallowing (199,206)

Clinical Manifestations

Dysphagia is the most common presentation of esophageal sarcoidosis. The severity of dysphagia depends on the underlying pathophysiology described above. Dysphagia can be mild with extrinsic compression of the esophagus (194) or severe with marked weight loss in direct esophageal infiltration with sarcoidosis (199) or secondary achalasia (200). In rare cases, dysphagia may be associated with nasal regurgitation, dysphonia, and dyspnea, if the larynx or cranial nerves are involved.

Diagnostic Features

A barium esophagram can identify areas of esophageal narrowing. Narrowing at the level of carina suggests extrinsic compression by subcarinal lymphadenopathy (194). A dilated esophagus and tapered gastroesophageal junction mimicking achalasia may be noted on esophagram or upper endoscopy (197,200). Mucosal irregularity and circumferential narrowing have been described in direct infiltration (196,202). Endoscopic biopsy may reveal the typical noncaseating, giant-cell granuloma and mononuclear infiltrates (200). However, special stains are needed to exclude tuberculosis and histoplasmosis. Manometric abnormalities may vary. Lower esophageal sphincter relaxation may be incomplete (193,200). Esophageal peristalsis can be decreased in amplitude (203) or nontransmitted (198), and aperistalsis has also been reported (198).

The chest radiograph is abnormal in nearly all cases of esophageal sarcoidosis. Chest-computed tomography may be needed to identify the mediastinal lymphadenopathy. Surgical mediastinal biopsy may be necessary to make the diagnosis, but recently, endoscopic ultrasound has been shown to be helpful in identifying the anatomy of the mediastinum and obtaining tissue with fine needle aspiration (207). Serum angiotensin-converting enzyme (ACE) level is elevated in two-thirds of patients with sarcoidosis, but approximately 5% of the positive tests can occur in other granulomatous disorders (191).

Treatment

Treatment with corticosteroids has been successful in relieving dysphagia (195,199,203), and manometric abnormalities may return to normal (198). Among the rare cases of secondary achalasia, botulinum toxin injection (200) and Heller myotomy (193,197) have improved dysphagia but residual symptoms may persist.

Eosinophilic Esophagitis

Eosinophilic esophagitis represents a distinct clinicopathologic entity with eosinophilic infiltration of the squamous epithelium or the deep layers of the esophagus. This disorder was once thought to be limited to children but is now being recognized in adults. There is a strong male predominance in children (208,209) and adults (210–213). Many descriptive diagnoses have been used in the literature for eosinophilic esophagitis, such as multiple esophageal rings (214), ringed esophagus (213), corrugated esophagus (215), and small-caliber esophagus (210). Endoscopic biopsy is required to make the diagnosis. Eosinophilic esophagitis should be differentiated from other disease states that can cause esophageal eosinophilia, such as GERD, collagen vascular syndromes, and infections.

Pathology and Pathophysiology

In animal experiments by Mishra et al. (216), it was reported that cytokine interleukin-5 (IL-5) has a major role in directing eosinophils to the esophagus. Esophageal eosinophilia can be induced by systemic IL-5 and allergen exposure (216). Straumann et al. (211) reported that T-lymphocytes and mast cells are increased in adults with eosinophilic esophagitis, along with an elevated expression of IL-5, tumor necrosis factor-α, and IgE-mediated inflammation. Eosinophilic esophagitis appears to be a selective inflammatory response that may be linked to allergic reactions (211).

The inflammation is usually limited to the mucosa with an eosinophilic inflammatory infiltrate (212), but submucosal thickening has been identified using endoscopic ultrasound (217). Besides the intraepithelial eosinophils, histology consists of basal layer hyperplasia and elongation of the papillae in the lamina propria (210,213,218,219). In rare cases, there is marked esophageal muscular hypertrophy with eosinophilic infiltration of the muscularis propria and the myenteric plexus (217,220). Multiple concentric strictures may develop throughout the esophagus. The underlying cause of the stricture formation is unclear. It may represent a progression of the inflammatory process in eosinophilic esophagitis (215) or a complication of acid reflux with esophageal shortening and infolding of redundant mucosa (213).

Clinical Manifestations

Dysphagia is the most common complaint in the adult patients (211,213,218). Dysphagia is usually chronic with multiple episodes of food impaction (210,211,213,221). The diagnosis of eosinophilic esophagitis may go unrecognized for many years (213,222). Attwood et al. (212) presented a series of 12 adult patients with prominent dysphagia but normal endoscopy. Morrow et al. (213) presented 19 adults with multiple concentric rings, and most patients reported long-standing dysphagia since childhood or adolescence. Chest and epigastric pain can also be the chief complaints in some patients in eosinophilic esophagitis (223,224).

Children with eosinophilic esophagitis have a different presentation consisting of dysphagia, vomiting, heartburn, regurgitation, chest pain, nausea, epigastric pain, slow growth, and respiratory symptoms (208,209,219,222,225). These children are often diagnosed initially with GERD and have persistent symptoms despite acid-suppression medication (208) and antireflux surgery (225). An allergic condition, such as asthma, allergic rhinitis, or atopic dermatitis, has been reported in over 80% of children with eosinophilic esophagitis (208,219).

Diagnostic Features

In the patients with dysphagia, a barium esophagram can detect the multiple strictures with narrowing of the lumen (210,213,224). However, the esophagram can be normal (213). Endoscopic findings consist of circumferential mucosa ridges along the length of the esophagus and diffuse narrowing of the lumen (Color Plates 37.5 and 37.6). The esophageal mucosa usually appears normal, emphasizing the need for biopsies. Barrett's esophagus has been reported in some patients with multiple concentric rings (213). The precise number of intraepithelial eosinophils per high power field (HPF) required to diagnose eosinophilic esophagitis is unknown. Most studies have used 15 to 20 as a threshold (209,210). In GERD, the number of eosinophils in the distal esophagus is less than five to ten cells per HPF (222). Finding eosinophils in the upper esophagus (219), eosinophils concentrated near the epithelial surface (212), aggregates of eosinophils (219), and scattered eosinophilic granules (212) are more indicative of eosinophilic esophagitis. Endoscopic biopsy can be nondiagnostic in rare cases, and eosinophilic esophagitis is discovered only after surgical resection (217).

Esophageal manometric findings are nonspecific. Reduced LES pressure, multipeaked waves, prolonged contraction duration, elevated peristaltic pressure, diffuse spasm, and vigorous achalasia have all been reported (212,217,220,223). Esophageal manometry can be normal, even in the patients with multiple concentric rings (210). Ambulatory pH monitoring may be needed to detect GERD (222). Spergel et al. (208) were able to identify potential food antigens, such as milk, egg, soy, wheat, beef and rye, in 24 children diagnosed with eosinophilic esophagitis using the skin prick or patch tests.

Treatment

Mechanical dilation is needed for multiple concentric rings causing dysphagia. However, deep mucosa tears occur frequently after dilation in adult patients with some patients requiring hospitalization for pain (210,213,215). Wire-guided dilation under fluoroscopic guidance can be performed safely, but the dilator sizes should progress gradually and cautiously. In a retrospective review by Morrow et al. (213), 18 of 19 adult patients with multiple concentric rings responded to esophageal dilations and proton pump inhibitors. Successful treatment with oral corticosteroids has been reported in adult patients refractory to dilations, but the data are very limited (212,213,226,227).

In children with eosinophilic esophagitis, dietary elimination of allergens was successful in 69% of patients in a prospective trial by Spergel et al (208). In a prospective study by Kelly et al. (228), ten children were fed elemental amino acid-based formulas for a minimum of 6 weeks. Symptoms were resolved in eight children but relapsed when the allergen was reintroduced (228). Successful treatment of eosinophilic esophagitis in children has been reported with oral corticosteroids (229). Topical corticosteroids have been tried by swallowing puffs of fluticasone inhalers, with a mixed treatment response (230).

Necrotizing Esophagitis

Necrotizing esophagitis represents an episode of acute esophageal necrosis resulting in a blackened esophageal mucosa at endoscopy. The prevalence of necrotizing esophagitis is reported to be 0.01% to 0.2% among patients undergoing upper endoscopies (231,232). Necrotizing esophagitis should be differentiated from other rare conditions that can cause a black esophagus without necrosis such as melanosis (233), pseudomelanosis from pigments of

lysosomal degradation (234), coal dust (235), and acanthosis nigricans (236).

The histologic findings of acute necrotizing esophagitis consist of severe acute inflammation, diffuse ulcerations, denuded epithelium, thrombosis of blood vessels, and extensive necrosis of the mucosa and submucosa (231). There are many proposed causes for necrotizing esophagitis. Ischemia is believed to be the most common etiology (231,234,237,238). Although the esophagus has a rich blood supply from the aorta, bronchial, intercostal, left gastric, and inferior thyroid arteries (239), a low-flow state during hypotension may cause mucosal ischemia and necrosis, which rapidly resolves after hemodynamic correction (231,234,238,240). Some cases have been reported after certain surgeries, which can compromise the blood supply to the esophagus (241,242). Cytomegalovirus (CMV) and herpes simplex virus (HSV) have been isolated (243,244), but it is unclear whether these organisms were the underlying cause. Severe acid reflux has been proposed as well (245). Hypersensitive drug reactions with antibiotics have been reported as a cause of necrotizing esophagitis (246).

Acute necrotizing esophagitis usually presents in seriously ill patients with multiple organ failure. In a prospective study by Soussan et al. (231), hypotension, acute renal failure, poor nutritional status, and other underlying conditions were common. Hematemesis is usually the presenting symptom (231). Upper endoscopy reveals the characteristic findings of extensive, circumferential, black appearance of the esophageal mucosa, sometimes with adherent yellow exudate (231,247). Mucosal bridges and submucosal lacerations have been noted (243). Biopsy findings are nonspecific, consisting of severe acute inflammation and extensive mucosal necrosis.

Conservative supportive treatment is successful in some patients with acute necrotizing esophagitis (234). Hemodynamic compromise must be corrected. Treating the underlying cause and using intravenous broad-spectrum antibiotics are recommended. If the patient survives the acute illness, the esophageal necrosis usually resolves (231), but stenosis may form causing significant dysphagia (240,247). Unfortunately, many patients die from the coexisting acute illness and not from necrotizing esophagitis (231).

NEUROMUSCULAR DISEASES

Neuromuscular diseases represent a category of acquired and primary disorders affecting the motor neurons, peripheral nerves, neuromuscular junctions, and muscles. Abnormalities involving the parasympathetic, sympathetic, and enteric nervous systems can potentially affect the esophagus. The degree of esophageal involvement varies significantly among the different neuromuscular diseases. Esophageal dysfunction can be debilitating or can occur with minimal or no symptomatology.

American Trypanosomiasis (Chagas Disease)

Brazilian Carlos Chagas first described the tropical protozoan parasitic infection caused by *Trypanosoma cruzi*. *T. cruzi* is a rural endemic disease in Central and South America, and an important public health problem in Brazil, Argentina, Venezuela, Bolivia, Chile, Peru, and Uruguay (248). Increasing incidence of *T. cruzi* infection has been noted in some regions of the United States with a concentrated population of immigrants from these endemic areas (249). The life cycle of *T. cruzi* involves insect vectors and mammalian hosts (250,251). Transmission to humans occurs when the feces of reduviid insects containing *T. cruzi* contaminate a bite, mucosal surface, or the conjunctiva. The parasite then spreads hematogeneously to internal organs. Infection can also be transmitted from the mother to her fetus, through blood transfusion, organ donation, and accidental exposure in laboratory workers (248,252).

Chagas disease often goes unrecognized in the acute phase, which involves four to six weeks of fever, malaise, and generalized lymphadenopathy. During the indeterminate phase, infected individuals are asymptomatic with low-grade parasitemia and detectable *T. cruzi* antibodies (248,251). Most people remain in the indeterminate phase, while 10% to 30% of individuals progress to chronic Chagas disease (251). The esophagus is affected in 7% to 10% of the chronic, *T. cruzi*–infected individuals in the endemic areas (253). The colon, small intestine, stomach, and biliary tract can be affected as well.

Pathology and Pathophysiology

Chagas disease was once thought to be an autoimmune illness, based on the observation that there was a tissue inflammatory reaction without discernible cause or identifiable parasites. Circulating autoantibodies against the M₂-musarinic acetylcholine receptors were subsequently reported in patients with Chagas disease associated with achalasia (254). With the advent of polymerase chain reaction, *T. cruzi* has been identified in nearly all affected organs, and high tissue parasitism is correlated with disease severity (255–257). The primary cause of Chagas disease may be infection-induced, immune-mediated tissue damage. The genetically diverse *T. cruzi* populations may determine specific organ involvement in Chagas disease (258). Esophageal histology reveals a hypertrophic muscular layer and marked decrease in the number of ganglion cells in the myenteric (Auerbach's) plexus (259).

Clinical Manifestations

Dysphagia is the most common symptom of Chagas disease and may develop within weeks to many years after the initial infection (253). Dysphagia is mostly intermittent in the early disease stages when the esophagus is not dilated. Complaints of odynophagia and chest pain can occur in the early stages. In the late stages of Chagas disease, dysphagia to solids will become more persistent. Nocturnal regurgitation, aspiration, pneumonia, and weight loss are usually present in patients with megaesophagus (251,260).

Diagnostic Features

The spectrum of esophageal motor dysfunction in Chagas disease varies from mild impairment of peristalsis to complete aperistalsis with megaesophagus. In a study by Dantas et al., 25% of asymptomatic individuals with a positive serology for *T. cruzi* had impaired esophageal function, as documented by barium esophagram or esophageal manometry (261). In early Chagas disease, a barium esophagram may be normal or consist of dysrhythmic contractions (260,262). In late Chagas disease, a dilated, atonic esophagus is present with a tapering *bird's beak*, similar to primary achalasia (Fig. 37.7).

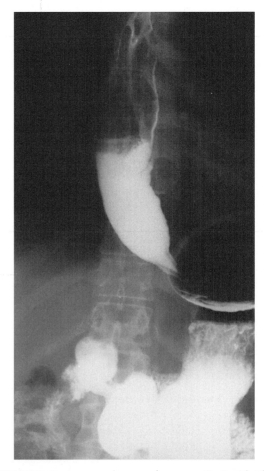

FIGURE 37.7. Barium esophagram from a patient with Chagas disease, which demonstrates a dilated esophagus with tapering at the gastroesophageal junction and an esophageal air–fluid level.

Esophageal manometric findings consist of diminished to normal LES pressures. The LES pressure does not correlate with the degree of esophageal peristaltic dysfunction (260,263). As the disease progresses, LES relaxation becomes impaired with a shorter duration of complete relaxation (260). The motility findings in the esophageal body vary from multipeaked waves, low peristaltic amplitude, and peristaltic failure to complete aperistalsis (260). Aperistalsis is a universal finding in those patients with megaesophagus (260). Chronic *T. cruzi* infection can be detected by finding serum antibodies to parasitic antigens by a variety of methods. However, false-positive reactions may occur in the patients with collagen vascular diseases, leishmaniasis, malaria, and syphilis (251).

Treatment

Medical treatment with benznidazole and nifurtimox can decrease the severity and duration of the acute infection. However, eradication of *T. cruzi* occurs in <50% of patients, and the chronic clinical course is not affected (251). The treatment of the esophageal disease is similar to that for primary achalasia. Sublingual isosorbide dinitrate can improve esophageal transit by scintigraphy (264) and alleviate dysphagia (265). Endoscopic pneumatic dilation is successful even in patients with a dilated esophagus (266). Injection of botulinum toxin into the LES has been reported, to cause transient improvement of dysphagia (267). Pinotti et al. (268) reported the surgical results of 840 patients treated with esophageal cardiomyotomy and an antireflux procedure (268). Surgical myotomy had a 95% success rate in patients with early disease and minimal esophageal dilation. In advanced cases, where there was an atonic and very dilated esophagus, surgical resection may have been required. However, it carries a 4% mortality rate, and a postoperative complication rate of 22% for pleural effusion and 8% for fistula at the anastomosis (268).

Amyloidosis

Amyloidosis is a group of disorders caused by the deposition of insoluble fibril proteins that are resistant to proteolysis. It can be a primary disorder or a secondary manifestation from other diseases. Amyloidosis is classified by the biochemical nature of the amyloid protein (269). The most common subtype is AL (light chain) from primary idiopathic amyloidosis or associated multiple myeloma. Clinical manifestations of amyloidosis are heterogeneous, depending on which organs are involved. The most common site of gastrointestinal involvement is the rectum, followed by the colon, small intestine, esophagus, and stomach.

Pathology and Pathophysiology

The typical histologic findings of amyloidosis consist of an amorphous material that stains positive with Congo red and

has a unique apple-green birefringence under polarized light. Amyloid deposits around the blood vessels are more common than deposits in the interstitial tissue (270,271). The amyloid protein has been found in the esophagus within the mucosa, submucosa, and smooth muscle (270–272). The myenteric plexus itself is usually intact histologically (273) but can be involved in rare cases (271).

Esophageal symptoms can result from either impairment of the autonomic nervous system (274) or from direct infiltration by the amyloid deposits (271). In a study by Bjerle et al. (274), the esophageal peristaltic response was reduced after neostigmine in patients with familial amyloidosis and polyneuropathy, suggesting a defective cholinergic innervation. Esophageal compliance appears to be similar between patients and controls, indicating that esophageal stiffness is not affected. Sensation with balloon distension is unaltered in familial amyloidosis (274).

Clinical Manifestations

Heartburn and dysphagia are reported in patients with amyloidosis (275). In rare cases, amyloidosis can mimic achalasia with persistent dysphagia and marked weight loss (276). Oropharyngeal dysphagia, hoarseness, and dysarthria can occur with amyloid deposition within the oropharynx producing profuse swelling of the tongue, hypopharynx, and larynx (277,278). An enlarged thyroid gland from amyloidosis can cause dysphagia from extrinsic compression of the esophagus (279). Hematemesis and esophageal perforation are other rare presentations (280).

Diagnostic Features

A barium esophagram may detect a dilated and atonic esophagus mimicking achalasia (276,281). Esophageal manometry is abnormal in more than half of patients with amyloidosis, but the manometric abnormalities vary and some patients have no symptoms (274,275). The amplitude of esophageal contraction is usually diminished with simultaneous activity (274,275). Esophageal aperistalsis may occur with or without impairment of LES relaxation (275,281). The elevation of esophageal baseline pressures compared to gastric pressures, as seen in primary achalasia, has been reported in amyloidosis (274,275). Sometime LES pressure is diminished (275). Endoscopic findings are subtle and nonspecific, consisting of mucosal granularity, erosions, and ulcerations (282). Congo red staining of the endoscopic biopsies from the esophagus and duodenum are often diagnostic. Rectal biopsy and abdominal fat pad aspirate can be obtained, if the biopsies of the upper gastrointestinal tract are nondiagnostic (269).

Treatment

Treatment of esophageal and gastrointestinal amyloidosis should be directed toward the primary cause, although effective treatments are not available. Pneumatic balloon dilation has been successful in patients with secondary achalasia caused by amyloidosis (276).

Paraneoplastic Syndromes

Paraneoplastic syndromes refer to the remote effects of neoplastic disorders on various organ systems. The underlying pathogenesis is believed to be that cancer cells express antigens mimicking the neuronal tissues, thus producing an autoimmune response (283). Small-cell lung cancer accounts for approximately 80% of the paraneoplastic syndromes, followed by breast, ovarian, and Hodgkin's lymphoma (284,285). Multiple paraneoplastic antineuronal antibodies and their targeting antigens have been identified (284). The most common antibody profile appears to be the anti-Hu antibody or antineuronal nuclear antibody 1 (ANNA-1) (285); however, it is not clear if these antibodies are pathogenic (284). In a review of 162 anti-Hu positive patients with paraneoplastic syndrome, Lucchinetti et al. (285) reported that 23% of the patients had gastrointestinal motility disturbances during their illness. Gastroparesis was the most common diagnosis in patients with a positive anti-Hu antibody (285). Nausea, vomiting, dehydration, and malnutrition from gastroparesis and chronic intestinal pseudo-obstruction (CIP) are usually the dominant symptoms (286,287). Esophageal manifestations of paraneoplastic syndrome are less often reported.

Pathology and Pathophysiology

The histology of paraneoplastic CIP has been reported. The myenteric plexus is infiltrated with lymphocytes and plasma cells associated with neuronal degeneration, marked loss of neurons, and axonal degeneration (287–289). Antibodies against the myenteric plexus neurons have been identified (288,289). Similar findings are noted in the esophagus. There is a loss of myenteric neurons in the esophagus with a predominant lymphocytic infiltrate within and surrounding the myenteric nerves (290). These histopathologic findings suggest that a visceral neuropathy may be the underlying cause. In rare cases, paraneoplastic cerebellar degeneration can cause impairment of oropharyngeal swallowing (291).

Clinical Manifestations

Symptoms of gastrointestinal dysmotility often precede the diagnosis of the neoplasm (285,286). The prevalence of esophageal manifestations is unknown. Dysphagia is the most commonly reported esophageal symptom. Some patients with esophageal involvement also have gastroparesis or CIP. Liu et al. (290) presented a retrospective clinicopathologic review of secondary achalasia associated with neoplasms. Out of 13 patients, 11 (85%) had direct metastatic invasion of the esophageal myenteric plexus (290). Secondary achalasia without neoplastic invasion was found in only one patient with a high titer for anti-Hu antibody (290). Oropharyngeal dysphagia associated with paraneoplastic neurologic syndrome usually presents with dysarthria, diplopia, nystagmus, and ataxia (291,292).

Diagnostic Features

The findings on esophageal manometry are nonspecific and include incomplete LES relaxation, simultaneous contractions, nonpropagated contractions (286), and in some cases, secondary achalasia (286,287,290). A comprehensive diagnostic panel of antineuronal antibodies is advocated for patients with new, onset-diffuse gastrointestinal dysmotility with an unclear etiology (286). Chest radiography is required to identify the presence of small-cell lung cancer, and computed tomography of the chest may be needed. However, radiograph studies can be normal on presentation, despite finding small-cell lung cancer later during the course of the illness (286).

Treatment

The treatment of the paraneoplastic esophageal symptoms depends on the severity of the esophageal disease compared to the stomach and the small bowel. Prokinetic drugs have been tried but are usually unsuccessful. A high index of suspicion is needed to achieve an early detection of the underlying cancer.

REFERENCES

1. LeRoy EC, Black C, Fleischmajer R, et al. Scleroderma (systemic sclerosis): classification, subsets and pathogenesis. *J Rheumatol* 1988;15:202–205.
2. Sjogren RW. Gastrointestinal motility disorders in scleroderma. *Arthritis Rheumatol* 1994;37:1265–1282.
3. Zaninotto G, Peserico A, Costantini M, et al. Oesophageal motility and lower oesophageal sphincter competence in progressive systemic sclerosis and localized scleroderma. *Scand J Gastroenterol* 1989;24:95–102.
4. D'Angelo WA, Fries JF, Masi AT, et al. Pathologic observations in systemic sclerosis (scleroderma). *Am J Med* 1968;46:428–440.
5. Abu-Shakra M, Guillemin F, Lee P. Gastrointestinal manifestations of systemic sclerosis. *Semin Arthritis Rheum* 1994;24:29–39.
6. Saladin TA, French AB, Zarafonetis CJ, et al. Esophageal motor abnormalities in scleroderma and related diseases. *Am J Dig Dis* 1966;11:522–535.
7. Åkesson A, Wollheim FA. Organ manifestations in 100 patients with progressive systemic sclerosis: a comparison between the CREST syndrome and diffuse scleroderma. *Br J Rheumatol* 1989;28:281–286.
8. Tuffanelli DL, Winklemann RK. Systemic scleroderma. *Arch Dermatol* 1961;84:359–371.
9. Poirer TJ, Rankin GB. Gastrointestinal manifestations of pro-

gressive systemic scleroderma based on review of 364 cases. *Am J Gastroenterol* 1972;58:30–44.

10. Altman RD, Medsger TA Jr, Bloch DA, et al. Predictors of survival in systemic sclerosis (scleroderma). *Arthritis Rheumatol* 1991;34:403–413.

11. Treacy WL, Baggenstoss AH, Slocumb CH, et al. Scleroderma of the esophagus: a correlation of histologic and physiologic findings. *Ann Intern Med* 1963;59:351–356.

12. Russell ML, Friesen D, Henderson RD, et al. Ultrastructure of the esophagus in scleroderma. *Arthritis Rheumatol* 1982;25: 1117–1123.

13. Atkinson M, Summerling MD. Oesophageal changes in systemic sclerosis. *Gut* 1966;7:402–408.

14. Cohen S, Fisher R, Lipshutz W, et al. The pathogenesis of esophageal dysfunction in scleroderma and Raynaud's disease. *J Clin Invest* 1972;51:2663–2668.

15. Bortolotti M, Pinotti R, Sarti P, et al. Esophageal electromyography in scleroderma patients with functional dysphagia. *Am J Gastroenterol* 1989;84:1497–1502.

16. Dessein PH, Joffe BI, Metz RM, et al. Autonomic dysfunction in systemic sclerosis: sympathetic overactivity and instability. *Am J Med* 1992;93:143–150.

17. Miller LS, Liu JB, Klenn PJ, et al. Endoluminal ultrasonography of the distal esophagus in systemic sclerosis. *Gastroenterology* 1993;105:31–39.

18. Yarze JC, Varga J, Stampfl D, et al. Esophageal function in systemic sclerosis: a prospective evaluation of motility and acid reflux in 36 patients. *Am J Gastroenterol* 1993;88:870–876.

19. Shoenut JP, Yamashiro Y, Orr WC, et al. Effect of severe gastroesophageal reflux on sleep stage in patients with aperistaltic esophagus. *Dig Dis Sci* 1996;41:372–376.

20. Basilisco G, Barbera R, Molgora M, et al. Acid clearance and oesophageal sensitivity in patients with progressive systemic sclerosis. *Gut* 1993;34:1487–1491.

21. Weihrauch TR, Korting GW, Ewe K, et al. Esophageal dysfunction and its pathogenesis in progressive systemic sclerosis. *Klin Wochenschr* 1978;56:963–968.

22. Bassotti G, Battaglia E, Debernardi V, et al. Esophageal dysfunction in scleroderma: relationship with disease subsets. *Arthritis Rheumatol* 1997;40:2252–2259.

23. Hurwitz AL, Duranceau A, Postlethwait RW. Esophageal dysfunction and Raynaud's phenomenon in patients with scleroderma. *Am J Dig Dis* 1976;21:601–606.

24. Dantas RO, Meneghelli UG, Oliveira RB, et al. Esophageal dysfunction does not always worsen in systemic sclerosis. *J Clin Gastroenterol* 1993;17:281–285.

25. Baron M, Arzoumanian A. Radionuclide esophageal transit studies in progressive systemic sclerosis: an analysis of longitudinal data. *J Rheumatol* 1991;18:1837–1840.

26. Johnson DA, Drane WE, Curran J, et al. Pulmonary disease in progressive systemic sclerosis: a complication of gastroesophageal reflux and occult aspiration? *Arch Intern Med* 1989; 149:589–593.

27. Troshinsky MB, Kane GC, Varga J, et al. Pulmonary function and gastroesophageal reflux in systemic sclerosis. *Ann Intern Med* 1994;121:6–10.

28. Zamost BJ, Hirschberg J, Ippoliti AF, et al. Esophagitis in scleroderma. Prevalence and risk factors. *Gastroenterology* 1987; 92:421–428.

29. Katzka DA, Reynolds JC, Saul SH, et al. Barrett's metaplasia and adenocarcinoma of the esophagus in scleroderma. *Am J Med* 1987;82:46–52.

30. Duncan SC, Winklemann RK. Cancer and scleroderma. *Arch Dermatol* 1979;115:950–955.

31. Segel MC, Campbell WL, Medsger TA Jr, et al. Systemic sclerosis (scleroderma) and esophageal adenocarcinoma: is

increased patient screening necessary? *Gastroenterology* 1985; 89:485–488.

32. Medsger TA Jr, Masi AT. The epidemiology of systemic sclerosis (scleroderma) among male U.S. veterans. *J Chronic Dis* 1978;31:73–85.

33. Kaye SA, Siraj QH, Agnew J, et al. Detection of early asymptomatic esophageal dysfunction in systemic sclerosis using a new scintigraphic grading method. *J Rheumatol* 1996;23:297–301.

34. Olivé A, Juncosa S, Evison G, et al. Air in the oesophagus: a sign of oesophageal involvement in systemic sclerosis. *Clin Rheumatol* 1995;14:319–321.

35. Weihrauch TR, Korting GW. Manometric assessment of oesophageal involvement in progressive systemic sclerosis, morphoea and Raynaud's disease. *Br J Dermatol* 1982;107: 325–332.

36. Wegener M, Adamek RJ, Wedmann B, et al. Gastrointestinal transit through esophagus, stomach, small and large intestine in patients with progressive systemic sclerosis. *Dig Dis Sci* 1994; 39:2209–2215.

37. Geatti O, Shapiro B, Fig LM, et al. Radiolabelled semisolid test meal clearance in the evaluation of esophageal involvement in scleroderma and Sjogren's syndrome. *Am J Physiol Imag* 1991; 6:65–73.

38. Drane WE, Karvelis K, Johnson DA, et al. Progressive systemic sclerosis: radionuclide esophageal scintigraphy and manometry. *Radiology* 1986;160:73–76.

39. Klein HA, Wald A, Graham TO, et al. Comparative studies of esophageal function in systemic sclerosis. *Gastroenterology* 1992; 102:1551–1556.

40. Schneider HA, Yonker RA, Longley S, et al. Scleroderma esophagus: a nonspecific entity. *Ann Intern Med* 1984;100:848–850.

41. Stentoft P, Hendel L, Aggestrup S. Esophageal manometry and pH-probe monitoring in the evaluation of gastroesophageal reflux in patients with progressive systemic sclerosis. *Scand J Gastroenterol* 1987;22:499–504.

42. Cameron AJ, Malcolm A, Prather CM, et al. Videoendoscopic diagnosis of esophageal motility disorders. *Gastrointest Endosc* 1999;49:62–69.

43. Hendel L, Svejgaard E, Walsøe I, et al. Esophageal candidiasis in progressive systemic sclersosis. *Scand J Gastroenterol* 1988; 23:1182–1186.

44. Johnson DA, Drane WE, Curran J, et al. Metoclopramide response in patients with progressive systemic sclerosis. Effect on esophageal and gastric motility abnormalities. *Arch Intern Med* 1987;147:1597–1601.

45. Hendel L, Stentoft P, Aggestrup S. The progress of oesophageal involvement in progressive systemic sclerosis during D-penicillamine treatment. *Scand J Rheumatol* 1989;18:149–155.

46. Henderson RD, Pearson FG. Surgical management of esophageal scleroderma. *J Thorac Cardiovasc Surg* 1973;66: 686–692.

47. Orringer MB, Orringer JS, Dabich L, et al. Combined Collis gastroplasty—fundoplication operations for scleroderma reflux esophagitis. *Surgery* 1981;90:624–630.

48. Poirier NC, Taillefer R, Topart P, et al. Antireflux operations in patients with scleroderma. *Ann Thorac Surg* 1994;58:66–72.

49. Mansour KA, Malone CE. Surgery for scleroderma of the esophagus: a 12-year experience. *Ann Thorac Surg* 1988;46: 513–514.

50. Hoffman RW, Greidinger EL. Mixed connective tissue disease. *Curr Opin Rheumatol* 2000;12:386–390.

51. Marshall JB, Kretschmar JM, Gerhardt DC, et al. Gastrointestinal manifestations of mixed connective tissue disease. *Gastroenterology* 1990;98:1232–1238.

52. Sharp GC, Irvine WS, Tan EM, et al. Mixed connective tissue disease—an apparently distinct rheumatic disease syndrome

associated with a specific antibody to an extractable nuclear antigen (ENA). *Am J Med* 1972;52:148–159.

53. Oxenhandler R, Hart M, Corman L, et al. Pathology of skeletal muscle in mixed connective tissue disease. *Arthritis Rheumatol* 1977;20:985–988.

54. Stacher G, Merio R, Budka C, et al. Cardiovascular autonomic function, autoantibodies, and esophageal motor activity in patients with systemic sclerosis and mixed connective tissue disease. *J Rheumatol* 2000;27:692–697.

55. Doria A, Bonavina L, Anselmino M, et al. Esophageal involvement in mixed connective tissue disease. *J Rheumatol* 1991;18:685–690.

56. Prakash UB, Luthra HS, Divertie MB. Intrathoracic manifestations in mixed connective tissue disease. *Mayo Clin Proc* 1985;60:813–821.

57. Gutierrez F, Valenzuela JE, Ehresmann GR, et al. Esophageal dysfunction in patients with mixed connective tissue diseases and systemic lupus erythematosus. *Dig Dis Sci* 1982;27:592–597.

58. Dalakas MC. Polymyositis, dermatomyositis, and inclusion-body myositis. *N Engl J Med* 1991;325:1487–1498.

59. Amato AA, Barohn RJ. Idiopathic inflammatory myopathies. *Neuro Clin* 1997;15:615–648.

60. Plotz PH. NIH conference: current concepts in the idiopathic inflammatory myopathies: polymyositis, dermatomyositis, and related disorders. *Ann Intern Med* 1989;111:143–157.

61. Kagen LJ, Hochman RB, Strong EW. Cricopharyngeal obstruction in inflammatory myopathy (polymyositis/dermatomyositis): report of three cases and review of the literature. *Arthritis Rheumatol* 1985;28:630–636.

62. Dietz F, Logeman JA, Sahgal V, et al. Cricopharyngeal muscle dysfunction in the differential diagnosis of dysphagia in polymyositis. *Arthritis Rheumatol* 1980;23:491–495.

63. O'Hara JM, Szemes G, Lowman RM. The esophageal lesions in dermatomyositis: a correlation of radiologic and pathologic findings. *Radiology* 1967;89:27–31.

64. de Merieux P, Verity MA, Clements PJ, et al. Esophageal abnormalities and dysphagia in polymyositis and dermatomyositis. *Arthritis Rheumatol* 1983;26:961–968.

65. Horowitz M, McNeil JD, Maddern GJ, et al. Abnormalities of gastric and esophageal emptying in polymyositis and dermatomyositis. *Gastroenterology* 1986;90:434–439.

66. Uthman I, Vazquez-Abad D, Senecal JL. Distinctive features of idiopathic inflammatory myopathies in French Canadians. *Semin Arthritis Rheum* 1996;26:447–458.

67. Jacob H, Berkowitz D, McDonald E, et al. The esophageal motility disorder of polymyositis: a prospective study. *Arch Intern Med* 1983;143:2262–2264.

68. Koh ET, Seow A, Ong B, et al. Adult onset polymyositis/dermatomyositis: clinical and laboratory features and treatment response in 75 patients. *Ann Rheum Dis* 1993;52:857–861.

69. Ramirez G, Asherson RA, Khamashta MA, et al. Adult-onset polymyositis-dermatomyositis: description of 25 patients with emphasis on treatment. *Semin Arthritis Rheum* 1990;20:114–120.

70. Maugars YM, Berthelot JM, Abbas AA, et al. Long-term prognosis of 69 patients with dermatomyositis or polymyositis. *Clin Exp Rheumatol* 1996;14:263–274.

71. Lotz BP, Engel AG, Nishino H, et al. Inclusion body myositis: observations in 40 patients. *Brain* 1989;112:727–747.

72. Tymms KE, Webb J. Dermatopolymyositis and other connective tissue diseases: a review of 105 cases. *J Rheumatol* 1985;12:1140–1148.

73. Palace J, Losseff N, Clough C. Isolated dysphagia due to polymyositis. *Muscle Nerve* 1993;16:680–681.

74. Wanamaker JR, Wanamaker HH, Lavertu P. Polymyositis pre-senting as a neck mass. *Arch Otolaryngol Head Neck Surg* 1992;118:318–320.

75. Kornizky Y, Heller I, Isakov A, et al. Dysphagia with multiple autoimmune disease. *Clin Rheumatol* 2000;19:321–323.

76. Sheikh SH, Shaw-Stiffel TA. The gastrointestinal manifestations of Sjogren's syndrome. *Am J Gastroenterol* 1995;90:9–14.

77. Rosztóczy A, Kovács L, Wittmann T, et al. Manometric assessment of impaired esophageal motor function in primary Sjogren's syndrome. *Clin Exp Rheumatol* 2001;19:147–152.

78. Grande L, Lacima G, Ros E, et al. Esophageal motor function in primary Sjogren's syndrome. *Am J Gastroenterol* 1993;88:378–381.

79. Anselmino M, Zaninotto G, Costantini M, et al. Esophageal motor function in primary Sjogren's syndrome: correlation with dysphagia and xerostomia. *Dig Dis Sci* 1997;42:113–118.

80. Kjellén G, Fransson SG, Lindström F, et al. Esophageal function, radiography, and dysphagia in Sjogren's syndrome. *Dig Dis Sci* 1986;31:225–229.

81. Palma R, Freire A, Freitas J, et al. Esophageal motility disorders in patients with Sjogren's syndrome. *Dig Dis Sci* 1994;39:758–761.

82. Tsianos EB, Chiras CD, Drosos AA, et al. Oesophageal dysfunction in patients with primary Sjogren's syndrome. *Ann Rheum Dis* 1985;44:610–613.

83. Sreebny LM. Saliva in health and disease: an appraisal and update. *Int Dental J* 2000;50:140–161.

84. ter Borg EJ, Groen H, Horst G, et al. Clinical associations of antiribonucleoprotein antibodies in patients with systemic lupus erythematosus. *Semin Arthritis Rheum* 1990;20:164–173.

85. Harvey A, Shulman L, Tumulty P, et al. Systemic lupus erythematosus: review of the literature and clinical analysis of 138 cases. *Medicine* 1954;33:291–437.

86. Sultan SM, Ioannou Y, Isenberg DA. A review of gastrointestinal manifestations of systemic lupus erythematosus. *Rheumatology (Oxford)* 1999;38:917–932.

87. Peppercorn MA, Docken WP, Rosenberg S. Esophageal motor dysfunction in systemic lupus erythematosus. Two cases with unusual features. *JAMA* 1979;242:1895–1896.

88. Ramirez-Mata M, Reyes PA, Alarcon-Segovia D, et al. Esophageal motility in systemic lupus erythematosus. *Am J Dig Dis* 1974;19:132–136.

89. Dubois EL, Tuffanelli DL. Clinical manifestations of systemic lupus erythematosus. *JAMA* 1964;190:104–111.

90. Lapadula G, Muolo P, Semeraro F, et al. Esophageal motility disorders in the rheumatic diseases: a review of 150 patients. *Clin Exp Rheumatol* 1994;12:515–521.

91. Geterud Å, Bake B, Bjelle A, et al. Swallowing problems in rheumatoid arthritis. *Acta Otolaryngol* 1991;111:1153–1161.

92. Bassotti G, Gaburri M, Biscarini L, et al. Oesophageal motor activity in rheumatoid arthritis: a clinical and manometric study. *Digest* 1988;39:144–150.

93. Lofgren RH, Montgomery WW. Incidence of laryngeal involvement in rheumatoid arthritis. *N Engl J Med* 1962;267:193–195.

94. Sørensen WT, Møller-Andersen K, Behrendt N. Rheumatoid nodules of the larynx. *J Laryngol Otol* 1998;112:573–574.

95. Erb N, Pace AV, Delamere JP, et al. Dysphagia and stridor caused by laryngeal rheumatoid arthritis. *Rheumatology (Oxford)* 2001;40:952–953.

96. Tsianos EB, Drosos AA, Chiras CD, et al. Esophageal manometric findings in autoimmune rheumatic diseases: is scleroderma esophagus a specific entity? *Rheumatol Int* 1987;7:23–27.

97. Bytzer P, Talley NJ, Leemon M, et al. Prevalence of gastrointestinal symptoms associated with diabetes mellitus: a population-based survey of 15,000 adults. *Arch Intern Med* 2001;161:1989–1996.

98. Maleki D, Locke GR, III, Camilleri M, et al. Gastrointestinal tract symptoms among persons with diabetes mellitus in the community. *Arch Intern Med* 2000;160:2808–2816.

99. Greene DA, Sima AA, Stevens MJ, et al. Complications: neuropathy, pathogenetic considerations. *Diabetes Care* 1992;15: 1902–1925.

100. Smith B. Neuropathology of the oesophagus in diabetes mellitus. *J Neurol Neurosurg Psych* 1974;37:1151–1154.

101. Westin L, Lilja B, Sundkvist G. Oesophagus scintigraphy in patients with diabetes mellitus. *Scand J Gastroenterol* 1986;21: 1200–1204.

102. Channer KS, Jackson PC, O'Brien I, et al. Oesophageal function in diabetes mellitus and its association with autonomic neuropathy. *Diabetic Med* 1985;2:378–382.

103. Hüppe D, Tegenthoff M, Faig J, et al. Esophageal dysfunction in diabetes mellitus: is there a relation to clinical manifestation of neuropathy? *Clin Invest* 1992;70:740–747.

104. Kinekawa F, Kubo F, Matsuda K, et al. Relationship between esophageal dysfunction and neuropathy in diabetic patients. *Am J Gastroenterol* 2001;96:2026–2032.

105. Horowitz M, Harding PE, Maddox AF, et al. Gastric and oesophageal emptying in patients with type 2 (non–insulin-dependent) diabetes mellitus. *Diabetologia* 1989;32:151–159.

106. Annese V, Bassotti G, Caruso N, et al. Gastrointestinal motor dysfunction, symptoms, and neuropathy in noninsulin-dependent (type 2) diabetes mellitus. *J Clin Gastroenterol* 1999;29: 171–177.

107. Holloway RH, Tippett MD, Horowitz M, et al. Relationship between esophageal motility and transit in patients with type I diabetes mellitus. *Am J Gastroenterol* 1999;94:3150–3157.

108. Verne GN, Sninsky CA. Diabetes and the gastrointestinal tract. *Gastroenterol Clin N Am* 1998;27:861–874.

109. Rayner CK, Samsom M, Jones KL, et al. Relationships of upper gastrointestinal motor and sensory function with glycemic control. *Diabetes Care* 2001;24:371–381.

110. De Boer SY, Masclee AA, Lam WF, et al. Effect of acute hyperglycemia on esophageal motility and lower esophageal sphincter pressure in humans. *Gastroenterology* 1992;103:775–780.

111. Rathmann W, Enck P, Frieling T, et al. Visceral afferent neuropathy in diabetic gastroparesis. *Diabetes Care* 1991;14: 1086–1089.

112. Kamath MV, Tougas G, Fitzpatrick D, et al. Assessment of the visceral afferent and autonomic pathways in response to esophageal stimulation in control subjects and in patients with diabetes. *Clin Invest Med* 1998;21:100–113.

113. Rayner CK. Effects of hyperglycemia on cortical response to esophageal distension in normal subjects. *Dig Dis Sci* 1999;44: 279–285.

114. Jackson AL, Rashed H, Cardoso S, et al. Assessment of gastric electrical activity and autonomic function among diabetic and nondiabetic patients with symptoms of gastroesophageal reflux. *Dig Dis Sci* 2000;45:1727–1730.

115. Lluch I, Ascaso JF, Mora F, et al. Gastroesophageal reflux in diabetes mellitus. *Am J Gastroenterol* 1999;94:919–924.

116. Talley NJ, Young L, Bytzer P, et al. Impact of chronic gastrointestinal symptoms in diabetes mellitus on health-related quality of life. *Am J Gastroenterol* 2001;96:71–76.

117. Keshavarzian A, Iber FL. Gastrointestinal involvement in insulin-requiring diabetes mellitus. *J Clin Gastroenterol* 1987;9: 685–692.

118. Feldman M, Schiller LR. Disorders of gastrointestinal motility associated with diabetes mellitus. *Ann Intern Med* 1983;98: 378–384.

119. Keshavarzian A, Iber FL, Nasrallah S. Radionuclide esophageal emptying and manometric studies in diabetes mellitus. *Am J Gastroenterol* 1987;82:625–631.

120. Murray FE, Lombard MG, Ashe J, et al. Esophageal function in diabetes mellitus with special reference to acid studies and relationship to peripheral neuropathy. *Am J Gastroenterol* 1987;82: 840–843.

121. Pozzi M, Rivolta M, Gelosa M, et al. Upper gastrointestinal involvement in diabetes mellitus: study of esophagogastric function. *Acta Diabetologica Latina* 1988;25:333–341.

122. Stewart IM, Hosking DJ, Preston BJ, et al. Oesophageal motor changes in diabetes mellitus. *Thorax* 1976;31:278–283.

123. The effect of intensive treatment of diabetes on the development and progression of long-term complications in insulin-dependent diabetes mellitus. *N Engl J Med* 1993;329:977–986.

124. Bassotti G, Pagliacci MC, Nicoletti I, et al. Intestinal pseudoobstruction secondary to hypothyroidism. Importance of small bowel manometry. *J Clin Gastroenterol* 1992;14:56–58.

125. Duret RL, Bastenie PA. Intestinal disorders in hypothyroidism: clinical and manometric study. *Am J Dig Dis* 1971;16:723–727.

126. Fournier JC, Navarro A. Étude de la musculature viscérale dans le myxedma. *Semin Hop Paris* 1960;3:211–217.

127. Wright RA, Penner DB. Myxedema and upper esophageal dysmotility. *Dig Dis Sci* 1981;26:376–377.

128. Urquhart AD, Rea IM, Lawson LT, et al. A new complication of hypothyroid coma: neurogenic dysphagia: presentation, diagnosis, and treatment. *Thyroid* 2001;11:595–598.

129. Eastwood GL, Braverman LE, White EM, et al. Reversal of lower esophageal sphincter hypotension and esophageal aperistalsis after treatment for hypothyroidism. *J Clin Gastroenterol* 1982;4:307–310.

130. Hohl RD, Nixon RK. Myxedema ileus. *Arch Intern Med* 1965;115:145–150.

131. Ritter FN. The effects of hypothyroidism upon the ear, nose, throat. *Laryngoscope* 1967;77:1427–1479.

132. Engel AG. Neuromuscular manifestations of Grave's disease. *Mayo Clin Proc* 1972;47:919–925.

133. Kammer GM, Hamilton CR Jr. Acute bulbar muscle dysfunction and hyperthyroidism: a study of four cases and review of the literature. *Am J Med* 1974;56:464–470.

134. Ming RH, Dreosti LM, Tim LO, et al. Thyrotoxicosis presenting as dysphagia: a case report. *S Afr Med J* 1982;61:554.

135. Noto H, Mitsuhashi T, Ishibashi S, et al. Hyperthyroidism presenting as dysphagia. *Intern Med* 2000;39:472–473.

136. Marks P, Anderson J, Vincent R. Thyrotoxic myopathy presenting as dysphagia. *Postgrad Med J* 1980;56:669–670.

137. Sweatman MC, Chambers L. Disordered oesophageal motility in thyrotoxic myopathy. *Postgrad Med J* 1985;61:619–620.

138. Joasoo A, Murray IP, Steinbeck AW. Involvement of bulbar muscles in thyrotoxic myopathy. *Aust Ann Med* 1970;19: 338–340.

139. Branski D, Levy J, Globus M, et al. Dysphagia as a primary manifestation of hyperthyroidism. *J Clin Gastroenterol* 1984;6: 437–440.

140. Meshkinpour H, Afrasiabi MA, Valenta LJ. Esophageal motor function in Grave's disease. *Dig Dis Sci* 1979;24:159–161.

141. Balcombe NR. Dysphagia and hypercalcemia. *Postgrad Med J* 1999;75:373–374.

142. Grieve RJ, Dixon PF. Dysphagia: a further symptom of hypercalcemia? *BMJ* 1983;286:1935–1936.

143. Mowschenson PM, Rosenberg S, Pallotta J, et al. Effect of hyperparathyroidism and hypercalcemia on lower esophageal sphincter pressure. *Am J Surg* 1982;143:36–39.

144. Iannello S, Belfiore F. Hypomagnesemia: a review of pathophysiological, clinical and therapeutical aspects. *Panminerva Med* 2001;43:177–209.

145. Iannello S, Spina M, Leotta P, et al. Hypomagnesemia and smooth muscle contractility: diffuse esophageal spasm in an old female patient. *Mineral Electrol Metab* 1998;24:348–356.

146. McLean RM. Magnesium and its therapeutic use: a review. *Am J Med* 1994;96:63–76.

147. Hamed IA, Lindeman RD. Dysphagia and vertical nystagmus in magnesium deficiency. *Ann Intern Med* 1978;89:222–223.

148. Flink EB. Dysphagia in magnesium deficiency. *Ann Intern Med* 1978;89:282.

149. Bujanda L. The effects of alcohol consumption upon the gastrointestinal tract. *Am J Gastroenterol* 2000;95:3374–3382.

150. Hogan WJ, Viegas DA, Winship DH. Ethanol-induced acute esophageal motor dysfunction. *J Applied Physiol* 1972;32:755–760.

151. Winship DH, Caflisch CR, Zboralske FF, et al. Deterioration of esophageal peristalsis in patients with alcoholic neuropathy. *Gastroenterology* 1968;55:173–178.

152. Mayer EM, Grabowski CJ, Fisher RS. Effects of graded doses of alcohol upon esophageal motor function. *Gastroenterology* 1978;75:1133–1136.

153. Keshavarzian A, Polepalle C, Iber FL, et al. Secondary esophageal contractions are abnormal in chronic alcoholics. *Dig Dis Sci* 1992;37:517–522.

154. Kaufman SE, Kaye MD. Induction of gastro-oesophageal reflux by alcohol. *Gut* 1978;19:336–338.

155. Vitale GC, Cheadle WG, Patel B, et al. The effect of alcohol on nocturnal gastroesophageal reflux. *JAMA* 1987;258:2077–2079.

156. Bor S, Caymaz-Bor C, Tobey NA, et al. Effect of ethanol on the structure and function of rabbit esophageal epithelium. *Am J Physiol* 1998;274:G819–G826.

157. Bor S, Bor-Caymaz C, Tobey NA, et al. Esophageal exposure to ethanol increases risk of acid damage in rabbit esophagus. *Dig Dis Sci* 1999;44:290–300.

158. Salo JA. Ethanol-induced mucosal injury in rabbit oesophagus. *Scand J Gastroenterol* 1983;18:713–721.

159. Shirazi SS, Platz CE. Effect of alcohol on canine esophageal mucosa. *J Surg Res* 1978;25:373–379.

160. Keshavarzian A, Muska B, Sundaresan R, et al. Ethanol at pharmacologically relevant concentrations inhibits contractility of isolated smooth muscle cells of cat esophagus. *Alcohol Clin Exp Res* 1996;20:180–184.

161. Keshavarzian A, Urban G, Sedghi S, et al. Effect of acute ethanol on esophageal motility in cat. *Alcohol Clin Exp Res* 1991;15:116–121.

162. Silver LS, Worner TM, Korsten MA. Esophageal function in chronic alcoholics. *Am J Gastroenterol* 1986;81:423–427.

163. Keshavarzian A, Iber FL, Ferguson Y. Esophageal manometry and radionuclide emptying in chronic alcoholics. *Gastroenterology* 1987;92:651–657.

164. Grande L, Monforte R, Ros E, et al. High amplitude contractions in the middle third of the oesophagus: a manometric marker of chronic alcoholism? *Gut* 1996;38:655–662.

165. Caygill CP, Johnston DA, Lopez M, et al. Lifestyle factors and Barrett's esophagus. *Am J Gastroenterol* 2002;97:1328–1331.

166. Avidan B, Sonnenberg A, Schnell TG, et al. Risk factors for erosive reflux esophagitis: a case–control study. *Am J Gastroenterol* 2001;96:41–46.

167. Gray MR, Donnelly RJ, Kingsnorth AN. The role of smoking and alcohol in metaplasia and cancer risk in Barrett's columnar lined esophagus. *Gut* 1993;34:727–731.

168. Eloubeidi MA, Provenzale D. Clinical and demographic predictors of Barrett's esophagus among patients with gastroesophageal reflux disease: a multivariable analysis in veterans. *J Clin Gastroenterol* 2001;33:306–309.

169. Gerson LB, Shetler K, Triadafilopoulos G. Prevalence of Barrett's esophagus in asymptomatic individuals. *Gastroenterology* 2002;123:461–467.

170. Fields JZ, Turk A, Durkin M, et al. Increased gastrointestinal symptoms in chronic alcoholics. *Am J Gastroenterol* 1994;89:382–386.

171. Geboes K, Janssens J, Rutgeerts P, et al. Crohn's disease of the esophagus. *J Clin Gastroenterol* 1986;8:31–37.

172. Decker GA, Loftus EV Jr, Pasha TM, et al. Crohn's disease of the esophagus: clinical features and outcomes. *Inflammat Bowel Dis* 2001;7:113–119.

173. Alcántara M, Rodriquez R, Potenciano M, et al. Endoscopic and bioptic findings in the upper gastrointestinal tract in patients with Crohn's disease. *Endoscopy* 1993;25:282–286.

174. D'Haens G, Rutgeerts P, Geboes K, et al. The natural history of esophageal Crohn's disease: three patterns of evolution. *Gastrointest Endosc* 1994;40:296–300.

175. Gheorghe C, Aposteanu G, Popescu C, et al. Long esophageal stricture in Crohn's disease: a case report. *Hepatogastroenterology* 1998;45:738–741.

176. Howden FM, Mills LR, Rubin JW. Crohn's disease of the esophagus. *Am Surgeon* 1994;60:656–660.

177. Miller LJ, Thistle JL, Payne WS, et al. Crohn's disease involving the esophagus and colon. *Mayo Clin Proc* 1977;52:35–38.

178. Ghahremani GG, Gore RM, Breuer RI, et al. Esophageal manifestations of Crohn's disease. *Gastrointest Radiol* 1982;7:199–203.

179. Mathis G, Sutterlutti G, Dirschmid K, et al. Crohn's disease of the esophagus: dilation of stricture and fibrin sealing of fistulas. *Endoscopy* 1994;26:508.

180. Honda S, Sugimoto K, Iwasaki H, et al. Multiple mucosal bridge formation in the esophagus in a patient with Crohn's disease. *Endoscopy* 1998;30:S37–S38.

181. Rholl JC, Yavorski RT, Cheney CP, et al. Esophagogastric fistula: a complication of Crohn's disease—case report and review of the literature. *Am J Gastroenterol* 1998;93:1381–1383.

182. LiVolsi VA, Jaretzki A. Granulomatous esophagitis: a case of Crohn's disease limited to the esophoagus. *Gastroenterology* 1973;64:313–319.

183. Levine MS. Crohn's disease of the upper gastrointestinal tract. *Radiol Clin North Am* 1987;25:79–91.

184. Sakane T, Takeno M, Suzuki N, et al. Current concepts: Behcet's disease. *N Engl J Med* 1999;341:1284–1291.

185. Bayraktar Y, Özaslan E, Van Thiel DH. Gastrointestinal manifestations of Behcet's disease. *J Clin Gastroenterol* 2000;30:144–154.

186. Kaklamani VG, Vaiopoulos G, Kaklamanis PG. Behcet's disease. *Semin Arthritis Rheum* 1998;27:197–217.

187. Mori S, Yoshihira A, Kawamura H, et al. Esophageal involvement in Behcet's disease. *Am J Gastroenterol* 1983;78:548–553.

188. Ikezawa K, Kashimura H, Hassan M, et al: a case of Behcet's syndrome with esophageal involvement treated with salicylazosulfapyridine and prednisolone. *Endoscopy* 1998;30:S52–S53.

189. Bottomley WW, Dakkak M, Walton S, et al. Esophageal involvement in Behcet's disease. Is endoscopy necessary? *Dig Dis Sci* 1992;37:594–597.

190. Yashiro K, Nagasako K, Hasegawa K, et al. Esophageal lesions in intestinal Behcet's disease. *Endoscopy* 1986;18:57–60.

191. Crystal RG. Sarcoidosis. In: Braunwald E, Fauci AS, Kasper DS, et al., eds. *Harrison's principles of internal medicine*. New York: McGraw-Hill, 2001;1969–1974.

192. Mayock RL, Bertrand P, Morrison CE, et al. Manifestations of sarcoidosis: analysis of 145 patients, with a review of nine series selected from the literature. *Am J Med* 1963;35:67–89.

193. Boruchowicz A, Canva-Delcambre V, Guillemont F, et al. Sarcoidosis and achalasia: a fortuitous association? *Am J Gastroenterol* 1996;91:413–414.

194. Cappell MS. Endoscopic, radiographic, and manometric findings in dysphagia associated with sarcoid due to extrinsic esophageal compression from subcarinal lymphadenopathy. *Am J Gastroenterol* 1995;90:489–492.

195. Cook DM, Dines DE, Dycus DS. Sarcoidosis: report of a case presenting as dysphagia. *Chest* 1970;57:84–86.

196. Davies RJ. Dysphagia, abdominal pain, and sarcoid granulomata. *BMJ* 1972;3:564–565.

197. Dufresne CR, Jeyasingham K, Baker RR. Achalasia of the cardia associated with pulmonary sarcoidosis. *Surgery* 1983;94:32–35.

198. Geissinger BW, Sharkey MF, Criss DG, et al. Reversible esophageal motility disorder in a patient with sarcoidosis. *Am J Gastroenterol* 1996;91:1423–1426.

199. Hardy WE, Tulgan H, Haidak G, et al. Sarcoidosis: a case presenting with dysphagia and dysphonia. *Ann Intern Med* 1967;66:353–357.

200. Lukens FJ, Machicao VI, Woodward TA, et al. Esophageal sarcoidosis: an unusual diagnosis. *J Clin Gastroenterol* 2002;34:54–56.

201. Polachek AA, Matre WJ. Gastrointestinal sarcoidosis: report of a case involving the esophagus. *Am J Dig Dis* 1964;9:429–433.

202. Wiesner PJ, Kleinman MS, Condemi JJ, et al. Sarcoidosis of the esophagus. *Am J Dig Dis* 1971;16:943–951.

203. Nidiry JJ, Mines S, Hackney R, et al. Sarcoidosis: a unique presentation of dysphagia, myopathy, and photophobia. *Am J Gastroenterol* 1991;86:1679–1682.

204. Benjamin B, Dalton C, Croxson G. Laryngoscopic diagnosis of laryngeal sarcoid. *Ann Otol Rhinol Laryngol* 1995;104:529–531.

205. Castroagudin JF, Gonzalez-Quintela A, Moldes J, et al. Acute reversible dysphagia and dysphonia as initial manifestations of sarcoidosis. *Hepatogastroenterology* 1999;46:2414–2418.

206. Vasan NR, Allison RS. Sarcoidosis presenting as hoarseness and dysphagia. *Aust N Z J Surg* 1999;69:751–753.

207. Wiersema MJ, Vazquez-Sequeiros E, Wiersema LM. Evaluation of mediastinal lymphadenopathy with endoscopic US-guided fine-needle aspiration biopsy. *Radiology* 2001;219:252–257.

208. Spergel JM, Beausoleil JL, Mascarenhas M, et al. The use of skin prick tests and patch tests to identify causative foods in eosinophilic esophagitis. *J Allergy Clin Immunol* 2002;109:363–368.

209. Orenstein SR, Shalaby TM, Di Lorenzo C, et al. The spectrum of pediatric eosinophilic esophagitis bfeyond infancy: a clinical series of 30 children. *Am J Gastroenterol* 2000;95:1422–1430.

210. Vasilopoulos S, Murphy P, Auerbach A, et al. The small-caliber esophagus: an unappreciated cause of dysphagia for solids in patients with eosinophilic esophagitis. *Gastrointest Endosc* 2002;55:99–106.

211. Straumann A, Bauer M, Fischer B, et al. Idiopathic eosinophilic esophagitis is associated with a T(H)2-type allergic inflammatory response. *J Allergy Clin Immunol* 2001;108:954–961.

212. Attwood SE, Smyrk TC, DeMeester TR, et al. Esophageal eosinophilia with dysphagia: a distinct clinicopathologic syndrome. *Dig Dis Sci* 1993;38:109–116.

213. Morrow JB, Vargo JJ, Goldblum JR, et al. The ringed esophagus: histological features of GERD. *Am J Gastroenterol* 2001;96:984–989.

214. Siafakas CG, Ryan CK, Brown MR, et al. Multiple esophageal rings: an association with eosinophilic esophagitis: case report and review of the literature. *Am J Gastroenterol* 2000;95:1572–1575.

215. Langdon DE. "Congenital" esophageal stenosis, corrugated ringed esophagus, and eosinophilic esophagitis. *Am J Gastroenterol* 2000;95:2123–2124.

216. Mishra A, Hogan SP, Brandt EB, et al. IL-5 promotes eosinophil trafficking to the esophagus. *J Immunol* 2002;168:2464–2469.

217. Stevoff C, Rao S, Parsons W, et al. EUS and histopathologic correlates in eosinophilic esophagitis. *Gastrointest Endosc* 2001;54:373–377.

218. Lee RG. Marked eosinophilia in esophageal mucosal biopsies. *Am J Surg Pathol* 1985;9:475–479.

219. Walsh SV, Antonioli DA, Goldman H, et al. Allergic esophagitis in children: a clinicopathological entity. *Am J Surg Pathol* 1999;23:390–396.

220. Landres RT, Kuster GG, Strum WB. Eosinophilic esophagitis in a patient with vigorous achalasia. *Gastroenterology* 1978;74:1298–1301.

221. Katzka DA, Levine MS, Ginsberg GG, et al. Congenital esophageal stenosis on adults. *Am J Gastroenterol* 2000;95:32–36.

222. Fox VL, Nurko S, Furuta GT. Eosinophilic esophagitis: it's not just kid's stuff. *Gastrointest Endosc* 2002;56:260–270.

223. Hempel SL, Elliott DE. Chest pain in an aspirin-sensitive asthmatic patient. Eosinophilic esophagitis causing esophageal dysmotility. *Chest* 1996;110:1117–1120.

224. Feczko PJ, Halpert RD, Zonca M. Radiographic abnormalities in eosinophilic esophagitis. *Gastrointest Radiol* 1985;10:321–324.

225. Liacouras CA. Failed Nissen fundoplication in two patients who had persistent vomiting and eosinophilic esophagitis. *J Pediatr Surg* 1997;32:1504–1506.

226. Van Rosendall GMA, Anderson MA, Diamant N. Eosinophilic esophagitis: case report and clinical perspective. *Am J Gastroenterol* 1997;92:1054–1056.

227. Ahmed A. A novel endoscopic appearance of idiopathic eosinophilic esophagitis. *Endoscopy* 2000;32:s33.

228. Kelly KJ, Lazenby AJ, Rowe PC, et al. Eosinophilic esophagitis attributed to gastroesophageal reflux: improvement with an amino acid–based formula. *Gastroenterology* 1995;109:1503–1512.

229. Liacouras CA, Wenner WJ, Brown K, et al. Primary eosinophilic esophagitis in children: successful treatment with oral corticosteroids. *J Ped Gastroenterol Nutrit* 1998;26:380–385.

230. Langdon DE. Corrugated (multiple) ringed esophagus, GERD versus allergy? *Am J Gastroenterol* 2002;5:1257–1258.

231. Soussan EB, Savoye G, Hochain P, et al. Acute esophageal necrosis: a 1-year prospective. *Gastrointest Endosc* 2002;56:213–217.

232. Moretó M, Ojembarrena E, Zabella M, et al. Idiopathic acute esophageal necrosis: not necessary a terminal event. *Endoscopy* 1993;25:534–536.

233. Sharma SS, Venkateswaran S, Chacko A, et al. Melanosis of the esophagus: an endoscopic, histochemical, and ultrastructural study. *Gastroenterology* 1991;100:13–16.

234. Geller A, Aguilar H, Burgart L, et al. The black esophagus. *Am J Gastroenterol* 1995;90:2210–2212.

235. Khan HA. Coal dust deposition—rare cause of "black esophagus". *Am J Gastroenterol* 1996;91:2256.

236. Kozlowski LM, Nigra TP. Esophageal acanthosis nigricans in association with adenocarcinoma from an unknown primary site. *J Acad Derm* 1992;26:348–351.

237. Haviv YS, Reinus C, Zimmerman J. "Black esophagus": a rare complication of shock. *Am J Gastroenterol* 1996;91:2432–2434.

238. Obermeyer R, Kasirajan K, Erzurum V, et al. Necrotizing esophagitis presenting as a black esophagus. *Surg Endosc* 1998;12:1430–1433.

239. Williams DB, Payne WS. Observations on esophageal blood supply. *Mayo Clin Proc* 1982;57:448–453.

240. Goldenberg SP, Wain SL, Marignani P. Acute necrotizing esophagitis. *Gastroenterology* 1990;98:493–496.

241. Gleysteen JJ, Condon RE. Danger of fundoplication after selective vagotomy and antrectomy. *Arch Surg* 1984;119:334–335.

242. Minatoya K, Okita Y, Tagusari O, et al. Transmural necrosis of the esophagus secondary to acute aortic dissection. *Ann Thorac Surg* 2000;69:1584–1586.

243. Barjas E, Pires S, Lopes J, et al. Cytomegalovirus acute necrotizing esophagitis. *Endoscopy* 2001;33:735.

244. Cattan P, Cuillerier E, Cellier C, et al. Black esophagus associated with herpes esophagitis. *Gastrointest Endosc* 1999;49:105–107.

245. Cummings DR. Acute necrotizing esophagitis. *Gastroenterology* 1990;99:1193.

246. Mangan TF, Colley AT, Wytock DH. Antibiotic-associated acute necrotizing esophagitis. *Gastroenterology* 1990;99:900.

247. Serna-Higuera C, Martinez J, Martin-Arribas MI, et al. Acute necrotizing esophagitis. *Gastrointest Endosc* 2001;54:225.

248. Prata A. Chagas' disease. *Infect Dis Clin North Am* 1994;8:61–76.

249. Galel SA, Kirchhoff LV. Risk factors for Trypanosoma cruzi infection in California blood donors. *Transfusion* 1996;36:227–231.

250. Villanueva MS. Trypanosomiasis of the central nervous system. *Semin Neurol* 1993;13:209–218.

251. Kirchhoff LV. American trypanosomiasis (Chagas' disease)—a tropical disease now in the United States. *N Engl J Med* 1993;329:639–644.

252. Wendel S, Gonzaga AL. Chagas' disease and blood transfusion: a New World problem? *Vox Sang* 1993;64:1–12.

253. de Oliveira RB, Troncon LE, Dantas RO, et al. Gastrointestinal manifestations of Chagas' disease. *Am J Gastroenterol* 1998;93:884–889.

254. Goin JC, Sterin-Borda L, Bilder CR, et al. Functional implications of circulating muscarinic cholinergic receptor autoantibodies in chagasic patients with achalasia. *Gastroenterology* 1999;117:798–805.

255. Lages–Silva E, Crema E, Ramirez LE, et al. Relationship between Trypanosoma cruzi and human chagasic megaesophagus: blood and tissue parasitism. *Am J Trop Med Hygiene* 2001;65:435–441.

256. Tarleton RL, Zhang L. Chagas disease etiology: autoimmunity or parasite persistence? *Parasitol Today* 1999;15:94–99.

257. Vago AR, Macedo AM, Adad SJ, et al. PCR detection of Trypanosoma cruzi DNA in oesophageal tissues of patients with chronic digestive Chagas' disease. *Lancet* 1996;348:891–892.

258. Vago AR, Andrade LO, Leite AA, et al. Genetic characterization of Trypanosoma cruzi directly from tissues of patients with chronic Chagas disease: differential distribution of genetic types into diverse organs. *Am J Pathol* 2000;156:1805–1809.

259. Koberle F. Chagas' disease and Chagas' syndromes: the pathology of American trypanosomiasis. *Adv Parasitol* 1968;6:63–116.

260. de Oliveira RB, Rezende FJ, Dantas RO, et al. The spectrum of esophageal motor disorders in Chagas' disease. *Am J Gastroenterol* 1995;90:1119–1124.

261. Dantas RO, Deghaide NH, Donadi EA. Esophageal manometric and radiologic findings in asymptomatic subjects with Chagas' disease. *J Clin Gastroenterol* 1999;28:245–248.

262. Mattoso LF, Reeder MM. Radiological diagnosis of Chagas' disease (American trypanosomiasis). *Semin Roentgenol* 1998;33:26–46.

263. Dantas RO, Godoy RA, Oliveira RB, et al. Lower esophageal sphincter pressure in Chagas' disease. *Dig Dis Sci* 1990;35:508–512.

264. Figueiredo MC, Oliveira RB, Iazigi N, et al. Short report: comparison of the effects of sublingual nifedipine and isosorbide dinitrate on oesophageal emptying in patients with Chagasic achalasia. *Aliment Pharmacol Ther* 1992;6:507–512.

265. Ferreira–Filho LP, Patto RJ, Troncon LE, et al. Use of isosorbide dinitrate for the symptomatic treatment of patients with Chagas' disease achalasia: a double-blind, crossover trial. *Braz J Med Biol Res* 1991;24:1093–1098.

266. Raizman RE, de Rezende JM, Neva FA. A clinical trial with pre- and post-treatment manometry comparing pneumatic dilation with bouginage for treatment of Chagas' megaesophagus. *Am J Gastroenterol* 1980;74:405–409.

267. Ferrari APJ. Treatment of achalasia in Chagas' disease with botulinum toxin. *N Engl J Med* 1995;332:824–825.

268. Pinotti HW, Felix VN, Zilberstein B, et al. Surgical complications of Chagas' disease: megaesophagus, achalasia of the pylorus, and cholelithiasis. *World J Surg* 1991;15:198–204.

269. Sipe JD, Cohen AS. Amyloidosis. In: Braunwald E, Fauci AS, Kasper DS, et al., eds. *Harrison's principles of internal medicine*. New York: McGraw-Hill, 2001;1974–1979.

270. Röcken C, Saeger W, Linke RP. Gastrointestinal amyloid deposits in old age. Report on 110 consecutive autopsical patients and 98 retrospective bioptic specimens. *Pathol Res Pract* 1994;190:641–649.

271. Gilat T, Revach M, Sohar E. Deposition of amyloid in the gastrointestinal tract. *Gut* 1969;10:98–104.

272. Tada S, Iida M, Yao T, et al. Intestinal pseudo-obstruction in patients with amyloidosis: clinicopathologic differences between chemical types of amyloid protein. *Gut* 1993;34:1412–1417.

273. Lefkowitz JR, Brand DL, Schuffler MD, et al. Amyloidosis mimics achalasia's effect on lower esophageal sphincter. *Dig Dis Sci* 1989;34:630–635.

274. Bjerle P, Ek B, Linderholm H, et al. Oesophageal dysfunction in familial amyloidosis with polyneuropathy. *Clin Physiol* 1993;13:57–69.

275. Rubinow A, Burakoff R, Cohen AS, et al. Esophageal manometry in systemic amyloidosis: a study of 30 patients. *Am J Med* 1983;75:951–956.

276. Suris X, Moya F, Panes J, et al. Achalasia of the esophagus in secondary amyloidosis. *Am J Gastroenterol* 1993;88:1959–1960.

277. Finsterer J, Wogritsch C, Pokieser P, et al. Light chain myeloma with oro-pharyngeal amyloidosis presenting as bulbar paralysis. *J Neurol Sci* 1997;147:205–208.

278. Loehrl TA, Smith TL. Inflammatory and granulomatous lesions of the larynx and pharynx. *Am J Med* 2001;111(suppl 8A):113S–117S.

279. Hamed G, Heffess CS, Shmookler BM, et al. Amyloid goiter: a clinicopathologic study of 14 cases and review of the literature. *Am J Clin Pathol* 1995;104:306–312.

280. Khan GA, Lewis FI, Dasgupta M. Beta 2-microglobulin amyloidosis presenting as esophageal perforation in a hemodialysis patient. *Am J Nephrol* 1997;17:524–527.

281. Estrada CA, Lewandowski C, Schubert TT, et al. Esophageal involvement in secondary amyloidosis mimicking achalasia. *J Clin Gastroenterol* 1990;12:447–450.

282. Tada S, Iida M, Iwashita A, et al. Endoscopic and biopsy findings of the upper digestive tract in patients with amyloidosis. *Gastrointest Endosc* 1990;36:10–14.

283. Levin KH. Paraneoplastic neuromuscular syndromes. *Neuro Clin* 1997;15:597–614.

284. Sutton I, Winer JB. The immunopathogenesis of paraneoplastic neurological syndromes. *Clin Sci* 2002;102:475–486.

285. Lucchinetti CF, Kimmel DW, Lennon VA. Paraneoplastic and oncologic profiles of patients seropositive for type 1 antineuronal nuclear autoantibodies. *Neurology* 1998;50:652–657.

286. Lee HR, Lennon VA, Camilleri M, et al. Paraneoplastic gastrointestinal motor dysfunction: clinical and laboratory characteristics. *Am J Gastroenterol* 2001;96:373–379.

287. Chinn JS, Schuffler MD. Paraneoplastic visceral neuropathy as a cause of severe gastrointestinal motor dysfunction. *Gastroenterology* 1988;95:1279–1286.

288. Lennon VA, Sas DF, Busk MF, et al. Enteric neuronal autoantibodies in pseudoobstruction with small-cell lung carcinoma. *Gastroenterology* 1991;100:137–142.

289. Briellmann RS, Sturzenegger M, Gerber HA, et al. Autoanti-

body-associated sensory neuronopathy and intestinal pseudo-obstruction without detectable neoplasia. *Eur Neurol* 1996;36: 369–373.

290. Liu W, Fackler W, Rice TW, et al. The pathogenesis of pseudo-achalasia: a clinicopathologic study of 13 cases of a rare entity. *Am J Surg Pathol* 2002;26:784–788.

291. Geomini PM, Dellemijn PL, Bremer GL. Paraneoplastic cerebellar degeneration: neurological symptoms pointing to occult ovarian cancer. *Gynecol Obstet Invest* 2001;52:145–146.

292. Wolfsthal SD, Benitez RM. A 56-year-old man with progressive dysphagia, dysarthria and ataxia. *Maryland Med J* 1996;45: 933–937.

THE ESOPHAGUS AND NONCARDIAC CHEST PAIN

JAN TACK
JOZEF JANSSENS

Angina-like chest pain is an alarming symptom, not only for the patient who is frightened by its cardiac connotations, but also for the physician who has to decide whether or not he or she is dealing with a life-threatening condition. An estimated 10% to 50% of patients presenting with chest pain sufficiently severe to perform more invasive examinations are reported to have no evidence of coronary artery disease (CAD) and no evidence of coronary spasm upon provocation (1–6). Even after cardiac disease has been ruled out, many patients continue to experience chest pain, anxiety, and compromised lifestyles. Hence, noncardiac chest pain remains a considerable clinical challenge.

PREVALENCE AND IMPACT OF NONCARDIAC CHEST PAIN

Chest pain of noncardiac origin is a frequent clinical entity in the Western world. On the basis of the number of cardiac catheterizations, it has been estimated that more than 100,000 new cases of noncardiac chest pain are identified yearly in the United States (7). The clinical relevance of the problem may well be underestimated, because not all patients with chest pain will undergo coronary arteriography. The vital prognosis of patients with angina-like chest pain and normal coronary angiograms is favorable. The incidence of myocardial infarction or death is almost zero in most long-term serial studies of patients with noncardiac chest pain (2–4,8–14). Myocardial infarction occurs in at most 1% of the cases (15,16) and cardiac death in 0.6% after follow-up of up to 10 years (16–19). In contrast, patients with coronary disease confined to a single vessel had a mortality of 15% at 48 months and 35% at 11 years (20).

Information on the functional disability of noncardiac chest-pain patients is sparse. However, about three-quarters continue to see a physician, one-half remain or become unemployed, and one-half regard their lives as significantly disabled after having been told that their coronaries were normal (3,4,8,9,11). Only about one-third to one-half appear reassured that they do not have a serious cardiac disorder (4,14). As many as half of the patients remain on cardiac medications. In 1989, it was estimated that each of these patients will spend on average approximately US$4,000 per year for medical expenses related to their chest pain syndromes (7).

It has been known for a long time that cardiac and esophageal symptoms can mimic each other. Depending on the criteria used, the esophagus has been implied as a possible source of the chest pain in 20% to 60% of patients characterized as having noncardiac chest pain (3–5,21–26). A positive diagnosis, establishing the esophageal origin of the noncardiac chest pain, resulted in a significant reduction in the need for medical facilities (4,27–29) and increased significantly the number of patients who were able to keep their job (28). Therefore, a good understanding of the causes of recurrent noncardiac chest pain is of major importance to the quality of life of many patients.

CLINICAL CHARACTERISTICS OF ESOPHAGEAL CHEST PAIN

The clinical history often does not distinguish between cardiac and esophageal causes of chest pain (6). Chest pain of esophageal origin is usually located retrosternally and may irradiate to the arms, neck, jaw, or back. The pain is often described as squeezing or burning. It can be triggered by swallowing or ingestion, but it may also be triggered by exercise. The pain may last for minutes up to hours or even be present intermittently for several days. The pain can be sufficiently severe to be accompanied by the patient turning ashen and perspiring.

J. Tack, J. Janssens: Department of Gastroenterology, Division of Internal Medicine, University Hospital Gasthuisberg, University of Leuven, Leuven, Belgium.

In patients with noncardiac chest pain, careful evaluation of esophageal symptoms, especially the presence of dysphagia, may increase the likelihood of an underlying motor disorder or gastroesophageal reflux (30). Unfortunately, as many as 50% of patients with a cardiac cause of chest pain may have one or more symptoms of esophageal pain, such as heartburn, regurgitation, or dysphagia (31). Furthermore, cardiac and esophageal disease may overlap and they may interact in the induction of chest pain. Hence, the existence of underlying cardiac or esophageal disease cannot be precluded on the basis of history and clinical presentation alone.

MECHANISMS OF ESOPHAGEAL CHEST PAIN

The mechanisms underlying chest pain of esophageal origin are incompletely understood. It is well known that patients with achalasia and symptomatic diffuse esophageal spasm may have retrosternal angina-like pain (32,33), and that some patients with gastroesophageal reflux do not feel typical heartburn, but angina-like chest pain (34,35). Thus, chest pain of esophageal origin may arise either from stimulation of acid-sensitive chemoreceptors, or from stimulation of mechanoreceptors during abnormal motility. A potential role for thermoreceptors in the induction of esophageal chest pain has received little attention. In addition, hypersensitivity to esophageal balloon distention has been found in a subset of patients with noncardiac chest pain, although studies have shown inconsistent results (36,37).

Reflux-Related Esophageal Chest Pain

Both acid perfusion tests and ambulatory pH and pressure monitoring in patients with noncardiac chest pain have confirmed that intraesophageal acid may trigger chest pain. The mechanism by which chest pain occurs after exposure of the esophageal mucosa to acid remains largely unknown. Earlier studies suggested that acid perfusion induced esophageal motor abnormalities (38). However, more recent studies have demonstrated that acid-induced pain is usually not accompanied by major changes in esophageal motility (6,34,37–43). Although structures acting as esophageal chemoreceptors have not formally been identified, it seems likely that intraepithelial free nerve endings may act as acid-sensitive nociceptors (44). On the other hand, topical anesthetics fail to alter the pain response to acid infusion (45).

It has been shown that intraesophageal acid infusion is able to trigger myocardial ischemia in patients with coronary disease or with microvascular angina (46,47). However, there is no convincing evidence that coronary ischemia underlies acid-induced pain in patients with noncardiac chest pain. In these patients, episodes of symptomatic acid reflux are not associated to changes in the electrocardiogram (48).

In gastroesophageal reflux disease, the duration and minimal pH of reflux episodes seem to be determinant factors in inducing the perception of heartburn (49,50). Hypersensitivity to acid seems to be a frequent finding in noncardiac chest pain. In these patients, pain frequently occurs after very brief and less acidic reflux episodes. Sensitization of nociceptors may play a role in the apparently lower threshold for acid-induced chest pain in these patients. Other factors, such as the acid clearance mechanism, the acid exposure during the period preceding a particular reflux event, and the contribution of other refluxed factors such as pepsin, bile acids, and trypsin may also modulate the occurrence of chest pain during reflux episodes.

Motility-Related Esophageal Chest Pain

It is well known that patients with symptomatic diffuse esophageal spasm may have retrosternal angina-like pain (33). In many patients with noncardiac chest pain, high-amplitude contractions of prolonged duration, and impaired peristaltic progression can be observed during esophageal manometry. The most frequent findings are nonspecific motor disorders, followed by nutcracker esophagus and diffuse esophageal spasm (37,51,52). Initially, a causal link between these abnormal patterns of contraction and the patient's symptoms seemed obvious.

One popular hypothesis has been that the high pressure occurring during these abnormal contractions would inhibit esophageal blood flow for a sufficiently long time to induce mucosal ischemia. MacKenzie et al. (53) used microthermistors to measure the rewarming time of the chilled esophagus. They observed a longer rewarming time in patients with nutcracker esophagus than in control subjects, suggesting esophageal ischemia as a possible cause of the pain. However, Gustaffson and Tibbling (54) observed that the rewarming times before and after edrophonium administration did not differ between patients with a positive or negative test. The authors concluded that esophageal chest pain, elicited by intravenous edrophonium, is not caused by a decreased blood flow in the esophageal wall, but is directly related to high-amplitude and long-lasting esophageal contractions.

The relationship, however, between the manometric findings and the chest pain has remained complex and incompletely understood. Patients are generally asymptomatic at the time when the motor disorders are identified. It has been assumed that these abnormal contractions might be a marker for even more severe motor disturbances during spontaneous episodes of chest pain. However, prolonged esophageal pressure monitoring studies have demonstrated that this is only rarely the case (34,37). Moreover, there is no relationship between the presence of a nutcracker esophagus and the response to provocation tests that stimulate motility (55). Finally, the reduction of the amplitude of contractions by pharmacotherapy does not correlate with a symptomatic improvement (56). More recently, it was also demonstrated that the nutcracker esophagus can be associated with gastroesophageal reflux disease (57).

Recent data suggest that psychological factors may contribute to the phenomenon. Psychological stress alone is able to increase the amplitude of esophageal contractions, and this is more marked in patients with a nutcracker esophagus (58).

In a preliminary report, using 24-hour esophageal pressure, and pH and intraluminal ultrasonograpy monitoring, the majority of episodes of chest pain were accompanied by a transient increase in esophageal muscle thickness on ultrasonography (59). These increases in esophageal muscle thickness, called sustained esophageal contractions, were not accompanied by sustained increases in intraluminal pressure. In addition, sustained esophageal contractions were associated with chest pain in all patients with a positive edrophonium test. They were not observed in subjects with a negative edrophonium test. These findings suggest that sustained esophageal contractions may be the motor correlate of both spontaneous and induced esophageal chest pain. As they are not detected by esophageal pressure recordings, it has been speculated that sustained esophageal contractions reflect contractions of the longitudinal esophageal muscle layer.

Visceral Hypersensitivity

Patients with noncardiac chest pain have significantly higher pain sensation scores during intraesophageal balloon distension than healthy control subjects (36). This abnormal sensory perception appears to be independent of esophageal contractions or esophageal wall tone. Studies by de Caestecker et al. (60) suggest that a stretch receptor, linked to the longitudinal muscle of the esophageal wall, mediates the sensory response, as edrophonium increases and atropine reduces the sensitivity to balloon distension (60).

In contrast to healthy subjects or patients with nonstructural dysphagia, patients with noncardiac chest pain report increasing pain sensation scores during repeated balloon distensions (61). These data suggest that patients with noncardiac chest pain exhibit a conditioning phenomenon during repeated distensions. The level at which this conditioning occurs is unknown.

Irritable Esophagus

The irritable oesophagus concept was derived from the observation that some patients with noncardiac chest pain, when studied by 24-hour pH and pressure measurements, sometimes developed pain associated with reflux alone (without motor disorders), and on other occasions during the same study experienced the same pain together with motility disorders alone (without acid reflux) (35). The esophagus of these patients appeared to be hypersensitive to a variety of stimuli. The diagnosis of irritable esophagus is therefore based on the demonstration that the patient's familiar chest pain can be elicited by both mechanical and chemical stimuli. Chest pain induced by mechanical stimuli can be observed during edrophonium provocation or balloon distension, or motility-related chest pain during ambulatory motoring. Chest pain induced by chemical stimuli can be observed during the Bernstein test or reflux-related chest pain during ambulatory monitoring.

The mechanism underlying this irritability is unclear. In order to elucidate an interaction between sensitivity to acid and sensitivity to mechanical stimulation, Mehta et al. (62) studied esophageal perception and pain thresholds to balloon distention and electrical stimulation before and after esophageal acid perfusion in patients with noncardiac chest pain and healthy controls. After acid perfusion, balloon perception and pain thresholds decreased in patients with noncardiac chest pain and negative provocation tests and in controls, but did not decrease further in patients who had positive provocation tests. These findings suggest that acid perfusion sensitized stretch-sensitive nociceptors in patients with negative provocation tests and controls. The failure to show such sensitization in patients with positive provocation tests suggests that these nociceptors may already have been sensitized. Mutual sensitization of acid-sensitive and mechanosensitive mechanisms may contribute to the development of irritability in the esophagus.

Other Causes of Esophageal Chest Pain

Ingestion of hot or cold liquids can trigger severe chest pain. This does not seem to be caused by accompanying esophageal motor disturbances (63).

A belching disorder may be the mechanism responsible for chest pain in some patients with abnormal sensitivity to intraesophageal balloon distention (64,65). Esophageal wall distension, mimicked during balloon distension, may occur spontaneously during eructation against a closed upper esophageal sphincter (65). A similar mechanism of esophageal distention may underlie chest pain induced by acute food impaction and ingestion of carbonated beverages. However, other factors are likely to be involved, as in patients with noncardiac chest pain, smaller volumes of esophageal balloon distention are required to produce pain than in asymptomatic subjects (36,65).

Almost 5% of patients taking the serotonin-1D receptor agonist sumatriptan for migraine have chest discomfort. These symptoms are most frequently not associated with changes in cardiac function or enzymes. In healthy subjects, administration of sumatriptan in supratherapeutic doses causes small but significant increases in the amplitude and duration of deglutitive contractions, and an increased frequency of repetitive contractions can be observed (66). These data suggest that sumatriptan might provoke diffuse esophageal spasm in susceptible patients. However, until now, no temporal association was observed between chest symptoms and abnormal esophageal motility after sumatriptan.

DIAGNOSTIC TOOLS IN CHEST PAIN OF ESOPHAGEAL ORIGIN

Gastrointestinal endoscopy reveals reflux esophagitis in up to 31% of the patients with noncardiac chest pain (67–69). Stationary manometry in patients with noncardiac chest pain is able to demonstrate abnormalities in up to 29% of the patients (37,51,52). As esophageal motor disorders and low-grade reflux esophagitis are a common finding in many patients, the mere presence of these disorders cannot be accepted as proof for the esophageal origin of the chest pain.

Therefore, the best way to accept the esophagus as the likely cause of noncardiac angina-like chest pain is to show a temporal correlation between the occurrence of chest pain and an abnormal esophageal event. To increase the chance of recording a pain episode during esophageal testing, one can use provocation tests or extend the recording period (24-hour intraesophageal pH and pressure recording).

The Bernstein acid-perfusion test, the ergonovine test, the edrophonium test (55,70), and the esophageal balloon distension test (36) are well-known and widely accepted provocation tests. Other tests, such as the use of hot and cold liquids, pentagastrin, vasopressin, solid food boluses, and bethanechol are less extensively studied, and are not discussed further.

Acid Perfusion Test

The acid perfusion test was first described by Bernstein et al. (71). When 0.1 N of hydrochloric acid infused into the middle third of the esophagus is able to induce the familiar chest pain, the test is called positive related. When acid induces only a retrosternal burning sensation, or another unfamiliar sensation, the test is called positive unrelated, and is not accepted as a proof that the chest pain has esophageal origin. Studies in patients with noncardiac chest pain show a wide range of sensitivity in the Bernstein test, probably related to differences in patient selection (Table 38.1). The Bernstein test is positive related in 10% to 38% of the patients with noncardiac chest pain (34,35,37,41, 42,52,72,73).

Ergonovine Test

Intravenous administration of ergonovine is used as a test to provoke coronary artery spasm. If administration of ergonovine causes chest pain in the presence of ischemic ST-T segment changes on the electrocardiogram, a diagno-

TABLE 38.1. DIAGNOSTIC ACCURACY OF ESOPHAGEAL PROVOCATION TESTS IN PATIENTS WITH NONCARDIAC CHEST PAIN

Study	Accuracy		
	Bernstein	Edrophonium	Balloon
Vantrappen (35)	11/33	6/12	—
De Caestecker (72)	21/60	12/60	—
Peters (34)	7/20	9/18	—
Soffer (41)	2/20	0/20	—
Hewson (42)	15/45	24/44	—
Ghillebert (37)	18/50	16/50	1/20
Humeau (82)	4/40	6/40	13/34
Nevens (6)	14/37	7/37	3/37
Goudot-Pernot (83)	—	19/78	33/78
Hewson (93)	18/95	15/78	—
Rokkas (73)	29/110	26/110	—
Mehta (62)	3/25	10/25	—
Ghillebert (102)	106/270	58/220	26/182
Frøbert (96)	10/63	9/63	—

sis of vasospastic angina (Prinzmetal's angina) is accepted (74). However, if ergonovine induces chest pain without ST-T segment changes, an esophageal origin of the chest pain is often accepted (75). As ergonovine is not superior to edrophonium in provoking abnormal motility and chest pain in patients with suspected esophageal pain, and as the drug may induce potentially fatal coronary artery spasm, ergonovine no longer has a place in the routine diagnostic work-up of chest pain patients, unless to exclude vasospastic angina.

Edrophonium Test

The cholinesterase inhibitor edrophonium has been shown to be the most reliable and safest pharmacological agent for routine provocative testing in the clinical setting (70). The test is positive if slow intravenous injection of $80\mu g/kg$ of edrophonium but not placebo induces the familiar chest pain within 5 minutes after the administration of the drug. Administration of edrophonium increases esophageal contraction amplitude and the number of repetitive waves after wet swallows in both age-matched control subjects and patients with noncardiac chest pain. The change in duration seems to be significantly higher in patients in whom edrophonium induces chest pain, but there is considerable overlap with patients without chest pain (70). Hence, only symptoms and no manometric criterion will determine a positive edrophonium test. However, the style of the test administration and the interaction of the tester and the patients may strongly influence the outcome of the provocation test (76). Hence, inclusion of a placebo IV injection when using edrophonium is advisable.

The test has been reported to be positive in 0% to 55% of the patients with noncardiac chest pain (Table 38.1)

(34,41,37,42,35,52,72). Lee et al. (55) and Dalton et al. (77) proposed the use of a higher dose of 10 mg, but this does not produce a higher response rate, although side effects are more pronounced.

Balloon Distension Test

In 1955, Bayliss et al. (78) proposed intraesophageal balloon distension as a diagnostic test to distinguish esophageal from cardiac chest pain. In 1986, the test was resurrected as a provocative test in the evaluation of patients with noncardiac chest pain. A small balloon is placed 10 cm above the lower esophageal sphincter and inflated at 1-ml increments to a total volume of 10 ml (36). The reproducibility of the balloon distension test has been confirmed in healthy subjects (79). Women have significantly lower pain thresholds to esophageal balloon distention than men (80). The rate of intraesophageal balloon inflation seems to determine the level of perception. With a rapid inflation rate, the mean volumes required to induce perception or discomfort are significantly lower (81). Sustained inflation seems to induce increasing sensation.

Richter et al. (36) observed that balloon distension with a volume of 8 ml reproduced chest pain in 15 out of 30 patients and had no effect in controls (36). In other studies, the sensitivity of the test has been reported to vary between 5% and 50% (6,36,37,82,83) (Table 38.1). The reasons for this discrepancy are incompletely understood. It has been shown that acid perfusion is able to decrease the thresholds for perception and pain to balloon distension in patients with noncardiac chest pain and negative provocation tests and in controls, but not in patients who had positive provocation tests (62). Thus, the examination sequence may explain some of the different results obtained with balloon distension.

Rao et al. (84) used impedance planimetry to perform esophageal balloon distensions. Impedance planimetry provides a way to assess the cross-sectional area of the lumen in a selected plane at a range of distending pressures in an intraesophageal balloon. The authors used this technique in 12 healthy controls and in 24 chest pain patients with negative cardiologic and conventional gastrointestinal studies. The balloon was used to carry out stepwise isobaric distensions of the esophagus, while the cross-sectional area was measured and grades of sensation were reported by the subject. Similar to previous studies, hypersensitivity to esophageal distention was found in the patients who had lower thresholds both for first perception and for pain. Especially at low inflating pressures, patients tended to have a larger cross-sectional area in response to stretching. Paradoxically, however, the reactivity of the esophageal wall to distention was greater in patients who had a higher frequency and amplitude of contractions and a higher motility index than controls. Furthermore, balloon distension normally induces an inhibition of contractions distal to the balloon. In patients, this distal inhibition of the amplitude of pressure waves was attenuated or absent, suggesting neuromuscular dysfunction. The greater reactivity to luminal distension may be partly attributable to the biomechanical properties of the esophageal wall: patients with noncardiac chest pain had a stiffer, less compliant esophageal wall than controls. This study seemed to at least partially resolve the inconsistencies of previous studies using balloon distensions to elicit chest pain of esophageal origin (36,37). In these studies, increasing balloon volumes were used as a stimulus to activate tension receptors in the esophagus, but the variable esophageal diameter among persons may result in a highly variable tension stimulus. Using isobaric distensions and simultaneously assessing the diameter of the esophagus, as performed in the study by Rao et al. (84), allows calculation of the wall tension that elicits typical sensations.

Prolonged Esophageal pH and Pressure Recordings

Ambulatory pH and pressure recordings allow the patient to record the occurrence of spontaneous chest pain episodes. This allows demonstration of a temporal relationship between chest pain and the occurrence of an abnormal esophageal event such as reflux, motor abnormalities, or both. Several systems for ambulatory pH and pressure recordings are now commercially available. They all record pressure for at least two levels in the esophagus and pH at 5 cm above the lower esophageal sphincter. They have an event marker for the patient to indicate the occurrence of symptoms. Data are collected on tape or on solid-state memory, and analyzed afterward.

Since the original development of prolonged esophageal pH and pressure recordings (40), several studies have reported the reproducibility of this technique (85,86). It has recently been suggested that the esophageal motor abnormalities observed after the onset of chest pain are the consequence rather than cause of the pain. Likewise, episodes of gastroesophageal reflux may be induced by pain. Lam et al. (87) analyzed the occurrence of reflux or esophageal motor abnormalities in a prepain and a postpain window of 2 minutes. During the prepain window, 24.7% of pain episodes were correlated with abnormal motility, compared with only 4.2% in the postpain window. Chest pain was followed by acid reflux in only 3.6% of the events. Therefore, in patients with noncardiac chest pain, gastroesophageal reflux and esophageal motor disorders are infrequently induced by pain (87). The optimal time window in symptom analysis of 24-hour esophageal pressure and pH data begins at 2 minutes before the onset of the pain and ends at the onset of the pain (88).

The diagnostic accuracy of 24-hour pH and pressure recordings in the diagnosis of an esophageal cause for chest pain ranges from 10% to 56% in several published studies (Table 38.2). These differences are likely to reflect differ-

TABLE 38.2. DIAGNOSTIC ACCURACY OF 24-HOUR PH AND PRESSURE RECORDINGS IN PATIENTS WITH NONCARDIAC CHEST PAIN

Study	No. of Patients	No. of Patients with Chest Pain Related to			
		Dysmotility	Acid	Both	Global
Janssens (40)	60	8	4	9	21
Peters (34)	24	3	5	5	13
Soffer (41)	20	0	6	4	10
Ghillebert (37)	50	4	12	3	19
Hewson (93)	45	6	11	4	21
Breumelhof (43)	44	2	2	4	8
Nevens (6)	37	1	4	1	6
Lam (87)	41	10	13	—	23
Lux (105)	30	4	5	1	10

ences in patient selection, which is also reflected in the variable proportion of patients experiencing chest pain during the recording. An additional problem is the many uncertainties that remain in the way in which 24-hour pH and pressure measurements should be analyzed.

The definition of abnormal motility or abnormal pH to be used in the analysis of the data is controversial. Abnormal motility can be defined as contraction complexes that significantly exceed in amplitude, duration, or peristaltic disorder the contraction waves that were observed during a control period, consisting of a number of 5-minute periods selected throughout the pain-free periods of the recording (34). Other authors have used shorter control periods (37), or have used nonparametric statistics based on an automatic analysis of the entire 24-hour recording (43). The definition of abnormal pH is even less well established. Most authors have used a threshold (pH<4) to accept a pain episode as pH associated. However, Weusten et al. suggested (89) that optimal pH thresholds varied, ranging from 5.0 to 6.4 in the upright position and from 4.5 to 5.7 in the supine position. The most reproducible parameter obtained during pH monitoring is the percentage of time at which the pH is less than 4 (90). This is often used as a criterion to determine whether pathological reflux is present. Esophageal pH monitoring is able to demonstrate pathological gastroesophageal reflux in up to 62% of the patients with noncardiac chest pain (6,22,34,40–43,52,67,82, 91–94). However, even in the absence of pathological reflux, reflux can still be the cause of a patient's symptoms of chest pain. In Shi et al. (95), a group of patients had a normal acid exposure, but still had a significant temporal relationship between reflux episodes and chest pain events. These patients were considered to have an acid-hypersensitive esophagus. Frøbert et al. (96) performed 24-hour esophageal manometry and pH monitoring and provocative testing with intravenous edrophonium chloride and esophageal acid perfusion in 63 patients with angina-like chest pain but normal coronary angiograms (96). Reflux indices and ambulatory recorded esophageal motor func-

tion did not differ significantly between patients and healthy controls. On the basis of these observations, the authors question the rationale for routine esophageal investigations in patients with angina-like chest pain but normal coronary angiograms. However, patients were discussed only as groups, and only the mean time of acid exposure during pH monitoring was taken into account as a marker for reflux disease. Esophageal acid perfusion was positive in 16% of the patients, suggesting that acid-sensitive esophagus might still be a cause of their symptoms.

To quantify a temporal relationship between symptoms and episodes of gastroesophageal reflux, several indices have been developed. The most frequently used is the symptom index, defined as the percentage of reflux-related symptom episodes (97). However, in contrast to patients with typical heartburn as a predominant symptom, in patients with noncardiac chest pain, receiver-operating-characteristic curve analysis failed to determine a discriminant threshold of the symptom index for use in noncardiac chest pain (98). In addition, the symptom index does not take into account the total number of reflux episodes.

To overcome these drawbacks, the symptom sensitivity index was defined as the percentage of symptom-associated reflux episodes (99). However, this index does not take into account the total number of symptoms.

More complex methods were proposed, such as the binomial symptom index, which is obtained using the values of esophageal acid exposure, total number of symptoms experienced, and number of reflux-related symptoms in a binomial mathematical formula (37). Emde et al. (100) presented a mathematical approach based on the Kolmogorov-Smirnov test to evaluate the significance of reflux episodes as a cause of pain.

The symptom-association probability is a new method to calculate the probability that the observed association between gastroesophageal reflux and symptoms is not caused by chance (101). The 24-hour signal is divided into consecutive 2-minute periods. These periods are analyzed for the presence of reflux. A contingency table can then be

TABLE 38.3. DIAGNOSTIC ACCURACY OF PROVOCATION TESTS COMPARED TO 24-HOUR PH AND PRESSURE RECORDINGS IN PATIENTS WITH NONCARDIAC CHEST PAIN

Study	No. of Patients	Positive Provocation Tests	Positive 24-Hour Recording	Positive 24-Hour and Negative Provocation	Positive Provocation and Negative 24-Hour
Peters (34)	18	13	8	3	7
Soffer (41)	20	2	10	8	0
Ghilleberg (37)	50	24	19	5	11
Hewson (93)	44	30	20	5	15
Nevens (6)	37	17	6	1	6
Ghillebert (102)	190	94	48	14	60

constructed, comprising all relevant variables, and the probability can be expressed that the associations of symptoms and events are not caused by chance. However, the method can only be applied to esophageal pH, and not to esophageal pressure events.

Relationship Between Provocation Tests and 24-Hour pH and Pressure Measurements

The usefulness of the acid perfusion test in predicting symptomatic reflux in patients who had pain during 24 hour pH monitoring is rather low. Ghillebert et al. found a sensitivity and specificity for the acid perfusion test of 57% and 62%, respectively (102). Similar observations were made by Richter et al. (103). Despite an excellent specificity (94%), the Bernstein test was found to be considerably less sensitive than pH monitoring in identifying an acid-sensitive esophagus (32%) (103). These data suggest that mucosal acid sensitivity and symptomatic reflux should be regarded as separate, although related, aspects of reflux disease (104). Moreover, a specificity of 62% implies that a positive acid perfusion test will be present in 38% of the patients in whom reflux could not be detected during a spontaneous pain attack. Therefore, acid perfusion is still useful, particularly in patients who have no symptoms during 24-hour pH monitoring.

The sensitivity and specificity of the edrophonium to find motility-related events during 24-hour recording were 50% and 71%, respectively. The sensitivity and specificity of a positive edrophonium test to find reflux-related events during 24-hour recording were 39% and 72%, respectively (102). These data support the idea that a positive edrophonium test mainly suggests the presence of an esophageal origin of chest pain, but often fails to identify the specific pathophysiological mechanism underlying spontaneous attacks.

Diagnostic Impact of Provocation Tests versus 24-Hour pH and Pressure Measurements

A number of studies performed edrophonium and Bernstein provocation tests and also prolonged ambulatory pH and pressure recording in patients with noncardiac chest pain (Table 38.3). In 50% of patients, at least one provocation test was positive. Twenty-four hour recording revealed an esophageal origin in 31% of the patients (Table 38.3).

A combination of the acid perfusion test and the edrophonium test revealed the esophageal origin of the chest pain in 105 patients who did not have painful abnormalities during prolonged monitoring (gain 29%). In contrast, the diagnostic gain of ambulatory pH and pressure monitoring in patients found to have positive provocation tests was only 10%. Hence, it seems logical to perform an acid perfusion and an edrophonium test first. However, if these provocation tests are negative, the chance to establish the esophageal origin by performing an ambulatory pH and pressure monitoring is still 20%.

As discussed above, positive provocation tests are indications that chest pain is of esophageal origin. They often fail to identify the specific pathophysiological mechanism underlying spontaneous attacks. Prolonged ambulatory pH and pressure recordings are presently the only method to demonstrate the mechanism underlying spontaneous pain attacks.

DIAGNOSTIC EVALUATION

The existence of CAD cannot be rule out on the basis of the history and the clinical presentation only (6). As this is a potentially life-threatening disorder, evaluation of patients with chest pain should always start with the exclusion of cardiac disease. Furthermore, esophageal disorders have been reported in up to 50% of patients with cardiac disease (105,106) and their coexistence may induce chest pain via complex interactions. In young patients, an electrocardiogram during chest pain as well as a negative exercise stress test may be sufficient. In older patients, in addition to the exercise stress test, a coronary angiogram, possibly with ergonovine provocation, may be mandatory. If the cardiologic work-up is negative, the patient may be considered to have chest pain of noncardiac origin.

Gastrointestinal work-up is aimed at demonstrating symptomatic gastroesophageal reflux, esophageal motor abnormalities or hypersensitivity of the esophagus to balloon distention. The examination sequence may consist of endoscopy, stationary esophageal manometry, esophageal provocation tests using acid infusion, balloon distention and edrophonium chloride IV, and 24-hour ambulatory esophageal pH testing with or without 24-hour ambulatory esophageal manometry. Alternatively, the physician may embark on a therapeutic trial. Endoscopy is the examination of choice to start with. If this shows esophagitis or an unusual cause of chest pain such as an ulcer, appropriate treatment can be started. As reflux is the most common esophageal cause of chest pain, an empiric trial of acid suppression with a high dose of a proton pump inhibitor can be considered if the endoscopy was negative. Alternatively, one may proceed to perform stationary esophageal manometry with provocation tests. In case of unrevealing provocative tests, 24-hour ambulatory esophageal pH and pressure monitoring can be performed to try and identify the factors that trigger spontaneously occurring episodes of chest pain. Finally, a psychiatric work-up may identify underlying psychological disorders that require appropriate treatment.

PSYCHOLOGICAL FACTORS

The perception and verbal report of pain constitute a complex process modulated by factors such as anxiety, depression, individual cultural values, and secondary gain. Clouse and Lustman (107) showed that psychiatric illnesses were associated with a specific cluster of esophageal contraction abnormalities (increase in mean wave amplitude, increase in mean wave duration, increased frequency of abnormal motor responses, and presence of triple-peaked waves), suggesting a relationship between emotional disturbances and esophageal motility (107). The relationship between emotional disturbances and esophageal motility probably also explains why patients with the nutcracker esophagus have a more pronounced increase in esophageal contraction amplitude during psychological stress as compared to controls (58).

Patients with noncardiac chest pain and nutcracker esophagus and patients with irritable bowel syndrome have significantly higher scores of gastrointestinal susceptibility and somatic anxiety than controls (108). Several studies found a high incidence of psychiatric diagnoses, such as panic disorder, generalized anxiety disorder or depression, and somatization disorder in patients with noncardiac chest pain (109–114). However, up to 50% of patients with noncardiac chest pain have no active psychiatric syndrome at the time of evaluation (107,110). Sexual or physical abuse seems to be less prevalent in patients with noncardiac chest pain than in patients with the irritable bowel syndrome or with gastroesophageal reflux (115).

Anxiety is an important factor that contributes to symptom perception in patients with chest pain. Up to 25% of patients presenting to the emergency department because of chest pain meet the diagnostic criteria for panic disorder (114). In patients with noncardiac chest pain, hyperventilation can cause altered esophageal motility, but is unlikely to cause chest pain through this mechanism (115).

It has been suggested that the psychological features of patients with noncardiac chest pain might be secondary to a long-standing painful medical illness. However, the degree of psychiatric comorbidity seems to be less in groups of patients with chronic organic esophageal or cardiac conditions.

The multiple interactions between psychological factors and chest pain may also explain why patients with contraction abnormalities and symptoms benefit from psychotropic drugs (114,116–118), even though the drugs do not influence the manometric parameters. In an uncontrolled study, symptomatic improvement was obtained with benzodiazepine treatment (119). In addition, a beneficial effect of cognitive-behavioral psychotherapy has been reported (120).

CARDIAC AND ESOPHAGEAL CHEST PAIN

It has been suggested that gastroesophageal reflux and esophageal motility disorders may elicit myocardial ischemia and chest pain, a phenomenon called linked angina. In patients admitted to a coronary care unit for a typical angina episode, ischemic pain episodes provoked by reflux or abnormal esophageal motility are rare (121).

Gastroesophageal reflux disease, a common cause of chest pain, and CAD are both highly prevalent in the population. Moreover, panic disorder has been reported to be highly prevalent both in patients with CAD and in patients with noncardiac chest pain. Hence, it seems likely that these disorders may coexist in some patients, thus creating confusion about the origin of chest pain.

Lux et al. (105) compared the frequency of esophageal disturbances in patients with normal coronary angiograms and patients with coronary heart disease. They observed that abnormal esophageal motility or gastroesophageal reflux correlated with chest pain episodes in 33% of patients with normal coronary arteries, but also in 26% of patients with pathologic coronary angiograms. In the latter group, reflux or dysmotility were often accompanied by ST-segment changes. Thus, in patients with CAD, a significant number of episodes of ST deviation correlate with gastroesophageal reflux or abnormal esophageal motility.

Ros et al. investigated causes of recurrent chest pain at rest in 18 patients with proven CAD who experienced recurrent rest pain despite appropriate revascularization and absence of ischemic ECG changes (the "problem group") (106). As a "control" group, 27 patients who had chest pain with ischemic ST segment changes in the ECG and who had obstructive coronary artery lesions without prior revascularization procedures were also studied. All patients underwent esophageal manometry, 24-hour pH studies, edrophonium provocation, and a psychiatric diagnostic interview. Based on these studies, in 44% of the patients in the problem group the esophagus was considered a likely cause of chest pain, and in 56% a probable cause. In the control group an esophageal cause of chest pain was thought unlikely in 48%, probable in 33%, and likely in only 19%. Panic disorder was diagnosed in 50% of the problem group and in 19% of the control group. The authors conclude that esophageal dysfunction and psychiatric disturbances are common in patients with CAD presenting with resting chest pain, and they may contribute to patients' symptoms; esophageal investigations may thus be beneficial in many of these patients because they can elucidate treatable causes of chest pain.

Esophageal disorders may not only coexist with CAD, but it has also been suggested that esophageal stimulation may elicit myocardial ischemia. Esophageal acid infusion reduces the threshold for exercise-induced angina in patients with CAD, and reduces coronary blood flow in patients with syndrome X and in patients with angiographically proven significant CAD (31,47,122). In 18 denervated cardiac transplant recipients, coronary blood flow was not affected by esophageal acid infusion. These observations suggest the involvement of a neural cardioesophageal reflex in the pathogenesis of so-called linked angina (122). The study raises the possibility that patients with CAD might benefit from acid-suppressive therapy.

MICROVASCULAR ANGINA

In 1973, Kemp used the term "syndrome X" to denote a group of patients with ischemic-appearing electrocardiograms during exercise, but with normal coronary angiograms during cardiac catheterization (123). A number of studies have subsequently shown that patients with chest pain and normal coronary angiograms had abnormal coronary flow dynamics during pharmacologically induced vasodilatation, suggestive of an impaired coronary flow reserve (124,125). It was hypothesized that the abnormality was due to dysfunction of the coronary microcirculation. Several studies reported that patients with syndrome X had an abnormal endothelial function (126–128) and an excessive sympathetic responsiveness (129–131). Most studies, however, failed to demonstrate metabolic evidence for ischemia (132,133). Moreover, even in the presence of some suggestion of ischemia, such as impaired left ventricular functional responses, or abnormal exercise thallium scintigraphy, the prognosis of these patients is excellent (134,135).

A number of groups observed that patients with chest pain and normal coronary angiograms would readily experience chest pain during cardiac catheterization, suggesting that abnormal cardiac pain perception might be present

(136–140). In patients with atherosclerotic or structural heart disease, chest pain is only rarely elicited during cardiac catheterization. Stimuli causing chest pain are catheter movement in the right atrium, intravenous administration of adenosine, intravenous dipyridamole, injection of saline or contrast medium, and right ventricular pacing. Cannon et al. (137) observed that right ventricular pacing was able to elicit characteristic chest pain in 85% of patients with chest pain and normal coronary angiograms, regardless of whether they had evidence of microvascular dysfunction. Thus, patients with increased cardiac perception may represent another manifestation of visceral hypersensitivity, present in several functional gastrointestinal disorders. The cause or mechanism underlying this hypersensitivity remains unclear.

The antidepressant drug imipramine is able to improve symptoms in patients with chest pain and normal coronary angiograms (114). The response to imipramine did not depend on the result of cardiac, esophageal, or psychiatric testing at baseline. It was shown that imipramine was able to improve cardiac sensitivity in this group of patients. Thus, the beneficial effect of imipramine may involve a visceral analgesic effect (114).

TREATMENT

The medical therapy of angina-like chest pain of esophageal origin remains controversial. Many patients may improve with confident reassurance alone, although it seems important for many patients not only to prove the absence of a cardiac disease or malignancy but also to establish a definite cause of the symptoms to avoid ongoing concern (4,141).

Anticholinergics have been suggested for the treatment of chest pain ascribed to underlying motility abnormalities, but at present there are no controlled studies to justify this therapy. In a single-blind acute study, cimetropium bromide produced a dramatic decrease in esophageal contraction amplitude in patients with the nutcracker esophagus, but data about pain relief were lacking (142). Nitroglycerin and long-acting nitrates have been shown to be beneficial in patients with symptomatic diffuse esophageal spasm (143,144), but to date no data have been published on the effect of these agents in patients with noncardiac chest pain without a manometric picture of diffuse spasm.

Several studies have examined the effect of the calcium channel blocker diltiazem on noncardiac chest pain, but the results are conflicting with regard to symptom relief as well as the effect on esophageal contraction amplitude (145–147). Nifedipine was shown to decrease the amplitude of esophageal contractions in patients with nutcracker esophagus, but it was no better than placebo in symptom relief after 6 weeks of treatment (56,148). A beneficial effect on symptom relief was obtained with a low dose of the antidepressant trazodone in symptomatic patients with esophageal contraction abnormalities (118).

A thoracic longitudinal myotomy has been reported to give symptomatic relief in some patients with chest pain due to esophageal motor abnormalities. More recently, it was reported that a thoracoscopic esophageal long myotomy is able to provide substantial or complete pain relief in a subset of patients with noncardiac chest pain with diffuse esophageal spasm or symptomatic hypertensive peristalsis (149). However, we feel that surgical management of esophageal chest pain is extremely rarely indicated.

In patients with noncardiac chest pain and proven gastroesophageal reflux, intensive antireflux therapy with high doses of H_2-blockers or with proton pump inhibitors, is able to improve symptoms (150,151). It is unclear whether acid suppression may improve symptoms in patients with coexisting motor disorders and pathologic acid reflux. Adamek et al. (152) performed prolonged manometric and pH recording in 95 patients with noncardiac chest pain. They observed a high rate of coexistence of hypermotility disorders and pathologic acid reflux. When patients with both disorders received omeprazole treatment, improvement in symptoms and reduction of pathologic acid reflux was observed, but the hypermotility disorder persisted, and patients did not become completely symptom-free, suggesting that the motor disorder did not depend on pathologic reflux.

The treatment of patients with an irritable or a hypersensitive esophagus is even more difficult. Acid-blocking agents will at best only partially relieve symptoms, while motor inhibitory drugs may aggravate reflux. Drugs that interfere with pain perception may well be indicated in these patients. Such a mechanism could explain the beneficial effect on symptom relief obtained with a low dose of the antidepressant trazodone in symptomatic patients with esophageal contraction abnormalities (118). Imipramine, a tricyclic antidepressant helpful in the management of patients with chronic pain syndromes, was evaluated in the treatment of patients with chest pain and normal coronary angiograms (114). Imipramine reduced by approximately 50% the number of chest pain episodes, and it also reduced the sensitivity to cardiac pain during electrical stimulation. Esophageal motility testing did not identify patients who were likely to respond to imipramine.

McDonald-Haile et al., evaluated the effect of muscle relaxation training on symptoms reports and esophageal acid exposure in patients with reflux disease (153). Subjects who received muscle relaxation had lower reflux symptoms and esophageal acid exposure. These data suggest that relaxation might be a useful adjunct to antireflux therapy.

FOLLOW-UP

More work needs to be done before an efficient treatment scheme for chest pain of esophageal origin can be established. The long-term follow-up of patients with noncardiac chest pain has been inadequately studied. The use of esophageal testing and diagnosis has been controversial. Rose et al. (154) studied prospectively the effect of esophageal testing on patient well-being in subjects with noncardiac chest pain. There was a decline in emergency room visits and patients tended to resume their normal activities, suggesting that esophageal testing by itself is useful in reassuring the patients of a noncardiac etiology of their symptoms. However, some patients did not fully comprehend the results of esophageal testing, and more than half of the patients who were found to have an esophageal abnormality still did not consider the esophagus as the source of the pain.

REFERENCES

1. Likoff W, Segel BL, Kasparian H. Paradox of normal selective coronary arteriograms in patients considered to have unmistakable coronary heart disease. *N Engl J Med* 1967;276: 1063–1066.
2. Waxler EB, Kimbiris D, Dreifus LS. The fate of women with normal coronary arteriograms and chest pain resembling angina pectoris. *Am J Cardiol* 1971;28:25–32.
3. Kemp HG, Vokonas PS, Cohn PF, et al. The anginal syndromes associated with normal coronary arteriograms: Report of a six year experience. *Am J Med* 1973;54:735–742.
4. Ockene IS, Shay MJ, Alpart JA, et al. Unexplained chest pain in patients with normal coronary arteriograms. A follow-up study of functional status. *N Engl J Med* 1980;303:1249.
5. Wilcox RG, Roland JM, Hampton JR. Prognosis of patients with "chest pain cause". *BMJ (Clin Res Ed)* 1981;282:431–433.
6. Nevens F, Janssens J, Piessens J, et al. Prospective study on the prevalence of esophageal chest pain in patients referred on an elective basis to a cardiac unit for suspected myocardial ischemia. *Dig Dis Sci* 1991;36:228–235.
7. Richter JE, Bradley LA, Castell DO. Esophageal chest pain: current controversies in pathogenesis, diagnosis and therapy *Ann Intern Med* 1989;110:66–78.
8. Bemiler CR, Pepine CJ, Rogers, AK. Long term observation in patients with angina and normal coronary arteries. *Circulation* 1973;47:36–43.
9. Day LJ, Sowton E. Clinical features and follow-up of patients with angina and normal coronary arteries. *Lancet* 1976;2: 334–337.
10. Marchandise B, Bourassa MG, Chaitman BR, et al. Angiographic evaluation of the natural history of normal coronary arteries and mild coronary atherosclerosis. *Am J Cardiol* 1978; 41:216–220.
11. Lavey EB, Winkle RA. Continuing disability of patients with chest pain and normal coronary arteriograms. *J Chron Dis* 1979;32:191–196.
12. Faxon DP, McCabe CH, Kreigel, et al. Therapeutic and economic value of a normal coronary angiogram. *Am J Med* 1982;73:500–505.
13. Bass C, Wade C, Hand D, et al. Patients with angina with normal and near normal coronary arteries: clinical and psychosocial state 12 months after angiography. *BMJ* 1983;287:1505–1508.
14. Lantinga LJ, Sprafkin RP, McCroskery JH, et al. One-year psychosocial follow-up of patients with chest pain and angiographically normal coronary arteries. *Am J Cardiol* 1988;62:209–213.
15. Pasternak RC, Thibault GE, Savoia M, et al. Chest pain with

angiographically insignificant coronary arterial obstruction. Clinical presentation and long-term follow-up. *Am J Med* 1980; 68:813–817.

16. Wielgosz AT, Fletcher RH, McCants CB, et al. Unimproved chest pain in patients with minimal or no coronary disease: a behavioural problem. *Am Heart J* 1984;108:67–72.

17. Brushke AVG, Proudfit WL, Sones FM. Clinical course of patients with normal, slightly or moderately abnormal coronary arteriogram. A follow-up study on 500 patients. *Circulation* 1973;47:936–945.

18. Proudfit WL, Bruschke AVG, Sones, FM. Clinical course of patients with normal or slightly or moderately abnormal coronary arteriograms:10 year follow-up of 521 patients. *Circulation* 1980;62:712–717.

19. Kemp HG, Kronmal RA, Vlietstra RE, et al. Seven year survival of patients with normal or near normal coronary arteriograms: a CASS registry study. *J Am Coll Cardiol* 1986;7:479–83.

20. Detre KM, Peduzzi P, Takaro T, et al. The Veterans Administration coronary Artery Bypass Surgery co-operative Study group. Eleven-year survival in the Veterans Administration randomized trial of coronary bypass surgery for stable angina. *N Engl J Med* 1984;311:1333–1339.

21. Dart AM, Davies AH, Dalal J, et al. Angina and normal coronary arteriograms: a follow-up study. *Eur Heart J* 1980;1:97–100.

22. DeMeester TR, O'Sullivan GC, Bermudez G, et al. Esophageal function in patients with angina-type chest pain and normal coronary angiograms. *Ann Surg* 1982;196:488–498.

23. Ferguson SC, Hodges K, Hersh T, et al. Esophageal manometry in patients with chest pain and normal coronary arteriograms. *Am J Gastroenterol* 1981;75:124–127.

24. Kubler W, Opherk D. Angina pectoris with normal coronary arteries. *Acta Med Scand* 1984;694:55–57.

25. Sax, F.L, Cannon SO, Henson L, et al. Impaired forearm vasodilator reserve in patients with microvascular angina. *N Engl J Med* 1987;317:1366–1370.

26. Cannon RO III, Epstein SE. Microvascular angina as a cause of chest pain with angiographically normal coronary arteries. *Am J Cardiol* 1988;61:1338–1343.

27. Ward B, Wu WC, Richter JE, et al. Long term follow-up of patients with non-cardiac chest pain: is diagnosis of esophageal etiology helpful? *Am J Gastroenterol* 1987;82:215–218.

28. Schofield PM. Follow-up study of morbidity in patients with angina pectoris and normal coronary angiograms and the value of investigation for esophageal dysfunction. *Angiology* 1990;41:286–296.

29. Swift GL, Alban-Davies N, McKirdy H, et al. A-long term clinical review of patients with esophageal pain. *Q J Med* 1991;295: 937–944.

30. Bak YT, Lorang M, Evans PR, et al. Predictive values of symptoms profiles in patients with suspected esophageal dysmotility. *Scand J Gastroenterol* 1994;29:392–397.

31. Alban Davies H, Page Z, Rush EM, et al. Oesophageal stimulation lowers exertional angina threshold. *Lancet* 1985;1: 1011–1014.

32. Vantrappen G, Hellemans J. Achalasia. In: Vantrappen G, Hellemans J, eds. *Diseases of the oesophagus.* Berlin, Heidelberg, New York: Springer–Verlag, 1975;287–354.

33. Vantrappen G, Hellemans J. Diffuse muscle spasm of the oesophagus and hypertensive oesophageal sphincter. *Clin Gastroenterol* 1976;5:59–72.

34. Peters L, Maas L, Petty D, et al. Spontaneous non-cardiac chest pain. Evaluation by 24-hour ambulatory esophageal motility and pH monitoring. *Gastroenterology* 1988;94:878–886.

35. Vantrappen G, Janssens J, Ghillebert G. The irritable esophagus—a frequent cause of angina-like pain. *Lancet* 1987;1: 1232–1234.

36. Richter JE, Barish CF, Castell DO. Abnormal sensory perception in patients with esophageal chest pain. *Gastroenterology* 1986;91:845–852.

37. Ghillebert G, Janssens J, Vantrappen G, et al. Ambulatory 24-hour intraoesophageal pH and pressure recordings vs provocation tests in the diagnosis of chest pain of oesophageal origin. *Gut* 1990;31:738–744.

38. Siegel CI, Hendrix TR. Esophageal motor abnormalities induced by acid perfusion in patients with heartburn. *J Clin Invest* 1963;42:686–695.

39. Richter JE, Johns DN, Wu WC, et al. Are esophageal motility abnormalities produced during the intra-esophageal acid perfusion test? *JAMA* 1985;253:1914.

40. Janssens J, Vantrappen G, Ghillebert G. 24-hour recording of esophageal pressure and pH in patients with non-cardiac chest pain. *Gastroenterology* 1986;90:1978–1984.

41. Soffer EE, Scalabrini P, Wingate DL. Spontaneous non-cardiac chest pain: value of ambulatory esophageal pH and motility monitoring. *Dig Dis Sci* 1989;24:1651–1655.

42. Hewson EG, Dalton CB, Richter, JE. Comparison of esophageal manometry, provocative testing and ambulatory monitoring in patients with unexplained chest pain. *Dig Dis Sci* 1990;35:302–309.

43. Breumelhof R, Nadorp JHSM, Akkermans LMA, et al. Analysis of 24-hour esophageal pH and pressure data in unselected patients with non-cardiac chest pain. *Gastroenterology* 1990; 99:1257–1264.

44. Lynn RB. Mechanisms of esophageal pain. *Am J Med* 1992;92: 11–19.

45. Hookman P, Siegel CI, Hendrix TR. Failure of oxethazine to alter acid induced esophageal pain. *Am J Dig Dis* 1966;11:811.

46. Mellow MH, Simpson AG, Watt L, et al. Oesophageal acid perfusion in coronary artery disease: induction of myocardial ischemia. *Gastroenterology* 1983;85:306–312.

47. Chauhan A, Petch MC, Schofield PM. Effect of oesophageal acid instillation on coronary blood flow. *Lancet* 1993;341: 1309–1310.

48. Wani M, Hishon S. ECG record during changes in oesophageal pH. *Gut* 1990;31:127–128.

49. Baldi F, Ferrarini F, Longanesi A, et al. Acid gastroesophageal reflux and symptom occurrence. Analysis of some factors influencing their association. *Dig Dis Sci* 1989;34:1890–1893.

50. Janssens J, Vantrappen G, Vos R, et al. The acid burden over and extended period preceding a reflux episode is a major determinant in the development of heartburn. *Gastroenterology* 1992;103:A90(abst).

51. Benjamin SB, Gerhardt DC, Castell DO. High amplitude, peristaltic esophageal contractions associated with chest pain and/or dysphagia. *Gastroenterology* 1979;77:478.

52. Cherian P, Smith LF, Bardhan DK, et al. Esophageal tests in the evaluation of non-cardiac chest pain. *Dis Esophagus* 1995;8: 129–133.

53. MacKenzie J, Belch J, Land JD, et al. Oesophageal ischemia in motility disorders associated with chest pain. *Lancet* 1988:529–595.

54. Gustafsson U, Tibbling L. The effect of edrophonium chloride-induced chest pain on esophageal blood flow and motility. *Scand J Gastroenterol* 1997;32:104–107.

55. Lee CA, Reynolds, JC, Ouyang A, et al. Esophageal chest pain: value of high-dose provocative testing with edrophonium chloride in patients with normal esophageal manometries. *Dig Dis Sci* 1987;32:682–688.

56. Richter JE, Dalton CB, Bradley LA, et al. Oral nifedipine in the treatment of non-cardiac chest pain in patients with the nutcracker esophagus. *Gastroenterology* 1987;93:21–28.

57. Achem SR, Kolts BE, Wears R, et al. Chest pain associated with

nutcracker esophagus: a preliminary study of the role of gastroesophageal reflux. *Am J Gastroenterol* 1993;93;88:187–192.

58. Anderson KO, Dalton CB, Bradley LA, et al. Stress induced alteration of esophageal pressures in healthy volunteers and non-cardiac chest pain patients. *Dig Dis Sci* 1989;34:89–91.

59. Balaban DH, Yamamoto, Y, Liu J, et al. Identification of a unique esophageal motor pattern by probe ultrasonography: a marker of spontaneous and induced esophageal chest pain. *Neurogastroenterol Motil* 1998;10:59(abst).

60. de Caestecker JS, Pryde A, Heading RC. Site and mechanism of pain perception with esophageal balloon distension and intravenous edrophonium in patients with esophageal chest pain. *Gut* 1992;33:580.

61. Patterson WG, Wang H, Vanner SJ. Increasing pain sensation to repeated esophageal balloon distension in patients with chest pain of undetermined etiology. *Dig Dis Sci* 1995;40:1325–1331.

62. Mehta AJ, De Caestecker JS, Camm AJ, et al. Sensitisation to painful distension and abnormal sensory perception in the esophagus. *Gastroenterology* 1995;95;108:311–319.

63. Meyer GW, Castell DO. Human esophageal response during chest pain induced by swallowing cold liquid. *JAMA* 1981;246: 2057.

64. Kahrilas PJ, Dodds WJ, Hogan WJ. Dysfunction of the belch reflex. A cause of incapacitating chest pain. *Gastroenterology* 1987;93:818–822.

65. Gignoux C, Bost R, Hostein J, et al. Role of upper esophageal reflex and belch reflex dysfunctions in non-cardiac chest pain. *Dig Dis Sci* 1993;38:1909–1914.

66. Houghton L, Foster JM, Whorwell PJ, et al. Is chest pain after sumatriptan esophageal in origin? *Lancet* 1994;344:985–986.

67. Voskuil JH, Cramer MJ, Breumelhof R, et al. Prevalence of esophageal disorders in patients with chest pain newly referred to the cardiologist. *Chest* 1996;109:1210–1214.

68. Hsia PC, Maher KA, Lewis JH, et al. Utility of upper endoscopy in the evaluation of noncardiac chest pain. *Gastrointest Endosc* 1991;37:22–26.

69. Frobert, O, Funch-Jensen P, Jacobsen, N.O, et al. Upper endoscopy in pateints with angina and normal coronary angiograms. *Endoscopy* 1995;27:365–370.

70. Richter JE, Hackshaw BT, Wu WC, et al. Edrophonium: a useful provocative test for esophageal chest pain. *Ann Intern Med* 1985;103:14–21.

71. Bernstein LM, Baker LA. A clinical test for esophagitis. *Gastroenterology* 1958;34:760–781.

72. De Caestecker JA, Pryde A, Heading RC. Comparison of intravenous edrophonium and esophageal acid perfusion during esophageal manometry in patients with non-cardiac chest pain. *Gut* 1988;29:1029–1034.

73. Rokkas T, Tanggiansah A, McCullagh M, et al. Acid perfusion and edrophonium provocation tests in patients with chest pain of undetermined etiology. *Dig Dis Sci* 1992;27:1212–1216.

74. Heupler FA, Prandit WL, Razavi M, et al. Ergonovine maleate provocation test for coronary artery spasm. *Am J Cardiol* 1978; 41:631–640.

75. London RL, Ouyang H, Snape WJ Jr, et al. Provocation of esophageal pain by ergonovine or edrophonium. *Gastroenterology* 1981;81:10–14.

76. Rose S, Achkar E, Falk GW, et al. Interaction between patient and test administrator may influence the results of edrophonium provocative testing in patients with non-cardiac chest pain. *Am J Gastroenterol* 1993;88:20–24.

77. Dalton CB, Hewson EG, Castell DO, et al. Edrophonium provocative test in non-cardiac chest pain. Evaluation of testing techniques. *Dig Dis Sci* 1990;35:1445–1451.

78. Bayliss JH, Komitz R, Trounce JR. Observation on distension of the lower end of the esophagus. *Q J Med* 1955;94:143–154.

79. Lasch H, DeVault KR, Castell DO. Intra-esophageal balloon distension in the evaluation of sensory thresholds: studies on reproducibility and comparison of balloon composition. *Am J Gastroenterol* 1994;89:1185–1190.

80. Nguyen P, Lee SD, Castell DO. Evidence of gender differences in esophageal pain threshold. *Am J Gastroenterol* 1995;90: 901–905.

81. Nguyen P, Castell DO. Stimulation of esophageal mechanoreceptors is dependent on rate and duration of distension. *Am J Physiol* 1994;267:G115–G118.

82. Humeau B, Cloarec D, Simon J, et al. Angina-like chest pain of esophageal origin. Results of functional tests and value of balloon distension. *Gastroenterol Clin Biol* 1990;14:334–341.

83. Goudot-Pernot C, Champignuelle B, Bigard MA, et al. Prospective study comparing the edrophonium test and the intra-esophageal balloon distension test in 78 non-cardiac chest pain patients and 12 healthy controls. *Ann Gastroenterol Hepatol* 1991;27:41–48.

84. Rao SSC, Gregersen H, Hayek B, et al. Unexplained chest pain: the hypersensitive, hyperreactive, poorly compliant esophagus. *Ann Intern Med* 1996;124:950–958.

85. Emde C, Armstrong D, Castiglione F, et al. Reproducibility of long tem ambulatory esophageal combined pH/manometry. *Gastroenterology* 1990;100:1630–1637.

86. Wang H, Beck IT, Paterson WG. Reproducibility and physiological characteristics of 24-hour ambulatory esophageal manometry/pH-metry. *Am J Gastroenterol* 1996;91:492–497.

87. Lam HGTH, Breumelhof R, Van Berge Henegouwen GP, et al. Temporal relationships between episodes of non-cardiac chest pain and abnormal oesophageal function. *Gut* 1994;35: 733–736.

88. Lam HGT, Breumelhof R, Roelofs JMM, et al. What is the optimal time window in symptom analysis of 24-hour esophageal pressure and pH data? *Dig Dis Sci* 1994;39: 402–409.

89. Weusten BLAM, Roelofs JMM, Akkermans LMA, et al. Objective determination of pH thresholds in the analysis of 24 hour ambulatory esophageal pH monitoring. *Eur J Clin Invest* 1996;26:151–158.

90. Wiener GJ, Richter JE, Copper JB, et al. Ambulatory 24-hour esophageal pH monitoring: reproducibility and variability of the pH parameters. *Dig Dis Sci* 1988;33:1127–1133.

91. de Caestecker JS, Blackwell JN, Brown J, et al. The oesophagus as a cause of recurrent chest pain: which patients should be investigated and which tests should be used? *Lancet* 1985;2: 1143.

92. Schofield PM, Bennett DH, Whorwell PJ, et al. Exertional gastroesophageal reflux: a mechanism for symptoms in patients with angina pectoris and normal coronary angiograms. *BMJ* 1987;294:1459.

93. Hewson EG, Sinclair JW, Dalton CB, et al. Twenty-four-hour esophageal pH monitoring: the most useful test for evaluating non-cardiac chest pain. *Am J Med* 1991;90:576–583.

94. Lam HGT, Dekker W, Kan G, et al. Acute non-cardiac chest pain in a coronary care unit. *Gastroenterology* 1992;102: 453–460.

95. Shi G, Bruley des Varannes S, Scarpignato C, et al. Reflux-related symptoms in patients with normal oesophageal exposure to acid. The acid hypersensitive oesophagus. *Gut* 1995;37: 457–464.

96. Frøbert O, Funch-Jensen P, Bagger JP. Diagnostic value of esophageal studies in patients with angina-like chest pain and normal coronary angiograms. *Ann Intern Med* 1996;124: 959–69.

97. Wiener GJ, Richter JE, Copper JB, et al. The symptom index: a clinically important parameter of ambulatory 24-hour

esophageal pH monitoring. *Am J Gastroenterol* 1988;83: 358–361.

98. Singh S, Richter JE, Bradley LA, et al. The symptom index. Differential usefulness in suspected acid-related complaints of heartburn and chest pain. *Dig Dis Sci* 1993;38:1402–1408.

99. Breumelhof R, Smout AJPM. The symptom sensitivity index: a valuable additional parameter in 24 hour esophageal pH recording. *Am J Gastroenterol* 1991;86:160–164.

100. Emde C, Armstrong D, Blum AL. Chest pain due to gastroesophageal reflux: presentation of a mathematical procedure to assess its significance. *J Gastrointest Motil* 1990;2:140.

101. Weusten BLAM, Roelofs JMM, Akkermans LMA, et al. The symptom association probability: an improved method for symptom analysis of 24 h esophageal pH data. *Gastroenterology* 1994;107:1741–1745.

102. Ghillebert G, Janssens J. Provocation tests versus 24-hour pH and pressure measurements. *Eur J Gastroenterol Hepatol* 1995;7: 1141–1146.

103. Richter JE, Hewson EG, Sinclair JW, et al. Acid perfusion test and 24-hour esophageal pH monitoring with symptom index. Comparison of tests for esophageal acid sensitivity. *Dig Dis Sci* 1991;36:565–571.

104. Howard PJ, Maher L, Pryde A, et al. Symptomatic gastroesophageal reflux, abnormal esophageal acid exposure, mucosal acid sensitivity are three separate, though related aspects of gastro-esophageal reflux disease. *Gut* 1991;32:128–132.

105. Lux G, Van Els J, The GS, et al. Ambulatory esophageal pressure, pH and ECG recording in patients with normal and pathological coronary angiography and intermittent chest pain. *Neurogastroenterol Motil* 1995;7:23–30.

106. Ros E, Armengol X, Grande L, et al. Chest pain at rest in patients with coronary artery disease. Myocardial ischemia, esophageal dysfunction, or panic disorder? *Dig Dis Sci* 1997;42: 1344–53.

107. Clouse RE, Lustman PJ. Psychiatric illnesses and contraction abnormalities of the esophagus *N Engl J Med* 1982;309: 1337–1342.

108. Richter JE, Obrecht WF, Bradley LA, et al. Psychological similarities between patients with the nutcracker esophagus and irritable bowel syndrome. *Dig Dis Sci* 1986;31:131–138.

109. Cornier LE, Katon W, Russo J, et al. Chest pain with negative cardiac diagnostic studies. Relationship to psychiatric illness. *J Nerv Ment Dis* 1988;176:351–358.

110. Katon W, et al. Chest pain: relationship of psychiatric illness to coronary arteriography results. *Am J Med* 1988;84:1–9.

111. Ayuso Mateos JL, Bayon Perez C, Santo-Domingo Carrasco J, et al. Atypical chest pain and panic disorder. *Psychother Psychosom* 1989;52:92–95.

112. Beitman BD, et al. Panic disorder in patients with chest pain and angiographically normal coronary arteries. *Am J Cardiol* 1989;63:1399–1403.

113. Kisely SR, Creed FH, Cotter L. The course of psychiatric disorder associated with non-specific chest pain. *J Psychosom Res* 1992;36:329–335.

114. Cannon RO, Quyyumi AA, Mincemoyer R, et al. Imipramine in patients with chest pain despite normal coronary angiograms. *N Engl J Med* 1994;19:1411–1417.

115. Scarinci IC, McDonald-Haile J, Bradley LA, et al. Altered pain perception and psychosocial features among women with gastrointestinal disorders and history of abuse: a preliminary report. *Am J Med* 1994;97:108–118.

116. Fleet RP, Dupuis G, Marchand A, et al. Panic disorder in emergency department chest pain patients: prevalence, comorbidity, suicidal ideation and physician recognition. *Am J Med* 1996; 101:371–380.

117. Cooke RA, Anggiansah A, Wang J, et al. Hyperventilation and esophageal dysmotility in patients with non-cardiac chest pain. *Am J Gastroenterol* 1996;91:480–484.

118. Clouse RE, Lustman PJ, Eckert TC, et al. Low dose trazodone for symptomatic patients with esophageal contraction abnormalities. *Gastroenterology* 1987;92:1027–1036.

119. Beitman BD, et al. Pharmacotherapeutic treatment of panic disorder in patients presenting with chest pain. *J Fam Pract* 1989; 28:177–180.

120. Klimes, I, Mayou RA, Pearce MJ, et al. Psychological treatment for atypical non-cardiac chest pain: a controlled evaluation. *Psychol. Med* 1990;20:605–611.

121. Lam HGTH, Dekker W, Kan G, et al. Esophageal dysfunction as a cause of angina pectoris ("linked angina"): does it exist? *Am J Med* 1994;96:359–364.

122. Chauhan A, Mullins PA, Taylor G, et al. Cardioesophageal reflex: a mechanism for `linked angina' in patients with angiographically proven coronary artery disease. *J Am Coll Cardiol* 1996;27:1621–1628.

123. Kemp HG. Left ventricular function in patients with the anginal syndrome and normal coronary arteriograms. *Am J Cardiol* 1973;32:375–376.

124. Opherk D, et al. Reduced coronary dilatory capacity and ultrastructural changes of the myocardium in patients with angina pectoris but normal coronary arteriograms. *Circulation* 1981; 63:817—825.

125. Cannon RO, Schenke WH, Leon MB, et al. Limited coronary flow reserve after dipyridamole in patients with ergonovine-induced coronary vasoconstriction. *Circulation* 1987;75:163–174.

126. Motz W, Vogt M, Rabenau P, et al. Evidence of endothelial dysfunction in coronary dysfunction in coronary resistance vessels in patients with angina pectoris and normal coronary angiograms. *Am J Cardiol* 1991;68:996–1003.

127. Egashira K, et al. Evidence of impaired endothelium-dependent coronary vasodilation in patients with angina pectoris and normal coronary angiograms. *N Engl J Med* 1993;328:1659–1664.

128. Quyyumi AA, Cannon RO, Panza JA, et al. Endothelial dysfunction in patients with angina pectoris and normal coronary arteries. *Circulation* 1992;86:1864–1871.

129. Chauhan A, Mullins PA, Taylor G, et al. Effect of hyperventilation and mental stress on coronary blood flow in syndrome X. *Br Heart J* 1993;69:516–524.

130. Galassi AR, Kaski JC, Crea F, et al. Heart rate response during exercise testing and ambulatory ECG monitoring in patients with syndrome X. *Am Heart J* 1991;122:458–463.

131. Rosano GMC, et al. Abnormal autonomic control of the cardiovascular system in syndrome X. *Am J Cardiol* 1994;73: 1174–1179.

132. Arbogast R, Bourassa MG. Myocardial function during atrial pacing in patients with angina pectoris and normal coronary arteriograms: comparison with patients having significant coronary artery disease. *Am J Cardiol* 1973;32:257–263.

133. Crake T, Canepa-Anson R, Shapiro L, et al. Continuous recording of coronary sinus oxygen saturation during atrial pacing in patients with coronary artery disease or with syndrome X. *Br Heart J* 1988;59:31–38.

134. Miller TD, Taliercio CP, Zinsmeister AR, et al. Prognosis in patients with an abnormal exercise radionuclide angiogram in the absence of significant coronary artery disease. *J Am Coll Cardiol* 1988;12:637–641.

135. Kaski, JC, Rosano GMC, Collins P, et al. Cardiac syndrome X: clinical characteristics and left ventricular function. *J Am Coll Cardiol* 1995;25:807–814.

136. Shapiro LM, Crake T, Poole-Wilson PA. Is altered cardiac sensation responsible for chest pain in patients with normal coronary arteries? Clinical observation during cardiac catheterization. *BMJ* 1988;6:170–171.

137. Cannon RO, et al. Abnormal cardiac sensitivity in patients with chest pain and normal coronary arteries. *J Am Coll Cardiol* 1990;16:1359–1366.

138. Lagerqvist B, Sylven C, Waldenstrom A. Lower threshold for adenosine-induced chest pain in patients with angina and normal coronary angiograms. *Br Heart J* 1992;68:282–285.

139. Chauhan A, Mullins PA, Thuraisingham SI, et al. Abnormal cardiac pain perception in syndrome X. *J Am Coll Cardiol* 1994; 24:329–335.

140. Rosen SD, Uren NG, Kaski JC, et al. Coronary vasodilator reserve, pain perception and sex in patients with syndrome X. *Circulation* 1994;90:50–60.

141. Van Dorpe A, Piessens J, Willems JL, et al. Unexplained chest pain with normal coronary arteriograms. A follow-up study. *Cardiology* 1987;74:436.

142. Bassotti G, Gaburri M, Imbimbo BP, et al. Manometric evaluation of cimetropium bromide activity in patients with nutcracker esophagus. *Scand J Gastroenterol* 1988;23:1079.

143. Orlando RC, Bozymski EM. Clinical and manometric effects of nitroglycerin in diffuse esophageal spasm. *N Engl J Med* 1973;289:23.

144. Swamy N. Esophageal spasm: clinical and manometric responses to nitroglycerine and long acting nitrites. *Gastroenterology* 1977;72:23.

145. Frachtman RL, Botoman VA, Pope CE. A double blind crossover trial of diltiazem shows no benefit in patients with dysphagia and/or chest pain of esophageal origin. *Gastroenterology* 1986;90:1420.

146. Richter JE, Spurling TJ, Cordova CM, et al. Effects of oral calcium blocker, diltiazem, on esophageal contractions. Studies in volunteers and patients with nutcracker esophagus. *Dig Dis Sci* 1984;29:649.

147. Spuring TJ, Cattau EL, Hirszel R, et al. A double blind crossover study of the efficacy of diltiazem in patients with esophageal motility dysfunction. *Gastroenterology* 1985;88:1596.

148. Richter JE, Dalton CB, Castell DO. Nifedipine: a potent inhibitor of esophageal contractions. Is it effective in the treatment of non-cardiac chest pain? *Dig Dis Sci* 1985;30:790.

149. Cuschieri A. Endoscopic esophageal myotomy for specific motility disorders and non-cardiac chest pain. *Endosc Surg Allied Technol* 1993;1:280–287.

150. Singh S, Richter JE, Hewson EG, et al. The contribution of gastro-esophageal reflux to chest pain in patients with coronary artery disease. *Ann Intern Med* 1992;117:824–830.

151. Stahl WG, Beton R, Johnson CS, et al. Diagnosis and treatment of patients with gastroesophageal reflux and non-cardiac chest pain. *South Med J* 1994;87:739–742.

152. Adamek RJ, Wegener M, Wienbeck M, et al. Esophageal motility disorders and their coexistence with pathologic acid reflux in patients with non-cardiac chest pain. *Scand J Gastroenterol* 1995;30:833–838.

153. McDonald-Haile J, Bradley LA, Bailey MA, et al. Relaxation training reduces symptom reports and acid exposure in patients with gastro-esophageal reflux disease. *Gastroenterology* 1994; 107:61–69.

154. Rose S, Achkar E, Easly KA. Follow-up of patients with non-cardiac chest pain: value of esophageal testing. *Dig Dis Sci* 1994; 39:2069–2073.

RUPTURE AND PERFORATION OF THE ESOPHAGUS

ANTHONY INFANTOLINO
ROLAND B. TER

Approximately 275 years ago, Hermann Boerhaave, a Dutch physician, reported the case of the Grand Admiral of Holland, who died as a result of a "spontaneous" rupture of the esophagus (1). It is doubtful that Boerhaave realized the number of people who had suffered or would suffer a similar, almost always fatal demise. However, most additional reported cases were not classified as "spontaneous," but rather as "iatrogenic," that is, secondary to either intraluminal or intraoperative injury. Recent improvements in early recognition, initiation of treatment, introduction of antibiotics, and improved surgical and endoscopic techniques have lowered the fatality statistics associated with "spontaneous" rupture of the esophagus. This chapter explores adult esophageal rupture and perforation from its etiology, pathophysiology, and clinical presentation through controversies associated with treatment.

DEFINITION

In order to clarify many of the different terms in the literature, one must agree on the definition of rupture and perforation. Boerhaave's syndrome has been called *barogenic perforation* and *postemetic perforation* (2). The term *spontaneous esophageal rupture* will be used interchangeably with *Boerhaave's syndrome*. However, most cases are not truly "spontaneous," since most are preceded by intense and prolonged vomiting. Esophageal perforation is similar in its consequence, that is, full-thickness tear in the wall; most are secondary to manipulation within the esophageal lumen, and the majority have preexisting esophageal pathology.

A. **Infantolino:** Division of Gastroenterology and Hepatology, Thomas Jefferson Medical College, and Division of Gastroenterology and Hepatology, Thomas Jefferson University Medical Center, Philadelphia, Pennsylvania.

R.B. Ter: Division of Gastroenterology, Graduate Hospital, Philadelphia, Pennsylvania.

Anastomotic leaks, which have also been called esophageal disruptions (3), often have poor outcomes, are postoperative complications, and will not be discussed. A complete list of etiologies is presented in Table 39.1.

HISTORICAL PERSPECTIVE

In 1946, N. R. Barrett summarized Hermann Boerhaave's description of the case of the Grand Admiral of Holland, Baron Wassenaer (1,4). In 1723, Boerhaave was called to the bedside of the admiral, who was complaining of a disagreeable feeling in the stomach. The admiral had overeaten 3 days before and complained of persistent stomach discomfort. He had taken multiple doses of ipecacuanha to induce vomiting, as well as almond seed oil. While vomiting violently, he complained of severe pain and exclaimed that something had burst, and he was sure he would die. Boerhaave found him doubled over, complaining of constant pain in the chest and epigastric area. Over 16 hours, the admiral became progressively tachycardic, tachypneic, and pale in color; he died shortly thereafter. The autopsy 24 hours later revealed a distended gastrointestinal tract, food and medicine in the chest cavity, and a rupture in the otherwise normal-appearing esophagus.

From 1723 through 1938, there were many reviews of additional, uniformly fatal cases without full explanation. According to Barrett, J. R. Meyer from Berlin in 1858 was the first to recognize this entity prior to death. Barrett described the first early diagnosis and surgical repair in 1946 (4), followed by Olson and Clagett (5) in 1947. From 1947 through the 1960s, early recognition improved, antibiotics became more widely available, and mortality rates decreased. However, as the use of technology expanded, instrumental perforation became more common, and the definitions of rupture, perforation, and esophageal disruption became blurred. In 1979, Cameron et al. (3) reported 0% mortality in a heterogeneous group of patients

TABLE 39.1. ETIOLOGY OF ESOPHAGEAL PERFORATIONS

Iatrogenic
  Instrumentation: esophagogastroduodenoscopy, flexible, rigid esophagoscopy
  Esophageal dilatation: Savory, pneumatic, Maloney, Eder-Puestow, through the scope
  Miscellaneous therapeutic tools: nasogastric tube, enteroclysis tube, overtube, band ligation/sclerotherapy, Sengstaken-Blakemore tube, endoprosthesis, Celestin, expandable metal stents, endotracheal tubes, obturator airway, intracavitary irradiation for esophageal cancer, laser, endoscopic ultrasonography, bicap, APC
  Surgical injury: antireflux, Heller myotony, vagotomy, leiomyoma/lipoma resection, pneumonectomy, tracheostomy, thoracic aneurysm repair, mediatinoscopy, thoracostomy tube, cervical spine surgery, thyroid resection
Boerhaave's syndrome
Trauma: blunt, penetrating
Tumor: lymphoma, primary esophageal, metastatic
Foreign body: meat, bone, pill, Angelchik prosthesis, other
Infection: tuberculosis, herpes simplex virus, cytomegalovirus, human immunodeficiency virus, syphilis
Acid related: Barrett's ulcer, Zollinger-Ellison syndrome
Vascular: aberrant right subclavian artery, aneurysm, anticardiolipin antibody syndrome
Other: esophageal diverticulum, radiation therapy, caustic injury

---

who were treated conservatively. In 1983, Larsen et al. (6) reported on 57 cases over a 19-year period (42 iatrogenic, 15 spontaneous) and concluded that early intervention decreased mortality by almost half. Overall, however, there was still a 25% mortality rate. In 1991, Pate et al. (7) retrospectively reviewed 34 cases of spontaneous rupture over 30 years and found an overall mortality of 41%; they concluded that early surgical repair, regardless of the time after onset, appears to be indicated. Fernandez et al. (8) in 1999 reported on their retrospective experience with 75 patients; whether management was surgical or medical, the mortality rate varied between 16% and 24%. From Boerhaave's original description in 1724 to the present, diagnosis remains difficult, management continues to be controversial, and the diagnosis carries significant morbidity and mortality.

IATROGENIC

Instrumental Perforation

Medical instrumentation in the esophagus is the most common cause of perforation. Flynn et al. (9) in a series of 69 patients reported that 48% of ruptures were iatrogenic, 33% were caused by external trauma, and only 8% occurred spontaneously (9). In a more recent retrospective series of 75 patients, 97.3% were attributed to therapeutic endoscopy (10). Diagnostic esophagogastroduodenoscopy is a common procedure worldwide, and risk of perforation is extremely low. Flexible esophagoscopy is associated with a lower incidence of perforation (0.03%) compared with rigid endoscopy (0.11%) (11,12).

The usual location of perforation from endoscopy is at the cricopharyngeus, but when esophageal dilatation is added to the procedure, the location is often proximal to or at the stricture. The risk of perforation increases tenfold when dilatation is performed at the time of endoscopy, and is dependent on the type of dilator. Cox and Bennett (13) reviewed the literature on esophageal perforation and found that the incidence of perforation related to conventional dilators varies from 0.09% (for Maloney-Hurst-type dilators) to as high as 2.2% (for the Celestin-type dilator) (13). The American Society of Gastrointestinal Endoscopy Survey estimated that the incidence of esophageal perforation for bougienage and metal-olive dilators was 0.4% and 0.6%, respectively (14). In a national survey, the incidence of perforation from hydrostatic balloon dilatation was 0.3% (15). Pneumatic dilatation of the esophagus is a well-established treatment for achalasia, and the most serious complication is perforation. Nair et al. (16) reported a 1.7% risk of perforation. Both higher inflation pressure and previous pneumatic dilatation increase this risk. The risk may increase up to 9.8% when inflation pressure exceeds 11 psi (16,17). A more recent review of pneumatic esophageal dilation for achalasia reported a perforation rate of 2% to 6% (18).

Endoscopic thermal therapy of gastrointestinal bleeding is associated with 1% to 2% incidence of perforation (19). Endoscopic variceal sclerotherapy-related perforations, in contrast to other endoscopic complications, occur in a delayed fashion, typically 5 to 7 days postprocedure. The incidence of perforation is 1% to 6% and is the result of transmural necroinflammatory injury to the esophagus (20,21). Perforation has also been reported as a complication of endoscopic variceal ligation (22,23). The injury is due to the pinching of the esophageal mucosa between the endoscope and the overtube (24).

Palliative endoscopic laser therapy for esophageal tumors is not uncommonly associated with esophageal perforation. It may occur during the procedure or be delayed up to 1 week after treatment. Its incidence is estimated to be about 5% (25). Photodynamic therapy is currently utilized for palliative treatment of esophageal neoplasm and can be complicated by esophageal perforation. In a multicenter phase III trial of photodynamic therapy (PDT), Lightdale et al. (26) found a perforation rate of 4.6%. With the introduction of multiband ligators and improvement in technique, overtubes are no longer required, markedly decreasing the risk of esophageal perforation. In its recent (2002) update on policy and procedures published by the American Society for Gastrointestinal Endoscopy, endoscopic band ligation has a perforation rate of 0.7%. Bipolar electrocoagulation has also been employed to thermally ablate esophageal neoplasm, and the incidence of perforation is similar to laser therapy (27). Another form of palliative endoscopic therapy is endoprosthesis, which includes expandable metal and plastic stents. Perforation has been reported to occur in 5% to 25% of cases following esophageal stent insertion (28). The perforation may occur during stent insertion or be delayed secondary to pressure necrosis. Knyrim et al. (29) compared complication rates of expandable metal wall stents and plastic stents. The authors found that 3 of 21 patients had perforation during plastic stent insertion, while there was no perforation in the expandable-wall-stent group. A survey of six centers with a substantial experience in performing endoscopic ultrasound revealed a perforation rate of about 0.1% (30).

Nonendoscopic esophageal instrumentation is rarely responsible for esophageal perforation. These include endotracheal intubation, Sengstaken-Blakemore or Minnesota tubes for tamponading variceal bleeding, and nasogastric tubes. Endotracheal tube intubation can result in perforation of the cervical esophagus, which is usually located in the posterior wall near the cricopharyngeal muscle (31). In a more recent review by Overholt et al. (32) in over 100 patients treated with PDT for Barrett's esophagus, no perforations were reported. Given the high morbidity and mortality associated with esophagectomy for Barrett's esophagus, new techniques, including endoscopic mucosal resection, by itself or combined with PDT, have been performed. In two recent reviews involving 81 patients, no esophageal perforations were reported (33,34).

Surgical Perforation

Esophageal perforation can occur following operations on the esophagus or its contiguous structures. These operations include vagotomy, radical pneumonectomy, Heller myotomy, antireflux surgery, leiomyoma enucleation, thyroid resection, tracheostomy, thoracic aneurysm repair, mediastinoscopy, thoracotomy tube, and anterior cervical spine surgery (31).

TRAUMATIC PERFORATION

Trauma can cause esophageal perforation and rupture and accounts for 8% to 15.3% of all causes (35,36). Trauma-related perforation can be separated into blunt or penetrating. Blunt trauma is an exceedingly rare cause of esophageal perforation, with an incidence of 0.001% (37). The most common scenario is a high-speed motor vehicle accident with a steering wheel injury where a rapid rise in intraesophageal pressure occurs leading to rupture at the level of the hypopharyngoesophageal junction (37). Esophageal perforation in the neck can also result from intratracheal disruption, second rib fracture, cervical spine fracture, or improper cervical hyperextension (38).

In contrast, penetrating injuries to the esophagus are more common and most often secondary to knife and gunshot wounds. The incidence of penetrating injury to the esophagus is approximately 11% to 17% (38). Penetrating injuries of the cervical esophagus are more common than injuries of the thoracic esophagus in surviving patients. Overall mortality remains high (15% to 40%); therefore, early diagnosis with emphasis on location and associated vascular injury is warranted (38).

TUMOR

Both primary and secondary esophageal cancer can be complicated by perforation. Invasion of the esophagus by contiguous primary or metastatic carcinomas has also been reported.

FOREIGN BODY

Perforation of the esophagus can occur secondary to foreign-body ingestion and during endoscopic removal. It accounts for 7% to 14% of esophageal perforations (39,40). The perforation most often occurs at areas of acute angulation or physiologic narrowing. The level of the cricopharyngeus muscle is the most frequent location. Patients having previous esophageal surgery are at increased risk of perforation (41). Perforations secondary to foreign bodies occur by a number of pathways. Penetrating injuries from sharp or pointed metallic objects, animal or fish bones, and toothpicks result in high rates of perforation (42,43). Pressure necrosis from a blunt foreign body such as a coin can also rarely occur and is more common in children (44). Clinical manifestation of foreign-body perforation may be seen within 48 hours or as late as 2 weeks with gradual erosion of the impacted foreign body through the esophageal wall.

CAUSTIC INJURY

Ingestion of caustic substances can result in devastating injuries to the esophagus. Liquefaction necrosis of the esophageal wall following ingestion of lye weakens the wall of the esophagus, leading to rupture. There is a high risk of perforation in the 3- to 5-day postingestion period associated with intense inflammatory response and further vascular thrombosis with ulceration and sloughing of superficial layers of the mucosa. Instrumentation in the esophagus may increase the risk of perforation.

PILL INDUCED

Pill-induced esophageal injury is common and may occur with a variety of medications. The most common medications are tetracycline preparations, potassium chloride, quinidine, and nonsteroidal antiinflammatory drugs. Sustained-released formulations are more likely to cause injury. Damage caused by prolonged contact of medication with esophageal mucosa may result in perforation (45).

INFECTION

Infectious esophagitis may occur with pathogens such as *Candida*, herpes simplex virus, or cytomegalovirus, usually in an immunocompromised host. Perforations from esophageal infections are extremely rare. Extensive herpes simplex virus esophagitis and *Candida* esophagitis have been reported to cause spontaneous perforations (46,47). Adkins et al. (48) reported a case of esophageal erosion and perforation secondary to mediastinal lymph node enlargement from *Mycobacterium* tuberculosis in an HIV-positive patient.

OTHERS

Barrett's ulceration and Zollinger-Ellison syndrome with peptic ulcerative esophagitis have also been reported as causal factors in esophageal perforation (31,41). Aneurysm and aberrant right subclavian artery have also resulted in esophageal rupture (31). Cappell et al. (49) reported a case of esophageal necrosis and perforation associated with anticardiolipin antibodies, apparently due to thromboemboli and ischemia.

CLINICAL PRESENTATION

The clinical presentation of esophageal rupture and perforation is largely dependent on location and size of the injury and the time course when the patient is encountered (50). Although Boerhaave's syndrome is classically postemetic, other causes of a sudden rise in intraesophageal pressure (bursting pressure 3.7 to 5.0 lb/in^2) can result in "spontaneous" rupture (42). These include weight lifting, laughing, hyperemesis gravidarum, and seizures, among others (Table 39.2). Spontaneous rupture almost always occurs on the left side of the esophagus in the distal third (14,51–54). In a review of 184 cases of spontaneous rupture, the vast majority were found in the lower third (166 cases), 15 in the middle, and 3 in the upper third of the esophagus (37). Other large series have confirmed this location distribution (15,23,51,55). Most tears occur along the longitudinal axis, varying from 0.6 to 8.9 cm in length (52,56–58). Often, the mucosal tear is longer than the muscle tear, which is important surgically. This predilection for the lower left side of the esophagus remains unclear, but weakening of the wall by entrance of nerves and vessels, lack of adjacent supporting structures, vertical orientation of the longitudinal

TABLE 39.2. BOERHAAVE'S SYNDROME: CHARACTERISTIC FEATURES

Classic presentation
  Middle-aged male (35–55 years old), often with a history of dietary and alcohol overindulgence presenting with *chest pain* and *subcutaneous emphysema* after recent *vomiting* or retching (*Mackler's triad*)
Other predisposing factors
  Heavy weightlifting
  Hyperemesis gravidarum
  Excessive coughing
  Inappropriate Heimlich maneuver
  Defecation
  Severe asthma
  Parturition
  Hiccups
  Neurologic disorders (seizures/tumors)
  Idiopathic
Clinical features
  Signs
  Fever
  Tachycardia
  Decreased breath sounds
  Subcutaneous emphysema
  Vascular collapse
  Tachypnea
  Cyanosis
  Abdominal pain
  Symptoms
  Extreme chest/upper abdominal pain
  Vomiting/nausea
  Dysphagia/odynophagia
  Dyspnea
  Palpitations
  Sweats
  Restlessness
  Hematemesis
Histopathology
  Predominantly lower one-third tears
  Longitudinal (0.6–8.9 cm)
  Left greater than right
Radiographic findings
  Chest x-ray
  Subcutaneous/mediastinal emphysema
  Pleural effusions
  Pneumothorax
  Mediastinal widening
  Subdiaphragmatic air
  Pneumomediastinum
  Hydrothorax
  Normal if taken early
  Computed tomography
  Air in soft tissue of mediastinum surrounding the esophagus
  Abscessed cavities in pleural space/mediastinum
  Communication of esophagus with mediastinal fluid collections

muscle bundles, and the anterior angulation of the esophagus have all been considered (23,40,58–61).

Given the above anatomic considerations, 80% to 100% of cases present with pain (4,51,52,59,62,63). The location is variable, but chest, epigastric, and upper abdominal pain are most common. Mackler's classic triad of vomiting, chest pain, and subcutaneous emphysema is less common than originally thought, and overreliance on this could lead to delayed diagnosis (64) (Table 39.2). Atypical signs and symptoms include back pain (47), shoulder pain (65), facial swelling, proptosis, dysphonia, polydipsia, and hematemesis (2). The hematemesis of perforation is usually of small volume relative to the more common Mallory-Weiss tear (66). Signs include an acutely ill-appearing patient with fever, subcutaneous or mediastinal emphysema, tachycardia, tachypnea, cyanosis, and upper abdominal rigidity. Hamman's sign, that is, mediastinal crunch sound as the heart beats against air-filled tissues, has also been reported (58). Depending on the time course, shock is common. Signs consistent with pericardial tamponade secondary to esophagopericardial fistula and food embolism have been reported, but are quite rare (67,68). Vomiting, the classic prerupture symptom, occurs in 67% to 100% of cases but is by no means required to suspect the diagnosis (14,40,51). Dyspnea is also common and may be secondary to pleural effusions, pneumothorax, or hydrothorax (51,52) (Table 39.2). If the perforation is thoracic and instrumental in its etiology, pain, fever, and subcutaneous emphysema predominate (69). Instrumental perforations continue to be predominantly thoracic, but when cervical perforations occur, the pain may initially localize in the neck and may have associated dysphonia, cervical dysphagia, hoarseness, and pain with cervical motion, sternocleidomastoid muscle spasm, and tenderness along with cervical emphysema (63,69).

DIAGNOSIS

The diagnosis of spontaneous rupture or perforation most often relies on radiographic findings, but the clinician must first consider the diagnosis. Up to 50% of cases are atypical in nature and lead to diagnostic errors (37,70). The diagnoses most often confused with Boerhaave's syndrome are reported in Table 39.3. In terms of instrumental perforation, if the normal anatomic structures are lost during the procedure, a perforation is likely (9,70). Patients complaining of pain after endoscopy should always be considered to have a perforation and the burden of proof lies with the physician. Regardless of the etiology of the perforation, the location and the time interval will determine the clinical features. Once suspected, urgent posteroanterior and lateral chest and upright abdominal radiography should be obtained (71). Experienced radiologists will suspect the diagnosis in 90% of cases (72,73). The lateral roentgenogram of the neck is useful in suspected cases of cervical perforation. Soft tissue edema and air dividing the trachea and esophagus from the cervical spine is known as the Minningerode sign. Some typical chest x-ray findings include pleural effusions, pneumomediastinum, subcutaneous emphysema, hydrothorax, and hydropneumothorax

TABLE 39.3. BOERHAAVE'S SYNDROME: MISDIAGNOSES

Pancreatitis
Tension pneumothorax
Mallory-Weiss tear
Spontaneous pneumothorax
Gastric volvulus
Mesenteric thrombosis
Pneumonia
Incarcerated diaphragmatic hernia
Perforated peptic ulcer disease
Myocardial infarction
Pulmonary embolism
Aortic dissecting aneurysm
Splenic infarction
Pericarditis
Renal colic

(5,74,75) (Table 39.2). If taken early, the chest x-ray may be normal. Soft tissue and mediastinal emphysema can take up to 1 hour to develop. Pleural effusions can take several hours to become evident. Panzini et al. (76) reported that 80% of instrumental perforation patients had abnormal chest x-ray findings. Pneumomediastinum was present in 60%, and 33% had a density adjacent to the descending aorta in the left cardiophrenic angle with a loss of descending aorta contour (5). The midthoracic esophagus lies next to the right pleura; therefore, perforations in this are associated with right-sided effusions, while distal perforations most often lead to left-sided effusions (74,76,77). Pneumoperitoneum may also be seen secondary to perforation of the intraabdominal esophagus.

Gastrografin and/or barium esophagography should follow plain radiography (78) (Figs. 39.1 and 39.2). If the patient has been sedated, contrast studies should be delayed, pending the return of the gag reflex. Studies should be performed in the upright supine and lateral decubitus position (79). If a thoracoesophageal fistula or free perforation into the lung is suspected, barium should not be utilized due to the possible risk of mediastinal inflammation. However, if the patient is at high risk for aspiration, barium is the first option due to reported cases of pulmonary edema from gastrografin. Others believe that barium should always be the first study (80). However, most agree that even if the gastrografin study is negative, it must be repeated with barium (81). The above technique will detect 60% of cervical and 90% of surgically confirmed perforations, but carries a false-negative rate of 10% to 36% (72,82,83). Esophageal dissections, which are rare, appear radiographically as a double-barreled esophagus (76) (Fig. 39.3). Sawyer et al. (68) stressed the importance of repeating the contrast study after several hours if a clinical scenario suggesting perforation persists, but the initial exam is negative. Spasm, tissue edema, and other factors may contribute to the false negatives (81).

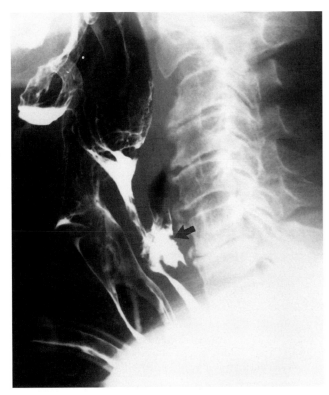

FIGURE 39.1. Sealed-off perforation of the cervical esophagus by endoscopy. Note the self-contained extraluminal collection of contrast in the prevertebral location (*black arrow*). (Courtesy S. Karasick, Thomas Jefferson University Hospital, Philadelphia, PA.)

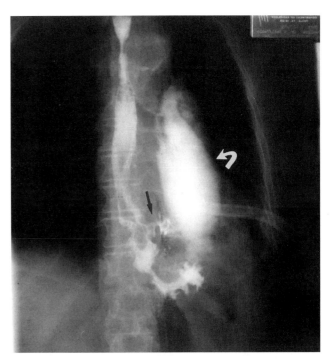

FIGURE 39.2. Spontaneous esophageal perforation or Boerhaave's syndrome. Water-soluble contrast study shows the presence of a localized perforation of the left lateral wall of the distal esophagus (*black arrow*) communicating with the left pleural cavity (*curved arrow*). (Courtesy of S. Karasick, Thomas Jefferson University Hospital, Philadelphia, PA.)

Computed tomography (CT) scanning may also be useful in cases where contrast esophagrams cannot be performed or are difficult to localize or diagnose (66,84–86). CT findings can include air in the soft tissues of the mediastinum surrounding the esophagus, abscess cavities adjacent to the esophagus in either the pleural space or mediastinum, and communication of the air-filled esophagus with adjacent mediastinal or paramediastinal air fluid collection (Fig. 39.4). Left-sided pleural effusion strengthens the suspected diagnosis. CT of the chest may be life saving in patients with atypical presentations (87). In patients who do not improve after initial therapy, CT is useful in localizing fluid collections and can assist in their drainage (55). Whether a CT scan can help predict who will benefit from operative versus nonoperative treatment remains to be determined (86).

Endoscopy has been utilized in some studies for diagnosis in difficult cases of perforation and has high accuracy for perforation secondary to external penetrating injuries. However, its role is highly questionable and is not recommended for acute, nonpenetrating perforations (82,88–91). Thoracentesis may aid in diagnosis of perforation. Acidic pH, elevated salivary amylase, purulent foul-smelling material, or the presence of undigested food helps make or confirm the diagnosis (65,92–94).

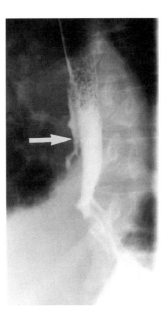

FIGURE 39.3. Intraluminal dissection with "double-barreled" esophagus. Note the longitudinal intraluminal tract (*arrow*) separated from the esophageal lumen by a radiolucent mucosal stripe. (Courtesy of S. Karasick, Thomas Jefferson University Hospital, Philadelphia, PA.)

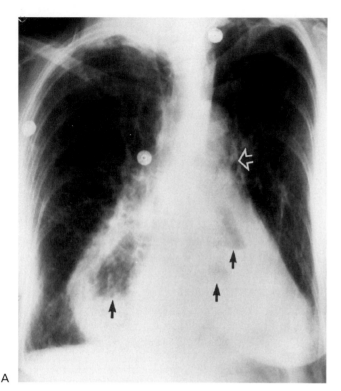

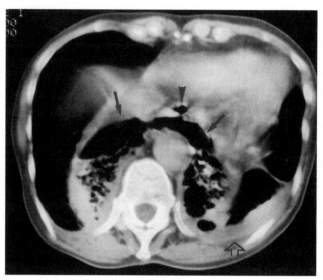

A   B

FIGURE 39.4. Patient with fever and chest pain 2 weeks following an illness with severe vomiting. Surgical exploration revealed a perforated esophagus. (Courtesy A. Salazar, Thomas Jefferson University Hospital, Philadelphia, PA.) **A:** Frontal chest radiograph demonstrates a mediastinal collection which extends on both sides of the midline with multiple air fluid levels (*arrows*). Pneumomediastinum is also present (*open arrow*). **B:** Contrast-enhanced computed tomography at the level of the heart demonstrates a large posterior mediastinal abscess with multiple loculations of fluid and air (*arrows*). There is air within the esophagus (*arrowhead*), and an accompanying left pleural effusion (*open arrow*).

PATHOPHYSIOLOGY

Lacking a serosal layer, the esophagus is naturally more vulnerable to rupture or perforation. Once a perforation occurs, retained gastric contents, saliva, bile, and so on enter the mediastinum, resulting in a necrotizing mediastinitis (95). The midesophagus lies adjacent to the right pleura and the distal esophagus to the left pleura; therefore, perforations in these locations lead to involvement of their respective pleural cavities. Mediastinal emphysema results, and eventually the parietal pleura is compromised, often resulting in hydropneumothorax. The degree of mediastinal contamination and location determines clinical presentation. Cervical perforation rarely leads to mediastinitis, unless the infection tracks down facial plains or the retroesophageal space into the posterior mediastinum (96). More commonly, a localized periesophageal abscess is noted (73). Due to negative intrathoracic pressure, thoracic perforations tend to disseminate mediastinal contamination of fluids and bacteria (62). Large-volume pleural effusions that contribute to cardiorespiratory difficulty are common (62).

Within 12 hours, a polymicrobial invasion of bacteria is noted with *Staphylococcus*, *Pseudomonas*, *Streptococcus*, and *Bacteroides* leading the way. The natural history of this process is fluid sequestration, sepsis, and death (39). Perforation of the intraabdominal esophagus rapidly progresses to peritonitis, shock, and death if left unchecked. If the perforation remains localized, signs of sepsis and shock may be absent. This subacute presentation (24 hours to 2 weeks) more often presents with chest pain and dyspnea as the predominant features (82).

MANAGEMENT

Medical Management

Esophageal perforation is a lethal condition with a high mortality rate. Therapy depends on the site and size of rupture, the time elapsed between rupture and diagnosis, and the overall health status of the patient. Traditionally, esophageal perforations are treated within 24 hours by surgery with primary closure and external drainage. However, a nonsurgical approach has been advocated by many authors. Medical treatment consists of parenteral nutrition, intravenous antibiotics, and nasogastric suction. In 1965, Mengoli and Klassen (91) reported 1 death among 15 patients treated without operation for instrumental perforation of the thoracic esophagus. They could not duplicate these results for spontaneous rupture of the esophagus, probably secondary to advanced mediastinitis. In 1975, Larriens and Kieffer (97) reported a successful conservative management and care of spontaneous perforation. Wesdorp et al. (98) treated 54 patients with instrumental perforation conservatively. They reported no deaths in 19 patients without malignancy and a mortality rate of 8.6% in those with carcinoma who sustained a perforation secondary to palliative intubation. These authors claimed that the key to successful conservative management is containment of the contamination of the mediastinum by nasogastric suction and control of local infection by massive doses of intravenous antibiotics. In a more recent review from Germany, 50 of 75 patients were treated conservatively; 16% of the conservative group versus 24% of the surgically treated group, died (8).

Criteria to select patients for conservative management were first recommended by Cameron et al. (3) in 1979. Eight patients with mid- and distal-esophageal perforations were managed without operation. The perforations of these patients were well contained with limited soilage. The authors suggested the following criteria for selection of patients for conservative therapy: absence of clinical sepsis, contained perforation, and drainage of perforation into the esophagus (3). In 1982, Sarr et al. (99) used these criteria for patients presenting more than 24 hours after instrumental perforation. They reported that one out of eight patients who were treated medically died, for a mortality of 13%, and concluded that nonoperative management might be entertained in minimally symptomatic patients with late, locally contained perforation and ongoing signs of minimal sepsis. Michel et al. (100) reported a mortality rate of 12.5% for patients with contained thoracic perforations treated conservatively. Other authors also reported favorable results obtained by conservative treatment for esophageal perforations (9,10,25,101).

In 1992, Shaffer et al. (102) reassessed Cameron's criteria (3) by comparing the results in 12 medically treated patients and 13 surgically treated patients. No mortality was seen in the medically treated group, but one surgically treated patient died postoperatively, indicating a nonsurgical approach as treatment for selected patients with esophageal perforation. They concluded that the most relevant of Cameron's criteria (3) was containment of the perforation within the mediastinum and the visceral plane. Patients with pain requiring narcotics, leukocytosis, fever, and the presence of retention or trapping of barium in the mediastinum did not preclude conservative therapy.

From these studies, it is concluded that a nonoperative approach may apply to specific situations. The guidelines

TABLE 39.4. CRITERIA TO SELECT PATIENTS FOR MEDICAL MANAGEMENT OF ESOPHAGEAL PERFORATION

Clinically stable, minimal sepsis
Elective instrumental perforations
Contained perforation
Absence of crepitus, pneumothorax, and pneumoperitoneum

for conservative therapy are (a) patients who are clinically stable with minimal signs of sepsis at the time of presentation and remain so; (b) instrumental perforations in which the patient had been on a regime of nothing by mouth and in which the perforation was detected early or the patient develops "tolerance" for the perforation without need for surgery; and (c) perforation contained within the neck or mediastinum with no extravasation and no signs of crepitus, pneumothorax, or pneumoperitoneum (Table 39.4) (3,102–104). The principles of medical treatment consist of nothing by mouth, parenteral alimentation, nasogastric suction, and broad-spectrum antibiotics covering anaerobes and both gram-negative and gram-positive aerobes. The decision to switch over to surgical management should always be considered. Cameron et al. (3) suggested that gastrograffin studies be performed every 3 to 5 days initially until it is evident that the patient is doing well. Deterioration of the patient's condition should prompt either contrast esophagography to look for leakage or a CT scan to detect an abscess. Surgical treatment should be considered early, as a delay in repair alters surgical approach and mortality.

Patients with esophageal cancer or disseminated malignancy who have had instrumental esophageal perforation represent a unique group. Conservative management with the use of endoprosthesis should be considered. Wesdorp et al. (98) reported 35 consecutive perforations in such patients, all treated medically with antibiotics, nutritional support, and protection of the perforation site. In ten of their patients, a prosthesis was inserted to seal the perforated sites. Only one patient developed mediastinitis. In 24 patients, an endoprosthesis was inserted within 1 week with no mortality. Hine and Atkinson (105) had similar results in 13 patients with disseminated esophageal cancer who underwent endoprosthesis placement for instrumental perforations. Covered self-expanding metal stents were also used in 18 patients with disseminated esophageal cancer with few complications (106,107). There have been a small number of case reports utilizing a fibrin sealant or endoscopic clips (10,76,86).

Surgical Management

Although conservative management of perforation can be applied successfully, it is only appropriate in a selected group of esophageal perforations. Most esophageal perfora-

TABLE 39.5. CRITERIA TO SELECT PATIENTS FOR SURGICAL MANAGEMENT OF ESOPHAGEAL PERFORATION

Boerhaave's syndrome
Clinically unstable with sepsis, shock, and respiratory failure
Contaminated mediastinum or pleural space
Perforation with retained foreign bodies
Perforation in esophageal diseases for which elective surgery is considered
Failed medical therapy

tions are not contained and require operative attention. Indications for surgery include Boerhaave's syndrome, clinically unstable patients with sepsis, respiratory failure or shock, contamination of the mediastinum or pleural space, associated pneumothorax, perforation with retained foreign bodies, and perforation in esophageal diseases for which elective surgery would be considered in the absence of a perforation (e.g., achalasia, stricture, cancer) (9,31,99,100, 108) (Table 39.5). Perforations caused by forceful vomiting, foreign bodies, and violent trauma are not optimal candidates for medical management because these cases are seldom recognized promptly and may have been grossly contaminated (31). Failed medical therapy or patients who become clinically unstable while on conservative treatment should be considered for urgent surgery. In general, surgical techniques used for esophageal perforation include drainage alone, drainage and repair, and drainage and diversion.

Cervical Perforations

Perforations in the hypopharynx and cervical esophagus that are contained can usually be managed conservatively (25,105,109). This usually includes selected patients with small instrumental perforations and perforations that are contained and well tolerated. Selection of the appropriate surgical approach is dependent on location, time period between perforation and diagnosis, and the presence of underlying esophageal disease. When the site of perforation cannot be found due to local inflammation, drainage only with intravenous antibiotics is adequate (77). An esophageal cervical fistula will close within a few days in the absence of distal obstruction. Some authors recommend primary surgical closure of the perforation with drainage of all perforations without delay, thereby avoiding mortality and reducing morbidity (64,99,100). However, there has been no clear evidence favoring one approach over the other.

Thoracoabdominal Perforations

In general, thoracic esophageal perforations are more lethal because of direct contamination of the mediastinum and eventually the pleural cavity. Conservative management for selected patients with thoracic perforations has been supported in recent literature (3,108,109). However, for uncontained thoracic esophageal leaks, debridement of necrotic tissue, generous irrigation, and complete mediastinal and pleural drainage are used. As in cervical perforations, care for thoracic perforations varies based on location, underlying disease, and overall condition of the patient. Treatment of choice for intrathoracic perforation within 24 hours is primary closure or reinforced primary closure in the absence of distal obstruction (3,92,110). Bufkin et al. (111) performed primary repair with or without reinforcement in 52% (28 of 54) of the patients with an 82% survival rate. The average time to diagnosis was 20 hours from the onset of perforation. Their success for primary closure was based on early diagnosis, careful intraoperative assessment, and meticulous repair.

The management of perforations diagnosed more than 24 hours later is more complicated and associated with higher mortality and morbidity. Delay in diagnosis results in inflamed and necrotic tissue around the site of the perforation. This tissue holds sutures poorly and results in a high incidence of recurrent leakage after direct closure. Thus, surgeons have included reinforced closure in the operation, even late after the perforation. Pleural flaps, diaphragm, adjacent muscle, and omentum have been employed to reinforce closures of perforations (31,112). Bufkin et al. (111) suggest that perforations beyond early repair require placement of an esophageal T-tube to divert all secretions and allow time for healing of the surrounding injury. Thapar et al. (112) reported on four cases of delayed perforation treated with paraesophageal mediastinal drainage with diversion. Esophageal resection is performed when a large perforation leads to continued leakage, as it may be the only method of controlling persistent mediastinal and pleural infection (112).

MORTALITY

The overall mortality of esophageal perforations is 15.5% to 29% (31). This rate is markedly increased, at 26% to 64% in patients in whom treatment is delayed more than 24 hours (6,7,39,40,72,82,100). In contrast, patients treated within 24 hours have mortality rates ranging from 0% to 30% (34,39,40,100). The outcome of esophageal perforation is also dependent on the location and etiology of the perforation. Cervical perforations have a lower mortality rate (0% to 14%) than thoracic perforations (13% to 59%) (6,9,12,31,82,104). The higher mortality rate in thoracic perforations is secondary to direct contamination of the mediastinum and pleural cavity (114). Boerhaave's syndrome has the highest mortality rate (ranging from 22% to 63%), while instrumental perforations have a lower mortality rate (5% to 26%) (31). Underlying esophageal disease increases the mortality rate by six times (100).

CONCLUSION

From Boerhaave's original description in 1724 to the present, esophageal rupture and perforation remain a diagnostic and therapeutic challenge. Although rare, spontaneous perforation must be considered in any acutely ill patient complaining of respiratory and gastrointestinal symptoms, especially after recent vomiting, and must not be confused with more common diagnoses. Instrumental perforation is far more common and must be suspected in any patient complaining of pain postprocedure. An immediate upright chest x-ray must be performed. If negative and the clinical presentation continues to suggest perforation, esophagram and/or chest CT should be considered. Thoracic site and delayed diagnosis and treatment are the main factors contributing to poor survival. Selecting patients carefully for conservative versus operative management is important and controversial. If surgery is performed, a 12- to 24-hour window is optimal. Ongoing advances in endoscopic technique and equipment may enhance our abilities to manage more patients safely with a nonoperative approach. Mortality unfortunately remains high (5% to 63%) under the best of circumstances, and therefore continued efforts to improve diagnostic and therapeutic approaches are important.

REFERENCES

1. Boerhaave H. *Atrocis, nec descripti prius, morbi historia: secundum medicae artis leges conscripta.* Lugduni Batavorum, Boutesteniana, 1724.
2. Henderson JA, Ploquin AJ. Boerhaave revisited: spontaneous esophageal perforation as a diagnostic masquerader. *Am J Med* 1989;86:559.
3. Cameron JL, Kieffer RF, Hendrix TR, et al. Selective nonoperative management of contained intrathoracic esophageal disruptions. *Ann Thorac Surg* 1979;27:404–408.
4. Barrett NR. Spontaneous perforation of the esophagus: review of the literature and report of 3 new cases. *Thorax* 1946;1:48.
5. Olson AM, Clagett OT. Spontaneous rupture of the esophagus. Report of a case with immediate diagnosis and successful surgical repair. *Postgrad Med* 1947;2:417.
6. Larsen K, Skov Jensen B, Axelsen F. Perforation and rupture of the esophagus. *Scand J Thorac Cardiovasc Surg* 1983;17:311.
7. Pate JW, et al. Spontaneous rupture of the esophagus: a 30-year experience. *Ann Thorac Surg* 1989;47:689.
8. Fernandez FF, et al. Treatment of endoscopic esophageal perforation. *Surg Endosc* 1999;13:962–966.
9. Flynn AE, Verrier ED, Way LW, et al. Esophageal perforation. *Arch Surg* 1989;124:1211.
10. Fleischer DF, Kessler F. Endoscopic Nd:YAG laser therapy for carcinoma of the esophagus: a new form of palliative treatment. *Gastroenterology* 1983;85:600.
11. Dawson J, Cockel R. Oesophageal perforation at fibreoptic gastroscopy. *BMJ* 1981;283:583.
12. Katz D. Morbidity and mortality in standard and flexible gastrointestinal endoscopy. *Gastrointest Endosc* 1967;14:134.
13. Cox JGC, Bennett JR. Benign esophageal strictures. In: Bennett JR, Hunt RH, eds., *Therapeutic endoscopy and radiology of the gut.* 2nd ed. Baltimore: Williams & Wilkins, 1990:11.
14. Silvis SE, et al. Endoscopic complications: results of the 1974 American Society for Gastrointestinal Endoscopy survey. *JAMA* 1976;235:928.
15. Kozarek RA. Hydrostatic balloon dilatation of gastrointestinal stenoses: a national survey. *Gastrointest Endosc* 1986;23:15.
16. Nair LA, et al. Complications during pneumatic dilatation for achalasia or diffuse esophageal spasm: analysis of risk factors, early clinical characteristics, and outcome. *Dig Dis Sci* 1993;38:1893.
17. Dellipani AW, Hewetson KA. Pneumatic dilation in the management of achalasia: experience with 45 cases. *Q J Med* 1986;58:253.
18. White RK, Morris DM. Diagnosis and management of esophageal perforations. *Am Surg* 1992;58:112.
19. Fleischer DE. Therapy for gastrointestinal bleeding. In: Geenen JE, Fleisher DE, Waye JD, eds. *Techniques in therapeutic endoscopy.* 2nd ed. New York: Gover Medical Publishing, 1992:25.
20. Clouse T, et al. Surgical repair of esophageal perforation in cirrhotic patients with varices. *Chest* 1994;105:1896.
21. Lee J, Lieberman D. Complications related to endoscopic hemostasis techniques. *Gastrointest Endosc Clin N Am* 1996;6:305.
22. Johnson P, et al. Complications associated with endoscopic band ligation of esophageal varices. *Gastrointest Endosc* 1993;39:181.
23. Perino LE, Gholson CF, Goff JS. Esophageal perforation after fiberoptic variceal sclerotherapy. *J Clin Gastroenterol* 1987;9:286.
24. Berkelhammer C, et al. "Pinch" injury during overtube placement in upper endoscopy. *Gastrointest Endosc* 1993;39:186.
25. Ell C, Riemann JF, Lux G, et al. Palliative laser treatment of malignant stenoses in the upper gastrointestinal tract. *Endoscopy* 1986;18(suppl 1):21.
26. Lightdale C, et al. A multi-center phase III trial of photodynamic therapy versus Nd:YAG laser in the treatment of malignant dysphagia. *Gastrointest Endosc* 1993;39:283A.
27. Johnston JH, Fleisher D, Pertrini J, et al. Palliative bipolar electrocoagulation of obstructing esophageal cancer. *Gastrointest Endosc* 1987;33:349.
28. Tytgat GN, den Hartos Jager FC, Bartelman JF. Endoscopic prosthesis for advanced esophageal cancer. *Endoscopy* 1986;18(suppl 3):32.
29. Knyrim K, et al. A controlled trial of an expansile metal stent for palliation of esophageal obstruction due to inoperable cancer. *N Engl J Med* 1993;329:1302.
30. ASGE Technical Assessment Committee. *Status evaluation: endoscopic ultrasound.* Chicago: American Society for Gastrointestinal Endoscopy, December 1991. Guidelines for training and practice 1997.
31. Williamson WA, Ellis FH. Esophageal perforation. In: Taylor MB, Gollan JL, Steer ML, et al., eds. *Gastrointestinal emergencies.* 2nd ed. Baltimore: Williams & Wilkins, 1997:31.
32. Overholt BF, et al. Photodynamic therapy for Barrett's esophagus: follow-up in 100 patients. *Gastrointest Endosc* 1999;49:1–7.
33. Christian ELL, et al. Endoscopic mucosal resection of early cancer and high-grade dysplasia in Barrett's esophagus. *Gastroenterology* 2000;118:670–577.
34. Buttar NS, et al. Combined endoscopic mucosal resection and photo dynamic therapy for esophageal neoplasia within Barrett's esophagus. *Gastrointest Endosc* 2001;54:682–688.
35. Pass LJ, et al. Management of esophageal gunshot wounds. *Ann Thorac Surg* 1987;44:253.
36. Symbar PN, et al. Penetrating wounds of the esophagus. *Ann Thorac Surg* 1972;13:552.
37. Beal SL, Pottmeyer EW, Spisso JM. Esophageal perforation following external blunt trauma. *J Trauma* 1988;28:1425.

38. Bjerke HS. Penetrating and blunt injury of the esophagus. *Chest Surg Clin N Am* 1994;4:811.

39. Ajalat GM, Mulder DG. Esophageal perforations: the need for individualized approach. *Arch Surg* 1984;119:1318.

40. Nesbitt JC, Sawyers JL. Surgical management of esophageal perforation. *Am Surg* 1987;53:183.

41. MacManus JE. Perforation of the intestine by ingested foreign body. *Am J Surg* 1941;53:393.

42. Selivanov V, Sheldon GF, Cello JP, et al. Management of foreign body ingestion. *Ann Surg* 1984;199:187.

43. Vizcarrando FJ, Brady PG, Nord HJ. Foreign bodies of the upper gastrointestinal tract. *Gastrointest Endosc* 1983;29:208.

44. Tucker J, Kim H, Lucas GW. Esophageal perforation caused by coin ingestion. *South Med J* 1994;87:269.

45. Yamaoka K, et al. A case of esophageal perforation due to a pill-induced ulcer successfully treated with conservative measures. *Am J Gastroenterol* 1996;91:1044.

46. Bauer TM, Dupont V, Zimmerli W. Invasive candidiasis complicating spontaneous esophageal perforation (Boerhaave's syndrome) *Am J Gastroenterol* 1996;91:1248.

47. Cronstedt JL, et al. Esophageal perforation in herpes simplex esophagitis. *Am J Gastroenterol* 1992;7:124.

48. Adkins MS, Raccuia JS, Acinapura AJ. Esophageal perforation in a patient with acquired immunodeficiency syndrome. *Ann Thorac Surg* 1990;50:299.

49. Cappell MS, Sciales C, Biempica L. Esophageal perforation at a Barrett's ulcer. *J Clin Gastroenterol* 1989;11:663.

50. Davis M, et al. Complications from enteroclysis tube insertion. *Am J Roentgenol* 1995;164:1–274.

51. Abbott OA, et al. Atraumatic so-called "spontaneous" rupture of the esophagus: a review of 47 personal cases with comments on a new method of surgical therapy. *J Thorac Cardiovasc Surg* 1970;59:67.

52. Anderson RL. Spontaneous rupture of the esophagus. *Am J Surg* 1957;93:282.

53. Baker RW, Spiro AH, Trinka YM. Mallory-Weiss tear complicating upper endoscopy: case reports and review of the literature. *Gastroenterology* 1982;82:140.

54. Bobo WO, Billups WA, Hardy JD. Boerhaave's syndrome: review of six cases of spontaneous rupture of the esophagus secondary to vomiting. *Ann Surg* 1970;172:1034.

55. Goldstein LA, Thompson WR. Esophageal perforations: a 15 year experience. *Am J Surg* 1992;143:495.

56. Anderson RL. Rupture of esophagus. *J Thoracic Surg* 1952;24:369.

57. Jones WG, Ginsber RJ. Esophageal perforation: a continuing challenge. *Ann Thorac Surg* 1992;53:534.

58. Kossick PR. Spontaneous rupture of the esophagus. *S Afr Med J* 1973;47:1807.

59. Borotto E, et al. Risk factors of oesophageal perforation during pneumatic dilatation for achalasia. *Gut* 1996;39:9.

60. Loop FD, Groves LK. Esophageal perforations. *Ann Thorac Surg* 1970;10:571.

61. Naclerio EA. The V-sign in the diagnosis of spontaneous rupture of the esophagus. *Am J Surg* 1957;93:291.

62. Barrett NR, Allison PR, Johnstone AS, et al. Discussion on unusual aspects of esophageal disease. *Proc R Soc Med* 1956;49:529.

63. Parkin FJS. The radiology of perforated esophagus. *Clin Radiol* 1973;24:234.

64. Mackler SA. Spontaneous rupture of the esophagus: experimental and clinical study. *Surg Gynecol Obstet* 1952;95:345.

65. Tesler MA, Eisenberg MM. Collective review: spontaneous esophageal rupture. *Surg Gynecol Obstet Int Abstr Surg* 1963;117:1.

66. Backer CL, et al. Computed tomography in patients with esophageal perforation. *Chest* 1990;98:1078.

67. Itabashi HH, Granada LO. Cerebral food embolism secondary to esophageal–cardiac perforation. *JAMA* 1972;219:373.

68. Sawyer R, Phillips C, Vakil N. Short- and long-term outcome of esophageal perforation. *Gastrointest Endosc* 1995;41:130.

69. Nobutsugu A, et al. Endoscopic nasomediastinal drainage followed by clip application for treatment of delayed esophageal perforation with mediastinitis. *Gastrointest Endosc* 2001;54:646–648.

70. Graeber GM, Niezgoda JA, Burton NA, et al. A comparison of patients with endoscopic esophageal perforation and patients with the Boerhaave's syndrome. *Chest* 1987;92:995.

71. Appleton DS, Sandrasagra FA, Flower CDR. Perforated esophagus: review of twenty-eight consecutive cases. *Clin Radiol* 1979;30:493.

72. Bladergroen MR, Lowe JE, Posthelwaite RW. Diagnosis and recommended management of esophageal perforation and rupture. *Ann Thorac Surg* 1986;42:235.

73. Reeder L, DeFilippi V, Ferguson M. Current results of therapy for esophageal perforation. *Am J Surg* 1995;169:615.

74. Han SY, McElvein RB, Aldrete JS, et al. Perforation of the esophagus: correlation of site and cause with plain film findings. *Am J Roentgenol* 1985;145:537.

75. O'Connell ND. Spontaneous rupture of the esophagus. *Am J Roentgenol* 1967;99:185.

76. Panzini L, Burrell MI, Traube M. Instrumental esophageal perforation: chest film findings. *Am J Gastroenterol* 1994;89:367.

77. Lafontaine E. Instrumentation injury of the oesophagus. In: Jaimieson GG, ed. *Surgery of the oesophagus.* London: Churchill Livingstone, 1988:387.

78. Brick SH, et al. Esophageal disruption: evaluation with iohexaol esophagography. *Radiology* 1988;169:141.

79. DeMeester TR. Perforation of the esophagus [Editorial]. *Ann Thorac Surg* 1986;42:231.

80. Foley MJ, Ghahremani GG, Rogers LF. Reappraisal of contrast media used to detect upper gastrointestinal perforations: comparison of ionic water-soluble media with barium sulfate. *Radiology* 1982;144:231.

81. Richter JE, Castell DO. Balloon dilatation for the treatment of achalasia. In: Bennet JR, Hunt RH, eds. *Therapeutic endoscopy and radiology of the gut.* 2nd ed. Baltimore: Williams & Wilkins, 1990:82.

82. Kim-Deobald J, Kozarek RA. Esophageal perforation: an 8-year review of a multispeciality clinic's experience. *Am J Gastroenterol* 1992;87:1112.

83. Snider DM, Crawford DW. Successful treatment of primary aorto-esophageal fistula resulting from aortic aneurysm. *J Thorac Cardiovasc Surg* 1983;85:457.

84. Fennerty B. Esophageal perforation during pneumatic dilatation for achalasia: a possible association with malnutrition. *Dysphagia* 1990;5:227.

85. Jaffe MH, Fleischer D, Zeman RK, et al. Esophageal malignancy: imaging results and complications of combined endoscopic radiologic palliation. *Radiology* 1987;164:623.

86. Stephanson SE Jr, Maness G, Scott HW Jr. Esophagopericardial fistula of benign origin. *J Thorac Cardiovasc Surg* 1958;36:208.

87. Jaworski A, Fischer R, Lippmann M. Boerhaave's syndrome: computed tomographic findings and diagnostic considerations. *Arch Intern Med* 1988;148:223.

88. Carter R, Hinshaw DB. Use of the esophagoscope in the diagnosis of rupture of the esophagus. *Surg Gynecol Obstet* 1965;120:1304–1306.

89. Coscia MG, Hormuth DA, Huang WL. Back pain secondary to esophageal perforation in an adolescent. *Spine* 1992;17:1256.

90. Horwitz B, et al. Endoscopic evaluation of penetrating esophageal injuries. *Am J Gastroenterol* 1993;88:1249.
91. Mengoli LR, Klassen KP. Conservative management of esophageal perforation. *Arch Surg* 1965;91:238.
92. Attar S, et al. Esophageal perforation: a therapeutic challenge. *Ann Thorac Surg* 1990;50:45.
93. Dubost C, et al. Esophageal perforation during attempted endotracheal intubation. *J Thorac Cardiovasc Surg* 1979;78:44.
94. Roufail WM, Brice BS. Esophago-pleural fistulae secondary to perforated esophageal ulcer. *Gastrointest Endosc* 1972;18:165.
95. Traumatic perforation of esophagus [Editorial]. *BMJ* 1972;2:524.
96. Burnett CM, Rosemurgy AS, Pfeiffer EA. Life-threatening acute posterior mediastinitis due to esophageal perforation. *Ann Thorac Surg* 1990;49:979.
97. Laurien AJ, Kieffer R. Boerhaave's syndrome: repeat of a case treated nonoperatively. *Ann Surg* 1975;181:452.
98. Wesdorp IC, et al. Treatment of instrumental esophageal perforation. *Gut* 1984;25:398.
99. Sarr MG, Pemberton JH, Payne WS. Management of instrumental perforations of the esophagus. *J Thorac Cardiovasc Surg* 1982;84:211.
100. Michel L, Grillo HC, Malt RA. Operative and nonoperative management of esophageal perforations. *Ann Surg* 1981;194:57.
101. Brewer LA III, Carter R, Mulder GA, et al. Options in the management of perforations of the esophagus. *Am J Surg* 1986;152:62.
102. Shaffer HA, Valenzuela G, Mittal RK. Esophageal perforation. A reassessment of the criteria for choosing medical or surgical therapy. *Arch Intern Med* 1992;152:757.
103. Altorjay A, Kiss J, Voros A, et al. Non-operative management of esophageal perforations. Is it justified? *Ann Surg* 1997;225:415.
104. White CS, Templeton PA, Attar S. Esophageal perforation: CT findings. *Am J Roentgenol* 1993;160:767.
105. Hine KR, Atkinson M. The diagnosis and management of perforations of the esophagus and pharynx sustained during intubation of neoplastic esophageal strictures. *Dig Dis Sci* 1986;31:571.
106. Nicholson AA, et al. Palliation of malignant esophageal perforations and proximal esophageal malignant dysphagia with covered metal stents. *Clin Radiol* 1995;50:11.
107. Watkinson A, et al. Plastic covered metallic endoprosthesis in the management of esophageal perforations in patients with esophageal carcinoma. *Clin Radiol* 1995;50:304.
108. Pasricha PJ, Fleischer DE, Kalloo AN. Endoscopic perforations of the upper digestive tract: a review of their pathogenesis, prevention, and management. *Gastroenterology* 1994;106:787.
109. Tilanus HW, et al. Treatment of oesophageal perforation: a multivariate analysis. *Br J Surg* 1991;78:852.
110. Sabanathan S, Eng J, Richardson J. Surgical management of intrathoracic esophageal rupture. *Br J Surg* 1994;81:863.
111. Bufkin BL, Muller JI, Mansour KA. Esophageal perforation: emphasis on management. *Ann Thorac Surg* 1996;61:1447.
112. Salo JA, et al. Management of delayed esophageal perforation with mediastinal sepsis: esophagectomy or primary repair? *J Thorac Cardiovasc Surg* 1993;106:1088.
113. Thapar VK, et al. Paraesophageal mediastinal drainage with diversion for delayed presentation of esophageal perforaton. *Indian J Gastroenterol* 2000;19:133–134.
114. Sundrasagra FA, English TAH, Milstein BB. The management and prognosis of esophageal perforations. *Br J Surg* 1978;65:629.

CUTANEOUS DISEASES AND THE ESOPHAGUS

CHARLES CAMISA
JOSEPH L. JORIZZO

A variety of dermatologic diseases are associated with esophageal involvement. This may occur because both skin and upper esophagus have stratified squamous epithelium. Table 40.1 summarizes dermatologic diseases that may be associated with dysphagia. Major examples of mucocutaneous diseases that can also affect the esophagus are epidermolysis bullosa, cicatricial pemphigoid, lichen planus, and pemphigus vulgaris. These and other dermatoses that may involve the esophagus are discussed in detail in this chapter.

Mucocutaneous signs may sometimes be helpful in the diagnosis of esophageal disease, such as infections, collagen vascular diseases, and neoplasms. These are covered more thoroughly in other chapters, but the cutaneous features of such diseases are briefly reviewed here.

Collaboration between specialists in dermatology and esophagology is important for the early recognition and optimal management of skin lesions associated with esophageal disease.

IMMUNOBULLOUS DISEASES

Epidermolysis Bullosa Acquisita

Epidermolysis bullosa acquisita (EBA) is a rare delayed-onset, blistering disease mediated by circulating IgG autoantibodies directed against type VII collagen, the major constituent of anchoring fibrils (1). It affects both the skin and mucosae and may be clinically indistinguishable from bullous and cicatricial pemphigoid. Linear deposits of IgG are found along the basement membrane zone of the skin and mucous membranes including esophagus in EBA using direct immunofluorescence testing (2). Immunoelectron microscopy reveals a distinct pattern of immunoreactant deposition below the lamina densa on biopsy specimens

from patients. The proximal third of the esophagus is involved, with the effect only seen in stratified squamous epithelium.

Blistering lesions with scarring occur at sites of trauma in EBA (Color Plate 40.1). Extensive oral, ocular, and esophageal scarring may also occur (3). EBA may rarely be associated with Crohn's disease and may resolve after resection of the involved intestine. Some patients with inflammatory bowel disease may have circulating IgG autoantibodies to type VII collagen, which is normally present in the skin and gut (4).

Bullous Pemphigoid and Cicatricial Pemphigoid

Bullous pemphigoid (BP) is an autoimmune blistering disease that affects people aged >60 years. Tense bullae arise on flexural skin, with or without inflammation and with intense pruritus (Color Plate 40.2).

Biopsy specimens of skin reveal a subepithelial blister with a mixture of inflammatory cells in the dermis including eosinophils (5). A linear pattern of IgG and complement deposition along the basement membrane zone is visualized on direct and indirect immunofluorescence microscopy in almost all cases. The BP antigens BPAG1 (230-kd) and BPAG2 (180-kd) are components of the epithelial adhesion complexes called *hemidesmosomes*.

Oral mucous membrane involvement occurs in about 40% of cases (Color Plate 40.3). Esophageal bullae may occur *de novo* or as a complication of endoscopy and can lead to complete sloughing of the esophageal mucosa. Direct immunofluorescence of esophageal biopsy specimens in patients with BP may show IgG and C3 in the basement membrane zone, even in the absence of gross mucosal lesions (6).

Cicatricial pemphigoid (CP), also known as benign mucous membrane pemphigoid, is a related but more heterogeneous disease of the elderly. The most common sites of blisters in CP are oral cavity (80% to 100%), ocular (50%

C. Camisa: Department of Dermatology, Cleveland Clinic Florida, Naples, Florida.

J.L. Jorizzo: Department of Dermatology, Wake Forest University School of Medicine, Winston-Salem, North Carolina.

TABLE 40.1. SELECTED DERMATOLOGIC DISEASES THAT MAY BE ASSOCIATED WITH DYSPHAGIA

Immunobullous diseases
  Epidermolysis bullosa acquisita
  Bullous pemphigoid
  Cicatricial pemphigoid
  Pemphigus vulgaris
Other bullous diseases
  Paraneoplastic pemphigus
  Stevens-Johnson syndrome/toxic epidermal necrolysis
Heritable syndromes
  Epidermolysis bullosa (several genetic subtypes)
  Hailey-Hailey disease (benign familial pemphigus)
  Darier's disease (keratosis follicularis)
  Cowden's disease (multiple hamartoma syndrome)
  Focal dermal hypoplasia (Goltz's syndrome)
  Ehlers-Danlos syndrome
  Hereditary hemorrhagic telangiectasia
    (Osler-Weber-Rendu syndrome)
Esophageal carcinomas
  Tylosis/Howel-Evans syndrome
  Paterson-Brown-Kelly syndrome (Plummer-Vinson syndrome)
  Acanthosis nigricans
  Acrokeratosis paraneoplastica (Bazex syndrome)
  Cutaneous metastases
Nonbullous immunologic diseases
  Lichen planus
  Aphthosis and Behçet's disease
  Dermatomyositis
  Scleroderma
  Other collagen vascular diseases
Miscellaneous diseases
  Candidiasis
  Herpes simplex
  Kaposi's sarcoma
  Tetracycline-induced injury

to 60%), and skin (25% to 30%). Pharyngeal, laryngeal, genital, nasal, esophagus, and anal involvement occur in decreasing order of frequency. Patients may present with desquamative gingivitis (Color Plate 40.4) or conjunctival scarring called symblepharon (7) (Color Plate 40.5).

The majority of sera from CP patients contain circulating IgG autoantibodies that recognize the BP 180-kd antigen (BPAG2) (8). Fewer sera recognize the BP 230-kd antigen (BPAG1), epiligrin (identical to laminin 5, formerly known as kalinin and nicein), and a 168-kd antigen expressed by buccal mucosa that is distinct from the BP antigens, laminin-5 subunits (9), and type VII collagen (the EBA antigen). Antiepiligrin CP is emerging as a potential paraneoplastic disease (10).

There is a tendency for CP lesions of the conjunctiva, larynx, and esophagus to form scars leading to potentially debilitating and life-threatening sequelae. Cicatricial pemphigoid manifestations include cervical esophageal webs, often multiple or complex, and frank strictures (11). Esophageal biopsy with direct immunofluorescence testing may be necessary for confirmation of the diagnosis of cicatricial pemphigoid unless more accessible sites are available

for study, such as the oral cavity, conjunctivae, or skin. In a series of 82 patients with CP evaluated at the Cleveland Clinic Foundation from 1986 to 2000, ten (12.2%) had symptomatic esophageal involvement (C. Camisa, unpublished data, 2001).

Therapy for BP and cicatricial pemphigoid is usually initiated with systemic corticosteroids (e.g., prednisone, 40 to 80 mg per day), with gradual tapering as the disease is controlled. BP, which is self-limited, usually responds to this treatment, but CP generally also requires immunosuppressive "steroid-sparing" therapy such as dapsone, azathioprine, mycophenolate mofetil, or cyclophosphamide. Secondary candidal or herpetic esophagitis should be sought in patients with persistent erosions who are on this therapy (12). Esophageal stenosis will require bougie dilation as it does not respond directly to medical therapy alone, however, the drugs may prevent re-stenosis if they are given after successful dilatation bougienage. Cyclophosphamide has emerged as a potentially remittive agent for severe CP when administered at 1 to 2 mg/kg/day for 12 to 18 months.

Pemphigus Vulgaris

Pemphigus vulgaris (PV) is another immunologically mediated bullous disease. It is less common than pemphigoid. The autoantigen is desmoglein 3, a transmembrane component of desmosomes that provide physical connections between cells. In contrast to BP, pemphigus affects the oral cavity in 100% of cases over the course of the disease and peaks at about age 45 (Color Plate 40.6). More severe cases show generalized flaccid bullae and erosions anywhere on the skin including the head and neck (Color Plate 40.7). Skin biopsy specimens reveal acantholysis of epidermal cells, and direct and indirect immunofluorescence microscopic findings show deposits of IgG and complement in the space between the epithelial cells (13). Symptomatic esophageal involvement in PV is uncommon; however, it is possible that frequent asymptomatic esophageal disease occurs. In a series of 56 consecutive patients with PV seen at the Cleveland Clinic Foundation from 1987 to 2000, four (7%) had symptomatic esophageal involvement (C. Camisa, unpublished data, 2001). A review of 11 symptomatic patients with esophageal pemphigus indicated that all were middle-aged women presenting with dysphagia or odynophagia. They experienced bleeding or vomiting of esophageal lining, and none of these patients had skin lesions at the time that their esophageal involvement was diagnosed (14). In two of these patients, esophageal disease was the initial presentation of PV. Diagnosis of esophageal pemphigus is suspected with endoscopic demonstration of flaccid bullae (Color Plate 40.8) and erosions, and confirmed with a biopsy specimen showing acantholytic blisters of the epithelium. Direct immunofluorescence (DIF) testing is more sensitive in esophageal specimens, even those lacking gross or histologic evidence of esophageal disease. DIF testing was positive in all 12 patients tested in one study; only 5 showed abnormalities by endoscopy, namely blisters and erosions in the proximal esophagus or longitudinal red lines (15) (Color Plate 40.9).

A patient may rarely vomit the entire mucosal lining of the esophagus in PV and other bullous diseases; this is termed *esophagitis dissicans superficialis* (16). The treatment of choice for control and possible remission of PV is moderate- to high-dose prednisone, 60 to 100 mg per day (17). In less responsive cases, the addition of a second immunosuppressive agent, such as dapsone, azathioprine, mycophenolate mofetil, or cyclophosphamide becomes necessary (18). Patients with a history of PV, even those in remission, should be evaluated endoscopically if they present with esophageal symptoms.

OTHER BULLOUS DERMATOLOGIC DISEASES

Paraneoplastic pemphigus is a distinct autoimmune vesiculobullous disease that was first described in 1990. It manifests mucocutaneous lesions that overlap clinically with PV, cicatricial pemphigoid, and lichen planus (19). It is most often associated with lymphoproliferative diseases such as chronic lymphocytic leukemia and non-Hodgkin's lymphoma. The patients' sera contain IgG antibodies against desmogleins, plakin proteins, and an unidentified 170-kd antigen. The prognosis is poor because the underlying disease is generally incurable.

Stevens-Johnson syndrome is a part of the spectrum of erythema multiforme and is characterized by fever, bullous cutaneous lesions (target or iris-like), and involvement of two or more mucous membrane surfaces (usually ocular and oral). More generalized epithelial sloughing, with or without prior bullous lesions in a much sicker patient, is called *toxic epidermal necrolysis* (TEN) (Color Plate 40.10). There is a wide range of precipitating factors associated with Stevens-Johnson syndrome or TEN (20), but infections and drug hypersensitivity reactions, respectively, are by far the main triggers (21). Hospitalization with supportive care, treatment of septic complications, and burn unit management of severe cases is indicated (22). Plasmapheresis and intravenous immunoglobulin may be of benefit (23,24).

Esophageal complications may occur with either Stevens-Johnson syndrome or TEN. Gastrointestinal hemorrhage may occur acutely from erosive involvement of the esophageal mucosa or from focal stress ulceration elsewhere in the gut (25). An immune-mediated pathogenesis of bullae in the esophagus in drug-induced Stevens-Johnson syndrome has been supported (26). Complications can include mucosal scarring with esophageal stricture or stenosis and web formation (27).

HERITABLE SYNDROMES WITH CUTANEOUS AND ESOPHAGEAL LESIONS

Heritable diseases or genodermatoses have been associated with blisters, erosions, or stricture of the esophagus.

Epidermolysis Bullosa

Epidermolysis bullosa (EB) is a family of inherited mechanobullous diseases with a spectrum of clinical presentations, which have as a major manifestation spontaneous or trauma-induced blisters of the skin (Color Plate 40.11). Mucous membranes are sometimes involved, with blisters, erosions, and scarring. In severe dystrophic types, deformities of the extremities may occur.

Classification of EB subtypes is based on inheritance pattern, the level of blistering within the dermal–epidermal junction as determined by immuno- and electron-microscopy, and molecular defects (28). In simplex EB, cleavage occurs through the basal keratinocytes and results from mutations of genes encoding keratins 5 and 14 and plectin. In junctional EB, the split occurs in the lamina lucida, and molecular defects are seen in the alpha 3, beta 3, or gamma 2-chain genes of laminin 5. In dystrophic EB, the split occurs below the lamina densa and results from abnormalities in the collagen VII gene coding for anchoring fibrils. Another form of EB associated with pyloric atresia and a homozygous mutation in the alpha-6, beta-4 integrin gene has recently been reported.

In patients with dystrophic EB, the onset of gastrointestinal manifestations, that is, oral blisters, dysphagia, constipation, and anal fissures, is often in the first 3 decades of life (29). One-third to two-thirds of patients may be affected; manifestations occur earlier and are more severe in the recessive types. In the esophagus, mechanical passage of food contributes to bullae, with subsequent scarring, stricture, shortening, stenosis, and atony (30). Proximal strictures are more common than distal ones. Not all patients with dysphagia demonstrate esophageal webs or strictures. Manometric studies of the esophagus in patients with EB have sometimes shown low baseline lower esophageal sphincter pressure even in the absence of strictures. Failure to thrive and nutritional deficiency are common in children (31).

Treatment of esophageal lesions in EB is symptomatic. Antireflux regimens may help when reflux is present. In infants with severe dysphagia, malnutrition may be treated by parenteral nutrition or feeding gastrostomies (32). Esophageal dilatation may be helpful but should be performed cautiously, particularly in children, since new bullae may be induced by the procedure (33). In severe cases, when strictured lesions no longer respond to dilatation, surgical treatment is indicated. Esophagectomy with colonic interposition is the procedure most often performed, and follow-up indicates successful results (34). Protection of mucosae and skin from trauma (surgical dressings, tape, etc.) must be emphasized to avoid perioperative induction of lesions.

Dystrophic EB may be inherited in a dominant or recessive fashion, and either type can involve the gastrointestinal tract. Onset of skin lesions occurs at or near the time of birth, and the diagnosis of EB may have been made prior to consultation for gastrointestinal symptoms. The major mucosal sites of involvement are the oral cavity, anal canal, and esophagus. In the mouth, blistering occurs and leads to scarring, a smooth tongue, and restricted tongue movement and mouth opening, resulting in compromise of chewing, swallowing, and speaking (35). Dental disease is common due to poor oral hygiene resulting from microstomia and pain from blisters. Esophageal perforation has been reported, requiring esophagectomy in some cases (36). The major cause of death in recessive dystrophic EB is squamous cell carcinoma, mainly of skin, but esophagus has also been reported.

Hailey-Hailey disease (benign familial pemphigus) usually presents with papulovesicular or superficial erosive lesions of intertriginous areas such as the axillae, groin, and submammary skin. Biopsy specimens of lesions reveal acantholysis. Esophageal involvement has rarely been reported in these patients (37). *Darier's disease* (keratosis follicularis) presents with pruritic hyperkeratotic papules of the neck and upper trunk, with characteristic nail changes, and has also been reported to involve the oral cavity and esophagus (38). Both diseases are inherited as autosomal dominant and result from mutations in two different adenosine triphosphate–dependent calcium transporter genes, ATP2C1 and ATP2A2, respectively (28). Acantholysis is likely to be seen in esophageal biopsy specimens in each of these diseases, and differentiation from pemphigus would require assessment of clinical and immunopathologic features.

There are other uncommon cutaneous syndromes that may rarely involve the esophagus. *Cowden's disease,* also called *multiple hamartoma syndrome,* is an autosomal dominant syndrome resulting from a deletion within the tumor suppressor PTEN gene at 10q22–23 (39). It manifests multiple facial trichilemmomas and oral mucosal fibromas that give a cobblestone appearance. The frequency of gastrointestinal involvement is approximately 70% to 85% and usually manifests as benign hamartomatous polyps of the rectum or sigmoid colon. Esophageal lesions have also been seen, and these are papillomas, fibromas, or diffuse glycogenic acanthosis (40). Recognition of Cowden's disease is important since up to one third of these patients develop a malignancy, usually of breast or thyroid (41).

Focal dermal hypoplasia (Goltz's syndrome) is characterized by skin atrophy and linear areas of hyper- or hypo-pigmentation, localized superficial fat deposits, and perioral and mucosal papillomas (42). Basement membrane zone disruption suggests abnormal type IV collagen formation, but the underlying chromosome abnormality has not been identified (43).

CARCINOMA OF ESOPHAGUS AND SKIN LESIONS

Tylosis (palmar and plantar keratoderma) is a nonspecific presentation of yellow hyperkeratosis of the palms and soles (Color Plate 40.12). In patients with long-standing thick palmar and plantar lesions and a strong family history of cancer, the question of gastrointestinal malignancy should be raised when presenting symptoms are suspicious. The strongest association has been with squamous cell carcinoma of the esophagus (44). This association is known as the Howel-Evans syndrome. It is transmitted in an autosomal dominant fashion, with up to 95% of family members who have palmar and plantar lesions developing esophageal carcinoma by age 65 (45). The "tylosis–esophageal cancer gene" locus has been mapped to 17q23 by linkage analysis (46). In such kindreds, regular follow-up with barium swallow and upper endoscopy is warranted (Color Plate 40.13).

Patients with the *Paterson-Brown-Kelly syndrome (Plummer-Vinson syndrome)* present with spoon-shaped, concave nails (koilonychia), iron deficiency anemia, angular stomatitis, smooth tongue, dysphagia caused by a postcricoid web, and an increased incidence of postcricoid carcinoma (47). Sjogren's syndrome may occur in association with *Plummer-Vinson syndrome.*

Acanthosis nigricans presents as a smooth, velvety, dark thickening of skin in the axillae and neck folds, which may become generalized (Color Plate 40.14). Palms may be thickened ("tripe palms"), and skin tags (acrochordons) may develop in intertriginous sites (48). Oral hyperkeratosis may occur in up to 40% of patients with acanthosis nigricans and may be quite verrucous or papillomatous, particularly in the malignant type (49). Esophageal involvement with acanthosis nigricans can occur and may cause dysphagia due to the thickened, papillated mucosa (50). Although the strongest association of malignant acanthosis nigricans is with gastric adenocarcinoma, esophageal carcinoma has also been reported.

Bazex syndrome or *acrokeratosis paraneoplastica* was first described in 1965. It is a rare psoriasiform eruption with a violaceous hue affecting helices of the ear, tip of the nose, tips of the fingers and toes (51). Severe nail dystrophy resembling onychomycosis and palmoplantar keratoderma may develop later (52). It is usually associated with squamous cell carcinoma of the upper airway and digestive tract including larynx and esophagus (53), although other neoplasms have been reported (51). The cutaneous signs of Bazex syndrome usually improve after successful eradication of the tumor.

Cutaneous metastases from carcinoma of the esophagus are rare, but present as smooth-surfaced, firm dermal to subcutaneous papules or nodules on the upper trunk (54). These metastases may rarely be the first manifestation of esophageal malignancy (55). Of primary dermatologic tumors, malignant melanoma is the type most reported to metastasize to the esophagus. This can occur many years after the cutaneous melanoma is excised and carries a dismal prognosis (56). Melanoma can arise primarily in the esophagus, but this is extremely rare (57). *Mycosis fungoides* (cutaneous T-cell lymphoma) or *Kaposi's sarcoma* may rarely involve the esophagus causing hoarseness and dysphagia (58).

NONBULLOUS CUTANEOUS IMMUNOLOGIC DISEASES

Lichen Planus

Lichen planus (LP) is a common mucocutaneous disease of unknown etiology that is believed to result from a cell-mediated immune response directed against the basal cell layer of the epithelium (59). Skin lesions are pruritic violaceous papules, usually acral and flexural in distribution (Color Plate 40.15). Oral and pharyngeal lesions are also common and range from asymptomatic lacy white striae on the buccal mucosa to the less common erosive form that causes buccal ulcerations, desquamative gingivitis, and tongue erosions (Color Plate 40.16). Genital and anal lesions have been well documented. Esophageal involvement with lichen planus has been reported occasionally but is likely unrecognized and underreported. In a survey of 584 patients with oral LP who were carefully questioned for dysphagia, eight were referred for endoscopy (60). Of these, four demonstrated erythema and erosions that were histologically confirmed to be LP. Chronic inflammation may lead to friable mucosa, easily stripped away by the endoscope, erosions, and strictures, usually in the upper third of the esophagus (Color Figure 40.17) (61), although stenosis may occur in the lower third (62,63). While endoscopy should be performed on any patient with LP complaining of odynophagia or dysphagia, clinicians should not be surprised to find lesions in asymptomatic patients. For example, in an endoscopic survey of 19 new patients with LP, 5 had esophageal lesions (64). The only patient with dysphagia demonstrated severe erosions throughout, and the others had subtle papules in the lower third.

Patients with symptomatic esophageal LP generally have preceding erosive oral LP as well as involvement in one or more other sites. Direct immunofluorescence testing is nonspecific in LP, but it helps to exclude pemphigus and pemphigoid, which may cause similar lesions.

The treatment of erosive oral LP most often requires potent topical corticosteroids and bursts of prednisone. For symptomatic esophageal LP, prednisone or sublesional triamcinolone injections may help temporarily, but endoscopic dilatation of strictures followed by chronic immunosuppressive therapy is necessary. Secondary candidiasis is common in the oral cavity and must be treated appropriately in the esophagus. Chronic oral erosive LP is associated with a slightly higher incidence of squamous carcinoma. The first case of squamous cell carcinoma developing in the setting of chronic esophageal LP was reported in 2003 (64a).

Aphthosis and Behçet's Disease

Aphthous stomatitis (canker sores) is a common ulcerative disease of the oral mucosa (Color Plate 40.18). *Complex aphthosis* manifests as multiple recurrent aphthae without any systemic manifestations (65). *Major aphthous stomatitis* has larger ulcerations that can cause severe discomfort, dysphagia, and scarring (66,67). In this condition, aphthae have been demonstrated endoscopically to occur in the stomach, esophagus, and at other sites in the gastrointestinal tract.

Behçet's disease is a complex multisystem disease diagnosed clinically by the presence of oral aphthae and at least two of the following clinical criteria: genital aphthae, synovitis, posterior uveitis, cutaneous pustular vasculitis (pathergy), and meningoencephalitis (68). Perivascular inflammation was the predominant histopathologic finding in a multicenter international analysis (69). Inflammatory bowel disease and Reiter's disease must be excluded. Esophageal aphthae may also occur in patients with Behçet's disease (70), which may predispose to the development of candidal esophagitis.

Treatment of Behçet's disease involves a therapeutic "ladder" that begins with aggressive topical and intralesional corticosteroids, colchicine, dapsone, methotrexate, and thalidomide. Systemic corticosteroids and potent immunosuppressives are reserved for severe systemic disease or ocular manifestations (71).

Dermatomyositis

Dermatomyositis (DM) is characterized by poikiloderma of upper trunk skin (i.e., the presence of telangiectasia, hyperpigmentation and hypopigmentation, and epidermal atrophy), with a violaceous hue affecting the periorbital skin (heliotrope sign), knuckles (Gottron's sign), scalp, and other extensor surfaces. Early involvement of the elbows and knees may be confused with psoriasis. Periungual telangiectasias and cuticular dystrophy are also seen (Color Plate 40.19). Patients are generally photosensitive. Weakness of the proximal muscles of the shoulder and hip girdles can usually be elicited. Involvement of the skeletal muscle lining the pharynx and upper esophagus may be a cause for dysphagia. Cricopharyngeal obstruction and distal esophageal dysmotility occur with dermatomyositis; the latter suggests overlap with scleroderma (72). Internal malignancy should be sought in adults aged >40 years with new onset DM because it may be paraneoplastic in a subset of patients.

Scleroderma

Scleroderma is a cutaneous or multisystem disease of unknown pathogenesis. Variants, which are believed to represent overlapping ends of a spectrum, include a localized cutaneous form called morphea, a milder systemic form called CREST (calcinosis, Raynaud's phenomenon, esophageal dysmotility, sclerodactyly, telangiectasia), and progressive systemic sclerosis (73). The important esophageal and systemic aspects of this disease are reviewed in Chapter 37 of this text and in an article by Sjogren (74). Cutaneous manifestations are variable. Calcinosis cutis occurs as firm papules or nodules, usually located over the joints. A chalky, white discharge may occur. Raynaud's phenomenon often results in trophic ("rat-bite") lesions on the digits as well as the typical white, blue, and red color changes that occur acutely in association with episodes of vasospasm (75). Peripheral gangrene is a later complication. Dermal sclerosis occurs acrally and periorally in the CREST variant of scleroderma, resulting in sclerodactyly and reduced oral aperture, but may be more proximal at the progressive systemic sclerosis end of the spectrum. A salt-and-pepper postinflammatory pigment change may overlie the area of dermal sclerosis in darker-skinned individuals. Telangiectasias are described as being box-like or mat-like (Color Plate 40.20). They occur over the face, neck, hands, oral mucosa, larynx, and esophagus and may bleed spontaneously (76).

Other Collagen Vascular Diseases

Dysphagia and other esophageal abnormalities are features of mixed connective tissue disease and a number of other connective-tissue disease overlap syndromes. A discussion of the cutaneous features of systemic lupus erythematosus, mixed connective tissue disease, and other collagen vascular diseases is beyond the scope of this chapter, given the limited primary association with esophageal disease (see Chapter 37).

MISCELLANEOUS CUTANEOUS DISEASES AND ESOPHAGUS

There are other mucocutaneous lesions that may be associated with esophageal disease; however, these are discussed in other chapters. Entities such as candidiasis, herpes simplex, and Kaposi's sarcoma have particular relevance in the setting of HIV infection. Heritable disorders of connective tissue, such as Ehlers-Danlos syndrome, and syndromes associated with gastrointestinal bleeding, such as hereditary hemorrhagic telangietctasia, may also initially present to a dermatologist due to their mucocutaneous lesions (77).

Treatment of dermatologic diseases may be associated with drug-induced esophageal injury. A familiar example is oral tetracycline antibiotics, which are commonly used for the treatment of inflammatory acne vulgaris (78,79). Failure to take the capsules with adequate oral liquids can produce esophageal erosion (see Chapter 34). Candidal esophagitis secondary to oral corticosteroids is commonly missed by clinicians and can be prevented with prophylactic clotrimazole troches and intermittent oral fluconazole.

REFERENCES

1. Wakelin SH, Bhogal B, Black MM, et al. Epidermolysis bullosa acquisita associated with epidermal-binding circulating antibodies. *Br J Dermatol* 1997;136:604–609.
2. Taniuchi K, Inaoki M, Nishimura Y, et al. Nonscarring inflammatory epidermolysis bullosa acquisita with esophageal involvement and linear IgG deposits. *J Am Acad Dermatol* 1997;36: 320–322.
3. Weinman D, Stewart MI, Woodley DT, et al. Epidermolysis bullosa acquisita (EBA) and esophageal webs: a new association. *Am J Gastroenterol* 1991;86:1518–1522.
4. Chen M, O'Toole EA, Sanghavi J, et al. The epidermolysis bullosa acquista antigen (Type VII collagen) is present in human colon and patients with Crohn's disease have autoantibodies to type VII collagen. *J Invest Dermatol* 2002;118:1059–1064.
5. Ahmed AR, Hameed A. Bullous pemphigoid and dermatitis herpetiformis. *Clin Dermatol* 1993;11:47–52.
6. Jorgensen BG, Pedersen AT, Gjertsen BT. Pemphigus vulgaris and benign cicatricial mucous membrane pemphigoid in the upper respiratory tract and esophagus. *Ugeskr Laeger* 1993;155: 2126–2129.
7. Camisa C, Meisler DM. Immunobullous diseases with ocular involvement. *Dermatol Clin* 1992;10:555–570.
8. Chan LS, Ahmed AR, Anhalt GJ, et al. The first international consensus on mucous membrane pemphigoid: Definition, diagnostic criteria, pathogenic factors, medical treatment, and prognostic indicators. *Arch Dermatol* 2002;138:370–379.
9. Ghohestani RF, Nicolas JF, Rouselle P, et al. Identification of a 168-kDa mucosal antigenin a subset of patients with cicatricial pemphigoid. *J Invest Dermatol* 1996;107:136–139.
10. Taniuchi K, Takata M, Matsui C, et al. Antiepiligrin (laminin 5) cicatricial pemphigoid associated with an underlying gastric carcinoma producing laminin 5. *Br J Dermatol* 1999;140:696–700.
11. Naylor MF, MacCarty RL, Rogers RS III. Barium studies in esophageal cicatricial pemphigoid. *Abdom Imaging* 1995;20: 97–100.
12. Vincent SD, Lilly GE, Baker KA. Clinical, historic, and therapeutic features of cicatricial pemphigoid. A literature review and open therapeutic trial with corticosteroids. *Oral Surg Oral Med Oral Pathol Oral Radiol Endod* 1993;76:453–459.
13. Sciubba JJ. Autoimmune aspects of pemphigus vulgaris and mucosal pemphigoid. *Adv Dent Res* 1996;10:52–56.
14. Goldberg NS, Weiss SS. Pemphigus vulgaris of the esophagus in women. *J Am Acad Dermatol* 1989;21:1115–1118.
15. Trattner A, Lurie R, Leiser A, et al. Esophageal involvement in pemphigus vulgaris: a clinical, histologic, and immunopathologic study. *J Am Acad Dermatol* 1991;24:223–226.
16. Schissel DJ, David-Bajar K Esophagitis dissecans superficialis associated with pemphigus vulgaris. *Cutis* 1999;63:157–160.
17. Scully C, Paes de Almeida O, Porter SR, et al. Pemphigus vulgaris: the manifestations and long-term management of 55 patients with oral lesions. *Br J Dermatol* 1999;140:84–89.
18. Woldegiorgis S, Swerlick RA. Pemphigus in the southeastern United States. *South Med J* 2001;94:694–698.
19. Camisa C, Helm TN, Liu Y-C, et al. Paraneoplastic pemphigus: a report of three cases including one long-term survivor. *J Am Acad Dermatol* 1992;27:547–543.
20. Dolan PA, Flowers FP, Arauj OE, et al. Toxic epidermal necrolysis. *J Emerg Med* 1989;7:65–69.
21. Schwartz RA. Toxic epidermal necrolysis. *Cutis* 1997;59: 123–128.
22. Yarbrough DR III. Experience with toxic epidermal necrolysis treated in a burn center. *J Burn Care Rehab* 1996;17:30–33.
23. Egan CA, Grant WJ, Morris SE, et al. Plasmapheresis as an

adjunct treatment in toxic epidermal necrolysis. *J Am Acad Dermatol* 1999;40:458–461.

24. Viard I, Wehrli P, Bullani R, et al. Inhibition of toxic epidermal necrolysis by blockade of CD 95 with human intravenous immunoglobulin. *Science* 1998;282:490–493.

25. Mahe A, Keita S, Blanc L, et al. Esophageal necrosis in the Stevens-Johnson syndrome. *J Am Acad Dermatol* 1993;29:103–104.

26. Guitart J. Immunopathology of Stevens-Johnson syndrome. *Allergy Asthma Proc* 1995;16:163–164.

27. Howell CG, Mansberger JA, Parrish RA. Esophageal stricture secondary to Stevens-Johnson syndrome. *J Pediatr Surg* 1987;22:994–995.

28. Pulkkinen L, Ringpfeil F, Uitto J. Progress in heritable skin diseases: Molecular bases and clinical implications. *J Am Acad Dermatol* 2002;47:91–104.

29. Horn HM, Tidman MJ. The clinical spectrum of dystrophic epidermolysis bullosa. *Br J Dermatol* 2002;146:267–274.

30. Wright JT, Fine JD. Hereditary epidermolysis bullosa. *Semin Dermatol* 1994;13:102–107.

31. Birge K. Nutrition management of patients with epidermolysis bullosa. *J Am Diet Assoc* 1995;95:575–579.

32. Haynes L, Atherton DJ, Ade-Aiayi N, et al. Gastrostomy and growth in dystrophic epidermolysis bullosa. *Br J Dermatol* 1996;134:872–879.

33. Fujimoto T, Lane GJ, Miyano T, et al. Esophageal strictures in children with recessive dystrophic epidermolysis bullosa: experience of balloon dilatation in nine cases. *J Pediatr Gastroenterol Nutr* 1998;27:524–529.

34. Touloukian RJ, Schonholz SM, Gryboski JD, et al. Perioperative considerations in esophageal replacement for epidermolysis bullosa: report of two cases successfully treated by colon interposition. *Am J Gastroenterol* 1988;83:857–861.

35. Wong WL, Entwisle K, Pemberton J. Gastrointestinal manifestations in the Hallopeau–Siemens variant of recessive dystrophic epidermolysis bullosa. *Br J Radiol* 1993;66:788–793.

36. Horan TA, Urschel JD, MacEachern NA, et al. Esophageal perforation in recessive dystrophic epidermolysis bullosa. *Ann Thorac Surg* 1994;57:1027–1029.

37. Kahn D, Hutchinson E. Esophageal involvement in familial benign chronic pemphigus. *Arch Dermatol* 1974;109:718–719.

38. Burge S. Darier's disease—the clinical features and pathogenesis. *Clin Exp Dermatol* 1994;19:193–205.

39. Nelen MR, Padberg GW, Peeters EA, et al. Localization of the gene for Cowden disease to chromosome 10q22–23. *Nature Genet* 1996;13:114–116.

40. Kay PS, Soetikno RM, Mindelzun R, et al. Diffuse esophageal glycogenic acanthosis: an endoscopic marker of Cowden's disease. *Am J Gastroenterol* 1997;92:1038–1040.

41. Mallory SB. Cowden syndrome (multiple hamartoma syndrome). *Dermatol Clin* 1995;13:27–31.

42. Kore-Eda S, Yoneda K, Ohtani T, et al. Focal dermal hypoplasia (Goltz syndrome) associated with multiple giant papillomas. *Br J Dermatol* 1995;133:997–999.

43. Lee IJ, Cha MS, Kim SC, et al. Electronmicroscopic observation of the basement membrane zone in focal dermal hypoplasia. *Pediatr Dermatol* 1996;13:5–9.

44. Ellis A, Field JK, Field EA, et al. Tylosis associated with carcinoma of the oesophagus and oral leukoplakia in a large Liverpool family—a review of six generations. *Eur J Cancer* 1994;30B:102–112.

45. Marger RS, Marger D. Carcinoma of the esophagus and tylosis. A lethal genetic combination. *Cancer* 1993;72:17–19.

46. Kelsell DP, Risk JM, Leigh IM, et al. Close mapping of the focal non-epidermolytic palmoplantar keratoderma (PPK) locus associated with oesophageal cancer (TOC). *Hum Mol Genet* 1996;5:857–860.

47. Hoffman RM, Jaffe PE. Plummer-Vinson syndrome. A case report and literature review. *Arch Int Med* 1995;155:2008–2011.

48. Gorisek B, Krajnc I, Rems D, et al. Malignant acanthosis nigricans and tripe plams in a patient with endometrial adenocarcinoma—a case report and review of literature. *Gynecol Oncol* 1997;65:539–542.

49. Tyler MT, Ficarra G, Silverman S Jr, et al. Malignant acanthosis nigricans with florid papillary oral lesions. *Oral Surg Oral Med Oral Pathol Oral Radiol Endod* 1996;81:445–449.

50. Kozlowski LM, Nigra TP. Esophageal acanthosis nigricans in association with adenocarcinoma from an unknown primary site. *J Am Acad Dermatol* 1992;26:348–351.

51. Hsu YS, Lien GH, Lai HH, et al. Acrokeratosis paraneoplastica (Bazex syndrome) with adenocarcinoma of the colon: report of a case and review of the literature. *J Gastroenterol* 2000;35:460–464.

52. Boudoulas O, Camisa C. Paraneoplastic acrokeratosis: Bazex syndrome. *Cutis* 1986;37:449–453.

53. Grimwood RE, Lekan C. Acrokeratosis paraneoplastica with esophageal squamous cell carcinoma. *J Am Acad Dermatol* 1987;17:685–686.

54. Tharakaram S. Metastases to the skin. *Int J Dermatol* 1988;27:240–242.

55. Farr P, Goens J, Herchuelz J, et al. Cutaneous metastasis as the first manifestation of adenocarcinoma in Barrett esophagus. *J Belge Radiol* 1987;70:329–332.

56. Schneider A, Martini N, Burt ME. Malignant melanoma metastatic to the esophagus. *Ann Thorac Surg* 1993;55:516–517.

57. Stranks GJ, Mathai JT, Rowe-Jones DC. Primary malignant melanoma of the oesophagus: case report and review of surgical pathology. *Gut* 1991;32:828–830.

58. Redleaf MI, Moran WJ, Gruber B. Mycosis fungoides involving the cervical esophagus. *Arch Otolaryngol Head Neck Surg* 1993;119:690–693.

59. Porter SR, Kirby A, Olsen I, et al. Immunologic aspects of dermal and oral lichen planus: a review. *Oral Surg Oral Med Oral Pathol Oral Radiol Endod* 1997;83:358–366.

60. Eisen D. The evaluation of cutaneous, genital, scalp, nail, esophageal, and ocular involvement in patients with oral lichen planus. *Oral Surg Oral Med Oral Pathol Oral Radiol Endod* 1999;88:431–436.

61. Holder PD, Wong WL, Pemberton J, et al. Diagnosis and treatment of an oesophageal stricture due to lichen planus. *Br J Dermatol* 1992;65:451–452.

62. Van Maercke P, Gunther M, Groth W, et al. Lichen ruber mucosae with esophageal involvement. *Endoscopy* 1988;20:158–160.

63. Jobard-Drobacheff C, Blanc D, Quencez E, et al. Lichen planus of the esophagus. *Clin Exp Dermatol* 1988;13:38–41.

64. Dickens CM, Heseltine D, Walton S, et al. The esophagus in lichen planus: an endoscopic study. *BMJ* 1990;300:84.

64a. Calabrese C, Fabbri A, Benni M, et al. Squamous cell carcinoma arising in esophageal lichen planus. *Gastrointest Endosc* 2003:47:596–599,

65. Schreiner DT, Jorizzo JL. Behcet's disease and complex apthosis. *Dermatol Clin* 1987;5:769–778.

66. Laccourreye O, Fadlallah JP, Pages JC, et al. Sutton's disease (periadenitis mucosa necrotica recurrens). *Ann Otol Rhinol Laryngol* 1995;104:301–304.

67. Ship JA. Recurrent aphthous stomatitis. An update. *Oral Surg Oral Med Oral Pathol Oral Radiol Endod* 1996;81:141–147.

68. O'Duffy JD. Behcet's disease. *Curr Opin Rheumatol* 1994;6:39–43.

69. Jorizzo JL, Abernethy JL, White WL, et al. Mucocutaneous criteria for the diagnosis of Behcet's disease: an analysis of clinicopathologic data from multiple international centers. *J Acad Dermatol* 1995;32:968–976.

70. Kemula M, Cabie A, Khuong MA, et al. Behcet's disease disclosed by recurrent meningitis and esophageal ulcers. *Ann Med Int* 1995;146:190–191.

71. Mangelsdorf HC, White WL, Jorizzo JL. Behcet's disease. Report of twenty–five patients from the United States with prominent mucocutaneous involvement. *J Acad Dermatol* 1996;34:745–750.

72. Kagen LJ, Hochman RB, Strong EW. Cricopharyngeal obstruction in inflammatory myopathy (polymyositis/dermatomyositis): report of three cases and review of the literature. *Arthritis Rheum* 1985;28:630–636.

73. van den Hoogen FH, de Jong EM. Clinical aspects of systemic and localized scleroderma. *Curr Opin Rheumatol* 1995;7:546–550.

74. Sjogren RW. Gastrointestinal features of scleroderma. *Curr Opin Rheumatol* 1996;8:569–575.

75. Wigley FM. Raynaud's phenomenon and other features of scleroderma, including pulmonary hypertension. *Curr Opin Rheumatol* 1996;8:561–568.

76. Ueda M, Abe Y, Fujiwara H, et al. Prominent telangiectasia associated with marked bleeding in CREST syndrome. *J Dermatol* 1993;20:180–184.

77. Solomon JA, Abrams L, Lichtenstein GR. GI manifestations of Ehlers-Danlos syndrome. *Am J Gastroenterol* 1996;91: 2282–2288.

78. Foster JA, Sylvia LM. Doxycycline-induced esophageal ulceration. *Ann Pharmacother* 1994;28:1185–1187.

79. Tankurt IE, Akbaylar H, Yenicerioglu Y, et al. Severe, long-lasting symptoms from doxycycline-induced esophageal injury. *Endoscopy* 1995;27:626.

41

ESOPHAGEAL DISEASE IN OLDER PATIENTS

KENNETH R. DEVAULT
SAMI R. ACHEM

The ageing population has become a major social, economic, and political issue. Whereas only 13% of the population was aged ≥65 years in 1990, it is estimated that 21% of the population will be aged ≥65 years by 2030. Currently, older individuals account for one third of total health care expenditures in the United States, and each year persons aged >75 years make six times as many office visits to an internist as do young adults. The old are more likely than the young to have multiple chronic and often terminal illnesses (1). They are also more likely to be on multiple medications, which may have unwanted side effects and drug–drug interactions.

Esophageal diseases are common in all age groups, including the old (2). In a survey in the Netherlands, 16% of a cohort of residents aged >87 years described symptoms of swallowing dysfunction (3). Some esophageal diseases are unique to the older patients, including Zenker's diverticulum, cervical osteophytes, and dysphagia aortica. Other disorders may pose special diagnostic considerations in the old (4). For example, in the older patient with achalasia the possibility of secondary achalasia due to a distal esophageal malignancy is more likely than in a young patient presenting with achalasia. In some cases, diagnosis may be made more complex because of atypical presentations or coexisting illnesses. Chest pain, due to chronic gastroesophageal reflux (GER), may be more difficult to diagnose because of associated coronary artery disease or lack of heartburn in older patients. Finally, there is a greater potential for older patients to develop complications of long-standing chronic diseases. For example, the frequencies of Barrett's esophagus and adenocarcinoma of the esophagus increase with the duration of chronic GER disease (GERD).

The diagnosis of esophageal disorders in older patients is complicated by changes brought about by "normal" ageing. The concept of presbyesophagus was proposed to explain age-related decreases in esophageal peristaltic pressures, abnormal contractions in the esophageal body, incomplete lower esophageal sphincter (LES) relaxation and dilation of the esophagus on barium examination in patients aged >90 (5). With the advent of esophageal manometry, this concept was challenged and the majority of older patients with abnormal peristalsis are now classified into one of the described motility disorders (achalasia, diffuse esophageal spasm, etc.), although a large number are labeled as "nonspecific" disorders or more recently as a disorder of ineffective peristalsis (6). The fate of esophageal peristalsis with ageing in both the normal population and in those with symptoms has been extensively debated. Although many have discarded the concept of presbyesophagus, there are certainly changes in the esophagus with ageing. These changes are manifest both in the physiology of the esophagus and in the presenting symptoms in older patients, which are often atypical to those seen in younger patients. Up to 10% of patients aged >50 have dysphagia, although they often do not report these symptoms to their healthcare provider (7). Another study found at least some swallowing difficulty in 15% of subjects aged >85 (3). In the older patient with esophageal disease, diagnosis is more likely to be delayed compared to younger patients because symptoms are often attributed to underlying cardiac and pulmonary disorders. Moreover, older patients are more likely than younger ones to experience complications resulting from aspiration and malnutrition, which often accompany inadequately treated esophageal diseases (8).

In this chapter, we review changes in pharyngoesophageal function with ageing and the unique aspects of esophageal diseases, including clinical presentation, diagnosis, and management, in older individuals.

K.R. DeVault, S.R. Achem: Department of Medicine, Mayo Clinic, Jacksonville, Florida.

CHANGES IN ESOPHAGEAL PHYSIOLOGY WITH AGEING

Motility

Upper Esophageal Sphincter/Pharynx

Dysfunction of the proximal aspects of swallowing—upper esophageal sphincter (UES) and pharynx—has been described with both normal ageing and with disease in older subjects. Reduction in lean muscle mass throughout the body occurs with age; therefore the skeletal muscles involved in the oral and pharyngeal phase of swallowing can be affected by ageing. In one autopsy study, an age-associated decrease in the number of type 1 (slow-acting) muscle fibers of the pharyngeal constrictor was found (9). In addition, the standard deviation of fiber diameters was significantly larger in patients aged >50 years than in younger patients; this was associated with a trend toward hypertrophy of individual muscle fibers and decreased fiber density.

These age-related changes may result in functional changes during the oropharyngeal phase of swallowing (10). Using videofluoroscopy, Ekberg and Feinberg (11) found swallowing to be normal, as defined in young persons, in only 16% of 56 older persons without dysphagia. In another study of 100 asymptomatic individuals aged >65 years, 22 had pharyngeal muscle weakness and abnormal cricopharyngeal relaxation on barium swallow, with pooling of barium in the valleculae and piriform sinuses. Some subjects also demonstrated tracheal aspiration of barium (12). Ageing has been reported to affect the coordination of swallowing in some (13), but not other (14) studies.

UES function is affected by ageing. Using a solid-state intraluminal transducer system, Fulp et al. (15) found that compared to persons aged <60 years, healthy persons aged >60 years have a lower resting UES pressure and delayed UES relaxation after swallowing (Fig. 41.1), as confirmed by others (14). On the other hand, Wilson et al. (16) found only marginally lower resting UES pressures, but higher pharyngeal contraction pressures and a reduction in the duration of upper esophageal contractions in older subjects than younger ones. We studied the function of the pharynx and UES in a group of asymptomatic patients aged >75 years in comparison to a younger control population aged 20 to 35 years (17). Both resting UES pressure and the ability of the UES to relax were decreased in the older "normal" population. These findings suggest that resistance to flow across the UES is increased because of decreased compliance with age (4). Indeed, the duration of oropharyngeal swallowing, as measured by videofluoroscopy, is significantly longer in older than in younger persons (14,18). The sensory threshold for initiating a swallow has also been reported to increase with age (19,20). It has been suggested that UES abnormalities, such as those described in the above studies may be causally related to GERD in some

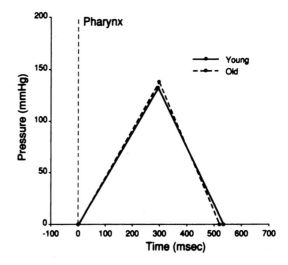

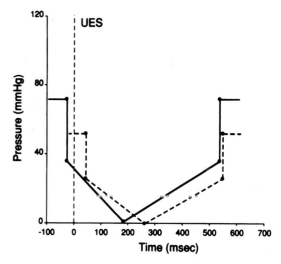

FIGURE 41.1. A simplified representation of pharyngeal and upper esophageal sphincter (UES) coordination based on computer analysis for pressure dynamics for wet swallows. There is a trend toward delayed UES relaxation in the normal elderly. (From Fulp S, et al. Aging-related alterations in human upper esophageal sphincter function. *Am J Gastroenterol* 1990;85: 1569, with permission.)

cases (21). Other authors have suggested that the reported changes in UES function with age reflect an increased frequency of concurrent illnesses in the old, rather than age-related physiologic changes per se (22,23). It would seem that the above data support age-related changes in both health and disease.

Esophageal Body

Although the effects of ageing on the esophageal body remain unclear, some data from pathology studies are available. In the human esophagus, the number of myenteric neurons decrease with ageing (24). This could result in dysmotility related to a relative deinnervation; producing disorders similar to idiopathic achalasia and diffuse spasm. In fact, the pathologic changes seen in the esophagus with ageing are very similar to the changes seen in patients with the more specific spastic esophageal motility disorders (25). Loss of esophageal innervation also most likely underlies the loss of balloon distention–induced secondary peristalsis in older healthy subjects (26). Secondary peristalsis is dependent on the sensory and motor function of the esophagus, either one of which could be affected with ageing. In a study by Hollis and Castell (27), edrophonium chloride did not increase pressures as readily in older compared to younger patients. They suggested that this indicated weakening in muscle, but not neurological function.

There has long been controversy as to whether "normal" ageing itself leads to disordered esophageal function. In 1964, Soergel et al. (5) found frequent nonpropulsive, tertiary contractions, delayed esophageal emptying, esophageal dilation, decreased LES relaxation, and an intrathoracic location of the LES (indicative of a hiatal hernia), in 15 nonagenarians studied with intraluminal manometry and barium radiography. They concluded that these abnormalities represented "presbyesophagus" and resembled diffuse esophageal spasm. In contrast, in 1974, Hollis and Castell (27) were unable to detect an increase in abnormal esophageal motility in a group of men aged 70 to 87 years when compared to a control group of young adults aged 19 to 27 years. However, in a subgroup of 80-year-old men, an age-related reduction in the amplitude of esophageal contractions was noted, implying that the neural system was intact, but that there was weakening of the smooth muscle (28).

In 1987, Richter et al. (29), using well-accepted modern manometric techniques, found an increase in distal esophageal amplitude and duration with age until age 50, after which values decreased. In this study, age had no effect on peristaltic velocity, basal LES pressure, or the frequency of double- and triple-peaked waveforms. In order to determine the utility of esophageal manometry in an older population, symptoms, manometric findings and diagnoses were compared between a group of patients aged >75 and another group <50 years (30). The older patients were more likely to be evaluated for dysphagia and less likely to be evaluated for chest pain. The LES was not different in the two groups, but the older patients were more likely to have ineffective peristalsis. Furthermore, when we evaluated patients referred for esophageal motility and pH testing, the only subgroup with frequent peristaltic failure was the older patients who had the highest percentage acid exposure (31).

Aperistalsis not otherwise explained by an underlying disease such as achalasia or scleroderma was found to be more common in older persons with dysphagia than in their younger counterparts (32). We have also made this observation in some of our patients (Fig. 41.2). If presbyesophagus truly exists, these patients with aperistalsis may represent its most advanced manifestation. On the other hand, it is often difficult to truly declare that patients without peristalsis do not actually have achalasia with a different onset or even different pathogenesis, since it has been long suggested that there is a second peak of achalasia in the later years. The differentiation of achalasia from other forms of aperistalsis (including "presbyesophagus") is often difficult and requires a careful comparison of the patient's history, manometry, and radiological and endoscopic studies. The prevalence of secondary achalasia related to malignancy seems to increase with age emphasizing the need for a careful endoscopy and, on occasion, other selected tests such as

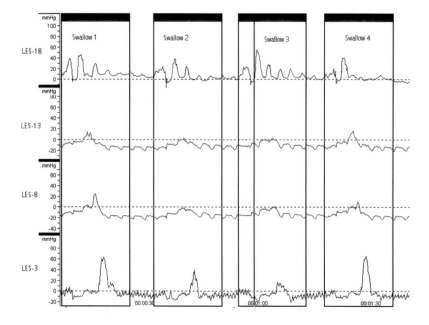

FIGURE 41.2. Weak, nontransmitted peristalsis from an older patient. The four channels are (top to bottom) 18, 13, 8, and 3 cm from the upper border of the lower esophageal sphincter. A weak peristaltic sequence is seen in the first and fourth swallow, whereas minimal to no activity is seen following the second and third swallows.

a computerized tomography (CT) scans and endoscopic ultrasound.

The clinical significance of the age-related esophageal manometric changes described above is unclear. An increased frequency of radiographic and scintigraphic transit abnormalities in older patients (e.g., "tertiary contractions") has not been shown to correlate with esophageal symptoms (33). The amount of gastric acid refluxed, as measured by an ambulatory pH system, was shown in one study to increase with age (34). However, another study found no difference in the frequency of spontaneous GER between a group of normal volunteers with a mean age of 49 years and a group with a mean age of 22 years (35). Moreover, Richter et al. (36) found no independent effect of age on ambulatory esophageal pH parameters, although older men experienced a significantly greater number of reflux episodes longer than 5 minutes than did women and younger men. The effect of age on GERD will be extensively discussed in a following section. Age-associated changes of the esophageal mucosa have not been studied critically, but the perception of pain on esophageal distention or infusion of acid has been reported to decline with age (37,38).

Thus, on the basis of the studies available, it appears that in normal healthy individuals, the physiologic function of the esophagus is preserved with increasing age, with the possible exception of the very old (>80 years), in whom the amplitude of esophageal contractions is decreased. In addition, there are some newer data that suggest an association of GERD with the peristaltic dysfunction that does occur. Finally, there is evidence to suggest that the perception of pain on distention of the esophagus or infusion of acid declines with age, which will be discussed below.

Lower Esophageal Sphincter

In 1977, Khan et al. (39) found an increased frequency of abnormal LES responses to deglutition, including a reduced amplitude of the after contraction, compared to results in a group of healthy persons aged <40 years. The older persons also showed reduced amplitude of peristaltic contractions in the upper and lower esophagus, reduced peristaltic velocity, and an increased frequency of simultaneous contractions. Basal LES pressures were similar between the two groups as has been the case in other manometric studies in healthy older patients. We confirmed this in our recent study that suggested a fall in LES pressure with increasing amounts of acid exposure that is independent of age (31). The length of the LES in addition to the pressure seems to be preserved with ageing. Paradoxically, hiatal hernias (both routine and paraesophageal) seem to increase in prevalence with age (40). We discuss specific issues related to the LES and GER in a following section, but the majority of the available evidence suggest minimal to no changes in LES pressure with ageing. Transient LES relaxations have not been adequately studied in an older population.

Sensory Function

Ageing has been noted to attenuate visual and gustatory sensation in healthy control subjects (41,42). The effect of ageing on the sensory function of the gastrointestinal tract has only partially been studied. As above noted, secondary peristalsis tends to fail with ageing, which could be due to a loss of the sensory function of the esophagus. Data to support this are provided in an elegant study by Lasch et al. (37). In this study, there was a clear distinction between the volume of balloon distention required to produce pain in a group of older patients compared to younger controls. In fact, in their 17 patients aged >65, 10 experienced no pain with at least one of the two trials performed even when the balloon was filled with 30 ml of air. No younger subject was able to tolerate this degree of distention. Weusten et al. (43) noted similar findings in a study where there were age-related alterations in cerebral potentials evoked by esophageal balloon distention. The new technique of impedance planimetry has been preliminarily reported to document reduced visceral pain perception from both the proximal and mid esophagus of a group of normal older subjects (44). When older patients undergo a modified Bernstein test of acid sensitivity, they have a longer lag time to symptoms and experience less intense symptoms that younger patients (45). This decreased esophageal acid sensitivity has also been noted in patients with Barrett's esophagus and a recent study suggested that these changes might be related to ageing and not just to the Barrett's esophagus (38).

It is reasonable to assume that much of the esophageal motility changes seen with ageing are related to nerve dysfunction. While some of these changes are probably intramural (within the wall of the esophagus), others are most certainly related to degeneration in central innervation. Failure of transmission of afferent, sensory information is most assuredly part of this equation. Since the afferent system is somewhat easier to investigate, we look forward to additional studies in these areas, which will add greatly to our understanding of the ageing esophagus. One can also assume that impaired sensory perception may lead to a delay in clinical presentation and the presentation at a more advanced or complicated stage of esophageal disease in the older patient.

GERD IN OLDER PATIENTS

Gastroesophageal reflux disease (GERD) is extremely common, with the prevalence of its major symptom—heartburn—ranging from 10% to 48% in large population-based studies (46). The estimated lifetime prevalence of GERD in the U.S. population is 25% to 30% (47). Yet, there is controversy as to whether GERD is more common in the old than the young. A Gallup survey (48) found that

22% of respondents aged >50 years used antacids and other antidyspeptic medications two or more times weekly compared to only 9% of those aged <50 years. In a Finnish survey of 487 older subjects aged >65 years (49), the frequency of daily symptoms suggestive of GERD was 8% in men and 15% in women, and 54% of men and 66% of women reported symptoms at least once per month. In a survey from the United States (50), heartburn at least once a week was reported by 22% of persons aged >65 years. On the other hand, among 476 predominantly male veterans who underwent upper endoscopy to evaluate upper gastrointestinal symptoms, the frequency and severity of esophagitis were similar in those aged >65 years and those under age 65 years (51). Moreover, in a random sample of 2,200 residents aged 25 to 74 years of Olmsted County, Minnesota, the overall prevalence of heartburn or acid regurgitation at least weekly was 20 per 100, and no significant increase in prevalence occurred with age. In fact, the prevalence of heartburn, but not acid regurgitation, declined with age, which supports the previously discussed concepts of impaired sensory function (52).

Could changes in physiology with ageing result in the paradox of more severe reflux disease with less severe symptoms? The risk of complications due to GERD seems to be higher in older patients. For example, Collen et al. (53) found erosive esophagitis in 81% of GERD patients aged >60 compared to 47% in those aged <60. Barrett's esophagus was also more common in older patients (25% vs. 15%). A recent case control study from the Veterans Administration found more erosions, ulcers, and strictures in older patients, particularly older, white males (54). In addition, in persons aged >80, esophagitis seems to account for a higher-than-expected proportion of patients with gastrointestinal bleeding (55). These older GERD patients are treated with both medical and surgical therapy, and in a study from Scotland, patients in their seventies decade were actually ten times more likely to undergo antireflux surgery than patients in their fifties (56).

Changes in GERD-Related Physiology with Aging

The change in esophageal physiology in disease and in normal older patients was discussed earlier. Many of the purported age-related changes in the esophageal body, LES, and anatomy (hiatal hernia) predispose to GERD. Transient LES relaxations are the single most common cause of reflux. The frequency of transient LES relaxations in older patients has not been evaluated. An age-dependent fall in salivary bicarbonate production has been reported, which may increase esophageal acid exposure due to a delay in acid clearance (57). The integrity of the esophageal mucosa resistance and the status of gastric emptying or duodenogastric reflux in older patients have also not been well evaluated.

The effect of aging on the LES has been previously examined in a series of 95 normal control subjects where age did not seem to adversely affect LES pressure (29). A hypotensive LES was suggested to be an uncommon finding in GERD especially in those with mild or moderate GERD (58), while other studies have suggested an inverse correlation between the severity of esophageal damage from GERD and LES pressures (59,60). These studies did not focus specifically on the effect of age on the LES while we recently demonstrated that LES pressure remains similar regardless of age even when patients were segregated by percentage of acid exposure (31). The lowest LES pressures occurred in those subjects with the most prolonged acid exposure independent of age.

An increased proportion of abnormal peristalsis and delayed esophageal acid clearance has been reported in older patients (61). It is possible that the variable changes in motility seen in older patients are more related to long-term esophageal acid exposure than to the effects of aging on esophageal smooth muscle. We have found that failed peristalsis occurs more commonly in the group of older patients with the most severe degree of acid exposure (31). These observations suggest that the increased prevalence of GERD complications may be due to impaired esophageal motility and hence delayed clearance. Additionally, older patients may fail to perceive esophageal reflux episodes due to a defective visceral sensory mechanism. Sustained and prolonged acid exposure experienced over time coupled with blunted sensory perception may be the most plausible explanations for the severity of GERD recognized in patients aged >65 years. This has not been documented in all studies, but was seen by Zhu et al. (62) when they observed that among patients with symptoms of GERD who underwent prolonged ambulatory esophageal pH monitoring, the mean percent time that the pH was <4 was 32.5% among 24 older patients with a mean age of 69 years, compared to 12.9% among 147 younger patients with a mean age of 45 years (62).

GERD in the elderly certainly could be influenced by coexisting diseases that affect the esophagus, including diabetes, Parkinson's disease, Alzheimer's disease, amyotrophic lateral sclerosis, and others. One factor likely to be important in the elderly is the use of medications known to decrease LES pressure and thereby increase GER. Drugs such as theophylline, nitrates, calcium antagonists, benzodiazepines, anticholinergics, antidepressants, lidocaine, and prostaglandins are more likely to be administered to the elderly than to the young and may therefore contribute to GER (63). An increase in body weight with age may also predispose to GER (64), which is important since our older population is now more likely to be obese than in the past.

In conclusion, it is clear that esophageal peristaltic dysfunction is common in older patients with more severe GERD while the fall in LES pressure seen with increased acid exposure does not seem to be age dependent. This impairment in esophageal function may result in a prolongation of acid exposure and potentially could increase older patients' risk for complications of GERD including ulcers, strictures, and Barrett's esophagus. Additional studies are needed to determine how these physiological abnormalities translate into differences in clinical outcome in older patients with GERD. It will also be important to determine whether these motility abnormalities are caused by acid reflux or are the cause of the reflux itself. This may be an unanswerable question, but perhaps a little of each is true. In some patients, reflux may impair motility, which subsequently worsens reflux and sets up a spiraling feedback loop that eventually results in both complications of GERD and impaired peristalsis. These events seem to be more common in older patients.

What Is the Role of *Helicobacter pylori* Infection and Other Gastric Factors?

The acid-peptic injury produced at the esophageal mucosa secondary to chronic GER is predominantly related to the acid content of the stomach and the resulting activation of pepsinogen. Although gastric acid secretion does not decrease because of aging per se (65), gastric acid secretion may decline in older persons with long-standing *Helicobacter pylori* infection in whom atrophic gastritis develops. Conversely, eradication of *H. pylori* has been reported to provoke reflux esophagitis, possibly by eliminating gastric ammonia, which is produced by *H. pylori* and may serve to neutralize acid in the esophagus (66). Thus, in the majority of older persons who are infected with *H. pylori*, refluxed material is less acidic than in the young, an observation that may explain in part a lower frequency of heartburn in older patients with GERD compared to young patients and the underrecognition of GERD in older people. Curing *H. pylori* infection may actually provoke reflux esophagitis in some patients (67). Since the prevalence of *H. pylori* seems to be decreasing in the Western world, one might hypothesize that more patients will retain their ability to secrete acid into old age. It is probable that this decrease in *H. pylori* prevalence has more to do with improved public health and increased use of antibiotics than it does with specific attempts at eradication. This increased acid secretion may result in a group of older patients with failing esophageal motility, who now have more acid gastric content and are at a greater risk for GERD and its complications.

Mold and Rankin (68) observed a surprisingly high frequency of distal esophageal alkalinity (>30%) among older patients undergoing ambulatory esophageal pH testing; such persons had a lower frequency of heartburn, but a higher frequency of pulmonary symptoms compared to those with acid reflux. A role for duodeno GER in more severe grades of reflux esophagitis has been suggested (69).

Differences in Presentation of GERD

Compared to younger patients, older patients with GERD are less likely to report heartburn, possibly because of a decline in esophageal sensitivity with age as previously discussed (37,38). On the other hand, dysphagia, chest pain, respiratory symptoms, and vomiting are common (70,71), and in persons aged >80 years, esophagitis may account for a greater percentage of cases of upper gastrointestinal bleeding than in younger persons (55). Because the severity of symptoms often does not correlate with the degree of esophagitis, diagnostic endoscopy should be considered in all older patients with a new onset of symptoms suggestive of GERD. It may be particularly challenging for the clinician to differentiate chest pain of cardiac origin from that of esophageal origin (72–74). Pulmonary and otolaryngologic manifestations of GER in the elderly, as in the young, include asthma, bronchitis, aspiration pneumonia, pulmonary fibrosis, hiccups, and laryngitis (75). In a study of 195 older patients with a mean age of 74 years, Raiha et al. (71) found that among those with esophagitis on endoscopy, heartburn was absent in 50% and the presence of heartburn did not correlate with the degree of reflux on ambulatory pH study. On the other hand, respiratory symptoms and dysphagia were common, and vomiting occurred in 25%. On surveying 487 subjects aged ≥65 years, these same investigators also found that typical symptoms of GERD were often associated with abdominal symptoms, chest pain, or respiratory symptoms (49). Restrictive ventilatory defects (76) and lung parenchymal scars and pleural thickening (77) in particular were more common in older patients with increased acid exposure on 24 hour esophageal pH studies than in those without abnormal results.

Special Considerations Related to Barrett's Esophagus in Older Patients

Because GERD is a chronic persistent disorder, it seems likely that the frequency of complications associated with GER increases with increasing duration of disease and thus with age. In 1969, Brunnen et al. (56) reported that in northern Scotland over an 11-year period (1951 to 1962), the incidence of patients referred for surgery for severe esophagitis was 18 per 100,000 in persons aged 60 to 69 years compared to only 1.7 per 100,000 in those aged 40 to 49 years. Despite milder heartburn, older patients may be more likely to have severe esophagitis, strictures, and Barrett's esophagus (62,78). The incidence of Barrett's esophagus rises with age. Moreover, older patients with Barrett's esophagus are less symptomatic than younger patients with Barrett's esophagus (38). On the other hand, older patients with GERD seem to need a greater degree of acid suppression to control symptoms and heal esophagitis than younger patients (53,79).

Once Barrett's is diagnosed in older patients, they usually are entered into a surveillance program. Many authors have advocated an end to Barrett's surveillance at some point as patients age. This was because of the unacceptable outcome of esophagectomy in older patients with high-grade dysplasia or cancer. The advent of less-invasive, albeit still experimental approaches to dysplastic Barrett's and early stage adenocarcinoma, such as photodynamic therapy and localized mucosal resection, has resulted in more older patients continuing with surveillance into advanced age. It is important to discuss the goals of Barrett's surveillance with all patients. If the patient does not agree to endoscopic or surgical treatment for high-grade dysplasia or cancer, continued surveillance is unreasonable.

Differences in Treatment of Older GERD Patients

Therapy of GERD is similar in the elderly and young. However, care must be taken in prescribing drugs to older patients with GERD, because certain medications are more likely to result in adverse effects in older patients. In addition, there is a greater frequency of adverse drug interactions in older patients, because they are more likely to take a variety of drugs for multiple medical conditions.

Lifestyle and Patient-Directed Therapy

Changes in lifestyle can be effective in controlling episodes of heartburn and dyspepsia in the elderly as in the young. In fact, emphasis on lifestyle therapy may be particularly appropriate in older patients, in whom additional drug therapy may be undesirable and difficult to afford (2). The patient should be instructed to eat three meals per day, with the evening meal taken at least 3 hours before bedtime, in order to avoid recumbency with a full stomach. Older patients may be more able to comply with these changes due to a more flexible lifestyle. Napping after lunch is common in older patients and may be refluxogenic, especially if lunch is the largest meal of the day. Obese patients should be advised to lose weight. For patients with nocturnal symptoms, the head of the bed should be elevated at least 6 inches by placing blocks or other elevators under the legs of the bed. Elevation of the head of the bed may be effective in decreasing nocturnal esophageal acid exposure, as assessed by overnight pH monitoring (80). Alternatively, placing a foam rubber wedge (10 in. high) on top of the mattress and under the patient's head may be as effective as elevating the entire head of the bed (81) and may be more convenient for some older patients.

Dietary recommendations include a decrease in the total fat content of the diet, because fat lowers esophageal sphincter pressure and thereby increases gastric acid reflux. Agents that may irritate the esophagus such as citrus juices, tomato products, coffee, and probably alcohol should be restricted. Smoking decreases LES pressure and should be discouraged. As noted earlier, medications that may decrease LES pressure should be avoided if possible. Dietary changes in older patients may be effective, but care should

be taken in prescribing an overly restrictive diet. Older patients may already be avoiding some foods due to advice on other medical conditions, may have decreased appetite and gustatory sensation, and may be living alone with little desire to prepare meals. Physician advice on diet can on occasion result in unwanted weight loss and contribute to malnutrition in an older patient who is zealous in following recommendations.

The intermittent use of antacids, alginic acid, or over-the-counter H_2-receptor antagonists is also appropriate. Antacids must be used with caution because of an increased risk of toxicity in older individuals, including salt overload, constipation, diarrhea, hypercalcemia, and interference with the absorption of other drugs. H_2-receptor antagonists (especially generic over-the-counter formulations) may provide attractive, low-cost therapy for older patients with mild reflux symptoms. An over-the-counter formulation of omeprazole has just been approved in the United States and may become an attractive alternative for some older reflux patients.

Medical Therapy

Acid suppression is the mainstay of GERD therapy in all age groups. Available agents include H_2-receptor antagonists (cimetidine, nizatidine, famotidine, ranitidine) and proton pump inhibitors (PPIs; esomeprazole, lansoprazole, omeprazole, pantoprazole, rabeprazole). The PPIs provide the greatest degree of acid suppression and are effective for the majority of patients, regardless of age, while H_2-receptor antagonists are effective in patients with milder disease.

The PPIs may be particularly useful in older patients with GERD, who seem to require a greater degree of acid suppression than younger patients to heal esophagitis (53,79,82). Analysis of controlled trials has suggested that, as in younger patients, therapy with PPIs is more effective than that with H_2-receptor antagonists in older patients with esophagitis (83,84). Although plasma clearance of PPIs decreases with age, no reduction in the dose of available PPIs is necessary in older patients, even those with impaired renal or hepatic function (85). Omeprazole and lansoprazole are metabolized by hepatic cytochrome P_{450} and may affect the metabolism of other drugs, but the effects have, thus far, been shown to be clinically insignificant (86,87). Long-term use of a PPI may lead to a reduction in protein-bound vitamin B_{12} absorption (88), but is unlikely to cause clinical B_{12} deficiency. Significant fat or carbohydrate malabsorption due to bacterial overgrowth is also not seen (89). Rabeprazole and pantoprazole have also been demonstrated to be highly effective in the therapy of GERD (90,91). Comparisons of clinical efficacy among agents are limited, although there have been several physiologic studies suggesting small benefits of one agent over another. A large study randomized patients with esophagitis to receive either omeprazole 20 mg or lansoprazole 30 mg daily. There were no significant differences between the outcomes of the two groups, with identical healing at 8 weeks (92). Similarly, approximately 200 patients with esophagitis were randomized to either omeprazole 20 mg or rabeprazole 20 mg and had identical healing at both 4 and 8 weeks (93). Finally, another trial of around 200 patients with esophagitis found no difference between omeprazole 20 mg daily and pantoprazole 40 mg daily (94). Esomeprazole (the s-isomer of omeprazole) has been purified and found to have superior activity to racemic omeprazole in physiology and gastric pH studies. In a large trial, this agent (esomeprazole 40 mg) was found to be clinically superior (symptoms and esophagitis) to omeprazole 20 mg, with an 8-week healing rate of 94% for esomeprazole and 87% for omeprazole ($p<0.05$) (95). This difference was particularly impressive in patients with more severe grades of esophagitis. Esomeprazole 40 mg has also been found to be superior to lansoprazole 20 mg in the healing of esophagitis (96). Agents with longer durations of action may be attractive when treating older patients who often need more aggressive acid control.

While PPIs have become the treatment of choice for GERD, some patients may be well managed on standard doses of H_2-receptor antagonists. For example, in maintenance trials, PPIs are usually superior to H_2-receptor antagonists, but up to 50% of patients can be successfully stepped down from PPI therapy. This will require twice-daily dosing, but can be considerably less expensive. Patients with severe or refractory GER or with complications of gastroesophageal disease may require higher-than-standard doses of H_2-receptor antagonists to promote relief of symptoms and heal esophagitis (97), and in fact are usually better served with PPI therapy. In the older patients, caution is required in using higher-than-standard doses of H_2-receptor antagonists. Mental status changes have been described in older patients, particularly those with renal and liver dysfunction, with both cimetidine and ranitidine (98). Cimetidine in particular may affect the metabolism of drugs by the hepatic cytochrome P_{450} system, including warfarin sodium (Coumadin), theophylline, and benzodiazepines. The addition of cimetidine to a regimen that already includes such a hepatically metabolized drug requires extreme care and a possible reduction in dose. Famotidine and nizatidine appear to be associated with low rates of side effects (97), but in patients with renal insufficiency, the doses of all H_2-receptor antagonists may need to be reduced (99).

The routine use of promotility agents for the treatment of GERD in this (or any) population should be discouraged. Metoclopramide, a dopamine antagonist that increases LES pressure and improves gastric emptying (100), must be used with great caution in older patients because of side effects in up to one-third of patients, including muscle tremors, spasms, agitation, anxiety, insomnia, drowsiness, and even frank confusion or tardive dyskinesia

(101). Domperidone is a similar agent, but with little to no CNS interactions, although it has not been proven to be very effective in GERD and is not available in the United States. Cisapride can cause cardiac arrhythmias and has been removed from the market in the United States. Bethanecol, which increases resting LES pressure, is rarely used and is associated with various side effects, including urinary frequency, abdominal pain, blurred vision, and worsening glaucoma. Finally, tegaserod is a promotility agent that has recently become available, although, like domeperidone, it has not been proven to be effective in GERD, nor has it been well studied in the older population.

Surgery

Surgery can be performed successfully in selected older patients who are reasonable operative risks, but should be avoided in patients with concomitant medical problems that make such surgery hazardous. A recent study found laparoscopic antireflux surgery to be safe and effective in both young and older patients with well-documented GERD (102). Large, paraesophageal hernias are an additional surgical problem in the older patient with GERD. Laparoscopic repair of these hernias is technically challenging and also associated with higher complication and recurrence rates (103). Regardless of the type of hernia (standard hiatal, paraesophageal, or mixed), older patients are at risk for weak peristalsis and are at risk for postoperative dysphagia. We continue to use the preoperative esophageal motility study to guide surgery, particularly in older patients.

DYSPHAGIA

Dysphagia may be caused by many of the diseases that can afflict the young as well as several others unique to the elderly. It is important to note that eating disorders in older patients may result not only from pharyngoesophageal disease, but also from disturbances not associated with the gastrointestinal tract, including cognitive or psychiatric problems, physical disability of the upper limbs, deterioration of the muscles of mastication, dental disease, and osteoporosis affecting the mandible (104–106).

Prevalence and Importance

Dysphagia is a frequently noted symptom in the geriatric population. Estimates of the prevalence of dysphagia in the elderly are variable. In studies from Europe, dysphagia occurs in 8% to 10% of persons aged >50 years, yet most do not consult a physician regarding this problem (7,107). In a survey in the U.S. Midwest, Talley et al. (108) estimated the prevalence at 6.9%. The prevalence of dysphagia is even higher in selected populations, such as patients residing in homes for the aged. Sibens et al. (109) reported that 30% to 40% of older nursing home residents have dysphagia. Studies from Singapore found that of a total of 211 patients in an acute geriatric unit assessed over a 3-month period, nearly 30% had swallowing impairment (110). Overall, difficulties at mealtime were observed in up to 87% of 349 residents in a home for the aged (105). Oropharyngeal dysphagia in particular may occur in up to 50% of nursing home residents (111). One study reported that even in older patients without dysphagia, video fluoroscopy shows abnormalities in up to 63% (11). Irreversible eating and swallowing disturbances are associated with a poor prognosis, regardless of the cause. In a study of 240 residents in a skilled nursing facility, persons who could eat without help had a significantly lower mortality rate at 6 months compared to those requiring assistance in eating (109). Determination of the cause of a patient's inability to maintain adequate nutrition may therefore be of vital prognostic importance.

As in the young, dysphagia in the elderly can be divided into two categories: abnormalities affecting the neuromuscular mechanisms controlling movements of the tongue, pharynx, and UES (oropharyngeal dysphagia), and disorders affecting the esophagus itself (esophageal dysphagia).

Oropharyngeal Dysphagia

Oropharyngeal dysphagia (OPD) refers to the inability to initiate the act of swallowing, so that food cannot be transferred from the mouth to the upper esophagus. Patients with OPD generally complain of food sticking in the throat, difficulty initiating a swallow, nasal regurgitation, and coughing during swallowing. Because of associated muscle weaknesses, they may also have dysarthria or nasal speech. In fact, OPD is usually one of several manifestations of a local, neurologic, or muscular disease (Table 41.1).

Central Nervous System Diseases

OPD can be caused by any disorder that affects the swallowing center in the brainstem or the nerves that modulate the swallowing process, including the fifth, seventh, ninth, tenth, and twelfth cranial nerves.

Stroke

Strokes are a common source of neurogenic dysphagia. At least 400,000 to 500,000 people in the United States are affected each year with a stroke, and approximately half of them die (112). The incidence of stroke rises with age and two-thirds of all strokes occur in people aged >65. It is estimated that up to one half of stroke survivors experience OPD (113–115). Patients with major strokes often manifest dysphagia as part of their neurologic deficit (116) (Fig. 41.3). In a study involving 128 patients with acute first-ever stroke, clinical and videofluoroscopic evidence of a swallowing disorder was noted in 51% (117). Notably, video-fluoroscopic evaluations have shown that a large proportion of these patients develop silent aspiration (118). Stroke-related swallowing difficulties lead to an increased rate of complications such as aspiration pneumonia, dehydration, malnutrition, and depression. Dysphagia is associated with pulmonary infections in 32% of stroke victims (117) and carries a high mortality rate at 90 days (119,120).

Strokes interrupt the normal neurophysiology of swallowing by affecting the transmission of impulses through the corticobulbar pathways, which extend from the inferior frontal region of the cortex to the lower brain stem nuclei. Although the corticobulbar pathways are bilateral, unilateral strokes can induce swallowing difficulties. In cortical strokes, lingual and pharyngeal paresis may be unilateral, thus allowing for a compensatory strategy of turning the head to the paretic side so as to exclude the weakened musculature from the path of the food bolus (116). Right cortical strokes affect the pharyngeal phase of swallowing resulting in pooling of secretions and possible aspiration. Left cortical strokes impair the oral phase of swallowing, resulting in pseudobulbar palsy due to disruption of the upper motor neuron. Symptoms include swallowing apraxia and impaired coordination of the oral mastication muscles. In anterior cortical strokes, the motor cortex controlling tongue movement may be affected and thereby result in poor oral control of a food bolus. Dysphagia is more likely with larger cortical strokes than with smaller

TABLE 41.1. CAUSES OF OROPHARYNGEAL DYSPHAGIA IN OLDER PATIENTS

Central nervous system disease
  Stroke
  Parkinson's disease
  Multiple sclerosis
  Wilson's disease
  Neoplasm
Other neurological and muscular disease
Peripheral neuropathy
Poliomyelitis and postpolio syndrome
Myasthenia gravis
Muscular dystrophy
Polymyositis and dermatomyositis
Amyotropic lateral sclerosis
Hyper and hypothyroidism
Hypercalcemia
Local lesions
  Oropharyngeal tumors
  Abscess
  Esophageal webs
  Thyromegally
  Cervical osteophytes
UES dysfunction
  Zenker's diverticulum
  Isolated cricopharyngeal (UES) dysfunction

UES, upper esophageal sphincter.

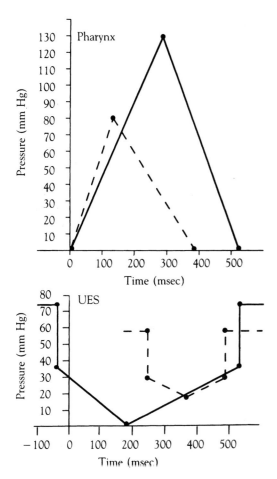

FIGURE 41.3. Schematic representation of pressures and timings obtained during computed manometry of the pharynx and upper esophageal sphincter in a normal person (*solid lines*) and in a patient following a stroke (*broken lines*). (From Castell DO. Esophageal diseases in the elderly. *Gastroenterol Clin North Am* 1990;19:227, with permission.)

ate the stroke victim but may not be sensitive enough to detect small infarctions (126).

There are little data regarding the effect of stroke on the tubular esophagus. In a study of 20 patients with a clinical diagnosis of stroke and no evidence of oropharyngeal dysphagia, the tubular esophagus was studied with manometry 3 to 5 days after the stroke and again at week 3. The major findings included an increase in velocity and peristaltic contractions following the second manometric study. Of interest is that these manometric findings were not associated with a symptomatic correlate. The evaluation of esophageal peristalsis by manometry can be challenging in stroke victims, since they often have enough oropharyngeal dysfunction to make initiation of swallows difficult. Repetitive swallowing often results in loss of peristalsis due to degultive inhibition.

Parkinson's Disease

Parkinson's disease is a disorder resulting from gradual degeneration of dopaminergic neurons in the central nervous system (CNS) that are thought to be replaced by cholinergic neurons leading to disorganized control of the central swallowing center (127). This disorder increases with age demonstrating an incidence of 12/100,00 for ages 55 to 64; 108/100,000 for ages 65 to 74; and 257/100,000 for ages 75 to 84 (128). Dysphagia develops in approximately 50% of patients and may be due to damage to both the central and enteric nervous systems (129,130). In patients with parkinsonism, OPD may result from tremor of the tongue or hesitancy in swallowing; dysfunction of the pharyngeal phase of swallowing is also likely (131,132). Abnormalities may be detected on videofluoroscopy even in the absence of symptoms (133). These patients not only experience dysfunction of the oral, pharyngeal, and esophageal phases of swallowing, but also have great difficulty in feeding themselves. Using a dynamic videoflurosocopic swallowing function study of 71 patients with Parkinson's disease (134), a variety of abnormalities have been reported. The most common abnormalities observed during the pharyngeal phase included impaired motility, vallecular and pyriform sinus stasis, supraglotic and glottic aspiration, and deficient epiglotic positioning and range of motion. Esophageal abnormalities included delayed transport, stasis, bolus redirection and tertiary contractions. Bassotti et al. (135) reported esophageal manometric abnormalities in 61% (n=18) patients with Parkinson's, including repetitive contractions, simultaneous contractions, reduced LES pressure, and high amplitude contractions. However, only 33% of patients had both symptoms and manometric abnormalities.

Multiple Sclerosis

Multiple sclerosis (MS) is the most common inflammatory demyelinating disease of the CNS. It affects between 25,000 and 350,000 people in the United States (136). It is a major

ones (121). Other symptoms associated with stroke include dysarthria, ataxia, vertigo, ipsilateral facial numbness, and contralateral body paresthesias. Dysphagia may occur in pseudobulbar palsy or in the Wallenberg syndrome, a lesion in the distribution of the posterior inferior cerebellar artery. Brainstem strokes may affect the swallowing center beneath the nucleus of the solitary tract, which coordinates pharyngeal swallowing, or the nucleus ambigus, which controls the muscles used in swallowing (22). Rarely, dysphagia has been observed as the sole manifestation of bilateral strokes (122) or an otherwise occult brainstem stroke (123). Lacunar strokes are small infarcts resulting from occlusion of penetrating arterioles into the brain and brain stem. These ministrokes are associated with aging, diabetes, and hypertension, and may produce dysphagia as sole manifestation (124,125). The diagnosis is based primarily on physical findings related to the deficits supplied by an artery. Magnetic resonance imaging (MRI) is frequently used to evalu-

cause of disability in both the young and elderly (137). In a study of 143 consecutive patients with MS, 34% reported dysphagia. The factors more closely correlating with the prevalence of dysphagia in MS are bulbar involvement and severity of the illness (138). A study of hospitalized patients with MS found documentable swallowing disturbances during a quantitative water test in up to 43%. However, almost half of these patients did not actually report swallowing difficulties (139). The diagnosis of MS rests on clinical grounds and has recently been revised by an international panel of MS experts in order to include the contribution of MRI and to involve progressive forms of the disease. Details are beyond of the scope of this review but the reader is referred to this source for more information (140).

Other Neuromuscular Disorders

OPD may also result from disorders affecting the peripheral nervous system or muscles involving the tongue, pharynx, or UES. In older patients, such disorders include peripheral neuropathy caused by diabetes mellitus, muscular dystrophies, polymyositis and dermatomyositis, hypothyroidism, and hyperthyroidism. In some cases, dysphagia may be the presenting or sole manifestation of the disorder. Depending on the degree of pharyngeal muscular involvement, polymyositis and dermatomyositis may result in weakness of the muscles controlling pharyngeal function and may lead to nasal regurgitation or aspiration, with abnormal pharyngeal transfer demonstrated on barium swallow (141). These abnormalities may reverse with treatment of the muscular inflammation. Occasionally, abnormal motility of the distal esophagus is also observed (142). An inflammatory myopathy isolated to the pharynx has also been described (143). Inclusion body myositis is an inflammatory myopathy distinguishable from other myopathic disorders by its characteristic histological feature: filamentous inclusions that may be intracytoplasmic or intranuclear. Clinical features include male preponderance, onset in the sixties or seventies, weakness of the distal musculature, absence of myalgias or connective tissue disease, a mixed pattern of myopathic/neurogenic process on electromyography, resistance to steroids, and a protracted course (144). Videofluoroscopy and motility studies usually disclose weak pharyngeal motility. In the elderly with OPD, it is particularly important to consider hyper- or hypo-thyroidism, since the clinical presentation may otherwise be occult. Postpolio muscular atrophy results from dysfunction of the residual motor neurons that were unaffected by the original viral infection. Up to 20% of the patients who experienced acute paralytic polio are now suffering from residual dysphagia (145).

Myasthenia Gravis

Myasthenia gravis (MG) is a disease of the neuromuscular junction affecting the motor end plate. MG is relatively rare with a reported annual incidence of 3 million to 4 million and a prevalence of about 4/100,000, although a recent report suggested a higher incidence of 9 million to 10 million (146). Although the disease is commonly seen in young women, recent data suggest that the elderly are also commonly affected. The disease is characterized by global fluctuating muscle fatigue. Typical clinical features include nasal regurgitation, a combination of strong jaw opening and weak closure, "jaw claudication" (progressive difficulty chewing with increasing discomfort that forces the patient to stop and rest), progressive fatigue, and ptosis or diplopia (147). Estimates of the prevalence of dysphagia are missing but some reports claim that up to 28% of patients may experience dysphagia at the outset (146). Unexplained dysphagia can be the first presenting symptom prior to the recognition of other clinical features of MG. Bulbar muscle weakness causes dysphagia and dysarthria labeled as "flaccid dysarthria" (hypernasality, imprecise articulation, and continuous breathiness with progression and an increase in severity with prolonged speaking). Some of these cases may not improve with treatment (148). In advanced MG, dysphagia may be profound. Atrophy of the tongue with paresis and eventually atrophy of other muscles of the palate and uvula have been described (149). Videofluoroscopic evaluation reveals a series of findings such as decreased pharyngeal motility, laryngeal penetration, and silent aspiration (148). Associated motility disturbances include decreased amplitude and duration of the peristaltic sequence and low cricopharyngeal sphincter pressures with normal coordination (150). Myasthenia-like symptoms might be induced by medications (procainamide, amynoglicosides, or penicillamine).

Amyotrophic Lateral Sclerosis

Amyotrophic lateral sclerosis (ALS), commonly called Lou Gehrig's disease, is a devastating condition and the most common degenerative motor neuron disorder in adults. It is estimated that 30,000 Americans currently have the disease with an annual incidence of 1 to 2/100,000 (151). At a specialized swallowing center (152), of 600 patients seen over a period of time, a third (n=211) suffered from ALS. The etiology remains unknown, although much research continues to focus on the potential role of glutamate, neurotoxins, and neurothrophic factors. The disease can begin at any time during adulthood but is most commonly diagnosed in middle age and affects more men than women. ALS is characterized by loss of motor neurons in the cortex, brain stem, and spinal cord, manifested by upper and lower motor neuron signs and symptoms affecting bulbar, limb, and respiratory muscles. It usually presents with problems in dexterity or gait resulting from muscle weakness. The bulbar phase is signaled by the appearance of dysarthria and dysphagia. OPD is characteristically progressive and severe, resulting in frequent aspiration, which usually indicates a preterminal phase of the disease (153). The patient eventually becomes paralyzed, and approximately 50 percent of patients die within 3 years after the onset of symptoms, usually due to respiratory failure (151). Two mechanisms have been described as source of OPD: delay in triggering the swallowing reflex for the voluntarily initiated swallow, and hyperreflexiveness and hypertension of the UES (154). Nutritional deficiency induced by OPD frequently requires supplemental gastrostomy feeding (155). The need for placement of a gastrostomy is a poor prognostic sign, in that median survival after gastrostomy placement, at least in one study, was confined to 185 days (156). In patients with ALS, a marked reduced forced vital capacity (FVC) predicts high mortality (within 30 days) for patients undergoing gastrostomy (157). A study in the Netherlands (158) found that provided the FEV was ≥ 1 L and PCO_2 ≤ 45 mm Hg, the success rate of gastrostomy placement and feeding in a group of patients with ALS was 89% (158).

Upper Esophageal Sphincter Dysfunction

The high-pressure zone of the UES results from contraction of the cricopharyngeus muscle and the adjacent hypopharyngeal musculature (159). Cricopharyngeal dysfunction may contribute to the development of OPD. As noted above, aging itself has been associated with a decrease in UES tone, although age-related decreases in UES tone do not appear to result in dysphagia (15). The term *cricopharyngeal achalasia* is often used inappropriately to describe putative cricopharyngeal dysfunction when the cricopharyngeal muscle is actually able to relax. The true abnormality is often an inability of the muscle to function in synchrony with other components of the swallowing mechanism or weakness of the pharyngeal muscles, resulting in inability to push the opening of the cricopharyngeus muscle (2). Other abnormalities in the UES that may result in OPD in the elderly include truly abnormal UES relaxation, a spectrum of disorders that includes oculopharyngeal muscular dystrophy (true cricopharyngeal achalasia) (160) and premature closure of the UES, or delayed relaxation of the sphincter, as in familial dysautonomia.

Local Structural Lesions

Various lesions may lead to OPD as a result of obstruction. In older patients, especially if they have been tobacco users, consideration must always be given to the possibility of head and neck tumors. Other obstructing lesions include inflammatory processes, such as an abscess, congenital web, prior surgical resection, an enlarged thyroid gland, and cervical hypertrophic osteoarthropathy. Although cervical osteoarthritis is frequent in the elderly, dysphagia secondary to compression of the esophagus by hypertrophic spurs of the anterior portion of cervical vertebrae is unusual. In a series of 116 patients evaluated for cervical ostheophytes,

only 7 reported dysphagia; the majority of patients complained of cervical and arm pain (161). The disease is most prevalent in men after age 50 and the typical clinical presentation includes difficulty swallowing solid foods, but on occasion, they may also have odynophagia, a foreign body sensation or globus, cough, hoarseness, and an urge to clear the throat. Compression by the osteophytes is most common at the C5–C7 levels, with 41% of reported cases occurring at the C5–C6 location (162). Barium swallow with lateral views makes the diagnosis, and since osteophytes are so common, dysphagia should not be blamed on the condition unless a solid bolus is documented to be delayed or stopped at the level of the osteophyte. Endoscopy should be performed to exclude an obstructing neoplasm, although the lesions may increase the difficulty of endoscopic intubation. This can be a particular problem with larger diameter and side-viewing instruments. Many patients respond to dietary modification and reassurance. For those with persistent symptoms, surgical excision of the osteophytes may be considered.

Diffuse idiopathic skeletal hyperostosis (DISH), also named Forestier disease, is characterized by new bone formation and especially new bone growth. The process begins with ossification of the anterior longitudinal ligament followed by cartilaginous metaplasia and ossification of the posterior longitudinal ligament. Spinal rigidity of a variable degree is the most common clinical presenting feature. Protrusion of hyperostotic formations causes esophageal compression and may lead to dysphagia (163). The diagnosis rests on plain radiographs of the spine showing a flowing ossification along the anterolateral aspect of at least four contiguous vertebrae in the absence of degenerative or inflammatory changes. Medical management includes anti-inflammatory medications, muscle relaxants, and reassurance, with surgical intervention only for those with unrelenting symptoms.

Zenker's Diverticulum

A Zenker's diverticulum is an outpouching in the posterior pharyngeal wall immediately above the UES (Killian's triangle), and is found almost exclusively in persons aged >50 years. The disorder is also more common in males than females (164). A community study from the UK estimates an annual incidence of two per 100,000/year (165). However, the true incidence may be difficult to evaluate since many patients with small pouches may not seek medical attention (166). The pathogenesis of Zenker's diverticulum is thought to relate to decreased compliance of the cricopharyngeus muscle, which results in increased resistance to the passage of a bolus (167,168). Intermittent OPD is often the earliest symptom. When the diverticulum becomes large enough to retain food, patients may develop more classic symptoms of cough, fullness and gurgling in the neck, postprandial regurgitation, and aspiration. A

Zenker's diverticulum may become large enough to produce a visible mass, which may gurgle on palpation (Boyce's sign) or to obstruct the esophagus by compression, thereby contributing to esophageal dysphagia. A sudden increase in the severity of symptoms, particularly progressive dysphagia or aphagia, pain, or hemoptysis may suggest the development of malignancy (169). The treatment of choice is surgical and the approach may be external or endoscopic. External surgical therapy consists of a diverticulectomy with myotomy. A staged approach (myotomy, diverticulectomy, and cervical esophagostomy, followed later by closure of the esophagostomy) is now being replaced by a single, definitive surgery (170). Endoscopic procedures involve division of the common muscular septum that separates the esophagus and the pouch. This approach is equivalent to performing an internal cricopharyngeal myotomy and creating a single lumen. Although the pouch has not been removed, it no longer fills and food passes into the esophagus resulting in symptomatic improvement (171). More recently endoscopic stapling devices have emerged as more popular treatment methods, but long-term outcome studies are still unavailable. Endoscopic therapies offer advantages over external surgical techniques: short procedure and anesthesia time, short hospital stay (1 to 2 days) with resumed oral intake within 24 hours and a lower complication rate. They can also be used for patients with recurrent diverticulum following a surgical approach. However, in some situations, such as an elderly, medically unfit patient with minimal symptoms, clinical observation might be the best therapeutic option.

Diagnostic Approach to Oropharyngeal Dysphagia

In evaluating the patient with OPD, a careful history and physical examination may provide clues to the diagnosis. For example, evidence of a systemic neurologic disorder should be sought. Careful examination of the head and neck for a neoplasm is also important. The diagnosis of Zenker's diverticulum may be suggested by a typical history. The major diagnostic study in the evaluation of OPD is a barium x-ray of the pharynx and UES with videofluoroscopy (also referred as the modified barium swallow). Rapid-sequence pictures must be obtained because bolus transfer from the mouth to the upper esophagus requires only approximately 1 second (172,173). Use of thick barium or a solid bolus is particularly helpful in assessing the ability of the patient to transfer food from the mouth to the esophagus (174). The main difference between videofluorscopy and the standard barium swallow is that the former is specifically aimed at analyzing functional impairment of the swallowing mechanism. Such an evaluation permits the detection of: (a) dysfunction or inability to initiate the pharyngeal swallow, (b) aspiration, (c) nasal regurgitation, (d) obstruction (mechanical or functional) to the

normal barium flow, and (e) residual bolus in the pharynx after swallowing. The development of improved computerized manometric techniques has simplified diagnostic testing, particularly in the evaluation of abnormalities of pharyngeal and UES coordination (15,174). However, manometry evaluation of UES dysfunction is limited due to catheter motion during swallowing necessitating the use of simultaneous radiography (manofluorography) to determine the location of the sensors (175). Electromyographic recordings of the cricopharyngeal muscle is a promising technique that might provide additional helpful information in the evaluation of patients with OPD. Larger studies are needed to determine the exact role of this test in patients with OPD (176).

Treatment

Treatment of OPD depends on the underlying cause. OPD associated with systemic illnesses, such as Parkinsonism, myasthenia gravis, polymyositis, and thyroid dysfunction often improves with treatment of the underlying disorder. Neoplasms require resection and, in some cases, chemotherapy or radiotherapy. Unfortunately, treatment itself may also result in dysphagia, because of the removal or loss of function of structures critical to normal swallowing. Dysphagia following a stroke may respond to techniques aimed at rehabilitation of the physical components of swallowing (177). Manipulation of the diet and proper positioning of the head may facilitate swallowing in these patients. There is less risk for aspiration with thickened liquids (honey-like consistency). In some cases, radiographic assessment of swallowing with various types of food (liquids, semisolids, and solids) in different head positions may permit recommendations that lead to improved swallowing. Consultation with a speech pathologist who is trained in swallowing therapy is helpful. There is some encouraging evidence showing that many patients will recover some swallowing function with this approach (116). To date, pharmacological therapy for the management of neurogenic dysphagia has received scant attention with the exception of Parkinson's disease. A small pilot study (n=17; double-blind, placebo-controlled) reported that nifedipine 30 mg orally resulted in improvement in swallowing in eight patients (five medication, three placebo) at the end of 4 weeks (178). The exact mechanism of action resulting in improved swallow in these patients remains speculative. For those with permanently impaired swallowing, a feeding gastrostomy or jejunostomy may be the only option.

In patients with neurologic disorders, including stroke and degenerative conditions, who present with pharyngeal dysphagia due to discoordination of the pharynx and UES, myotomy should also be considered, particularly in those with inadequate incomplete sphincter relaxation and "adequate" tongue/pharyngeal propulsion and laryngeal/hyoid elevation. Studies in small groups of patients with pharyngeal dysphagia have revealed good to excellent results with cricopharyngeal myotomy in patients with strokes, motor neuron disease, head trauma, poliomyelitis, and neoplastic or postsurgical nerve injury (179–181). Obstruction to thick or solid barium at the UES or hypopharyngeal bar ≥50% of the lumen throughout the swallow would indicate a defective opening UES. Additionally, the "adequacy" of tongue/pharyngeal and laryngeal/thyroid peristalsis should be established during this study. Cineradiographic studies have shown that myotomy produces improvement in the motor function of the entire pharyngoesophageal segment, not just the UES (182). Injection of botulinum toxin may provide an alternative approach to cricopharyngeal dysfunction, but its exact role in therapy remains to be defined (183). In a recent trial, in ten patients with well-defined UES dysfunction (incomplete or delayed opening primarily), OPD was improved but not resolved (184). Passing a large-diameter dilator (18 to 20 mm) may improve dysphagia, particularly in patients in whom manometric studies show high UES pressure or impaired relaxation.

Esophageal Dysphagia

Esophageal dysphagia is characterized by difficulty in the transport of ingested material down the esophagus and can result from a variety of neuromuscular (motility) disorders or mechanically obstructing lesions. A careful history usually allows the physician to place a patient into one of these two main categories of esophageal dysphagia. In approaching the patient with esophageal dysphagia, the three most important questions to answer are: (a) Is swallowing liquids or solids associated with dysphagia? (b) Is the dysphagia intermittent or progressive? (c) Is there associated heart-burn? The presence of additional associated symptoms, including chest pain, and nocturnal symptomatology and/or weight loss may also provide helpful clues to the diagnosis (see Chapter 2 for details) (185).

The major neuromuscular (motility) disorders to be considered in older patients include achalasia, diffuse esophageal spasm and related disorders, and scleroderma. As noted above, in some elderly patients with dysphagia, the principal manometric finding is aperistalsis not associated with a classic primary motility disorder (32). The major mechanical causes of esophageal dysphagia in the elderly include esophageal carcinoma, peptic strictures, rings or webs, vascular lesions, and medication-induced esophageal injury (Table 41.2). In general, motility disorders are characterized by dysphagia for both solids and liquids, whereas mechanical obstructing lesions initially cause dysphagia for solids only.

Achalasia

Achalasia is an esophageal disorder of undetermined etiology with an estimated annual incidence of 0.3 to 1/100,000, depending on the country where the disease is studied (186). Achalasia is characterized by slowly progressive dysphagia for solids and liquids and gradual weight loss (see Chapter 11). The onset of achalasia is usually between ages 20 and 40 years, but there is clear evidence that the incidence of the disease increases with age with a second peak occurring in the elderly. In general, the clinical and manometric presentation of achalasia in the elderly is similar to that observed in younger counterparts. However, Clouse et al. (60) found in a small study (n=13) of older patients with idiopathic achalasia (mean age 79, ±2years) that fewer complained of chest pain (27% vs. 53%), and the pain was less severe. In addition the LES residual pressure was significantly lower (60). In a large retrospective study in older patients, achalasia was associated with a significant increase in risk for pulmonary complications, malnutrition, and gastroesophageal cancer (187). In the older patient with long-standing achalasia, extreme dilatation and tortuosity of the esophagus as seen on barium x-ray may result in the so-called sigmoid esophagus.

In an older patient with apparent achalasia, it is important to perform an upper endoscopy (including a retroflexed view of the gastroesophageal junction), with biopsy of any suspicious area to exclude the possibility of secondary achalasia caused by a cancer that may produce the clinical, radiographic, and manometric abnormalities associated with idiopathic achalasia (188). Tumors most likely to be associated with secondary achalasia are proximal gastric cancers and distal esophageal cancers. Occasionally, pancreatic cancer, lung cancer, breast cancer, mesothelioma, hepatocellular carcinoma, sarcoma, and lymphoma can present in this manner (189–191). Secondary achalasia should be suspected in a patient with the clinical triad of age >50

TABLE 41.2. ESOPHAGEAL CAUSES OF DYSPHAGIA IN OLDER PATIENTS

Motility disorders
  Achalasia
  Spastic disorders
  Scleroderma
  GERD-related dysmotility
  Diabetic dysmotility
  Nonspecific aperistalsis or weak esophagus
    (presbyesophagus)
Structural lesions
  GERD-related strictures
  Lower esophageal ring
  Carcinoma
  Esophageal webs
  Medication injury
  Neoplasms
  Dysphagia aortica
  Adenopathy
  Mild and distal esophageal diverticula

GERD, gastroesophageal reflux disease.

years, dysphagia of <1 year duration, and weight loss of >15 lb (188). However, this triad is not diagnostic and can also be associated with idiopathic achalasia. Moreover, squamous cell carcinoma may develop as a consequence of long-standing achalasia (192). Endoscopic ultrasonography may be particularly sensitive in detecting small neoplasms before they are visible at endoscopy (193). The role of routine endoscopic ultrasound to exclude malignancy in achalasia has not been established.

As in the young patient with achalasia, treatment of the older patient can be medical or surgical, and the choice depends on the preference and expertise of the treating physicians, the overall health of the patient, and the patient's preference after being properly apprised of the techniques, risks, and expected outcomes. The principal options are pneumatic dilatation, surgical myotomy, and injection of botulinum toxin. Pneumatic dilation is a safe procedure in the older patient. One report has suggested that pneumatic dilatation may be particularly suitable for older patients in whom improvement in dysphagia is often sustained after pneumatic dilatation and the need for surgical myotomy is infrequent (194). In fact, patients aged <40 years had a significantly poorer response to pneumatic dilatation (2-year remission rate of 29%) than did patients aged >40 years (2-year remission rate of 67%) (195). The more prolonged relief in older patients may be related to a weaker tissue resistance with aging, which allows for easier disruption of the smooth muscle fibers. On the other hand, an esophageal perforation after pneumatic dilation may be particularly devastating in an older patient with a risk of considerable morbidity and potential mortality. Myotomy of the abnormal sphincter (Heller procedure) has also been followed by a good outcome in carefully selected older patients, although surgery is generally associated with a higher frequency of side effects, including GER, compared to pneumatic dilatation (196). In 1991, Shimi et al. (197) described the first case of achalasia treated by a minimally invasive approach. In 1992, Pellegrini et al. (198) published the first series in the English literature including 17 cases treated via a thoracoscopic approach. Recent data suggest that minimally invasive surgery via the abdominal laparoscopic approach provides effective short-term improvement in achalasia that compares favorably with the open surgical approach (199). The abdominal approach allows for an easier to perform antireflux procedure and offers several other technical advantages over the thoracoscopic approach (200). Therefore, laparoscopic myotomy has emerged as a preferred technique for the surgical management in achalasia, although long-term data regarding the durability, success, and potential complications of the procedure are eagerly awaited. Furthermore, patient selection remains influenced by the ability of the older patient to tolerate general anesthesia (although the same can be said of pneumatic dilation with its inherent risk of perforation, which usually requires a thoracotomy).

In the older patient with other serious medical problems in whom both pneumatic dilatation and surgery are high risk (American Society of Anesthesiology class ≥III) or those with challenging anatomical risk factors such as a tortuous megaesophagus or epiphrenic diverticulum, injection of botulinum toxin into the LES provides effective symptomatic relief, at least temporarily (201,202). Unfortunately, treatment frequently has to be repeated due to symptom recurrence resulting in increasing costs. The noninvasive nature of botulinum toxin injection compared to traditional therapies makes this a particularly attractive first-line approach in the surgically unfit older patient. Although botulinum toxin is devoid from major side effects (203), recent troubling reports described a death in a patient suffering from a fatal heart block following therapy with this agent and urinary retention in another case (204,205). On the other hand, conservative therapy with smooth-muscle–relaxing agents, such as isosorbide dinitrate or nifedipine given sublingually before meals, has not proven to be very effective (206). Sildenafil (Viagara) prescribed for the treatment of impotence has recently emerged as a drug that may have a potential application for the treatment of achalasia. In a preliminary study of 14 patients with achalasia, sildenafil caused a significant decrease in LES pressure lasting for <1 hour. No data were provided regarding the effects on clinical parameters (207). Further studies are needed to determine the clinical efficacy and the safety of this agent in patients with achalasia. For the rare patient with refractory dysphagia to repeated attempts at balloon dilation and/or surgical myotomy and botulinum toxin injection, experienced surgeons at tertiary centers have resorted, as a last option, to esophagectomy through a transhiatal approach using the stomach as esophageal substitute (208). This is a major operation of last resort that must be reserved only for the medically fit patient; gastrostomy feeding may be a better alternative for the older patient, particularly if they have considerable comorbidities.

Diffuse Esophageal Spasm and Related Disorders

Esophageal motility testing in patients with chest pain and/or dysphagia commonly reveals a spectrum of abnormal patterns whose cause, pathophysiology, and importance remain to be determined. In an effort to provide a critical frame of reference that may serve as a tool to clinicians and investigators alike, Spechler and Castell have proposed a new system (applicable to all ages) to classify the esophageal motility abnormalities as discussed in Chapter 5 (209).

Diffuse esophageal spasm is characterized by intermittent dysphagia for both solids and liquids, often in association with chest pain. Esophageal manometry shows normal peristalsis interrupted by simultaneous (nonperistaltic) contractions. The etiology of diffuse spasm has not been established. Rao et al. (210), using esophageal impedance planimetry and balloon distension studies, found that a disturbed esophageal sensory processing is more likely to correlate with symptoms than abnormal esophageal motility. These findings support the theory that esophageal dysmotility may represent a marker associated with patient's symptoms rather than the cause. Others argue that the abnormal esophageal motility originates in deeper layers of the muscularis that are not amenable to detection by conventional manometry but can be observed during esophageal intraluminal sonography (211). The structural basis for these abnormal esophageal motility patterns has been difficult to study since most of these subjects do not require surgery and the benign nature of the disease does not result in death and subsequent autopsy. Whether these patients represent an early spectrum of achalasia is unclear. Support to the role of a disorder of the autonomic nervous system has also been noted in some patients (212,213). Increased frequency of psychiatric diagnoses has been reported in patients with spastic esophageal disorders (214,215). To this date, no single explanation has provided a satisfactory basis for these patients' abnormal motility, although many of the changes noted could be explained by a loss of innervation or loss of muscle function, which may be particularly important in the older patient with a motility disorder.

The aim of treatment of spastic esophageal disorders is to decrease esophageal pressure or the patient's response to the pain. Agents such as nitrates, calcium antagonists (nifedipine or diltiazem), sedatives, and anticholinergic compounds may be helpful; however, there is poor correlation between improvement in motility changes and clinical response. These agents should be used carefully in older patients who may be taking other drugs that could predispose them to orthostatic changes and put them at risk of falling. We, as well as others, have reported the frequent coexistence of GERD in patients with spastic dysmotility, underscoring the importance of an initial therapeutic antireflux trial in this population (216,217). Occasionally, esophageal dilatation provides relief, and in severe, refractory cases, esophageal myotomy may be considered (218). Many patients improve after being reassured that their chest pain is esophageal, not cardiac, in origin.

Nitric oxide (NO) is a major inhibitory neurotransmitter in the gastrointestinal tract. *In vivo* studies in humans have shown that by removing NO or inhibiting its production with N-monomethyl-L-arginine, the simultaneous contractions characteristic of diffuse esophageal spasm can be induced (219,220). Therefore, pharmacological agents that result in augmentation of NO may improve the clinical and manometric patterns of patients with hypercontractile responses. In a recent small study of 6 healthy volunteers and 11 patients with a variety of spastic motility disorders, sildenafil (Viagra) significantly reduced LES pressure vector volume and distal esophageal amplitude in healthy controls. Manometric improvement was also observed in 9 of 11 patients with hypercontractile esophageal motility; however, only four of these reported

symptomatic improvement and two of these four discontinued drug therapy due to side effects (221). Larger, placebo-controlled trials are needed to determine whether this compound or other related agents may be of benefit to patients with hypercontractile disorders. Contraindications for use of this agent may be more common in older patients and include use of nitrates, cardiovascular disease, bleeding disorders, and active peptic ulcer disease.

Recently, Miller et al. (222) completed an open label trial of botulinum toxin in 29 patients with spastic motility disorders other than achalasia. They found that 72% of the patients experienced symptomatic improvement. No information was provided regarding the effects of botulinum toxin on esophageal manometry. The mean duration of response was 6.2 (standard deviation, 4.8) months and six of nine responders required a third dose to sustain remission (222). Placebo-controlled trials are also needed to confirm the results of this study, although the risk of botulinum toxin therapy is low enough that offering it to patients with spastic dysmotility of the esophagus seems reasonable.

Scleroderma

Esophageal involvement occurs in >80% of patients with scleroderma and correlates with the presence of Raynaud's phenomenon (see Chapter 37) (223). Those with a positive anti-centromere antibody have more pronounced esophageal involvement when compared to those who are positive for other markers commonly observed in scleroderma, such as anti-Scl70 antibodies (also known as anti-RNA polymerase antibodies) or antinuclear antibodies (224). Patients with scleroderma often experience slowly progressive dysphagia for both solids and liquids, as in achalasia. However, in scleroderma, unlike achalasia, heartburn is a prominent symptom of severe GER, and up to 40% of patients with GER due to scleroderma develop a peptic esophageal stricture; many develop Barrett's esophagus (225). Manometric findings include decreased LES pressure and feeble peristalsis in the lower esophagus with preserved peristalsis in the upper esophagus. Videoradiology and manometry can demonstrate abnormalities in up to 80%, but a full third of these patients may be asymptomatic, again underscoring the lack of relationship between tests and symptoms (226). Any patient with aperistalsis of the distal esophagus and a weak LES should be examined for signs of systemic scleroderma, and selected patients should have antibody testing to exclude the disease. This is particularly important in older patients where these motility changes may be inaccurately ascribed to presbyesophagus. The treatment of esophageal involvement in scleroderma includes measures to treat severe GER as discussed above.

Esophageal Cancer

In any older patient with a new onset of dysphagia, cancer should be the primary initial diagnostic consideration. In esophageal cancer, dysphagia is usually progressive, initially for solids and then for liquids, and is associated with weight loss. In patients with squamous cell carcinoma of the esophagus, there is often a history of tobacco and alcohol use. The principal risk factor for adenocarcinoma is Barrett's esophagus as a result of long-standing GER, and over the past 2 decades, the incidence of adenocarcinoma of the esophagus (as well as the gastric cardia) has risen faster than that of most other cancers (227). The diagnosis of esophageal cancer may be suggested by a barium x-ray study, but confirmation with tissue diagnosis requires endoscopy with biopsy and cytology, which is safe and well tolerated in the elderly (228).

The treatment of choice for esophageal cancer is surgical resection, which can be performed successfully in selected older patients with no or few coexisting medical problems (229–232). Studies in the 1980s showed a higher surgical mortality for patients aged >80 years when compared to younger counterparts (233). More contemporary, albeit small series, suggest that age alone should not be used as a selection criteria not to undergo esophageal resection (234). Unfortunately, many older patients are poor operative risks, and often the disease is unresectable at the time of diagnosis. CT scanning and endoscopic ultrasonography should be used to determine resectability. Endoscopic ultrasonography with biopsy of any suspicious lymph nodes may be even more important in the older patient, since accurate staging may avoid unnecessary surgery in these patients with greater risk of operative morbidity and mortality. Laser ablation and photodynamic therapy also have shown promise in the treatment of Barrett's esophagus, with or without dysplasia or early cancer (235–238). In patients who are poor operative risks or who have unresectable disease, palliation with radiotherapy, chemotherapy, or both may be considered. For relief of dysphagia, bougienage or laser photocoagulation of obstructing esophageal lesions, photodynamic therapy, or endoscopic insertion of an expandable mesh stent or silastic prosthesis are options (see Chapter 13). In general, the prognosis of esophageal cancer is poor, with a 5-year survival rate of <5%. The prognosis is much better when cancer is detected early as part of endoscopic surveillance in Barrett's esophagus.

Peptic Stricture

Peptic strictures are estimated to occur in 7% to 23% of patients with untreated reflux disease, especially older men (239). Patients with peptic strictures usually present with progressive dysphagia for solids in the setting of a long history of heartburn and other symptoms of GER. Patients with strictures are usually older than patients with GER but no stricture, presumably because stricture formation results over a long period of time (240). Peptic strictures can be demonstrated by barium radiography, but endoscopy is mandatory to exclude carcinoma. The strictures are typically smooth, tapered, and of varying lengths. If they are located above the distal esophagus, Barrett's esophagus may be found.

Most patients with a peptic stricture can be managed with intermittent dilatation using standard Maloney or Savary dilators in combination with aggressive long-term antireflux therapy. Recurrence of esophageal stricture necessitating repeated dilation treatment has been linked to those patients reporting a history of weight loss and less likely to those reporting heartburn at initial presentation (241). Recent data indicate that following dilation of peptic esophageal strictures, treatment with omeprazole in place of an H$_2$-blocker significantly decreases the need for esophageal dilation and maybe more cost-effective (242, 243). These observations, coupled with the successful healing rates of PPIs in erosive disease, have led to the replacement of H$_2$-receptor antagonists by PPIs as standard therapy for the management of patients with reflux-related complications such as esophageal stricture. If the stricture does not respond to conservative therapy, intralesional endoscopic steroid injection may be a useful adjunctive therapy to esophageal dilation (244). A number of studies have shown the benefits of laparoscopic antireflux surgery in patients with refractory peptic strictures. For instance, Klinger et al. (245) noted a significant decrease in the need for esophageal dilation after surgery when compared to preoperative intervention.

Rings or Webs

Rings or webs usually present with intermittent dysphagia for solids. Unlike dysphagia associated with esophageal cancer, dysphagia caused by rings or webs is typically nonprogressive. Most symptomatic rings present after age 50, and there is no difference in the prevalence of rings based on gender. These rings are seen in 6% to 14% of routine barium exams, while symptomatic rings occur in about 0.5% of these exams (246). The first episode of dysphagia frequently occurs while the patient is eating steak or bread, so the disorder has been termed the "steakhouse syndrome." Often the bolus can be forced down by drinking liquids, but occasionally it must be regurgitated, after which the meal can usually be finished without difficulty. Barium swallow with a solid bolus makes the best diagnosis, and endoscopy is indicated to facilitate dilation and if there is any question about the diagnosis.

The most common type of ring is Schatzki's ring, which is composed of invaginated mucosa located at the gastroesophageal mucosal junction (247). The cause of lower esophageal ring remains a subject of debate. Theories range from a congenital lesion to pill-induced esophageal inflammation. There is conflicting information about the association of these rings with GERD (248,249). On barium swallow, these rings are seen approximately 3 to 4 cm above the diaphragm. They produce symptoms when the lumen is narrowed to <12 or 13 mm. Treatment usually consists of dilatation of the esophagus with a large-caliber bougie. If symptoms occur infrequently, careful chewing of food may suffice. In patients who do not respond to standard bougienage, electrocautery incision and even Neodynium:yttrium-aluminnum-garnet (ND:YAG) has been reported to provide successful outcome in small number of cases (see Chapter 15). Hiatal hernias predispose to Schatzki's ring and are more common with age. Other factors that may increase the incidence of symptomatic rings in older patients include oropharyngeal and dental difficulties, which decrease mastication and weaken peristaltic pressures.

Vascular Compression

The term dysphagia aortica was first used by Pape (250) in 1932 to describe difficulty in swallowing caused by external compression from a tortuous or aneurysmal aorta (Fig. 41.4). Dysphagia aortica is a disorder of the elderly hypertensive patient who is more often female (251). Radi-

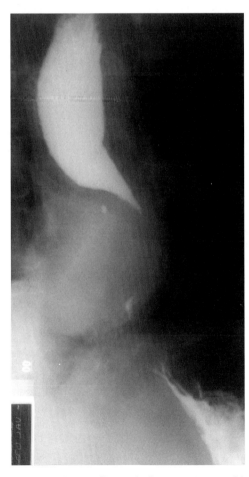

FIGURE 41.4. Barium radiograph from a 72-year-old patient with dysphagia aortica from a thoracic aortic aneurysm. Compression of the barium-filled distal esophagus produces a pseudoachalasia appearance.

ographic findings include a prominent indentation of aortic arch on a plain chest radiograph. On barium swallow, features include a partial esophageal obstruction at the aortic arch area, pulsatile movement of barium synchronous with aortic pulsation, and a flattened contour of the left margin of the esophagus (252). Endoscopic findings include stenosis, band-like pulsatile extrinsic compression, or kinking of the esophagus (253). Esophageal manometry may reveal a localized high-pressure barrier with superimposed oscillations synchronous with aortic pulsation confined to one transducer (254). This manometric finding is interesting, but lacks specificity. Mittal et al. (254) and Nguyen et al. (255) reported similar patterns in healthy controls and in dysphagia lusoria (compression of the esophagus by an aberrant subclavian vessel) (254,255). Surprisingly, CT has not been found as helpful in the evaluation of dysphagia aortica; vascular MRI may prove to be a more useful diagnostic technique.

Occasionally, the esophagus may be compressed by a markedly enlarged left atrium (256). Rarely, exsanguinating hemorrhage may result from penetration of an esophageal ulcer into an adjacent major blood vessel (257). Several cases have been identified of aorta-esophageal fistulas. This is a rare and lethal complication caused by fistulization of an expanding atherosclerotic thoracic aortic aneurysm into the esophagus, or less commonly, by a reflux-associated ulcer into the aorta (258). Aorta-esophageal fistulas can be also caused by a penetrating carcinoma of the esophagus after esophageal surgery, following radiation to the mediastinum, tuberculosis of the mediastinum, mycotic aneurysm, pseudoaneurysm, foreign bodies, and after repair of a thoracic aortic aneurysm. All of these disorders disproportionately affect older individuals.

Medication-Induced Esophageal Injury

Medication-induced esophageal injuries occur when caustic medicinal preparations dissolve in the esophagus rather than passing into the stomach as intended. Injury of this type has been termed pill esophagitis or pill-induced esophageal injury. This is a common disorder with nearly 1000 documented cases reported in the world's literature and an estimated 10,000 cases per year occurring in the United States (259). Elderly patients are at particular risk of medication-induced esophageal injury for several reasons: They take more medications than younger patients, are more likely to have anatomic or motility disorders or the esophagus, spend more time in a recumbent position, and may have reduced salivary production and/or impaired esophageal motility. Women appear to suffer from pill-induced injury at twice the rate of men, which is possibly related to the more common use of agents to treat osteoporosis (alendronate) and bladder disturbances (emepronium bromide) in women, although the precise reason has not been critically appraised. Patients with scleroderma and neurological diseases may also be more predisposed to pill esophagitis.

Acute esophageal injury may result from ingestion of a variety of medications (see also Chapter 34). Several observations indicate that sustained-release preparations may be more injurious than standard preparations of the same medications (260). Large pills or those with sticky surfaces are most likely to induce injury (261). Other factors that predispose to drug-induced esophageal injury include the patient's position at the time the drug is ingested and the volume of fluid ingested with the drug. It has been well established that the likelihood of passage of a pill through the esophagus is reduced when the medication is ingested by a patient in a recumbent position and with <15 ml of water. It is thus particularly ill advised to administer medications at bedtime with small sips of water, as is common practice. The majority of patients with medication-induced esophageal lesions do not have underlying esophageal abnormalities. The site of injury probably relates primarily to anatomic factors, as injury occurs most frequently in the mid-esophagus at the level of the aortic arch or distally in the area adjacent to the left atrium or above the LES.

The most commonly reported cause of pill esophagitis in the current medical literature is alendronate. There are nearly 100 documented cases, of which nine are complicated with the development of a stricture and three with hemorrhage (262). Other commonly reported cases have been associated with emepronium bromide (an anticholinergic agent used to relax the urinary bladder and not available in the United States), tetracycline derivatives, potassium chloride, quinidine, and nonsteroidal antiinflammatory drugs (NSAIDs) (263–265). Other medications have been implicated less frequently (see tables in chapter 34). A double-contrast barium swallow may identify the lesion and may provide information about possible extrinsic esophageal compression. Endoscopy also may confirm the diagnosis. Lesions vary from an erythematous patch to an ulcer or stricture. Most strictures tend to occur in the proximal esophagus (266). Occasional deaths from hemorrhage and perforation have even been reported in patients with potassium chloride–induced esophagitis (263). However, most medication-induced esophageal lesions heal with discontinuation of the causative agent and short-term therapy with antacids. Occasionally, more aggressive antireflux therapy is required and, in rare instances, resulting strictures must be dilated (267). Strictures are most likely to occur with esophageal injury from potassium chloride and quinidine preparations (47% of patients exposed to these agents), and older age has been shown to be a significant risk factor for the development of such strictures.

NSAIDs, which are very commonly used by older patients, account for about 8% of reported cases of pill esophagitis. Recent experience suggests that as many as 20% of patients on NSAID therapy have coexisting esophagitis (268). Whether this is the result of a direct effect of the medications on the esophagus or underlying chronic GERD remains to be determined. In one report (269), evidence of recent aspirin or NSAID use was found in 62% of patients with endoscopically verified esophagitis, compared to 26% of control subjects. Patients with a hiatal hernia taking NSAIDS appear to be at particular risk of developing esophageal ulcers (270). NSAIDs have been frequently associated with the development of esophageal strictures (271,272). Concomitant therapy with PPIs is very protective against gastric injury caused by NSAID use, but the effect of this combination on esophageal disease has not been studied.

Miscellaneous Lesions

Spontaneous intramural hematoma of the esophagus is a rare condition usually affecting middle-aged and older women, and presents with acute substernal or epigastric pain and dysphagia or hematemesis. The pathogenesis is uncertain, and symptoms usually resolve with conservative therapy (273). In other cases, endoscopy or a forced Valsalva maneuver have also been identified as precipitating events (274,275). The endoscopic appearance may resemble an esophageal neoplasm.

Acute esophageal necrosis (AEN) is another rare disorder that tends to occur more commonly in older individuals. Of 25 recognized cases in the literature, only three occurred in subjects aged <50 (in two additional cases age was not reported) (276). AEN was first described in 1990 at endoscopy, although two postmortem cases had previously been reported (277,278). The etiology is unknown although spontaneous rupture of the thoracic aorta, hypercoagulable state, Stevens-Johnson syndrome, and gastric outlet obstruction have been noted associations. Ischemic esophageal infarction due to shock has been described in the elderly (279). For patients undergoing endoscopy, the appearance of the esophageal mucosa is that of a black, necrotic-appearing esophagus with a pink transition zone at the gastroesophageal junction. Biopsies confirm mucosa and submucosa necrosis.

Spontaneous hemorrhage into a parathyroid adenoma has also been reported to cause acute dysphagia (280). Intramural esophageal pseudodiverticulosis is another disease associated with dysphagia in persons aged >60 years. The disorder is characterized by multiple small circumferential invaginations of the esophageal wall, either diffusely or focally, presumably as a result of dilatation of the secretory ducts of the submucosal glands (281). In addition to pseudodiverticulosis, stenoses or areas of reduced distensibility are found, usually in the upper esophagus. The etiology is unknown, but many affected patients have associated *Candida albicans* colonization of the esophageal mucosa. Another entity termed chronic esophagitis dessicans, characterized by chronic dysphagia, shedding of the esophageal mucosa, and localized esophageal strictures, has been described in five older patients with a mean age of 66 years (282).

CONCLUSIONS

In general, the classic symptoms of dysphagia, heartburn, and chest pain are the presenting manifestations of esophageal disorders in the elderly, as in the young. Several unique conditions may occur in the elderly, including Zenker's diverticulum and vascular compression of the esophagus. Certain disorders increase in frequency with age, such as oropharyngeal dysphagia due to neurologic disorders. Treatment approaches are similar in older and younger patients, but the potential for adverse drug effects and drug interactions is greater in the elderly than in the young. Endoscopy and surgery can also be used to treat esophageal disease, although procedure-related complications may be more devastating in older patients. GERD may present differently and be more difficult to treat in the older patient.

The special psychosocial, economic, and humanistic aspects of caring for the aged are just as important as medical ones. Factors that may have an impact on illness in an older person include the losses and disability associated with aging; feelings of isolation; a reticence to discuss certain embarrassing problems; and the variety of settings for health care, including nursing homes, home care communities, geriatric units, geropsychiatric units, rehabilitation units, and hospices. The multiplicity of medical problems that often lead to contradictory and mutually exclusive management options and the frequency of multiple-drug use and adverse drug reactions may pose great challenges to treatment of an older patient. In addition, many older patients have a limited income and may not be able to afford expensive medications. Clearly, just as children are not "little adults," the elderly are not "big adults," and the delivery of care to the older patients requires special expertise and sensitivity.

REFERENCES

1. Gastrointestinal disorders in the elderly. *Gastroenterol Clin North Am* 1990;19:227–457.
2. Castell DO. Esophageal disorders in the elderly. *Gastroenterol Clin North Am* 1990;19:235–54.
3. Bloem BR, Lagaay AM, van Beek W, et al. Prevalence of subjective dysphagia in community residents aged over 87. *BMJ* 1990;300:721–2.
4. Tack J, Vantrappen G. The aging oesophagus. *Gut* 1997;41:422–4.
5. Soergel KH, et al. Presbyesophagus: Esophageal motility in nonagenarians. *J Clin Invest* 1964;43:1472.
6. Leite LP, Johnston BT, Barrett J, et al. Ineffective esophageal motility (IEM): the primary finding in patients with nonspecific esophageal motility disorder. *Dig Dis Sci* 1997;42:1859–65.
7. Lindgren S, Janzon L. Prevalence of swallowing complaints and clinical findings among 50–79-year-old men and women in an urban population. *Dysphagia* 1991;6:187–92.
8. Gorman RC, Morris JB, Kaiser LR. Esophageal disease in the elderly patient. *Surg Clin North Am* 1994;74:93–112.
9. Leese G, Hopwood D. Muscle fibre typing in the human pharyngeal constrictors and oesophagus: the effect of ageing. *Acta Anat* 1986;127:77–80.
10. Nelson JB, Castell DO. Aging of the gastrointestinal system. In: Hazzard WR, et al. *Principles of geriatric medicine and gerontology.* New York: McGraw-Hill, 1990:593.
11. Ekberg O, Feinberg MJ. Altered swallowing function in elderly patients without dysphagia: radiologic findings in 56 cases. *Am J Roentgenol* 1991;156:1181–1184.
12. Piaget F, Fouillet J. Le pharynx et l'oesophage seniles: etude clinique radiologique et radiocinematographique. *J Med Lyon* 1959;40:951.
13. Nilsson H, Ekberg O, Olsson R, et al. Quantitative aspects of swallowing in an elderly nondysphagic population. *Dysphagia* 1996;11:180–184.
14. Shaw DW, Cook IJ, Gabb M, et al. Influence of normal aging on oral-pharyngeal and upper esophageal sphincter function during swallowing. *Am J Physiol* 1995;268:G389–G396.
15. Fulp SR, Dalton CB, Castell JA, et al. Aging-related alterations in human upper esophageal sphincter function. *Am J Gastroenterol* 1990;85:1569–1572.
16. Wilson JA, Pryde A, Macintyre CC, et al. The effects of age, sex, and smoking on normal pharyngoesophageal motility. *Am J Gastroenterol* 1990;85:686–691.
17. DeVault KR, Klingler PJ, Bammer T, et al. Manofluorographic evaluation of swallowing and pharyngeal function in the young and aged. *Gastroenterology* 1998;116:A985.
18. Robbins J, Hamilton JW, Lof GL, et al. Oropharyngeal swallowing in normal adults of different ages. *Gastroenterology* 1992;103:823–829.
19. Aviv JE, Martin JH, Jones ME, et al. Age-related changes in pharyngeal and supraglottic sensation. *Ann Otol Rhinol Laryngol* 1994;103:749–752.
20. Shaker R, Ren J, Zamir Z, et al. Effect of aging, position, and temperature on the threshold volume triggering pharyngeal swallows. *Gastroenterology* 1994;107:396–402.
21. Shaker R. Protective mechanisms against supraesophageal GERD. *J Clin Gastroenterol* 2000;30:S3–S8.
22. Ergun GA, Kahrilas PJ. Oropharyngeal dysphagia in the elderly. *Pract Gastroenterol* 1993;17:9.
23. Feinberg MJ, Ekberg O, Segall L, et al. Deglutition in elderly patients with dementia: findings of videofluorographic evaluation and impact on staging and management. *Radiology* 1992;183:811–814.
24. Eckhardt VF, LeCompte PM. Esphageal ganglia and smooth muscle in the elderly. *Am J Dig Dis* 1978;23:443.
25. Adams CW, Brain RH, Trounce JR. Ganglion cells in achalasia of the cardia. *Virchows Arch A Pathol Anat Histol* 1976;372:75–79.
26. Ren J, Shaker R, Kusano M, et al. Effect of aging on the secondary esophageal peristalsis: presbyesophagus revisited. *Am J Physiol* 1995;268:G772–G779.
27. Hollis JB, Castell DO. Esophageal function in elderly man. A new look at "presbyesophagus". *Ann Intern Med* 1974;80:371–374.
28. Goekas MD, Conteas CN, Majumdar AP. The aging gastrointestinal tract, liver, and pancreas. *Clin Geriatr Med* 1985;1:177.
29. Richter JE, Wu WC, Johns DN, et al. Esophageal manometry in 95 healthy adult volunteers. Variability of pressures with age and frequency of "abnormal" contractions. *Dig Dis Sci* 1987;32:583–592.

30. Ribeiro AC, Klingler PJ, Hinder RA, et al. Esophageal manometry: a comparison of findings in younger and older patients. *Am J Gastroenterol* 1998;93:706–710.

31. Achem AC, Achem SR, Stark ME, et al. Failure of esophageal peristalsis in older patients: association with esophageal acid exposure. *Am J Gastroenterol* 2003;98:35–39.

32. Meshkinpour H, Haghighat P, Dutton C. Clinical spectrum of esophageal aperistalsis in the elderly. *Am J Gastroenterol* 1994; 89:1480–1483.

33. Grishaw EK, Ott DJ, Frederick MG, et al. Functional abnormalities of the esophagus: a prospective analysis of radiographic findings relative to age and symptoms. *Am J Roentgenol* 1996; 167:719–723.

34. Smout AJ, Breedijk M, van der Zouw C, et al. Physiological gastroesophageal reflux and esophageal motor activity studied with a new system for 24-hour recording and automated analysis. *Dig Dis Sci* 1989;34:372–378.

35. Spence RA, Collins BJ, Parks TG, et al. Does age influence normal gastro-oesophageal reflux? *Gut* 1985;26:799–801.

36. Richter JE, Bradley LA, DeMeester TR, et al. Normal 24-hr ambulatory esophageal pH values. Influence of study center, pH electrode, age, and gender. *Dig Dis Sci* 1992;37:849–856.

37. Lasch H, Castell DO, Castell JA. Evidence for diminished visceral pain with aging: studies using graded intraesophageal balloon distension. *Am J Physiol* 1997;272:G1–G3.

38. Grade A, Pulliam G, Johnson C, et al. Reduced chemoreceptor sensitivity in patients with Barrett's esophagus may be related to age and not to the presence of Barrett's epithelium. *Am J Gastroenterol* 1997;92:2040–2043.

39. Khan TA, Shragge BW, Crispin JS, et al. Esophageal motility in the elderly. *Am J Dig Dis* 1977;22:1049–1054.

40. Stilson WL, Sanders I, Gardiner GA, et al. Hiatal hernia and gastroesophageal reflux. A clinicoradiological analysis of more than 1,000 cases. *Radiology* 1969;93:1323–1327.

41. Gray LS, Heron G, Cassidy D, et al. Comparison of age-related changes in short-wavelength–sensitive cone thresholds between normals and patients with primary open-angle glaucoma. *Optom Vis Sci* 1995;72:205–209.

42. de Graaf C, Polet P, van Staveren WA. Sensory perception and pleasantness of food flavors in elderly subjects. *J Gerontol* 1994; 49:93–99.

43. Weusten BL, Lam HG, Akkermans LM, et al. Influence of age on cerebral potentials evoked by oesophageal balloon distension in humans. *Eur J Clin Invest* 1994;24:627–631.

44. Patel R, Rao S. Biochemical and sensory parameters of the human oesophagus vary with age. *Am J Gastroenterol* 1995;90: 1567(abst).

45. Fass R, Pulliam G, Johnson C, et al. Symptom severity and oesophageal chemosensitivity to acid in older and young patients with gastro-oesophageal reflux. *Age Ageing* 2000;29: 125–130.

46. Heading RC. Prevalence of upper gastrointestinal symptoms in the general population: a systematic review. *Scand J Gastroenterol Suppl* 1999;231:3–8.

47. Scott M, Gelhot AR. Gastroesophageal reflux disease: diagnosis and management. *Am Fam Physician* 1999;59:1161–1169, 1199.

48. Gallup Organization. *A Gallup survey on heartburn across America.* Princeton, NJ: Gallup Organization, 1988.

49. Raiha IJ, Impivaara O, Seppala M, et al. Prevalence and characteristics of symptomatic gastroesophageal reflux disease in the elderly. *J Am Geriatr Soc* 1992;40:1209–1211.

50. Talley NJ, O'Keefe EA, Zinsmeister AR, et al. Prevalence of gastrointestinal symptoms in the elderly: a population-based study. *Gastroenterology* 1992;102:895–901.

51. Triadafilopoulos G, Sharma R. Features of symptomatic gastroesophageal reflux disease in elderly patients. *Am J Gastroenterol* 1997;92:2007–2011.

52. Locke GR 3rd, Talley NJ, Fett SL, et al. Prevalence and clinical spectrum of gastroesophageal reflux: a population-based study in Olmsted County, Minnesota. *Gastroenterology* 1997;112: 1448–1456.

53. Collen MJ, Abdulian JD, Chen YK. Gastroesophageal reflux disease in the elderly: more severe disease that requires aggressive therapy. *Am J Gastroenterol* 1995;90:1053–1057.

54. El-Serag HB, Sonnenberg A. Associations between different forms of gastro-oesophageal reflux disease. *Gut* 1997;41: 594–599.

55. Zimmerman J, Shohat V, Tsvang E, et al. Esophagitis is a major cause of upper gastrointestinal hemorrhage in the elderly. *Scand J Gastroenterol* 1997;32:906–909.

56. Brunnen PL, Karmody AM, Needham CD. Severe peptic oesophagitis. *Gut* 1969;10:831–837.

57. Sonnenberg A, Steinkamp U, Weise A, et al. Salivary secretion in reflux esophagitis. *Gastroenterology* 1982;83:889–895.

58. Dent J, Holloway RH, Toouli J, et al. Mechanisms of lower oesophageal sphincter incompetence in patients with symptomatic gastrooesophageal reflux. *Gut* 1988;29:1020–1028.

59. Iascone C, DeMeester TR, Little AG, et al. Barrett's esophagus. Functional assessment, proposed pathogenesis, and surgical therapy. *Arch Surg* 1983;118:543–549.

60. Clouse RE, Abramson BK, Todorczuk JR. Achalasia in the elderly. Effects of aging on clinical presentation and outcome. *Dig Dis Sci* 1991;36:225–228.

61. Ferriolli E, Oliveira RB, Matsuda NM, et al. Aging, esophageal motility, and gastroesophageal reflux. *J Am Geriatr Soc* 1998;46: 1534–1537.

62. Zhu H, Pace F, Sangaletti O, et al. Features of symptomatic gastroesophageal reflux in elderly patients. *Scand J Gastroenterol* 1993;28:235–238.

63. Richter JE, Castell DO. Gastroesophageal reflux. Pathogenesis, diagnosis, and therapy. *Ann Intern Med* 1982;97:93–103.

64. Wajed SA, Streets CG, Bremner CG, et al. Elevated body mass disrupts the barrier to gastroesophageal reflux. *Arch Surg* 2001; 136:1014–1019.

65. Hurwitz A, Brady DA, Schaal SE, et al. Gastric acidity in older adults. *JAMA* 1997;278:659–662.

66. Vakil NB. Review article: gastro-oesophageal reflux disease and Helicobacter pylori infection. *Aliment Pharmacol Ther* 2002;16 (suppl 1):47–51.

67. Labenz J, Blum AL, Bayerdorffer E, et al. Curing Helicobacter pylori infection in patients with duodenal ulcer may provoke reflux esophagitis. *Gastroenterology* 1997;112:1442–1447.

68. Mold JW, Rankin RA. Symptomatic gastroesophageal reflux in the elderly. *J Am Geriatr Soc* 1987;35:649–659.

69. Champion G, Richter JE, Vaezi MF, et al. Duodenogastroesophageal reflux: relationship to pH and importance in Barrett's esophagus. *Gastroenterology* 1994;107:747–754.

70. Nano M, Ferrara L, Camandona M. Sliding hiatal hernia in the elderly: a clinical entity. *J Am Geriatr Soc* 1981;29:463–464.

71. Raiha I, Hietanen E, Sourander L. Symptoms of gastro-oesophageal reflux disease in elderly people. *Age Ageing* 1991; 20:365–370.

72. Browning TH. Diagnosis of chest pain of esophageal origin. A guideline of the Patient Care Committee of the American Gastroenterological Association. *Dig Dis Sci* 1990;35:289–293.

73. Castell DO. Chest pain of undetermined origin: overview of pathophysiology. *Am J Med* 1992;92:2S–4S.

74. Richter JE, Bradley LA, Castell DO. Esophageal chest pain: current controversies in pathogenesis, diagnosis, and therapy. *Ann Intern Med* 1989;110:66–78.

75. Deschner WK, Benjamin SB. Extraesophageal manifestations of

gastroesophageal reflux disease. *Am J Gastroenterol* 1989;84: 1–5.

76. Raiha IJ, Ivaska K, Sourander LB. Pulmonary function in gastro-oesophageal reflux disease of elderly people. *Age Ageing* 1992;21:368–373.

77. Raiha I, Manner R, Hietanen E, et al. Radiographic pulmonary changes of gastro-oesophageal reflux disease in elderly patients. *Age Ageing* 1992;21:250–255.

78. Richter JE. Gastroesophageal reflux disease in the elderly. *Geriatr Med Today* 1989;8:27.

79. James OF, Parry-Billings KS. Comparison of omeprazole and histamine H2-receptor antagonists in the treatment of elderly and young patients with reflux oesophagitis. *Age Ageing* 1994;23:121–126.

80. Johnson LF, DeMeester TR. Evaluation of elevation of the head of the bed, bethanechol, and antacid form tablets on gastroesophageal reflux. *Dig Dis Sci* 1981;26:673–680.

81. Hamilton JW, Boisen RJ, Yamamoto DT, et al. Sleeping on a wedge diminishes exposure of the esophagus to refluxed acid. *Dig Dis Sci* 1988;33:518–522.

82. Garnett WR, Garabedian-Ruffalo SM. Identification, diagnosis, and treatment of acid-related diseases in the elderly: implications for long-term care. *Pharmacotherapy* 1997;17:938–958.

83. Hetzel DJ, Dent J, Reed WD, et al. Healing and relapse of severe peptic esophagitis after treatment with omeprazole. *Gastroenterology* 1988;95:903–912.

84. Skoutakis VA, Joe RH, Hara DS. Comparative role of omeprazole in the treatment of gastroesophageal reflux disease. *Ann Pharmacother* 1995;29:1252–1262.

85. McTavish D, Buckley MM, Heel RC. Omeprazole. An updated review of its pharmacology and therapeutic use in acid-related disorders. *Drugs* 1991;42:138–170.

86. Andersson T. Pharmacokinetics, metabolism and interactions of acid pump inhibitors. Focus on omeprazole, lansoprazole and pantoprazole. *Clin Pharmacokinet* 1996;31:9–28.

87. Petersen KU. Review article: omeprazole and the cytochrome P450 system. *Aliment Pharmacol Ther* 1995;9:1–9.

88. Saltzman JR, Kemp JA, Golner BB, et al. Effect of hypochlorhydria due to omeprazole treatment or atrophic gastritis on protein-bound vitamin B12 absorption. *J Am Coll Nutr* 1994;13:584–591.

89. Saltzman JR, Kowdley KV, Pedrosa MC, et al. Bacterial overgrowth without clinical malabsorption in elderly hypochlorhydric subjects. *Gastroenterology* 1994;106:615–623.

90. Cloud ML, Enas N, Humphries TJ, et al. Rabeprazole in treatment of acid peptic diseases: results of three placebo-controlled dose–response clinical trials in duodenal ulcer, gastric ulcer, and gastroesophageal reflux disease (GERD). The Rabeprazole Study Group. *Dig Dis Sci* 1998;43:993–1000.

91. Dettmer A, Vogt R, Sielaff F, et al. Pantoprazole 20 mg is effective for relief of symptoms and healing of lesions in mild reflux oesophagitis. *Aliment Pharmacol Ther* 1998;12:865–872.

92. Castell DO, Richter JE, Robinson M, et al. Efficacy and safety of lansoprazole in the treatment of erosive reflux esophagitis. The Lansoprazole Group. *Am J Gastroenterol* 1996;91: 1749–1757.

93. Dekkers CP, Beker JA, Thjodleifsson B, et al. Double-blind comparison of rabeprazole 20 mg vs. omeprazole 20 mg in the treatment of erosive or ulcerative gastro-oesophageal reflux disease. The European Rabeprazole Study Group. *Aliment Pharmacol Ther* 1999;13:49–57.

94. Mossner J, Holscher AH, Herz R, et al. A double-blind study of pantoprazole and omeprazole in the treatment of reflux oesophagitis: a multicentre trial. *Aliment Pharmacol Ther* 1995; 9:321–326.

95. Richter JE, Kahrilas PJ, Johanson J, et al. Efficacy and safety of esomeprazole compared with omeprazole in GERD patients with erosive esophagitis: a randomized controlled trial. *Am J Gastroenterol* 2001;96:656–665.

96. Castell DO, Kahrilas PJ, Richter JE, et al. Esomeprazole (40 mg) compared with lansoprazole (30 mg) in the treatment of erosive esophagitis. *Am J Gastroenterol* 2002;97:575–583.

97. Colin-Jones DG. Histamine-2-receptor antagonists in gastro-oesophageal reflux. *Gut* 1989;30:1305–1308.

98. Lipsy RJ, Fennerty B, Fagan TC. Clinical review of histamine2 receptor antagonists. *Arch Intern Med* 1990;150:745–751.

99. Hatlebakk JG, Berstad A. Pharmacokinetic optimisation in the treatment of gastro-oesophageal reflux disease. *Clin Pharmacokinet* 1996;31:386–406.

100. Lieberman DA, Keeffe EB. Treatment of severe reflux esophagitis with cimetidine and metoclopramide. *Ann Intern Med* 1986; 104:21–26.

101. Verlinden M. Review article: a role for gastrointestinal prokinetic agents in the treatment of reflux oesophagitis? *Aliment Pharmacol Ther* 1989;3:113–131.

102. Richardson WS, Hunter JG, Waring JP. Laparoscopic antireflux surgery. *Semin Gastrointest Dis* 1997;8:100–110.

103. Trus TL, Bax T, Richardson WS, et al. Complications of laparoscopic paraesophageal hernia repair. *J Gastrointest Surg* 1997;1: 221–228.

104. Gutmann E. Muscle. In: CE Finch and L Hayflick, eds. *Handbook of the biology of aging*. New York: Van Nostrand Reinhold, 1977:709.

105. Steele CM, Greenwood C, Ens I, et al. Mealtime difficulties in a home for the aged: not just dysphagia. *Dysphagia* 1997;12: 43–51.

106. Wickal KE, Swoope CC. Studies of residual ridge resorption: II. The relationship of dietary calcium and phosphorus to residual ridge resorption. *J Prosthet Dent* 1974;32:13.

107. Tibbling L, Gustafsson B. Dysphagia and its consequences in the elderly. *Dysphagia* 1991;6:200–202.

108. Talley NJ, Weaver AL, Zinsmeister AR, et al. Onset and disappearance of gastrointestinal symptoms and functional gastrointestinal disorders. *Am J Epidemiol* 1992;136:165–177.

109. Siebens H, Trupe E, Siebens A, et al. Correlates and consequences of eating dependency in institutionalized elderly. *J Am Geriatr Soc* 1986;34:192–198.

110. Lee A, Sitoh YY, Lieu PK, et al. Swallowing impairment and feeding dependency in the hospitalised elderly. *Ann Acad Med Singapore* 1999;28:371–376.

111. Trupe EH, et al. Prevalence of feeding and swallowing disorders in a nursing home. *Arch Phys Med Rehabil* 1984;65:651.

112. American Heart Association. *1992 Heart and stroke facts*. Dallas, American Heart Association, 1991.

113. Buchholz DW. Dysphagia associated with neurological disorders. *Acta Otorhinolaryngol Belg* 1994;48:143–155.

114. Horner J, Massey EW, Riski JE, et al. Aspiration following stroke: clinical correlates and outcome. *Neurology* 1988;38: 1359–1362.

115. Palmer JB, DuChane AS. Rehabilitation of swallowing disorders due to strokes. *Phys Med Rehabil Clin N Am* 1991;2:259.

116. Gordon C, Hewer RL, Wade DT. Dysphagia in acute stroke. *Br Med J (Clin Res Ed)* 1987;295:411–4.

117. Mann G, Hankey GJ, Cameron D. Swallowing disorders following acute stroke: prevalence and diagnostic accuracy. *Cerebrovasc Dis* 2000;10:380–386.

118. Daniels SK, Brailey K, Priestly DH, et al. Aspiration in patients with acute stroke. *Arch Phys Med Rehabil* 1998;79:14–19.

119. Sharma JC, Fletcher S, Vassallo M, et al. What influences outcome of stroke—pyrexia or dysphagia? *Int J Clin Pract* 2001;55:17–20.

120. Smithard DG, O'Neill PA, Parks C, et al. Complications and

outcome after acute stroke. Does dysphagia matter? *Stroke* 1996;27:1200–1204.

121. Alberts MJ, Horner J, Gray L, et al. Aspiration after stroke: lesion analysis by brain MRI. *Dysphagia* 1992;7:170–173.

122. Celifarco A, Gerard G, Faegenburg D, et al. Dysphagia as the sole manifestation of bilateral strokes. *Am J Gastroenterol* 1990; 85:610–613.

123. Buchholz DW. Neurogenic dysphagia: what is the cause when the cause is not obvious? *Dysphagia* 1994;9:245–255.

124. Domenech E, Kelly J. Swallowing disorders. *Med Clin North Am* 1999;83:97–113, ix.

125. Schroeder PL, Richter JE. Swallowing disorders in the elderly. *Semin Gastrointest Dis* 1994;5:154–165.

126. Buchholz DW. Clinically probable brainstem stroke presenting primarily as dysphagia and nonvisualized by MRI. *Dysphagia* 1993;8:235–238.

127. Bramble MG, Cunliffe J, Dellipiani AW. Evidence for a change in neurotransmitter affecting oesophageal motility in Parkinson's disease. *J Neurol Neurosurg Psychiatry* 1978;41:709–712.

128. van de Vijver DA, Roos RA, Jansen PA, et al. Estimation of incidence and prevalence of Parkinson's disease in the elderly using pharmacy records. *Pharmacoepidemiol Drug Saf* 2001;10: 549–554.

129. Edwards LL, Quigley EM, Pfeiffer RF. Gastrointestinal dysfunction in Parkinson's disease: frequency and pathophysiology. *Neurology* 1992;42:726–732.

130. Pfeiffer RF. Gastrointestinal dysfunction in Parkinson's disease. *Clin Neurosci* 1998;5:136–146.

131. Logemann JA, Blonsky ER, Boshes B. Dysphagia in parkinsonism [Editorial]. *JAMA* 1975;231:69–70.

132. Silbiger ML, Pikielney R, Donner MW. Neuromuscular disorders affecting the pharynx. Cineradiographic analysis. *Invest Radiol* 1967;2:442–448.

133. Bird MR, Woodward MC, Gibson EM, et al. Asymptomatic swallowing disorders in elderly patients with Parkinson's disease: a description of findings on clinical examination and videofluoroscopy in sixteen patients. *Age Ageing* 1994;23:251–254.

134. Leopold NA, Kagel MC. Pharyngo-esophageal dysphagia in Parkinson's disease. *Dysphagia* 1997;12:11–20.

135. Bassotti G, Germani U, Pagliaricci S, et al. Esophageal manometric abnormalities in Parkinson's disease. *Dysphagia* 1998;13: 28–31.

136. Anderson DW, Ellenberg JH, Leventhal CM, et al. Revised estimate of the prevalence of multiple sclerosis in the United States. *Ann Neurol* 1992;31:333–336.

137. Rodriguez M, Siva A, Ward J, et al. Impairment, disability, and handicap in multiple sclerosis: a population-based study in Olmsted County, Minnesota. *Neurology* 1994;44:28–33.

138. Calcagno P, Ruoppolo G, Grasso MG, et al. Dysphagia in multiple sclerosis—prevalence and prognostic factors. *Acta Neurol Scand* 2002;105:40–43.

139. Thomas FJ, Wiles CM. Dysphagia and nutritional status in multiple sclerosis. *J Neurol* 1999;246:677–682.

140. McDonald WI, Compston A, Edan G, et al. Recommended diagnostic criteria for multiple sclerosis: guidelines from the International Panel on the diagnosis of multiple sclerosis. *Ann Neurol* 2001;50:121–127.

141. Grunebaum M, Salinger H. Radiologic findings in polymyositis-dermatomyositis involving the pharynx and upper oesophagus. *Clin Radiol* 1971;22:97–100.

142. Jacob H, Berkowitz D, McDonald E, et al. The esophageal motility disorder of polymyositis. A prospective study. *Arch Intern Med* 1983;143:2262–4.

143. Shapiro J, Martin S, DeGirolami U, et al. Inflammatory myopathy causing pharyngeal dysphagia: a new entity. *Ann Otol Rhinol Laryngol* 1996;105:331–335.

144. Darrow DH, Hoffman HT, Barnes GJ, et al. Management of dysphagia in inclusion body myositis. *Arch Otolaryngol Head Neck Surg* 1992;118:313–317.

145. Dalakas MC, Elder G, Hallett M, et al. A long-term follow-up study of patients with post-poliomyelitis neuromuscular symptoms. *N Engl J Med* 1986;314:959–963.

146. Schon F, Drayson M, Thompson RA. Myasthenia gravis and elderly people. *Age Ageing* 1996;25:56–58.

147. Hopkins LC. Clinical features of myasthenia gravis. *Neurol Clin* 1994;12:243–261.

148. Kluin KJ, Bromberg MB, Feldman EL, et al. Dysphagia in elderly men with myasthenia gravis. *J Neurol Sci* 1996;138:49–52.

149. De Assis JL, Marchiori PE, Scaff M. Atrophy of the tongue with persistent articulation disorder in myasthenia gravis: report of 10 patients. *Auris Nasus Larynx* 1994;21:215–218.

150. Huang MH, King KL, Chien KY. Esophageal manometric studies in patients with myasthenia gravis. *J Thorac Cardiovasc Surg* 1988;95:281–285.

151. Walling AD. Amyotrophic lateral sclerosis: Lou Gehrig's disease. *Am Fam Physician* 1999;59:1489–1496.

152. Hillel A, Dray T, Miller R, et al. Presentation of ALS to the otolaryngologist/head and neck surgeon: getting to the neurologist. *Neurology* 1999;53:S22–S25, S35–S36.

153. Robbins J. Swallowing in ALS and motor neuron disorders. *Neurol Clin* 1987;5:213–229.

154. Ertekin C, Aydogdu I, Yuceyar N, et al. Pathophysiological mechanisms of oropharyngeal dysphagia in amyotrophic lateral sclerosis. *Brain* 2000;123:125–140.

155. Borasio GD, Voltz R, Miller RG. Palliative care in amyotrophic lateral sclerosis. *Neurol Clin* 2001;19:829–847.

156. Chio A, Finocchiaro E, Meineri P, et al. Safety and factors related to survival after percutaneous endoscopic gastrostomy in ALS. ALS Percutaneous Endoscopic Gastrostomy Study Group. *Neurology* 1999;53:1123–1125.

157. Kasarskis EJ, Scarlata D, Hill R, et al. A retrospective study of percutaneous endoscopic gastrostomy in ALS patients during the BDNF and CNTF trials. *J Neurol Sci* 1999;169:118–125.

158. Mathus–Vliegen LM, Louwerse LS, Merkus MP, et al. Percutaneous endoscopic gastrostomy in patients with amyotrophic lateral sclerosis and impaired pulmonary function. *Gastrointest Endosc* 1994;40:463–469.

159. Gerhardt DC, Shuck TJ, Bordeaux RA, et al. Human upper esophageal sphincter. Response to volume, osmotic, and acid stimuli. *Gastroenterology* 1978;75:268–274.

160. Fradet G, Pouliot D, Robichaud R, et al. Upper esophageal sphincter myotomy in oculopharyngeal muscular dystrophy: long-term clinical results. *Neuromuscul Disord* 1997;7(Suppl 1): S90–S95.

161. Saffouri MH, Ward PH. Surgical correction of dysphagia due to cervical osteophytes. *Ann Otol Rhinol Laryngol* 1974;83:65–70.

162. Ladenheim SE, Marlowe FI. Dysphagia secondary to cervical osteophytes. *Am J Otolaryngol* 1999;20:184–189.

163. Ebo D, Goethals L, Bracke P, et al. Dysphagia in a patient with giant osteophytes: case presentation and review of the literature. *Clin Rheumatol* 2000;19:70–72.

164. Maran AG, Wilson JA, Al Muhanna AH. Pharyngeal diverticula. *Clin Otolaryngol* 1986;11:219–225.

165. Laing MR, Murthy P, Ah-See KW, et al. Surgery for pharyngeal pouch: audit of management with short- and long-term follow-up. *J R Coll Surg Edinb* 1995;40:315–318.

166. Siddiq MA, Sood S, Strachan D. Pharyngeal pouch (Zenker's diverticulum). *Postgrad Med J* 2001;77:506–511.

167. Cook IJ, Blumbergs P, Cash K, et al. Structural abnormalities of the cricopharyngeus muscle in patients with pharyngeal (Zenker's) diverticulum. *J Gastroenterol Hepatol* 1992;7: 556–562.

168. Cook IJ, Gabb M, Panagopoulos V, et al. Pharyngeal (Zenker's) diverticulum is a disorder of upper esophageal sphincter opening. *Gastroenterology* 1992;103:1229–1235.

169. Bradley PJ, Kochaar A, Quraishi MS. Pharyngeal pouch carcinoma: real or imaginary risks? *Ann Otol Rhinol Laryngol* 1999;108:1027–1032.

170. Louie HW, Zuckerbraun L. Staged Zenker's diverticulectomy with cervical esophagostomy and secondary esophagostomy closure for treatment of massive diverticulum in severely debilitated patients. *Am Surg* 1993;59:842–845.

171. Ishioka S, Felix VN, Sakai P, et al. Manometric study of the upper esophageal sphincter before and after endoscopic management of Zenker's diverticulum. *Hepatogastroenterology* 1995; 42:628–632.

172. Dodds WJ, Logemann JA, Stewart ET. Radiologic assessment of abnormal oral and pharyngeal phases of swallowing. *Am J Roentgenol* 1990;154:965–974.

173. Dodds WJ, Stewart ET, Logemann JA. Physiology and radiology of the normal oral and pharyngeal phases of swallowing. *Am J Roentgenol* 1990;154:953–963.

174. Castell JA, Castell DO. Upper esophageal sphincter and pharyngeal function and oropharyngeal (transfer) dysphagia. *Gastroenterol Clin North Am* 1996;25:35–50.

175. McConnel FM. Analysis of pressure generation and bolus transit during pharyngeal swallowing. *Laryngoscope* 1988;98:71–78.

176. Jaradeh SS, Shaker R, Toohill RB. Electromyographic recording of the cricopharyngeus muscle in humans. *Am J Med* 2000; 108(suppl 4a):40S–42S.

177. Elmstahl S, Bulow M, Ekberg O, et al. Treatment of dysphagia improves nutritional conditions in stroke patients. *Dysphagia* 1999;14:61–66.

178. Perez I, Smithard DG, Davies H, et al. Pharmacological treatment of dysphagia in stroke. *Dysphagia* 1998;13:12–16.

179. Bonavina L, Khan NA, DeMeester TR. Pharyngoesophageal dysfunctions. The role of cricopharyngeal myotomy. *Arch Surg* 1985;120:541–549.

180. David VC. Relief of dysphagia in motor neurone disease with cricopharyngeal myotomy. *Ann R Coll Surg Engl* 1985;67: 229–231.

181. Ellis FH Jr, Crozier RE. Cervical esophageal dysphagia: indications for and results of cricopharyngeal myotomy. *Ann Surg* 1981;194:279–289.

182. Ekberg O, Lindgren S. Effect of cricopharyngeal myotomy on pharyngoesophageal function: pre- and postoperative cineradiographic findings. *Gastrointest Radiol* 1987;12:1–6.

183. Schneider I, Thumfart WF, Pototschnig C, et al. Treatment of dysfunction of the cricopharyngeal muscle with botulinum A toxin: introduction of a new, noninvasive method. *Ann Otol Rhinol Laryngol* 1994;103:31–35.

184. Alberty J, Oelerich M, Ludwig K, et al. Efficacy of botulinum toxin A for treatment of upper esophageal sphincter dysfunction. *Laryngoscope* 2000;110:1151–1156.

185. Cattau EL, Jr., Castell DO. Symptoms of esophageal dysfunction. *Adv Intern Med* 1982;27:151–181.

186. Mayberry JF. Epidemiology and demographics of achalasia. *Gastrointest Endosc Clin N Am* 2001;11:235–248, v.

187. Sonnenberg A, Massey BT, McCarty DJ, et al. Epidemiology of hospitalization for achalasia in the United States. *Dig Dis Sci* 1993;38:233–244.

188. Tucker HJ, Snape WJ, Jr., Cohen S. Achalasia secondary to carcinoma: manometric and clinical features. *Ann Intern Med* 1978;89:315–318.

189. Herrera JL. Case report: esophageal metastasis from breast carcinoma presenting as achalasia. *Am J Med Sci* 1992;303:321–323.

190. Kahrilas PJ, Kishk SM, Helm JF, et al. Comparison of pseudoachalasia and achalasia. *Am J Med* 1987;82:439–446.

191. Subramanyam K. Achalasia secondary to malignant mesothelioma of the pleura. *J Clin Gastroenterol* 1990;12:183–187.

192. Meijssen MA, Tilanus HW, van Blankenstein M, et al. Achalasia complicated by oesophageal squamous cell carcinoma: a prospective study in 195 patients. *Gut* 1992;33:155–158.

193. Dancygier H, Classen M. Endoscopic ultrasonography in esophageal diseases. *Gastrointest Endosc* 1989;35:220–225.

194. Robertson CS, Fellows IW, Mayberry JF, et al. Choice of therapy for achalasia in relation to age. *Digestion* 1988;40:244–250.

195. Eckardt VF, Aignherr C, Bernhard G. Predictors of outcome in patients with achalasia treated by pneumatic dilation. *Gastroenterology* 1992;103:1732–1738.

196. Csendes A, Velasco N, Braghetto I, et al. A prospective randomized study comparing forceful dilatation and esophagomyotomy in patients with achalasia of the esophagus. *Gastroenterology* 1981;80:789–795.

197. Shimi S, Nathanson LK, Cuschieri A. Laparoscopic cardiomyotomy for achalasia. *J R Coll Surg Edinb* 1991;36:152–154.

198. Pellegrini C, Wetter LA, Patti M, et al. Thoracoscopic esophagomyotomy. Initial experience with a new approach for the treatment of achalasia. *Ann Surg* 1992;216:291–299.

199. Sharp KW, Khaitan L, Scholz S, et al. 100 consecutive minimally invasive Heller myotomies: lessons learned. *Ann Surg* 2002;235:631–639.

200. Berreca M, Oelschlager BK, Pellegrini CA. Minimally invasive surgery for the treatment of achalsia. *Endoscopia* 2002;14: 59–66.

201. Gordon JM, Eakcr EY. Prospcctive study of csophagcal botulinum toxin injection in high-risk achalasia patients. *Am J Gastroenterol* 1997;92:1812–1817.

202. Pasricha PJ, Rai R, Ravich WJ, et al. Botulinum toxin for achalasia: long-term outcome and predictors of response. *Gastroenterology* 1996;110:1410–1415.

203. Schiano TD, Parkman HP, Miller LS, et al. Use of botulinum toxin in the treatment of achalasia. *Dig Dis* 1998;16:14–22.

204. Malnick SD, Metchnik L, Somin M, et al. Fatal heart block following treatment with botulinum toxin for achalasia. *Am J Gastroenterol* 2000;95:3333–3334.

205. Khurana V, Nehme O, Khurana R, et al. Urinary retention secondary to detrusor muscle hypofunction after botulinum toxin injection for achalasia. *Am J Gastroenterol* 2001;96:3211–3212.

206. Ghosh S, Heading RC, Palmer KR. Achalasia of the oesophagus in elderly patients responds poorly to conservative therapy. *Age Ageing* 1994;23:280–282.

207. Bortolotti M, Mari C, Lopilato C, et al. Effects of sildenafil on esophageal motility of patients with idiopathic achalasia. *Gastroenterology* 2000;118:253–257.

208. Devaney EJ, Lannettoni MD, Orringer MB, et al. Esophagectomy for achalasia: patient selection and clinical experience. *Ann Thorac Surg* 2001;72:854–858.

209. Spechler SJ, Castell DO. Classification of oesophageal motility abnormalities. *Gut* 2001;49:145–151.

210. Rao SS, Hayek B, Summers RW. Functional chest pain of esophageal origin: hyperalgesia or motor dysfunction. *Am J Gastroenterol* 2001;96:2584–9.

211. Balaban DH, Yamamoto Y, Liu J, et al. Sustained esophageal contraction: a marker of esophageal chest pain identified by intraluminal ultrasonography. *Gastroenterology* 1999;116:29–37.

212. Achem SR, Percy R, Burton L, et al. Autonomic dysfunction in patients with noncardiac chest pain. *Gastroenterology* 1994;106 (suppl 4):A36.

213. Pirtniecks A, Smith LF, Thorpe JA. Autonomic dysfunction in nonspecific disorders of oesophageal motility. *Eur J Cardiothorac Surg* 2000;17:101–105.

214. The oesophagus and chest pain of uncertain cause. *Lancet* 1992; 339:583–584.

215. DeVault KR, Achem SR, Stark ME, et al. Nutcracker esophagus: a statistical aberrancy associated with psychopathology? *Am J Gastroenterol* 2002;97:S33.

216. Achem SR, Kolts BE, MacMath T, et al. Effects of omeprazole versus placebo in treatment of noncardiac chest pain and gastroesophageal reflux. *Dig Dis Sci* 1997;42:2138–2145.

217. Borjesson M, Pilhall M, Rolny P, et al. Gastroesophageal acid reflux in patients with nutcracker esophagus. *Scand J Gastroenterol* 2001;36:916–920.

218. Champion JK, Delisle N, Hunt T. Laparoscopic esophagomyotomy with posterior partial fundoplication for primary esophageal motility disorders. *Surg Endosc* 2000;14:746–749.

219. Murray JA, Ledlow A, Launspach J, et al. The effects of recombinant human hemoglobin on esophageal motor functions in humans. *Gastroenterology* 1995;109:1241–1248.

220. Konturek JW, Thor P, Lukaszyk A, et al. Endogenous nitric oxide in the control of esophageal motility in humans. *J Physiol Pharmacol* 1997;48:201–209.

221. Eherer AJ, Schwetz I, Hammer HF, et al. Effect of sildenafil on oesophageal motor function in healthy subjects and patients with oesophageal motor disorders. *Gut* 2002;50:758–764.

222. Miller LS, Pullela SV, Parkman HP, et al. Treatment of chest pain in patients with noncardiac, nonreflux, nonachalasia spastic esophageal motor disorders using botulinum toxin injection into the gastroesophageal. *Am J Gastroenterol* 2002;97: 1640–1646.

223. Zamost BJ, Hirschberg J, Ippoliti AF, et al. Esophagitis in scleroderma. Prevalence and risk factors. *Gastroenterology* 1987;92: 421–428.

224. Gonzalez R, Storr M, Bloching H, et al. Autoantibody profile in progressive systemic sclerosis as markers for esophageal involvement. *J Clin Gastroenterol* 2001;32:123–127.

225. Katzka DA, Reynolds JC, Saul SH, et al. Barrett's metaplasia and adenocarcinoma of the esophagus in scleroderma. *Am J Med* 1987;82:46–52.

226. Ipsen P, Egekvist H, Aksglaede K, et al. Oesophageal manometry and video-radiology in patients with systemic sclerosis: a retrospective study of its clinical value. *Acta Derm Venereol* 2000; 80:130–133.

227. Kelsen D. Multimodality therapy for adenocarcinoma of the esophagus. *Gastroenterol Clin North Am* 1997;26:635–645.

228. Bannister P, Stanners AJ, Mountford RA. Dysphagia in the elderly: what does it mean to the endoscopist? *J R Soc Med* 1990;83:552–553.

229. Adam DJ, Craig SR, Sang CT, et al. Esophagectomy for carcinoma in the octogenarian. *Ann Thorac Surg* 1996;61:190–194.

230. Jougon JB, Ballester M, Duffy J, et al. Esophagectomy for cancer in the patient aged 70 years and older. *Ann Thorac Surg* 1997;63:1423–1427.

231. Muehrcke DD, Kaplan DK, Donnelly RJ. Oesophagogastrectomy in patients over 70. *Thorax* 1989;44:141–145.

232. Thomas P, Doddoli C, Neville P, et al. Esophageal cancer resection in the elderly. *Eur J Cardiothorac Surg* 1996;10:941–946.

233. Wong J. Management of carcinoma of oesophagus: art or science? *J R Coll Surg Edinb* 1981;26:138–149.

234. Kuwano H, Morita M, Baba K, et al. Surgical treatment of esophageal carcinoma in patients eighty years of age and older. *J Surg Oncol* 1993;52:36–39.

235. Ertan A, Zimmerman M, Younes M. Esophageal adenocarcinoma associated with Barrett's esophagus: long-term management with laser ablation. *Am J Gastroenterol* 1995;90: 2201–2203.

236. Overholt BF, Panjehpour M. Barrett's esophagus: photodynamic therapy for ablation of dysplasia, reduction of specialized mucosa, and treatment of superficial esophageal cancer. *Gastrointest Endosc* 1995;42:64–70.

237. Salo JA, Salminen JT, Kiviluoto TA, et al. Treatment of Barrett's esophagus by endoscopic laser ablation and antireflux surgery. *Ann Surg* 1998;227:40–44.

238. Sampliner RE. Ablation of Barrett's mucosa. *Gastroenterologist* 1997;5:185–188.

239. Richter JE. Gastroesophageal reflux disease in the older patient: presentation, treatment, and complications. *Am J Gastroenterol* 2000;95:368–373.

240. Marks RD, Richter JE. Peptic strictures of the esophagus. *Am J Gastroenterol* 1993;88:1160–1173.

241. Agnew SR, Pandya SP, Reynolds RP, et al. Predictors for frequent esophageal dilations of benign peptic strictures. *Dig Dis Sci* 1996;41:931–936.

242. Barbezat GO, Schlup M, Lubcke R. Omeprazole therapy decreases the need for dilatation of peptic oesophageal strictures. *Aliment Pharmacol Ther* 1999;13:1041–1045.

243. Marks RD, Richter JE, Rizzo J, et al. Omeprazole versus H2–receptor antagonists in treating patients with peptic stricture and esophagitis. *Gastroenterology* 1994;106:907–915.

244. Zein NN, Greseth JM, Perrault J. Endoscopic intralesional steroid injections in the management of refractory esophageal strictures. *Gastrointest Endosc* 1995;41:596–598.

245. Klingler PJ, Hinder RA, Cina RA, et al. Laparoscopic antireflux surgery for the treatment of esophageal strictures refractory to medical therapy. *Am J Gastroenterol* 1999;94:632–636.

246. DeVault KR. Lower esophageal (Schatzki's) ring: pathogenesis, diagnosis and therapy. *Dig Dis* 1996;14:323–329.

247. Schatzki R. The lower esophageal ring. *Am J Roentgenol* 1963; 90:805.

248. Marshall JB, Kretschmar JM, Diaz-Arias AA. Gastroesophageal reflux as a pathogenic factor in the development of symptomatic lower esophageal rings. *Arch Intern Med* 1990;150: 1669–1672.

249. Ott DJ, Ledbetter MS, Chen MY, et al. Correlation of lower esophageal mucosal ring and 24-h pH monitoring of the esophagus. *Am J Gastroenterol* 1996;91:61–64.

250. Pape R. Uber einen abnormen verlauf ("tiefe Rechtslage") der mesa aortitischen aorta descendes. *Fortschr Roetgenstr* 1932;46: 257–269.

251. Sundaram U, Traube M. Radiologic and manometric study of the gastroesophageal junction in dysphagia aortica. *J Clin Gastroenterol* 1995;21:275–277.

252. Birnholz JC, Ferrucci JT, Wyman SM. Roentgen features of dysphagia aortica. *Radiology* 1974;111:93–96.

253. Hanna A, Derrick JR. Dysphagia caused by tortuosity of the thoracic aorta. *J Thorac Cardiovasc Surg* 1969;57:134–137.

254. Mittal RK, Siskind BN, Hongo M, et al. Dysphagia aortica. Clinical, radiological, and manometric findings. *Dig Dis Sci* 1986;31:379–384.

255. Nguyen P, Gideon RM, Castell DO. Dysphagia lusoria in the adult: associated esophageal manometric findings and diagnostic use of scanning techniques. *Am J Gastroenterol* 1994;89:620–623.

256. Kress S, Martin WR, Benz C, et al. Dysphagia secondary to left atrial dilatation. *Z Gastroenterol* 1997;35:1007–1011.

257. Mo KM, Craig GM, Clark JV, et al. Sudden death from perforation of a benign oesophageal ulcer into a major blood vessel. *Postgrad Med J* 1988;64:687–689.

258. Luketich JD, Sommers KE, Griffith BP, et al. Successful management of secondary aortoesophageal fistula. *Ann Thorac Surg* 1996;62:1852–1854.

259. Kikendall JW. Pill esophagitis. *J Clin Gastroenterol* 1999;28: 298–305.

260. Hiraoka T, Okita M, Koganemaru S, et al. [Hemorrhagic esophageal ulceration associated with slow-release morphine sulfate tablets]. *Nippon Shokakibyo Gakkai Zasshi* 1991;88: 1231–1234.

261. Hey H, Jorgensen F, Sorensen K, et al. Oesophageal transit of six commonly used tablets and capsules. *Br Med J (Clin Res Ed)* 1982;285:1717–1719.

262. de Groen PC, Lubbe DF, Hirsch LJ, et al. Esophagitis associated with the use of alendronate. *N Engl J Med* 1996;335:1016–1021.

263. Bott S, Prakash C, McCallum RW. Medication-induced esophageal injury: survey of the literature. *Am J Gastroenterol* 1987;82:758–763.

264. Delpre G, Kadish U, Stahl B. Induction of esophageal injuries by doxycycline and other pills. A frequent but preventable occurrence. *Dig Dis Sci* 1989;34:797–800.

265. Kikendall JW, Friedman AC, Oyewole MA, et al. Pill-induced esophageal injury. Case reports and review of the medical literature. *Dig Dis Sci* 1983;28:174–182.

266. McCord GS, Clouse RE. Pill-induced esophageal strictures: clinical features and risk factors for development. *Am J Med* 1990;88:512–518.

267. Bonavina L, DeMeester TR, McChesney L, et al. Drug-induced esophageal strictures. *Ann Surg* 1987;206:173–183.

268. Semble EL, Wu WC, Castell DO. Nonsteroidal antiinflammatory drugs and esophageal injury. *Semin Arthritis Rheum* 1989; 19:99–109.

269. Lanas A, Hirschowitz BI. Significant role of aspirin use in patients with esophagitis. *J Clin Gastroenterol* 1991;13:622–627.

270. Shallcross TM, Wyatt JI, Rathbone BJ, et al. Non-steroidal anti-inflammatory drugs, hiatus hernia, and Helicobacter pylori, in patients with oesophageal ulceration. *Br J Rheumatol* 1990;29: 288–290.

271. Heller SR, Fellows IW, Ogilvie AL, et al. Non-steroidal anti-inflammatory drugs and benign oesophageal stricture. *Br Med J (Clin Res Ed)* 1982;285:167–168.

272. Wilkins WE, Ridley MG, Pozniak AL. Benign stricture of the oesophagus: role of nonsteroidal anti–inflammatory drugs. *Gut* 1984;25:478–480.

273. Ackert JJ, Sherman A, Lustbader IJ, et al. Spontaneous intramural hematoma of the esophagus. *Am J Gastroenterol* 1989;84: 1325–1328.

274. McIntyre AS, Ayres R, Atherton J, et al. Dissecting intramural haematoma of the oesophagus. *QJM* 1998;91:701–705.

275. Thomson A, Fleischer DE, Epstein B. Submucosal hemorrhage of the esophagus associated with endoscopy in a patient with cervical osteophytes. *J Clin Gastroenterol* 1998;27:267–268.

276. Lacy BE, Toor A, Bensen SP, et al. Acute esophageal necrosis: report of two cases and a review of the literature. *Gastrointest Endosc* 1999;49:527–532.

277. Goldenberg SP, Wain SL, Marignani P. Acute necrotizing esophagitis. *Gastroenterology* 1990;98:493–496.

278. Lee KR, Stark E, Shaw FE. Esophageal infarction complicating spontaneous rupture of the thoracic aorta. *JAMA* 1977;237: 1233–1234.

279. Haviv YS, Reinus C, Zimmerman J."Black esophagus": a rare complication of shock. *Am J Gastroenterol* 1996;91:2432–2434.

280. Korkis AM, Miskovitz PF. Acute pharyngoesophageal dysphagia secondary to spontaneous hemorrhage of a parathyroid adenoma. *Dysphagia* 1993;8:7–10.

281. Medeiros LJ, Doos WG, Balogh K. Esophageal intramural pseudodiverticulosis: a report of two cases with analysis of similar, less extensive changes in "normal" autopsy esophagi. *Hum Pathol* 1988;19:928–931.

282. Ponsot P, Molas G, Scoazec JY, et al. Chronic esophagitis dissecans: an unrecognized clinicopathologic entity? *Gastrointest Endosc* 1997;45:38–45.

SUBJECT INDEX